Psychiatric & Mental Health Nursing

for Canadian Practice

Psychiatric & Mental Health Nursing

for Canadian Practice

SECOND EDITION

Wendy Austin, RN, MEd (Counselling), PhD

Professor and Canada Research Chair (Relational Ethics in Health Care)
Faculty of Nursing and the Dossetor Health Ethics Centre
University of Alberta
Edmonton, Alberta, Canada

Mary Ann Boyd, PhD, DNS, APRN, BC

Professor and Associate Dean
Southern Illinois University Edwardsville
Edwardsville, Illinois

Wolters Kluwer | Lippincott Williams & Wilkins
Health

Philadelphia · Baltimore · New York · London
Buenos Aires · Hong Kong · Sydney · Tokyo

Senior Acquisitions Editor: Jean Rodenberger
Product Manager: Michelle Clarke
Director of Nursing Production: Helen Ewan
Art Director, Design: Joan Wendt
Manufacturing Manager: William Alberti
Compositor: SPi Technologies
Printer: C&C

Second Edition

9 8 7 6 5 4 3 2

Printed in China

Library of Congress Cataloging-in-Publication Data
Austin, Wendy, 1947–
   Psychiatric & mental health nursing for Canadian practice / Wendy Austin,
Mary Ann Boyd.—2nd ed.
      p. ; cm.
   Rev. ed. of: Psychiatric nursing for Canadian practice / Wendy Austin, Mary Ann Boyd.
   Includes bibliographical references and index.
   ISBN 978-0-7817-9593-7 (alk. paper)
   1. Psychiatric nursing—Canada. I. Boyd, M. (Mary Ann) II. Austin, Wendy, 1947–
Psychiatric nursing for Canadian practice. III. Title. IV. Title: Psychiatric and mental health
nursing for Canadian practice.
   [DNLM: 1. Psychiatric Nursing—methods—Canada. 2. Mental Disorders—nursing—
Canada. WY 160 A9375p 2010]
   RC440.A87   2010
   616.89'0231—dc22

                                                                        2009050578

Care has been taken to confirm the accuracy of the information presented and to describe generally accepted practices. However, the author, editors, and publisher are not responsible for errors or omissions or for any consequences from application of the information in this book and make no warranty, express or implied, with respect to the content of the publication.

The author, editors, and publisher have exerted every effort to ensure that drug selectin and dosage set forth in this text are in accordance with the current recommendations and practice at the time of publication. However, in view of ongoing research, changes in government regulations, and the constant flow of information relating to drug therapy and drug reactions, the reader is urged to check the package insert for each drug for any change in indications and dosage and for added warnings and precautions This is particularly important when the recommended agent is a new or infrequently employed drug.

Some drugs and medical devices presented in this publication have Food and Drug Administration (FDA) clearance for limited use in restricted research settings. It is the responsibility of the health care provider to ascertain the FDA status of each drug or device planned for use in his or her clinical practice.

LWW.com

This book is dedicated to all those who strive and struggle to improve psychiatric and mental health care, whether it be in their own communities or beyond.

Canadian Contributors

Geertje Boschma, RN, PhD
Associate Professor
School of Nursing
University of British Columbia
Vancouver, British Columbia, Canada

Freida S. Chavez, RN, BScN, MHSc, CHE
Senior Lecturer
Faculty of Nursing
University of Toronto
Toronto, Ontario, Canada

Diana Clarke, RN, PhD
Associate Professor and Associate Dean (Research)
Faculty of Nursing
University of Manitoba
Winnipeg, Manitoba, Canada

Anne Marie Creamer, RN, MSN, PhD(c)
Nurse Practitioner Primary Health care
Saint Joseph's Community Health Centre
Horizon Health Network
Saint John, New Brunswick, Canada

Christine Davis, RN, MEd, MN(c), CPMHN(C)
Coordinator
Collaborative BScN Program
St. Lawrence College
Laurentian University
Brockville, Ontario, Canada

Charl Els, MBChB, FCPsych, MMedPsych, ABAM, MROCC
Clinical Assistant Professor
Faculty of Medicine and Dentistry
University of Alberta
Edmonton, Alberta, Canada

Carol Ewashen, RN, PhD
Associate Professor
Faculty of Nursing
University of Calgary
Calgary, Alberta, Canada

Cheryl Forchuk, RN, PhD
Professor
Arthur Labatt Family School of Nursing
Faculty of Health Sciences
University of Western Ontario
London, Ontario, Canada

Julia Gajewski-Noel, RN, BA, MN
Certificate in Mental Health Nursing
Senior Teaching Associate – Retired 2009
Faculty of Nursing
University of New Brunswick
Fredericton, New Brunswick, Canada

Ruth Gallop, RN, PhD
Professor Emerita
Faculty of Nursing
University of Toronto
Toronto, Ontario, Canada

Marlee Groening, RN, MSN
Lecturer
School of Nursing
University of British Columbia
Vancouver, British Columbia, Canada

Mary Haase, RPN, RN, BScN, PhD
Faculty Member
BScN Program
Grant MacEwan University
Edmonton, Alberta, Canada

Brad Hagen, RN, R. Psych, PhD (Nsg)
Associate Professor
Faculty of Health Sciences
University of Lethbridge
Lethbridge, Alberta, Canada

Sandy Harper-Jaques, RN, MN, RMFT
Clinical Nurse Specialist
Adult Mental Health
CHR South Calgary Health Centre
Calgary, Alberta, Canada

Yvonne R. Hayne, RN, PhD
Psychiatric and Mental Health Nursing
Faculty of Nursing
University of Calgary
Calgary, Alberta, Canada

Marion Healey-Ogden, RN, RCC, BSN, MEd, MA, PhD
Assistant Professor
Faculty of Nursing
Thompson Rivers University
Kamloops, British Columbia, Canada

Kathleen Hegadoren, RN, BScN, MSc, PhD
Professor
Canada Research Chair in Stress Disorders in Women
Faculty of Nursing
University of Alberta
Edmonton, Alberta, Canada

L. Elizabeth Hood, RN, MSN, PhD
Clinical Nurse Specialist (Mental Health)
Regional Mental Health Program
Alberta Hospital Edmonton
Edmonton, Alberta, Canada

Jean Robinson Hughes, RN, PhD
Associate Professor
School of Nursing
Dalhousie University
Halifax, Nova Scotia, Canada

Arlene Kent-Wilkinson, RN, MN, PhD
Assistant Professor
College of Nursing
University of Saskatchewan
Saskatoon, Saskatchewan, Canada

Diane Kunyk, RN, MN, PhD(c)
Graduate Student
Faculty of Nursing
University of Alberta
Edmonton, Alberta, Canada

Annette M. Lane, RN, PhD
Assistant Professor
Faculty of Nursing
University of Calgary
Calgary, Alberta, Canada

Gerri Lasiuk, RN, BA, PhD, CPMHN(C)
Assistant Professor
Faculty of Nursing
University of Alberta
Edmonton, Alberta, Canada

Lori Houger Limacher, RN, PhD, RMFT
Private Practice
Calgary, Alberta, Canada

Elizabeth A. McCay, RN, PhD
Associate Professor
School of Nursing
Ryerson University
Toronto, Ontario, Canada

Sharon L. Moore, RN, BA, MEd, PhD
Associate Professor
Centre for Nursing and Health Studies
Athabasca University
Athabasca, Alberta, Canada

B. Lee Murray, RN, MN, PhD(c)
Clinical Nurse Specialist
Associate Professor
College of Nursing
University of Saskatchewan
Saskatoon, Saskatchewan, Canada

Ginette Pagé, RN, PhD
Clinical Nurse Specialist, Consultant in Nursing
Private Practice
Dunham, Québec, Canada

Cindy Peternelj-Taylor, RN, MSc, PhD(c), DF-IAFN
Professor
College of Nursing
University of Saskatchewan
Saskatoon, Saskatchewan, Canada

Cheryl Pollard, RN, PhD (c)
Faculty Member
Health and Community Stuides, BScN Program
Grant MacEwan University
Edmonton, Alberta, Canada

Hélène Provencher, RN, PhD
Professor
Faculty of Nursing
Laval University
Québec City, Québec, Canada

Yvonne Savard, RPN, RN, BScN, MA Ed/CI
Instructor/Year II Facilitator
Faculty of Health Sciences
Department of Psychiatric Nursing
Douglas College
Coquitlam, British Columbia, Canada

Peggy (Margaret) Simpson, RN, PhD
Lecturer
School of Nursing
University of British Columbia
Vancouver, British Columbia, Canada

Nicole Snow, RN, MN, CPMHN(C)
Faculty
Centre for Nursing Studies
St. John's, Newfoundland and Labrador, Canada

Michel A. Tarko, RPN, PhD
Vice President Education
Justice Institute of British Columbia
New Westminster, British Columbia, Canada

Tracey Tully, RN, PhD
Clinical Nurse Specialist
Sunnybrook and Women's College Health Sciences Centre
Toronto, Ontario, Canada

Stephen VanSlyke, RN, MN
Senior Teaching Associate
Faculty of Nursing
University of New Brunswick
Fredericton, New Brunswick, Canada

Kathryn Weaver, RN, PhD
Associate Professor
University of New Brunswick
Fredericton, New Brunswick, Canada

Jane Hamilton Wilson RN, MHSc, PhD(c)
Professor
Conestoga College Institute of Technology and Advanced Learning
McMaster Mohawk Conestoga BScN Program
Kitchener, Ontario, Canada

Olive Yonge, RN, PhD, R Psych
Professor
Faculty of Nursing
Vice Provost (Academic Programs)
University of Alberta
Edmonton, Alberta, Canada

American Contributors

Marjorie Baier, PhD, RN
Associate Professor
School of Nursing
Southern Illinois University Edwardsville
Edwardsville, Illinois

Doris E. Bell, PhD, APRN, BC
Professor of Nursing
Southern Illinois University Edwardsville
Edwardsville, Illinois

Ann R. Bland, PhD, APRN, BC
Associate Professor
Department of Baccalaureate & Graduate
  Nursing
Eastern Kentucky University
Richmond, Kentucky

Andrea C. Bostrom, PhD, RN, APRN, BC
Associate Professor and Dean of Academic
  Programs
Kirkhof College of Nursing
Grand Valley State University
Allendale, Michigan

Mary R. Boyd, PhD, RN
Associate Professor
College of Nursing
University of South Carolina
Columbia, South Carolina

Stephanie Burgess, PhD, APN-BC
Clinical Professor and Associate Dean for
  Nursing Practice
College of Nursing
University of South Carolina
Columbia, South Carolina

Rita Canfield, RN, MSN, DNSc
School of Nursing
Southern Illinois University Edwardsville
Edwardsville, Illinois

Jeanne A. Clement, EdD, APRN, BC, FAAN
Associate Professor and
Director of Graduate Specialty Program in
  Psychiatric-Mental Health Nursing
College of Nursing
The Ohio State University
Columbus, Ohio

Harvey Davis, RN, PhD, CARN, PHN
School of Nursing
San Francisco State University
San Francisco, California

Denise M. Gibson, MSN, APRN, BC
Instructor
Southern Illinois University School of Nursing
  Edwardsville
Edwardsville, Illinois

Catherine Gray Deering, PhD, RN, APRN, BC
Professor
Clayton State College
Morrow, Georgia

Peggy El-Mallakh, PhD, RN
Post-Doctoral Scholar
College of Nursing
Chandler Medical Center
University of Kentucky
Lexington, Kentucky

Barbara G. Faltz
Clinical Nurse Specialist
Addiction Treatment Services, Veterans
    Administration
Palo Alto Healthcare System
Palo Alto, California

Judith E. Forker, PhD, APRN, BC
Associate Dean for Academic Affairs
School of Nursing
Adelphi University
Garden City, New York

Vanya Hamrin, RN, MS, APRN, BC
Assistant Professor
School of Nursing
Yale University
New Haven, Connecticut

Beverly Gilliam Hart, RN, PhD
Associate Professor of Baccalaureate and
    Graduate Nursing
Eastern Kentucky University
Richmond, Kentucky

Emily J. Hauenstein, PhD, APRN, LCP, BC
Professor
School of Nursing
University of Virginia
Charlottesville, Virginia

Nancy Anne Hilliker, MA, RN, ANP, CS
Nurse Practitioner
Barnes-Jewish Hospital
St. Louis, Missouri

Gail L. Kongable, MSN, RN, FNP
Associate Professor
Neurological Surgery
University of Virginia Health Systems
Charlottesville, Virginia

Kathy Lee, MS, RN, APRN, BC
Associate Professor & Psychiatric Mental Health Nurse
    Practitioner
School of Nursing – SNSN
Oregon Health & Science University
Center for Women's Health
Portland, Oregon

Susan McCabe, EdD, APRN, BC
Associate Professor, College of Nursing
East Tennessee State University
Johnson City, Tennessee

**Ruth Beckmann Murray, MSN, EdD, N-NAP,
    FAAN**
Professor Emerita
Doisy College of Health Sciences
School of Nursing
St. Louis University
St. Louis, Missouri

Robert B. Noud, MS, APRN, BC
Adjunct Faculty
Staff, University of Missouri St. Louis
St. Louis University Hospital
St. Louis, Missouri

Maryellen C. Pachler, MSN, APRN
Child Psychiatric Nurse Practitioner
Child Study Center
School of Medicine
Yale University
New Haven, Connecticut

Nan Roberts, MS, APRN, BC
Director of Clinical Trials
Advent Research Institute
St. Peters, Missouri

Lawrence Scahill, PhD, MSN, FAAN
Professor of Nursing and Child Psychiatry
Child Study Center
Yale University
New Haven, Connecticut

Victoria Soltis-Jarrett, PhD, APRN-BC
Clinical Associate Professor and MSN Coordinator,
    Psychiatric Mental Health
Family Psychiatric Nurse Practitioner and Clinical
    Nurse Specialist
School of Nursing
University of North Carolina at Chapel Hill
Chapel Hill, North Carolina

Mickey Stanley, PhD, RN
Associate Professor
School of Nursing
Southern Illinois University Edwardsville
Edwardsville, Illinois

Roberta Stock, MS, APRN, BC
Advanced Practice Nurse
Comtrea, Inc
Festus, Missouri

Sandra P. Thomas, PhD, RN, FAAN
Professor and Director, PhD Program
College of Nursing
The University of Tennessee
Knoxville, Tennessee

Barbara Jones Warren, PhD, APRN, BC
Associate Clinical Professor
College of Nursing
The Ohio State University
Executive Nurse
Ohio Department of Mental Health
Columbus, Ohio

Jane White, PhD, DNSc, APRN, BC
Vera E. Bender Professor of Nursing and
Associate Dean for Research and Graduate Programs
Adelphi University
Garden City, New York

Lorraine D. Williams, RN, PhD, APRN, BC
Associate Professor
School of Nursing
Southern Illinois University Edwardsville
Edwardsville, Illinois

Rhonda Kay Wilson, RN, BSN, MS
Quality Manager
Chester Mental Health Center
Chester, Illinois

Richard Yakimo, PhD, APRN, BC
Assistant Professor
School of Nursing
Southern Illinois University Edwardsville
Edwardsville, Illinois

Reviewers

Hudson T. Andrews, RPN, BSc, MSc
Douglas College
New Westminster, British Columbia, Canada

Susan Ashton, RN, PHN, BScN
Health Programs Instructor
Aurora College
Yellowknife, Northwest Territories, Canada

Amy Bender, RN, PhD
Assistant Professor
Lawrence S. Bloomberg Faculty of Nursing
University of Toronto
Toronto, Ontario, Canada

Marilynn J. Berg, BScN, MEd, RN
Clinical Teaching Faculty
Grant MacEwan University
Edmonton, Alberta, Canada

Leigh S. Blaney, RN, BScN, MA, CFMHN(C)
Professor, Bachelor of Science in Nursing Program
Vancouver Island University
Nanaimo, British Columbia, Canada

Florence Budden, BN, RN, CPMHN(c)
Faculty
Centre for Nursing Studies
St. John's, Newfoundland and Labrador, Canada

Anu Chiarelli, RN, BA, MA
Instructor, Health & Community Care
Bow Valley College
Calgary, Alberta, Canada

Sharon Chin, RN, MHScN, CPMHN(c)
Professor, Nursing
Nipissing University/Canadore College, Collaborative
    BScN Program
North Bay, Ontario, Canada

Linda Hopper Cook, RN, BSN, MN, PhD
Faculty Member, Baccalaureate Nursing Program
Grant MacEwen University
Edmonton, Alberta, Canada

Doreen Dawe, BN, MSc
Associate Professor
School of Nursing, Memorial University
St. John's, Newfoundland and Labrador, Canada

Adrianna D'Ilio, RN, BSN, MSN
Nursing Instructor
British Columbia Institute of Technology
Burnaby, British Columbia, Canada

Karen Fraser, BN, MScN
Professor
Loyalist College
Belleville, Ontario, Canada

Julia Gajewski-Noel, RN, BA, MN
Certificate in Mental Health Nursing
Senior Teaching Associate – Retired 2009
Faulty of Nursing
University of New Brunswick
Fredericton, New Brunswick

Elizabeth E. Harris, RN, BScN, MEd
Professor, Nursing Studies
Algonquin College
Ottawa, Ontario, Canada

Anna M. Helewka, RPN, RN, BSN, MSN
Curriculum and Program Evaluation Coordinator
Department of Psychiatric Nursing, Faculty of Health
    Sciences
Douglas College, David Lam Campus
New Westminster, British Columbia, Canada

Barney Hickey, RN, BScN, MScN
Nursing Faculty
Langara College
Vancouver, British Columbia, Canada

Linda Hopkins
Centennial College
Vancouver, British Columbia, Canada

Angela Hyden, RN, BScN, MN
Professor of Nursing
Sault College
Sault Ste. Marie, Ontario, Canada

Sonya Jakubec, RN, BHScN, MN, PhD(c)
Associate Professor
School of Nursing
Mount Royal University
Calgary, Alberta, Canada

Elsabeth Jensen, RN, PhD
Assistant Professor
York University, School of Nursing
Toronto, Ontario, Canada

Jane Karpa, BA, RPN, CMHW(C/A), MMFT
Assistant Professor
Bishop's University, Winnipeg Campus, School of
    Health Studies, Department of Psychiatric Nursing
Winnipeg, Manitoba, Canada

Robert Lockhart, Dip.SW, RPN, RN, BScN, MA
Site Coordinator, Psychiatric Nursing
Grant MacEwan University, Ponoka Campus
Edmonton, Alberta, Canada

Pat Mac Phail-Darrach, RN, BN
Clinical Coordinator, School of Nursing
University of Prince Edward Island
Charlottetown, Prince Edward Island, Canada

Karen Maddox, RN, BScN, MA(N)
Associate Professor
Lakehead University, School of Nursing
Thunder Bay, Ontario, Canada
Paula Maisonville, RN, BSN, MEd
Nurse Educator/College Instructor
Langara College
Vancouver, British Columbia, Canada

Paula Maisonville, RN, BSN, MEd
Nurse Educator/College Instructor
Langara College
Vancouver, British Columbia, Canada

Maureen Makepeace-Dore, RN, Med, BScN
Nursing Professor
Vancouver Island University
Nanaimo, British Columbia, Canada

Lynn McCleary, RN, BScN, MSc, PhD
Assistant Professor
Brock University
St. Catharines, Ontario, Canada

Robert J. Meadus, PhD, MSc, BN, BVocEd, RN
Assistant Professor
Memorial University, School of Nursing
St. John's, Newfoundland and Labrador, Canada

Sherri Melrose, RN, MEd, PhD
Assistant Professor
Athabasca University
Athabasca, Alberta, Canada

Marilyn Merritt-Gray, RN, MN
Professor
University of New Brunswick, Faculty of Nursing
Fredericton, New Brunswick, Canada

Phyllis Montgomery, RN, MScN, PhD
Associate Professor,
School of Nursing, Laurentian University
Sudbury, Ontario, Canada

**Sue Myers, RPN, Advanced Diploma in Psychiatric
    Nursing, BSW, M Voc/Tech Ed**
Program Head, Psychiatric Nursing Program
Saskatchewan Institute of Science and Technology,
    Wascana Campus
Regina, Saskatchewan, Canada

Linda Nykolyn, RN, BScN
Coordinator – Curriculum Development
NorQuest College
Edmonton, Alberta, Canada

Judy Osborne, RN, BN(c)
Clinical Faculty, Mental Health
Fleming College
Peterborough, Ontario, Canada

Norma Poirier, MN, PhD
Professeure titulaire
Université de Moncton
Moncton, New Brunswick, Canada

Catherine Pugnaire Gros, RN, MSc(A)
Faculty Lecturer
McGill University, School of Nursing
Montreal, Quebec, Canada

Iris Rudnisky, RN, BScN, MEd
Faculty Lecturer
Nursing Faculty, University of Alberta
Edmonton, Alberta, Canada

Yvonne Savard, RPN, RN, BScN, MA Ed/CI
Year II Facilitator, Nursing Instructor
Faculty of Health Sciences, Department of Psychiatric
   Nursing
Douglas College, David Lam Campus
Coquitlam, British Columbia, Canada

Andrew C. Sharpe, RN, MN, CPMHN(c)
Part-time Professor, School of Nursing
Faculty of Health Sciences, University of Ottawa
Ottawa, Ontario, Canada

Nicole Snow, MN, RN, CPMHN(c)
Faculty, Centre for Nursing Studies
St. John's, Newfoundland and Labrador, Canada

Wendy Stanyon, RN, BN, MA Ed, EdD
Associate Professor
University of Ontario Institute of Technology
Oshawa, Ontario, Canada

John Stone, RN, BScN, BA, MA, CPMHN(c)
Professor, Bachelor of Nursing Program
University of New Brunswick – Humber
Toronto, Ontario, Canada

Beth Swart, RN, MES
Professor
Daphne Cockwell School of Nursing
Ryerson University
Toronto, Ontario, Canada

Landa Terblanche, RN, MSN, PhD
Dean, School of Nursing
Trinity Western University
Langley, British Columbia, Canada

James Thomson, RPN, RN, CPMHN(c), MSN
Nursing Lecturer
Thompson Rivers University, School of Nursing
Kamloops, British Columbia, Canada

Judith Toth, RN, MN
Faculty of Nursing
University of Manitoba
Winnipeg, Manitoba, Canada

Barb Walsh, RPN, RN, BScN, MEd
Instructor
Douglas College
New Westminster, British Columbia, Canada

Wendy M. Wheeler, RN, BScN, MN
Nursing Instructor
Red Deer College
Red Deer, Alberta, Canada

Bernadine Wojtowicz, RN, BN
Academic Assistant II
University of Lethbridge
Lethbridge, Alberta, Canada

Preface

*I*t is an exciting time in Canada for the field of mental health. We now have a national mental health strategy aimed at improving the health and social outcomes of people living with mental illness. There is increasing recognition that mental health is not only an integral component of every individual's health and well-being but also a key aspect of a society's capacity to flourish. Nurses are well situated to contribute to the development and implementation of quality mental health care, as well as to the promotion of mental health and the prevention of mental illness. All professional nurses in this country are expected to bring a generalist level knowledge and skill in psychiatric and mental health (PMH) nursing to their practice. It is hoped that *Psychiatric and Mental Health Nursing for Canadian Practice*, now in its second edition, will be a prime resource for students in their efforts to gain that knowledge and skill. It would be very gratifying to the contributors to this book if it inspired, even in a small way, some students to pursue PMH as their specialty.

A major change from the first edition is the evolution of the bio/psycho/social model to a model that acknowledges more fully the spiritual domain of nursing. The spiritual domain is envisioned as encompassing the bio/psycho/social domains and as significant to the way individuals, families, and communities ascribe meaning and purpose to life. Our discipline has roots deeply embedded in the spiritual care of the sick and the wounded. Contemporary nursing is recognizing spirituality as an area for increased exploration, understanding, and skill development. Research suggests that many nurses are hesitant regarding their ability to provide appropriate spiritual care. The bio/psycho/social/spiritual model will, hopefully, provide nurses with a broader framework for holistic practice.

There is one completely new chapter in this edition: Chapter 5: *Mental Health in the Workplace*. Nurses must understand workplace health issues if they are to help address the psychosocial hazards and work-related stress that affect one fifth of the global working population. It is also necessary to nurses' own health and well-being. Canadian nurses' absenteeism rate, the time lost to injury and illness, is well above the national average. How can we provide safe, compassionate, competent, and ethical nursing care if we are not healthy ourselves? This chapter includes examination of what constitutes a healthy workplace, discusses work-life balance, describes ways to accommodate persons with mental health problems in the workplace, and explores workplace violence and bullying. It offers students a basis for understanding their own workplace issues.

As in the first edition, the terminology used to identify individual recipients of nursing care—patient, client, consumer, user, person—has been left to the preference of the chapter authors, as no term, as yet, predominates in the nursing literature. The many pedagogical features of the first edition have been retained, as well. The **Movies** feature has evolved to include novels and biographies in some chapters while retaining movies in all chapters. See below for a listing of features and information about the teaching-learning package.

■■ FEATURES

- Chapters open with **Learning Objectives**, **Key Terms**, and **Key Concepts** that cue students to the material they will encounter.
- **Summary of Key Points** encapsulates core chapter content to facilitate assimilation and review.
- **Critical Thinking Challenges** are grounded in chapter content and aimed at stimulating both analytical and reflective thinking about it on the part of students.
- In the **Movies**, **Novels**, and **Biographies** feature, movies and books are suggested as a rich, evocative means of raising and exploring complex ideas. Points to consider are offered. Students can use the suggested works to stimulate discussion with their family and friends, as well as their classmates and teachers.
- **Web Links** are listed to direct students to excellent sources of supplemental information.
- **CRNE Notes** are the Canadian authors' suggestions regarding important areas of preparation for the national registration examination.
- The **In a Life** feature illustrates the way the topic of the chapter has shaped or been played out in a particular person's life.
- **Research Boxes** focus on specific studies that contribute to improving PMH nursing practice. Most are recent Canadian nursing research projects and some reflect the work of the chapter's author(s). When a less recent study is highlighted, it is because of its significance to the topic.
- **Therapeutic Dialogue Boxes** encourage the comparison of therapeutic and nontherapeutic communication by giving relevant examples of both.
- **Clinical Vignette Boxes** present reality-based clinical portraits of persons with symptoms of interest to the chapter topic. Questions are posed to help students consider solutions to issues presented.
- **Drug Profile Boxes** present a profile of specific psychotropic medication, commonly prescribed in the treatment of mental disorders.
- **Psychoeducation Checklists** identify content areas for the education of persons with specific disorders and their families.
- **Key Diagnostic Characteristics**, tables, and summaries outline diagnostic criteria for disorders as standardized in the *Diagnostic and Statistical Manual of Mental Disorders*, 4th ed., Text revision (*DSM-IV-TR*) authored by the American Psychiatric Association.
- **Line, art, photo, scan images, and flow charts** illustrate the interrelationship of the biologic, psychological, social, and spiritual domains of mental health and illness.

■■ TEACHING-LEARNING PACKAGE

Student Resources

Students can find rich online multimedia resources at thePoint.lww.comAustin2e.

Free and bound in the book, this DVD-ROM supplies the following learning tools:

- *Movie Viewing Guides* that highlight films depicting individuals with mental health disorders and provide students the opportunity to approach nursing care related to mental health illness in a novel way.
- *Clinical Simulations* on schizophrenia, depression, and the acutely manic phase that walk students through case studies and put them in real-life situations.

These and other valuable student resources are also available on the Point. The DVD-ROM included with the book is designed to accompany the US edition of *Psychiatric Nursing*. As such, there may be slight differences between the materials provided here and the Canadian edition of the textbook.

Instructor Resources

The Instructor's Resources DVD-ROM contains additional information and activities that will help you engage your students from the semester's beginning to its end including

- PowerPoint slides
- Image Bank
- Test Generator
- WebCT, Blackboard, and Angel-Ready Material

This DVD-ROM is designed to accompany the US edition of *Psychiatric Nursing*. As such, there may be slight differences between the materials provided here and the Canadian edition of the textbook.

Wendy Austin
RN, MEd (Counselling), PhD,
Professor and Canada Research Chair
(Relational Ethics in Health Care)
University of Alberta

Contents

UNIT VIII Care Challenges in Psychiatric and Mental Health Nursing ... 851

UNIT *I*

The Landscape of Mental Health, Mental Illness, and Mental Health Care

1

Psychiatric and Mental Health Nursing: From Past to Present

Geertje Boschma and Marlee Groening

Adapted from the chapter "Psychiatric and Mental Health Nursing: From Past to Present" by Mary Ann Boyd

LEARNING OBJECTIVES

After studying this chapter, you will be able to:

- Identify the historical influences and social changes that affect the delivery of mental health care.
- Relate the concept of social change to the history of psychiatric and mental health care.
- Discuss the history of psychiatric and mental health (PMH) nursing and its place within nursing history.
- Analyze the theoretical arguments that shaped the development of contemporary scientific thought about PMH nursing practice.
- Summarize the impact of current social, economic, and political forces on the delivery of mental health services.

KEY CONCEPT

- social change

KEY TERMS

- biologic view • deinstitutionalization • moral treatment • psychiatric and mental health nursing education • psychiatric hospitals • psychiatric pluralism • psychoanalytic movement • psychosocial theory

*U*ntil the 19th century, mentally ill people were kept mostly at home, cared for by their families. Sometimes, their legal guardians boarded them with other families for a fee, as part of a broader poor relief system. Only the most seriously afflicted people whose behaviour was severely disturbing or dangerous, to either themselves, their families, or other citizens, were locked in, often in prisons or a separate wing of a local poor house. Indigent mentally ill people were grouped with other old, sick, orphaned, or convicted people, and the circumstances in these scanty public facilities were most basic and often harsh (Boschma, 2003; Shorter, 1997). For those who could afford it, privately maintained institutions emerged as well (McKenzie, 1992; Warsh, 1989).

EARLY FORMS OF INSTITUTIONAL CARE

As of the 1400s, the beginning of the Renaissance, some European towns established small-scale asylums as charitable enterprises, initially housing about 10 people. Most often they were civilian, charitable initiatives in which neither the church nor doctors were involved. Bedlam in London, Britain, founded in 1371, and the Reinier van Arkel asylum, founded in 1442, in the Dutch town of Den Bosch, are early examples of insane asylums or "mad houses" spreading throughout Europe, and, in the wake of colonialism, in other parts of the world over the next centuries. These asylums were managed as a

FIGURE 1.1 Interior of Bethlehem Asylum, London. (From U.S. National Library of Medicine. Images from the history of medicine. National Institutes of Health, Department of Health and Human Services.)

large household, like other guest houses or poor houses, administered by a board of noted citizens, with a steward and matron, often a married couple, taking charge of the day-to-day management, assisted by a few servants. In the changing social and economic context of the 18th and 19th centuries, these homes grew into larger institutions (Boschma, 2003) (Fig. 1-1).

Religious orders, often under the protection or authority of the church, also involved themselves with charitable work and poor relief. Roman Catholic orders, for example, reemerged in 17th-century France during the Counter Reformation, and many of them managed the care in small-scale, premodern hospitals. Sometimes, the orders themselves owned the houses. Influential cases in point were the male order of the Congregation of Lazarists and the female congregation of the Sisters of Mercy (or Daughters of Charity), founded by Vincent the Paul in 1625 and 1633, respectively (Jones, 1989). These orders generated the early models for nursing work as a socially respectable endeavour at a time when medical care was hardly available nor developed (Nelson, 1999, 2001; Porter, 1993). In the Americas, one of the first institutions that took in mentally ill people was San Hipólito in Mexico City, which opened as a hospital for the insane in 1589, under the auspices of the Roman Catholic Church. It was run by the brothers of the order of La Caridad y San Hipólito, founded a few decades earlier in 1566. Living by the vows of poverty and charity, the brothers relied on alms to support themselves, and working as attendants in the institution was one of their activities (Leiby, 1992). In Canada, the earliest forms of institutional treatment date back to the 19th century.

Diverse approaches to deal with mental illness or attempts to treat it have been employed throughout history and reflect the beliefs of the time. Spiritual, biologic, and social explanations commonly were intertwined in popular perceptions of causes of mental illness. Evil spirits, sin, demonic possession, contagious environments, or brain disturbances figured in explanations of mental disorders and shaped people's responses and medical treatments accordingly. The various ways of caring for mentally ill people typically depended on a community's perceived notions and fears of those with mental disorders as well as communities' resources.

History reflects that, generally, in periods of relative social stability, there are fewer fears and more tolerances for deviant behaviour, and it is easier for individuals with mental disorders to live safely within their communities. During periods of rapid **social change** and instability, there are more general anxieties and fears and, subsequently, more intolerances and ill treatments of people with mental disorders. As industrialization and urbanization increased during the 18th and 19th centuries, the rising middle class became concerned about a growing number of poor and deviant people who were not able to work and sustain themselves. Moreover, under the influence of the Enlightenment, medical and social ideas about mental illness changed during this time, and medical concern with the treatment of mental illness increased. Insight gained ground so that, rather than being afflicted by a loss of reason, the mentally ill were perceived as rational beings with a human nature just like all human beings. The idea that spirits or demons kept the insane in a bestial stage and, therefore, that restraints or enchainment seemed a reasonable approach, was rejected in favour of the view that mentally afflicted people should be treated humanely. Hence, the idea of a moral, pedagogical treatment emerged that would help these sufferers to restore their innate capacity for self-control (Boschma, 2003; D'Antonio, 2006; Tomes, 1994).

KEY CONCEPT **Social change**, the structural and cultural evolution of society, is constant and, at times, erratic. Psychiatric and mental health care has evolved within the social framework and cannot be separated from economic, sociocultural, and political realities.

A REVOLUTIONARY IDEA: HUMANE TREATMENT

By the height of the French Revolution in 1792, **moral treatment** became a most influential idea, dramatically altering the care of the mentally ill and generating important reform initiatives in which reform-minded physicians had an influential role. During this time Philippe Pinel (1745–1826) was appointed physician to Bicêtre, a hospital for men, which had a very poor reputation. Pinel, influenced by enlightened ideas, believed that the

Boarding Mentally Ill People With Families (12th to 19th Centuries)

The Geel Lunatic Colony, Belgium

The Legend of Saint Dymphna

According to the legend, Dymphna, an Irish princess, came to Geel in the 6th century. Disappointed that she was not a son, her father, king of Ireland, had left her and her mother in the care of a priest who converted them to Christianity. After Dymphna's mother died, the king became filled with grief and wanted another woman, just like his former wife. His advisors decided that only his own daughter could match the queen. However, when her pagan father wanted to marry Dymphna, she fled out of fear with her priest and came to Geel. When the Irish king eventually found Dymphna and the priest, he beheaded both. In some sources, the legend tells that several lunatics witnessing this frightful scene suddenly became cured. Symbolic for her resistance to the spirit of evil, Dymphna became patron of lunatics, and the site of her death, a place of miraculous healing. Some sources tell how the Saint Dymphna Guesthouse and chapel were built at this place, evolving into a place of pilgrimage.

A Powerful Example of Family Care in Geel, Belgium

Since the Middle Ages (1286), the Saint Dymphna Guesthouse and chapel have existed in Geel, Belgium, eventually with a separate sick room for lunatic pilgrims. Chronically mentally ill patients who came to the Guesthouse as pilgrims seeking healing were often boarded out to families, and the Geel Lunatic Colony came into being. In the 19th century, the place evolved into a formal institution with a strong emphasis on boarding out patients with foster families, which became a model for many countries to follow. The legend of Saint Dymphna illustrates mythical and religious beliefs, explanations, and practices that have lost their meaning today. However, the cultural heritage of the Geel Colony demonstrates how powerful past ideas and beliefs can be in structuring creative and humane solutions to the care of mentally ill people.

From Parry-Jones, W. L. L. (1981). The model of the Geel Lunatic Colony and its influence on the nineteenth-century asylum system in Britain. In A. Scull (Ed.), *Madhouses, mad-doctors, and madmen. The social history of psychiatry in the Victorian Era* (pp. 201–217). London, UK: The Athlone Press; Boschma, G. (2003). *The rise of mental health nursing: A history of psychiatric care in Dutch asylum, 1890–1920* (pp. 182–183, 277–278). Amsterdam, the Netherlands: Amsterdam University Press; and Goldstein, J. L., & Godemont, M. M. L. (2003). The legend and lessons of Geel, Belgium: A 1500-year-old legend, a 21st century model. *Community Mental Health Journal, 39*(5), 441–458.

FIGURE 1.2 The perspective view of the north front of the retreat near York. (From U.S. National Library of Medicine. *Images from the history of medicine.* National Institutes of Health, Department of Health and Human Services.)

humane, moral treatment, a pedagogical approach of kind supervision, proper medical treatment, and meaningful activities and distractions. Reform-minded physicians believed that such a purposefully designed asylum provided the proper environment to indeed cure the mentally ill (D'Antonio, 2006; Tomes, 1994).

Based on these influential examples, initiatives emerged throughout the Western world to establish purposefully designed asylums that provided sympathetic care in quiet, pleasant surroundings with some form of industrial occupation such as weaving or farming. In the United States, the Quaker Friends Asylum was proposed in 1811 and opened 6 years later in Frankford, Pennsylvania (now Philadelphia) to become the second asylum in the United States. The humane and supportive rehabilitative attitude of the Quakers was seen as an extremely important influence in changing techniques of caring for those with mental disorders (D'Antonio, 2006).

THE 19TH AND EARLY 20TH CENTURIES: AN ERA OF ASYLUM BUILDING

In Canada, New Brunswick was the first of the old British North American provinces to open a mental institution. In 1835, a committee was appointed to prepare a petition to the provincial legislature proposing the establishment of a provincial lunatic asylum. Until that time, counties had carried the responsibility under the Poor Laws system to confine indigent insane who could no longer be managed within the family, in local jails, or in poor houses. Yet, as the population rapidly increased in the early 1800s, the number of mentally ill in the need of publicly provided care grew. In 1835, the provincial government approved

insane were sick patients who needed humane treatment, and, once installed in his position, ordered the removal of the chains, stopped the abuses of drugging and bloodletting, and placed the patients under the care of more adequately prepared physicians. Three years later, the same standards were extended to Salpetrière, the asylum for female patients. At about the same time in England, William Tuke (1732–1822), a Quaker tea-merchant in York and a member of the Society of Friends, raised funds for a retreat for members of his Quaker community who had mental disorders. The York Retreat, which opened in 1796, became an evenly influential example for reform initiatives (Fig. 1-2). Tuke also introduced a regimen of

FIGURE 1.3 Canada's first hospital for the mentally ill, Saint John, New Brunswick, ca. 1885. (From Provincial Archives of New Brunswick, Saint John Stereographs—P86–67.)

the conversion of a building in Saint John, formerly a hospital for cholera patients a few years before, in 1832, to a Provincial Lunatic Asylum until a new facility could be built. By 1848, this new facility was ready for use

(Fig. 1-3) (Heritage Resources Saint John, 2000; Hurd, 1973/1916–17; Sussman, 1998).

During the latter half of the 19th century and beginning of the 20th century each Canadian province established an asylum (Table 1-1). Up until the mid-20th century, involuntary confinement and institutional care became the most dominant treatment modality for mentally ill people, replacing older forms of familial care and Poor Law–based approaches (Moran, 2000; Moran & Wright, 2006). In-depth historical analyses of admission patterns, one of the Ontario-based Homewood Retreat, for example, showed that gender differences were reflective of the social situation of the time (Warsh, 1989). Another analysis of the British Columbian psychiatric system revealed that many Aboriginal patients died soon after being admitted to the asylum, often from tuberculosis (Menzies & Palys, 2006).

The Legal Basis for Mental Health Care

Following the terms established by the British North America Act of 1867, the organization of mental health care became provincially based in Canada and each province developed its own legislation to deal with problems created by mental illness. In the late 19th century, all provinces passed legislation, most often called an Insanity Act, to provide a legal basis to publicly supported confinement of the mentally ill. In the course of the 20th century, the legislation has been changed and updated several times

Table 1.1	The First Asylums in British North America and Canada	
Province	**Date**	**Notes**
Quebec	1845	• Beauport, or the Quebec Lunatic Asylum, was opened.
		• A small dwelling for 12 mentally ill women was erected by Bishop St. Vallier.
	1714	• The Hotel Dieu cared for indigents, the crippled, and "idiots."
New Brunswick	1848	• The Provincial Lunatic Asylum was erected.
	1835	• Canada's first mental hospital opened in a small wooden building, a former cholera hospital, and was used as a temporary asylum.
Ontario	1850	• The Provincial Lunatic Asylum in Toronto admitted patients.
	1841	• Mentally ill people were placed in county jails until 1841 after which the Old York Jail served as a temporary asylum.
Newfoundland	1854	• An asylum for mentally ill patients was erected and admitted its first patients.
Nova Scotia	1857	• The first patients were admitted to the Provincial Hospital for the Insane.
British Columbia	1872	• A remodelled provincial general hospital (the old Royal Hospital) was opened as the Asylum for the Insane in British Columbia.
Prince Edward Island	1877	• The Prince Edward Island Hospital for the Insane was built.
Manitoba	1886	• The Selkirk Lunatic Asylum was opened.
Saskatchewan	1914	• The Saskatchewan Provincial Hospital admitted the first patients.
Alberta	1911	• The Provincial Asylum for the Insane opened in Ponoka.
Yukon and North West Territories		• These districts had no asylums in the early 20th century. The Royal North West Mounted Police assisted in transporting mentally ill patients to asylums in neighbouring provinces.

Adapted from Sussman, S. (1998). The first asylums in Canada: A response to neglectful community care and current trends. *Canadian Journal of Psychiatry, 43*, 260–264; Hurd, H. M. (Ed.). (1973, originally printed 1916–17). *The institutional care of the insane in the United States and Canada* (Vol. IV). New York, NY: Arno Press.

and eventually renamed into a provincial Mental Health Act, reflecting changing views and a stronger medical influence on the care and treatment of the mentally ill. In the beginning of institutional psychiatric care in Canada, all patients admitted to public institutions were certified patients. Today, patients are being admitted to an institutional facility on either a voluntary or a certified basis. A carefully designed legal process has to be followed for patients admitted as certified patients under the terms of a mental health act, although criteria may differ between provinces. In several provinces, the use of community treatment orders is a new development under the mental health act. (See Chapter 3 for the current legal context of mental health care.)

A Social Reformer: Dorothea Lynde Dix

An ardent advocate for establishing state-supported, public care of the mentally ill was Dorothea Lynde Dix (1802–1887). Her crusade for more humane treatment was responsible for much of the reform of mental health care systems in North America in the 19th century (Fig. 1-4). Almost 40 years of age, Dix, a retired school teacher living in Massachusetts, was solicited by a young theology student to help in preparing a Sunday School class for women inmates at the East Cambridge jail. Dix herself led the class and was shocked by the filth and dirt in the jail. She was particularly struck by the treatment of inmates with mental disorders. It was the dead of winter, and the jail provided no heat. When she questioned the jailer about the lack of heat, his answer was that "the insane need no heat." The prevailing myth was that the insane were insensible to extremes of temperature. Dix's outrage initiated a long struggle in the reform of care (Lightner, 1999).

Influenced by a wider social reform movement that had a strong cultural influence throughout the Western world, drawing men and women into a wide range of reform activities, Dix followed patterns of new women's activism, also employed by social reformers such as Elizabeth Fry in prison reform and Josephine Butler in protecting women against prostitution (Van Drenth & De Haan, 1999). She diligently investigated the conditions of jails and the plight of the mentally ill. Dix's solution to improving mental health care was to promote the building of more hospitals. In Canada, she was instrumental in advocating for mental institutions in Halifax, Nova Scotia, and St. John, Newfoundland (Hurd, 1973/1916–17; Lightner, 1999). Eventually, Dix expanded her work into Great Britain and other parts of Europe. During the Civil War, she was appointed superintendent of women nurses, the highest position held by a woman during the war.

Life Within Early Institutions

Despite the good intentions of early reformers, the approach inside the institution was one of custodial care and practical management, and treatment rarely occurred. The major concern was the management of a large number of people, many displaying disruptive behaviours. Patient numbers rapidly grew from the time provinces became legally responsible for financing care of the mentally ill. Soon, institutions experienced severe overcrowding and had little more than food, clothing, pleasant surroundings, and perhaps some means of employment and exercise to offer. Limited resources made life in the institutions difficult. Although a medical superintendent usually directed an institution, overcrowded wards and few resources created rowdy, dangerous, and unbearable situations. Quiet patients were involved in work as institutions grew into self-contained communities that produced their own food and made their own clothing. Day-to-day care was in the hands of lay personnel who shared with the patients the same routines of eating, sleeping, and working. Once admitted, many patients had little hope of reentering society.

Ontario psychiatrist Charles K. Clarke (1857–1924) had an influential role in bringing about new models of care that would influence change of this situation. As superintendent of various Ontario provincial **psychiatric hospitals** (e.g., Rockwood Hospital, 1881–1905), he was aware of the enormous problems that asylums experienced (Brown, 2000). He continuously brought improvement to the asylums that he directed, including the introduction of nurse training for asylum personnel. To find better treatments and approaches, he sought to start an urban centre for the treatment of acute mental illness under the best possible conditions and supported by university-based scientific research. Eventually, his dream came through in the establishment of the Toronto Psychiatric Hospital (TPH), which opened in 1925. Clarke's name was commemorated in Toronto's Clarke Institute of Psychiatry, the 1966 successor of TPH (Greenland, 1996) and now

FIGURE 1.4 Dorothea Lynde Dix. (From U.S. National Library of Medicine. *Images from the history of medicine.* National Institutes of Health, Department of Health and Human Services.)

known, after a merger with other Ontario institutions, as the Centre for Addiction & Mental Health.

Soon, the deplorable state of large mental institutions generated public commotion. In 1908, Clifford Beers (1876–1943) published an autobiography, *A Mind That Found Itself*, depicting his 3-year experience in three different types of hospitals: a private for-profit hospital, a private nonprofit hospital, and a state institution. In all these facilities, he reported that he was beaten, choked, imprisoned for long periods in dark, dank, padded cells, and confined for many days in a straight jacket. He became an ardent advocate of the reform of psychiatric care. Beers' cause was supported by a prominent neuropathologist, Adolf Meyer (1866–1950), who suggested the term "mental hygiene" for bringing about improvement of people's mental health similar to public health initiatives. By 1909, Beers formed a National Committee for Mental Hygiene. Through the committee's efforts, child guidance clinics, prison clinics, and industrial mental health approaches developed. In Canada, Beers and Meyer found a close ally in Clarence Hincks, a leading Toronto psychiatrist, who was instrumental in founding the Canadian National Committee for Mental Hygiene (CNCMH) in 1918, together with his colleague Charles Clarke.

The appalling situation of Canadian provincial mental hospitals triggered particular political concern when returning veterans suffering from shell shock had to rely on existing psychiatric facilities in their home provinces. A new belief in scientific approaches and reliance on expert knowledge in the prevention of mental illness and so-called weak-mindedness gained ground. These views were intertwined with class-based concern about the alleged excessive growth of the weak minded and betterment of the human race, influenced by eugenic ideas of the time. This context of change provided a climate for expanding professionalism of many groups, including psychiatrists, psychologists, and nurses. The CNCMH clearly promoted the transformation of asylums into mental hospitals, introducing a trained nursing staff as part of its strategy. Voluntary admission controlled by physicians was supported, thus advancing the view that mental illness was similar to any physical illness.

Development of Psychiatric and Mental Health Nursing

Early Developments

In its many surveys of institutional facilities, the CNCMH recommended the enhancement of asylum personnel and suggested the introduction of training schools for mental nurses, later called psychiatric nurses, similar to nurse training schools in general hospitals (Boschma, Yonge, & Mychajlunow, 2005; MacLennan, 1987; Tipliski, 2004). Charles K. Clarke, psychiatrist and superintendent of

Rockwood Mental Hospital in Ontario (1881–1905), was instrumental in establishing one of the first training schools for nurses.

Clarke's initiative to implement nurse training for female personnel in mental hospitals occurred first at Rockwood Hospital and later at the Provincial Hospital in Toronto (Brown, 2000). Well-educated women with a sense of order and compassion had been essential in the introduction of training schools in general hospitals. In their efforts to model psychiatric asylums after the general hospitals, psychiatrists took that ideal and geared the training of mental nurses toward women. The trained nurses provided them with the assistance they needed for new therapies and enhanced the hospital's reputation (Boschma, 2003; Brown, 2000; Connor, 1996). It was thought that women had the right moral, feminine characteristics for good patient care. Whereas in general hospitals, the care of male patients was put in the hands of female nurses assisted by male orderlies, in psychiatry, this shift was less easily made, owing to the nature of difficult patient behaviour. Male attendants retained a prominent place in the care of the mentally ill, but their training obtained a lower status, or, in the Ontario mental hospitals, they initially did not receive any training at all (Tipliski, 2002). See Box 1-1 for historical highlights.

BOX 1.1
Highlights From PMH Nursing History

1888	The first mental nurse training school established at Kingston's Rockwood Asylum
1918	Foundation of the Canadian National Committee of Mental Hygiene
1920	First psychiatric nursing text published, *Nursing Mental Disease*, by Harriet Bailey
1922	First Registration of Nurses Act passed in Ontario including nurse training schools at the mental hospitals
1930s	Mental hospitals in western Canada established schools for mental nurses and attendants
1950	Psychiatric Nurses Association of Canada (PNAC) founded
1952	Publication of Hildegard E. Peplau's *Interpersonal Relations in Nursing*
1963	*Perspectives in Psychiatric Care* and *Journal of Psychiatric Nursing* published
1979	*PNAC Working paper on Standards of Practice for Psychiatric Nurses* published
1986	The Canadian Nurses Association establishes a national certification program for specialty nursing practice
1988	Canadian Federation of Mental Health Nurses (CFMHN) founded
1995	*CFMHN Standards of Psychiatric and Mental Health Nursing Practice* published
2006	*Canadian Standards for Psychiatric-Mental Health Nursing*, 3rd edition published

Regional Influences

In western Canada, which had a stronger orientation to British traditions of institutional care, the introduction of mental nurse training also followed the Training School model, except that men were trained as well. In western provinces, mental hospitals began implementing training schools in the 1930s. In Alberta, for example, in 1932, the Alberta Department of Health hired psychiatrist Charles A. Barager, initially as acting superintendent and soon as commissioner of mental health service, to implement reform. Barager came from Manitoba, where he had introduced a nurse training school as superintendent at the Brandon Asylum. He had a strong belief in the ability of female compassion: "The nursing of mental patients requires women of finer personality, of wider sympathies, greater self-control and higher intelligence than even the nursing of those who are physically ill" (Boschma et al., 2005; Dooley, 2004; Tipliski, 2002, p. 95).

Barager's term in Alberta was short lived; he died suddenly in 1936. However, the training for nurses and attendants that he initiated in the Alberta Hospital at Ponoka had a lasting influence. Despite opposition to his ideas from the Registered Nurses Association in Alberta, which had controlled the registration of nurses since 1916, he was able to secure approval for a new diploma in mental nursing through the Alberta Department of Health. Creatively, he established arrangements with general hospitals in the province, so that, after 2 years of training in the mental hospital, female nurse students could undertake an additional 18 months of training at a general hospital and take licensing exams for registered nurses, after which they would return to the mental hospital. For male attendants, a 3-year certificate course was implemented, leading to a diploma in mental nursing. Male graduates did not obtain registered nursing status, reflective of the gendered context in which mental nurse training emerged. Skilled nursing was essential for new therapies, such as electroshock and insulin coma therapy introduced in the 1930s and 1940s. Alberta Hospital at Ponoka had, as well, a large infirmary with many frail and sick patients (Boschma et al., 2005).

This climate of change created many new opportunities for working and middle-class women to pursue a career as psychiatric nurses, and nursing thought continued to develop. The first psychiatric and mental health (PMH) nursing textbook that appeared in North America, *Nursing Mental Disease*, was written by Harriet Bailey in 1920. The content of the book reflected an understanding of mental disorders of the times and set forth nursing care in terms of appropriate procedures.

◼◼ MODERN THINKING

As PMH nursing began to develop as a profession in the early part of the 20th century, modern perspectives on mental illness were emerging. These new theories would profoundly shape the future of mental health care for all practitioners. Chapter 8 examines the underlying ideologies, but it is important to understand their development within the social and historical context to appreciate fully their impact on treatment approaches.

Evolution of Scientific Thought

In the early 1900s, two opposing views were held regarding mental illnesses: the belief that mental disorders had biologic origins and the belief that the problems were attributed to environmental and social stresses. **Psychosocially oriented ideas** proposed that mental disorders resulted from environmental and social deprivation. Moral treatment grew out of this idea, and the notion of prevention advocated by the mental hygiene movement also reflected a psychosocial orientation. The **biologic view** held that mental illnesses had a biologic cause and could be treated with physical interventions. However, biologic approaches and physical treatments such as bed rest; wet packs, which entailed wrapping patients in wet sheets; and prolonged baths became popular as new treatments around 1900 as part of the rise of scientific psychiatry. They were grounded in the idea that overstrained nerves should obtain rest. This turned out to be largely ineffective.

Meyer and Psychiatric Pluralism

Adolf Meyer bridged the ideologic gap between the two approaches by introducing the concept of **psychiatric pluralism**, an integration of human biologic functions with the environment. He focused on investigating how organic functions related to the person and how the person, constituted of these organs, related to the environment (Neill, 1980). Unfortunately, this included the surgical treatment of psychosis by one of his disciples, Henry Cotton, who believed infection caused insanity and, thus, removed sites of sepsis (e.g., teeth, tonsils, colon) from his patients in an effort to cure them (Scull, 2005). Meyer's ideas had little chance to evolve and flourish as the emerging psychoanalytic theories soon dominated the psychiatric world in North America for a long time to come.

Freud and the Psychoanalytic Theory

Sigmund Freud (1856–1939) and the **psychoanalytic movement** of the early 1900s promised a radically new approach to PMH care. Freud, trained as a neuropathologist, developed a personality theory based on unconscious motivations for behaviour, or drives. Using a new technique, psychoanalysis, he delved into the patient's feelings and emotions regarding past experiences, particularly early childhood and adolescent memories, to explain the basis of aberrant behaviour. He showed that symptoms of hysteria could be produced and made to disappear while patients were in a subconscious state of hypnosis.

According to the Freudian model, normal development occurred in stages, with the first three—oral, anal, and genital—being the most important. The infant progressed through the oral stage, experiencing the world through symbolic oral ingestion; into the anal stage, in which the toddler developed a sense of autonomy through withholding; and on to the genital stage, in which a beginning sense of sexuality emerged within the framework of the Oedipal relationship. If there was any interference in normal development, such as psychological trauma, psychosis or neurosis would develop.

Primary causes of mental illnesses were now viewed as psychological, and any physical manifestations or social influences were considered secondary (Malamud, 1944). Psychoanalysts believed that mental illnesses originated from disturbed personality development and faulty parenting. They categorized mental illnesses either as a psychosis (severe) or neurosis (less severe). A psychosis impaired daily functioning because of breaks in contact with reality. A neurosis was less severe, but individuals were often distressed about their problems. The terms *psychosis* and *neurosis* entered common, everyday language and added credibility to Freud's conceptualization of mental disorders. Soon, Freud's ideas represented the forefront of psychiatric thought and shaped society's view of mental health care. Freudian ideology dominated psychiatry well into the 1970s. Intensive psychoanalysis, aimed at repairing the trauma of the original psychological injury, was the treatment of choice. Psychoanalysis was costly and time-consuming and required lengthy training. Few could perform it. Thus, thousands of patients in state institutions with severe mental illnesses were essentially ignored.

Integration of Biologic Theories into Psychosocial Treatment

Until the 1940s, the biologic understanding of mental illness was unsophisticated and misguided. Early biologic treatments often were unsuccessful because of the lack of understanding and knowledge of the biologic basis of mental disorders. For example, the use of hydrotherapy, or baths, was an established procedure in mental institutions. The use of warm baths and, in some instances, ice cold baths were thought to produce calming effects for patients with mental disorders. However, the treatment's success was ascribed to its effectiveness as a form of restraint because the physiologic responses that hydrotherapy produced were not understood. Baths often ended up as a form of restraint, rather than as a therapeutic practice. Other examples of biologic procedures applied either indiscriminately or inappropriately included psychosurgery and electroconvulsive therapy (see Chapters 14 and 21).

Thanks to modern technology, neurosurgical techniques and electroconvulsive therapy can now be applied more humanely with positive therapeutic outcomes for some psychiatric disorders.

Support for the biologic approaches received an important boost as successful symptom management with psychopharmacologic agents became a more wide-spread possibility in the early 1950s. Psychopharmacology revolutionized the treatment of mental illness and led to an increased number of patients discharged into the community, and the eventual focus on the brain became a key to understanding psychiatric disorders. Chlorpromazine was an early neuroleptic drug that became widely used. Profound behavioural changes, observed as a result of this medication in long-term mentally ill patients, created an enormous enthusiasm about the potential of new medications. However, the knowledge about the working of the drugs was in infancy, and side effects of the new medications soon became serious drawbacks. As knowledge increased, and the management of side effects improved, psychopharmacotherapeutics obtained a central place in the treatment of mental illness. The introduction of lithium in the early 1970s brought a lasting change in the treatment of bipolar disorder, as did antidepressants in the treatment of mood disorders (LaJeunesse, 2000). Nurses obtained an essential role in administering medication, in monitoring its effect, and in teaching clients about their working.

New Trends in Post–World War II Mental Health Care

Following the experiences of World War II, insight grew among governments, as well as health professionals, that psychiatric services had to be placed on a new footing. By the end of the 1940s, patients in overcrowded, isolated psychiatric hospitals outnumbered the number of patients in other health care facilities, including general hospitals. Increased federal funding for health services and training of health care personnel created new opportunities. The implementation of universal health insurance for hospital care and medical services during the 1950s and 1960s, based on a 50%/50% cost sharing between federal and provincial governments, generated funding for the establishment of psychiatric departments in general hospitals, shifting the focus of services away from large provincial institutions. The Canadian Mental Health Association (CMHA), renamed from the earlier CNCMH, had an instrumental role in policy development for integrated services in general hospitals and the community. In its influential 1963 report, *More for the Mind*, the CMHA argued that mental illness had to be dealt with in similar ways to physical illness, and it argued for the application of multiple perspectives—medical, social, and familial—in multidisciplinary services and community treatment. A shift in mental health policy resulted in **deinstitutionalization**, the downsizing of the large provincial psychiatric hospitals, and a new orientation on community-based services. Biologic approaches, such as use of psychopharmacology and safer application of electroconvulsive therapy, were complemented by new rehabilitative services, the use of group therapy and other psychotherapies, as well as the provision of day treatment (Greenland, Griffin, & Hoffman, 2001; Shorter, 1997).

Because of these policies and trends, Canadian developments in psychiatric care differed substantially from post–World War II changes in the United States, where after the passage of the 1946 National Mental Health Act and the subsequent 1963 Mental Retardation Facilities and Community Mental Health Centres Construction Act, the emphasis was placed on newly built community mental health centres. In Canada, funding for mental health care became part of the larger health care system, with a strong emphasis on general hospital–based psychiatric care. Although the services in the new general hospital units improved treatment opportunities, the needs of the former provincial hospital population were not always adequately met, and it became apparent that problems created by persistent and severe mental illness were not resolved (Hector, 2001; Shorter, 1997).

In the late 1970s, the federal government shifted to a new funding structure for health care, reducing its share in the cost. Provinces developed different models and strategies to fund specialized services, for example, alcohol and substance abuse treatment programs, a pressing post–World War II mental health care need. To address the needs of different population groups, subspecialties such as child psychiatry, forensic, and geriatric services also emerged. The perception of health care as a right enhanced consumer and volunteer involvement, as well as public education on mental illness, and it increased the demand for patient autonomy. The 1981 Charter of Rights and Freedoms was a reflection of this social change (Greenland et al., 2001).

Continued Evolution of Psychiatric and Mental Health Nursing

The new multidisciplinary services generated an enormous need for more and better trained mental health care personnel, including nurses. The changes created a context for new developments in **PMH nursing education**. Organized responses of provincial professional nurses organizations, as well as efforts of hospital administrators and psychiatrists, who traditionally had a central role in hospital-based nurse training programs to staff the psychiatric hospitals and new health care facilities, resulted in a diverse pattern of PMH nurse education. As of the 1950s, Canada entertained two models of education for PMH nursing, resulting in the preparation of two different professional nursing groups for nursing care in mental

health services. Regional influences played a large role in the generation of the two models. On the one hand, general hospital–based schools of nursing, especially in eastern Canada, began to integrate psychiatric nursing into their curriculum. In Ontario, for example, under the influence of the mental hygiene movement, as of the 1930s, general hospital training schools began to include care of mentally ill patients into their training. Student nurses attended the provincial psychiatric hospitals for a brief period of training, called an *affiliation program*. Conversely, mental nurse trainees, mostly women, from the psychiatric hospital–based nurse training programs opted for an affiliation to the general hospital, resulting in both groups' obtaining the title of registered nurse. After World War II, the provincial government and the provincial association of registered nurses in Ontario formalized this pattern into a permanent structure. Gradually, the psychiatric hospital–based programs decreased in number and size, and the registered nurse became the main nursing care provider in mental health services (Tipliski, 2004).

In the less densely populated western Canadian provinces, the pattern that general hospital nurse trainees chose affiliation experiences at the psychiatric hospitals also emerged, but the bulk of nursing care in the provincial hospitals continued to be provided by nurses and attendants graduated from psychiatric hospital–based training programs. As noted previously, some western provinces, such as Alberta Hospital in Ponoka, established an affiliation program for female mental nurse trainees, and its graduates obtained the title of registered nurse. Yet, the program was limited in size, and many women worked in the institution as untrained attendants until the 1960s. Male trainees received a diploma in mental nursing. In British Columbia a training school for mental nurses, later called psychiatric nurses, was established in 1930 at Essondale, which eventually became Riverview Hospital (Fig. 1-5).

FIGURE 1.5 Graduation ceremony, School of Psychiatric Nursing, Essondale (Riverview Hospital), ca. 1950s. (From Historical collection, Riverview Hospital Historical Society, Coquitlam, BC.)

In the western provinces, the government had less control over nurse training than in neighbouring Ontario. Provincial associations of registered nurses in western provinces failed to support affiliation for psychiatric hospital–based nurse trainees, while medical superintendents of psychiatric hospitals retained much of their influence over psychiatric nurse education (Boschma et al., 2005; Tipliski, 2004).

In the late 1940s, attendants in the province of Saskatchewan took the lead in obtaining political support for a different pattern of nurse education that would lead to a separate Psychiatric Nurses Act and subsequent training acts, independent of provincial registered nurse practice acts. Their action resulted in a distinct professional group of psychiatric nurses. During the 1950s, all four western Canadian provinces passed such acts, which entitled graduates of psychiatric hospital–based nurse training programs in the West to receive the title of psychiatric nurse. In Saskatchewan, registered nurses had never successfully integrated into the mental hospitals. The very dominant medical superintendent, James Mac-Neill, who held sway over North Battleford hospital until the 1940s, strongly believed that general hospital training had little relevance for mental hospitals. In the 1930s, a psychiatric training program emerged for Saskatchewan asylum attendants, which was expanded after World War II to address the new need for psychiatric expertise, but it never resulted in registration as a nurse. Dissatisfied with their exclusion from any professionally recognized nursing title, provincial hospital attendants, who in Saskatchewan had obtained the right to unionize after the election of the new Co-operative Commonwealth Federation government in 1944, became instrumental in generating union support, as well as backing from the new government, for legislation of a separate psychiatric nurses act, which passed Parliament in 1948. Soon, the other western provinces followed suit, and in 1950, the Psychiatric Nurses Association of Canada was formed (Dickinson, 1989; Tipliski, 2002, 2004). The two separate models of psychiatric nursing education exist until today and have been integrated into the regular education system over the past decades.

■ THE LATE 20TH AND EARLY 21ST CENTURY

In the post–World War II era, nurses continued their central role in facilitating the therapeutic climate within psychiatric hospitals (Fig. 1-6). The community mental health movement and deinstitutionalization advocated with much enthusiasm during the 1960s and 1970s generated many new functions for PMH nurses (Boschma et al., 2005; Church, 1987). Nurses became involved in preparing and guiding persons with chronic, yet stabilized mental illness for discharge and living into the community. In the psychiatric hospitals and general hospital units, nurses obtained new therapeutic roles in group therapies, and their work in community mental health services expanded. New theoretical models became available that emphasized building therapeutic nurse–patient relationships and holistic nursing approaches. Hildegard Peplau, in recent scholarship recognized as "Psychiatric Nurse of the Century," proved to be a strong leader in the field (Boschma et al.; Calaway, 2002).

Expansion of Holistic Nursing Care

In 1952, Peplau published the landmark work, *Interpersonal Relations in Nursing*. It introduced PMH nursing practice to the concepts of interpersonal relations and the importance of the therapeutic relationship. In fact, the nurse–patient relationship was defined as the very essence of PMH nursing and supported a holistic perspective on patient care (see Chapters 7 and 9). Peplau's view was also important in its conceptualization of nursing care as truly independent of physicians. The nurse's use of self as a nursing tool was outside the dominance of both hospital administrators and physicians.

By 1963, two U.S.-based nursing journals, the *Journal of Psychiatric Nursing* (now the *Journal of Psychosocial Nursing and Mental Health Services*) and *Perspectives in Psychiatric Care*, as well as the *Canadian Journal of Psychiatric Nursing* (*1975–1990*), focused on psychiatric nursing. Also, the *Canadian Journal for Nursing Research* began to publish PMH nursing research. During the 1980s, the Canadian Federation of Mental Health Nurses (CFMHN) formed as an interest group of the Canadian Nurses Association with the view to promote the interests of mental health nurses and to bring matters of mental health nursing interest and psychiatric patient care to the attention of the public at large. In 1995, this group

FIGURE 1.6 Sports Day on Riverview Hospital grounds, nurses and patients, 1966. (From Historical collection, Riverview Hospital Historical Society, Coquitlam, BC.)

published the *Canadian Standards of Psychiatric and Mental Health Nursing Practice*. Based on the influential work of Patricia Benner (1984), the standards were written within a "domains of practice" framework. It promoted a holistic perspective on nursing care, with PMH nurses practicing in a variety of settings with a variety of clientele. The emphasis was on activities ranging from health promotion to health restoration. The standards reflected the belief that PMH nursing should be research driven, continually incorporating new findings into nursing practice. Relying on these standards, the Canadian Nurses Association created the opportunity to become certified in mental health nursing as part of their larger certification program of specialty nursing areas established during the 1980s. Recently, the CFMHN revised and updated the standards, incorporating the most recent perspectives on psychiatric care (CFMHN, 2006).

Contemporary Issues

During the 1980s, wrinkles in the social fabric of mental health care emerged. The mixed results of deinstitutionalization became apparent and generated a series of government-commissioned reports in all provinces to improve mental health services. Enormous variation existed among provinces in the extent and timing in which they implemented deinstitutionalization policies. People with mental disorders were discharged into communities that were often ill prepared to offer sufficient support in the way of community support programs, housing, or vocational opportunities. These communities were also sometimes hesitant in accepting people with persistent mental illness in their midst, and stigma remained attached to mental health services (Hector, 2001; Sealy & Whitehead, 2004).

Self-help groups and family and consumer organizations, such as the Schizophrenia Society of Canada and the Mood Disorder Society of Canada, have become active participants in mental health care services during the past decades. Outreach and mobile crisis response teams emerged to address problems created by severe mental illness in the community. A new category of "revolving door" patients signified that long-term, severe mental illness remained a persistent problem, with patients continuously moving in and out of the acute care system. Also, the interconnected issues of severe mental illness, substance dependency, and inadequate community resources and housing have resulted in a growing number of homeless people with mental illness, as well as a large population of mentally ill winding up in the criminal justice systems. Within these groups, the specific mental health needs of women remain poorly addressed. Moreover, there exists a growing awareness that diverse cultural populations have distinctive mental health needs. Aboriginal mental health is a pressing issue in Canada because Aboriginal communities experience disproportionate rates of both physical and mental illness due to an unbalanced health care system that has not been adaptive to the specific health needs of Aboriginal peoples (see Chapter 3). Today mental health services are still fragmented and not sufficiently developed to meet the need. Millions of adults and children are disabled by mental illness every year. When compared with all other diseases, mental illness ranks first in terms of causing disability in North America and Western Europe (Greenland et al., 2001; Hart Wasekeesikaw, 2006; Hector, 2001; Morrow, 2002; World Health Organization [WHO], 2001).

The New Era of Health Care Reform

Both public and private expenditures for health care services have increased in North America. Financial and social barriers continue to affect the overall funding for mental health. Now, large networks of public and private organizations share responsibility for mental health care, with the state remaining as the major decision maker for resource allocation. Emphasis is on reducing expensive institutional care and increasing the resources devoted to community-based care for the mentally ill, such as those in clinics, homes, schools, and treatment centres. With so many organizations involved in mental health services, the voice of mental health care has become fragmented. It became clear during the 1990s that new federal initiatives in mental health policy were urgently needed. In 1998, the Canadian Alliance on Mental Illness and Mental Health (CAMIMH) was formed as a conjoint initiative of the Canadian Psychiatric Association, the Canadian Mental Health Association, the Mood Disorder Association of Canada, the National Network for Mental Health, and the Schizophrenia Society of Canada. Jointly, consumers and service providers began to lobby the federal government to come to an action plan and a new national agenda for mental health care (Beauséjour, 2001). Two years later, the CAMIMH joined the Canadian Collaborative Mental Health Initiative (CCMHI) which was formed to focus more strongly on the improvement of mental health care in the primary health care setting. Consumers and caregivers were actively involved in this collaborative initiative (see Chapters 7 and 12).

In 2002, the CAMIMH published its first report, a collation of the latest Canadian data on mental illness, with assistance from Health Canada. The report revealed that currently 86% of hospitalizations for mental illness in Canada occur in general hospitals. Twenty percent of Canadians will personally experience mental illness over their lifetime. Approximately 8% of adults will experience major depression. Bipolar disorder and schizophrenia each affect 1% of the Canadian population. The hospitalization rates in general hospitals of anxiety disorders, affecting 12% of the population, are twice as high among women as men. Suicide accounts for 24% of all deaths among 15- to 24-year-olds and for 16% among 25- to 44-year-olds. Although the report also found that mental illness can be treated more effectively, the data clearly reveal the need for continued, integrated mental health policy development (Health Canada, 2002). In 2001, the WHO focused its annual *World Health Report* on mental health, also emphasizing the importance of mental health to the well-being of individuals (WHO, 2001).

• CRNENOTE

CRNENOTE
Current mental health policy's focus on community-based care and integration aims at moving away from older, more stigmatizing approaches of long-term institutionalization and custodial care.

Developing a National Mental Health Strategy

Between 2003 and 2006, the Senate Standing Committee on Social Affairs, Science and Technology, chaired by Senator Michael Kirby, completed a systematic review of the Canadian mental health system in an attempt to explore and address the significant and universal service gaps. The committee published four reports (Kirby, 2004; Kirby & Keon 2006). The first report detailed the personal stories of individuals and families afflicted by mental illness, which highlighted the fragmented and often difficult to access mental health and addiction services. The second report drew attention to Canada's lack of a national mental health strategy through the examination and comparison of the mental health services of four G8 countries (New Zealand, Australia, England, and the United States). The third report summarized and set options for mental health and addiction services in Canada. "Out of the Shadows at Last: Transforming Mental Health, Mental Illness and Addiction Services in Canada," was the fourth and final report (Kirby & Keon, 2006). It summarized the previous reports and proposed 118 recommendations, all with the primary intention of promoting mental health and recovery as opposed to focusing on mental illness alone. See Box 1-2 for a summary of the key principles and key initiatives proposed in this report.

Woven throughout the stories of Canadians suffering from mental illness, the complex issues of stigmatization and discrimination are highlighted. Their far-reaching social, economic, and policy effects impact not only on health care but also on housing, employment, social welfare, as well as the justice system (Kirby & Keon, 2006). The reality of this discrimination is epitomized by the "national health policy in Canada, the *Canada Health Act* (CHA), [which] explicitly excludes coverage

BOX 1.2

Key Principles and Initiatives of the Kirby Report, "Out of the shadows at last"

Key principles of the proposed mental health reform: Working toward a recovery and prevention focused system resting upon three pillars:

- **Choice:** Access to a wide range of publicly funded services and supports that offer people living with mental illness the opportunity to choose those that will benefit them most.
- **Community:** Making these services and supports available in the communities where people live, and orienting them toward supporting people living in the community.
- **Integration:** Integrating all types of services and supports across the many levels of government and across both the public/private divide and the professional/nonprofessional dichotomy.

Key initiatives that need to become a primary focus in the proposed mental health reform:

- Initiate a 10-year national antistigma campaign.
- Establishment of a national Knowledge Exchange Centre.
- Develop a national strategy to address mental illness with all stakeholders involved.

Kirby, M. J. L., & Keon, W. J. (2006). Out of the shadows at last: Transforming mental health, mental illness and addiction services in Canada. Ottawa, ON: Government of Canada. Retrieved September 17, 2008, from http://www.parl.gc.ca/39/1/parlbus/com-mbus/senate/com-e/soci-e/rep-e/rep02may06-e.htm

for treatment in psychiatric hospitals" (Kirby, 2005, p. 9). The review also highlights disparities in access to care between urban and rural Canada, which are further complicated by unique regional multicultural needs. Much of this regional discrepancy is blamed on the lack of a nationwide mental health strategy and the inconsistent provincial jurisdictions that determine mental health policies and the allocation and delivery of services (Kirby, 2004).

While the report has been embraced by many mental health care consumers and caregivers, it is not without its critics. Some of the criticisms are related to being "prevalence focused," with not enough emphasis on "preventative determinants," as well as the lack of recognition of the depth of disability caused by mental illness (Arboleda-Flórez, 2005). Some women's advocate groups have also challenged the report's "silence" on the disparities between mental health and addiction services for men and women, while others have critiqued the report's "neutrality to ownership" as erosive of our publically funded health care system and condoning of privatization in health care (Canadian Women's Health Network, 2006).

Despite these criticisms, it is clear that the report spotlighted mental health issues of Canadians and has

BOX 1.3

The Mental Health Commission of Canada: Four Main Goals (2007)

Goal 1 Be a catalyst for the reform of mental health policies and improvements in service delivery

Goal 2 Act as a facilitator, enabler, and supporter of a national approach to mental health issues

Goal 3 Work to diminish the stigma and discrimination faced by Canadians living with mental illness

Goal 4 Disseminate evidence-based information on all aspects of mental health and mental illness to governments, stakeholders, and the public

From www.mentalhealthcommission.ca/mhcc.en.html

offered options for mental health care reform. To that end, the report recommended a national (not federal) initiative in the form of a Mental Health Commission of Canada to direct policy on mental health and addiction services across Canada, minimize fragmentation of mental health services, and to develop research and strategies around best practices to achieve equitable care (Kirby & Keon, 2006). In 2007 the federal government established such a Commission and appointed Kirby as its Chair. Currently the Commission is working toward a national mental health policy and has articulated four main goals (Box 1-3).

The challenge before Canadian nurses is to strive to address these goals while working within the existing constraints to provide cost-effective services. To address the pressing mental health care needs in the 21st century, nurses must continue to participate in devising and implementing a continuum of mental health services that provides access for all and to develop appropriate partnerships with other health professionals and consumer groups.

SUMMARY OF KEY POINTS

☐ Throughout history, attitudes and treatment toward those with mental disorders have drastically changed as a result of the changing socioeconomic backdrop of our society and the development of new theories and study by key individuals and groups.

☐ During the 1800s, as mental illness began to be viewed as an illness, more humane and moral treatments began to develop.

☐ Social reformers, such as Dorothea Dix, C. K. Clarke, Clifford Beers, and C. Hincks, dedicated their efforts to raising society's awareness and to advocating public responsibility for the proper treatment of persons with mental illness.

☐ Theoretic arguments characterized the evolution of scientific thought and psychiatric practice. Gradually, the importance of the biologic aspect of mental disorders has been recognized while psychosocial approaches were also developed.

☐ Although the need for PMH nursing was recognized near the end of the 19th century, initially there was resistance to training attendants for the care of the insane. At the initiative of C. K. Clarke, medical superintendent of Rockwood Hospital (1881–1905), the first Training School for Mental Nurses was established in 1888.

☐ Gradually, all provinces adapted to education for PMH nurses. By the 1930s, all provinces had established training schools for asylum attendants and nurses. In the post–World War II era, two models of education for psychiatric nurses emerged, leading to two distinct professional groups.

☐ Through key federal and state legislative initiatives, mental health services were funded, but remain inadequate in meeting the needs.

☐ Recent initiatives and reports, such as the CAMIMH (1998), the CCMHI (2001), and the 2006 Kirby Report highlight the continued need for resource planning and mental health policy specifically devoted to the care of persons with mental illness and their families.

CRITICAL THINKING CHALLENGES

1 Compare the ideas of psychiatric care during the 1800s with those of the 1990s and 2000s and identify some major political and economic forces that influenced care.

2 Analyze the social, political, and economic changes that influenced the transition to community mental health.

3 Explain how training and education of nurses became essential in psychiatric care.

4 Present an argument for the moral treatment of people with mental disorders.

5 Trace the history of biologic psychiatry and highlight major ideas and treatments.

6 Identify the strengths and challenges of accessible community-based care.

WEB LINKS

www.saintjohn.nbcc.nb.ca/Heritage/LunaticAsylum/ index.htm This website provides interesting historical information about Canada's first asylum for the mentally ill. The website also includes a personal account of a staff member who worked in the asylum in the 20th century and a story about a day in the life of a patient.

www.cpa-apc.org/index.php   This is the website of the Canadian Psychiatric Association and houses clinical practice guidelines and position papers.

www.phac-aspc.gc.ca/mh-sm/   This mental health website at the Public Health Agency of Canada has information on mental disorders and mental health promotion. The website also includes links.

www.hc-sc.gc.ca/hl-vs/pubs/adp-apd/bp_disorder-mp_concomitants/index-eng.php   This government report provides best practice in the management of substance use and mental illness.

www.phac-aspc.gc.ca/publicat/mh-sm/mhp02-psm02/index.html   This government site discusses mental health promotion in Canada.

www.parl.gc.ca/37/2/parlbus/commbus/senate/com-e/soci-e/rep-e/repoct02vol6-e.htm   This website has the original Health of Canada survey Kirby report (2004).

www.mentalhealth.com   This website has information on disorders and diagnoses and provides links to other sites.

cna-aiic.ca/cna/resources/default_e.aspx   The website of the Canadian Nurses Association (CNA) offers a listing of CNA publications, including the 1992 report on mental health care reform.

www.cfmhn.ca   This is the website of the Canadian Federation of Mental Health Nurses.

www.cmha.ca   The website of the Canadian Mental Health Association has information on mental health and a variety of resources.

www.samhsa.gov/index.aspx   This Substance Abuse and Mental Health Statistics website provides national statistics on alcohol, tobacco, and illegal drug use, substance abuse treatment, and mental health.

www.who.int/mental_health/en/   The website of the World Health Organization has information on mental health disability and programs.

www.mentalhealthcommission.ca/   This is the website of the Mental Health Commission of Canada, established in response to Kirby's "Out of the Shadows" report.

www.nmhac.ca   This is the Native Mental Health Association of Canada, whose mission is to promote mental wellness.

www.phac-aspc.gc.ca/publicat/human-humain06/pdf/human_face_e.pdf   The Human Face of Mental Health and Mental Illness in Canada 2006. The purpose of this report is to raise awareness and increase knowledge and understanding about mental health and mental illness in Canada.

www.parl.gc.ca/39/1/parlbus/commbus/senate/com-e/soci-e/rep-e/rep02may06-e.htm   This is the Senate Committee's mental health of Canada report "Out of the Shadows at Last: Transforming mental Health in Canada" (Kirby & Keon, 2006).

MOVIES, NOVELS, AND BIOGRAPHIES

Virginia Holman 2003 Rescuing Patty Hearst: Memories from a decade gone mad. NY: Simon & Schuster. A work of nonfiction. A memoir of a daughter about her mother, who suffered from schizophrenia.

VIEWING POINTS: Why was 1974 a bad year to go crazy, according to the author?

Beautiful Dreamers: 1992. This Canadian film is based on a true story about poet Walt Whitman's visit to an asylum in London, Ontario. Whitman, played by Rip Torn, is shocked by what he sees and persuades the hospital director to offer humane treatment. Eventually, the patients wind up playing the townspeople in a game of cricket.

VIEWING POINTS: Observe the stigma that is associated with having a mental illness.

An Angel at My Table: 1989. This thought-provoking, three-part television mini-series from New Zealand, based on Janet Frame's autobiography, traces her life from a shy, socially inept little girl to New Zealand's most famous writer/poet. Produced by Jane Campion and starring Kerry Fox, the story is told in three stages of the main character's life: childhood, young adulthood, and adulthood. During the second period, Janet Frame receives an inaccurate diagnosis of schizophrenia and is hospitalized for 8 years. She barely avoids a leukotomy.

VIEWING POINTS: Observe how the role of the woman in society influenced Janet Frame's admission to the hospital. Do you observe any changes in the perspective on women by today's standards?

One Flew Over the Cuckoo's Nest: 1975. This classic film, starring Jack Nicholson as Randle P. McMurphy, who challenges the state hospital establishment, won all five of the top Academy Awards: Best Picture, Best Actor, Best Actress, Best Director, and Best Adapted Screenplay. The film depicts life in an inpatient psychiatric ward of the late 1960s and offers increased public awareness of the potential human rights violations inherent in a large, public mental system. However, the portrayal of electroconvulsive therapy is stereotyped and inaccurate, and the suicide of Billy appears to be linked simplistically to his domineering mother. You might want to discuss whether this film probably contributes to the stigma of mental illness.

VIEWING POINTS: This film should be viewed from several different perspectives: What is the basis of McMurphy's admission? How does Nurse Ratchet interact with the patients? What is missing? What is different in today's public mental health systems?

The Cobweb: 1955. This movie, based on the novel by William Gibson, is set at a private psychiatric centre in the 1950s. It captures a psychiatrist's attempt to introduce a patient-centred approach to care, including a system of self-government for the residents. The issue of new drapes for the centre's library becomes a focal point for power struggles among the staff, residents, and even the family of the staff (the psychiatrist's wife intends to redecorate the library herself). The ensuing drama illustrates how professionals' behaviour can impact the therapeutic milieu. It has a star-studded cast, including Lauren Bacall as an occupational therapist and Richard Widmark as the psychiatrist.

VIEWING POINTS: Consider how the nurse changes in her behaviour and attitude toward the patients as she begins to embrace a less paternalistic and more patient-centred approach.

REFERENCES

Arboleda-Flórez, J. (2005). The epidemiology of mental illness in Canada. *Canadian Public Policy: Analyse de Politique, 31*(s1), 13–16.

Bailey, H. (1920). *Nursing mental diseases.* New York, NY: Macmillan.

Beauséjour, P. (2001). Advocacy and misadventures in Canadian Psychiatry. In Q. Rae-Grant (Ed.), *Psychiatry in Canada: 50 years, 1951–2000* (pp. 137–148). Ottawa, ON: Canadian Psychiatric Association.

Beers, C. (1908). *A mind that found itself.* New York, NY: Longmans, Green, & Co.

Benner, P. (1984). *From novice to expert: Excellence and power in clinical nursing practice.* Menlo-Park, CA: Addison-Wesley.

Boschma, G. (2003). *The rise of mental health nursing: A history of psychiatric care in Dutch asylum, 1890–1920.* Amsterdam, the Netherlands: Amsterdam University Press.

Boschma, G., Yonge, O., & Mychajlunow, L. (2005). Gender and professional identity in psychiatric nursing practice in Alberta, Canada, 1930– 1975. *Nursing Inquiry, 12*(4), 243–255.

Brown, W. H. (2000). Dr. C. K. Clarke and the Training School for Nurses. In E. Hudson (Ed.), *The provincial asylum in Toronto: Reflections on social and architectural history* (pp. 167–180). Toronto, ON: Toronto Region Architectural Conservancy.

Calaway, B. J. (2002). *Hildegard Peplau: Psychiatric nurse of the century.* New York, NY: Springer.

Canadian Federation of Mental Health Nurses. (2006). *Canadian standards for psychiatric-mental health nursing* (3rd ed.) Toronto, ON: Canadian Federation of Mental Health Nurses.

Canadian Women's Health Network. (2006). Women, Mental Health, Mental Illness and Addiction in Canada. Response to "Out of the Shadows At Last." Retrieved June 23, 2008, from http://www.cwhn.ca/resources/cwhn/mentalHealth.html

Church, O. (1987). From custody to community in psychiatric nursing. *Nursing Research, 36*(1), 48–55.

Connor, P. J. (1996). "Neither courage nor perseverance enough": Attendants at the Asylum for the Insane, Kingston, 1877–1905. *Ontario History, 88*(4), 251–272.

D'Antonio, P. (2006). *Founding friends: Families, staff, and patients at the Friends Asylum in early nineteenth century Philadelphia.* Bethlehem, PA: Lehigh University Press.

Dickenson, H. D. (1989). *The two psychiatries: The transformation of psychiatric work in Saskatchewan, 1905–1984.* Regina, SK: University of Regina Canadian Plains Research Centre.

Dooley, C. (2004). "The gave their care, but we gave loving care": Defining and defending boundaries of skill and craft in the nursing service of a Manitoba Mental Hospital during the Great Depression. *Canadian Bulletin of Medical History, 21*(2), 229–251.

Goldstein, J. L., & Godemont, M. M. L. (2003). The legend and lessons of Geel, Belgium: A 1500-year-old legend, a 21st century model. *Community Mental Health Journal, 39*(5), 441–458.

Greenland, C. (1996). Origins of the Toronto Psychiatric Hospital. In E. Shorter (Ed.), *TPH: History and memories of the Toronto Psychiatric Hospital, 1925–1966.* Toronto, ON: Wall & Emerson.

Greenland, C., Griffin, J., & Hoffman, B. F. (2001). Psychiatry in Canada from 1951–2000. In Q. Rae-Grant (Ed.), *Psychiatry in Canada: 50 years, 1951–2001* (pp. 1–16). Ottawa, ON: Canadian Psychiatric Association.

Hart Wasekeesikaw, F. (2006). Challenges for the new millennium: Nursing in First Nations. In M. McIntyre, E. Thomlinson, & C. McDonald (Eds.), *Realities of Canadian nursing: Professional, practice and power issues* (pp. 415–433). Philadelphia, PA: Lippincott Williams & Wilkins.

Health Canada. (2002). *A report on mental illnesses in Canada.* Ottawa, ON: Author.

Hector, I. (2001). Changing funding patterns and the effect on mental health care in Canada. In Q. Rae-Grant (Ed.), *Psychiatry in Canada: 50 years, 1951–2001* (pp. 59–76). Ottawa, ON: Canadian Psychiatric Association.

Heritage Resources Saint John. (Updated 2000). Retrieved August 22, 2005, from http://www.saintjohn.nbcc.nb.ca/Heritage/LunaticAsylum/index.htm

Hurd, H. M. (Ed.). (1973, originally printed 1916–17). *The institutional care of the insane in the United States and Canada* (Vol. IV). New York, NY: Arno Press.

Jones, C. (1989). *The charitable imperative: Hospitals and nursing in ancient régime and revolutionary France.* London, UK: Routledge.

Kirby, M. J. L. (2004). *Mental health, mental illness and addiction: Reports 1, 2, & 3.* Interim Report of the Standing Committee on Social Affairs, Science and Technology. Retrieved September 29, 2005, from http://www.parl.gc.ca/38/1/parlbus/commbus/senate/com-e/soci-e/rep-e/repintnov04-e.htm

Kirby, M. J. L. (2005). Mental health reform for Canada in the 21st century: Getting there from here. *Canadian Public Policy: Analyse de Politique, 31*(s1), 5–12.

Kirby, M. J. L., & Keon, W. J. (2006). Out of the shadows at last: Transforming mental health, mental illness and addiction services in Canada. Ottawa, ON: Government of Canada. Retrieved September 17, 2008, from http://www.parl.gc.ca/39/1/parlbus/commbus/senate/com-e/soci-e/rep-e/rep02may06-e.htm

LaJeunesse, R. A. (2000). *Political asylums.* Edmonton, AB: Muttart Foundation.

Leiby, J. S. (1992). San Hipólito's treatment of the mentally ill in Mexico City, 1589–1650. *The Historian, 54*(3), 491–498.

Lightner, D. L. (1999). *Asylum prison and poorhouse: The writings and reform work of Dorothea Dix in Illinois.* Carbondale and Edwardsville, IL: Southern Illinois University Press.

MacLennan, D. (1987). Beyond the asylum: Professionalization and the Mental Hygiene Movement in Canada, 1914–1928. *Canadian Bulletin of Medical History, 4*, 7–23.

Malamud, W. (1944). The history of psychiatric therapies. In J. K. Hall, G. Zilboorg, & H. Bunker (Eds.), *One hundred years of American psychiatry* (pp. 273–323). New York, NY: Columbia University Press.

McKenzie, C. (1992). *Psychiatry for the rich: A history of Ticehurst Private Asylum, 1792–1917.* London, UK: Routledge.

Menzies, R., & Palys, T. (2006). Turbulent spirits: Aboriginal patients in the British Columbia psychiatric system, 1879–1950. In J. E. Moran, & D. Wright (Eds.). *Mental health and Canadian society: Historical Perspectives* (pp. 149–175). Montreal and Kingston: McGill-Queen's University Press.

Moran, J. E. (2000). *Committed to the state asylum: Insanity and society in nineteenth-century Quebec and Ontario.* Montreal and Kingston: McGill-Queen's University Press.

Moran, J. E., & Wright, D. (Eds.). (2006). *Mental health and Canadian society: Historical Perspectives.* Montreal and Kingston: McGill-Queen's University Press.

Morrow, M. (2002). *Violence and trauma in the lives of women with serious mental illness: Current practices in service provision in British Columbia.* Vancouver, BC: Centre of Excellence for Women's Health.

Neill, J. (1980). Adolf Meyer and American psychiatry today. *American Journal of Psychiatry, 137*(4), 460–464.

Nelson, S. (1999). Entering the professional domain: The making of the modern nurse in 17th century France. *Nursing History Review, 7*, 171– 187.

Nelson, S. (2001). *Say little, do much: Nursing, nuns, and hospitals in the nineteenth century.* Philadelphia, PA: University of Pennsylvania Press.

Parry-Jones, W. L. L. (1981). The model of the Geel Lunatic Colony and its influence on the nineteenth-century asylum system in Britain. In A. Scull (Ed.), *Madhouses, mad-doctors, and madmen. The social history of psychiatry in the Victorian Era* (pp. 201–217). London, UK: The Athlone Press.

Peplau, H. (1952). *Interpersonal relations in nursing.* New York, NY: Putnam.

Porter, R. (1993). Disease, medicine and society in England 1550–1860. Houndmills, UK: Macmillan Education.

Scull, A. (2005). *Madhouse: A tragic tale of megalomania and modern medicine.* New Haven, CT: Yale University Press.

Sealy, P., & Whitehead, P. C. (2004). Forty years of deinstitutionalization of psychiatric services in Canada: An empirical assessment. *Canadian Journal of Psychiatry, 49,* 249–257.

Shorter, E. (1997). *A history of psychiatry: From the era of the asylum to the age of Prozac.* New York, NY: John Wiley & Sons.

Sussman, S. (1998). The first asylums in Canada: A response to neglectful community care and current trends. *Canadian Journal of Psychiatry, 43,* 260–264.

Tiplisky, V. M. (2002). Parting at the crossroads: The development of education for psychiatric nursing in three Canadian provinces, 1909–1955 (Ph.D. thesis, University of Manitoba).

Tipliski, V. M. (2004). Parting at the crossroads: The emergence of education for psychiatric nursing in three Canadian provinces, 1909–1955. *Canadian Bulletin of Medical History, 21*(2), 253–279.

Tomes, N. (1994). *The art of asylum-keeping: Thomas Story Kirkbride and the origins of American psychiatry.* Philadelphia, PA: University of Pennsylvania Press.

Van Drenth, A., & De Haan, F. (1999). *The rise of caring power: Elizabeth Fry and Josephine Butler in Britain and the Netherlands.* Amsterdam, the Netherlands: Amsterdam University Press.

Warsh, C. K. (1989). *Moments of unreason: The practice of Canadian psychiatry and the Homewood Retreat, 1883–1923.* Montreal and Kingston: McGill-Queens University Press.

World Health Organization. (2001). *The world health report: Mental health 2001. Mental health: New understanding, new hope.* Geneva, Switzerland: Author.

CHAPTER 2

Mental Health and Mental Illness

Marion Healey-Ogden

Adapted from the chapter "Mental Health and Mental Illness" by Mary Ann Boyd

LEARNING OBJECTIVES

After studying this chapter, you will be able to:

- Differentiate the concepts of mental health, mental illness, and mental disorder.
- Explain the conceptual foundation of mental health in Canada.
- Discuss the universality of mental health.
- Discuss mental health promotion strategies.
- Differentiate the five axes used in making a psychiatric diagnosis.
- Discuss the significance of epidemiology in understanding the impact of mental disorders.
- Differentiate prevention from treatment approaches.
- Explain the role of evidence-based care in psychiatric and mental health nursing.

KEY CONCEPT

- mental disorder

KEY TERMS

• epidemiology • evidence-based care • health promotion • incidence • mental disorder • mental health • mental illness • multiaxial diagnostic system • point prevalence • prevalence • primary health care • rate • risk factors • social determinants of health • well-being

Mental health and mental illness are not polar opposites; rather, they can be viewed as separate concepts on two separate and simultaneously occurring continua. More than 20 years ago, a significant Canadian government document, *Mental Health for Canadians: Striking a Balance* (Epp, 1988), framed **mental health** as separate from mental disorder. (Note that **mental disorder** is the medical term for **mental illness** and refers to a diagnosable condition based on criteria delineated in the American Psychiatric Association's [2000] *Diagnostic and Statistical Manual of Mental Disorders* or in the World Health Organization's [WHO; 2007] *International Classification of Diseases and Related Health Problems*.) In *Mental Health for Canadians*, optimal mental health and minimal mental health represent the extremes on one continuum. Maximal mental disorder and absence of mental disorder represent the extremes on the other continuum (Fig. 2-1). Optimal mental health involves "individual, group, and environmental factors [that] work together effectively, ensuring subjective well-being; optimal development and use of mental abilities; achievements of goals consistent with justice; and conditions of fundamental equality" (Epp, p. 9). By contrast, minimal mental health is defined as "individual, group, and environmental factors [that] conflict, producing subjective distress; impairment or underdevelopment of mental abilities; failure to achieve goals; destructive behaviours; and entrenchment of inequalities" (Epp, p. 9). It is possible

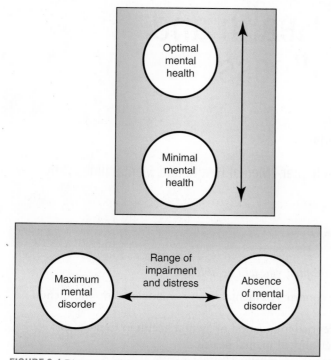

FIGURE 2.1 Diagrams of the mental health and mental disorder continua. (Epp, J. [1988]. *Mental health for Canadians: Striking a balance* [p. 9] [Cat. H39–128/1988E]. Ottawa, ON: Supply and Service Canada.)

that a person with a mental disorder can experience optimal mental health and a person without a mental disorder can experience minimal mental health. As a result of the way these factors interrelate, a person's mental health can vary across his or her lifespan. Maximal mental disorder on the mental illness continuum includes the "greatest severity; frequency and range of psychiatric symptoms" (Epp, p. 9). Absence of mental disorder on the other end of this continuum includes "freedom from psychiatric symptoms; effective prevention or cure" (Epp, p. 9). Like the mental health continuum, the severity of a person's mental disorder can vary over his or her lifetime.

■ UNIVERSALITY OF MENTAL HEALTH

A person who is mentally healthy is able to deal effectively with human emotions, is productive, has successful relationships with others, can adapt to change, and can positively cope with adversity. Everyone has the potential to be mentally healthy. Mental health is a universal condition that shapes the way people think, feel, and communicate. Physical health or physical illness does not necessarily lead to mental health or mental illness. A person with a mental illness can learn to cope with the symptoms and treatment of a disorder in order to live a mentally and physically healthy life and experience well-being.

The concept of **well-being** is not well defined in health-related literature and specifically in mental health literature. Beginning understanding can come from reviewing a lay dictionary definition of this word: Well-being is "the state of being healthy, happy, and free from want" (Cayne, 1988, p. 1117). Additional insight comes from health literature. WHO (2001) defined mental health as "a state of well-being in which the individual realizes his or her own abilities, can cope with the normal stresses of life, can work productively and fruitfully, and is able to make a contribution to his or her community" (Section 2, bullet 1). These definitions, in addition to the continua described by Epp (1988), highlight the possibility that well-being can exist within health and illness and, specifically, within mental health and mental disorder. Views of health often seem to refer to the existence of "something more" (Kikuchi, 2004, p. 30). It is possible that this something more is well-being. The centenary edition of the *Code of Ethics for Registered Nurses* (Canadian Nurses Association, 2008b) included, for the first time, "*well-being*" in its glossary, defining it as "a person's state of being well, content and able to make the most of his or her abilities" (p. 28).

Healey-Ogden (2008) found that well-being is not experienced in a purposeful way. Rather, like happiness, if directly sought, a sense of well-being can be elusive. Although it involves a personal drive to exist, well-being is experienced in a self-forgetful way as feelings of being orientated to one's world, including acceptance of the inherent vulnerability of that world. Well-being is interwoven with one's self-identity and relationships. Nurses must cultivate their understanding of well-being and be mindful that, as suggested by definitions of mental health, mental illness, and the continua by Epp (1988), it is possible for people living with mental disorders to experience well-being (see Box 2-1).

Health of Canadians

This Canadian text is built on an understanding of health derived from the definition used in Epp's (1986, p. 2) report, *Achieving Health for All: A Framework for Health Promotion*. Specifically, this report stated that "health is a basic and dynamic force in our daily lives, influenced by our circumstances, our beliefs, our culture and our social, economic and physical environments." This broad approach to health encompasses biologic, psychological, social, and spiritual well-being. (See Chapter 7 for the conceptual framework used in this text.) In particular, the Epp report identified three challenges in maintaining the health of Canadians: reducing inequalities, increasing the prevention effort, and enhancing people's capacity to cope. The strong link between mental health and mental disorder that this report highlights gives equal weight to assisting people with mental illnesses and assisting people in maintaining their mental health.

BOX 2.1

Research for Best Practice: Uncovering the Mystery of Well-Being

From Healey-Ogden, M. J. (2008). The experience of well-being: Uncovering the mystery. *Unpublished doctoral dissertation, University of Alberta, Edmonton.*

THE QUESTION: What is the nature of the lived experience of well-being?

METHOD: A hermeneutic phenomenological study of people's experiences of well-being involved interviewing five Canadians identified through public descriptions of their lives (e.g., newspaper articles, autobiography) as exemplifying the phenomenon of well-being. Interviews were analyzed and interpreted during ongoing writing and rewriting that wove the exemplars' stories together with data from a range of other sources, such as prose, poetry, and art. The result of this type of study is a written description of a human phenomenon that brings us as close as possible to understanding what it is like, including its mystery.

FINDINGS: This study revealed that well-being lies on the journey through life events. It involves dwelling in spaces of well-being, (e.g., spaces of play, creativity, nature, and spirituality) while embracing life's journey wherever it goes. Well-being was shown as different from health and wellness, experienced in a relational space where people are self-forgetful about how to live and, instead, engage in living well. It is coming home to self where the notion of home is critical.

IMPLICATIONS FOR NURSING: Nurses need to understand well-being, as well as health, wellness, and illness, and, in their nursing relationships, to honour the well-being experiences of others as they dwell in their homes, including their bodily homes.

Health Promotion

The Ottawa Charter for Health Promotion (WHO, 1986) defined **health promotion** as "the process of enabling people to increase control over, and to improve, their health" (p. 1). Rather than being a goal toward which a person strives, the Ottawa Charter stated that health is "a resource for everyday life… [that] goes beyond healthy lifestyles to well-being" (p. 1). This statement is reflected in the health promotion framework advocated in the 1986 Epp report.

Health promotion is built on the concept of **primary health care** outlined in the Alma-Ata Declaration (WHO, 1978), which identified primary health care as including the main concepts of "equity, community involvement/participation, intersectorality, appropriateness of techniques and affordable costs" (p. 3). Although the concept of primary health care is well defined, it is apparent that much work remains to improve primary care and thereby the mental health and care of Canadians (Kirby & Keon, 2004). Kirby and Keon (2006) took a significant step forward in this regard with their report, *Out of the Shadows at*

IN A LIFE

Margot Kidder (1948–)
Actor

Public Persona

Margot Kidder is a Canadian actor who has starred in many movies and television shows. The *Superman* series in which she played Lois Lane stands out among her most well-known movies. Kidder's ongoing accomplishments extend to her far-reaching advocacy work.

Personal Realities

Kidder documented her experiences with bipolar disorder in her autobiography, *Calamities*. In the midst of writing that book in 1996, her bipolar disorder swung out of control. In the 1990s, she had been experiencing an overwhelming amount of stress that was coupled with the near loss of her autobiographical documents from her computer. This loss was the ultimate catalyst that sent Kidder into a psychotic break with extreme paranoia, leading her into a brief period of homelessness.

Kidder was born in Yellowknife, Northwest Territories (NWT). During her childhood and adolescence, she lived with her parents and four siblings in various mining towns in the NWT and in Newfoundland. Her experience of living with bipolar disorder initially was evident when she attempted suicide during her adolescence.

Mental illness awareness groups benefit from Kidder's ongoing support. Often, she is the keynote speaker at mental health conferences. She attributes her recovery and mental health to holistic treatment and to a balanced lifestyle.

Source: Carlson, J. (2000). *Margot Kidder speaks up for mental health.* Retrieved May 26, 2008, from http://www.networkwomen.com/archives/coverstory01_00.html; Nunes, J., & Simmie, S. (2002). *Beyond crazy.* Toronto, ON: McClelland & Stewart.

Last: Transforming Mental Health, Mental Illness, and Addiction Services in Canada, which described mental health, mental illness, and addictions in Canada from a vast range of perspectives. It reviewed then-current initiatives and provided recommendations to transform the Canadian approach to mental illness such that mental disorder is considered to be as significant as other health concerns. Health education is one of the key primary health care activities that, when applied to mental health, becomes a catalyst for each person to work toward experiencing optimal mental health. The global nature of mental illness is another key aspect of primary health care. It is important that health practitioners, such as nurses, honour and develop local cultural responses to meet an extensive range of mental health needs (Adelson, 2005; Beiser, 2005). The nursing care described in this text reflects primary health care and health promotion approaches.

CRNENOTE

The CRNE is based on a primary health care framework (Canadian Nurses Association, 2008a, 2008b).

Social Determinants of Health

The **social determinants of health** lie at the forefront of health promotion. In a 2002 conference at York University, a broad spectrum of social determinants of health were discussed in view of developing policies to address the following key social determinants in Canada:

- Income inequality
- Social inclusion and exclusion
- Employment and job security
- Working conditions
- Contributions of the social economy
- Early childhood care
- Education
- Food security
- Housing

Mental health is contingent on policies and actions that address these social determinants of health across all sectors (Public Health Agency of Canada, 2004).

Mental Health Promotion

A person's mental health can be challenged by a variety of factors such as biologic changes or illnesses, psychological pressures, social tension, and spiritual distress. Healthy life span development includes formulating strategies to eliminate or reduce the impact of these destructive factors throughout one's life. For example, relaxation, proper nutrition and sleep, and trusting relationships can support a person's mental health. Following the model upon which this text is based, mental health promotion is underpinned by the promotion of one's spirituality.

Mental Illness Prevention

Specific **risk factors,** or characteristics that increase the likelihood of developing a mental illness, can contribute to minimal mental health and influence the development and severity of a mental disorder. Risk factors do not cause the disorder and are not symptoms of the illness but, rather, are factors that influence the likelihood that the symptoms will appear. The existence of a risk factor does not always mean the person eventually will have the disorder; it does, however, increase the person's chances. There are many different kinds of risk factors, including genetic, biologic, environmental, cultural, and occupational. Gender, too, is a risk factor for some disorders. For example, more women experience depression than men (Government of Canada, 2006b; Health Canada, 2002; WHO, n.d.).

Some risk factors can be controlled or changed through mental health promotion activities, whereas others cannot. The genetic predisposition of a person, for instance, cannot be altered at this time; although gene therapy research may provide ways to do so in the future. Risk factors that can be changed include those related to lifestyle behaviours or environment. Someone who is genetically at high risk for bipolar disorder (i.e., one or more family members have the disorder), for example, can modify his or her lifestyle and environment to decrease the impact of these factors. Similarly, decreasing stress in one's life, such as selecting a minimally stressful job, can reduce the likelihood of developing an anxiety disorder. However, even if it is possible to change behaviours, occupations, and environmental conditions, the actual change can be difficult. Many risky behaviours are physically, psychologically, socially, or spiritually rewarding and/or pleasurable, such as eating a high-calorie meal, engaging in unprotected sexual intercourse, or focusing on spiritual experiences to the exclusion of other healthy behaviours. One of the challenges of nursing is helping people identify, monitor, and reduce their risk factors and live a balanced life. Although people's risk factors vary according to individuals' circumstances, the impact of homelessness and cultural factors have been highlighted in the mental health literature as significantly contributing to the occurrence of mental illness (Adelson, 2005; Beiser, 2005; Government of Canada, 2006b; Kirby & Keon, 2006).

Homelessness and Mental Health

Mental illness and homelessness are not always linked; although, when homelessness is explored in Canada, it is apparent that there are significant connections between mental illness and homeless lifestyles (Government of Canada, 2006b; Kirby & Keon, 2006). Until the early 21st century, little attention was paid to the impact of homelessness on a person's mental health. By focusing on the social determinants of health, it is not surprising to note that when a person is homeless, his or her mental health is at risk. In 1999, the Canadian government announced a National Homelessness Initiative (NHI) that would identify key areas of research and consultation needed to address homelessness across the country (Government of Canada, 2003, 2006a). The National Research Group (NRG) that grew out of the NHI is focusing on a range of research areas such as the Aboriginal population and other cultural groups; youth and seniors; health, education, employment, and income; justice issues; cycles of homelessness; and the impact of living in the north (Government of Canada, 2003, 2006a). The NRG identified mental illness as a significant health concern. *Housing, Health & Mental Health*, a comprehensive report by the Canadian Mental Health Association (2004), described homelessness across Canada and its significant impact on mental health. This document pointed out a distinction between homelessness and houselessness. Challenges exist, globally, when attempting to agree on the definition of homelessness (Springer, 2000), especially when a home is considered to include more than a shelter. By contrast, there is greater agreement on what houselessness involves when referring only to housing (Springer). Progress must be made throughout Canada in order for all citizens to meet the basic human needs of having both a shelter and a home (Canadian Mental Health Association, 2004).

Culture and Mental Health

Mental health and mental disorder often are defined by cultural norms of and beliefs about mentally healthy behaviours (see Chapter 3). Canadians represent a blend of people from a vast array of cultures. Some people strictly maintain their cultural practices when living in Canada. Other people assimilate into the general Canadian culture. The collective impact of a variety of factors, such as exposure to trauma in one's country of origin, the stress of acculturation, limited resources, and resilience, challenges the mental health of people who are immigrants or refugees (Beiser, 2005). Aboriginal people in Canada experience many cultural factors that contribute to mental illness and related concerns such as addictions. Their marginalization and historical context, which includes residential school experiences and a loss of their original lands, are examples of cultural factors that can negatively affect their mental health (Adelson, 2005). The Canadian Mental Health Association's (2008) policy statement highlights the importance of cultural sensitivity and appropriateness when serving the public.

■■■ MENTAL ILLNESS

Mental illnesses, in other words, diagnosable mental disorders, are considered syndromes or clusters of symptoms that occur together and that could have multiple causes.

Importance of Epidemiology

The occurrence of mental disorders is studied through epidemiologic research, as it is for any other disorder. **Epidemiology** is the study of patterns of disease distribution in time and space. It focuses on the health status of population groups, or aggregates, rather than of individuals, and it involves quantitative analysis of the occurrence of illnesses in population groups. Epidemiologic approaches are useful in understanding the occurrence of mental disorders. Throughout this text, mental disorders are described using epidemiologic data. See Box 2-2 for an explanation of terms. Refer to various chapters in this text and to federal, provincial, and municipal government websites for the incidence and prevalence of particular mental disorders in specific regions and communities in Canada.

BOX 2.2

Epidemiologic Terms

In *epidemiology*, certain terms have specific meanings relative to what they measure. When expressing the number of cases of a disorder, population rates, rather than raw numbers, are used.

Rate is a *proportion* of cases in the population when compared with the total population of cases and noncases. Rate usually refers to new cases. It is expressed as a fraction, in which the numerator is the number of cases and the denominator is the total number in a defined population. The term *average rate* is used for measures that involve rates over specified time periods:

$$\text{Rate} = \frac{\text{Cases in the population}}{\text{Defined total population}}$$

Prevalence refers to the total number of people who have a particular disorder within a given population at a *specified* time, regardless of how long ago the disorder started.

Point prevalence is the basic measure that refers to the proportion of individuals in a given population who have the disorder at a specified point in time (cases at *t*) when compared with the population at the same point in time. This point can be a day on the calendar, such as April 1, 2010, or a point defined in relation to the study assessment, such as the day of the interview.

$$\text{Point prevalence rate} = \frac{\text{Cases at } t}{\text{Given population at } t}$$

Incidence refers to the number of *new* cases that have occurred within a clearly defined time period, most commonly 1 year. The study of incidence cases requires at least two measurements to be taken, one at the start of the prescribed time period and another at the end of it.

Mental Disorders Overview

KEY CONCEPT Mental disorders are health conditions characterized by alterations in a variety of factors that include mood and affect, behaviour, and thinking and cognition. The disorders are associated with various degrees of distress and impaired functioning.

These alterations are unexpected and are outside the limits of expected psychological states, such as sadness, grief, and mild depression normally associated with the death of a spouse. Cultural definitions of "normal" responses also are taken into consideration. If a behaviour is considered normal within a specific culture, it is not viewed as a symptom of a mental disorder by members of that group. For example, it is common in some religious groups to "speak in tongues." To an observer, it may appear that the individuals are experiencing hallucinations (see Chapter 11), a psychiatric symptom, but this behaviour is usual for this group within a particular setting.

Diagnosing Mental Disorders

In Canada, the American Psychiatric Association's (2000) *Diagnostic and Statistical Manual of Mental Disorders*, 4th ed., Text Revision (*DSM-IV-TR*) is used in the diagnosis of mental disorders. The *DSM-IV-TR* system contains subtypes and other specifiers to further describe the characteristics of the diagnosis as exhibited by a given individual. Some disorders are influenced by cultural factors. Other disorders are culture-bound syndromes that are present only in a particular setting (see Box 2-3). Although the *DSM-IV-TR* provides criteria for diagnosing mental disorders, there are no absolute boundaries separating one disorder from another, and similar disorders may have different manifestations at different points in time.

The *DSM-IV-TR* diagnostic criteria are based on a **multiaxial diagnostic system** that includes five axes, or domains of information. Axis I includes most *clinical disorders* and other conditions that may be a focus of clinical attention, such as relational problems or those related to abuse or neglect. Axis II contains *personality disorders* and *mental retardation*. Axis III includes *general medical conditions* that must be considered in the diagnosis and treatment of primary psychiatric disorders. Each of the first three axes is essential to understanding and treating an individual with psychiatric concerns. For example, a person with major depression (Axis I) may meet the criteria for having a dependent personality disorder (Axis II) and also may have diabetes (Axis III). See Table 2-1 for a listing of diagnostic classes included under each axis and Box 2-4 for a clinical example. (Refer to Appendix A for *DSM-IV-TR* classifications: Axis I and II categories and codes.)

Although the first three axes appear to contain all of the diagnostic information, a truly accurate picture of the individual is complete only when considering other factors such as life stressors and current level of functioning. Axis IV relates to any *psychosocial and environmental problems* that may produce additional stress and confound the diagnosis and that are important aspects of treating the primary psychiatric disorder. For example, a range of life events such as the death of a spouse, a recent divorce, or job discrimination may exacerbate symptoms of clinical depression or prompt the symptoms to emerge, as may stressors such as starting a new job, getting married, or having a baby. Using the *DSM-IV-TR* suggestions for identifying areas of concern, the prudent clinician making the diagnosis would clearly describe the individual's specific response on this axis.

Ratings given on Axis V provide a *Global Assessment of Functioning* (GAF) that is an estimate of *overall functioning* in psychological, social, and occupational spheres of life excluding limitations related to physical or environmental factors (American Psychiatric Association, 2000). These data are useful in planning treatment and determining their impact. The GAF *scale* is scored from low functioning (0 to 10) to high functioning (91 to 100;

BOX 2.3

DSM IV

Selected Culture-Bound Syndromes

DEFINITION: Behaviours limited to specific cultures that have meaning within that culture.

BRAIN FAG: A condition experienced by high school or university students in response to the challenges of schooling. Symptoms include difficulties in concentrating, remembering, and thinking. This term was originally used in West Africa.

FALLING OUT OR BLACKING OUT: An episode of sudden collapse that is sometimes preceded by feelings of dizziness. Individuals' eyes are usually open, but the person claims an inability to see. It occurs primarily in southern United States and Caribbean groups.

SHENJING SHUAIRUO (NEURASTHENIA): This condition is recognized in the Chinese equivalent to the *DSM-IV-TR*. It involves difficulties with concentration and memory and includes physical symptoms such as dizziness, headaches, sleep disturbances, gastrointestinal difficulties, and irritabilities.

For more information, see American Psychiatric Association. (2000). *Diagnostic and statistical manual of mental disorders* (4th ed., Text revision). Washington, DC: Author.

BOX 2.4

DSM IV

Diagnostic Axes and Their Disorders and Conditions

CLINICAL EXAMPLE

Axis I: 300.21* Panic Disorder With Agoraphobia
Axis II: 301.4 Obsessive-Compulsive Personality Disorder
Axis III: 250.00† Diabetes Mellitus
Axis IV: Occupational Problems: Frequent Absences From Work
Axis V: Global Assessment of Function
            GAF = 55 (current)
                    90 (potential)

*In this example, code numbers are used and can be found in the DSM-IV-TR. To improve readability, these code numbers are not used when discussing the various disorders, although the code numbers are commonly used in the clinical setting.

†The medical conditions in Axis III are coded according to the *International Classification of Diseases (ICD)*.

For more information, see American Psychiatric Association. (2000). *Diagnostic and statistical manual of mental disorders* (4th ed., Text revision). Washington, DC: Author.

Table 2.1 *DSM-IV-TR* Multiaxial Diagnoses for Persons With Mental Disorders

Diagnostic Axes and Their Main Diagnostic Classes

Axis I: Clinical Disorders and Other Conditions That May Be a Focus of Clinical Attention

Disorders Usually First Diagnosed During Infancy, Childhood, or Adolescence

Delirium, Dementia, Amnestic Disorder, and Other Cognitive Disorders

Mental Disorders due to General Medical Conditions

Substance-Related Disorders

Schizophrenia and Other Psychotic Disorders

Mood Disorders

Anxiety Disorders

Somatoform Disorders

Factitious Disorders

Dissociative Disorders

Sexual and Gender Identity Disorders

Eating Disorders

Sleep Disorders

Impulse Control Disorders (Not Elsewhere Classified)

Adjustment Disorders

Other Conditions That May Be a Focus of Clinical Attention

Axis II: Personality Disorders and Mental Retardation

Personality Disorders:

Paranoid Personality Disorder

Schizoid Personality Disorder

Schizotypal Personality Disorder

Antisocial Personality Disorder

Borderline Personality Disorder

Histrionic Personality Disorder

Narcissistic Personality Disorder

Avoidant Personality Disorder

Dependent Personality Disorder

Obsessive-Compulsive Personality Disorder

Personality Disorder Not Otherwise Specified

Mental Retardation

Axis III: General Medical Conditions

Infectious and Parasitic Diseases

Neoplasms

Endocrine, Nutritional, and Metabolic Diseases and Immunity Disorders

Diseases of the Blood and Blood-Forming Organs

Diseases of the Nervous and Sense Organs

Diseases of the Circulatory System

Diseases of the Respiratory System

Diseases of the Digestive System

Diseases of the Genitourinary System

Complications of Pregnancy, Childbirth, and the Puerperium

Diseases of the Skin and Subcutaneous Tissue

Diseases of the Musculoskeletal System and Connective Tissue

Congenital Anomalies

Certain Conditions Originating in the Perinatal Period

Symptoms, Signs, and Ill-Defined Conditions

Injury and Poisoning

Axis IV: Psychosocial and Environmental Problems

Problems With Primary Support Group

Problems Related to the Social Environment

Educational Problems

Occupational Problems

Housing Problems

Economic Problems

Problems With Access to Health Care Services

Problems Related to Interaction With the Legal System/ Crime

Other Psychosocial and Environmental Problems

Axis V: Global Assessment of Functioning (GAF)

Current = After separately rating the person's level of functioning and level of symptoms, the person's current GAF score represents the lower level of the two ratings at the time of assessment.

Psychological, social, and occupational functioning on a hypothetical continuum of mental health illness.

Scores

91–100	Superior functioning, no symptoms
81–90	Absent or minimal symptoms, good functioning in all areas
71–80	If symptoms are present, they are transient and expectable reactions to psychosocial stressors; no more than slight impairment in social, occupational, or school functioning
61–70	Some mild symptoms or some difficulty in social, occupational, or school functioning, but generally functioning well; has some meaningful interpersonal relationships
51–60	Moderate symptoms or moderate difficulty in social, occupational, or school functioning
41–50	Serious symptoms or any serious impairment in social, occupational, or school functioning
31–40	Some impairment in reality testing or communication or major impairment in several areas, such as work or school, family relations, judgment, thinking, or mood
21–30	Behaviour is considerably influenced by delusions or hallucinations or serious impairment in communication or judgment or inability to function in almost all areas
11–20	Some danger of hurting self or others or occasionally fails to maintain minimal personal hygiene or gross impairment in communication
1–10	Persistent danger of severely hurting self or others or persistent inability to maintain minimal personal hygiene or serious suicidal act with a clear expectation of death

GAF scores can be recorded at specific times, for example, on admission or at the time of discharge. These scores also can show the highest level of GAF over a specified time period.

GAF scales are written as: GAF = rating (time period)

For example: GAF = 30 (current) or GAF = 75 (at discharge)

American Psychiatric Association. (2000). *Diagnostic and statistical manual of mental disorders* (4th ed., Text revision). Washington, DC: Author.

see Table 2-1). Each 10-point rating reflects the severity of symptoms and of functioning; each component is assessed separately in a variety of settings. The rating is based on observations and specific assessments of mood; affect; behaviour; and a full range of cognitive functioning, including thinking ability, judgment, and communication. The appropriate GAF is an expression of the lowest of the two assessments with additional flexibility to rate the person within the most fitting 10-point rating. This rating may be made at the beginning of or during treatment, at discharge from the clinical setting, or at any point thereafter. The point of time should be indicated, such as "on admission," "current," or "at discharge from the hospital" (American Psychiatric Association, 2000).

Consequences of Labelling

A diagnosis becomes a way of labelling a particular person's illness. However, negative consequences of labelling can include, for example, loss of personal identity when the labelled person becomes a disease and experiences stigma associated with mental illness. To avoid labelling a person, refer to individuals using person-first language. For example, refer to someone with diabetes mellitus as a "person with diabetes" rather than as a "diabetic." Likewise, someone with a mental disorder would be referred to as a "person with schizophrenia" or as a "person with bipolar disorder" rather than as a "schizophrenic" or as a "bipolar." It is important for nurses and other health care professionals to avoid the pitfalls of negative labelling and stigmatization (Austin, 2000; Kirby & Keon, 2004). The Mental Health Commission of Canada was formed in March 2007 as a result of the work described in the Kirby and Keon (2004, 2006) reports (Mental Health Commission of Canada, n.d.). A goal of this Commission is to reduce stigmatization and resultant discrimination of people with mental illnesses in Canada. The focus of a currently funded Health Canada project is the exploration of the mental health literacy (MHL) of Canadians. MHL was defined as "knowledge, beliefs and abilities that enable the recognition, management or prevention of mental health problems" (Canadian Alliance on Mental Illness and Mental Health, 2007, p. 4). This project is revealing that stigma and discrimination are negatively influencing Canadians' responses to people with mental illnesses, especially serious mental illnesses, and Canadians' disclosure of mental illnesses, especially at work. Focus group participants point to a variety of sources of stigmatization, including that by health professionals. Improving MHL can positively influence the mental health of Canadians (Canadian Alliance on Mental Illness and Mental Health).

Similar troubling results emerged from the Canadian Medical Association's (2008) *8th Annual Report Card on Health Care*. In this Ipsos Reid survey, a significant number of Canadians reported actual or perceived barriers associated with mental illness. Stigma was present in a broad range of life events, such as seeking treatment for mental illness, socializing with people with mental illnesses, and utilizing the professional services of someone with mental illness (Canadian Medical Association). It is critical that nurses take a key role in raising the social consciousness of Canadians, such that mental illness and physical illness become equally acceptable.

Individualizing Diagnoses and Care

A *DSM-IV-TR* diagnosis is useful in identifying a disorder but is limited in that it does not provide information regarding individual responses to the disorder and specific needs. For example, two individuals may acquire the same flu virus, but one may experience a high fever; an upset stomach; and a dry, harsh cough. The other may have only a mild fever, a slight cough, and no nausea. Similarly, of two individuals who are diagnosed with clinical depression, one person may be unable to carry on with day-to-day activities and be hospitalized because of a suicide attempt, whereas the other person may continue to maintain home and family responsibilities. A person's response to a mental disorder also ranges in degree. For example, aggression can range from verbal anger to physical assault; anxiety, from mild to panic; self-destruction, from indirect to direct; and depression, from grief to major depression. Human responses to illness provide direction for the health care team to guide people toward mental health and successful coping with mental disorders. The Canadian Federation of Mental Health Nurses' (2006) standards for nursing practice support the individualization of nursing care and provide direction for achieving excellence in psychiatric and mental health (PMH) nursing practice.

▰ EVIDENCE-BASED CARE

Traditionally, interventions have been developed in response to clinicians' own experiences and have not necessarily been subjected to rigorous testing. One of the challenges in PMH nursing is to generate interventions for **evidence-based care**. Today, the focus is on developing and refining clinical questions and finding evidence on which practice can be based, thereby providing direction for treatment guidelines (Canadian Nurses Association, 2008a, 2008b). These guidelines may include decision trees that can be used in making treatment decisions. Research-supported interventions are included throughout this text along with several treatment guidelines.

The best guidelines are evidence-based and combined with an individualized approach to health care.

SUMMARY OF KEY POINTS

☐ Mental health and mental illness can be viewed as separate concepts on two separate and simultaneously occurring continua.

☐ Mentally healthy people are able to deal effectively with normal human emotions. Mental illnesses are diagnosable mental disorders that follow the *DSM-IV-TR* criteria.

☐ The 1988 Epp report gives equal weight to assisting people who are mentally ill and to assisting people to maintain their mental health.

☐ Health promotion is built on the concept of primary health care that forms the basis for PMH nursing. A focus on social determinants of health and on health education promotes optimal mental health.

☐ Risk factors include factors that can and cannot be changed. Genetic predisposition cannot be changed; however, lifestyle and behaviour are amenable to change.

☐ Cultural norms and beliefs contribute to the identification of mentally healthy behaviour.

☐ Epidemiology is important in understanding the distribution of mental illness within a given population. The rate of occurrence refers to the proportion of the population that has the disorder. The prevalence is the rate of occurrence of all cases at a specified time. Point prevalence refers to the proportion of individuals in the population who have the disorder at a specified point in time. The incidence is the rate of new cases within a specified time.

☐ The use of diagnoses in mental health can be problematic because of the negative association of the label *mental illness* or of the name of a specific mental disorder. The diagnoses outlined in the *DSM-IV-TR* are the standardized, accepted language in the mental health field. There are five diagnostic axes: clinical disorders, personality disorders and mental retardation, general medical conditions, psychosocial and environmental problems, and overall functioning.

CRITICAL THINKING CHALLENGES

1 Distinguish between the terms *mental health*, *mental illness*, and *mental disorder*.
2 Describe the framework on which the Canadian approach to mental health is based.
3 Relate homelessness to *mental health* and *mental illness*.
4 Define the epidemiologic terms *prevalence*, *incidence*, and *rate*.
5 Define *risk factors* and identify the various types of risk factors related to mental illness.
6 State the differences between the five axes of the *DSM-IV-TR* and explain the importance of considering all five axes as they apply to every individual.
7 Discuss the negative impact of labelling someone with a psychiatric diagnosis.
8 Discuss the value of *evidence-based care*. Discuss the value of individualized care.

WEB LINKS

www.bcmhas.ca   This is the site of the BC Mental Health & Addiction Services.

www.ccmhi.ca   This is the site of the Canadian Collaborative Mental Health Initiative.

www.ciw.ca/en/Home.aspx   This is the site of Canada's Institute of Wellbeing that oversees the development and implementation the Canadian Index of Wellbeing (CIW), a tool to measure Canadians' quality of life. The Institute aims to promote a vision of wellbeing that encompasses regional and cultural differences and increases understanding of what contributes to wellbeing and what detracts from it. Their 2009 report, *The Economic Crisis through the Lens of Economic Wellbeing* is available at this site.

www.cna-nurses.ca   This is the site of the Canadian Nurses Association.

www.gov.ns.ca/health/mhs   This Nova Scotia government site includes links to Canadian mental health resources and a variety of databases.

www.hc-sc.gc.ca   This is the site of Health Canada, which provides information on the Canadian health care system and primary health care, including information on First Nations and Inuit health and on mental health and wellness.

www.ornl.gov/sci/techresources/Human_Genome/ medicine/genetherapy.shtml   This is the site of the Human Genome Project, which contains information about gene therapy research.

www.parl.gc.ca   This is the site of the Parliament of Canada, which contains Senate reports related to mental health, mental illness, and addictions.

www.phac-aspc.gc.ca   This is the site of the Public Health Agency of Canada, which provides various links to mental health reports and best practices.

www.who.int/en   This is the site of the WHO, which includes links to related mental health sites. It also includes documents such as *The World Health Report 2001—Mental Health: New Understandings, New Hope.*

www.who.int/hpr/NPH/docs/hp_glossary_en.pdf   This *Health Promotion Glossary* is published by the WHO.

MOVIES, NOVELS, AND BIOGRAPHIES

People Say I'm Crazy: 2004. This autobiographical film documents a 10-year period of artist John Cadigan's life and experience of schizophrenia and societal labelling. It reveals his struggle with psychosis and his attempt to discern what is real in his life. His world of creativity and many healthy human emotions are woven into his struggle of living with mental illness. With the support of his family, John shows how having schizophrenia does not exclude mental health.

VIEWING POINTS: Identify the societal labels that John experienced. How is spirituality significant in his life? According to Epp's (1988) mental health and mental disorder continua, how is John's experience viewed differently over the 10-year period as shown in this film? Describe well-being within his experience of living with paranoid schizophrenia.

REFERENCES

Adelson, N. (2005). The embodiment of inequity: Health disparities in Aboriginal Canada. *Canadian Journal of Public Health, 96*, S45–S61.

American Psychiatric Association. (2000). *Diagnostic and statistical manual of mental disorders* (4th ed., Text revision). Washington, DC: Author.

Austin, W. (2000, February). Ethics and the stigma of mental illness. *Health Ethics Today, 2*(12), 1–2. Retrieved May 26, 2007, from http://www.phen.ab.ca/materials/intouch/vol2/intouch2–12.html

Beiser, M. (2005). The health of immigrants and refugees in Canada. *Canadian Journal of Public Health, 96*, S30–S44.

Canadian Alliance on Mental Illness and Mental Health. (2007). *Mental health literacy in Canada: Phase one draft report, metal health literacy project*. Retrieved August 20, 2008, from http://www.camimh.ca/files/literacy/MHL_REPORT_FINAL.pdf

Canadian Federation of Mental Health Nurses. (2006). *Standards of practice: Canadian standards for psychiatric-mental health nursing* (3rd ed.). Toronto, ON: First Stage Enterprises.

Canadian Medical Association. (2008, August). *8th annual national report card on health care*. Retrieved August 26, 2008, from http://www.cma.ca/multimedia/CMA/Content_Images/Inside_cma/Annual_Meeting/2008/GC_Bulletin/National_Report_Card_EN.pdf

Canadian Mental Health Association. (2004). *Housing, health & mental health*. Retrieved June 17, 2008, from http://www.cmha.ca/citizens/ENG_Housing_FINAL.pdf

Canadian Mental Health Association. (2008). *CMHA Policy Statements*. Retrieved May 26, 2008, from http://www.cmha.ca/bins/content_page.asp?cid=5–33&lang=1

Canadian Nurses Association. (2005). *CRNE bulletin: A new milestone for nursing in Canada*. Retrieved May 26, 2008, from http://www.cna-aiic.ca/CNA/documents/pdf/publications/CRNE_Bulletin_October_2005_e.pdf

Canadian Nurses Association. (2008a). *Canadian registered nurse examination: Competencies*. Retrieved May 20, 2008, from http://cna-aiic.ca/CNA/nursing/rnexam/competencies/default_e.aspx

Canadian Nurses Association. (2008b). *Code of ethics for registered nurses*. Ottawa, ON: Author. Available at http://www.cna-nurses.ca/CNA/documents/pdf/publications/Code_of_Ethics_2008_e.pdf

Carlson, J. (2000, January). *Margot Kidder speaks up for mental health*. Retrieved May 26, 2008, from http://www.networkwomen.com/archives/coverstory01_00.html

Cayne, B. (Ed.). (1988). *The new lexicon Webster's encyclopedic dictionary of the English language* (Canadian ed.). New York, NY: Lexicon.

Epp, J. (1986). *Achieving health for all: A framework for health promotion* (Cat. H39–102/1986E). Ottawa, ON: Supply and Services Canada.

Epp, J. (1988). *Mental health for Canadians: Striking a balance* (Cat. H39–128/1988E). Ottawa, ON: Supply and Services Canada.

Government of Canada. (2003). *Evaluation of the national homelessness initiative: Implementation and early outcomes of the HRDC-based components. Final report*. Retrieved May 27, 2008, from http://www.hrsdc.gc.ca/en/cs/sp/hrsdc/edd/reports/2003–002435/spah203_03_e.pdf

Government of Canada. (2006a). *National homelessness initiative. Report of the Treasury Board of Canada Secretariat*. Retrieved March 16, 2009, from http://www.tbs-sct.gc.ca/rma/eppi-ibdrp/hrdb-rhbd/dep-min/hrdc-rhdsc/nhi-ins/description_e.asp

Government of Canada. (2006b). *The human face of mental health and mental illness in Canada, 2006*. Retrieved May 27, 2008, from http://www.phac-aspc.gc.ca/publicat/human-humain06/pdf/human_face_e.pdf

Healey-Ogden, M. J. (2008). *The experience of well-being: Uncovering the mystery*. Unpublished doctoral dissertation, University of Alberta, Edmonton, Alberta.

Health Canada. (2002). *A report on mental illnesses in Canada*. Retrieved May 27, 2008, from http://www.phac-aspc.gc.ca/publicat/miic-mmac/

Kikuchi, J. F. (2004). 2002 CNA code of ethics: Some recommendations. *Nursing Leadership, 17*(3), 28–38.

Kirby, M. J., & Keon, W. J. (2004). *Report 3. Mental health, mental illness and addiction: Issues and options for Canada*. Interim Report of the Standing Committee on Social Affairs, Science and Technology. Retrieved May 27, 2008, from http://www.parl.gc.ca/38/1/parlbus/commbus/senate/com-e/soci-e/rep-e/report3/repintnov04vol3-e.pdf

Kirby, M. J., & Keon, W. J. (2006). *Out of the shadows at last: Highlights and recommendations*. Final Report of the Standing Committee on Social Affairs, Science and Technology. Retrieved May 20, 2008, from http://www.parl.gc.ca/39/1/parlbus/commbus/senate/com-e/soci-e/rep-e/pdf/rep02may06high-e.pdf

Mental Health Commission of Canada. (n.d.). *The mental health commission of Canada*. Retrieved March 16, 2009, from http://www.mentalhealthcommission.ca/English/Pages/Background.aspx

Nunes, J., & Simmie, S. (2002). *Beyond crazy*. Toronto, ON: McClelland & Stewart.

Public Health Agency of Canada. (2004). *Social determinants of health: An overview of the implications for policy and the role of the health sector*. Retrieved May 27, 2008, from http://www.phac-aspc.gc.ca/ph-sp/oi-ar/01_overview-eng.php

Springer, S. (2000). Homelessness: A proposal for a global definition and classification. *Habitat international, 24*, 475–484. Retrieved March 16, 2009, from http://action.web.ca/home/housing/resources.shtml?x=66864&AA_EX_Session=34800adbfe34db2f12f35212d3d63967

World Health Organization. (1978). *Primary health care: Report of the international conference on primary health care*. Alma-Ata, USSR. Geneva, Switzerland: Author.

World Health Organization. (1986). *Ottawa charter for health promotion*. Retrieved May 27, 2008, from http://www.who.int/hpr/NPH/docs/ottawa_charter_hp.pdf

World Health Organization. (2001). *Mental health: Strengthening mental health promotion*. Retrieved May 28, 2008, from http://www.who.int/mediacentre/factsheets/fs220/en/

World Health Organization. (2007). International classification of diseases (10th rev. ed.). Retrieved September 14, 2008, from http://www.who.int/classifications/icd/en/

World Health Organization. (n.d.). *Gender and women's mental health*. Retrieved May 26, 2008, from http://www.who.int/mental_health/prevention/genderwomen/en/

The Context of Mental Health Care: Cultural, Socioeconomic, and Legal

Arlene Kent-Wilkinson

Adapted from the chapter "The Context of Mental Health Care" by Mary Ann Boyd

KEY CONCEPTS

- culture
- cultural competence
- Mental Health Act
- poverty

LEARNING OBJECTIVES

After studying this chapter, you will be able to:

- Explore the cultural roots of mental illness and its relationship to beliefs of religion and spirituality.
- Relate the concept of cultural competence to the role of the psychiatric and mental health (PMH) nurse.
- Consider the unique culture of Aboriginal peoples in Canada and their mental health beliefs.
- Identify the influence of socioeconomic factors (poverty, geographic) on the mental health of Canadians.
- Describe the mental health care delivery issues related to providing services to culturally diverse populations in Canada's many geographic areas.
- Identify and explain the mental health legislation enacted to help protect, promote, and improve the lives and mental well-being of Canadians.

KEY TERMS

• Aboriginal health • assimilation • best interests • colonialism • community treatment order • competent • cultural competence • cultural dissonance • cultural safety • discrimination • displacement • ethnocentrism • mandatory outpatient treatment • prejudice • religion • spirituality • stereotyping • stigma • substitute decision maker • telehealth

*H*ealth, including the mental health, of any human population is the product of a complex web of cultural, environmental, historical, physiologic, psychological, spiritual, socioeconomic, and legislative factors. This chapter examines three contexts of mental health and illness in Canada: *cultural, socioeconomic,* and *legal.* Culture will be examined with regard to cultural roots, spirituality, and religion. Then, socioeconomic factors that influence mental health (poverty, geographic access to services) will be explored. Finally,

international agreements and Canadian legislation enacted to protect, promote, and improve the lives and mental well-being of citizens will be discussed.

CULTURAL CONTEXT OF MENTAL HEALTH CARE

All people have a culture. It reflects the basic values and biases through which we interpret the world around us and make decisions about our own behaviour and our relationships with others. Our culture shapes our perceptions and attitudes, from our personal-space comfort zones to our attitudes toward mental health and mental illness.

Culture

Geertz (1973) described humans as animals who have spun "webs of significance" for themselves. These webs are culture. Understanding mental health and culture is not about finding its "laws" but about interpreting its meaning. The metaphor of a complex web is strong as webs show intricacy and interconnectedness, creativity and skill that can only be seen close-up. Each individual thread contributes to the strength of the web.

"Culture is commonly understood as learned traditions and unconscious rules of engagement that people use to interpret experience and to generate social behaviour" (Srivastava, 2007, p. 324). Members of a culture rarely have insight into their own culturally learned ideas and values regarding normal and abnormal behaviours; typically, these values are seen as correct and proper for everyone. This is termed **ethnocentrism**.

KEY CONCEPT Culture is not only a way of life for people who identify or associate with one another on the basis of some common purpose, need, or similarity of background but also the totality of learned, socially transmitted beliefs, values, and behaviours that emerge from its members' interpersonal transactions.

Cultural Diversity in Canada

In 1971, Canada was the first country to develop a *multiculturalism policy*, a policy that states that Canadians should be able to maintain and develop their own cultural identities if they so wish, be willing to share their cultures with other Canadians, and be free from prejudice and discrimination (Government of Canada, 2004a). This policy challenges Canadians to accept cultural pluralism, while encouraging them to participate fully and equally in Canadian society.

Canada's approach to diversity has evolved over the years and is embedded within a broad policy and legislative framework. The *Canadian Multiculturalism Act* was passed in 1988, and in 1997, the renewed *multiculturalism program* was announced (Government of Canada, 2004b).

Culture is one of the 12 key determinants of health (Canadian Nurses Association [CNA], 2004), and nurses are responsible to provide culturally competent care (some nurses prefer the term culturally sensitive care) to diverse populations with different cultural beliefs. Nurses must

BOX 3.1

Mental Health and Culturally Sensitive Services

There are numerous mental health and inner city clinics across Canada that offer mental health and culturally sensitive services. Although too many to cite here, a few great examples are

Calgary—8th & 8th Community Health Centre	http://www.calgaryhealthregion.ca/hospitals/calgary/calgary-public_health_8th-8th.htm?noheader&nofooter
Edmonton—Boyle Street Coop, "Street Works"	Professionals: http://www.streetworks.ca/pro/aswstaff.html Clients: http://www.streetworks.ca/client/contactinfo.html
Regina—Four Directions Community Health Centre	http://www.rqhealth.ca/programs/comm_hlth_centres/four_directions/four_directions_programs.shtml
Toronto—Inner City Health Program at St. Michaels Hospital	http://www.stmichaelshospital.com/programs/ich/index.php
Vancouver—Native Health Society	http://www.vnhs.net/index.php?option=com_content&task=view&id=22&Itemid=54
CMHA—Locations (select on the map of Canada for locations in each province or territory)	http://www.cmha.ca/bins/loc_page.asp?cid=58–85&lang=1

strive to understand the way people of various cultures think, feel, behave, and respond when it comes to matters of health. This can be especially difficult because the cultural face of Canada continues to change, and we have a larger range of ethnicity, language, and country of origin than ever before. Those new to Canada have health needs related to their migration, particularly refugees who may have been exposed to war or other trauma (Khanlou, 2008). See Box 3-1 for Internet links to examples of mental health and culturally sensitive services in Canada.

The culture of Aboriginal peoples has been chosen as a focus in this discussion on culture as Canadian psychiatric and mental health (PMH) nurses have identified a pressing need for such knowledge and understanding (Austin, Gallop, McCay, Peternelj-Taylor, & Bayer, 1999).

Aboriginal Peoples

According to the 2006 Canadian census, the number of people who identified themselves as an Aboriginal person surpassed the one-million mark, reaching 1,172,790 or almost 4% of the Canadian population (Statistics

BOX 3.2

Aboriginal Peoples

FIRST NATIONS

The term *First Nation* replaces the term *Indian* (Royal Commission on Aboriginal Peoples, 1996). This term began to be used in the 1970s as a substitute for Indians, a term that has fallen into disfavour with Aboriginal people. The term does not mean the same as *Aboriginal people* or *First Peoples* because it does not include Inuit and Métis (Public Health Agency of Canada, 2006). *Indian Band Member* or *First Nation* refers to those people who reported being a member of an Indian band or a First Nation of Canada. Band membership is 554,860 (Statistics Canada, 2003).

INUIT

The term *Inuit* replaces the term *Eskimo* (Royal Commission on Aboriginal Peoples, 1996). The Inuit are Aboriginal people in northern Canada, who live above the tree line in Nunavut, the Northwest Territories, Northern Quebec, and Labrador. The word means *people* in the Inuit language—*Inuktitut*. The singular of Inuit is Inuk (Aboriginal Health Glossary, 2004).

MÉTIS

The term *Métis* refers to Aboriginal people of mixed First Nation and European ancestry who identify themselves as Métis people, as distinct from First Nations people, Inuit, or non-Aboriginal people. The Métis have a unique culture that draws on their diverse ancestral origins, such as Scottish, French, Ojibway, and Cree (Government of Saskatchewan, 2003).

Canada, 2008a). Aboriginal peoples in Canada are the descendants of the original inhabitants of North America. The Canadian Constitution under section 35(2) recognizes three groups of Aboriginal peoples: North American Indians (First Nations), Métis people, and Inuit. These represent three separate peoples with unique heritages, languages, multiple cultural practices, and spiritual beliefs (Aboriginal Health Glossary, 2004; Public Health Agency of Canada, 2006). See Box 3-2 for definitions of the three groups of Aboriginal peoples in Canada.

Cultural Diversity Within Aboriginal Peoples in Canada

The 2006 census recorded over 60 different Aboriginal languages or dialects spoken by First Nations People in Canada, grouped into distinct language families. These include Algonquian, Athapascan, Siouan, Salish, Tsimshian, Wakashan, Iroquoian, Haida, Kutenai, and Tlingit.

Of the 596 First Nations bands and 2,284 reserves, only 40% live on reserve, while 60% reside in nonreserve areas (54% urban, 6% rural; Statistics Canada, 2008a). The cultural and linguistic differences among the groups are greater than the differences that divide European nations. In addition to intergroup social, cultural, and environmental differences, there is an enormous diversity of values, lifestyles, and perspectives within any community or urban Aboriginal population (Kirmayer, Brass, & Tait, 2000).

Cultural Roots of Mental Health and Illness

The expression of mental illness is heavily determined by culture. Symptoms of a disorder that are prominent in one culture may be insignificant or absent in another and may even be interpreted as normal in a third (Health Canada, 2003; Public Health Agency of Canada, 2003). Some disorders may be exotic and specific to a particular culture, for example, Windigo among the Cree and Ojibwa and Pibloktog among the Inuit are native myths about rare types of mental illness (Waldram, 2004).

Diagnostic Cultural Formulations

The American Psychiatric Association (APA; 2000) *Diagnostic and Statistical Manual of Mental Disorders (DSM-IV-TR)* is used to set the boundaries, conditions, and criteria for psychiatric diagnosis throughout North America. Culture was not specifically addressed until the fourth edition of the manual (*DSM-IV*) (APA, 1994). After exploring different ways of facilitating the application of a cultural perspective to the process of clinical interviewing, a cultural formulation outline was adopted for use in the fourth edition. However, it was relegated to the back of the book, in the ninth appendix along with a glossary of cultural terms and idioms of distress. This was a problematic solution for many, who believe that culture must be more central to the process of clinical evaluation and treatment (Austin et al., 1999). It has been argued that psychiatric researchers, focused on a biologic model of mental disorders, tend to ignore cultural factors. For instance, in a review of psychiatric drug studies, it was found that only 8% of patient subjects were from minority groups (Vedantam, 2005). (See Chapter 2 for further information on the *DSM-IV-TR*.)

Some new disorders may be a recent development in response to cultural change. The *totally discouraged syndrome* (depression, alcoholism, lack of social responsibility, neglect of family, suicidal behaviour), described for the Sioux, may be such a disorder (Johnson & Johnson, 1965). *Residential school syndrome* as discussed by Brasfield (2001) suggests that this syndrome is similar to posttraumatic stress disorder (see Chapter 21) yet different due to the cultural impact. First-line health care workers see the impact that the residential schools have had on the Aboriginal communities. It presents itself today in a variety of ways through social issues and psychological problems. Addressing these requires understanding of the cultural causes and culturally sensitive approaches to healing.

Aboriginal Mental Health

"**Aboriginal health** is influenced by the rich diversity of social, economic, and political circumstances that give rise to a variety of health problems and healing strategies in Aboriginal communities" (Waldram, Herring, & Young, 2006, p. 3). Many Aboriginal people are raised to believe the body is affected by four elements comprising the spiritual, emotional, mental, and physical. Aboriginal peoples have adopted a holistic view of mental health with mental health seen as part of full health.

The traditional Aboriginal healing system encompasses a holistic view of manifestations of illness in an individual. There is little evidence of a clear distinction between what science would call somatic disorders and disorders of the psyche. The mind, body, and spirit are seen as an integrated whole. Notions of *sanity* and *insanity* and of *personality disorders* are not strictly defined, as in the case of the biomedical tradition. The Western approach, in contrast, separates the body from the mind and spirit, and the emphasis is on disease and treatment (Waldram, 2004). It is necessary to recognize the historical, socioeconomic, and political circumstances of Aboriginal people in Canada in order to understand the mental health problems or disorders of a person from this culture because they may be related to factors that have historically confronted them.

Less than 1% of health care workers in Canada are of Aboriginal ancestry, affecting the provision of health services to this population (Health Canada, 2003). In response to the Royal Commission of Aboriginal Peoples' (1996) recommendation that the number of Aboriginal health care workers be increased, federal and provincial initiatives were implemented. The First Nations University of Canada in Regina, opened in 2003, is one example. Programs to promote Aboriginal medical and nursing education, such as the Native Access Program to Nursing (NAPN) at the University of Saskatchewan (NAPN, 2008), are increasing the number of physicians and nurses who are of Aboriginal descent.

The Romanow Report in 2002 recognized that social problems among Aboriginal people are a legacy of history, a result of the repeated assaults on their culture and identity. The foundation of their society has been weakened and has resulted in the alienation that drives some to self-destruction and antisocial behaviour (Health Canada, 2004b). Abuse of alcohol and drugs, family violence, youth crime, poverty, suicide, and sexual abuse are all social/health issues that require attention if the mental health of Aboriginal peoples is to be promoted.

Colonialism, Assimilation, and Displacement

Colonialism is the institutionalized political domination of one nation over another. There is direct political administration by the colonial power, control of all economic relationships, and a systematic attempt to transform the culture. Before Confederation and up through the first half of the 20th century, the strategy of the Government of Canada toward First Nations was a colonial one. Government policy was to *Canadianize* Aboriginal people and *assimilate* them into the majority culture (Public Health Agency of Canada, 2004; Thira, 2005).

Part of making Native peoples into *Canadians* was to convert them to Christianity: while traditional Aboriginal practices served spiritual, economical, social, and personal purposes essential to the survival of the community, legislation was passed to control these traditional practices (Thira, 2005). Government and several churches and religious orders cooperated to run residential schools in which Aboriginal children, often as young as 6 years of age, were displaced from their parental homes, families, culture, language, and traditions and placed into boarding schools for 10 months of the year. Over 130 residential schools in Canada were located in every province and territory except Newfoundland, New Brunswick, and Prince Edward Island. It is estimated that about 80,000 Aboriginal people living today experienced residential schools (Health Canada, 2007). In the 1980s students of the residential schools began to come forward with allegations of abuse. Corrado and Cohen (2003) described four forms of abuse: physical, sexual, psychological, and spiritual, indicating that 30% to 83% of children in residential schools fell victim to some form of abuse.

In 2001, the Canadian government, after acknowledging the negative effects of this past policy, established the Indian Residential Schools Resolution Canada, a department dedicated to working with First Nations, Inuit, and Métis peoples to address and resolve issues arising from the legacy of residential schools (Indian Residential Schools Resolution Canada, 2005). On June 11, 2008, the official historic apology was given by the Government of Canada to residential school survivors (CBC-news, 2008).

Religion as a Culture System

Religion can be seen as a cultural system, in that it is a system of meanings that shapes our experience. People who have shared common experiences over time develop commonalities of culture. (*Religion* comes from *re-ligare*: to bind together.) Family traditions are a commonality that develops over a generation or two. Religion is a commonality that develops over a longer time in groups of peoples. Prior to the advent of modern Western medicine, health care was often inexorably linked with spirituality or faith (Skip Knox, 2004). Often, there was little that could be done about a medical condition except to pray or give offerings (Srivastava, 2007).

Religious Beliefs and Approaches to Mental Illness

Religious beliefs often define an individual's relationship within a family and community. Many different religions are practiced throughout the world. Although Judeo-Christian beliefs tend to dominate Western societies and other religions such as Islam, Hinduism, and Buddhism dominate Eastern and Middle Eastern cultures, it is likely that all religions are represented among Canadians. (See Web Links for religions in Canada.)

Beliefs about mental illness are intimately linked with concepts of religion, social values, norms, and ideals of human relationships. These shared beliefs determine the nature of traditional medicine and provide the framework for interpreting symptoms and guiding action in response to them. Western medicine and psychiatry are premised on the belief that mental illness is caused by biologic and experiential events; many other cultures ascribe a metaphysical or spiritual cause as well (Health Canada, 2003).

Aboriginal Spirituality and Culture

Spirituality is an important aspect to the Aboriginal culture. Medical practices of Aboriginal people are closely related to other aspects of the culture, especially their spirituality (Waldram et al., 2006). For some there is no distinction between spiritual life and cultural life. Getting in touch with one's own spirituality is identified as a key to recovery or healing. Spirituality is linked to a sense of life purpose and personal identity and is seen as a key element for individuals to find their place in the world. To most Aboriginal people, the concept of spirituality refers to a sense of direction: it is not a religion but a way of life.

Though the rites have been modified throughout the years, Aboriginal spirituality remains alive and continues to be practiced. Interest in Aboriginal spirituality has grown recently, attracting both Aboriginal and non-Aboriginal followers. Many people admire the holistic aspect of Aboriginal spirituality and are drawn to this expression of faith, seeking inner peace and wellness. This renewed interest has created a unique opportunity for the preservation of Aboriginal spirituality and culture.

Prejudice, Discrimination, Stereotyping, and Stigma

It is often difficult for one cultural group to understand the values, beliefs, and patterns of accepted behaviour of a different cultural group. This is especially true in regard to mental illness—some cultures view it as a condition for which the ill person must be punished, banished or ostracized from society, whereas other cultures are more tolerant and believe that family and community members are key to the care and treatment of the mentally ill (Health Canada, 2003). Mental illness indirectly affects all Canadians through a family member, friend, or colleague. Arboleda-Florez (2005) notes that families may also become casualties under the stress of caring for acutely mentally ill relatives, especially within a rejecting community. The concepts of stereotyping, prejudice, discrimination, and stigma are important in understanding the life of people with mental disorders and cultural groups.

Stereotyping is expecting individuals to act in a characteristic manner that conforms to a usually negative perception of their cultural group. Individual characteristics are not considered. Stereotyping occurs because of lack of exposure to enough people in a particular group. "Health professionals who make unsubstantiated assumptions and have stereotypical attitudes about those who differ from themselves not only place the health and well-being of their patients at risk, they also seriously impair service delivery" (Richardson, 2008, p. 40).

Prejudice is a hostile attitude toward others simply because they belong to a particular group that is considered to have objectionable characteristics. Srivastava (2007) notes that everybody has some biases and prejudices, but that health care providers need to acknowledge and examine their biases in preparation for competent, sensitive care for all patients and families. If health care providers do not address their biases in a meaningful way, their ability to form trusting, healing relationships will be affected. **Discrimination** is the differential treatment of others because they are members of a particular group or identified as being negatively different. It can include ignoring, derogatory name calling, denying services, and threatening. Discrimination arises from a lack of understanding and appreciation of differences among people but can be overcome.

Nurses, too, can experience subtle discrimination from patients and families: patients may express a desire to have a nurse "more like them" assigned to their care. Alberta Pasco's (2004) study of Filipino Canadians' experience of hospital care found that her participants initially desired nurses who were "one of us" (*hindi ibang tao*). However, non-Filipino nurses became "one of us" as the patient came to know the nurse as a caring person who was kind, respectful, and trustworthy.

Stigma is the mark of a spoiled identity. In ancient Greece, stigma was literally a sign cut or burnt into a person's body to indicate low moral status (Goffman, 1963). In the correctional facilities in this country, there are now more *culturally sensitive programs* available. However, it has been observed that Aboriginal offenders have not always taken advantage of these programs, because being "different" in prison is not a good thing. Many were ashamed to be Aboriginal. Stigma has been very present in prisons (Office of the Correctional Investigator, 2006, 2007). Sometimes the programs have been utilized (e.g., sweet grass) only for the purpose of getting out of their cells. The programs were there, but the teaching and the installment of pride (of who you are) were sometimes absent. This is just beginning to change as more Aboriginals across Canada are valuing their identity.

The Stigma of Mental Illness

People with mental illnesses or mental health problems often are stigmatized by society in which they live, a phenomenon that has occurred across history (see Chapter 1). In his work, *Madness and Civilization*, Foucault (1967) argues that in the Middle Ages, madness came to occupy the position leprosy once held. Individuals deemed mad were excluded from society as lepers had been. Even with today's more enlightened view of mental illness, a stigma remains attached to those with mental disorders or those who seek help for mental illness (Arboleda-Florez, 2003). Individuals with mental illnesses can be cruelly characterized as "crazy" or "nuts."

Despite the fact that only 5% to 7% of violent crimes are committed by individuals with some form of mental illness, the most prevalent misconceptions about mental illness is the belief that persons with a mental disorder are dangerous (Arboleda-Florez, 2003). Representations of people with mental illness in the media (e.g., movies, television, magazines, newspapers) can perpetuate this negative stereotype. Webster (2005) compared Canadian media coverage of a death due to domestic violence with that of the killing of an Royal Canadian Mounted Police officer by a man with schizophrenia. She found the latter act received much greater coverage.

Stigmatization is an obstacle to progress in mental health care and a powerful force to influence the treatment and rehabilitation of people with a mental disorder. It is a barrier to seeking help. Despite availability of treatment, nearly two thirds of people with a known mental disorder never seek help from a health professional (World Health Organization [WHO], 2001). Persons affected with a mental disorder that is chronic and incapacitating may have the additional burden of dealing with negative social attitudes and even social exclusion that prevents full engagement in their communities (Arboleda-Florez, 2003).

Cultural Competence

Health care professionals at every level need to add **cultural competence** to their repertoire of skills. When patients and nurses come together in situations where one person is in need of care and often vulnerable, and the other is providing the care from a position of strength, "the obligation is on the health care provider to understand patients and their culture, whether the nurse is from the majority or minority culture" (Xu & Flaskerud, 2007, p. 1191). The CNA (2004) position paper, *Promoting Culturally Competent Care*, outlines this obligation in relation to nursing.

KEY CONCEPT **Cultural competence** is the application of knowledge, skills, attitudes, and personal attributes required by nurses to provide appropriate care and services in relation to cultural characteristics of their patients (CNA, 2004).

Cultural competence includes valuing diversity, knowing about cultural mores and traditions of the populations being served, and being sensitive to these while caring for the individual. Nurses are responsible for acquiring, maintaining, and continually enhancing cultural competencies in relation to their patients. They are responsible for incorporating culture into all phases of the nursing process and in all domains of nursing practice (CNA, 2004).

To be culturally competent one does not have to have extensive knowledge of all cultures—this would be impossible. Rather, one must be aware that cultural differences exist, be aware that one's own culture is not superior to that of others, be careful to avoid imposing one's cultural beliefs on others, be willing to learn about and understand other people's cultures, and be willing to incorporate that knowledge into practice and educational curricula. An important first step is to recognize the influence of one's own culture on one's belief system and practice (Srivastava, 2007). Culturally competent care allows for a cultural safe environment, one that respectfully acknowledges a person's cultural identity (Smylie, 2007).

CRNENOTE

Cultural competence of the nurse impacts many aspects of care, including assessment and the meaning of signs and symptoms to patients and families.

Cultural dissonance between nurse and patient is particularly significant in PMH nursing because of culture's influence on values, beliefs, and norms that form the foundation for people's behaviours (Xu & Flaskerud, 2007). It may affect communication as the elements of communication, such as tone, rhythm, pace, and accent, affect persons' ability to comprehend one another and engage in meaningful interaction. For instance, the

---

BOX 3.3

Research for Best Practice: Cultural Competence

Petrucka, P., Bassendowski, S., & Bourassa, C. (2007). Seeking paths to culturally competent health care: Lessons from two Saskatchewan Aboriginal communities. Canadian Journal of Nursing Research, 39(2), 166–182.

Seeking paths to culturally competent health care: Lessons from Saskatchewan Aboriginal communities.

THE QUESTION:

1. How can curricula of health profession's education programs become more culturally respectful for Aboriginal people?
2. How can health service delivery systems become more culturally respectful for Aboriginal people?

METHOD: Taking a community-based research approach, two Saskatchewan Aboriginal communities and the Southern Saskatchewan/Urban Aboriginal Health Coalition, an interdisciplinary, intersectoral team of researchers and communities used sharing circles to determine what key elements are seen as requisite for culturally competent care. Thematic analysis was carried out with the resulting data.

FINDINGS: Four broad thematic groupings were derived: trust, respect, communication, and understanding. Findings indicated that cultural competence requires a caring, respectful nurse–patient relationship in order to assure care that accommodates the beliefs, values, and practices of the patient related to regaining and maintaining health. Respect of traditional medicines and healers and recognition of the importance of family and community are significant components of care in these communities.

IMPLICATIONS: Study findings can inform not only the practice within these Aboriginal communities but also further research. Cultural competency needs to be studied with the involvement of the community itself.

---

direct style of communication favoured in health care can seem confrontational to persons of Asian and Aboriginal cultures (Xu & Flaskerud). Confusion regarding cultural meaning can influence diagnosis to the extent that misdiagnosis can occur (Foster, 2006). Other factors affected by cultural dissonance are access, quality, and availability of care (Flaskerud, 2007). It is important that patients and their families feel comfortable sharing cultural needs, feelings, and concerns with nurses and other health care providers and that they experience their care as sensitive and respectful (Srivastava, 2007). See Box 3-3 for research on culturally competent care.

▅▅ SOCIOECONOMIC CONTEXT OF MENTAL HEALTH CARE

The determinants of health, factors that influence our health status, are greatly affected by sociocultural and socioeconomic circumstances. Factors such as income and social status, social support networks, education, employment and working conditions, physical environment, and health services affect one's well-being. In 2000, the United Nations (UN) rated Canada the best country in the world in which to live. In subsequent years, it remained consistently in the top five. This assessment is based on a country's Human Development Index. Not everyone in Canada, however, enjoys the advantages of living in a highly developed country (Kendall, 2001). Canada ranked fourth in the world on the 2007 United Nations Human Development Index. Yet, if Aboriginals were viewed separately, *Aboriginal Canada* would slip to 78th, a rank currently held by Kazakhstan (World Vision Canada, 2005).

Poverty in Canada

Poverty changes a population's ability to make choices. Poverty chooses your life for you. Poverty in the North American context is primarily relative rather than absolute. The measurement of poverty in Canada has been a challenge as there is no official government measure. There is an ongoing debate about whether a relative measure of poverty or an absolute measure is more valid. According to Statistics Canada, in 2004, about 3.5 million people were living below the low-income cutoff line (Ligaya, 2007). In 1989, the House of Commons unanimously resolved to "seek to achieve the goal of eliminating poverty among Canadian children by the year 2000." Yet, the *2006 Report card on child and family poverty* indicates that close to 1.2 million children, almost one child out of every six in Canada, still live in poverty (Campaign 2000, 2006).

> **KEY CONCEPT Poverty** can be measured as absolute or relative. Absolute poverty is calculated by comparing a person's total income against the cost of goods and services essential to daily life. Relative poverty is measured by comparing total income and spending with those of the general population (see http://canadianeconomy.gc.ca).

Poverty and Mental Illness

Families living in poverty are under tremendous financial and emotional stress, which may trigger or exacerbate mental problems. Along with the daily stressors of trying to provide food and shelter for themselves and their families, lack of time, energy, and money prevents them from attending to their psychological needs. Often, these families become trapped in a downward economic spiral, as tension and stress mount. The inability to gain employment and the lack of financial independence only add to the feelings of powerlessness and low self-esteem. Being self-supporting gives one a feeling of control over life and bolsters self-esteem. Dependence on others or the government causes frustration, anger, apathy, and feelings of depression and meaninglessness (Axelson, 1999). Alcoholism, depression, and child and partner abuse may become a means of coping with such hopelessness and despair. The homeless population is the group most at risk for being unable to escape this spiral of poverty. The number of homeless people with mental illness in Canada is causing great concern, and adequate societal responses are being sought (see Chapter 2).

The chances of becoming poor are greater if someone is mentally ill. Three percent of Canadians suffer from severe and chronic mental disorders that can cause serious functional limitations and social and economic impairment (Kirby Report, 2002). Still, many people with mental illness hold down well-paid jobs. A key factor for many of these people is a strong support network of family and friends. The World Health Organization (WHO), in a three-decade study, found that people with schizophrenia living in less-developed nations typically do better than those in industrialized countries like Canada. The reason may be that people with schizophrenia in those countries are included in social events, family obligations, and work (WHO, 2001).

● CRNENOTE

Mental illness puts a person at greater risk for poverty and homelessness which, in turn, places serious constraints on regaining and maintaining health.

Socioeconomic Influences on Aboriginal Mental Health

Although Canada is considered to have one of the finest publicly funded health care systems, Aboriginal populations continue to exhibit morbidity and mortality rates in some dimensions in excess of some Third World countries. Shamefully, the gap in life expectancy between First Nations individuals and other Canadians is 7 years for men and 5 years for women. Life expectancy for Inuit is also believed to be lower, although statistics are not available for all northern regions (Health Canada, 2005a). While one in six was the estimate for Canadian children living in poverty, this figure does not include the appalling situation for First Nations communities where one in every four children is growing up in poverty (Campaign 2000, 2006). Aboriginal peoples experience lower education levels and are seriously underrepresented in the labour force. Those living in rural areas also contend with inadequate housing. Many Aboriginals' homes do not have a telephone, computer, or Internet access. Aboriginal peoples also experience higher rates of suicide especially among youth, which is five to six times higher than the national average for First Nations youth and 11 times higher for Inuit youth. Suicide is the single greatest cause of injury-related deaths for Aboriginal people. In addition, there are higher rates of infant mortality and an increasing number of First Nations children born addicted to drugs (Health Canada, 2004b, 2005a, 2005b). Aboriginal health status has been improving over the past 20 years in some areas, such as life expectancy and reduction of infant mortality. Although Aboriginal people are enjoying better health today, it still remains less than the health status of non-Aboriginal Canadians (Health Canada, 2004b).

There is a connection between socioeconomic status and involvement with the criminal justice system, and Aboriginal peoples are overrepresented in that system. Although they represent about 3% of the population, they form about 16% of the offender population (Canadian Criminal Justice Association, 2000; Canadian Centre for Justice Statistics, 2006; Office of the Auditor General of Canada, 2008). Social and health problems, along with the effects of rapid culture change, cultural oppression, and marginalization (Kirmayer, Simpson, & Cargo, 2003), are reflected in high rates of mental health problems among Aboriginal populations (Kirmayer et al., 2000; Waldram, 2004).

Epidemiologic studies have documented high levels of mental health problems in many Canadian Aboriginal communities (Kirmayer, 1994; Royal Commission on Aboriginal Peoples, 1996). These studies indicate rates of psychiatric disorders varying from levels comparable to those found in the general population to up to twice those of neighbouring non-Aboriginal communities (Kirmayer et al., 2000). Most estimates of the prevalence of psychiatric disorders are based on service utilization records, but because many Aboriginal people never come for treatment, service utilization is at best only a lower estimate of the true prevalence of distress in the community.

As noted, there is a tendency of First Nations individuals not to use the mental health services provided by the dominant culture. If services are accessed, approximately 50% drop out, and for many, treatments are not effective (Smye & Browne, 2002), partly because mental health services ignore the unique cultural identities, histories, and sociopolitical contexts of the everyday lives of Aboriginal peoples. Many indigenous communities are doing well despite the challenges they face. Transforming attitudes, policies, and practice principles by gaining an awareness of the political and historical forces shaping the health and social status of indigenous peoples is vital (Browne & Fiske, 2001). Culturally sensitive mental health services and health promotion could contribute to greater well-being.

Geographic Location and Access to Mental Health Services

Although comprehensiveness, universality, portability, and accessibility are key components of the Canada Health Act (Health Canada, 2004a; Lewis, Donaldson, Mitton, & Currie, 2001), getting mental health services to rural and isolated communities continues to be a challenge. Most mental health services are located in urban areas, with access for people in the far North being very different from that of people living in the more highly populated areas of Canada. All age groups in rural areas have limited access to health care, but the lack of resources is particularly problematic for children and elderly people, who have specialized needs.

According to the 2006 census, up to one third of Canadians and one half of Atlantic Canadians live in rural areas (Statistics Canada, 2008b). Transportation is a major barrier to the receipt of health services in rural areas. For instance, past reports of the Auditor General have noted that 121 First Nations communities have no road access, and an additional 75 communities with road access were more than 90 km from the nearest physician. Costs of travel and accommodation for patients and families can be high, in dollars and energy. Services should be delivered in communities where possible, but the small population of some rural communities can be a deterrent. As well, specialized services are located in large urban centres (Office of the Auditor General of Canada, 2008). Mobile service delivery and specialist circuits are one option used to address this issue.

Telehealth also holds promise. Telehealth is the use of electronic information and communication technologies to support health care services over distance. It ranges from the retrieval of laboratory results or other health records posted on a network to the assessment of a person by a psychiatrist through videoconferencing.

Although it is often assumed that treatment approaches are effective across urban and rural environments, this may not always be the case (Haddon, Merritt-Gray, & Wuest, 2004). The way in which a rural environment influences social and health needs, as well as help-seeking behaviours, is only beginning to be explored.

Role of PMH Nurses in Rural and Remote Areas and in the North

The role of nurses takes on new dimensions in rural and remote areas or in Canada's north, where they are often the only or the most accessible health care professionals, and thus the primary health care providers. Nurses in these regions often practice in expanded roles, acting as the first point of contact in the health system. These nurses may be advocates, collaborators, or mediators in encouraging the development of public policies and resources for their region.

■ LEGAL CONTEXT OF MENTAL HEALTH CARE

Every society needs laws to achieve its objectives. According to WHO (2005b), the fundamental aim of mental health legislation is to protect, promote, and improve the lives and mental well-being of citizens.

Human Rights and Mental Illness

In accordance with the objectives of the UN Charter and international agreements, a fundamental basis for mental health legislation is human rights. Key rights and principles include equality and nondiscrimination, the right to privacy and individual autonomy, freedom from inhuman and degrading treatment, the principle of the least restrictive environment, and the rights to information and participation.

In most parts of the world, according to the Romanow Report in 2002, mental health and mental illness are not given the same degree of importance as physical health (Health Canada, 2004b). Global resources for people suffering from mental and neurologic disorders are grossly insufficient to address the growing burden of mental health needs (WHO, 2005b). The WHO (2005a) *Mental Health Atlas—2005* shows no substantial change in global mental health resources since 2001 and a growing gap between allocations in high- and low-income countries (CNA, 2005). Currently, more than 40% of countries have no mental health policy and more than 30% have no mental health program. About 25% of countries have no mental health legislation (WHO, 2001). Canada has been one of the few industrialized countries without a national mental health strategy; however, in 2007, the Commission on Mental Health and Mental Illness was established with the development of a national strategy as a prime responsibility (Mental Health Commission of Canada, 2008). An initial framework, *Toward Recovery and Well-being* (January, 2009), proposes eight goals for a mental health system:

1. The hope of recovery is available to all.
2. Action is taken to promote mental health and well-being to prevent mental health problems and illnesses.
3. The mental health system is culturally safe and responds to the diverse needs of Canadians.
4. The importance of families in promoting recovery and well-being is recognized and their needs are supported.
5. People of all ages have equitable access to a system of appropriate and effective programs, services, and supports that is seamlessly integrated around their needs.

BOX 3.4

Canadian and International Agreements Relevant to Culture and to Mental Health

1948	Universal Declaration of Human Rights (United Nations, 1948)
1957	The Indigenous and Tribal Populations Convention, 1957 (No. 107)
1965	The International Convention on the Elimination of All Forms of Racial Discrimination (Canadian ratification in 1969)
1966	The International Covenant on Economic, Social, and Cultural Rights (ICESCR; Canadian ratification in 1976)
1966	The International Covenant on Civil and Political Rights (Canadian ratification in 1976)
1971	Multiculturalism policy (Canada) (Government of Canada, 2004a)
1976	International Covenant on Economic, Social, and Cultural Rights (ICESCR)
1982	Canadian Charter of Rights and Freedoms (Department of Justice Canada, 2005)
1984	Canada Health Act (Department of Justice Canada, 2008)
1988	Multiculturalism Act (Canada) (Government of Canada, 2004b)
1989	Indigenous and Tribal (Peoples Populations) Convention (Revised)
1990	Declaration of Caracas (WHO, 1990)
1991	Principles of Protection of Persons With Mental Illness (United Nations, 1991)
1997	Renewed Multiculturalism Program in Canada
2001	Immigration and Refugee Protection Act (IRPA, 2001)

BOX 3.5

Rights of Persons With Mental Illness

- Right to medical care (Principle 1.1)
- Right to be treated with humanity and respect (Principle 1.2)
- Equal protection right (Principle 1.4)
- Right to be cared for in the community (Principle 7)
- Right to provide informed consent before receiving any treatment (Principle 11)
- Right to privacy (Principle 13)
- Freedom of communication (Principle 13)
- Freedom of religion (Principle 13)
- Right to voluntary admission (Principles 15 and 16)
- Right to judicial guarantees (Principle 17)

From United Nations. (1991). *Principles for the protection of persons with mental illness and the improvement of mental health care.* Adopted by General Assembly resolution 46/119 of 17 December 1991, Office of the United Nations High Commissioner for Human Rights. Retrieved October 15, 2005, from http://www.unhchr.ch/html/menu3/b/68.htm

6. Actions are based on appropriate evidence, outcomes are measured, and research is advanced.
7. Discrimination against people living with mental health problems and illnesses is eliminated, and stigma is not tolerated.
8. A broadly based social movement keeps mental health issues out of the shadows—forever.

International Agreements

There are many significant international agreements to help protect people with mental illness. The most significant are listed in Box 3-4. Mental health principles, adopted by the UN in 1991, are outlined in Box 3-5. See Web Links at the end of the chapter for Internet access information regarding national and international advocacy organizations.

Mental Health Legislation

Mental health legislation is a powerful tool for codifying and consolidating these fundamental values and principles,

for protecting the rights of people with mental disorders, and for promoting the mental health of populations. It offers an important mechanism to ensure adequate and appropriate care and treatment. Being unable to access treatment and care is an infringement of a person's right to health and right to access can be included in legislation (WHO, 2005c).

Mental Health Acts in Canada

Legislation in Canada strongly influences the context of our mental health care. Each province and territory is guided by its own Mental Health Care Act. Each act must be congruent with the rights stipulated under the *1982 Charter of Rights and Freedoms* (Department of Justice Canada, 2005) and the resources to enforce the act must be in place. See Box 3-6 for Internet access information on the various mental health acts.

KEY CONCEPT   A **Mental Health Act** is a law that gives certain powers, and sets the conditions (including time limits) for those powers, to stipulated health care professionals and designated institutions regarding the admission and treatment of individuals with a mental disorder.

Gray and O'Reilly (2001) reviewed the Mental Health Act provisions in all Canadian jurisdictions. They found significant differences among the provinces and territories and raised a concern that some provisions might prevent people from receiving appropriate care.

BOX 3.6

Mental Health Acts

Province/Territory	Website Address
Alberta	http://download.cmha.ab.ca/alberta/mha.pdf
British Columbia	www.qp.gov.bc.ca/statreg/stat/m/96288_01.htm
Manitoba	http://web2.gov.mb.ca/laws/statutes/ccsm/m110e.php
New Brunswick	www.gnb.ca/0062/PDF-acts/m-10.pdf
Newfoundland and Labrador	www.cmhanl.ca/
Northwest Territories	http://action.attavik.ca/home/justice-gn/attach-en_conlaw_postdiv/consRSNWT1988cM-10.pdf
Nova Scotia	www.gov.ns.ca/legislature/legc/bills/59th_1st/1st_read/b109.htm
Nunavut	www.iijcan.org/nu/laws/sta/m-10/20061207/whole.html
Ontario	www.elaws.gov.on.ca/html/statutes/english/elaws_statutes_90m07_e.htm
Prince Edward Island	http://govpe.ca/law/statutes/pdf/m-06_1.pdf
Quebec	www.amiquebec.org/TreatmentServices.htm
Saskatchewan	www.qp.gov.sk.ca/index.cfm?fuseaction=publications.details&p=626
Yukon	www.gov.yk.ca/legislation/acts/mehe.pdf

BOX 3.7

Involuntary Admission Criteria in Provincial and Territorial Mental Health Acts

Is not suitable as a voluntary inpatient: A person who is willing and capable of consenting to a voluntary admission cannot be admitted with an involuntary status anywhere in Canada.

Meets the definition of mental disorder: The person must have a mental disorder. In many, but not all of the jurisdictions, it is specified that the disorder must seriously impair the person's functioning.

Meets the criteria for harm: In most jurisdictions, this is not limited to serious bodily harm; nonbodily harms are acceptable. The criterion of "danger" stipulated in some acts, however, has been interpreted by the courts to mean bodily harm.

Likely to suffer substantial mental or physical deterioration: This is included in some provinces (British Columbia, Saskatchewan, Manitoba, and Ontario) as an alternative to the harm criterion.

In need of psychiatric treatment: This is a criterion in British Columbia, Saskatchewan, and Ontario. It is possible in other jurisdictions to commit a person with a mental disorder who is dangerous, but for whom there is no treatment (e.g., antisocial personality disorder) for the purpose of preventative detention.

Refusal of treatment: By the person after admission: This is allowed in some jurisdictions but not others. In some jurisdictions, a refusal can be overruled in the person's best interests.

Review and appeal procedures regarding the validity of involuntary hospitalization: These are found in all jurisdictions.

From Gray, J., & O'Reilly, R. (2001). Clinically significant differences among Canadian Mental Health Acts. *Canadian Journal of Psychiatry, 46*, 315–321.

See Box 3-7 for an overview, based on their work, of basic criteria for involuntary admission in the various jurisdictions. It is the responsibility of PMH nurses to understand the Mental Health Act of their province or territory. Nurses need to be able to explain the act's basic provisions to people with mental illness and their families.

Mental Health Acts within Canada may allow involuntary treatment of a person admitted under such an act if the person is not considered **competent** to make decisions regarding treatment. Competence, in this respect, means being able to understand (at a basic level) matters relevant to the decision and to understand the consequences of the decision. Competence is not a fixed capacity; it changes over time. There are specific provisions within mental health acts regarding the evaluation of competency and what action may be taken if a person is deemed not competent. When a person is unable to consent to treatment, consent from a **substitute decision maker** may be sought. Depending on the jurisdiction, these substitute decision makers can be state appointed, appointed by the person when competent, or be a guardian or relative. There are different criteria

to guide substitute decision making: **best interests** (e.g., treatment will make the person less ill, the person will get more ill without treatment, the benefits outweigh any risks), *capable wishes* (what the person expressed while capable, even if not in current best interests), and *modified best interests* (follow expressed wishes except if they would endanger the person or others; Gray & O'Reilly, 2001).

Mandatory Outpatient Treatment

In some jurisdictions, an involuntary patient may return to the community on a *conditional leave* if the admission criteria are still met and if stipulations for treatment are followed. If the stipulations (e.g., taking medication and meeting with a physician) are not followed, the person can be returned to the hospital. **Mandatory outpatient treatment** (MOT) involves legal provisions

BOX 3.8

Community Treatment Orders

Province	Website Address
Alberta	www.cmha.ab.ca/bins/site_page. asp?cid = 284–285–1247&lang = 1 www.alberta.ca/home/News-Frame.cfm?ReleaseID = / acn/200712/22685AC9BDE06-A5B9-DF6F-D6AE78CB7D8D2A61.html&\;
British Columbia	www2.parl.gc.ca/Content/HOC/ Committee/392/SECU/Web-Doc/WD3420686/392_SECU_ SpeakingNotes/392_SECU_ SpeakingNotes_B.C.%20Schyzophre-nia%20Society-e.pdf
Manitoba	http://ww1.cpa-apc.org:8080/publica-tions/archives/cjp/2005/january/obrien. asp
New Brunswick	www.law.ualberta.ca/centres/hli/pdfs/ hlj/v11_2003/Trueman.pdf
Newfoundland and Labrador	www.assembly.nl.ca/Legislation/sr/ Annualstatutes/2006/M09–1.c06.htm
Nova Scotia	www.law.ualberta.ca/centres/hli/pdfs/ hlj/v11_2003/Trueman.pdf
Ontario	www.health.gov.on.ca/english/public/ pub/mental/treatment_order.html
Saskatchewan	www.health.gov.sk.ca/mental-health-personal-rights

requiring people with a mental illness to comply with a treatment plan while living in the community (O'Reilly et al., 2003). **Community treatment orders** (CTOs) are a type of MOT, existing in such provinces as Saskatchewan, Ontario, and Newfoundland, that are usually initiated by a physician. People who do not meet involuntary admission criteria and who are not necessarily in a hospital at the time of the CTO can be required to comply with the stipulated treatment. See Box 3-8 for websites that will provide provincial information regarding CTOs.

CTOs are meant to ensure that people with serious mental illness get the care and treatment they need in a community-based system. The intent is to remove barriers to help from families, police, and health care professionals in getting people at risk for harm to self or others the care and treatment they need (Canadian Mental Health Association [CMHA], 2008a; Canadian Centre on Substance Abuse, 2006; Government of Ontario, 2006). It is, perhaps, unfortunate that there is a tendency to name MOT legislation, such as Brian's Law in Ontario, after an individual killed by a person who acted on the basis of psychotic delusions. This emphasizes protection of society rather than the health of the ill person.

MOT remains a somewhat controversial concept in Canada, although it has existed for more than 20 years in some states in the United States. The concern is that a person's right to autonomy should not be infringed on unless absolutely necessary (Snow & Austin, 2009). In Alberta, for instance, it was argued that while CTOs may have utility with a small number of persons with severe and persistent mental illness, the potential for abuse, the lack of clear outcome evidence, and the availability of less coercive options indicate that there should be a far greater priority in improving community resources than putting in place CTOs (CMHA, 2008b). Szasz (1961, 2005), who challenges the legitimacy of any psychiatric treatment, argues that CTOs have "turned all of society into a kind of mental hospital" (2005, p. 81). A recent study on the use of CTOs in Ontario found that CTOs were helpful in assisting individuals who historically refused services to remain engaged with treatment and support services (Hunt, da Silva, Lurie, & Goldbloom, 2007).

CRNENOTE

In Canada, the laws governing mandated commitment and treatment for major mental disorders are at the provincial level. Nurses need to understand, and be able to communicate to patients and their families, the core provisions of the Mental Health Act of the province in which they practice.

Separate from mental health legislation are the legal provisions that can require people to follow treatment as a condition of probation. The law allows for persons to be found *Not Criminally Responsible due to a Mental Disorder* (NCRMD) for an offence if they are suffering from a mental disorder that makes them incapable of appreciating the nature of the act or knowing that what they did was wrong. In these cases the mentally ill offender needs to comply with treatment monitored by Criminal Code Review Boards (see Chapter 34).

RESEARCH AND THE CONTEXT OF MENTAL HEALTH CARE

Many health professionals, advocacy groups, and policy analysts believe that greater support for research on the context of mental health issues is urgently required. Unresolved, these issues pose a serious threat to the survival and health of Canadian communities. Such research should include studies on methodologies to identify the determinants of mental health disorders, to explore the prevalence of preventable causative factors related to mental illness, to determine the nature and extent of barriers to access to mental health treatment and care, and to determine whether mental health legislation is effective (Arboleda-Florez, 2005). Longitudinal studies are needed. For instance, although there is much research on the abuse that occurred at residential schools for Aboriginal children, the long-term effects and subsequent mental health issues have not been sufficiently studied (Söchting, Corrado, Cohen, Ley, & Brasfield, 2007).

SUMMARY OF KEY POINTS

◻ The term *culture* is defined as a way of life that manifests the learned beliefs, values, and accepted behaviours that are transmitted socially within a specific group.

◻ Cultural competence consists of cultural awareness, cultural knowledge, cultural skills, and cultural encounters. It is an obligation of all Canadian nurses.

◻ Aboriginal mental illness and disorders encompass the recognition of the historical, socioeconomic, and political circumstances of Aboriginal people in Canada. Mental imbalance as experienced by Aboriginal peoples may be related to one or all of the life experiences historically confronting Aboriginal people.

◻ Stigmatization occurs as a result of prejudice, discrimination, and stereotyping. Cultural groups and people with mental illness are often stigmatized.

◻ Religious beliefs are closely intertwined with beliefs about health and mental illness.

◻ Mental health services should be integrated as completely as possible into the helping systems currently accepted by the culture.

◻ Access to mental health treatment is particularly limited for those living in rural, remote, and northern areas or those living in poverty.

◻ Progressive legislation can be an effective tool to promote access to mental health care as well as to promote and protect the rights of people with mental disorders.

CRITICAL THINKING CHALLENGES

1 Discuss to what extent culture matters in the treatment of mental illness and Aboriginal health in Canada.

2 Explore the Aboriginal understanding of mental health through conversations with people of Aboriginal cultures or by reading books such as *Revenge of the Windigo: The Construction of the Mind and Mental Health of North American Aboriginal Peoples* (Waldram, 2004).

3 Compare the access to mental health services in rural areas to urban areas in your province or territory.

4 Discuss the goals of the national mental health strategy. What, if anything, would you add or change?

5 What does poverty look like in your local community?

6 Discuss the influence of social and socioeconomic factors on the mental health of Canadians.

7 Compare Canada's mental health legislation to international initiatives.

8 Outline the basic tenets of the Mental Health Act of your province or territory.

9 In 1996, a pregnant Aboriginal woman with a history of solvent abuse (see Chapter 24) was ordered by a Winnipeg judge to undergo treatment. This court decision raised a number of issues regarding the use of the legal system to mandate treatment. Discuss these issues with your classmates. Consider the dangers of substance abuse to the fetus, the need for women to feel safe in accessing health care (including prenatal care), and the efficacy of involuntary treatment of an addiction.

10 Identify the type of research needed to improve the context of Canadian mental health care.

WEB LINKS

www.camimh.ca The Canadian Alliance on Mental Illness and Mental Health (CAMIMH) is the largest mental health advocacy group in Canada. It is an alliance of mental health organizations comprised of health care providers as well as of the mentally ill and their families.

www.cmha.ca The Canadian Mental Health Association (CMHA) is a national, voluntary organization that promotes mental health and serves consumers and others through education, public awareness, research, advocacy, and direct services.

www.mdri.org Mental Disability Rights International (MDRI) is an advocacy organization dedicated to the recognition and enforcement of rights of people with mental disabilities.

www. mentalhealthcommission.ca The Mental Health Commission of Canada (MHCC) is a nonprofit organization created to focus national attention on mental health issues, to work to improve the mental health of Canadians, and to reduce the stigma associated with this disease.

www.who.int/about/en The World Health Organization (WHO) is the United Nations agency for health. The WHO's objective is, as set out in its Constitution, the attainment, by all peoples, of the highest possible level of health.

www.wfmh.org The World Federation for Mental Health (WFMH) is the only international, multidisciplinary, grassroots advocacy and education mental health organization.

www.forces.gc.ca/hr/religions/engraph/ religions00_e.asp Religions in Canada is a resource by the National Defense to provide general information and awareness about the various religious and spiritual practices in Canada.

MOVIES, NOVELS, AND BIOGRAPHIES

Saint Monica: 2002. Set in Toronto's Portuguese-Canadian community, this film tells the story of Monica, a lonely 10-year-old girl fixated on things spiritual: she fantasizes and plays with toy angels and Blessed Virgin Mary figurines the way other kids play with Barbies or read Harry Potter. When Monica is denied the role of an angel in her church's holy day procession because her family moves to a new neighbourhood, she steals the angel wings, only to lose them. The wings are found by a mentally ill, homeless woman, Mary. The story evolves as Monica attempts to recover the wings and develops a unique relationship with Mary.

VIEWING POINTS: Consider how the religious beliefs of others may be difficult to understand initially. Did Monica's and Mary's behaviours gain meaning for you by the end of the film? Note the settings of the drop-in centre and the psychiatric hospital.

Where the Spirit Lives: 1989. This Canadian movie reveals the oppression of Aboriginal culture in residential schools through the story of a young girl, Komi. It is 1937 and Komi, along with others, is abducted to a Catholic residential school (based on Shubenacadie Indian Residential School in Nova Scotia). This movie captures, in a thoughtful way, the experience of the children and their families. It shows the complex motivations of those enacting this coercive policy.

VIEWING POINTS: Reflect on what is revealed about self-identity and the role culture plays within its development. How does the film reveal "the tyranny of the majority?"

Nuts: 1987. A strong-willed, high-priced prostitute, played by Barbra Streisand, is accused of manslaughter. Her family and attorney want her to plead guilty by reason of insanity. The movie revolves around their attempts to have her declared incompetent to stand trial, which would commit her to a mental health facility and deny her a trial, and her anger and rebellion against this type of plea.

VIEWING POINTS: Consider the complexities of the concept of "competence" and "incompetence" as illustrated in this film.

REFERENCES

Aboriginal Health Glossary. (2004). *Aboriginal health and cultural diversity online glossary*. Compiled by A. Kent-Wilkinson (assistant professor) & technology by M. Tomtene (programmer analyst)., Saskatoon, SK: College of Nursing, University of Saskatchewan. Retrieved August 1, 2008, from http://www.usask.ca/nursing/aboriginalglossary

American Psychiatric Association. (1994). *Diagnostic and statistical manual of mental disorders (DSM IV)* (4th ed.). Washington, DC: Author.

American Psychiatric Association. (2000). *Diagnostic and statistical manual of mental disorders (DSM IV-TR)* (4th ed., Text revision). Washington, DC: Author.

Arboleda-Florez, J. (2003). Considerations on the stigma of mental illness. *Canadian Journal of Psychiatry, 48*(10), 645–650. Retrieved August 1, 2008, from http://server03.cpa-apc.org:8080/Publications/Archives/CJP/2003/november/guesteditorial.pdf

Arboleda-Florez, J. (2005). The epidemiology of mental illness in Canada. *Canadian Public Policy-Analyse de Politiques, 31*, S13–S16. Retrieved August 1, 2005, from Special Electronic Supplement on Mental Health Reform for the 21st Century: http://economics.ca/cgi/jab?journal = cpp&view = v31s1/CPPv31s1p013.pdf&\;http://www.afn.ca/Programs/Health%20Secretariat/health.htm

Austin, W., Gallop, R., McCay, E. Peternelj-Taylor, C., & Bayer, M. (1999). Culturally competent care for psychiatric patients who have a history of sexual abuse. *Clinical Nursing Research, 8*(1), 5–25.

Axelson, J. A. (1999). *Counseling and development in a multicultural society* (3rd ed.). Belmont, CA: Wadsworth, Brooks/Cole.

Brasfield, C. R. (2001). Residential school syndome. *BC Medical Journal, 43*(2), 78–81.

Browne, A. J., & Fiske, J. (2001). First Nations women's encounters with mainstream health care services. *Western Journal of Nursing Research, 23*(2), 126–147. Retrieved August 1, 2008, from Sage Publications, http://wjn.sagepub.com/cgi/reprint/23/2/126.pdf

Campaign 2000. (2006). *Oh Canada! Too many children in poverty for too long… 2006 Report card on child and family poverty in Canada.* Retrieved August 1, 2008, from http://www.campaign2000.ca/rc/rc06/06_C2000NationalReportCard.pdf

Canadian Centre for Justice Statistics. (2006). Crime statistics for 2006. *Juristat, 27*(5). Retrieved August 1, 2008, from http://dsp-psd.pwgsc.gc.ca/collection_2007/statcan/85-002-X/85-002-XIE2007005.pdf

Canadian Centre on Substance Abuse. (2006). *Fact sheet – mandatory and coerced treatment. CCSA-CCLAT.* Retrieved August 1, 2008, from http://www.ccsa.ca/nr/rdonlyres/379bfb 3a-02a1-49b3-9abb-ccef7ef9a811/0/ccsa0036482006.pdf

Canadian Criminal Justice Association. (2000). *Aboriginal people and the criminal justice system.* Retrieved February 5, 2005, from http://www.ccja-acjp.ca/en/abori.html

Canadian Mental Health Association. (2008a). *Community treatment orders (CTO).* Retrieved August 1, 2008, from http://www.cmhaottawa.ca/services.htm

Canadian Mental Health Association. (2008b). *Community treatment orders [Position statement].* Alberta Division http://www.cmha.ab.ca/bins/site_page.asp?cid = 284–285–1247&lang = 1

Canadian Nurses Association. (2004). *Promoting culturally competent care [Position Statement].* Retrieved August 1, 2005, from http://cna-aiic.ca/CNA/documents/pdf/publications/PS73_Promoting_Culturally_Competent_Care_March_2004_e.pdf

Canadian Nurses Association. (2005). Global mental health care. *CNA Review*, October 10–23.

CBCnews.ca (2008, June). *PM cites 'sad chapter' in apology for residential schools.* Retrieved June 11, 2008, from http://www.cbc.ca/canada/story/2008/06/11/aboriginal-apology.html

Corrado, R. R., & Cohen, I. M. (2003). *Mental health profiles for a sample of British Columbia's Aboriginal survivors of the Canadian residential system.* Ottawa, ON: Aboriginal Healing Foundation.

Department of Justice Canada. (2005). *Canadian Charter of Rights and Freedoms.* Constitution Act, 1982(79). Constitution Acts 1967–1982. Retrieved August 1, 2005, from http://canada.justice.gc.ca/Loireg/charte/const_en.html

Department of Justice Canada. (2008). *Canada Health Act, 1984. c. 6, s. 1.* Retrieved August 1, 2008, from http://laws.justice.gc.ca/en/C-6

Flaskerud, J. H. (2007). Cultural dissonance: Therapist and client. *Issues in Mental Health Nursing, 28*, 1081–1083.

Foster, C. H. (2006). What nurses should know when working in Aboriginal communities. *Canadian Nurse, 102*(4), 28–31.

Foucault, M. (1967). *Madness and civilization: A history of insanity in the age of reason.* (R. Howard, Trans.). London, UK: Tavistock Publications (original work published 1961).

Geertz, C. (1973). *The interpretation of cultures: Selected essays.* New York, NY: Basic Books.

Goffman, I. (1963). *Stigma: Notes on the management of spoiled identity.* Englewood Cliffs, NJ: Prentice Hall.

Government of Canada. (2004a). Multiculturalism: Policy and legislative framework. *Canadian heritage.* Retrieved August 1, 2008, from http://www.canadianheritage.gc.ca/progs/multi/policy/framework_e.cfm

Government of Canada. (2004b). Multiculturalism: Canadian Multiculturism Act. *Canadian heritage.* Retrieved August 1, 2008, from http://www.canadianheritage.gc.ca/progs/multi/policy/act_e.cfm

Government of Ontario. (2006). *Community treatment orders.* Brian's Law (Mental Health Legislative Reform), 2000. Ministry of Health and Long Term care. Retrieved August 1, 2008, from http://www.health.gov.on.ca/english/public/pub/mental/brianslaw.html

Government of Saskatchewan. (2003). *Glossary.* Government Relations and Aboriginal Affairs (GS-GRAA). Regina, SK: Author.

Gray, J., & O'Reilly, R. (2001). Clinically significant differences among Canadian Mental Health Acts. *Canadian Journal of Psychiatry, 46,* 315–321.

Haddon, A., Merritt-Gray, M., & Wuest, J. (2004). Private matters and public knowledge in rural communities: The paradox. In M. L. Stirling, C. A. Cameron, N. Nason-Clark, & B. Miedema (Eds.), *Understanding abuse: Partnering for change* (pp. 249–266). Toronto, ON: University of Toronto Press.

Health Canada. (2003). *What determines health? Sante de la population health?* Retrieved August 1, 2005, from http://www.hcsc.gc.ca/hppb/phdd/determinants/determinants.html

Health Canada. (2004a). *Canada's health care system (Medicare).* Retrieved August 1, 2008, from http://www.hc-sc.gc.ca/hcs-sss/medi-assur/index-eng.php

Health Canada. (2004b). Commission on the future of health care in Canada: The Romanow Commission. *Romanow Report, November 28, 2002.* Retrieved August 1, 2008, http://www.hc-sc.gc.ca/hcs-sss/hhr-rhs/strateg/romanow-eng.php

Health Canada. (2005a). *Regional health surveys. First Nations, Inuit, and Aboriginal health.* Retrieved August 1, 2008, from http://www.hc-sc.gc.ca/fniah-spnia/pubs/services/_home-domicile/2000_cp-pc_rev-exam/31_region_surveys-enquetes-eng.php

Health Canada. (2005b). Suicidal behaviour. Mental health. In *Clinical guidelines for nurses in primary care.* Nursing in First Nations Communities. Retrieved August 1, 2008, from http://www.hc-sc.gc.ca/fniah-spnia/pubs/services/_nursing-infirm/2000_clin-guide/chap_15e-eng.php#15–35 (Chapter 15).

Health Canada. (2007). *First Nations, Inuit and Indian health: Indian residential schools.* Retrieved May 20, 2008, from http://www.hc-sc.gc.ca/fniah-spnia/services/indiresident/index-eng.php

Hunt, A. M., da Silva, A., Lurie, S., & Goldbloom, D. S. (2007). Community treatment orders in Toronto: The emerging data. *The Canadian Journal of Psychiatry, 52*(10), 647–656. Retrieved August 1, 2008, from http://publications.cpa-apc.org/media.php?mid = 529

Immigration and Refugee Protection Act, S. C. 2001, C.27. (2001). Retrieved October 23, 2009, from http://www.canlii.org/en/ca/laws/stat/sc-2001-c-27/latest/sc-2001-c-27.html

Indian Residential Schools Resolution Canada. (2005). *Government of Canada reaches historic Agreement in Principle—November 23, 2005.* Retrieved August 1, 2005, from http://www.irsr-rqpi.gc.ca/english/index.html

Johnson, D. L., & Johnson, C. A. (1965). Totally discouraged: A depressive syndrome of the Dakota Sioux. *Transcultural Psychiatry, 2*(2), 140–143.

Kendall, J. (2001). Circles of disadvantage: Aboriginal poverty and underdevelopment in Canada. *American review of Canadian studies* (p. 43). Retrieved August 1, 2003, from Expanded Academic ASAP database.

Khanlou, N. (2008). Young and new to Canada: promoting the mental well-being of immigrant and refugee female youth. *International Journal of Mental Health and Addiction, 6,* 514–516.

Kirby Report. (2002). *The health of Canadians—The federal role: Final report.* Volume Six: Recommendations for reform. The Standing Senate Committee on Social Affairs, Science and Technology. Retrieved August 1, 2005, from http://www.parl.gc.ca/37/2/parlbus/commbus/senate/com-e/soci-e/rep-e/repoct02vol6-e.htm

Kirmayer, L. J. (1994). Is the concept of mental disorder culturally relative? In S. A. Kirk, & S. Einbinder (Eds.), *Controversial issues in mental health* (p. 1–20). Boston, MA: Allyn & Bacon.

Kirmayer, L. J., Brass, G. M., & Tait, C. L. (2000). The mental health of Aboriginal peoples: Transformations of identity and community. *Canadian Journal of Psychiatry, 45*(7), 607–616.

Kirmayer, L., Simpson, C., & Cargo, M. (2003). Indigenous populations healing traditions: Culture, community and mental health promotion with Canadian Aboriginal peoples. *Australasian Psychiatry, 11*(Suppl.), S15.

Lewis, S., Donaldson, C., Mitton, C., & Currie, G. (2001). The future of health care in Canada. *British Medical Journal, 323*(7318), 926–929. Retrieved August 1, 2008, from http://www.pubmedcentral.nih.gov/articlerender.fcgi?artid = 1121447

Ligaya, A. (2007). *The debate over Canada's poverty line.* CBCnews Online. Retrieved August 1, 2008, from http://www.cbc.ca/news/background/economy/poverty-line.html

Mental Health Commission of Canada. (2008). Retrieved August 1, 2008, from http://www.mentalhealthcommission.ca/background-en.php

Mental Health Commission of Canada (2009, Janurary). *Toward recovery and well-being: A framework for a mental health strategy for Canada.* Available at http://www.mentalhealthcommission.ca/SiteCollectionDocuments/Key_Documents/en/2009/Mental_Health_ENG

Native Access Program to Nursing/Medicine. (2008). *About NAPN/M.* Retrieved August 1, 2008, from http://www.usask.ca/nursing/napn/about.htm

Office of the Auditor General of Canada. (2008). *First Nations Child and Family Services Program. 2008 May Report of the Auditor General of Canada.* Retrieved August 1, 2008, from http://www.oag-bvg.gc.ca/internet/English/aud_ch_oag_200805_04_e_30700.html#ex1

Office of the Correctional Investigator. (2006, October). *Report finds evidence of systemic discrimination against Aboriginal inmates in Canada's prisons.* Retrieved August 1, 2008, from http://www.oci-bec.gc.ca/newsroom/releases/20061016_e.asp

Office of the Correctional Investigator. (2007, September). *Annual Report of the Office of the Correctional Investigator of Canada, 2006–2007.* Available at: www.oci-bec.gc.ca

O'Reilly, R., Brooks, S., Chaimowitz, G., Neilson, G., Carr, P., Zikos, E., et al. (2003, January). Mandatory outpatient treatment. *Canadian Psychiatric Association Position Paper.* Retrieved May 20, 2006, from http://www.psychdirect.com/forensic/PsychLaw/cto/pos_paper_mandatory_treat.htm

Pasco, A. (2004). Cross-cultural relationships between nurses and Filipino Canadian patients. *Journal of Nursing Scholarship, 36*(3), 239–246.

Petrucka, P., Bassendowski, S., & Bourassa, C. (2007). Seeking paths to culturally competent health care: Lessons from two Saskatchewan Aboriginal communities. *Canadian Journal of Nursing Research, 39*(2), 166–182.

Public Health Agency of Canada. (2003). *What makes Canadians healthy or unhealthy?* Retrieved August 1, 2008, from http://www.phac-aspc.gc.ca/ph-sp/determinants/determinants-eng.php

Public Health Agency of Canada. (2004). *Is mental illness related to poverty? Canadian Health Network.* Retrieved August 1, 2005, from http://www.canadian-healthnetwork.ca/servlet/Content-Server?cid=1001871&pagename=CHNRCS%2FCHNResource%2FFAQCHNResourceTemplate&c=CHNResource& lang =En

Public Health Agency of Canada. (2006). *Appendix 1: Using the right terms. Division of Aging and Seniors.* Retrieved August 1, 2008, from http://www.phac-aspc.gc.ca/seniors-aines/pubs/communicating_aboriginal/appendix_e.htm#ab

Richardson, D. (2008). Cultural safety: An introduction. *Paediatric Nursing, 20*(2), 39–43.

Royal Commission on Aboriginal Peoples. (1996). *Final report.* Ottawa, ON: Communication Group.

Skip Knox, E. L. (2004). *History of western civilization.* Retrieved August 1, 2008, from http://history.boisestate.edu/westciv/plague/10.shtml

Smylie, J. (2007). Cultural competency starts with respect. *Canadian Nurse, 103*(8), 48.

Smye, V., & Browne, A. (2002). "Cultural safety" and the analysis of health policy affecting Aboriginal people. *Nurse Researcher, 9*(3), 42–56.

Snow, N., & Austin, W. (2009). Community treatment orders: the ethical balancing act in community mental health. *Journal of Psychiatric and Mental Health Nursing, 16,* 177–186.

Söchting, I., Corrado, R., Cohen, I. M., Ley, R., & Brasfield, C. (2007). Traumatic pasts in Canadian Aboriginal people: Further support for a complex trauma conceptualization? *BC Medical Journal, 49*(6), 320–326.

Statistics Canada. (2003, January). *Aboriginal peoples of Canada: A demographic profile.* 2001 Census: Analysis series. Report No. 96F0030XIE2001007. Ottawa, ON: Author. Retrieved August 1, 2008, from http://www12.statcan.ca/english/census01/products/analytic/companion/abor/pdf/96F0030XIE2001007.pdf

Statistics Canada. (2008a). *Aboriginal Peoples in Canada in 2006: Inuit, Métis and First Nations, 2006 Census.* Ottawa, ON: Author. Retrieved August 1, 2008, from http://www12.statcan.ca/english/census06/analysis/aboriginal/pdf/97-558-XIE2006001.pdf

Statistics Canada. (2008b). *Report on the demographic situation in Canada: 2005 and 2006*. Retrieved August 1, 2008, from http://www.statcan.ca/english/freepub/91–209-XIE/91–209-XIE2004000.htm

Srivastava, R. H. (Ed.). (2007). *The healthcare professional's guide to clinical cultural competence*. Toronto, ON: Mosby/Elsevier.

Szasz, T. (1961). *The myth of mental illness: Foundations of a theory of personal conduct*. New York, NY: Hoeber-Harper.

Szasz, T. (2005). "Idiots, infants, and the insane": Mental illness and legal incompetence. *Journal of Medical Ethics, 31*(2), 78–81.

Thira, D. (2005). *Beyond the four waves of colonization*. Retrieved August 1, 2008, from http://www.swaraj.org/fourwaves.htm

United Nations. (1948). *Universal declaration of human rights*. Geneva, Switzerland: Author. Available at: http://www.un.org/Overview/rights.html

United Nations. (1991). *Principles for the protection of persons with mental illness and the improvement of mental health care. Adopted by General Assembly resolution 46/119 of 17 December 1991, Office of the United Nations High Commissioner for Human Rights*. Retrieved August 1, 2005, from http://www.unhchr.ch/html/menu3/68.htm

Vedantam, S. (2005, June). Patients' diversity is often discounted: Alternatives to mainstream medical treatment call for recognizing ethnic, social differences. Mind and culture: Psychiatry's missing diagnosis. *Washington Post*, A01. Retrieved August 1, 2008, from http://www.washingtonpost.com/wp-dyn/content/article/2005/06/25/AR2005062500982.html

Waldram, J. B. (2004). *Revenge of the Windigo: The construction of the mind and mental health of North American Aboriginal peoples*. Toronto, ON: University of Toronto Press.

Waldram, J. B., Herring, D. A., & Young, T. K. (2006). *Aboriginal health in Canada: Historical, cultural and epidemiological perspectives* (2nd ed.). Toronto, ON: University of Toronto Press.

Webster, C. (2005, November). News media critique: "Crazies in the Streets." *International Journal of Mental Health & Addiction, 3*(2), 64–68.

World Health Organization. (1990). *Declaration of Caracas*. Adopted by WHO in 1990. Geneva, Switzerland: Author.

World Health Organization. (2001, October). *The world health report 2001. Mental health: New understanding, new hope*. Geneva, Switzerland: Author. Retrieved August 1, 2008, from http://www.who.int/whr/2001/en

World Health Organization. (2005a). *Mental Health Atlas—2005*. A project of the Department of Mental Health and Substance Abuse, Geneva, Switzerland: Author. Retrieved August 1, 2008, from http://www.who.int/mental_health/evidence/atlas

World Health Organization. (2005b, October). *New WHO mental health atlas shows global mental health resources remain inadequate*. Geneva, Switzerland: Author. Retrieved August 1, 2008, from http://www.who.int/mediacentre/news/notes/2005/np21/en/index.html

World Health Organization. (2005c). *WHO Resource book on mental health, human rights and legislation*. Geneva, Switzerland: Author. Retrieved August 1, 2008, from http://whqlibdoc.who.int/publications/2005/924156282X.pdf

World Vision Canada. (2005). *End child poverty in Canada*. Retrieved August 1, 2008, from http://www.worldvision.ca/home/get-involved/make-poverty-history/end-child-poverty-in-canada

Xu, Y., & Flaskerud, J. H. (2007). Cultural dissonance between nurse and patient: The other side of the coin. *Issues in Mental Health Nursing, 28*, 1089–1092.

CHAPTER 4

The Continuum of Psychiatric and Mental Health Care

Cheryl Pollard

Adapted from the chapter "The Continuum of Psychiatric and Mental Health Care" by Freida Chavez, Denise M. Gibson, and Robert B. Noud

LEARNING OBJECTIVES

After studying this chapter, you will be able to:

- Identify the different treatment settings and associated programs along the continuum of care.
- Discuss the role of the nurse along the continuum of care.
- Describe current health care trends in psychiatric services.
- Describe the importance of integrated services for people with mental illness or mental health concerns.

KEY CONCEPTS

- collaborative mental health care
- continuum of care

KEY TERMS

- case management • collaborative mental health care • community-based residential services • continuum of care • consultation • crisis response • empowerment • integrated approach • intensive outpatient program • intensive residential services • mental health promotion • partnership • primary care • primary health care • referrals • relapse • reintegration • self-help • stabilization • supportive employment

*H*ealth care systems need to have well-integrated psychiatric and mental health care across the continuum, from health promotion to rehabilitation. Most mental illnesses are not caused by a single factor, but are a result of a combination of factors. These causative factors relate to the complex interactions between biological, social, psychological, and spiritual aspects of people's lives. Effective psychiatric and mental health services and supports must be able to address people's needs in all of these areas. As a result, the continuum of psychiatric and mental health care incorporates a range of resources.

Across all aspects of the Canadian health care, health professionals, such as nurses, are expected to provide appropriate care to persons with mental health problems and/or mental illness. Psychiatric and mental health services offer more specialized expertise in meeting the needs of persons related to a mental illness. Extending beyond such formal health services are other resources, such as community organizations that deliver social supports to people with and without a diagnosed mental illness and groups that facilitate peoples' connections to the community, including religious organizations, educational institutions and recreational associations, as well as family and peer groups. Resources that foster people's sense of self, of social inclusion and belonging, of having a sense of meaning and purpose and that empower individuals to develop their capacity for well-being are important components of the psychiatric and mental health care continuum.

PRIMARY HEALTH CARE APPROACH

It is important to situate the continuum of care in an over-all approach to health services: **primary health care**. Primary health care (not to be confused with "primary care") adopted by the World Health Organization in 1978 as the basis for the delivery of health services (WHO, 2008b), is an approach that encompasses five types of care: promotive; preventive; curative; rehabilitative; and supportive/palliative. It is based on the principles of accessibility, public participation, health promotion, appropriate technology (i.e., adapted to the community's social, economic, and cultural developments), and intersectoral cooperation (necessary as health and well-being are linked to social and economic policies). Nurses are expected to apply these principles in their practice across the continuum of care (Canadian Nurses Association, 2000).

DEFINING THE CONTINUUM OF CARE

The Mental Health Commission of Canada (2009) defines recovery as "a journey of healing that builds on individual, family, cultural and community strength, and enables people living with mental problems and illnesses to lead meaningful lives in the community, despite any limitations imposed by their condition" (p. 8). In order to facilitate recovery for individuals, family, groups or communities, the approach of the services or supports provided must be founded on the principles of hope, **empowerment**, choice and responsibility (Mental Health Commission of Canada, 2009). The **continuum of care** represents the complex, integrated system of services provided by health professionals in general and by those with specialized psychiatric and mental expertise, as well as the supports provided by informal providers and organizations within the community.

The continuum begins with health promotion strategies that look for ways of keeping people from experiencing mental health problems or becoming mentally ill, as well as improving the mental health status of the whole population. Beyond health promotional activities, service and support providers work with individuals with mental health problems or mental illness, their family member, peers, other services providers to determine what services or supports are most appropriate to meet their identified needs. Further components of the continuum of care range from supportive interventions by informal support providers in the community to professional service providers delivering clinical treatment in the community, to professional services being provided in a hospital setting. There are also components of the continuum that are focused on the psychiatric and mental health care needs of specific patient populations, such as children and families, seniors, military personnel, people with brain injuries, people who are involved with the legal system, people with addictions, and people with developmental challenges. These specialized services are sustained by mental health professionals with the necessary expertise.

KEY CONCEPT A **continuum of care** consists of an integrated health system of supports and services designed to maximize people's health and well-being that is provided by professional health care clinicians (some who offer specialized services, such as psychiatric mental health services), as well as by non-professional caregivers.

In Canada, most of the services to people who experience a mental health problem or mental illness are situated in community settings. Inpatient care (hospitalization) may be periodically necessary, but is typically of very short duration. The goal of the system is to deliver the appropriate medical, nursing, psychological, social, and spiritual services by the right person, to the right person or family, at the right time, and in the right place. By doing so, the continuum facilitates the stability, continuity, and comprehensiveness of service provision to an individual over the period of time in which services and supports are required. Due to the complexity of the continuum of care, individuals and families may require assistance with the coordination of their care, services, and supports.

Coordination of Care

Coordination of care is the integration of appropriate services so that individualized person-centred care and treatment is provided. Appropriate services are those that are tailored to promote recovery through holistic care that supports and develops an individual's strengths, addresses vulnerabilities, promotes cultural safety, inspires hope, facilitates empowerment, and offers choice and responsibility. The Health Quality Council of Alberta (2006), based on a survey designed to measure satisfaction with health care services, has identified an improvement of coordination in meeting patient needs as a priority. The move toward increasing professional coordination of services and social supports has occurred consistently across the Canadian health care system. There are many terms that are used to describe these types of coordinating services. They include the following: **case management**, service coordination, care management, care coordination, service navigation, and transition care services. Although the terms may be different, the services provided can be described as a collaborative, client-driven

---

BOX 4.1
Guiding Principles of Case Management

- **Client-centred**
  Case management is client/caregiver centred and is sometimes driven or provided by the client. Generally, case management services benefit complex care clients the most.

- **Navigation**
  Case management provides navigation and networks through the wide spectrum of services to meet client needs. It moves beyond the boundaries of programs and service sectors.

- **Collaboration/coordination**
  Case management strategies build upon clinical expertise and the collaborative relationships/formalized partnerships amongst health care professionals, clients, and their caregivers. Health professionals work as interdisciplinary teams.

- **Health promotion/prevention**
  Case management strategies enhance health promotion, illness prevention, and risk mitigation through client education and emphasis on enhancing client self-care capacity. Case management incorporates the principles of population health and the broad determinants of health.

- **Quality of care**
  Case management incorporates evidence-based practice to promote quality of care (Quality of Care Matrix; Health Quality Council of Alberta, 2006).

- **Resources management**
  Case management engages the family and organizes available resources.

- **Communication**
  Case management requires effective communication among health care providers, clients, and caregivers.

- **Advocating**
  Case management advocates on behalf of clients, and promotes self-advocacy and independence. The challenge is that case management must balance client focused services with effective use of resources for system sustainability.

- **Discretionary judgment**
  Professionals are empowered to use discretionary judgment, within the context of their own profession's accountability framework, in performing case management to meet a client's unique needs.

- **Flexibility**
  Degree of intensity, type of case management and who the case manager is, varies based on client characteristics, varying levels of service complexity, and the sectors/environment/programs involved in the partnerships.

- **Education**
  Case management provides clients and their families with the education and support that enables clients to understand their care needs and to be confident in providing self-care.

From Alberta Health and Wellness. (2006). *System case management for continuing care clients.* Prepared for Continuing Care Leaders Council. Edmonton, AB: Author.

---

process designed to support the patient's achievement of goals within a complex health, social and fiscal environment. To meet patient goals, the coordinator of services for patients and families may need to liaise with several agencies: **primary care** services, public health, mental health, social services, housing, education, the workplace, and the criminal justice system, to name a few. For health professionals to be effective in this role, they must develop collaborative and cooperative relationships among many different service partners. See Box 4-1 for guiding principles of case management and Box 4-2 for Canadian Standards of Practice for Case Management.

The Nurse as Case Manager

Because of the often cyclical nature of serious mental illness, psychiatric and mental health nurses serve in various pivotal functions across the continuum of care. These functions can involve both direct care and coordination of the care delivered by others. The case manager or care coordination role is one in which the nurse must have commanding knowledge of the patient's/family's needs and areas of strengths, as well as the available community resources. In order for nurses to be successful in this role,

they must practice with the philosophy that recovery is defined by the patient, not the service provider, and that well-being is possible for all people living with a mental illness. The nurse must have expertise in working with the family as a unit. The repertoire of required skills includes collaborative, teaching, management, leadership, group, and research skills. The nurse as case manager probably is the most diverse role within the psychiatric continuum.

■ COMPREHENSIVE MENTAL HEALTH SYSTEM: CORE PROGRAMS AND SERVICES

Each province within Canada has slightly different services available to promote mental health, prevent mental illness, to provide treatment services and/or community supports to people with a mental health problem or mental illness. All, however, should be based on a commitment to patient-centred care. Patient-centred care is care that establishes a **partnership** among practitioners, patients, and their families (when appropriate) to ensure that decisions respect patients' wants, needs and preferences. Patients' input needs to

---

BOX 4.2

Canadian Standards of Practice for Case Management

1. Clients who meet the eligibility for case management services are identified.
   This is the first step in establishing an appropriate case management service relationship.
2. In conjunction with the client, the case manager conducts and documents an individualized assessment using a structured process.
   Assessment is a dynamic and ongoing collaborative process that actively involves the client and others to secure information in a timely manner and to identify the client's values, goals, functional and cognitive capacity, strengths, abilities, preferences, resources, supports, and needs.
3. Client goals and priorities are documented and are reflected in the strategy for action agreed upon between the client and the case manager.
   The planning is designed to document the actions to achieve client's short-term and long-term goals and optimal health care outcomes. The ultimate goal is returning the client to optimal self-care and functional recovery. The plan of care explains the use of formal and informal services and resources.

4. Planned services, resources, and supports are initiated, coordinated, and adjusted as necessary.
   Implementation reflects the case manager's accountability to ensure that the client's individualized plan of care is being implemented. Implementation is the process in which all parties involved in the services/resource plan collaborate to carry out the mutually agreed-upon activities.
5. A periodic reassessment to identify the client's current needs and progress within the client's individualized plan.
   Evaluation is a part of the monitoring process and includes information from clients and others to determine the progress made by clients against the identified goals within the case management plan.
6. Transformation process that supports disengagement or shift in the mechanisms for achieving client goals.
   A redefinition of the client/case manager relationship in the evolution of the client's journey toward meeting his/her goals.

From National Case Management Network of Canada. (2009). *Canadian standards of practice for case management.* Ottawa, ON: Author.

---

be solicited, including what they require in terms of knowledge, skills, and support to make decisions and participate in their own care.

Mental Health Promotion and Illness Prevention

Effective and efficient mental health service delivery systems have integrated **mental health promotion** and illness prevention into all aspects of the system. Mental health promotion strategies are directed toward addressing the determinants of health that can impact the population's mental health. Several mental health promotion policies and programs have been mainstreamed into the government and business sectors in Canada. A few examples of these include the following: early childhood intervention programs, such as home visiting for high risk pregnant women; nutritional and psychosocial interventions for vulnerable populations; mental health interventions in the workplace (e.g., stress prevention programs); and community-based violence prevention that involve community policing initiatives. See Box 4-3 for a summary of Best Practices related to mental health promotion.

Mental illness prevention strategies are designed to keep something from happening. This something may be the illness itself, the severity or duration of the illness, or may be a disability associated with the illness or disease. The World Health Organization has identified three categories of prevention strategies that will reduce the risk of experiencing the illness itself: (1) universal prevention: targets the general population; (2) selective prevention: targets groups or individuals at higher risk, than the general population, for a specific illness; and (3) indicated prevention: targets people at high risk for mental illness (WHO, 2002). An important example of illness prevention services is respite services for family caregivers of persons with a mental illness. The goals of respite programs are typically threefold:

- To validate and reinforce the necessity and value of informal caregiving within the continuum of care
- To provide support and advocacy to informal caregivers
- To prevent unnecessary long-term care placements and hospitalizations due to informal caregiver burnout. Respite services can be provided within the home,

---

BOX 4.3

Best Practices: Mental Health Promotion

1. Enhances capacity to take control of life and health
2. Promotes resiliency
3. Relies on intersectoral linkages
4. Takes a positive perspective

From Canadian Mental Health Association. (2008). *Mental health promotion: A framework for action by the Canadian Mental Health Association.* Ottawa, ON: Author.

within a community living option (group home or supportive living setting), or may be provided within an inpatient setting.

Another example of a mental illness prevention strategy is the practice of providing critical incident stress debriefings. For example, if a volunteer fire crew responded to the scene of a very gruesome accident that involved one of their own members and his family, in which there was only one survivor who was severely injured and disfigured, the community mental health services may offer a critical incident stress debriefing. This intervention strategy is provided as a means to help the fire crew members avoid the potential onset of posttraumatic stress disorder.

Consumer Self-Help and Consumer/ Survivor Initiatives

During the past two decades, there has been tremendous growth in the number of **self-help** groups and organizations of people who have experienced mental illness (Segal, Silverman, & Temkin, 1993, 1994, 1995) and who refer to themselves as "consumers." Some consider themselves as "survivors"—not survivors of their illness, but survivors of their health care experience. Consumer/survivor initiatives (CSIs) are self-help organizations that are operated exclusively by and for people with serious mental illness. CSIs are not treatment services, rather they are self-help groups that operate on the values that include member empowerment, participation, social justice, and community.

CSIs are a unique component of the mental health system. Participation in CSIs provides personal empowerment, utilization of mental health care, social support and friendship, community integration, access to valued resources (work, education, finances, housing). In Ontario, there are more than 50 CSIs funded by the Ministry of Health and Long-Term Care (Centre for Community Based Research, 2004). In a longitudinal study of CSIs in Ontario, the CSI participants demonstrated a significant reduction in the number of hospitalizations; symptom distress; and significant improvements in social support, quality of life (daily activities), and employment/education (Nelson, et al., 2007). The qualitative data also showed that the active participants had improved mental health, more social support, and fewer relationship difficulties. See Box 4-4 for Best Practices related to consumer self-help initiatives.

Crisis Response Systems and Psychiatric Emergency Services

An organized approach is required to treat individuals in crisis, including a mechanism for rapid access to care (24/7), telephone crisis services, mobile **crisis response**, access to crisis emergency residential services, or psychiatric emergency services in hospitals. Crisis response systems emphasize crisis supports that are flexible, portable, and person centred. This type of short-term intervention care focuses on de-escalation, **stabilization**, symptom reduction, and prevention of **relapse** requiring inpatient services.

Crisis intervention units can be found in the emergency department of a general or psychiatric hospital or in crisis centres within a community mental health centre. Patients

---

BOX 4.4

Best Practices: Consumer Self-Help and Consumer Initiatives

RESEARCH EVIDENCE

Although there is variability in the quality of studies conducted to evaluate self-help and consumer initiatives, there is consistency in findings.

Participation in self-help is associated with the following:

- Reduced hospitalization
- Reduced use of other services
- Increased knowledge, information, and coping skills
- Increased self-esteem, confidence, sense of well-being, and sense of being in control
- Stronger social networks and support

Compared with professionally led groups, self-help groups emphasize experiential knowledge and social support and tend to be more spontaneous, unstructured, and unconstrained by time.

KEY ELEMENTS OF BEST PRACTICE

There are growing numbers of funded organizations that utilize nonservice models to engage in

- Mutual support
- Advocacy
- Cultural activities
- Knowledge development and skills training
- Public education
- Educating professionals
- Economic development

Evaluation of the effectiveness of these initiatives that uses appropriate, alternative methods is supported. The general public and mental health professionals are educated about the value of self-help. Steps are taken to attract and train strong leaders for self-help groups.

From Health Canada. (1998). *Review of best practices in mental health reform.* Prepared for the Federal/Provincial/Territorial Advisory Network on Mental Health.

in crisis demonstrate severe symptoms of acute mental illness, including labile mood swings, suicidal ideation, or self-injurious behaviours. Therefore, this treatment option commands a high degree of nursing expertise. Patients in crisis usually require medications such as anxiolytics or benzodiazepines for symptom management. Key nursing roles include an assessment of short-term therapeutic interventions and medication administration. Nurses also facilitate **referrals** for increased community services or support, admission to the hospital or for outpatient services.

Crisis Stabilization

When the immediate crisis does not resolve quickly, crisis stabilization is the next step. The primary purpose of stabilization is the control of precipitating symptoms through medications, behavioural interventions, and coordination with other agencies for appropriate aftercare. The major focus of nursing care in a short-term inpatient setting is symptom management. Ongoing assessment; short-term, focused interventions; and medication administration and monitoring of efficacy and side effects are major components of nursing care during stabilization. Nurses also may provide focused group psychotherapy designed to develop and strengthen the personal management strategies of patients. When treating aggressive or violent patients, the nurse monitors the appropriate use of seclusion and restraints. See Box 4-5 for a summary of Best Practices related to crisis response systems and psychiatric emergency services.

Primary Care

Primary care is the term used regarding the first point of access to the health care system. The Canadian health care system has typically partitioned the services for physical illness and mental illness. This has resulted in a system that fragments people's needs, which is both counterproductive and harmful. An **integrated approach** to assist people in managing their illnesses, regardless of its origin, is required. The integrated approach begins with ensuring that the services and supports that are delivered are done so in a patient-centred manner. This means that people are empowered: choice is promoted, they remain in control, and community integration is facilitated. A patient-centred approach emphasizes the partnership that the person with mental illness has with the service providers. It does not shift responsibility on people to "get themselves together," "get over it," or "deal with it"; this model does not blame the affected individual. People who experience a mental illness need to be involved in their own recovery, albeit, the degree of involvement will depend on the person. Paternalistic approaches to services—for example, the traditional medical model still used by many mental

---

BOX 4.5

Best Practices: Crisis Response Systems and Psychiatric Emergency Services

RESEARCH EVIDENCE
Nonexperimental and descriptive studies suggest that

- Crisis housing provides a viable alternative to hospitalization for people with serious mental illness
- Diversion programs are effective
- Crisis centres can serve people with psychosocial problems

KEY ELEMENTS OF BEST PRACTICE
Services are established that resolve crises for people with serious mental illness using minimally intrusive options. Crisis programs are in place to divert people from inpatient hospitalization. Evaluation and research protocols are incorporated into crisis programs. Examples of crisis programs are

- Telephone crisis services
- Mobile crisis units
- Crisis residential services (e.g., supervised apartments/houses, foster homes)
- Psychiatric emergency/medical crisis services in hospitals

From Health Canada. (1998). *Review of best practices in mental health reform.* Prepared for the Federal/Provincial/Territorial Advisory Network on Mental Health.

---

health care professionals—encourage passive consumer involvement (Ryan-Nicholls & Haggarty, 2007). Such an approach, given the importance of the principle of autonomy, is ethically questionable.

Collaborative mental health care models have been established in response to specialist mental health service provider shortages, access issues, and the recognition that family physicians are the first point of contact for approximately 85% of people with mental illness (Kirby, 2008). These models have been described using a variety of terms: integrated care, shared care, collaborative care, managed care among others. In essence, collaborative care recognizes that primary care for mental health is essential, but to be fully effective it must be supported by additional levels of care as no single service setting, or provider, can meet everyone's mental health needs (World Health Organization, 2008a). See Box 4-6 for Best Practices related to the goals and potential activities of collaborative mental health care services. See Box 4-7 related to the benefits of integrating mental health into primary care.

KEY CONCEPT **Collaborative mental health care** refers to activities or initiatives that strive to strengthen links between primary care and specialized mental health services (Ryan-Nicholls & Haggarty, 2007).

BOX 4.6

Goals and Potential Activities of Collaborative Mental Health Care Services

GOALS

- Improve access to a comprehensive range of high-quality and effective health care services.
- Improve outcomes for people that use the mental health system.
- Integration of community services across sectors.

POTENTIAL ACTIVITIES

- Regular visits by a mental health care worker to a primary care setting.
- Unified programs that offer mental health and physical health care through one administration and financial entity.
- Regular telephone consultation between primary care and mental health providers.

- Integration of specialized care providers such as psychiatrists, psychologists, nurse, social workers, pharmacists, occupational therapists, and dietitians within primary care settings.
- Joint development of treatment plans by consumers and providers.
- Incorporation of mental health interventions into the management of general medical conditions (e.g., diabetes).
- Meeting the primary health care needs of individuals with severe and persistent mental illness.
- Strategies to improve access to community mental health services.
- Development of more formal partnerships with specialized service providers.

From Ryan-Nicholls, K., & Haggarty, J. (2007). Collaborative mental health care in rural and isolated Canada: Stakeholder feedback. *Journal of Psychosocial Nursing, 45*(12), 37–45.

BOX 4.7

Benefits of Integrating Mental Health into Primary Care

1. **The burden of mental disorders is great.** Mental disorders are prevalent in all societies. They create a substantial personal burden for affected individuals and their families, and they produce significant economic and social hardships that affect society as a whole.
2. **Mental and physical health problems are interwoven.** Many people suffer from both physical and mental health problems. Integrated primary care services help ensure that people are treated in a holistic manner, meeting the mental health needs of people with physical disorders, as well as the physical health needs of people with mental disorders.
3. **The treatment gap for mental disorders is enormous.** In all countries, there is a significant gap between the prevalence of mental disorders, on one hand, and the number of people receiving treatment and care, on the other hand. Primary care for mental health helps close this gap.
4. **Primary care for mental health enhances access.** Integrating mental health into primary care is the best way of ensuring that people get the mental health care they need. When mental health is integrated into primary care, people can access mental health services closer to their homes, thus keeping their families together and

maintaining their daily activities. Primary care services also facilitate community outreach and mental health promotion, as well as long-term monitoring and management of affected individuals.
5. **Primary care for mental health promotes respect of human rights.** Mental health services delivered in primary care minimizes stigma and discrimination. This also removes the risk of human rights violations that occur in psychiatric hospitals.
6. **Primary care for mental health is affordable and cost effective.** Primary mental health care services are less expensive than psychiatric hospitals, for patients, communities, and governments alike. In addition, patients and families avoid indirect costs associated with seeking specialist care in distant locations. The treatment of common mental disorders is very cost effective, and even small investments by governments can bring important benefits.
7. **Primary care for mental health generates good health outcomes.** The majority of people with mental health disorders treated in primary care have good outcomes, particularly, when linked to a network of services at secondary level and in the community.

From World Health Organization. (2008a). *Integrating mental health into primary care: A global perspective.* Geneva, Switzerland: Author.

The other levels of care required to support primary care providers include secondary service components. These components include opportunities for **consultation** and support through referrals regarding patient care needs outside the primary care provider's current competency level, as well as supervision and support to facilitate further skill development and education of the primary care provider.

Collaborative mental health care also extends to include formal and informal community supports for people with mental illness, such as housing, education and recreational organizations. It has been demonstrated that people with mental illness who receive good community care services and support have better health and mental health outcomes, and better quality of life than those people who were treated in psychiatric hospitals (World Health Organization, 2008a). However, there is a small proportion of the population that require very specialized services. These are people who have treatment-resistant or very complex presentations of illness, those who lack community support, and/or those requiring forensic services.

Outpatient Care

Outpatient care is a level of care that occurs outside of a hospital or institution. Outpatient services usually are less intensive and are provided to patients who do not require inpatient services. Many patients enrol in outpatient services immediately upon discharge from an inpatient setting. This promotes community **reintegration**, medication management and monitoring, and symptom management. Patients gain the right to choose home as a placement option, become more involved in aftercare support services individualized to the care they need, and become more socially integrated into society (Friedrich, R., Hollingsworth, Hradek, Friedrich, H.B., & Culp, 1999). Outpatient services are provided by private practices, clinics, and community mental health centres.

Intensive Outpatient Programs

The primary focus of **intensive outpatient programs** is on stabilization and relapse prevention for highly

vulnerable individuals who function autonomously on a daily basis. People who meet these criteria have returned to their previous lifestyle (e.g., interacting with family, resuming work, or returning to school). Attendance in this type of program benefits individuals who still require frequent monitoring and support within a therapeutic milieu that enables them to remain connected to the community. The duration of treatment and level of services rendered are based on the patient's immediate needs. Treatment duration usually is time limited, with sessions offered 3 to 4 hours per day and 2 to 3 days per week. See Box 4-8 for Best Practices related to inpatient care and outpatient care.

Housing and Community Support

With the focus on community-based care, there has been an increasing attention to housing and community support. New approaches and philosophies about housing have emerged for those with serious mental illness. Patients with psychiatric disabilities who are homeless are a vulnerable population. One of the largest hurdles to overcome in treating the severely mentally ill patient is finding appropriate housing that will meet the patient's immediate social, financial, and safety needs. The course of chronic mental illness, as symptoms wax and wane, preys on the stamina of families and caregivers. The prevalence of

---

BOX 4.8

Best Practices: Inpatient and Outpatient Care

RESEARCH EVIDENCE

Well-designed follow-up studies show that

- Discharge of long-stay patients is associated with improved social functioning over time
- Individuals and families prefer community care to hospitalization
- Clinical and social outcomes are at least as good for discharged patients receiving community care as for matched counterparts remaining in hospital

Numerous controlled trials show that

- Day hospitalization is less costly than inpatient care with comparable outcomes
- Day hospitalization offers more intensive treatment in a less restrictive and more homelike environment
- Shorter length of stay is generally not associated with increased readmission and achieves similar outcomes to longer-stay admissions
- Home-based treatment is an effective alternative to admission for many patients

Preliminary descriptive studies show that integrating mental health professionals in primary care settings can

- Enhance continuity of care
- Increase accessibility to mental health services
- Lead to more efficient use of mental health services
- Provide new opportunities for continuing education for physicians
- Improve communication between mental health services and family practitioners

KEY ELEMENTS OF BEST PRACTICE

- Long-stay patients in provincial psychiatric hospitals are moved into the community with carefully planned transitions to alternative care models.
- Inpatient stays are kept as short as possible without harmful effects on patient outcomes.
- Partial hospitalization programs are available as an alternative to inpatient admission.
- Day treatment is an option for those with nonpsychotic diagnosis.
- Home treatment programs (that are either assertive community treatment teams or adjuncts to intensive case management) are available as an alternative for inpatient admission.
- New service delivery models that link family physicians with mental health specialists are in place.

From Health Canada. (1998). *Review of best practices in mental health reform.* Prepared for the Federal/Provincial/Territorial Advisory Network on Mental Health.

mental illness among homeless people may range as high as 35% (Tsemberis & Eisenberg, 2000). Most individuals live in some form of supervised or supported community living situation, which ranges from highly supervised congregate settings to independent apartments. Those who lack the resources to find housing suffer higher rates of substance abuse, physical illness, incarceration, and victimization (Tsemberis & Eisenberg).

Supported Housing

There has been a paradigm shift from a reliance on the residential continuum to what is now known as supported housing. This model incorporates the use of generic housing in the community, provision of individualized support at varying degrees at different times, consumers' choice, and assistance in finding and maintaining their homes (Health Canada, 1998). **Community-based residential services** provide a place for people to reside during a 24-hour period or any portion of the day, on an ongoing basis. A residential facility can be publicly or privately owned. **Intensive residential services** are intensively staffed for patient treatment. These services may include medical, nursing, psychosocial, vocational, recreational, or other support services. Combining residential care and mental health services, this treatment form offers rehabilitation and therapy to people with serious and persistent mental illnesses, including chronic schizophrenia, bipolar disorder, and unrelenting depression. These services may provide short-term treatment for stays from 24 hours to 3 or 6 months or long-term treatment for several months to years.

As a result of deinstitutionalization, there has been an increasing attention on housing and community support for those with serious and persistent mental illness. Many patients who were unable to live independently were placed in nursing homes and other types of privately operated boarding homes. Over time, a number of residential and housing services evolved.

Nursing plays an important role in the care of people who have severe and persistent mental illnesses and who require long-term stays at residential treatment facilities. Nurses provide basic psychiatric nursing care with a focus on psychoeducation, basic social skills training, aggression management, activities of daily living (ADLs) training, and group living. Education on symptom management, understanding mental illnesses, and medication is essential to recovery. *The Scope and Standards of Psychiatric–Mental Health Nursing Practice* guides the nurse in delivering patient care (Canadian Federation of Mental Health Nurses, 2005) (see Chapter 6).

Supportive Employment

Supportive employment services assist individuals to find work; assess individuals' skills, attitudes, behaviours, and interest relevant to work; offer vocational rehabilitation or other training; and provide work opportunities. Supportive employment programs are new, highly individualized, and competitive. They provide on-site support and job-coaching services on a one-to-one basis. They occur in real work settings and are used for patients with severe mental illnesses. The primary focus is to maintain attachment between the mentally ill person and the work force. Transitional employment programs offer the same support as supported employment programs, but the employment is temporary. This type of work has a time frame agreed on by the employer and the participant. The person works at the temporary position until he or she can find permanent, competitive employment (Bustillo, Laurillo, Horan, & Keith, 2001).

Acute Inpatient Care

Acute inpatient hospitalization involves the most intensive treatment and is considered the most restrictive

---

BOX 4.9

Research for Best Practices: Therapeutic Relationships: From Psychiatric Hospital to Community

Forchuk, C., Martin, M., Chan, Y., & Jensen, E. (2005). Therapeutic relationships: From psychiatric hospital to community. Journal of Psychiatric and Mental Health Nursing, 12(5), 556–564.

QUESTION: What is the cost effectiveness of a transitional discharge model of care compared to those of a standard model of discharge for persons with serious and persistent mental illness?

METHOD: The study used a cluster-randomized design that included four Canadian provincial psychiatric hospitals and patients from 26 units. The *control group* received discharge care as per usual practices. The *experimental group* had an overlap of inpatient and community staff involvement (i.e., the inpatient staff continued their relationship with the patients until a relationship was established with a community service provider), as well as the option of peer support for at least 1 year.

FINDINGS: Although the *quality of life after discharge* of the participants in the experimental group was not significantly better than the participants who received traditional discharge care, their *length of hospitalization* was significantly reduced.

IMPLICATIONS: When community support is readily available to people who have required hospitalization due to a serious and persistent mental illness, the need for hospitalization and for being away from family and community supports can be reduced. Nurses working in both inpatient and community settings can facilitate earlier discharges by maintaining supportive relationships with patients and facilitating community connections.

setting in the continuum. Inpatient treatment is reserved for acutely ill patients who, because of a mental illness, meet one or more of three criteria: high risk for harming oneself, high risk for harming others, or inability to care for one's basic needs. The delivery of inpatient care can occur in a psychiatric hospital or psychiatric unit within a general hospital. Admission to inpatient environments can be voluntary or involuntary (see Chapter 3). Provincial legislation mental health acts describe conditions that warrant hospitalization. Length of inpatient stay is kept as short as possible without harmful effects on patient outcomes. See Box 4-9 Research for Best Practices on therapeutic relationships from psychiatric hospital to community.

SUMMARY OF KEY POINTS

☐ The continuum of psychiatric and mental health care must be well integrated within the overall health care system and shaped by the principles of primary health care: accessibility, public participation, health promotion, appropriate technology, and intersectoral cooperation.

☐ The continuum of care is a comprehensive system of services and programs spanning the range from mental health promotion and illness prevention to very specialized services designed to match the needs of the individuals and populations with the appropriate care and treatment, which vary according to levels of service, structure, and intensity of care.

☐ The psychiatric and mental health nurse's specific responsibilities vary according to the setting. In most settings, nurses function as members of a multidisciplinary team. Consumers of mental health services and their families should be considered as core members of that team.

☐ An integrated approach to delivering a patient-centred mental health care is required to ensure effective and efficient services.

CRITICAL THINKING CHALLENGES

1 Define the continuum of care and discuss the importance of using a patient-centred approach.

2 Differentiate the role of the nurse across the continuum of care.

3 Consider, in light of recommended Best Practices, the housing and community supports for people with mental disorders that are available in your community.

4 Envision an integration of services that you believe would best serve patients and their families in your community.

WEB LINKS

www.hc-sc.gc.ca This is the Health Canada website. Use the "search" feature to explore information on Best Practices.

www.cmha.ca/bins/index.asp The Canadian Mental Health Association advocates leadership by federal and provincial governments to ensure equitable access to services and treatment across Canada.

www.recovery-inc.org This is the website of Recovery, Inc., a self-help mental health program active since 1937 that is nonprofit, nonsectarian, and completely member managed. Groups meet every week around the world.

www.mind.org.uk This is the website of Mind, the leading mental health charity in England and Wales. Among its objectives is to inspire the development of quality services that reflect expressed need and diversity.

MOVIES, NOVELS, AND BIOGRAPHIES

The Soloist: 2008. Based on a true story, this movie tells of the friendship between a journalist, Steve Lopez (played by Robert Downey Jr.), and a homeless man, Nathaniel Ayers (played by Jamie Foxx), that begins on the streets of Los Angeles. Nathaniel was once a dynamic musical prodigy headed for fame. This fame was not to be realized as life—and schizophrenia—intervened. Lopez embarks on a mission to find Ayers a home and to improve Ayer's life; he finds that his own life is enhanced.

VIEWING POINTS: What were the community supports that were available to Mr. Ayers? How do you think that Mr. Ayers would describe his recovery? How has Mr. Ayers been empowered or disempowered in his recovery journey? Consider how health services require flexibility in order to meet the needs of people living with a severe and persistent mental illness.

REFERENCES

Alberta Health and Wellness. (2006). *System case management for continuing care clients.* Prepared for Continuing Care Leaders Council. Edmonton, AB: Author.

Bustillo, J. R., Laurillo, J., Horan, W. P., & Keith, S. J. (2001). The psychosocial treatment of schizophrenia. *American Journal of Psychiatry, 158*(2), 163–175.

Canadian Federation of Mental Health Nurses. (2005). *Canadian standards of psychiatric and mental health nursing practice* (3rd ed.). Ottawa, ON: Author.

Canadian Mental Health Association. (2008). *Mental health promotion: A framework for action by the Canadian Mental Health Association.* Ottawa, ON: Author.

Canadian Nurses Association. (2000, June). *Fact sheet: The primary health care approach*. Ottawa, ON: Author. Available at: www.cna-nurses.ca

Centre for Community Based Research. (2004). *A longitudinal study of consumer/survivor initiatives (CSIs) in community mental health in Ontario: Individual-level and system-level activities and impacts—Fact sheet*. Available at http://www.communitybasedresearch.ca/resources/crehs.on.ca/downloads/CSDI%20fact%20sheet.pdf

Forchuk, C., Martin, M., Chan, Y., & Jensen, E. (2005). Therapeutic relationships: From psychiatric hospital to community. *Journal of Psychiatric and Mental Health Nursing, 12*(5), 556–564.

Friedrich, R., Hollingsworth, B., Hradek, E., Friedrich, H. B., & Culp, K. R. (1999). Family and client perspectives on alternative residential settings for persons with severe mental illness. *Psychiatric Services, 50*(4), 509–514.

Health Canada. (1998). *Review of best practices in mental health reform*. Prepared for the Federal/Provincial/Territorial Advisory Network on Mental Health.

Health Quality Council of Alberta. (2006). *Satisfaction with health care services: A survey of Albertans 2006*. Calgary, AB: Author.

Kirby, M. (2008). Mental health in Canada: Out of the shadows forever. *Canadian Medical Association Journal, 178*(10), 1320–1322.

Mental Health Commission of Canada. (2009). *Toward recovery and well-being: A framework for a mental health strategy for Canada*. Available at http://www.mentalhealthcommission.ca/SiteCollectionDocuments/Key-Documents/en/2009/Mental_Health_ENG.pdf

National Case Management Network of Canada. (2009). *Canadian standards of practice for case management*. Ottawa, ON: Author.

Nelson, G., Ochocka, J., Janzen, R., Trainor, J., Goering, P., & Lomorey, J. (2007). A longitudinal study of mental health consumer/survisor initiatives: Part V – outcomes at 3-year follow-up. *Journal of Community Psychology, 35*(5), 655–665.

Ryan-Nicholls, K., & Haggarty, J. (2007). Collaborative mental health care in rural and isolated Canada: Stakeholder feedback. *Journal of Psychosocial Nursing, 45*(12), 37–45.

Segal, S., Silverman, C., & Temkin, T. (1993). Empowerment and self-help agency practice for people with mental disabilities. *Social Work, 38*(6), 705–712.

Segal, S., Silverman, C., & Temkin, T. (1994). Issues in self-help agency research. *Innovations and Research, 3*(1), 47–49.

Segal, S., Silverman, C., & Temkin, T. (1995). Characteristics and service use of long term members of self-help agencies for mental health clients. *Psychiatric Services, 46*(3), 269–274.

Tsemberis, S., & Eisenberg, R. (2000). Pathways to housing: Supported housing for street-dwelling homeless individuals with psychiatric disabilities. *Psychiatric Services, 51*(4), 487–493.

World Health Organization. (2002). *Prevention and promotion in mental health*. France: Author.

World Health Organization. (2008a). *Integrating mental health into primary care: A global perspective*. Geneva, Switzerland: Author.

World Health Organization. (2008b). *The world health report 2008: Primary health care – now more than ever*. Geneva, Switzerland: Author.

CHAPTER 5

Mental Health in the Workplace

Wendy Austin and Marion Healey-Ogden

LEARNING OBJECTIVES

After studying this chapter, you will be able to:

- Identify the relationship between work and mental health.
- Describe a healthy workplace.
- Identify the work content and context factors that affect mental health.
- Explain work-life balance.
- Discuss workplace mental health support strategies.
- Determine ways to accommodate persons with mental health problems in the workplace.
- Analyze a health care environment for healthy workplace attributes.

KEY CONCEPTS

- work
- workplace health
- workplace violence

KEY TERMS

- bullying • burnout • compassion fatigue • individual placement and support (IPS) • job strain • mobbing • role overload • unemployed • underemployed • work content • work context • work-life balance • work-life conflict

The World Health Organization (WHO, 2009) finds that each year 160 million new cases of work-related illness and 1.7 million work-related deaths occur. Furthermore, research in industrial nations shows that psychosocial hazards and work-related stress affect one fifth of the working population. In Canada, mental health issues are the leading cause of disability claims (Watson Wyatt, 2007), with mental health and addiction problems estimated at costing the Canadian economy nearly $30 billion a year (Public Health Agency of Canada, 2001). Also in Canada, nurses' absenteeism rate is much higher than the national average, with more than 16 million nursing hours lost to injury and illness annually, equivalent to a loss of nearly 9,000 full-time nursing positions per year (Registered Nurses' Association of Ontario, 2008). Workplace health is a pressing issue.

Fortunately, the workplace has a great potential as a setting in which the health of workers and their families can be protected and promoted. It offers a venue for health education, for workers to access preventive health services, and for links to primary health care (WHO, 2009). WHO's *Global plan of action on workers' health* (2008–2017) aims at strengthening the links between workplace health, public health, and health systems development and at improving working conditions everywhere. The health and well-being of the health workforce is a particular area of interest, as the health of all others depends upon it (WHO, 2006).

Nurses need to understand workplace health issues not only to better care for patients, families, and communities but also to better address their own health and well-being and that of their colleagues. How can safe, compassionate, competent, ethical care be provided by individuals who, themselves, are not healthy and who feel fatigued and burned out? Similar to airplane passengers who are advised to put on their own oxygen mask before helping others, nurses have a responsibility to attend to their own health and well-being.

This chapter is focused on mental health in the workplace, with the acknowledgment that physical health and mental health are essentially integrated. The relation of work to health and well-being is addressed, as are the attributes of a healthy workplace. Outlined are some ways in which workplaces may support and accommodate individuals at risk for, or who have, mental health concerns. Health care environments are considered as workplaces, particularly from the perspective of nurses, and workplace violence is discussed.

■ WORK

Work is the term used to signify our paid employment, the job or task we perform to earn a living. In the lives of most people, however, work in its broadest sense is not restricted to places of employment. Some individuals work entirely within their homes, are not employees of any organization, and do not receive any monetary remuneration for their contribution to family, home, and community life. Work shapes the way individuals perceive themselves, including their sense of worth as a member of their society (WHO, 2005). In *The Psychology of Working*, Blustein (2008) argues that "work plays a central role in the development, expression, and maintenance of psychological health" (p. 228).

 KEY CONCEPT Work is "the job, occupation, or task one performs as a means of providing a livelihood" (Venes, 2009, p. 2502).

The Changing Nature of Work

The Tokyo Declaration (1998), an international document created over a decade ago by occupational health experts, describes the increasing employee stress arising from economic and technological changes to the workplace aimed at short-term productivity and profit. These changes include organizational restructuring and downsizing, decreased job stability, the frantic pace of work and life, and decreases in leisure time. The landscape of work continues to be transformed by factors such as the increasing turnover of work to machines and robotic devices, digital technology that allows production to occur anywhere on the globe while managed from a central location, and a decline in the need for middle management that contributes to downsizing (Blustein, 2008). This transformation of the nature of work is having direct effects on the work life of Canadians.

One out of every three Canadians says that he or she is a "workaholic" (Statistics Canada, 2007). Comparisons of the 1991 and 2001 National Work-Life Conflict Surveys reveal that time in work seems to have increased across all job groups (Duxbury & Higgins, 2009). Where one in ten survey respondents worked 50 or more hours per week in 1991, one in four did so in 2001. The number of employees performing unpaid overtime has nearly doubled. It appears that employees find it increasingly difficult to complete their work during regular hours. Unsurprisingly, the survey comparisons reveal that the perceived level of stress and depression among workers has increased, as well.

The world entered a time of economic crisis in 2009 that had serious consequences for workers. Sharp and/or sustained rise in unemployment negatively impacts a community's well-being as people lose jobs, acquire debt, and become unable to maintain their current lifestyle. If appropriate measures are not in place, such as adequate unemployment benefits, social services, and community support, the level of stress and mental health problems in a community will rise (Gunnell, Platt, & Hawton, 2009). Work has the potential to be a positive factor in sustaining health and well-being, but work, or the lack of it, can have a negative effect on existing health problems or can contribute to the development of new ones.

Unemployment

Most governments identify an individual as **unemployed** when the person does not have paid employment, wants to be employed, and is actively seeking work. This definition, however, does not encompass individuals who are **underemployed** (those with insufficient work relative to hours, skills, income, or status) nor "discouraged workers," individuals who want to work but have given up seeking it (Dooley, 2003; Dooley & Catalano, 2003; Friedland & Price, 2003). When considering a person's employment status, it may be more useful to consider employment along a continuum rather than as a dichotomous state of employed or unemployed.

Unemployment places individuals at risk for adverse health effects. The research support for this claim is substantial (Fryer & Fagan, 2003). For instance, a meta-analysis of the unemployment literature by McKee-Ryan, Song, Wanberg, and Kinicki (2005) found that the unemployed had lower psychological and physical well-being than their employed counterparts. The World Health Organization (2008) identifies the adverse effects of unemployment as including:

- Elevated blood pressure
- Increased depression and anxiety
- Increased visits to general medical practitioners
- Increased symptoms of coronary disease
- Greater stress
- Increased psychological morbidity

- An increase in the number of health problems
- An increase in family problems, particularly financial hardships

Research indicates that obtaining permanent employment after being in an unstable employment situation can be health promoting: the probability of psychological symptoms decreases (Reine, Novo, & Hammarström, 2008).

Given the changing nature of work, it is increasingly important to understand that the adverse effects of job change go beyond those who have lost jobs (Dooley & Catalano, 2003). Underemployed workers, for example, report lower levels of health and well-being than adequately employed workers (Friedland & Price, 2003). Others affected include survivors of downsizing who must take on the work of those who have left while dealing with the guilt of keeping their jobs; family members of those who have lost their jobs can face hardship and stigma; and individuals who failed to find an adequate job after leaving school and face an uncertain future (Dooley & Catalano). Insecurity regarding one's job contributes to a sense of insecurity regarding the future.

HEALTHY WORKPLACES

Workplace health has been conceived in competing ways, as *safety* and as *lifestyle* (Allender, Colquhoun, & Kelly, 2006). Conceiving workplace health as safety tends to limit it to the relationship with workers and their physical safety, while a lifestyle approach encourages links between employees' work and their private lives. This lifestyle approach seems more congruent with the idea of well-being as defined by the Canadian Nurses Association (2008): "a person's state of being well, content and able to make the most of his or her abilities" (p. 28). It fits with Healey-Ogden's (2008) findings on the experience of well-being as interwoven with one's self-identity and relationships (see Chapter 2).

> **KEY CONCEPT Workplace health** is the promotion and maintenance of the health and well-being of workers through policies, programs, and practices that promote safety, minimize risk, and create a positive, responsive, equitable workplace culture and a supportive workplace climate.

Healthy workplaces are those that have policies, practices, and programs in place to provide workers with the conditions necessary to protect and promote their health and well-being. These workplaces offer a safe and healthy physical environment and a positive, supportive psychosocial climate that does not tolerate harassment or violence. A survey of over 4,000 Canadians conducted for the Global Business and Economic Roundtable on Addictions and Mental Health (Ipso Reid, 2007) found that seven in ten employed individuals considered their workplaces as healthy and found their employer to be supportive of their personal needs.

Workplace constraints can contribute independently to psychological stress. It has been found that family structure, social network outside the workplace, and the personality of the worker do not moderate the influence of the workplace, with the exception of strained marital relations (Marchand, Demers, & Durand, 2006). When Winkelmann (2009) explored whether social capital (i.e., social networks and social activities) mediated the effect of unemployment on well-being, he found no evidence that it does.

Mental Health Problems in the Workplace

WHO (2005) declares that mental health problems evolve from "a complex interplay between biological, psychological, social and environmental factors" (p. 2) and that both the content and the context of work play a role in the development of mental health problems (see Boxes 5-1 and 5-2 for **work content** and **work context** factors, respectively, that affect mental health). High job demands and low decision-making latitude are particularly significant to workplace mental health problems (Lowe, 2003). (See Chapter 2 regarding mental health problems.)

Work-Life Balance

A challenge for many people is to balance the demands of their paid employment with other aspects of their lives, such as family and community. Individuals have many roles beyond that of an employee: they may be a spouse, parent, or a caregiver of a parent. Nonwork roles, such as educational, cultural, recreational, and volunteer activi-

---

BOX 5.1

Content Factors of Work That Affect Mental Health

WORKLOAD: Excessive workload (e.g., too much to do, too little time, insufficient resources)

PARTICIPATION AND CONTROL: Unable to influence work life or participate in decisions that affect it

JOB CONTENT: Unpleasant or monotonous tasks, dangerous tasks, exposure to traumatic events

Adapted from World Health Organization. (2005). *Mental health policies and programmes in the workplace.* Geneva, Switzerland: Author.

BOX 5.2

Context Factors of Work That Affect Mental Health

ROLE IN ORGANIZATION: role conflict (incompatible demands) and role ambiguity (uncertainty regarding expectations)

REWARD: perception of one's worth at work; not just salary, but respect and esteem. Adequate social support at work

EQUITY: being fairly or justly treated (e.g., workload, promotions, involvement in decisions)

INTERPERSONAL RELATIONSHIPS: quality of relationships with coworkers and supervisors; leadership style; harassment, bullying, or isolation

WORKING ENVIRONMENT: physical environment (e.g., noise, light, pollution) and working hours (e.g., shift work, excessive hours)

WORKPLACE CULTURE: communication, leadership, and organizational structure

HOME-WORK INTERFACE: tensions between home and work; lack of support at home for work commitments or at work for home commitments

Sources: World Health Organization. (2005). *Mental health policies and programmes in the workplace.* Geneva, Switzerland: Author; Marchand, A., Demers, A., & Durand, P. (2006). Social structures, agent personality and workers' mental health: A longitudinal analysis of the specific role of occupation and of workplace constraints-resources on psychological distress in the Canadian workforce. *Human Relations, 59*(7), 875–901.

ties, are important to life satisfaction and contribute to the cohesion of a society (Lero, Richardson, & Korabik, 2009). **Work-life balance** is achieved when an individual finds a satisfactory interaction among all the domains of his or her life. This balance will not be the same for everyone but will differ based on personal values, family structure, life situations and expectations, and societal norms.

Work-life conflict occurs when the demands of work and nonwork roles directly interfere with an individual's ability to meet one or more of the roles and upset his or her work-life balance. Many workplaces operate under "the myth of separate worlds" (Duxbury & Higgins, 2005; Kantor, 1977). For instance, about 40% of employee respondents stated that it was difficult to arrange their work schedules to meet personal or family commitments; about 75% noted that it was very difficult to be at home from work when their children arrived after school; and about 25% either delayed or decided not to start a family or had fewer children because they did not believe that they could balance the demands of work and family (Duxbury & Higgins, 2009). Lero et al.'s (2009) review of work-life balance practices notes that the research literature associates work and family conflicts with such health issues as stress, anxiety, depression,

sleep disturbances, suppressed immune functioning, poor dietary habits, lack of exercise, hypertension, and medication use, among others.

Heavy job demands (e.g., heavy workload; multiple and/or time-pressured tasks) are a primary antecedent of work-life conflict. In an attempt to meet job demands, workers may stay on the job after regular hours, take work home, or work on days off. **Role overload** occurs when an individual is unable to satisfy role demands. Both the number of demands and the control the individual feels regarding the demands are factors in work-life conflict (Duxbury & Higggins, 2009; Lero et al., 2009). The quality and availability of community supports, such as day care or dependent care, can mitigate pressures on individuals and families, as can flexible working practices (e.g., varied hours of work, telecommuting, opportunity for leave, and "family-friendly" workplaces) (Canadian Council on Social Development, 1999; Lero et al., 2009). Employees, however, may not take advantage of work-family policies if they believe that doing so will have negative consequences for their career (Lowe, 2003). Research is being conducted to determine ways to measure employees' appraisal of organization-level stress management interventions (Randall, Nielsen, & Tvedt, 2009).

Stress in the Workplace

Stress at work does not necessarily have a negative effect on employees but rather depends on the nature, intensity, and duration of the stress and whether or not protective factors (e.g., employees feel some control regarding their work situation) are present (WHO, 2005). Indications that an individual's stress is work related include an awareness that he or she functions without any difficulty outside of the workplace and that stress is experienced when preparing for work or when thinking primarily about workplace issues (see Chapter 35 for information regarding stress). Factors that contribute to workers taking leave for mental health concerns include perceived lack of support from employers and coworkers, workplace stress, and fear of failure (Raderstorf & Kurtz, 2006). Human Resources and Skills Development Canada (2002), responding to increases in stress-related illness, developed a project that focuses on individual well-being through a "toolkit" that employees and managers may use to assist in the improvement of their well-being. *Physical* (e.g., exercise, nutrition, sleeping habits), *emotional* (e.g., humour, assertiveness, forgiveness, dealing with anger), *intellectual* (e.g., creativity, continuous learning activities), *social* (e.g., time with family and colleagues, recreation, life balance), and *spiritual* (e.g., reflection on one's sense of meaning, of connection to something greater than oneself) components are addressed in the toolkit.

Depression, Anxiety, and Substance-Related Disorders

Mental disorders, such as depression, anxiety, and substance-related disorders, affect individuals during their working years. WHO expects, for instance, that depression will become the leading cause of disability by 2020 (WHO, 2001). The workplace can play a role in the prevention and early detection of disorders by improving the knowledge of mental health problems and disorders within the organization, by supporting work-life balance, and by helping employees develop protective factors such as coping and stress management skills (Couser, 2008). Organizations can ensure the availability of leave for treatment.

Use of tobacco products is a major substance-related issue in the workplace. Supportive policies regarding assistance with cessation of tobacco use seem more effective than a narrow focus on the enforcement of "no smoking policies" and can have a positive impact. It is important to understand the workplace factors that affect smoking and cessation. Nurses, for example, describe taking a smoking break to relieve stress during shifts—"if you don't smoke, you don't get a break"—and find that workplace stress makes it difficult to quit smoking (Sarna, Bialous, Wewers, Froelicher, & Danao, 2004, p. 85). Paradoxically, the effect of nicotine is short acting and, within 30 minutes of using tobacco, the individual will experience withdrawal that can include symptoms such as anxiety, restlessness, irritability, impaired task performance, and diminished concentration (Fiore et al., 2008). Important to workplace climate, smoking can be a source of dissention. Nonsmoking nurses can perceive their colleagues who smoke as taking more breaks, spending less time with their patients, and being less committed to their profession (Sarna et al.). (See Chapter 20 for information about mood disorders, Chapter 21 for anxiety disorders, and Chapter 24 for substance-related disorders.)

At-Risk Employees

Awareness of the potential for mental health issues among employees is an important component of a healthy workplace. This includes awareness that some employees may be more vulnerable, in the short or long term, to stress and other work-related threats to mental health than other employees. Such vulnerability may be associated with factors such as gender, age, health status, family situation, or life history. See Box 5-3 for research that examined the work environment's influence on the psychological health of the latest generation of nurses.

Workplace strategies can be put in place to assist and support specific workers or groups of workers (WHO, 2005). Examples of such strategies include workshops

---

BOX 5.3

Research for Best Practice: A Healthy Workplace for Gen-Next Nurses

Lavoie-Tremblay, M., Wright, D., Desforges, N., Gélinas, C., Marchionni, C., & Drevniok, U. (2008). Creating a healthy workplace for new-generation nurses. *Journal of Nursing Scholarship, 40*(3), 290–297.

THE QUESTION: How do dimensions of the psychosocial work environment influence the psychological health of the latest generation of nurses?

METHOD: In a quantitative study using correlational description, participants were recruited from among Quebec nurses born after 1981 (Generation Y, or "Nexters"); sociodemographic data (age, gender, education, etc.) were collected. Using validated self-report questionnaires specifically targeting the variables selected to define psychosocial dimensions of the workplace, respondents reported personal experience of psychological demands, decision latitude, job strain, social support from colleagues and superiors, and effort/reward. The outcome variable was *psychological distress*. Cross tabulations were performed to describe the relationship between the psychosocial work environment and the psychological distress.

FINDINGS: Of 309 respondents, 96.4% were females; the mean age was 22.6 years. More than half had held current positions for 2 years or less. Results showed among other things that 53% of respondents reported high psychological demand, 58% low decision latitude, 58% low social support, and 29% high job strain. Nurses who were exposed to a level of psychological distress higher than the provincial median perceived an imbalance between effort expended and reward received, high psychological demand, and elevated job strain. The study showed the influence of social support from colleagues and superiors as well as of decision latitude on levels of psychological distress. High levels of psychological demand and an imbalance between effort and reward were shown to increase the level of psychological distress. Nearly half of all respondents were found to experience high psychological distress—twice the percentage of health care providers of all ages reported in a similar survey in Quebec.

IMPLICATIONS: The responses of Quebec's Generation Y nurses reflected the pressures of poor practice environments and working conditions contributing to global recruitment and retention of nurses. Strategies are needed that address the psychological health of new-generation nurses by targeting the psychosocial work environment. The results indicate the importance of creating a stable work environment where new nurses can cope with their workload and work with the same team members to promote socialization and deliver safe care, both of which are sources of reward for nurses. Research is needed on the ways that the organization of care can be changed to improve the perception of reward by health care providers in an environment affected by shortages and limited financial resources.

for workers nearing retirement, counselling for workers exposed to traumatic events, interventions for employees with substance-related problems, and support groups for single parents. Individuals with chronic health problems may require individually negotiated support, such as an adaption of work hours to include rest periods. Strategies can also include education for managers regarding particular topics (e.g., cross-cultural issues to enable them to assist new immigrant employees).

Accommodation

Employers in Canada are expected to provide reasonable accommodation to special needs of current or potential employees. While an employer can show that a discriminatory policy or standard is necessary for a particular job, for example, good vision for ambulance drivers, this expectation is a legal requirement under labour laws and human rights acts and prevents discrimination in employment practices. Accommodation involves primarily simple, low-cost strategies. Examples of reasonable accommodation for people with mental health problems and disorders include (WHO, 2005):

- Changes in communication (e.g., requests put in writing for a clerk who becomes anxious with verbal instructions; positive feedback given, not just criticisms; opportunities for self-appraisal prior to evaluation; planning sessions with a coworker as needed)
- Modifications to the physical environment (e.g., quiet work space provided)
- Job modifications (e.g., opportunities to work at home; hiring an assistant)
- Schedule modification (e.g., flexible working hours; rest periods or recuperation time; time allowed for medications or for treatment appointments; opportunity to start part-time work and move to full time)

Work and Persons Living With a Mental Disorder

Individuals living with mental disorders want self-determination and life satisfaction through work as others do (Gold & Waghorn, 2007). (See Chapter 2 regarding mental disorders.) Work can help achieve relief from poverty, diminish reliance on social assistance, and promote social inclusion. Work can play an important role in recovery from mental illness and is a means to integrate persons with mental disorders back into their community (WHO, 2001). In Canada, the Standing Senate Committee on Social Affairs, Science and Technology (2006), in examining the situation of mental health, the workplace, and employment, has made several recommendations, including the development of best management practices to encourage mental health in the workplace, the creation of a Pan-Canada Knowledge Exchange Centre to foster

management of mental illness in the workplace, and the creation of support for the development of alternative businesses both owned and operated by persons with a mental illness. To date, good progress has been made toward fulfilling these recommendations. Nevertheless, finding appropriate employment remains difficult for persons with a mental disorder diagnosis: individuals with severe mental disorders have higher unemployment rates than people with physical disabilities (WHO).

Individual placement and support (IPS) employment programs are a way to assist individuals with severe mental disorders to enter the workplace. IPS involves a rapid job search that is based on the individual's personal preferences and then continuing support to both the individual and the employer from an employment specialist working with the mental health service team (Burns et al., 2007; Gold & Waghorn, 2007). It has been an effective approach in improving employment for young people with first episode psychosis (Lauber, 2009) and shown to be more effective than traditional vocational services (Burns et al., 2007). Research done at Douglas Hospital in Montreal found this approach to be more successful for persons with severe mental illness: 47% of those in the supported employment group obtained at least some competitive employment versus 18% in the control group (Latimer et al., 2006).

NURSES AND WORKPLACE MENTAL HEALTH

"At the heart of every health system, the workforce is central to advancing health" (WHO, 2006, p. xv). In 2006, the health workforce was selected as the focus of the World Health Report, *Working together for Health* (WHO, 2006), because the education, recruitment, and retention of workers in the health sector are now pressing global concerns. The Commission on the Future of Health Care in Canada (2002), in presenting its final report, raised serious concerns regarding the quality of work life in the health sector, particularly that of nurses. It noted the effects of poor working conditions not only on nurses' health but also on the quality of patient care. It is apparent that the quality of work life in health care environments needs urgent attention due to heavy workloads, excessive overtime, inflexible scheduling, safety hazards, poor management, and lack of opportunity for professional development. These factors have the potential to negatively impact the Canadian health workforce (Shamian & El-Jardali, 2007). Nurses are the largest component of the health care workforce. They work across a wide range of settings, primarily on shift-work schedules, engaging with patients and families and all other members of the health care workforce (Kerr & Mustard, 2007). Nurses' health is a barometer of workplace health in the health sector.

The first Canadian *National Survey of the Work and Health of Nurses* reveals that psychosocial and interpersonal factors (e.g., work stress, low autonomy, and lack of respect) are more closely associated with health problems among nurses than work overtime (Statistics Canada, 2006). In this survey of approximately 19,000 regulated nurses, nearly one third had high **job strain**, defined as what happens when the psychological demands of a job exceed the worker's discretion of how to enact it. Many nurses (45% of female nurses and 51% of male nurses) believed that they had only low support from coworkers. This percentage compares unfavourably with employed Canadians in general among whom approximately 33% describe low support. About one in five nurses indicated that his or her mental health made it difficult to handle his or her workload in the past month.

In a Canadian study examining the processes by which nurses' mental health was "weakened," Alderson (2008) concluded that there was a perception on the part of nurses that they had responsibility but not professional recognition, autonomy, and decisional power (p. 161). Further, she found that nurses' burnout and mental health problems did not come from their empathic engagement with patients, but rather in the way their work was organized, so that nurses found their sense of identity, self-esteem, and worth to be compromised. Alderson points out the problems with an organizational paradigm in which nurses' work is framed from an industrial perspective of growth and productivity. Nurses find meaning in their work in their relationships with patients and families and need the time to provide comfort and personalized care. It is here, Alderson argues, that nurses "reinforce their identity and preserve their mental health" (p. 171). The Canadian Nurses Association (CNA) and the Canadian Federation of Nurses Unions (CFNU) (2006) have a joint policy statement on practice environments that will maximize client, nurse, and system outcomes. See Box 5-4 for the characteristics of quality practice environments as identified by CNA and CFNU.

The Registered Nurses' Association of Ontario (2008) has developed an evidence-based best practice guideline for healthy work environments for nurses, based on the assumption that such environments are essential for quality care. The model underpinning the guideline presents the workplace as a product of individual, organizational, and external system determinants that are connected and interdependent. The key recommendations for workplace health, safety, and well-being of the nurse can be found in Table 5-1. When nurses' work environments are not healthy places to be, nurses are put at risk for burnout and compassion fatigue.

Burnout

Burnout is a term used to indicate "exhaustion due to chronic job stress" (Venes, 2009, p. 332).

It has been conceived further as "a psychological syndrome in response to chronic interpersonal stressors on the job with three dimensions: exhaustion, cynicism and detachment, and lack of a sense of accomplishment" (Maslach, Schaufeli, & Leiter, 2001, p. 399). The stressors can include unresolved ethical distress (Severinsson, 2003). Initially, the individual may experience physiological arousal (e.g., anxiety, high blood pressure, insomnia), then enter a phase of energy conservation (e.g., tiredness,

---

BOX 5.4

Characteristics of Quality Practice Environments for Nurses

Communication and collaboration	Effective and across the system
Responsibility and accountability	Participation in decision making that affects nursing, including policies, resource allocation, and patient
Realistic workload	Time for safe, competent, compassionate, and ethical care. For maintaining competence, developing therapeutic relationships, and creating work-life balance
Leadership	Important in all nursing roles, including roles as mentors, role models, visionaries, and advocates
Support for information and knowledge management	Technologies available that support optimal information and knowledge management
Professional development	Opportunities for developing and maintaining competence, including continuing education, online learning, formal education, and mentoring
Workplace culture	Values the well-being of clients and employees. Is continually assessed

Source: CAN & CFNU. (2006). Joint Position Statement. Practice environments: Maximizing Client, Nurse and System Outcomes. Available at www.cna-aiic.ca

Table 5.1	Recommendations for Workplace Health, Safety, and Well-being of the Nurse
Organization Practice Recommendations	Organizations/nursing employers create and design environments and systems that promote safe and healthy workplaces, including such strategies as: Creating a culture, climate, and practices that support, promote, and maintain staff health, well-being, and safety. Ensuring that the organization's annual budget includes adequate resources (human and fiscal) to implement and evaluate health and safety initiatives. Establishing organizational practices that foster mutual responsibility and accountability by individual nurses and organizational leaders to ensure a safe work environment. Organizations/nursing employers are aware of the impact of organizational changes (such as restructuring and downsizing) on the health, safety, and well-being of nurses and be responsible and accountable for implementing appropriate supportive measures. Organizations/nursing employers implement and maintain education and training programs aimed at increasing awareness of health and safety issues for nurses (e.g., safe-lift initiative, employee rights, hazard awareness, etc.). Workplace health and safety best practices be embedded/integrated across all sectors of the health care system.
Research Recommendations	Researchers actively collaborate with health care partners to demonstrate the effectiveness of interventions aimed at improving nurse health, safety, and well-being using rigorous research and evaluation methodologies. Researchers make full use of existing databases on nurse health, including the National Survey on the Work and Health of Nurses, in order to improve understanding of the key factors contributing to healthy work environments for nurses and to develop and test best practice indicators.
Education Recommendations	Nursing education institutions model the integration of health, safety, and well-being into their own workplace culture. Nursing education institutions incorporate information about the health, safety, and well-being of the nurse into the core curriculum of nursing education programs.
System Recommendations	Governing/accreditation bodies incorporate the Organization Practice Recommendations from this Healthy Work Environments Best Practice Guideline in their quality health and safety standards for health care service and education organizations.

Registered Nurses' Association of Ontario. (2008). *Workplace health, safety and well-being of the nurse.* Toronto, ON: Registered Nurses' Association of Ontario.

apathy) leading to exhaustion (e.g., headaches, depression) (Pompili et al., 2006). Burnout has been associated with diseases of the circulatory, musculoskeletal, and respiratory systems (Toppinen-Tanner, Ojajärvi, Väänänen, Kalimo, & Jäppinen, 2005). Although WHO (2005) finds that burnout is a "long-term exposure to a work situation that is beyond the person's capacity to cope" (p. 18), burnout may occur more quickly than anticipated: Cho, Laschinger, and Wong (2006) found that, of the new (under 2 years of practice) graduate nurses studied, 66% had symptoms of burnout.

Compassion Fatigue

Once used to describe the reduced public empathy toward social problems or crises, **compassion fatigue** is now the term applied to disengagement on the part of care-giving professionals and equated frequently with burnout. Compassion fatigue has been primarily conceived at the level of the individual: a state arising from an interaction of the psychology of the person affected, the nature of his or her work, and his or her capacity to mediate engagement with others. More recently, compassion fatigue is being considered at the macro level as a phenomenon shaped by conditions of the environment (Austin, Goble, Leier, & Byrne, 2009). Risk factors for compassion fatigue include continued exposure to patients' experiences and family members' emotions, burnout and stress, lack of self-care, and empathy. In a study of sexual assault counsellors in northern Ontario, it was found that location (isolation, community attitudes, lack of privacy) was also a factor (Coholic & Blackford, 2005). Protective factors include contributing to patients' recovery, compassion satisfaction, and personal and professional support

---

BOX 5.5

Research for Best Practice: Nurses and Compassion Fatigue

Austin, W., Goble, E., Leier, B., & Byrne, P. (2009). Compassion fatigue: The experience of nurses. Ethics & Social Welfare, 3(2), 195–214.

THE QUESTION: What is it like to have compassion fatigue as a nurse?

METHOD: In this pilot study, interpretive description, a human science research approach developed by nurse theorist Sally Thorne, was used to understand the phenomenon of compassion fatigue as lived by nurses. Registered nurses (RNs) and registered psychiatric nurses (RPNs) who identified themselves as having compassion fatigue were invited to participate in the study. Five nurses from various service areas were interviewed about their experiences by the RN member of the research. The interviews were audiotaped and transcribed verbatim. The researchers reflected upon the transcripts, using collected materials to clarify questions of institutional procedures and nursing practice. Themes were identified.

FINDINGS: Six interconnected themes were found: running on empty; shielding myself; being impotent as a nurse;

losing balance; the kind of nurse I was; and trying to survive. Nurses used phrases such as "my emotional tank is empty" to denote feeling unable to give holistic care to their patients and described acting like "a robot." This disconnection from patients was much different from the way they nursed in the past. They felt discouraged and hopeless about being able to influence their practice or the health care system in any meaningful way. Compassion fatigue overwhelmed their home life, as well. Strategies used for "survival" included attending workshops and educational opportunities, changing jobs or hours of work, remembering times when they "made a difference," and actively seeking balance in their lives.

IMPLICATIONS: Can it be that caring work like nursing is dangerous to one's well-being? It may be, rather, that being unable to provide care to patients in a holistic, engaged way puts one at risk for compassion fatigue. Compassion fatigue can lead nurses to quit their employment or even leave the discipline itself. Addressing nurses' compassion fatigue is important if safe, competent, compassionate, ethical care is to occur.

(e.g., good team relationships and sufficient resources) (Austin et al.) (see Box 5-5).

WORKPLACE VIOLENCE

Studies show that 80% to 90% of health care providers have experienced workplace violence (Felblinger, 2008; Sofield & Salmond, 2003). Violence in the workplace gained attention as a serious health, safety, organizational, and economic problem when the International Labour Organization began publishing its reports on violence at work in 1998. The reports reveal that violence occurs, not as many isolated, individual incidents, but as an institutional issue rooted in socioeconomic and other broader cultural factors (Chappell & Di Martino, 2000).

Describing and defining workplace violence is itself difficult given the diversity of perceptions in different contexts and cultures of what constitutes violence. Nor is violence strictly physical. Beyond the obvious violence of homicide, battery, or rape, there is a wide and overlapping range of physical and psychological violence: racial and sexual harassment, bullying, mobbing, stalking, intimidation, ostracism, robbery, vandalism, rude or aggressive behaviour, and using profanity are among its many forms, and there are few individuals who will not, at one time or another, experience some form of violence in the workplace. A study by the European Union indicated the relationship of a number of factors to workplace violence, including gender, age, job precariousness, rank, and industry of occupation. A study in Sweden of occupations

at risk showed workplace violence to be particularly concentrated (nearly half of total cases) in the areas of health care and social services, more so than in law (Chappell & Di Martino, 2000).

KEY CONCEPT Workplace violence is the intimidation, harassment, or abuse of an individual in his or her place of employment.

It is becoming increasingly evident that preventive and systematic approaches to the causes of workplace violence are needed. In particular, early intervention measures that raise awareness of the full range of violent behaviours, improve working relationships, and recognize that workers' health, safety, and well-being are integral parts of the economic sustainability of workplaces are required (Chappell & Di Martino, 2000).

Bullying

The ILO (Chappell & Di Martino, 2000) reports that workplace **bullying** is among the fastest-growing forms of workplace violence. Researchers have suggested that bullying be seen on a spectrum of abuse, with general incivility in the workplace establishing conditions in which more aggressive behaviours such as harassment and bullying can emerge (Felblinger, 2008; Namie, 2003). It seems that tolerance of competitive and abusive behaviours increases the possibilities for psychological and physical violence. The normalization of incivility and bullying and the subsequent shame of the victims have adverse professional and clinical outcomes (Felblinger, 2008). Incivility consists in a lack of empathy and social support; in the workplace, it may involve gossip, name-calling, taking credit for another's work or refusing collaboration, withholding important information or discounting input from others, verbal attacks or the "silent treatment," angry outbursts, condescending remarks, etc. Bullying escalates competitive, aggressive tendencies and concentrates their effects upon a selected target for sustained attack. The repeated, persistent, and intended physical or psychological harm is inflicted on an individual, and through tactics of intimidation and shaming, the target feels powerless to stop the abuse (Felblinger, 2008; Zapf & Gross, 2001). Targets of bullying can suffer from posttraumatic stress disorder and symptoms of low self-esteem, anxiety, sleep disturbance, recurrent nightmares, somatic problems, concentration difficulties, irritability, depression, and feelings of self-hatred (Felblinger, 2008; Mikkelsen & Einarsen, 2002). It has been noted that absenteeism and the extensive use of sick time frequently indicate workplace bullying (MacIntosh, 2005). As targets, they might also feel isolated and that they have no one to turn to for understanding.

A separate term, **mobbing**, is often used to refer to several people ganging up on a selected target for bullying. Research has shown that the bully's power advantage tends to gather allies, either through the organizational hierarchy or through the social network of peers, and the "campaign of hate" spreads; thus, the significance of the difference between bullying and mobbing tends to disappear (Namie, 2003). This also suggests that bullying is less an issue of "personality" and more a problem of workplace culture. The target of bullying is often chosen for their show of independence or of not quite "fitting in"; often, a bully is threatened by a show of job competence. Some participants in a study of workplace bullying said that they may have been singled out as whistle-blowers for having a strong sense of ethics; while others felt picked out for their submissive or nonconfrontational character (MacIntosh, 2005). In general, the reasons are as numerous as the opportunities, suggesting again that causes are situated in accepted practice.

Violence in Health Care Settings

Canadian studies have also shown that nursing is a comparatively high-risk occupation; most Canadian nurses have experienced some form of violence during the course of their career, and nurses and physicians rarely report violent incidents. A study of workplace violence in Alberta and British Columbia hospitals showed that a nurse can expect several incidences of violence in a given work week, particularly in the emergency, psychiatric, and medical-surgical settings (Hesketh et al., 2003). While most violence and abuse are committed by patients, a significant portion—particularly emotional abuse and sexual harassment—is committed by coworkers.

It is crucial to address violence in health care settings. In fact, Standard IV of the Canadian Federation of Mental Health Nurses practice standards, *Effectively Manages Rapidly Changing Situations*, requires the PMH nurse to utilize safety measures to protect client, self, and colleagues from potentially abusive situations in the work environment (see Chapter 6).

The place to start is to identify sources of violence in the workplace, then discussions can begin and strategies can be adopted for its prevention. Strategies may be as simple as providing timely information to patients and their friends and family, as this effectively lessens the risk of assault in health care settings, particularly in cases involving distress and long waiting periods (Chappell & Di Martino, 2000). A person on the brink of physical aggression can be swayed by those around him or her to take a more measured, thoughtful approach to the situation. Staying calm; speaking gently, slowly, and clearly; and avoiding aggressive or confrontational body language are important in dealing with aggressive individuals. It is also critical that organizational pressures are identified in a preventive strategy: ensuring that staff levels and shift lengths are appropriate can reduce stress and avert aggression among staff and between workers and the public. Identifying competencies and experience and assigning tasks accordingly are also important in reducing contributing factors.

Hesketh and colleagues (2003) found that PMH nurses, when asked about experiences of abuse within their past five shifts, reported that the majority of violence was committed by patients, although family and other visitors, physicians, fellow nurses, and other staff members also were at fault, particularly in experiences of emotional abuse, where nearly a third of the violence committed came from someone other than a patient. The study also showed that emotional abuse, particularly that by a coworker, was especially underreported on the job, possibly because it is not always considered a form of violence. Hesketh and colleagues further suggest that an environment in which emotional abuse is tolerated, or not considered a form of violence, plays a role in making other forms of violence, such as physical and sexual assault, more acceptable. If emotional abuse is tolerated on the job, an environment is created that is more conducive to abuse and violence. Patients, visitors, and all involved tend to respond in kind.

Rather than simply adopting an antiviolence stance, the health care setting needs to be an environment where practice is infused with courtesy, decency, and civility (Hesketh et al., 2003). It is essential that workplace violence be recorded and reported, as establishing patterns of behaviour is helpful in a preventive strategy

(Chappell & Di Martino, 2000). Victims experience a wide range of reactions, some of them disabling, and need a wide range of psychosocial and professional support, depending on the extent to which trauma has been sustained: a debriefing involving as many people possible who were involved in the incident can help to foster an environment in which "petty crimes" are not tolerated. Counselling by qualified staff or outside specialists may be deemed necessary in more serious cases, while in the case of major incidents of violence, victims may need more long-term support and rehabilitation.

• CRNENOTE

Nurses who are the victims of violence in the workplace may need support to deal with their reaction to the incident. A debriefing with those involved in the incident is important to the resolution of the violence and to the prevention of further incidences.

Nurses, in particular, may accept workplace abuse as endemic, that it "comes with the territory," a by-product of having high stress and responsibility. When nurses are the targets of bullying, personal and professional dissatisfaction grows and clinical effectiveness diminishes. The energy needed for safe patient care can be consumed by personal insecurity, dissatisfaction, hopelessness, and hostility.

Interventions are needed to help nurses confront incivility in a professional manner and identify bullying behaviours and the ensuing cycle of shame and insecurity. Acceptable behaviours may require definition, and their internalization requires systemic recognition and support. Bullying may best be understood as an organizational problem rather than explained by individual characteristics of either the "target" or the "bully" (Lewis, 2006).

SUMMARY OF KEY POINTS

□ Work influences self-identity, as well as provides an income, and plays a significant role in an individual's health and well-being. Unemployment and underemployment can cause psychological distress and negatively affect an individual's mental health. As well, there are adverse effects related to job change that go beyond those who have lost jobs.

□ The nature of work has been changing across the globe due to economic and technological developments; these changes are affecting the mental health of workers.

□ Nurses need to understand workplace health, not only as it relates to those in their care but also as it relates to the health workforce. Workplaces are excellent settings for health protection and promotion.

□ Achieving work-life balance among the domains of one's life can be difficult: work-life conflict occurs when one role interferes with meeting the demands of another.

□ The content and the context of work affect mental health.

□ There are identified strategies and programs for creating a healthy workplace, including those to accommodate employees at risk for stress and/or mental health problems.

□ Work can help persons with mental disorders in their recovery and in the improvement of their well-being. Independent placement and support facilitates acquiring and maintaining employment for persons with severe mental disorders.

□ Workplace violence is a serious threat to workers' mental health and that needs to be discussed, addressed, and eliminated.

CRITICAL THINKING CHALLENGES

1   Imagine your "dream" workplace as a practicing nurse. What would it be like? What would be the barriers to making this dream come true?

2   Identify the strategies in place at your educational institution for the support of the mental health of students, faculty, and staff. Are there additional strategies that you believe should be in place?

3   Consider your experience as a student in a health care environment. What factors do you find cause or increase stress for you? What factors mitigate stress for you?

4   Have you been affected by an incident of workplace violence? Consider the immediate and long-term influences that may have influenced the occurrence of this incident. What was done, if anything, to prevent it from happening again?

WEB LINKS

www.cmha.ca   This is the website of the Canadian Mental Health Association where information about their work in workplace mental health, including the employment of persons with mental health problems, can be found.

www.mentalhealthworks.ca   The website of Mental Health Works, an initiative of the Canadian Mental Health Association, Ontario, that began in 2001 as a partnership among the voluntary sector, government, and business. It has links and articles regarding mental health in the workplace, including accommodation of employees with mental health problems and mental disorders.

www.canoshweb.org/en/   This is the website of Can Osh: Canada's National Occupational Health and

Safety (CanOSH) and a source of helpful information regarding healthy workplaces.

www.hc-sc.gc.ca/index_e.html   This is Health Canada's website.

workplacebullying.org   The Workplace Bullying Institute is an American organization dedicated to the eradication of workplace bullying through public education, help for individuals, employer solutions, and legislative advocacy.

www.who.int/en/   Important documents about global initiatives can be found at the World Health Organization's website.

MOVIES, NOVELS, AND BIOGRAPHIES

Nurse Jackie: 2009. This Showtime television show is about a New York emergency room nurse who, addicted to analgesics related to her chronic back pain, struggles daily to face work and family demands. The depiction of this nurse is outrageous in many ways, but poignant moments with patients, colleagues, and family are also portrayed.

VIEWING POINTS: What do you think about the representation of nurses' work life in *Nurse Jackie*? Of the situation of the student nurse character? The New York State Nurses Association has voiced concern about the effect this show will have on nurses' public image. What do you think?

(See http://www.nysna.org/general/communications/nursejackie.htm.)

The Weather Man: 2005. This comedy-drama stars Nicholas Cage as Dave Spritz, a Chicago weather man who gets paid very well for spending 2 hours a day, as he puts it, "basically reading prompts." Dave's father, Robert, played by Michael Caine, is a Pulitzer Prize–winning writer. Dave feels that he disappoints and fails his father, as well as the rest of his family: his estranged wife, his teenage son, and daughter. When Dave learns that his father has a terminal illness, his reaction (to himself) is "Don't die yet, Robert; let me get it together." The movie follows Dave as he tries to do just that.

VIEWING POINTS: What do you think Dave means by "getting it together"? How does his work (and his comparison of it with that of his father) affect his self-identity? What does the movie, through Dave and his "American accomplishment," say about work and status in Western nations?

Waydowntown: 2000. This dark comedy, set in Calgary's interconnected downtown core, opens on the 28th day of a wager among four young office workers. The winner of their wager will be the one who can stay indoors the longest; each has bet a month's salary and the winner will take all. When we meet them on day 28, they are struggling, not only to stay indoors but also to stay sane.

VIEWING POINTS: How does this movie heighten the sense of the workplace as the ultimate influence on a person's everyday life? What do you think Tom, Sandra, Curt, and Randy are discovering about themselves and about living meaningfully as they exist within the confines of their wager?

Norma Rae: 1979. An Academy award–winning film about a woman working in a textile mill in the southern United States who fights to organize a union for workers to address low wages, long hours, and unsafe workplace conditions. It was inspired by a true story.

VIEWING POINTS: Consider how the environment of the textile mill impacted the mental health of the workers. Do you think the struggle for better conditions affected workers' mental health in positive ways? Negative ways? Explain your position.

REFERENCES

Alderson, M. (2008). Work structure in the chronic care setting: Possible consequences for nurses' mental health. *Canadian Journal of Nursing Research, 40*(3), 160–178.

Allender, S., Colquhoun, D., & Kelly, P. (2006). Competing discourses of workplace health. *Health: An Interdisciplinary Journal for the Social Study of Health, Illness and Medicine, 10*(1), 75–93.

Austin, W., Goble, E., Leier, B., & Byrne, P. (2009). Compassion fatigue: The experience of nurses. *Ethics & Social Welfare, 3*(2), 195–214.

Blustein, D. (2008). *The psychology of working: A new perspective for career development, counseling, and public policy*. Mahwah, NJ: Lawrence Erlbaum Associates Inc.

Burns, T., Catty, J., Becker, T., Drake, R., Fioritti, A., Knapp, M., et al. (2007). The effectiveness of supported employment for people with severe mental illness: A randomized controlled trial. *The Lancet, 370*, 1146–1152.

Canadian Council on Social Development. (1999, April). *Work, family and community: Key issues and directions for future research*. Prepared for the Labour Program Human Resources and Skills Development Canada. Retrieved from http://www.hrsdc.gc.ca/eng/lp/spila/wlb/wfc/01presentation.shtml

Canadian Federation of Mental Health Nurses. (2006, January). *Canadian Standards of Psychiatric-Mental Health Nursing* (3rd ed.). Available at http://www.cfmhn.ca/standards.html

Canadian Nurses Association. (2008). *Code of ethics for registered nurses*. Ottawa, ON: Author.

Chappell, D., & Di Martino, V. (Eds.) (2000). *Violence at work* (2nd ed.). Geneva: International Labour Organization, Programme on Safety and Health at Work and the Environment. Available at: http://www.ilo.org/public/english/protection/safework/violence/index.htm

Cho, J., Laschinger H., & Wong C. (2006). Workplace empowerment, work engagement and organizational commitment of new graduate nurses. *Canadian Journal of Nursing Leadership, 19*(3), 43–60.

Coholic, D., & Blackford, K. (2005). Exploring secondary trauma in sexual assault workers in northern Ontario locations: The challenges of working in the northern Ontario context. In K. Brownlee & J. R. Graham (Eds.), *Violence in the Family* (pp. 1–15). Toronto, ON: Canadian Scholar's Press Inc.

Commission on the Future of Health Care in Canada. (2002, February). *Shape of the future of health care*. Ottawa, ON: Author.

Couser, G. (2008). Challenges and opportunities for preventing depression in the workplace: A review of the evidence supporting workplace factor and interventions. *Journal of Occupational and Environmental Medicine, 50*(4), 411–427.

Dooley, D. (2003). Unemployment, underemployment, and mental health: Conceptualizing employment status as a continuum. *American Journal of Community Psychology, 32*(1/2), 9–20.

Dooley, D., & Catalano, R. (2003). Introduction to underemployment and its social costs. *American Journal of Community Psychology, 32*(1/2), 1–7.

Duxbury, L., & Higgins, C. (2005). Saying "No" in a culture of hours, money and non-support. *Ivey Business Journal Online.* Retrieved October 24, 2009, from http://www.iveybusinessjournal.com/view_article.asp?intArticle_ID=566

Duxbury, L., & Higgins, C. (2009). *Work-life conflict in Canada in the new millennium: Key findings and recommendations from the 2001 National Work-Life Conflict Study.* Ottawa, ON: Public Health Agency of Canada.

Fiore, M., Bailey, W., Cohen, S., Dorfman, S., Goldstein, M., Gritz, E., et al. (2008). *Treating tobacco use and dependence.* Clinical practice guideline. Rockville, MD: U.S. Department of Health and Human Services. Public Health Service.

Felblinger, D. M. (2008). Incivility and bullying in the workplace and nurses' shame responses. *Journal of Obstetric, Gynecologic & Neonatal Nursing, 37*(2), 234–241.

Friedland, D. S., & Price, R. H. (2003). Underemployment: Consequences for the health and well-being of workers. *American Journal of Community Psychology, 32*(1/2), 33–45.

Fryer, D., & Fagan, R. (2003). Toward a critical community psychological perspective on unemployment and mental health research. *American Journal of Community Psychology, 32*(1/2), 89–96.

Gold, P., & Waghorn, G. (2007). Comment: Supported employment for people with severe mental illness. *The Lancet, 370,* 1108–1109.

Gunnell, D., Platt, S., & Hawton, K. (2009). Editorial: The economic crisis and suicide: Consequences may be serious and warrant early attention. *British Medical Journal, 338,* 1456–1457.

Healey-Ogden, M. J. (2008). *The experience of well-being: Uncovering the mystery.* Unpublished doctoral dissertation, University of Alberta, Edmonton.

Hesketh, K. L., Duncan, S. M., Estabrooks, C. A., Reimer, M. A., Giovanetti, P., Hyndman, K., et al. (2003). Workplace violence in Alberta and British Columbia hospitals. *Health Policy, 63,* 311–321.

Human Resources and Skills Development Canada. (2002). *Addressing Work-life balance in Canada.* Available at: http://www.hrsdc.gc.ca/eng/lp/spila/wlb

Ipso Reid. (2007, November). Mental Health in the Workplace: Largest Study Ever Conducted of Canadian Workplace Mental Health and Depression. Public Release. Available at: http://www.ipsos-na.com

Kantor, R. (1997). *Work and family in the United States: A critical review and agenda for research and policy.* New York, NY: Russell Sage Foundation.

Kerr, M., & Mustard, C. (2007). The challenge of effective workplace change in the health sector. *HealthcarePapers, 7*(Sp), 69–73. Available at: www.healthcarepapers.com

Latimer, E., Lecomte, T., Becker, D., Drake, R., Duclos, I., Piat, M., et al. (2006). Generalisability of the individual placement and support model of supported employment: Results of a Canadian randomized controlled trial. *British Journal of Psychiatry, 189,* 65–73.

Lauber, C. (2009). Individual placement and support improves employment of young people with first episode psychosis. *Evidence Based Mental Health, 12,* 53.

Lavoie-Tremblay, M., Wright, D., Desforges, N., Gélinas, C., Marchionni, C., & Drevniok, U. (2008). Creating a healthy workplace for new-generation nurses. *Journal of Nursing Scholarship, 40*(3), 290–297.

Lero, D., Richardson, J., & Korabik, K. (2009). *Cost-benefit review of work-life balance practices—2009.* Gatineau, QC: Canadian Association of Administrators of Labour Legislation.

Lewis, S. (2006). Recognition of workplace bullying: A qualitative study of women targets in the public sector. *Journal of Community & Applied Social Psychology, 16,* 119–135.

Lowe, G. (2003). *Healthy workplaces and productivity: A discussion paper.* Ottawa, ON: Economic Analysis and Evaluation Division, Health Canada. Available at: http://www.grahamlowe.ca/documents/48/Healthy%20workplaces8

MacIntosh, J. (2005). Experiences of workplace bullying in a rural area. *Issues in Mental Health Nursing, 26,* 893–910.

Marchand, A., Demers, A., & Durand, P. (2006). Social structures, agent personality and workers' mental health: A longitudinal analysis of the specific role of occupation and of workplace constraints-resources on psychological distress in the Canadian workforce. *Human Relations, 59*(7), 875–901.

Maslach, C., Schaufeli, W. B., & Leiter, M. P. (2001). Job burnout. *Annual Review of Psychology, 52,* 397–422.

McKee-Ryan, F. M., Song, Z., Wanberg, C. R., & Kinicki, A. J. (2005). Psychological and physical well-being during unemployment: A meta-analytic study. *Journal of Applied Psychology, 90*(1), 53–76.

Mikkelsen, E. G., & Einarsen, S. (2002). Basic assumptions and symptoms of post-traumatic stress among victims of bullying at work. *European Journal of Work and Organizational Psychology, 11,* 87–111.

Namie, G. (2003). *The Workplace Bullying Institute 2003 report on abusive workplaces.* Retrieved June 26, 2009, from http://www.workplacebullying.org/res/2003results.pdf

Pompili, M., Rinaldi, G., Lester, D., Girardi, P., Ruberto, A., & Taterelli, R. (2006). Hopelessness and suicide risk emerge in psychiatric nurses suffering from burnout and using specific defense mechanisms. *Archives of Psychiatric Nursing, 20*(3), 135–143.

Public Health Agency of Canada. (2001). *A Report on Mental Illnesses in Canada.* Ottawa, ON: Author. Available at: http://www.phac-aspc.gc.ca/index-eng.php

Raderstorf, M., & Kurtz, J. (2006). Mental health issues in the workplace: Maintaining a productive work force. *American Association of Occupational Health Nurses Journal, 54*(8), 360–365.

Randall, R., Nielsen, K., & Tvedt, S. (2009). The development of five scales to measure employees' appraisals of organization-level stress management interventions. *Work & Stress, 23*(1), 1–23.

Registered Nurses' Association of Ontario. (2008). *Workplace health, safety and well-being of the nurse.* Toronto, ON: Author.

Reine, I., Novo, M., & Hammarström, A. (2008). Does transition from an unstable labour market position to permanent employment protect mental health? Results from a 14-year follow-up of school-leavers. *BMC Public Health, 8.* Retrieved July 21, 2009, from *http://www.biomedcentral.com/1471-2458/8/159*

Sarna, L., Bialous, S. A., Wewers, M. E., Froelicher, E. S., & Danao, L. (2004). Nurses, smoking, and the workplace. *Research in Nursing & Health, 28,* 79–90.

Severinsson, E. (2003). Moral stress and burnout: Qualitative content analysis. *Nursing and Health Sciences, 5*(1), 59–66.

Shamian, J., & El-Jardali, F. (2007). Healthy workplaces for health workers in Canada: Knowledge transfer and uptake in policy and practice. *HealthcarePapers, 7*(Sp), 6–25.

Sofield, L., & Salmond, S. W. (2003). Workplace violence: A focus on verbal abuse and intent to leave the organization. *Orthopaedic Nursing, 22,* 274–283.

Standing Senate Committee on Social Affairs, Science and Technology. (2006, May). *Out of the shadows at Last: Transforming mental health, mental illness and addiction services in Canada. Final report.* Ottawa, ON: The Committee.

Statistics Canada. (2006, December). National survey of the work and health of nurses. *The Daily.* Retrieved from http://www.statcan.gc.ca/daily-quotidien/061211/dq061211b-eng.htm

Statistics Canada. (2007, May). Study: Workaholics and time perception. *The Daily.* Retrieved from http://www.statcan.gc.ca/daily-quotidien/070515/dq070515c-eng.htm

The Tokyo Declaration. (1998). *The Tokyo Declaration on work-related stress and health in three postindustrial settings—The European Union, Japan and the United States.* Adopted at a "triangular" Conference at the Tokyo Medical University. Available at: http://www.workhealth.org/news/tokyo.html

Toppinen-Tanner, S., Ojajärvi, A., Väänänen, A., Kalimo, R., & Jäppinen, P. (2005). Burnout as a predictor of medically certified sick-leave absences and their diagnosed causes. *Behaviorial Medicine, 31,* 18–27.

Venes, D. (Ed.). (2009). *Taber's cyclopedic medical dictionary* (21st ed.). Philadelphia, PA: F.A. Davis Company.

Watson Wyatt. (2007, December). Workers' *Mental Health and Stress Affecting Business Results in Canada.* Toronto, ON: Authors. Available at: http://www.watsonwyatt.com/canada-english/

Winkelmann, R. (2009). Unemployment, social capital, and subjective well-being. *Journal of Happiness Studies, 10*(4), 421–430.

World Health Organization. (2001). *World Health Report 2001: Mental Health: New understanding, new hope.* Geneva, Switzerland: Author.

World Health Organization. (2005). *Mental health policies and programmes in the workplace.* Geneva, Switzerland: Author.

World Health Organization. (2006). *World Health Report 2006: Working together for health.* Geneva, Switzerland: Author.

World Health Organization. (2008). *World Health Report 2008: Primary health care: now more than ever.* Geneva, Switzerland: Author.

World Health Organization. (2009). Occupational health. Retrieved July 20, 2009, from http://www.who.int/occupational_health/en/index.html

Zapf, D., & Gross, C. (2001). Conflict escalation and coping with workplace bullying: A replication and extension. *European Journal of Work and Organizational Psychology, 10,* 497–522.

UNIT *II*

Foundations of Psychiatric and Mental Health Nursing

Contemporary Psychiatric and Mental Health Nursing Practice

Olive Yonge and Wendy Austin

Adapted from the chapter "Contemporary Psychiatric and Mental Health Nursing Practice" by Mary Ann Boyd

LEARNING OBJECTIVES

After studying this chapter, you will be able to:

- Explain the bio/psycho/social/spiritual model as a conceptual framework for understanding and treating mental health problems and disorders.
- Delineate the scope and standards of psychiatric and mental health nursing practice.
- Identify the seven domains of practice used to structure the *Canadian Standards of Psychiatric-Mental Health Nursing*.
- Describe the competencies associated with each domain.
- Discuss the basic tools of psychiatric and mental health nursing.
- Discuss identified challenges of psychiatric and mental health nursing.
- Discuss the impact of professional organizations on psychiatric and mental health nursing.

KEY CONCEPTS

- bio/psycho/social/spiritual model
- standards of practice

KEY TERMS

•clinical decision making•competencies•critical pathways•domains of practice•interdisciplinary approach•multidisciplinary approach

*T*his chapter introduces the bio/psycho/social/spiritual model as the organizational thread for the rest of the book. The scope of psychiatric and mental health (PMH) nursing is explained, followed by a discussion of the standards of practice expected of Canadian nurses working in PMH care settings. These standards are integral to the understanding of day-to-day practice and should be familiar to all students involved in PMH nursing. The discussion of the challenges of PMH nursing sets the stage for the rest of the text through an overview of the dynamic nature of this specialty.

THE BIO/PSYCHO/SOCIAL/ SPIRITUAL MODEL OF PMH NURSING

Contemporary PMH nursing uses theories from the biologic, psychological, and social sciences as a basis of practice. As well, PMH nurses are increasingly informed by knowledge from the spiritual domain of human health (Barker & Buchanan-Barker, 2004). This holistic approach, referred to as the bio/psycho/social/spiritual model of PMH nursing, is necessary to truly understand

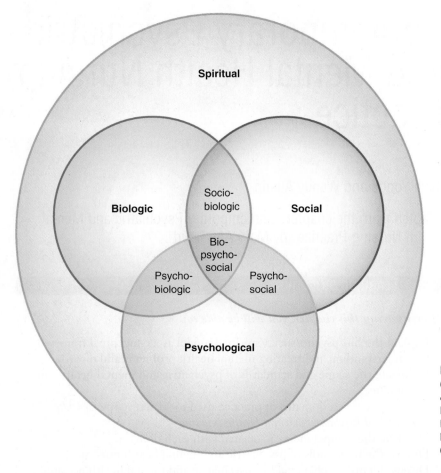

FIGURE 6.1 Bio/psycho/social/spiritual model. (Originally adapted from Abraham, I., Fox, J., & Cohen, B. [1992]. Integrating the bio into the bio/psycho/social: Understanding and treating biological phenomena in psychiatric mental health nursing. *Archives of Psychiatric Nursing*, 6[5], 296–305.)

the individual who is experiencing mental health problems or a mental disorder. Holism joins the biological, psychological, social, and spiritual domains in an integrated, dynamic, evolutionary, and vital conceptualization of human health (Hood Morris, 1996). The model is ideal for organizing nursing care and is used throughout this text for organizing theoretic knowledge and the nursing process (Fig. 6-1).

> **KEY CONCEPT** The **bio/psycho/social/spiritual model** consists of separate but interdependent domains: biologic, psychological, social, and spiritual. Each domain can be understood independently but can interact and be mutually interdependent with the other domains.

Biologic Domain

The *biologic* domain consists of the biologic theories related to mental disorders and problems as well as *all* of the biologic activity related to other health problems. Today, there is evidence of neurobiologic changes in most psychiatric disorders. Within this domain, there are also theories and concepts used as a basis of interventions focusing on the client's physical functioning, such as exercise, relaxation,

sleep, and adequate nutrition. In addition, the neurobiologic theories also serve as a basis for understanding such biologic treatments as pharmacologic agents and electroconvulsive therapy (see Chapter 10).

Psychological Domain

The *psychological* domain contains the theoretical basis of the psychological processes—thoughts, feelings, and behaviour (intrapersonal dynamics) that influence one's emotion, cognition, and behaviour. The psychological and nursing sciences generate theories and research that are critical to understanding a client's symptoms and responses to mental disorders. Although mental disorders have a biologic component, they are often manifested in psychological symptoms and physical changes. The person with a thought disorder may have bizarre behaviour that needs to be interpreted within the context of the neurobiologic dysfunction of the mental disorder.

Many PMH nursing interventions are based on knowledge generated within this domain. Cognitive approaches, behaviour therapy, and client education are all based on the use of theories from the psychological domain. These interventions are explained in Unit III. PMH interventions are also based on the use of interpersonal communication techniques, which require nurses to develop awareness of their own, as well as their client's, internal thoughts, feelings, and behaviour. For PMH nurses, exploring their own and coming to understand their client's intrapersonal dynamics and motivation is critical to the development of a therapeutic relationship that motivates clients to learn about and understand their disorders and participate in their management. Motivating clients to engage in learning activities best occurs within the context of a therapeutic relationship (see Chapter 9).

Social Domain

The *social* domain includes theories that account for the influence of social forces (including cultural forces) encompassing the client, family, and community. This knowledge base is generated from social and nursing sciences and delineates the connections within families and communities that affect the health and treatment of people with mental disorders. Understanding family factors, including origin, extended family, and other significant relationships, contributes to the total understanding and treatment of individual clients. Family-based interventions can reduce rates of relapse and improve the recovery of the client, as well as positively influence family well-being (Heru, 2006). Psychiatric disorders and their treatment can be significantly affected by the society in which the client lives. Public attitudes and beliefs about mental illness can be supportive or stigmatizing, making individuals with mental disorders vulnerable to prejudice and discrimination. Community forces, including cultural and ethnic groups within larger communities, shape clients' manifestation of disorders, response to treatment, and overall experience of living with a mental illness. Community-based issues such as housing, employment opportunities, and access to health and social services have a broad impact on both mental health and recovery from mental illness. Nurses need to understand these forces within the communities where they practice. (See Chapter 3 for the cultural, legal, and socioeconomic context of mental health care.)

The Spiritual Domain

The spiritual domain encompasses the bio/psycho/social domains. Spirituality is about the core of whom we are and the connections within and among self, others, and the universe over time and space. Spirituality is a complex, even mysterious, concept involving the thoughts, feelings, beliefs, and values that give meaning and purpose to one's life. One definition of spirituality is "the essence of our being, which permeates our living and infuses our unfolding awareness of who and what we are, our purpose in being, and our inner resources; and shapes our life journey" (Dossey, Keegan, & Guzzetta, 2004, p. 91). Spirituality may also be regarded as the driving force that pervades all aspects of and gives meaning to an individual's life. It creates a set of beliefs and values that influence the way that people conduct their lives. Spiritual activity involves introspection, reflection, and a sense of connectedness to others or to the universe. For many people, this connectedness focuses ultimately on a supreme being who is sometimes called God. (Catalano, 2006, p. 396)

Although there remains a lack of agreement concerning the way spirituality should be defined, a review of the interdisciplinary literature on spirituality reveals common themes: Everyone has the potential for spirituality and spiritual growth; the way one lives one's life is reflective of spirituality; spirituality is relational in nature; and there is a link among religion, spirituality, and moral norms (Catalano). Religion differs, nevertheless, from spirituality. Religion involves organized systems of rituals, patterns of beliefs, and groups of people usually congregating around the worship of a deity. A person may be spiritual but not religious, both religious and spiritual, or religious but not spiritual (Mauk & Schmidt, 2004).

Spiritual growth may be stimulated by pivotal life events, even distressing ones like being diagnosed with a mental disorder. It can be very difficult, however, to transcend one's current reality and the suffering it may entail. O'Reilly (2004) noted that mentally ill individuals often struggle with the loss of meaning and purpose. They may wonder "Why has this happened to me?" and be affected by religious or cultural beliefs that view mental illness as a form of punishment. The nurse can help individuals experiencing spiritual distress by supporting their efforts to find meaning in their circumstances, which may include meditation, contemplation, prayer, and other spiritual practices that may give comfort. The relationship of the body, mind, relation, and spirit in the content of human health is holistic, synergistic, and unifying. The bio/psycho/social/spiritual model of PMH nursing is used as the framework for assessment and nursing care planning in this Canadian text.

■ STANDARDS OF PROFESSIONAL PRACTICE

As a regulated health profession, nurses are given the authority to practice under provincial or territorial laws that set out governance, registration, and discipline requirements as a means of protecting the public. These laws require the provincial or territorial nursing regulatory bodies to set, monitor, and enforce standards of practice that, along with the Code of Ethics for Registered Nurses (see Chapter 7), articulate the profession's values, knowledge, and skills. Such standards facilitate the profession's self-governance because they make explicit the profession's expectations of its members' **competencies**

BOX 6.1

Canadian Federation of Mental Health Nurses

Formed in 1988, the Federation's initial endeavour was to achieve national credentialing in PMH nursing. It did so in 1995.

A strong voice for this specialty practice, today the Federation's objectives are to:

- Assure national leadership in the development and application of nursing standards that inform and affect PMH nursing practice.
- Examine and influence government policy and address national issues related to mental health and mental illness.
- Communicate and collaborate with national and international groups that share professional interests.
- Facilitate excellence in PMH nursing by providing our members with educational and networking resources.

From Canadian Federation of Mental Health Nurses. (2006). *The Canadian standards for psychiatric-mental health nursing* (3rd ed.). Toronto, ON: Author. Available at: http://www.cfmhn.ca/resources/multimedia/PDF/28065-singles.pdf

and performance. In Canada, specialty areas of nursing practice are designated by the Canadian Nurses Association (CNA). The CNA requires any specialty group desiring designation to establish its own standards of practice. The Canadian Federation of Mental Health Nurses (CFMHN), an associate group with CNA, created the first Canadian PMH nursing standards and achieved designation in 1995 (see Box 6-1).

KEY CONCEPT **Standards** are used by nurses to guide their own actions and to communicate to others the desired and achievable level of performance in providing nursing care (CNA, 1998).

Canadian Standards of PMH Nursing

The *Canadian Standards of Psychiatric-Mental Health Nursing* (the Standards) were developed by expert PMH nurses in 1996 (Austin, Gallop, Harris, & Spencer, 1996), revised in 1998 (CFMHN, 1998) with a greater community focus, and revised again in 2006 (CFMHN, 2006). For the 2006 revision, input was sought from consumer groups through focus groups across Canada. The facilitators of the focus groups noted how powerful this experience was for them, and the current standards have been markedly influenced by their input, particularly in the area of forming partnerships. (Note: In the third edition of the Standards, the term *psychiatric-mental health nursing* became hyphenated; however, this text continues to use the term without a hyphen.)

CRNENOTE

Use the *Canadian Standards for Psychiatric-Mental Health Nursing* (CFMHN, 2006) as one guide to studying for the CRNE.

Domains of Practice

The Standards are organized by a **"domains of practice"** framework (Benner, 1984), with competencies classified within seven domains. In the Standards, each domain is described, and the specific competencies necessary to meet that standard are listed (see Boxes 6-2 to 6-8.).

Nurses' achievement of competent practice is shaped by the nursing model they utilize, as well as by the social, cultural, economic, and political factors that act on the health care environment (Health and Welfare Canada, 1988). Beliefs underlying the Standards include the belief that the therapeutic use of self, based on trust and mutual respect, is at the core of PMH nursing practice and that continual advances in knowledge necessitate the incorporation of new research-based findings into practice. Also foundational to the Standards is a belief in holistic, reflective, ethical practice that includes the protection of human rights and the alleviation of the stigma and discrimination associated with mental illness. The importance of equitable access to culturally competent care is acknowledged. A belief in quality practice environments is also espoused. PMH nurses usually practice in multidisciplinary settings and need to be aware of the impact of team dynamics on care. In interdisciplinary settings, there may be an overlapping of professional roles, with nurses being accountable for both the discrete and shared functions within their practice. Within the Standards, it is acknowledged that supporting these identified beliefs can involve sociopolitical action to promote awareness of issues and to influence health policy (CFMHN, 2006).

TOOLS OF PMH NURSING PRACTICE

Clinical Decision Making

Decision making involves critical thinking and is at the core of clinical practice. **Clinical decision making** focuses on the choices made in clinical settings. In addition to the complex decisions, such as collecting, processing, and organizing information and formulating nursing approaches, many moment-to-moment decisions are made, such as deciding whether a client should receive a PRN medication. The development and implementation of efficacious interventions involves critical analysis of client, family, and community data and making decisions about care. Such decision making should involve the client, family, and other significant stakeholders as

BOX 6.2

Canadian Standards of Psychiatric-Mental Health Nursing

STANDARD I: *Provides Competent Professional Care Through the Development of a Therapeutic Relationship*

A primary goal of PMH nursing is the promotion of mental health and the prevention or diminution of mental disorder. The development of a therapeutic relationship is the foundation from where the PMH nurse can "enter into partnerships with clients, and through the use of the human sciences, and the art of caring, develop helping relationships" (CNA, 1997, p. 43).

The nurse is expected to demonstrate competence in therapeutic relationships by the following:

1. Assesses and clarifies the influences of personal beliefs, values, and life experience on the therapeutic relationship and distinguishes between social and therapeutic relationships.
2. Works in partnership with the client, family, and relevant others to determine goal-directed needs and establishes an environment that is conducive to goal achievement.
3. Uses a range of therapeutic verbal and nonverbal communication skills that include empathy, active listening, observing, genuineness, and curiosity.
4. Recognizes the influence of culture, class, ethnicity, language, stigma, and social exclusion on the therapeutic

process and negotiates care that is sensitive to these influences.
5. Mobilizes and advocates for resources that increase clients' and families' access to mental health services and that improve community integration.
6. Understands and responds to human reactions to distress and loss of control that may be expressed as anger, anxiety, fear, grief, helplessness, hopelessness, and humour.
7. Guides the client through behavioural, developmental, emotional, or spiritual change while acknowledging and supporting the client's participation, responsibility, and choices in self care.
8. Supports the client's and family's sense of resiliency, self-esteem, power, and hope through continuity of a therapeutic relationship, on a 1:1 basis or within a group context.
9. Fosters mutuality of the relationship by reflectively critiquing therapeutic effectiveness through client and family responses, clinical supervision, and self-evaluation.
10. Understands the nature of chronic illness and applies the principles of health promotion and disease prevention when working with clients and families.

BOX 6.3

Canadian Standards of Psychiatric-Mental Health Nursing

STANDARD II: *Performs/Refines Client Assessments Through the Diagnostic and Monitoring Function*

Effective assessment, diagnosis, and monitoring is central to the nurse's role and is dependent on theory, as well as on understanding the meaning of the health or illness experience from the perspective of the client. This knowledge, integrated with the nurse's conceptual model of nursing practice, provides a framework for processing client data and for developing client-focused plans of care. The nurse makes professional judgments regarding the relevance and importance of these data and acknowledges the client as a valued and respected partner throughout the decision-making process.

The nurse is expected to demonstrate competence in the mental health assessment tools in various workplaces, for example, mental status exam and recovery principles.

The nurse explains to the client the assessment process and content and provides feedback for all of the following:

1. Collaborates with clients and with other members of the health care team to gather holistic assessments through observation, examination, interview, and consultation, while being attentive to issues of confidentiality and pertinent legal statutes.
2. Documents and analyzes baseline data to identify health status, potential for wellness, health care deficits,

potential for danger to self and others; alterations in thought content or process, affect behaviour, communication and decision-making abilities; substance use and dependency; and history of trauma or abuse (emotional, physical, neglect—sexual or verbal).
3. Formulates and documents a plan of care in collaboration with the client and with the mental health team, recognizing variability in the client's ability to participate in the process.
4. Refines and extends client assessment information by assessing and documenting significant change in the client's status and by comparing new data with the baseline assessment and intermediate client goals.
5. Continuously assesses status and anticipates potential problems and risks. Collaborates with the client to examine his or her environment for risk factors: self-care, housing, nutrition, economic, psychological, and social. Utilizes assessment data to identify potential risks to client and others. Advocates and practices for interventions that are appropriate to risk type and level.
6. Determines most appropriate and available therapeutic modality that will potentially best meet client's needs, and assists the client to access these resources.

BOX 6.4

Canadian Standards of Psychiatric-Mental Health Nursing

STANDARD III: *Administers and Monitors Therapeutic Interventions*

Due to the nature of mental health problems and mental disorders, there are unique practice issues confronting the PMH nurse in the assessment phase and the administration of therapeutic interventions. Safety in PMH nursing has unique meaning because many clients are at risk for harm to self or others and self-neglect. Clients may not be mentally competent to participate in all aspects of decision making. However, every effort must be made to include the client. In collaboration with the client, the PMH nurse needs to be alert to adverse reactions as clients' ability to self-report may be impaired.

The PMH nurse uses evidence-based and experiential knowledge from nursing, health sciences, and related mental health disciplines to both select and tailor nursing interventions. The nurse

1. Utilizes and evaluates evidence-based interventions to provide safe, effective, and efficient nursing care.
2. Provides information to clients and families/significant others, ensuring that the client consents to such information being shared, on an on-going basis about care and treatment.
3. Assists, educates, and empowers clients to select choices that will support positive changes in their affect, cognition, behaviour, and relationships, even when some of these choices may involve a level of risk as assessed by the clinical team (CNA, 1997, p. 68).
4. Supports clients to draw on own assets and resources for self-care, activities of daily living, mobilizing resources, and mental health promotion (CNA, 1997, p. 68).

5. Makes discretionary clinical decisions, using knowledge of client's unique responses and paradigm cases as the basis for the decision (e.g., frequency of client contact in the community).
6. Uses appropriate technology to perform safe, effective, and efficient nursing intervention (CNA, 1997, p. 68).
7. Administers medications accurately and safely, monitoring therapeutic responses, reactions, untoward effects, toxicity, and potential incompatibilities with other medications or substances. Provides medication education with appropriate content and in accordance with workplace policies.
8. Assesses client responses to deficits in activities of daily living, mobilizes resources in response to client's capabilities, and offers alternatives when appropriate.
9. Provides support and assists with protection for clients experiencing difficulty with self-protection.
10. Utilizes therapeutic elements of group process.
11. Incorporates knowledge of family dynamics and cultural values and beliefs about families in the provision of care.
12. Collaborates with the client, health care providers, and community to access and coordinate resources and seeks feedback from the client and others regarding interventions.
13. Incorporates knowledge of community needs or responses in the provision of care.
14. Encourages and assists clients to seek out support groups for mutual aid and support.
15. Assesses the client's response to, and perception of, nursing and other therapeutic interventions.

much as possible. Reflective thinking about the client's illness experience and personal response to the treatment and care situation is an important aspect of choosing interventions as well. The nurse needs to have a thorough understanding of the rationale and the theoretical underpinnings of the client's care plan.

Critical Pathways in Care Planning

Many psychiatric facilities use **critical pathways** to ensure a quality level of care in a cost-effective way. These care paths are similar to individual treatment plans in that all the disciplines' interventions are included on one plan. Critical pathways, however, are designed for a hypothetical client who has typical symptoms and who follows an expected course of treatment. Care paths are not developed for each individual client. This unification of care can be helpful if it means that best practices shape the care received by all clients and if it facilitates the use of expert knowledge by all those providing care. It is not helpful if the unique needs and situation of each client

and family are ignored, or if nurses are restrained in their provision of thoughtful, sensitive care.

■ INTERDISCIPLINARY APPROACH AND THE NURSE'S ROLE

Several professionals other than nurses and physicians provide mental health services. These professionals come from a variety of disciplines and provide services based on their training and licensure, which may vary from province to province. PMH care has a long tradition of using a **multidisciplinary approach**, with several disciplines providing services to a client. In the hospital, a client may be seeing a psychiatrist for the management of the disorder symptoms and for prescribed medications; a psychiatric social worker for individual psychotherapy; a psychiatric nurse for the management of responses related to the mental disorder, administration of medication, and monitoring side effects; and an occupational therapist for transition into the workplace. In the community clinic,

BOX 6.5

Canadian Standards of Psychiatric-Mental Health Nursing

STANDARD IV: *Effectively Manages Rapidly Changing Situations*

The effective management of rapidly changing situations is essential in critical circumstances that may be termed psychiatric emergencies. These situations include self-harm and assaultive behaviours and rapidly changing mental health states. This domain also includes evidence-based assessment and screening for risk factors and referral related to psychiatric illnesses and social problems (e.g., substance abuse, violence/abuse, and suicide/homicide; Society for Education and Research in Psychiatric-Mental Health Nursing, 1996, p. 41).

The nurse

1. Utilizes the therapeutic relationship throughout the management of rapidly changing situations.
2. Assesses the client using a comprehensive holistic approach for actual or potential health problems, issues, and risk factors and for crisis/emergency/catastrophic situations (e.g., psychotic episode, neuroleptic malignant syndrome, acute onset of extra pyramidal side effects, substance abuse, violence/abuse and suicide/homicide, drug toxicity, and delirium).
3. Knows resources required to manage actual and potential crisis/emergency/catastrophic situations and plans access to these resources.
4. Monitors client safety and utilizes continual assessment to detect early changes in client status, and intervenes accordingly.
5. Implements timely, age-appropriate, client-specific crisis/emergency/catastrophic interventions as necessary.

6. Commences critical procedures: In an institutional setting, for example, suicide precautions, emergency restraint, elopement precautions, infectious disease management, when necessary; in a community setting, uses appropriate community support systems, such as police, ambulance services, and crisis response resources.
7. Coordinates care to prevent errors and duplication of efforts where rapid intervention is imperative.
8. Utilizes a "least restraint" approach to care.
9. Develops and adequately documents the crisis/emergency/catastrophic intervention/plan.
10. Evaluates the effectiveness of the rapid responses and modifies critical plans as necessary.
11. In collaboration with the client, facilitates the involvement of the family and significant others to assist in the identification of the precipitates of the crisis/emergency event and plans to minimize risk for recurrence.
12. Participates in "debriefing" process with team (including client and family) and other service providers (e.g., reviews of critical event and emergency situation).
13. Utilizes safety measures to protect self, colleagues, and clients from potentially abusive situations in the work environment (e.g., harassment, psychological abuse, and physical aggression).
14. Implements appropriate protocols for disasters.
15. Participates in educational, organizational, and institutional activities, which improve client safety in the practice setting.

BOX 6.6

Canadian Standards of Psychiatric-Mental Health Nursing

STANDARD V: *Effectively Manages Rapidly Changing Situations*

All nurse–client interactions are potentially teaching/learning situations. The PMH nurse attempts to understand the life experience of the client and uses this understanding to support and promote learning related to health and personal development. The nurse provides health promotion information to individual, family, and group populations and communities.

The nurse

1. In collaboration with clients determines clients' learning needs.
2. Plans and implements, with the client, health promotion education while considering the context of the client's life experiences andconsiders readiness, culture, literacy, language, preferred learning style, and resources available.
3. Engages with the client to explore available options and resources to build knowledge to make informed choices

related to health needs and to navigate the system as needed.
4. Facilitates the client's search for ways to find meaning of their experience.
5. Incorporates knowledge of a wide variety of learning models and principles when creating opportunities for clients, for example, health promotion models, adult-learning principles, stages of development, cultural competence, and health beliefs models.
6. Provides relevant information guidance and support to the client's significant others.
7. Documents the teaching/learning process (assessment, plan, implementation, client involvement, and evaluation).
8. Determines, with the client, the effectiveness of the educational process and collaboratively develops or adapts the ways to meet learning needs.
9. Engages in teaching/learning opportunities as partners with community agencies and consumer and family groups.

BOX 6.7

Canadian Standards of Psychiatric-Mental Health Nursing

STANDARD VI: *Monitors and Ensures the Quality of Health Care Practices*

The nurse has a responsibility to advocate for the client's right to receive the least restrictive form of care and to respect and affirm the client's right to self-determination in a safe, fair, and just manner. Mental health care occurs under the provisions of provincial or territorial mental health acts and related legislation. It is essential for the PMH nurse to be informed regarding the interpretation of relevant legislation and its implications for nursing practice.

The nurse

1. Identifies workplace cultures (philosophy, attitudes, values, and beliefs) that affect the nurse's ability to perform with skill, safety, and compassion and takes action as appropriate.
2. Explores how the determinants of health that affect the health of the community (e.g., poverty, malnutrition, and unsafe housing) affect mental health nursing practice.

3. Understands current and relevant legislation and the implications for nursing practice, for example, privacy laws.
4. Expands and incorporates knowledge of innovations and changes in mental health and psychiatric nursing practice to ensure safe and effective care.
5. Ensures and documents ongoing review and evaluation of PMH nursing care activities.
6. Understands and questions the interdependent functions of the team within the overall plan of care.
7. Advocates for the client within the context of organizational and professional parameters and family and community interests.
8. Advocates for changes and improvements to the system/organizational structures in keeping with the principles of delivering safe, ethical, and competent care.
9. Recognizes the dynamic changes in health care locally and globally and, in collaboration with stakeholders, develops strategies to manage these changes. For example, considers changes in determinants of health that affect the community (e.g., terrorism, decline of industries).

BOX 6.8

Canadian Standards of Psychiatric-Mental Health Nursing

STANDARD VII: *Practices Within Organizational and Work-Role Structure*

The PMH nursing role is assumed within organizational structures, in both community and institutional contexts, through the provision of PMH care. For the PMH nurse, the ethics of care is based on reflective and evidence-based practice judgments within complex and dynamic situations. The increasing move of mental health and psychiatric treatment into the community necessitates the PMH nurse to be knowledgeable and skillful in collaborative care planning and implementation, mental health promotion, social action, and community consultation.

The nurse

1. Works in collaborative partnerships with clients, families, and other stakeholders to facilitate healing environments that ensure the safety, support, and respect of all individuals.
2. Understands quality outcome indicators and strives for continuous quality improvement.
3. Actively participates with nurses to sustain and promote a climate that supports ethical practice and the

establishment of a moral community (Varcoe, Rodney, & McCormick, 2003).
4. Participates in supporting a climate of trust that sponsors openness, encouraging questioning of the status quo, and the reporting of incompetent care (CNA, 2002).
5. Seeks to utilize constructive and collaborative approaches to resolve differences affecting care among members of the health care team (CNA, 2002).
6. Actively participates in developing, implementing, and critiquing mental health policy for community and institutional settings.
7. Supports the contribution of leadership, as it occurs within the advanced practice role, to effective care and treatment.
8. Practices independently within legislated scope of practice.
9. Supports and participates in mentoring and coaching new graduates.
10. Utilizes knowledge of collaborative strategies for social action in working with consumer and advocacy groups.

From Canadian Federation of Mental Health Nurses. (2006). *The Canadian standards for psychiatric-mental health nursing* (3rd ed.). Toronto, ON: Author.

---

a client may meet weekly with a therapist, monthly with a physician or nurse practitioner who reviews response to prescribed medication, and twice a week with a group leader in a day treatment program. All of these professionals bring a specialized skill to the client's care.

However, a multidisciplinary approach may lead to fragmented care when approaches are independent of each other. An **interdisciplinary approach**, in which interventions from the different disciplines are integrated in the delivery of care, can be more effective. In this model, a nurse and a psychologist may simultaneously intervene with a client on changing a behaviour related to medication compliance. An interdisciplinary approach requires close collaboration among the care team.

When an interdisciplinary approach is taken, it involves the creation and implementation of an integrated care plan. Nursing care will be a component of the plan, and aspects of collaboration should be outlined. It is often the nurse who coordinates the delivery of care by the various disciplines.

CHALLENGES OF PMH NURSING

The challenges of PMH nursing are increasing in the 21st century. New knowledge is being generated, technology is shaping health care into new dimensions, and nursing practice is becoming more specialized and autonomous. This section discusses a few of the challenges.

Knowledge Development, Dissemination, and Application

Results of new research efforts continually redefine our knowledge base relative to mental disorders and their treatment. For instance, there have been significant advances in neurobiologic knowledge. In the 1970s, the cause of schizophrenia was hypothesized to be overactivity of dopamine. Later, it was discovered that other neurotransmitters seemed to play a role as well. Such knowledge resulted in new medications with various side-effect profiles becoming available, requiring nurses to redefine their monitoring and interventions related to medication administration.

The presence of comorbid medical disorders is gaining importance in the treatment of mental disorders. For example, hypertension, hypothyroidism, hyperthyroidism, and diabetes mellitus all affect the treatment of psychiatric disorders. In some settings, the nurse may be the only one who has a background in medical disorders, such as human immunodeficiency viral illness, acquired immunodeficiency syndrome, and other somatic health problems.

The challenge for nurses today is to stay abreast of the advances in total health care in order to provide safe, competent care to individuals with mental disorders. Nurses must strive to provide evidence-based nursing care, developing their knowledge on an ongoing basis. Accessing up-to-date information through journals, electronic databases, and continuing education programs is a recognized responsibility.

Not only do nurses need to access current research studies but they also must evaluate the usefulness of the studies. For instance, one research project supporting a particular treatment approach may not be as meaningful as several statistically significant studies. The results of qualitative research studies, although not generalizable, may have important implications for practice, for instance, insights that can deepen our understanding of client experiences. Nurses practicing in PMH settings are challenged to improve care by integrating knowledge into a bio/psycho/social/spiritual model that includes all human responses to potential or actual health problems.

Health Care Delivery System Challenges

Additional continuing challenges for Canadian PMH nurses include supporting the integration of mental health care within primary health care, articulating the influence of the determinants of health on mental health, and supporting the development of a national strategy for mental health and mental illness. Competent, ethical PMH nursing care provided within integrated hospital and community health services is needed to meet the emerging needs of the Canadian population. Assertive community treatment, for instance, reduces inpatient service use, promotes continuity of outpatient care, and increases the stability and quality of life of clients with serious mental illnesses. Nurses have a role making the Canadian health care system more responsive to the mental health needs of individuals, families, and the community.

Consumers of mental health services are gaining voice and calling for changes in the delivery of services. Inequities in health care for marginalized populations, such as those living with a chronic mental illness, are being challenged. Paternalistic approaches to the delivery of care are being actively rejected, and the use of partnership models is being advocated. Nurses and other health professionals are collaborating with consumers to effect these positive changes.

Impact of Technology

The impact of technologic advances on PMH nursing is unprecedented. Nurses are challenged to gain and develop the skills to use this technology in improving care. Telemedicine, for example, takes many forms, from communicating with remote sites to completing educational programs. Technology can facilitate clients and families in learning about disorders, treatment, and resources. Software programs can make daily functioning easier for some, and e-mail and the Internet are effective forms of communication. Advocacy groups for consumers of mental health services use these means to organize and lobby for change locally, nationally, and internationally.

A significant challenge related to new technology is maintaining client confidentiality. Client records, once stored in remote areas and rarely viewed, are now readily available and easily accessed. Nurses need to be vigilant in maintaining privacy and confidentiality. Moreover, documentation skills need to be updated continually to reflect quality client care within the changing health care environment.

Advances in neuroimaging and genetic technologies further challenge nurses to stay up to date on the evolution of neuroscience assessment techniques and new understandings regarding the etiology of mental disorders. Nurses need to be well-informed if they are to respond appropriately to clients' questions about new directions in mental health care.

PMH NURSING ORGANIZATIONS

Whereas the establishment and reinforcement of standards go a long way toward legitimizing PMH nursing, it is professional organizations that provide leadership in shaping mental health care. They do so by providing a strong voice for meaningful legislation that promotes quality client care and advocates for the maximal use of nursing skills.

The CNA is one such organization. Although its focus is on addressing the emergent needs of nursing in general, the CNA supports PMH nursing practice through such activities as advocating for PMH nursing at the national and provincial levels and working closely with PMH nursing organizations. The CNA is a federation of 11 provincial and territorial registered nurses associations. The CNA speaks for Canadian registered nurses; represents Canadian nursing to other organizations on national and international levels; and advocates for healthy public policy within a quality, publicly funded health care system. The membership of more than 136,200 registered nurses is broad and diverse and reflects the face of nursing today.

Canadian Certification as a PMH Nurse

Nurses with a current registration and license in Canada who have completed a minimum of 3,900 hours in PMH nursing practice within the past 5 years (Option A) *or* who have a nursing degree or post–basic course/program in the specialty (of at least 300 hours) and have accumulated a minimum of 1,950 hours of PMH nursing practice during the past 3 years (Option B) are eligible to apply for national certification by the CNA, provided they have endorsement by a supervisor or consultant in the specialty. Upon achieving a Pass on the PMHN Certification examination, the nurse is certified for 5 years and can use CPMHN(C) after their name. Recertification is possible if 100 hours of continuous learning activities in the specialty were completed during the 5 years or by retaking the Certification examination.

The Registered Psychiatric Nurse

In the four western provinces of British Columbia, Alberta, Saskatchewan, and Manitoba, PMH nursing is also practiced by registered psychiatric nurses (RPNs). These nurses have provincial regulatory bodies (separate from those of registered nurses) that register graduates from psychiatric nursing programs (ranging from diploma, to postdiploma, to degree).

Other Associations

The American Psychiatric Nurses Association (APNA) is the equivalent of the CFMHN in the United States. Its primary mission is advancing the PMH nursing practice; improving mental health care for culturally diverse individuals, families, groups, and communities; and shaping health policy for the delivery of mental health services.

The International Society of Psychiatric-Mental Health Nurses (ISPN) is an organization that works to unite and strengthen the presence and the voice of PMH nurses and to promote quality care for individuals and families with mental health problems. The ISPN consists of three specialist divisions: the Association of Child and Adolescent Psychiatric Nurses, the International Society of Psychiatric Consultation Liaison Nurses, and the Society for Education and Research in Psychiatric-Mental Health Nursing. Student memberships are available.

In Canada, there is a close relationship between mental health providers and those receiving care. One example of this relationship is the Canadian Alliance on Mental Illness and Mental Health (CAMIMH). CAMIMH, created in 1998, consists of consumers, their families, researchers, and care providers from numerous professions. Their mission is to influence national policy, to speak in a unified voice, and to focus strategically on mental health and mental illness. CAMIMH is also a member of the Canadian Collaborative Mental Health Initiative (CCMHI). The CCMHI has received national funding from Health Canada's Primary Health Care Transition Fund. Their primary goal is to improve the mental health of Canadians by strengthening relationships and enhancing collaboration among consumers, families, communities, and health care providers. They believe that consumers require access to services from the appropriate providers, in a timely manner, at an accessible location, and with the fewest obstacles.

PMH NURSING IN A GLOBAL COMMUNITY

Professional associations and alliances with advocacy groups can support PMH nurses in responding to their responsibilities as health professionals in a global community. These responsibilities include opposing the stigma and discrimination associated with mental illness around the world and the inequities experienced by people with mental disorders in their daily lives and within the health care systems upon which they rely for treatment and care (Desjarlais, Eisenberg, Good, & Kleinman, 1995).

Capacity building among health care practitioners to enable them to promote mental health, to prevent mental illness, and to provide quality mental health care is a pressing priority for the World Health Organization (WHO; 2001), as outlined in their report, *Mental Health: New Understanding, New Hope.* The nursing faculty at the University of Alberta is a WHO Collaborating Centre in Nursing and Mental Health, with capacity building for mental health care being a prime objective of the Centre. Through such local, national, and international organizations, the individual PMH nurse can make a significant contribution in bringing mental health to all.

An international association to which nurses belong is the World Federation for Mental Health (WFMH), an organization whose mission, since 1948 when it was founded, has been to advance mental health promotion and mental disorder prevention and care among all peoples and nations. It works with governments from more than 100 countries and nongovernment groups. WFMH sponsors World Mental Health Day, which occurs annually on October 10.

Mental Disability Rights International (MDRI) is another advocacy group dedicated to the enforcement of rights of people with mental disabilities. Examples of their country reports on human rights, mental health, and psychiatric care include Turkey (2005), Romania (2006), Argentina (2007), and Serbia (2007).

SUMMARY OF KEY POINTS

▫ The bio/psycho/social/spiritual model focuses on separate but interdependent dimensions of biologic, psychological, social, and spiritual factors in the assessment and treatment of mental disorders. This comprehensive and holistic approach to mental disorders is the foundation for effective PMH nursing practice and is used as the basic organizational framework for this text.

▫ The framework of the *Canadian Standards of Psychiatric-Mental Health Nursing* is based on the seven domains of practice delineated in Patricia Benner's research on nursing practice. Expected competencies are associated with each domain.

▫ PMH nurses interact with other disciplines and many times act as a coordinator in the delivery of care.

▫ PMH nurses need to be aware of team dynamics and their impact on care. When nurses practice in interdisciplinary settings, there may be an overlapping of professional roles. Nurses are accountable for both discrete and shared functions that they perform in their practice.

▫ New challenges for PMH nurses are emerging. Using technology well, including the protection of privacy and confidentiality; applying research findings to practice; and working to make the health care system more responsive to the mental health needs of Canadians are some of these challenges.

▫ Nurses and other health professionals practicing in PMH settings need to collaborate with patients, families, and communities in all aspects of care.

▫ Several organizations provide leadership in shaping local, national, and international mental health care, providing an avenue for the PMH nurse to make a significant, positive difference.

CRITICAL THINKING CHALLENGES

1 Explain the bio/psycho/social/spiritual model and apply it to the following three clinical examples:
   a. A first-time father is extremely depressed after the birth of his child, who is perfectly healthy.
   b. A child is unable to sleep at night because of terrifying nightmares.
   c. An older woman is resentful of moving into a senior citizens' residence even though the decision was hers.
2 Identify some mental health needs of the Canadian population. Consider such needs across factors such as age, location, general health, and socioeconomic status.
3 Visit the CFMHN website (http://www.cfmhn.ca) to access a complete version of the *Canadian Standards for Psychiatric-Mental Health Nursing.* Review the Beliefs/Values and the brief description of the history of PMH nursing included in the document.
4 Visit the websites of the organizations listed in the Web Links section of this chapter and discover the role of each in promoting quality mental health care or supporting nursing practice.
5 Contrast *multidisciplinary* and *interdisciplinary* practice. Describe how and when nursing care plans and integrated care paths should be used.

WEB LINKS

www.cna-nurses.ca Canadian Nurses Association website

www.cfmhn.ca Canadian Federation of Mental Health Nurses website

www.rpnaa.ab.ca Registered Psychiatric Nurses of Canada website with links to provincial RPN association websites

www.miaw-ssmm.ca Canadian Alliance on Mental Illness and Mental Health website

www.cpa-apc.org   Canadian Psychiatric Association website

www.ccmhi.ca   Canadian Collaborative Mental Health Initiative website

www.apna.org   American Psychiatric Nurses Association website

www.ispn-psych.org   International Society of Psychiatric–Mental Health Nurses website

www.who.int   World Health Organization website

www.mdri.org   Mental Disability Rights International website

www.wfmh.com   World Federation for Mental Health website

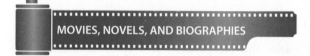

MOVIES, NOVELS, AND BIOGRAPHIES

Awakenings: (1990). Based on the book by Oliver Sacks, this film is the story of victims of an encephalitis epidemic who have remained in a catatonic state for years. A new physician arrives at the hospital where they "reside" and, desperate to help them, gets permission to try a potential chemical cure. His clients begin to awaken. We see the nurses engaging with the awakened individuals in a deeper way than they did when the clients were comatose. One client, played by Robert DeNiro, becomes paranoid and aggressive from too much of the dopamine treatment. This client, however, has much to teach the physician and nurses about living life fully.

VIEWING POINTS: Nurses practicing in PMH settings strive to engage therapeutically with those in their care. Consider the challenge of engaging with an unresponsive, catatonic person and with a person who is suspicious and aggressive. What ideas does this movie offer you in terms of meeting such challenges?

REFERENCES

Abraham, I., Fox, J., & Cohen, B. (1992). Integrating the bio into the biopsychosocial: Understanding and treating biological phenomena in psychiatric–mental health nursing. *Archives of Psychiatric Nursing, 6*(5), 296–305.

Austin, W., Gallop, R., Harris, D., & Spencer, E. (1996). A domain of practice approach to the standards of psychiatric and mental health nursing. *Journal of Psychiatric and Mental Health Nursing, 3,* 111–115.

Barker, P. J., & Buchanan-Barker, P. (2004). *Spirituality and mental health breakthrough.* London, UK: Whurr Publishers.

Benner, P. (1984). *From novice to expert: Excellence and power in clinical nursing practice.* Menlo Park, CA: Addison-Wesley.

Canadian Federation of Mental Health Nurses. (1998). *The Canadian standards of psychiatric and mental health nursing* (2nd ed.). Toronto, ON: Author.

Canadian Federation of Mental Health Nurses. (2006). *The Canadian standards for psychiatric-mental health nursing* (3rd ed.). Toronto, ON: Author. Available at: http://www.cfmhn.ca/resources/multimedia/PDF/28065-singles.pdf

Canadian Nurses Association. (1998, April). *A national framework for the development of standards for the practice of nursing: A discussion paper for Canadian Registered Nurses* (ISBN 1–55119–033–8). Ottawa, ON: Author.

Canadian Nurses Association. (2002). *Code of ethics for registered nurses.* Ottawa, ON: Author.

Catalano, J. T. (2006) *Nursing now: Today's issues, tomorrow's trends.* Philadelphia, PA: F. A. Davis Company.

Desjarlais, R., Eisenberg, L., Good, B., & Kleinman, A. (1995). *World mental health: Problems and priorities in low-income countries.* New York, NY: Oxford University Press.

Dossey, B. M., Keegan, L., & Guzzetta, C. E., (2004). *Holistic nursing: A handbook for practice* (4th ed.). Frederick, MD: Aspen.

Health and Welfare Canada. (1988). Mental health for Canadians: Striking a balance (Cat. H39–128/1988E). Ottawa, ON: Minister of Supply and Service Canada.

Heru, A., & Drury, L. (2006). Overcoming barriers in working with families. *Academic Psychiatry, 30,* 379–384.

Hood Morris, L. E. (1996). A spiritual well-being model: Use with older women who experience depression. *Issues in Mental Health Nursing, 17*(5), 439–455.

Mauk, K., & Schmidt, N. (2004). *Spiritual care in nursing practice.* New York, NY: Lippincott Williams & Wilkins.

Society for Education and Research in Psychiatric-Mental Health Nursing [SERPN]. (1996). *Educational preparation for psychiatric-mental health nursing practice.* Pensacola, FL: Author.

O'Reilly, M. (2004). Spirituality and mental health clients. *Journal of Psychosocial Nursing and Mental Health Service, 42*(7), 44–59.

Varcoe, C., Rodney, P., & McCormick, J. (2003). Health care relationships in context: An analysis of three ethnographies. *Qualitative Health Research, 13*(7), 957–973.

World Health Organization. (2001). *The World Health report 2001. Mental health: New understanding, new hope.* Geneva, Switzerland: Author.

CHAPTER 7

Ethical Psychiatric and Mental Health Nursing Practice

Wendy Austin

LEARNING OBJECTIVES

After studying this chapter, you will be able to:

- Define ethics.
- Distinguish between the domains of ethics and law.
- Describe the nurse as a moral agent.
- List and describe the seven values and related responsibilities of the Canadian Nurses Association *Code of Ethics for Registered Nurses*.
- Identify the most common approaches to ethics that inform health ethics.
- Distinguish between a moral dilemma and a moral distress.
- Outline examples of ethical decision-making frameworks.
- Discuss the five ethical issues in psychiatric and mental health nursing.
- Identify the ethical responsibilities of nurses related to psychiatric research.

KEY CONCEPTS

- ethics
- everyday ethics
- moral agent
- moral dilemma
- moral distress

KEY TERMS

- beneficence • casuistry • confidentiality • conscientious objection
- deontology • ethics of care • feminist ethics • human rights • justice
- nonmaleficence • practical wisdom • principlism • relational ethics
- respect for autonomy • telehealth • utilitarianism • virtue

WHAT IS ETHICS?

Ethics is about how we should live; it is *"aiming at the 'good life' with and for others in just institutions"* (Ricouer, 1992, p. 172, original italics). Ethics is about learning how to reach our potential as human beings, and so it is about values, relationships, principles, duties, rights, and responsibilities. In writing about ethics in *On Equilibrium*, Saul (2001) noted that, although we may think about ethics as something exotic or romantic, for heroes or saints, ethics is actually down to earth and practical: it needs to be an everyday part of our lives and built into our society.

In this chapter, the nurse as a moral agent will be described, common approaches to ethics identified, and moral dilemmas and moral distress defined. Several ethical issues common to psychiatric and mental health (PMH) settings will be discussed. Although some philosophers differentiate ethics from morality, ethics and morals can be used as interchangeable terms (*ethics* comes from *ethos*, Greek for *custom*; *morals* comes from *mores*, Latin for *custom*) and will be so used here.

KEY CONCEPT Ethics is the consideration of the way a person should act in order to live a good life with and for others.

The Legal Domain as Separate From Ethics

Law and ethics are separate domains. In a perfect world, societal laws would be totally compatible with ethical behaviours in every situation. In the real world, however, this is not always the case. Citizens may need to work to change laws that they believe to be unethical. Nurses need to be vigilant about laws that affect their practice. PMH nurses, for instance, must understand the legal context of mental health care in Canada (see Chapter 3). Nurses in forensic psychiatric settings must understand how the competing demands of the health care and justice systems affect their practice (see Chapter 34).

Health Ethics

Somerville (2000), at the McGill Centre for Ethics, Medicine and Law, describes Canada as a secular society, with diverse religious groups: we have no common, external, absolute moral authority. She asks, how can we know, as a society, how to respond to new approaches to science, technology, and health care? The landscape of contemporary ethics is shaped by factors such as intense individualism (the individual coming before the common good), corporatism (dominance of business interests), unprecedented advances in science and technology, the power of the media, the increased use of law as a means to resolve disputes that are inherently about values, and a loss of a sense of the sacred. She proposes that two absolute values, *profound respect for life* and *commitment to the human spirit*, will allow us to make ethical societal choices. We need, she argues, to act so as to protect these values.

Somerville (2000, p. xii) uses the metaphor of a canary to signify key issues that "test the ethical air in our societal mineshaft". As canaries once served to detect toxic gas in underground mines (i.e., sick or dead canaries warned miners that the air was unsafe), these issues warn us that the ethical tone of our society is putting us at risk. Many of these issues are situated in health care. The way in which Canadians address the well-being of those living with mental illness is recognizable to PMH nurses as an ethical canary.

The Ethical Nurse

For nurses, ethics is foundational: "All nursing practice is ethical practice" (Tschudin, 2003, p. ix). Stating that "I am a nurse" is a type of moral claim. Nurses have a fiduciary relationship with the public. (*Fiducial* comes from the Latin, *fidere*, to trust.) Nurses, as professionals, profess or claim that they will use their specialized knowledge and skills for the benefit of the public in a trustworthy way. Nurses are trusted to be ethical (Austin, 2006). In polls, nurses are consistently rated the most honest and ethical professionals (Gallup, 2005). Whenever nurses enact their professional responsibilities, they are active as **moral agents**. Being ethical as a nurse requires more than having moral courage in times of crises (although it may require this); it requires the everyday expression of a commitment to the well-being of those in their care (Levine, 1977; Tschudin, 2003).

> **KEY CONCEPT** A **moral agent** is a person engaged in determining or expressing a moral (ethical) choice.

> **KEY CONCEPT** **Everyday ethics** is "the way nurses approach their practice and reflect on their ethical commitments to the people they serve. It involves nurses' attention to a common ethical event such as protecting a person's physical privacy" (Canadian Nurses Association [CNA], 2002, p. 5).

The Canadian Nurses Association *Code of Ethics for Registered Nurses*

To guide nurses in enacting their moral agency, codes of ethics have been developed by nursing associations. These are statements of the shared values and recognized duties and commitments of the profession. They set the ethical standards for practice and inform other disciplines and the public about the ethical commitments of nurses. In 1954, CNA adopted the *International Council of Nurses Code of Ethics* (created in 1953; revised in 2002). This code delineates nurses' primary responsibilities to the people they serve, to the profession, and to their coworkers (see Web Links for access to the International Council of Nurses code). In 1980, Canadian registered nurses (RNs) created their own code.

The CNA code (CNA, 2008) is framed by seven values and their related ethical responsibilities, grounded in nurses' professional relationships (Box 7-1). The code document includes, as well, "ethical endeavours," an outline of ways nurses may endeavour, on their own and collectively, to change systems and social structures in order for greater equity for all. It has a glossary of pertinent terms and advice on responding to incompetent, noncompassionate, unsafe, or unethical care. It stipulates a provision for **conscientious objection**, defined as "a situation in which a nurse requests permission from his or her employer to refrain from providing care because a practice of procedure conflicts with the nurse's moral or religious beliefs" (CRNBC, 2007). Although the CNA is

Canadian Code of Ethics: Nursing Values and Ethical Responsibilities

The code is organized around seven primary values and accompanying responsibilities, central to the ethical nursing practice:

PROVIDING SAFE, COMPASSIONATE, COMPETENT, AND ETHICAL CARE: Nurses value the ability to provide safe, COMPASSIONATE, competent, and ethical care.

PROMOTING HEALTH AND WELL-BEING: Nurses work with people to enable them to attain their highest possible level of health and well-being.

PROMOTING AND RESPECTING INFORMED DECISION-MAKING: Nurses recognize, respect, and promote a person's right to be informed and make decisions.

PRESERVING DIGNITY: Nurses recognize and respect the intrinsic worth of each person.

MAINTAINING PRIVACY AND CONFIDENTIALITY: Nurses recognize the importance of privacy and confidentiality and safeguard personal, family, and community information obtained in the context of a professional relationship.

PROMOTING JUSTICE: Nurses uphold principles of justice by safeguarding human rights, equity, and fairness and by promoting the public good.

BEING ACCOUNTABLE: Nurses are accountable for their actions and answerable for their practice.

Source: Canadian Nurses Association. (2008). *Code of ethics for registered nurses*. Ottawa, ON: Author.

IN A LIFE

Jan Storch (1940–)
Canadian Nurse Ethicist

Public Persona

Dr. Jan Storch's laudatory leadership in nursing ethics in Canada includes helping launch a centre of health ethics (at the University of Alberta), a provincial health ethics network (in Alberta), being the President of the Canadian Bioethics Society and the National Council on Ethics in Human Research, doing research in ethics, publishing widely (including the ethics text, *Toward a Moral Horizon*), and speaking passionately about ethics to diverse audiences. Her guidance of the 2008 centenary revision of CNA's Code of Ethics was the fourth time she has contributed to CNA in this way. She has received awards as an outstanding nurse from the nursing associations of both Alberta and British Columbia and has been recognized as a leading public intellectual.

Personal Realities

Jan Storch is a wife and mother, a nurse, and a professor at the University of Victoria. Her deep commitment to ethical health care and to nurses' role in it is truly inspirational.

Source: Sibbald, B. (2005) Nurse to know: Ethics in action. *Canadian Nurse, 101*(5), 44.

---

for RNs, it is expected by the nursing profession that students of nursing comply with the code. Those cared for by students should know the status of the student caregiver, and their care should be congruent with the code. Professional nurses are expected to share their knowledge, provide feedback, and treat students with respect (CNA, 2008). Guidelines for relationships with nursing students are provided.

To provide further support for ethical practice, CNA has developed an *Ethics in Practice* resource with topics such as advance directives, whistle-blowing, ethical distress, and public health ethics. (See Web Links for access to CNA.) *Canadian Nurses Interested in Ethics* is a CNA interest group.

APPROACHES TO ETHICS

There are a number of theoretical approaches to ethical knowledge that inform ethical action in health care. Some are based on moral philosophy and others on concepts such as human rights. A brief outline of the most common approaches follows. See Table 7-1 for a summary.

Virtue Ethics

Virtue ethics, emphasizing the character of the moral agent, was the earliest approach to ethics used in nursing (Fowler, 1997). A virtuous person is one who, without strict reliance on rules, is sensitive and wise enough to perceive how to act well in a particular situation. The virtuous person *wants* to behave well. Lists of the virtues vary, but they can include compassion, courage, tolerance, prudence, honesty, humility, and trustworthiness. Aristotle (1996), the Greek philosopher whose works most inform virtue theory, believed that acquiring the virtues would assist a person to flourish as a human being. He found our moral upbringing to be important: we learn the virtues through our relationships. Observing compassion in others, for instance, can help us to develop a compassionate disposition. To acquire a virtue, it must become habitual; it is not enough, for instance, to be occasionally honest. Aristotle's concept of the virtue of *phronesis* or **practical wisdom** seems particularly relevant to nurses. It means having the sensitivity, imagination, and experience to do what is ethically fitting in difficult situations (Austin, 2007a).

In a profession with role-specific duties and responsibilities (evidenced by such things as a code of ethics), a trait that supports the good of that practice acquires the status of a moral virtue. A professional's virtues, in that sense, are necessary to his or her role (Radden & Sadler, 2008). Nevertheless, virtue ethics is not as influential

Table 7.1	Approaches to Ethics		
Approach	**Core Elements**	**Proponents**	**Critiques**
Virtue ethics	Character of the moral agent Some virtues: honesty, courage, compassion, practical wisdom	Aristotle Alasdair MacIntyre	Exclusive focus on the agent
Deontology	Duty based Some acts are wrong in themselves Universality Do not treat others as a means to an end (respect)	Immanuel Kant	Disregard of consequences Impartiality over relationship Emotion = Irrationality
Utilitarianism	Consequence based Actions are right if they promote the best outcome (e.g., happiness, pleasure, satisfaction) for most people	Jeremy Bentham John Stuart Mill	Utility as the only principle Majority rules
Casuistry	Case based Use of paradigm cases to identify issues and courses of action for a new case	Albert Jonsen Stephen Toulmin	Keeps the status quo Can miss the broad issues
Principlism	Based on a set of principles compatible with most moral theories Nonmaleficence, beneficence, respect for autonomy, justice	Tom Beauchamp James Childress	Too abstract Which principle has a priority when different principles compete?
Ethics of care	Care based Connection/responsibility for others Emotional responsiveness	Carol Gilligan Nel Noddings	Creates a dichotomy between "care" (feminine) and "justice" (masculine) approaches to ethics Valorizes women as caregivers
Feminist ethics	Addresses power inequities, dominance, and oppression	Annette Baier Susan Sherwin	Lacks impartiality Lacks universal norms
Relational ethics	Ethical action involves relationships Context matters; emotion accepted Dialogue is supported Aims for the "fitting" response	Vangie Bergum John Dossetor	Too relativistic Lacks impartiality Lacks universality
Human rights	Rights based (negative and positive) Every person is entitled to certain basic rights	John Locke Thomas Paine United Nations	As a concept is "nonsense" Too legalistic Too individualistic

as it once was. Research indicates that, for some, the character of a PMH nurse does not matter. Armstrong, Parsons, and Barker (2000) explored moral virtues (especially compassion) and PMH nurses. Nearly half of their sample in a Delphi study did not believe that the moral character of a PMH nurse is important in ethical decision making, and most of their round-one sample thought virtues could not be acquired. Others, however, consider virtue ethics as "especially well suited to understanding and promoting ethical psychiatric practice" (Radden & Sadler, p. 373). Lützén and da Silva (1996) used examples of practice situations to discuss the place of virtue ethics in PMH nursing, illustrating that ethical action can mean compassionately transcending the rules in the best interest of the patient. This is one of their examples: a nurse in an emergency may restrain a patient without the necessary physician's order to protect the patient from harming himself. To stand aside

as a confused, acutely ill person injures himself may be correct according to rules or policies, but it does not seem ethical.

Scott (2003), a nurse philosopher who finds virtue ethics relevant to practice and a rationale for good role models in nursing education, also warns that focusing naively on the individual without attending to the context and collective responsibility is dangerous. A renewed interest in virtue ethics is occurring, stimulated by the work *After Virtue* by MacIntyre (1984). A paraphrase of his question, "What would a nurse (person) lack, who lacked the virtues?" is worth reflecting on.

Deontology

Deontology (from the Greek *deon* or *duty*) postulates duty or obligation as the basis of doing right. This is not duty as in following external orders, but as self-imposed obligation. This approach is also termed *Kantian ethics* because the work of Kant (1996), an 18th century philosopher, laid its foundation. Kant believed that we should use reason alone to determine how to act. Reason, unhampered by emotions or desires, allows us to determine the types of acts that are wrong in themselves, no matter how good their consequences might be. Kant stipulated a criterion (a *categorical imperative*) for judging the reason (or "maxim") for one's actions: universality. One should act only on a choice that one can conceive of as a universal law. Is a lie acceptable if it saves someone from danger? No, because lying cannot be willed as a universal principle. If we lie to help a person in trouble, truth will be subverted and society corrupted. In Kantian ethics, the moral worth of a person's action is determined by the intent of the person, not the effects of the action. If you act rightly, you are not responsible for bad effects.

Kant stipulated a second imperative: act so that you treat others always as an end and never as a means. Kant argued that we must treat one another with dignity and respect: it is wrong to use other people for our own purposes. Informed consent is grounded on this belief. For instance, individuals should not be used as research subjects unless they understand what will happen and agree to it. Nor should we, according to Kantian ethics, place individuals at risk in research by depriving them of the best known treatment in order to carry out a placebo-controlled study, even though this would provide the most valid evidence.

Kant's emphasis on the individual's rational capacity as the facilitator of moral action can be seen as highly relevant to psychiatric ethics, as it is the impairment of rational capacity alone that justifies coercive or involuntary psychiatric treatment (Robertson, Morris, & Walter, 2007). Kantian ethics supports the quest for universal ethical principles, such as the United Nations Educational, Scientific, and Cultural Organization's (UNESCO's) efforts (see "Human Rights"). It upholds that, from a moral standpoint, all persons should be treated the same. A major problem, however, is its disregard for the role of consequences in ethical action. Consequences, however, are the sole focus of the next approach.

Utilitarianism

The principle of utility is the foundation of utilitarianism: actions are right in proportion to their tendency to promote happiness. What is right to do is what gives the best consequences (e.g., happiness, pleasure, preference, satisfaction) for the greater number of people. Bentham (1983) and Mill (2002), philosophers of the 18th and 19th centuries, originated this theory that uses a type of cost/benefit analysis to determine the moral worth of an action.

The principle of utility can also be applied to determining which moral rules to follow. This is termed **rule utilitarianism** and holds that once we decide on the best rules, we should follow them, even if in some situations happiness is not maximized. A rule utilitarian might determine that a good rule for a PMH nurse is not to go against hospital policies except if it is necessary for the best interests of a patient. Covertly putting an antipsychotic medication in an acutely ill person's food, for instance, might be regarded as ethically acceptable in a special circumstance when such an action causes the least suffering to the ill person (Ipperciel, 2003; Scott, 1998). A Kantian would never approve of this, and, despite ethical justification from a utilitarian perspective, such an act can result in a disciplinary or legal action (Wong, Poon, & Hui, 2005).

Principlism

In the principles approach, it is believed that a few moral principles (ethical norms) can provide a basis for moral reasoning in health ethics (Beauchamp, 1994). Such a set of principles would be compatible with most moral theories (e.g., deontology, utilitarianism). A widely accepted set of principles is that articulated by Tom Beauchamp and James Childress of the Kennedy Institute of Ethics, Georgetown University. They identified four *prima facie* (at first sight) principles: nonmaleficence, beneficence, respect for autonomy, and justice (Beauchamp & Childress, 2008). **Nonmaleficence** as a principle means that one should do no harm; **beneficence** means that one should do, or attempt to do, good and make things better (promote benefit) for others when one can. **Respect for autonomy** (also considered as respect for persons) means an obligation to respect a person's right to be self-governing and his or her ability to make decisions. **Justice**, as conceived by Beauchamp and Childress, is about obligations of fairness in the distribution of benefits and risks. One criticism of **principlism** is that four principles cannot sufficiently capture moral norms (Walker, 2009). Another common criticism is that when principles compete, as they will in complex situations, there is no framework for settling the conflict.

The nature of mental illness creates situations in which there is a conflict between respect for autonomy and beneficence. How should one act when a person with a mental illness chooses to act in a way that brings harm to himself or herself? For instance, what if a person with schizophrenia is living homeless on the streets? Should respect for autonomy be upheld, or should there be an intervention to bring the person to shelter? Respect for autonomy is dependent on a person's competence to make his or her own informed decisions. Evaluating such competence can be difficult.

Casuistry or Case-Based Ethics

Casuistry (pronounced kăzh' ū-ĭ;-strē), from the Latin *casus* for *case*, is the use of case comparisons to facilitate moral reasoning and decision making. It is a bottom-up approach. One starts with the details of the present case and locates that case in a taxonomy of cases as a way to identify the pertinent ethical concerns and responses (Jonsen, 1991; Jonsen & Toulmin, 1988). The focus in casuistry is on agreement about cases, not necessarily principles or theories, and precedents are central to this approach. Past decisions about what was right or wrong in significant cases serve to inform decisions about the new case. (This is similar to what happens in legal judgments.) The PMH nurse using this approach will need to decide how the "case" fits and does not fit paradigmatic cases. There are suggested steps to use (Strong, 2000):

1. Identify the main ethical values and concerns relevant to the case.
2. Identify the main alternative courses of action that can be taken.
3. Identify the casuistic factors (i.e., the morally relevant ways the cases of this type differ).
4. Compare the case with relevant paradigm cases that have been identified.

Casuistry seems congruent with the way nurses think in practice. When a clinical situation confronts us, we often think of similar situations that we have experienced, or we turn to paradigm cases to guide us. A criticism of casuistry is that there is a risk that one will miss the broad issues and that prevalent beliefs and practices will not be sufficiently questioned.

The Ethics of Care and Feminist Ethics

The **ethics of care** can be seen as a feminine approach to ethics (Sherwin, 1992). Gilligan (1982), in researching moral development, found that females seemed to differ from males in their approach to ethical decision making. Females focused on caring, connectedness, and responsibility rather than the deductive reasoning and abstract principles preferred by males. She argued that women are different from men in their approach to moral decisions, not inferior to them. (Aristotle and Kant both assumed that the moral agent was male.) Canadian philosopher Sherwin (1992), in *No Longer Patient: Feminist Ethics and Health Care*, argues that women's perspective of the world as a web of interdependent relationships in which our responsibility to one another is implicit needs to be incorporated into a contemporary ethical theory. Noddings (1984), the author of *Caring: A Feminine Approach to Ethics and Moral Education*, says that the ethics of care should be *the* theory. For her, receptivity, relatedness, and responsiveness with values and emotions, like compassion, are the important components of ethical responses.

Feminist ethics differs from the ethics of care in that it comes from a political perspective, offering insight into oppression (unjust, unwarranted use of power) and dominance in individual and societal-level relationships. Using understandings gained from the analysis of women's oppression, feminist ethicists illuminate negative power differentials that may be so inherent as to be invisible and remain unquestioned. For instance, some feminist ethicists are concerned that the ethics of care valorizes the caregiving traits of women, even when such traits can be viewed as self-defeating (Sherwin, 1992).

Race, religion, class, and disability are factors other than gender that have affected people's ability to flourish within their society. Such discriminations are morally wrong in feminist ethics (Liaschenko & Peter, 2003). Baier's (1985, 1994) feminist approach has been proposed as useful for nursing ethics. It combines political dimensions with the core values of care and commitment (Peter & Morgan, 2001). It may offer a constructive framework for challenging the oppression of people with mental illness (Martin, 2001).

Relational Ethics

Relational ethics is based on the assumption that all ethical actions are situated in relationship. Ideas of duty and utility, principles, and the character of the moral agent are accepted as important in informing action, but relationship is taken as foundational. Ethics is about how we treat one another, individually and within society, as well as how we resolve moral problems. Ethical situations are encompassed by complexity and uncertainty, and an understanding of the "messiness" of life needs to be cultivated.

Within this perspective, one strives to be responsive to the situation at hand in such a way that genuine dialogue is opened and mutual respect fostered among those involved. Feelings and emotions are viewed as a component of rational thinking and are explored, not ruled out as too subjective or confusing. Context matters. Not anything goes, but one's actions need not only to be shaped by ethical knowledge but also to be adapted to the specific circumstances of the situation. In relational ethics, one aims for the fitting response (Niebuhr, 1963). Questions can be raised within this approach (e.g., issues of power and control) that may not be raised in approaches that focus primarily on moral reasoning.

In Canada, this approach to ethics was developed through research at the University of Alberta. Vangie Bergum (a nurse) and John Dossetor (a physician) questioned the dominance of the principle of autonomy in health care ethics. To explore what a different focus, one of relationship and responsibility, might be like in health care, they brought together an interdisciplinary research team of health professionals and scholars (Austin, Bergum, & Dossetor, 2003; Bergum & Dossetor, 2005). Using interpretive inquiry methods, the team explored existing cases and described each case in terms of relational ethics. Core elements were identified as mutual respect, engagement, embodied knowledge, attention to the interdependent environment, and uncertainty/vulnerability. Although there is not enough space to discuss these themes here, this research is described in *Relational Ethics: The Full Meaning of Respect* (Bergum & Dossetor). An article about relational ethics in forensic psychiatric settings with examples from an undergraduate nursing practicum may be also helpful to students who want to better understand this approach (Austin, 2001a). A relational ethics decision-making framework is outlined in Box 7-2.

Relational ethics seems congruent with PMH nursing practice. In a study of PMH nurses' use of ethical principles, Garritson (1988) found that nurses were greatly influenced by situational variables. Nurses did not act consistently on their stated priority of ethical principles. Their specific concerns about the persons in their care and their obligation to keep them and others safe shaped their ethical decisions (Garritson).

Human Rights

Using human rights as an approach to health ethics is a fairly recent phenomenon (Austin, 2001b). The idea of human rights, however, goes back to 1215 and Britain's Magna Carta, to the rights language of the philosopher John Locke (Sumner, 2000) in the 17th century, and to Thomas Paine's *Rights of Man* (1996) in the 18th century. The central assumption of **human rights** is that every person has certain claims or entitlements because he or she is a human. Rights can be conceived as negative or positive. Negative rights are usually civil or political in nature, with the State or others required to refrain from obstructing these rights (e.g., freedom of speech, freedom to worship). Positive rights are obligations of the state or others to provide a right (e.g., right to health, right to education). These rights are typically social, cultural, or economic in nature.

Rights relating to health are included in many international documents, beginning with the constitution

---

BOX 7.2

A Relational Ethics Decision-Making Framework

KEY QUESTIONS
1. What is happening here?
2. What are the alternatives for ethical action?
3. What is the most fitting thing to do?
Action
4. What happened as the result of our action?

Question 1: What is happening here?
- What are the ethical questions?
- Their context?
- Who is involved? (Who are the moral agents?) What are their commitments to one another?
- What further information do we need?
- Is there legal, organizational, professional, cultural, religious, or any other aspect to consider? Are values in conflict?
- What resources do we have? Need?
  - Patient and family resources (e.g., personal directive)
  - Health care resources (e.g., access to home care)
  - Ethics resources: principles, precedents, codes, policies, guidelines, ethicists/ethics committees, etc.
- To what, in particular, do we need to attend?

Question 2: What are the alternatives for ethical action?
- What are the consequences for each alternative?
- What might constrain ethical action?
- What, if anything, makes me or others uncomfortable in regard to a potential action?
- Remember: refraining from making a decision is still a decision.

Question 3: What is the most fitting thing to do?
- What is the best way to make it (the plan) happen?
- Who is affected? Who needs to be involved?
- How do we bridge disparate views?

Question 4: What happened as the result of our action?
- What concerns remain?
- Is anyone distressed about the result?
- Is further action desirable?
- Do we need to address systemic factors that gave rise to the situation?
- Would we act in the same way again?
- What did we learn?

Copyright: Wendy Austin, University of Alberta, Canada.

of the World Health Organization (WHO) in 1946 and the *Universal Declaration of Human Rights (UDHR)* adopted by the General Assembly of the United Nations in 1948. In 1991, the United Nations declared *Principles for the Protection of Persons With Mental Illness and for the Improvement of Mental Health Care* (see Chapter 3 for Web Links). Human rights law allows for international scrutiny of a nation's health policies and practices (Gostin, 2001).

In October 2005, a *Universal Declaration on Bioethics and Human Rights* was adopted by the UNESCO. Among other things, the principles uphold respect for autonomy, the solidarity among human beings, and the need for sharing the benefits of scientific research and for protecting future generations and the planet itself.

"Health" as a human right means that every person has a right to the highest attainable level of health (including a standard of living that is adequate for health) and to access to health care and social services as needed. Health conceptualized as a right is very different from health as a commodity for purchase. There are important connections between health and human rights that nurses and other health professionals must consider (Mann et al., 1999). First, *health policies and practices have an impact on human rights*. For instance, mandatory outpatient treatment for persons with a mental illness is an infringement on individual rights. This infringement can only be justified if it is in the best interests of the person or for the necessary protection of the public. Second, *human rights violations impact health*. Torture, for instance, may have long-lasting effects on an individual's mental health. The International Council of Nurses not only supports the United Nation's *UDHR* but also stipulates in *Torture, Death Penalty and Participation by Nurses in Executions* that nurses may not voluntarily participate in any deliberate infliction of physical or mental suffering. The World Psychiatric Association's (1996) *Madrid Declaration on Ethical Standards for Psychiatric Practice* stipulates the same for psychiatrists. Third, *health professionals have a responsibility to protect human rights by helping the public identify rights violations*. Mental Disability Rights International (MDRI), a rights advocacy group, reports that in Kosovo, women were raped in psychiatric facilities despite the presence of local staff and international relief workers (MDRI, 2002). Such terrible rights violations must be made public.

Human rights approach to ethics requires action not only to end inhumane treatment and conditions but also to stop discrimination that prevents persons with mental illness from fully participating in their communities. The idea that humans are born with "rights" strikes some philosophers as "nonsense" (Waldron, 1987). There is also an argument that universal rights cannot exist because there is no universal human community, every culture being different. A rights approach has been criticized as too legalistic and the law as a slow, ineffective means of addressing rights violations. A final criticism is that human rights are too individualistic, placing the person in an antagonistic position against his or her community (Austin, 2001b). Nevertheless, human rights as an approach to health ethics underscores the point that health is a social good, not merely a medical issue. It reminds us of the need for human dignity and equality and of our obligations to one another (Leary, 1994).

◼◼◼ MORAL DILEMMAS AND MORAL DISTRESS

A **moral dilemma** is a conflict that is morally relevant (Audi, 1995). It may be defined more narrowly as a situation in which one has an obligation to act but must choose between two incompatible alternatives. In health ethics, frameworks have been developed to facilitate the decision-making process. See Box 7-3 for an example of a framework developed by Michael McDonald at the University of British Columbia. For an illustration of its application, see Peternelj-Taylor's (2003) analysis of a nurse's decision to whistle blow on a colleague.

The CNA Code of Ethics for RNs includes other examples of ethical decision-making frameworks. One example is Oberle's and Bouchal's (2009) Framework for Ethical Decision Making, outlined in detail in their work, *Ethics in Canadian Nursing Practice*. Their framework has five steps: assessing the ethics of the situation (relationships, goals, beliefs, and values), reflecting on and reviewing potential actions (recognizing available choices and how those choices are valued), selecting an ethical action (maximizing good), engaging in ethical action, and reflecting on and reviewing the ethical action

---

BOX 7.3

A Framework for Ethical Decision Making

This is the outline of a guide for making ethical decisions developed by Michael McDonald, W. Maurice Young Centre for Applied Ethics (CAE) at the University of British Columbia. The full framework is much more complex; be certain to access it at the CAE website: http://www.ethics.ubc.ca/people/mcdonald/decisions.htm

- Collect information and identify the problem(s).
- Specify feasible alternatives for treatment and care.
- Use your ethical resources to evaluate alternatives (principles/concepts, standards, personal judgments and experiences, and organized procedures for ethical consultation).
- Propose and test possible resolutions.
- Make your choice.

(p. 62). Refer to Box 7-2 for a framework based on relational ethics. Decision-making frameworks are simply tools to guide ethical deliberation, based on particular or composite approaches.

KEY CONCEPT A **moral dilemma** is a conflict in which one feels a moral obligation to act but must choose between incompatible alternatives.

Moral distress is the anger, frustration, or anguish we feel when we are unable to fulfill our ethical obligations in the way we believe we should. We feel a sense of responsibility and make a moral judgment about the right response, but some constraint prevents us from enacting that response (Austin, Lemermeyer, Goldberg, Bergum, & Johnson, 2005; CNA, 2002; Nathaniel, 2002). A constraint may be internal (e.g., a lack of moral courage) or external (e.g., the inability to influence the actions of the care team).

Jameton (1993) has identified two types: the *initial distress* when obstacles to right action are first experienced and the *reactive distress* that occurs when we do not act on the initial distress. Reactions include headaches, loss of appetite or sleep, heart palpitations, and loss of confidence (Fry, Harvey, Hurley, & Foley, 2002). When we do not act, we may feel like we participated in a moral wrongdoing (Nathaniel, 2002). An action on the issue can reduce moral distress and prevent *moral residue*, what we experience when our integrity feels compromised (Webster & Baylis, 2000). A Canadian qualitative study of the moral distress of mental health practitioners found that nurses experienced moral distress related to being "unable to answer the call of their patients." They lacked the resources to do so, particularly time for individualized care. Several participants described leaving a nursing position due to moral distress (Austin, Bergum, & Goldberg, 2003).

KEY CONCEPT **Moral distress** occurs when one is unable to act on one's moral choices because of internal or external constraints.

Sources of nurses' moral distress include harm to patients (pain, suffering), treatment of patients as objects, effects of cost containment, policy constraints, and inadequate staffing (Corley, 2002). For many PMH nurses, the lack of time to engage with patients (including suicidal patients) appears to be a common source of distress (Box 7-4) (Austin, Bergum, & Goldberg, 2003; McLaughlin, 1999; Midence, Gregory, & Stanley, 1996; Sjöstedt, Dahlstrand, Severinsson, & Lützén, 2001).

It is helpful to identify the source of distress, to refer to the CNA *Code of Ethics* and other documents for guidance, and to seek support. Support may be available from peers, the health care team, or the ethics committee of one's institution or agency. It is available from one's nursing regulatory body, association, or union. For more information, refer to CNA's *Ethical Distress in Health Care Environments* that is part of its *Ethics in Practice* series (CNA, 2003a).

BOX 7.4

Research for Best Practice: Being Good Enough: Coping With a Troubled Conscience

Dahlqvist, V., Soderberg, A., & Norberg, A. (2009). Facing inadequacy and being good enough: Psychiatric care providers' narratives about experiencing and coping with troubled conscience. *Journal of Psychiatric and Mental Health Nursing, 16*, 242–247.

QUESTION: What is it like, as a provider of psychiatric care, to have a troubled conscience?

METHOD: Ten therapists (nine nurses and one social worker), representing a variety of perceptions of conscience, were selected for interviews from among psychiatric personnel who completed a series of questionnaires of conscience in health care. All had over 23 years of experience. In individual interviews, participants were asked to describe situations in their work that have troubled their conscience. The interviews were tape recorded, transcribed verbatim, and analyzed using a phenomenological-hermeneutic method inspired by Paul Ricouer's three-step, circular interpretation approach. The steps are naïve reading, structural analysis, and critical interpretation. The researchers discussed emerging interpretations until consensus was reached.

FINDINGS: The process of coping with a troubled conscience involves wavering, doubting, and wondering how to handle feelings of being the one who sometimes betrays. Two themes emerged: *facing inadequacy* and *struggling to view oneself as being "good enough."* Facing inadequacy encompassed the subthemes of exercising one's power over the patient, being unable to satisfy claims of the conscience, and blaming oneself and being blamed. Struggling to view oneself as being "good enough" entailed sharing feelings of guilt and powerlessness and reconciling shortcomings.

IMPLICATIONS: Ethical demands can be experienced as overwhelming, especially when one is unable to ease the suffering of those in one's care. Nurses in PMH settings may live an ongoing struggle to reconcile what they wished they could do with morally acceptable limits on their abilities and responsibilities. They must come to accept being "good enough."

SOME ETHICAL ISSUES IN PMH SETTINGS

It is not possible to identify in this chapter all the complex ethical issues of PMH settings; rather, a few significant ones are discussed. Although some issues are not unique to this specialty area (e.g., confidentiality), all are shaped by the PMH context.

Behaviour Control and Restraint

Some users of mental health care systems call themselves "survivors." They are not saying that they survived their illness, as one might say "I have survived cancer." Rather, they are saying that they survived their treatment and care (Gallop, 1993). "We need to recover from being in hospital" (Roper, 2003, p. 14). Such claims are, and should be, very disturbing to PMH nurses. We need to ask, What is it like to use our mental health services? What is it like to be our patient or our patient's family member?

In PMH settings, some patients may be involuntary, committed to care without their consent. They may be treated against their will, as they have been deemed unable to make informed treatment decisions due to a mental disorder. A person significantly out of touch with reality can require help to survive and recover. Most societies have legal provisions that allow some form of intervention when this is so or if the person is at risk for harming self or others (see Chapter 3). This type of legitimated coercion must be monitored and used with great care. There is abiding potential for its abuse (subtle or otherwise), and this potential is a major concern of persons living with mental illness (Campbell, 1997). Szasz (1961, 1993, 2005), among others, questions any use of this type of power. Szasz argues, in the *Myth of Mental Illness* and other works, that mental illness is not a true illness but a societal label for "deviant" behaviour. To Szasz, psychiatry is merely a means to control that deviance. Involuntary patients may be restrained (physically, chemically, or by being placed "in seclusion") if they put self or others (including staff) at risk for harm. To use restraint is a decision dilemma for nurses (Marangos-Frost & Wells, 2000).

Such measures must be used only when absolutely necessary and then with sensitivity and great caution. They can have serious relational consequences. A review of the empirical literature on locked doors in acute care psychiatry indicates that locked units are associated with increased patient aggression and poorer satisfaction with treatment (Van der Merwe et al., 2009).

Holmes, Kennedy, and Perron (2004) found, in a Canadian study of seclusion from the patient's perspective, that seclusion was perceived as punitive and as a method of control. Feelings of exclusion, rejection, abandonment, and isolation were intensified, not from the seclusion per se, but from the lack of contact with nurses.

A qualitative study of Canadian nurses' decision-making process in regard to the use of seclusion suggests that its use is shaped by a complex interaction of personal, professional, and organizational factors that includes peer pressure (Holmes & Jacob, 2007). Nurses need to be very attentive to what is influencing such practice decisions and ensure that ethical responsibilities are primary. Larue, Dumais, Ahern, Bernheim, and Mailhot (2009), in examining aggression- and agitation-management measures used in Québec health care settings, note that patient traits can provoke anxiety and a premature expectation of the risk of violence and that informal norms regarding the relations with patients, as well as the solidarity of team members, are factors in an intervention. They are researching seclusion practices with the aim of determining best practices.

Gallop, McCay, Guha, and Khan (1999), in another Canadian study, explored the experience of restraint of women with histories that included childhood sexual abuse. Many of the restraint situations were triggered by self-harm behaviours, but no participant viewed the restraint as necessary or helpful in keeping her safe. It was traumatic, terrifying, and degrading. They suggested clinical responses that they preferred: empathic engagement rather than aloof professionalism, constant observation, comfort measures (e.g., hot milk), and outlets for aggression (e.g., punching bag). They suggested an orientation to the consequences of uncontrolled behaviour to increase the awareness of its risks. Other solutions, such as good staffing and better environmental design of PMH settings, can reduce the frequency and extent of restraint interventions (Marangos-Frost & Wells, 2000).

Practitioners justify coercive measures as beneficent, for the protection and welfare of patients, when failing to act would seem unethical. Nevertheless, practitioners find these measures difficult to use (McCain & Kornegay; 2005; Slomka, Agisch, Stango, & Smith, 1998; Vuckovich & Artinian, 2005). Psychiatric staff in a Swedish study termed them "unpleasant," "hard," and "detestable" (Eriksson & Kjellin, 1989). In "volatile" rather than "violent" conflict situations with patients (prevention of fights or damage to property, protection of visitors, diffusing demands on nursing time, etc.), PMH nurses have been found to use a variety of maneuvers (e.g., body block positions, bear hugs, a show of force) that were rarely charted or evaluated (Ryan & Bowers, 2005). Nurses seem reluctant to question the use of coercion and, rather than do so, try to be as gentle and humane as possible (Olofsson, Gilje, Jacobsson, & Norberg, 1998) and use coercion only as a last resort (Vuckovich & Artinian, 2005).

Being open to questioning and discussing the use of coercive measures, however, seems important (Austin, Begum, & Nuttgens, 2004; Breggin, 1997; Kjellin et al., 1993). It reduces the risk for becoming desensitized to such measures and allowing them to become "routinized" out of awareness (Brody, 1995). Nurses need to question the "taken-for-granted" institutional practices whenever those practices place the rights and dignity of patients in jeopardy (Holmes, 2001). Ethical action in PMH settings can be so complex that the nurse philosopher Scott (1998) asks if, at times, as nurses, we must choose to do the "least bad thing" (p. 484). In such situations, she urges nurses to confront the question openly and honestly.

Other types of behavioural control in PMH care can raise ethical concerns, including electroconvulsive therapy, behaviour modification, medication, and psychosurgery. Discharge from hospital and care centres can also be a form of coercion if premature and unsupported (Eriksson & Westrin, 1995). Psychotherapy, too, can have ramifications for one's autonomy, as when therapists expect their interpretations of clients' experiences to be accepted and acted upon (Austin, Bergum, & Nuttgens, 2004). Research with PMH nurses (Muller & Poggenpoel, 1996) indicates that persons receiving care may encounter a lack of empathy and patronizing and paternalistic attitudes. Some professionals too readily dismiss concerns raised by a person with mental illness as faulty thinking (Davis, Liaschenko, Aroskar, & Drought, 1997). Margot Kidder, Canadian actor and mental health advocate, has described her psychiatric hospitalization as "You're completely invalidated as a human being. You're treated like a naughty child who must be taught a lesson" (Moore, 1999, p. A12). Yet, PMH settings should be healing places with sufficient numbers of competent and caring staff members who are able to offer respectful, person-centred care. When this is not so, it is an ethical issue that must be addressed.

Relational Engagement

Engagement in therapeutic relationships is an important aspect of most, if not all, PMH care, and complex ethical issues are situated in the boundaries of these relationships (see Chapter 9). Although "boundary," the term that is commonly used to describe the limits of such relationships, implies clear borders that should not be crossed, actual practice can be more complicated. Gift giving is an example. Although accepting a gift from a person with whom one is in a therapeutic relationship can be seen as an initial step down the "slippery slope" toward a boundary violation and to be always avoided, it may be more complicated than that (Austin, Bergum, Nuttgens, & Peternelj-Taylor, 2006). Gallop (1997) has shared her experience as a student nurse who received a gift (handmade woolen slippers) from her patient, a young woman with schizophrenia. She kept the gift a secret from her clinical teacher. "Although we were not permitted to accept gifts, I accepted the slippers, deciding the wrath of my instructor was easier to endure than the injury I would inflict by refusing her gift" (p. 28). Nurses need to be thoughtful about the meaning of a gift and be able to receive knowledgeable advice from members of the team and clinical supervisors.

Campbell (2002), in a survey of Albertan Mental Health nurses, found that nurses did cross boundaries. PMH nurses working in child and adolescent settings or in geriatric settings were more likely to do so than nurses working as group therapists or in forensic settings. The latter were the nurses most likely to have received boundary education. Although some nurses in the study admitted to dating a patient after discharge, it was less than 1% (eight nurses).

One of the most serious types of boundary violation is the sexual harassment and abuse of patients. Despite policies of zero tolerance, abuse occurs and is known to be significantly underreported (Rodgers, 2004). Professionals who commit serious boundary violations at times argue that it was a mutual decision, made with the patient. Given the power differentials in therapeutic relationships, this "defence" is unacceptable.

Transgressions of boundaries are most often discussed as "over" involvement. "Under" involvement can also be an ethical issue given the definition of a boundary violation as being "any behaviour that infringes upon the primary goal of providing care" (Epstein, 1994, p. 2). There may be times in which a patient evokes a negative response from a nurse, for example, if the patient rejects care, is abusive, or is guilty of a morally reprehensible act, such as child abuse (Liaschenko, 1994). A nurse may, for instance, find engaging with patients with self-harming behaviours more difficult than engaging with other patients (Loughrey, Jackson, Molla, & Wobbleton, 1997). Liaschenko found that when nurses had difficulty connecting with a patient, they chose among three options: to emotionally distance themselves from the patient, to transfer the patient to another nurse, or to make a conscious effort to be respectful and provide good care. The nurses in this study recognized difficulties in "bridging the gap" to a patient as an ethical issue.

In order to engage ethically with patients, nurses need to attend to their own personal and professional boundaries, as well as to respect those of others. Education about boundaries is helpful, as are strategies such as clinical supervision and resources such as *Professional Boundaries for Registered Nurses: Guidelines for the Nurse–Client Relationship* (Alberta Association of Registered Nurses, 1998).

Confidentiality and Privacy

CNA's *Code of Ethics* defines **confidentiality** as the ethical obligation to keep someone's personal and private information secret or private duty to preserve a person's privacy. (See CNA's [2003b] "Privacy and Health Information: Challenges for Nurses and for the Nursing Profession" in their *Ethics in Practice* series.) As individuals, there is information about ourselves we do not wish to have disclosed to others, and we may not want others to intrude on our personal space. This may be particularly important in PMH settings, given the stigma attached to mental disorders and to psychiatric care. Consent is a central factor in decisions related to privacy and confidentiality, and this factor becomes more complicated when the person involved has an illness that affects his or her ability to give consent. Overall, nurses safeguard the information learned in the context of their professional relationships, sharing it outside the health care team only with the patients' permission or as legally required.

Disclosure of information within the team, however, seems standard, with the team considered as one entity. Nurses should inform persons in their care about this sharing of health information within the team (CNA, 2002). This is particularly important because studies of public perceptions about confidentiality in mental health services reveal the belief that what is said remains in absolute confidence (e.g., similar to confession with a priest; Ormrod & Ambrose, 1999).

In Campbell's survey of Albertan PMH nurses, 94.4% of respondents said that they never kept a confidence regarding the safety of a person in their care from the treatment team at that person's request (Campbell, Yonge, & Austin, 2005). One nurse wrote that if patients want to tell him or her something that they do not want disclosed to anyone else, "I decline and state my role and responsibilities." When patients confide information that is peripheral to treatment, however, this type of information is not shared. Nurses have identified "patient privacy" as an ethical issue in PMH home care visits, including the use of various persuasive techniques to gain entrance (Magnusson & Lützén, 1999). Too strict observation of privacy and confidentiality rules can also be problematic (Kirby, 2004). When a person with a mental disorder is not competent to give consent for information to be shared, family members and caregivers may be excluded from knowing what is occurring, and this lack of knowledge can place them and the person at risk.

There are, of course, occasions that legally require the reporting of information received in a patient care situation. Mandatory reporting of child abuse and abuse of adults in care is an example. (Refer to provincial and territorial legislation for reporting requirements.) Nurses are expected to intervene if others within the health care system fail to meet obligations regarding confidentiality and privacy (CNA, 2008).

Advances in Technology as a Threat to Privacy

Electronic health record systems, costing millions of dollars, are being established across Canada in an effort to improve health care services. These information systems require nurses and others to go beyond questioning whether or not to share patient information. Health care staff members need to question their own perusal of information: it must be on a need-to-know basis only (Griener, 2005). Other uses of technology, such as **telehealth**—"any use of technology for health purposes"—may affect privacy through security breaches and data mining, as well as involve other issues such as inaccurate data (Kaplan & Litewka, 2008, p. 401).

Surveillance devices employed in some mental health care services (e.g., closed circuit television) are giving new meaning to patient observation. Nurses need to consider the use of such technology and whether it jeopardizes their patients' rights and dignity, as well as care relationships (Holmes, 2001). Advances in neurotechnology may bring new threats to privacy. Imaging technology may increasingly predict mental events and behaviours with far-reaching ramifications, including such areas as insurance, employment, education, immigration, and counterterrorism (Kirby, 2004). Illes and Racine (2005), for instance, postulate that brain scans might one day be used to screen passengers at airports for their propensity to violence.

Advances in genetics raise other concerns, some based on past experience (Appelbaum, 2004; Cox, 2005). Eugenics (Greek for "well-born") was once a worldwide movement, beginning at the onset of the 20th century, that aimed at improving the human race. In 1939 in Nazi Germany, a program was initiated that lead to the killing of thousands of "incurable" psychiatric patients (useless eaters), who were deemed to have a life "not worth living" and to weaken their society. Nurses actively participated in this program (Aly & Roth, 1984; Benedict & Kuhla, 1999; McFarland-Icke, 1999). For the most part, however, eugenics involved preventing the physically and mentally disabled from reproducing; sterilization was a favoured strategy. Alberta and British Columbia had laws that sanctioned forced sterilization of the mentally ill and the intellectually disabled until the early 1970s (Cox).

With contemporary advances in genetic engineering, a new eugenics may arise. In the future, genetic testing may allow prenatal selection and termination of a pregnancy when the fetus is at risk for a mental disorder. (Even though it is doubtful that straight linkages between a given gene and a psychiatric disorder exist; see Chapter 8.) Genetic profiles of individuals may lead to discrimination and to "genetic essentialism" (i.e., a person is defined by his or her genes; Kirby, 2004). In considering the ethical acceptability of clinical genetic testing in a particular situation, such questions as What is the purpose of the test? How predictive is the test? How stigmatized is the condition being tested for? Do effective interventions exist for it? Will the testing affect third parties, such as family members? should be asked (Hoop, 2008). As genetic research evolves, its risks and benefits will need to be continually assessed.

Ethical Practice Environments

Ethical practice environments need to be developed and supported (Austin, 2007b). Research has identified nurses' environmental problems to include an inability to engage in ethical deliberations, receive administrative support, and have policies consistent with practice (McDaniel, 1997). Environment is predictive of nurses' moral distress (Corley, Minick, Elswick, & Jacobs, 2005). Relationships (with patients, peers, physicians, and administration) are a key issue (Olson, 1998).

Fisher (1995) discovered that when PMH nurses balanced their desire to "do the right thing" with the need to "get along with colleagues," colleagues won out. Carpenter (1991) also found that power structures and concern for relationships were the reasons for PMH nurses' rejection of a first choice of the right thing to do. Forchuk (1991), in her descriptive study of the ethical conflicts of Canadian PMH nurses, learned that staff conflict played a major role in inpatient settings. It must be asked, "In what types of environments can doing the right thing and getting along coexist (Fisher, 1995, p. 203)?"

It should be safe for nurses, including students, to raise their ethical questions and concerns (Dwyer, 1994). Nurses' ethical assertiveness (i.e., trying to influence ethical deliberation, even when not invited) is, unfortunately, least likely to occur when nurses do not expect the acceptance of their input—exactly when assertiveness is needed (Dodd et al., 2004). For our PMH settings to be morally habitable, a "culture of questioning" must be actively nurtured (Austin, Bergum, & Nuttgens, 2004). CNA, the Canadian Medical Association, and the Boards of Directors of the Canadian Healthcare Association and the Catholic Health Care Association have developed a joint statement on preventing and resolving ethical conflicts involving health care. It is available at the CNA website, as is their position on quality professional practice environments and what is needed for nurses to provide safe, competent, and ethical care to the trusting public (see Web Links).

Research Ethics in PMH Nursing

Psychiatric research in Canada has a tainted history. In the 1950s and early 1960s, the "depatterning" experiments of Dr. Ewen Cameron at the Allen Memorial Institute, McGill University (partially funded by the U.S. Central Intelligence Agency), were an attempt to erase the memories of patients before the insertion of new "positive" ideas. Without their consent, patients were "brainwashed," with many permanently losing their memories. Although Dr. Cameron was an international leader in psychiatric medicine with the reputation of being a humanitarian, his research caused great harm to his patients (Collins, 1988; see Movies at the end of the

chapter). His research is a strong example of the necessity for vigilance regarding the ethics of research.

At the same time, there must be adequate support for mental health and addictions research. Although persons with a mental disorder may be at times more vulnerable because of their illness, they are no more vulnerable than other groups of research participants, as long as the research is conducted in an ethically sensitive way (Adshead, 2008; Usher & Holmes, 1997). DuVal (2004) analyzed study designs in psychiatric research and identified three types that raise particular ethical concerns: (1) placebo-controlled studies may deprive participants in the placebo arm of the research from needed existing treatment; (2) washout studies (in which patients' or subjects' medications are discontinued) can put persons at risk for illness; and (3) challenge studies (a pharmaceutical or psychological challenge is administered under controlled conditions, usually with some deception, and the subject's response observed) may cause adverse effects.

These risks need to be attended to in the planning, conducting, and evaluating of research projects, ensuring that persons with mental illness, addiction, or neurologic impairment are never exploited.

CNA (2003a, 2003b) has developed *Ethical Research Guidelines for Registered Nurses* that speak to nurse researchers and research assistants, to staff nurses who are caring for people who are research subjects or who are collecting research information, to nurses who serve on research ethics committees, to nurse administrators who monitor research activities, and to nurses who are teaching research ethics. The guidelines are in accordance with the *Tri-Council Policy Statement on the Ethical Conduct of Research Involving Humans* (Medical Research Council of Canada, Natural Sciences and Engineering Research Council of Canada, & Social Sciences and Humanities Council of Canada, 1998) that delineates the ethics policy of Canada's federal research funding agencies.

Social Justice

Conditions of fundamental equality and justice are seen as important to optimal mental health (Epp, 1988, p. 9; see Chapter 2). Justice, a principle of fair treatment of individuals and groups within society, is a core value underpinning the CNA *Code of Ethics*. "Social justice involves attention to those who are most vulnerable in society, e.g., those who have been excluded or forgotten due to handicap, limited education or failing health" (CNA, 2002, p. 20). In Canada, the inequality of resources mandated to mental health care within the overall health care system may be identified as a social justice issue. The stigma and discrimination associated with mental illness negatively affect resource allocation. The nature of mental health problems and mental disorders means that a quality response to them involves more than the

FIGURE 7.1 *Untitled.* Sylvester Kantontoka. (Originally published in *Denied Citizens* [2005], World Health Organization.)

health care system itself. Teachers, social workers, clergy, police, and others also contribute to a complex system of supports and services. Unfortunately, this complex system seems to be poorly coordinated—to the extent that it increases the chance for homelessness and incarceration of the mentally ill (Kirby, 2004). To address these and other issues, the government of Canada announced, in November 2005, the formation of a Canadian Mental Health Commission. Canada is one of the few industrialized nations without a national mental health strategy.

The social injustices related to mental illness exist worldwide (Desjarlais, Isenberg, Good, & Kleinman, 1995). When, in 2001, the WHO report focused on mental health, its findings were disturbing. Only a small percentage of the 450 million people who suffer from a behavioural disorder receive even minimal treatment; 40% of countries have no mental health policy; 30% have no mental health program; and 90% have no mental health policy that includes children and adolescents. Although mental and behavioural disorders account for 12% of the global burden of diseases, mental health receives less than 1% in health spending for most countries (WHO, 2001). In some low-income countries, there are few practitioners trained in PMH care; there is limited access to medications and treatment, and stigma and discrimination against persons with mental illness and their families abound (see Chapter 3). In some communities, people with mental disorders are tied or chained to trees or poles, deprived of clothing, and kept in places that lack clean water and toilet facilities (WHO, 2005) (see Fig. 7-1).

Canadian nurses have an ethical responsibility to address the social, economic, and political issues that affect health and well-being (CNA, 2002). Their continued contributions to the mental health of Canadians are important. A new ethical question, however, is arising. As members of a global community, what can and should Canadian nurses do to address the inequities and injustices experienced by persons with mental illness living in other parts of the world (Austin, 2001c)?

SUMMARY OF KEY POINTS

☐ Ethics is the consideration of the way a person should act in order to live a good life with and for others.

☐ Ethics and law are separate domains. Nurses must be vigilant about the laws that affect their practice.

☐ Key issues can warn us about the ethical tone of our society; many of these issues are situated in health care. The way in which Canadians address the well-being of persons living with mental illness is one of these issues.

☐ Whenever nurses enact their professional responsibilities, they are active as moral agents. Nursing practice involves "everyday ethics," an attentiveness and responsiveness to their duties and commitments.

☐ CNA supports ethical practice through the *Code of Ethics for Registered Nurses* and *Ethical Research Guidelines for Registered Nurses*, as well as the development of various position statements (e.g., on torture, conflict resolution) and resources such as *Ethics in Practice*.

☐ There are theoretical approaches to ethical knowledge (based on moral philosophy and concepts such as human rights) that inform health ethics. These include virtue ethics, deontology, utilitarianism, principlism, casuistry, ethics of care, feminist ethics, relational ethics, and human rights.

☐ A moral dilemma is a morally relevant conflict in which one must choose between incompatible alternatives. Frameworks for ethical decision making are available to assist in such a choice. Moral distress is the anger, frustration, or anguish experienced when one is unable to fulfill one's ethical obligations as one believes one should.

☐ There are many complex ethical issues in PMH settings. These include issues related to behaviour control and restraint, relational engagement, confidentiality and privacy, ethical practice environments, research ethics, and social justice.

CRITICAL THINKING CHALLENGES

1 Identify a PMH nursing situation that involves an ethical dilemma. Use a decision-making framework to decide how the nurse should act in the situation.

2 Recall an experience of moral distress. What were the barriers to doing what you believed was right? Did you discuss your concerns with others? How was the situation resolved? Was it ever resolved for you? Is there anything that you would do differently?

3 Who is your moral hero? What are his or her heroic characteristics? What, for you, constitutes moral courage?

4 In their anthology, *The Moral of the Story*, Singer and Singer (2005) have collected works that raise issues of ethics. Use this resource or select your own stories to help you explore the question of how we should live together.

5 In his "sci-phi" book, *The Philosopher at the End of the Universe*, Mark Rowlands (2004) addresses such issues as good and evil (Star Wars), the question of why one should be moral (*Hollow Man*), and the problem of free will (*Minority Report*). View two films in the science fiction genre. Identify the philosophical themes they raise.

WEB LINKS

www.cna-nurses.ca The website of the Canadian Nurses Association includes the *Code of Ethics*, *Guidelines for Research*, position statements, and the *Ethics in Practice* series. At the website, select the "Nursing Practice" tab and then select "Nursing Ethics."

www.bioethics.georgetown.edu The National Reference Center for Bioethics Literature (Kennedy Institute of Ethics, United States), on the Georgetown University website, can be accessed to search for articles and books and to request a customized bibliography.

The following are the websites of Canadian health ethics centres:

www.ethics.ubc.ca The W. Maurice Young Centre for Applied Ethics, University of British Columbia.

www.ualberta.ca/bioethics Dossetor Health Ethics Centre, University of Alberta.

www.utoronto.ca/jcb University of Toronto Joint Centre for Bioethics.

www.mcgill.ca/biomedicalethicsunit McGill University Biomedical Ethics Unit.

bioethics.medicine.dal.ca Dalhousie University, Department of Bioethics.

The following are websites of health ethics organizations:

www.phen.ab.ca The Provincial Health Ethics Network (PHEN) of Alberta is a nonprofit organization that provides resources on addressing ethical issues related to health.

www.bioethics.ca Canadian Bioethics Society.

www.fabnet.org International Network Feminist Approaches to Bioethics.

www.bioethics-international.org International Association of Bioethics.

www.unesco.org/shs/bioethics This is the quick link to UNESCO's bioethics page, where the UNESCO Declaration of Bioethics and Human Rights can be found.

www.pre.ethics.gc.ca This is the website of the Interagency Advisory Panel on Research Ethics where you can access the *Tri-Council Policy Statement on Ethical Conduct for Research Involving Humans*. Check the "Links" at this site for more research ethics websites.

MOVIES, NOVELS, AND BIOGRAPHIES

The Terminal: 2004. Although it is unlikely that this movie was meant to be an illustration of virtue, it is. The main character, Viktor Navorski, is on a quest to fulfill a promise to his father and arrives in New York from his homeland, Krakozia. Because a coup occurred in Krakozia during his journey, Viktor becomes a citizen of nowhere, stranded in the airport. It is during his struggles to survive in the terminal that Viktor reveals what it means to be a virtuous man. Other characters, Gupta (a cleaner), Amelia (a flight attendant), and Frank (the airport manager), are lacking in virtue and act as foils to Viktor's "practical wisdom."

VIEWING POINTS: In one scene, Viktor refuses to lie even though it will help him; yet in another, he does tell a lie. Explain this inconsistency using virtue theory.

Virtue is learned in relationship with others. How is this illustrated in the movie?

The first line of *The Terminal*, "What is the purpose of your visit?" seems to echo a theme of virtue theory, what is the purpose of your life? Imagine how each of the characters might answer such a question. How would you answer it?

Wit: 2001. Vivian Bearing, a professor of English literature, learns that she has ovarian cancer with little hope of recovery. She agrees to take part in a research project. Based on a Pulitzer Prize winning play, *Wit* reveals the nuances of relationships between patient/research subject and caregiver/researcher.

VIEWING POINTS: Do you think Professor Bearing gave informed consent for her participation in the research? On what do you base your response? Using the core elements of relational ethics, deconstruct the scene between patient and nurse that occurs in the early hours of the morning.

The Sleep Room: 1998. This 4-hour CBC miniseries is based on the true story of Dr. Ewen Cameron's CIA-funded "depatterning" experiments in Montreal in the 1950s and early 1960s. It is based on the book, *In the Sleep Room* (Collins, 1988).

VIEWING POINTS: What factors, in your opinion, allowed this research to happen? Could something similar happen today? Imagine that you are a student nurse in the 1950s, assigned to a practicum on Dr. Cameron's ward. How might you react? What pressures might shape your reaction to participating in the research?

REFERENCES

Adshead, G. (2008). Studying the mind: Ethical issues and guidance in mental health research. *Clinical Ethics, 3,* 141–144.

Alberta Association of Registered Nurses. (1998). *Professional boundaries for registered nurses: guidelines for the nurse–client relationship.* Edmonton, AB: Author.

Aly, G., & Roth, K. H. (1984). The legalization of mercy killings in medical and nursing institutions in Nazi Germany from 1938 to 1941. *International Journal of Law and Psychiatry, 7,* 145–163.

Appelbaum, P. (2004). Ethical issues in psychiatric genetics. *Journal of Psychiatric Practice, 10*(6), 343–352.

Aristotle. (1996). *Nicomachean ethics.* H. Rackham (Trans.). Ware, UK: Wordsworth Classics.

Armstrong, A., Parsons, S., & Barker, P. (2000). *Journal of Psychiatric and Mental Health Nursing, 7,* 297–306.

Audi, R. (Ed.). (1995). *The Cambridge dictionary of philosophy.* Cambridge, UK: Cambridge University Press.

Austin, W. (2001a). Relational ethics in forensic settings. *Journal of Psychosocial Nursing, 39*(9), 12–17.

Austin, W. (2001b). Using the human rights paradigm in health ethics: The problems and the possibilities. *Nursing Ethics, 8*(13), 183–195.

Austin, W. (2001c). Nursing ethics in an era of globalization. *Advances in Nursing Science, 24*(2), 1–18.

Austin, W. (2006). Toward an understanding of trust. In J. Cutcliff & H. McKenna (Eds.), *The essential concepts of nursing* (pp. 317–330). London, UK: Churchill Livingstone.

Austin, W. (2007a). The ethics of everyday practice: Healthcare environments as moral communities. *Advances in Nursing Science, 30*(1), 81–88.

Austin, W. (2007b). The terminal: A tale of virtue. *Nursing Ethics, 14*(1), 54–61.

Austin, W., Bergum, V., & Dossetor, J. (2003). Relational ethics: An action ethic as foundation for health care. In V. Tschudin (Ed.), *Approaches to ethics* (pp. 45–52). Woburn, MA: Butterworth-Heinemann.

Austin, W., Bergum, V., & Goldberg, L. (2003). Unable to answer the call of our patients: Mental health nurses' experiences of moral distress. *Nursing Inquiry, 10*(3), 177–183.

Austin, W., Bergum, V., & Nuttgens, S. (2004). Addressing oppression in psychiatric care: A relational ethics perspective. *Ethical Human Psychology and Psychiatry, 6*(1), 69–78.

Austin, W., Bergum, V., Nuttgens, S., & Peternelj-Taylor, C. (2006). A revisioning of boundaries in professional helping relationships: Exploring other metaphors. *Ethics & Behaviour, 16*(2), 77–94.

Austin, W., Lemermeyer, G., Goldberg, L., Bergum, V., & Johnson, M. (2005). Moral distress in healthcare practice: The situation of nurses. *HealthCare Ethics Committee Forum: An Interprofessional Journal on Healthcare Institutions' Ethical and Legal Issues, 17*(1), 33–48.

Baier, A. (1985). What do women want in a moral theory? *Nous, 19,* 53–65.

Baier, A. (1994). *Moral prejudices: Essays on ethics.* Cambridge, MA: Harvard University Press.

Bentham, J. (1983). *Deontology together with a table on the springs of action and the article on utilitarianism.* Oxford, UK: Oxford University Press.

Beauchamp, T. (1994). The "four principles" approach. In R. Gillon (Ed.), *Principles of health care ethics* (pp. 3–12). New York, NY: John Wiley & Sons.

Beauchamp, T., & Childress, J. (2008). *Principles of biomedical ethics* (6th ed.). New York, NY: Oxford University Press.

Benedict, S., & Kuhla, J. (1999). Nurses' participation in the euthanasia programs of Nazi Germany. *Western Journal of Nursing Research, 21*(2), 246–263.

Bergum, V., & Dossetor, J. (2005). *Relational ethics: The full meaning of respect.* Hagerstown, MD: University Publishing Group.

Breggin, P. (1997). Coercion in voluntary commitment. In R. Edwards (Ed.), *Ethics of psychiatry.* Amherst, NY: Prometheus Books.

Brody, E. (1995). Editorial: The humanity of psychotic persons and their rights. *Journal of Nervous and Mental Disease, 183*(4), 193–194.

Campbell, J. (1997). How consumer/survivors are evaluating the quality of psychiatric care. *Evaluation Review, 21*(3), 357–363.

Campbell, R. J. (2002). *Attitudes and behaviours of Alberta mental health nurses toward professional boundaries, boundary crossings and boundary violations in patient care.* Unpublished Masters Thesis. University of Alberta.

Campbell, R. J., Yonge, O., & Austin, W. (2005). Intimacy boundaries between mental health nurses and psychiatric patients. *Journal of Psychosocial Nursing and Mental Health Services, 43*(5), 239.

Canadian Nurses Association. (2002). *Code of ethics for registered nurses.* Ottawa, ON: Author.

Canadian Nurses Association. (2003a, October). Ethical distress in health care environments. *Ethics in Practice for Registered Nurses.* Retrieved February 20, 2006, from http://www.cna-nurses.ca/cna/documents/pdf/publications/Ethics_Pract_Ethical_Distress_Oct_2003_e.pdf

Canadian Nurses Association. (2003b, October). Privacy and health information: Challenges for nurses and for the nursing profession. *Ethics in Practice for Registered Nurses.* Retrieved February 20, 2006, from www.cna-nurses.ca/cna/documents/pdf/publications/Ethics_Pract_Privacy_Health_Nov_2003_e.pdf

Canadian Nurses Association. (2008). *Code of ethics for registered nurses.* Ottawa, ON: Author.

Carpenter, M. (1991). The process of ethical decision making in psychiatric nursing practice. *Issues in Mental Health Nursing, 12,* 179–191.

College of Registered Nurses of British Columbia. (2007). *Practice standard for Registered Nurses and Nurse Practitioners: Duty to provide care.* Vancouver, BC: Author.

Collins, A. (1988). *In the sleep room: The story of the CIA brainwashing experiments in Canada.* Toronto, ON: Lester & Orpen Dennys.

Corley, M. (2002). Nurse moral distress: A proposed theory and research agenda. *Nursing Ethics, 9*(6), 636–650.

Corley, M., Minick, R., Elswick, R., & Jacobs, M. (2005). Nurse moral distress and ethical work environment. *Nursing Ethics, 12*(4), 381–390.

Cox, S. (2005). Human genetics, ethics and disability. In J. Storch, P. Rodney, & R. Starzomski (Eds.), *Toward a moral horizon: Nursing ethics for leadership and practice* (pp. 378–395). Toronto, ON: Pearson Education.

Dahlqvist, V., Soderberg, A., & Norberg, A. (2009). Facing inadequacy and being good enough: Psychiatric care providers' narratives about experiencing and coping with troubled conscience. *Journal of Psychiatric and Mental Health Nursing, 16,* 242–247.

Davis, A., Liaschenko, J., Aroskar, M., & Drought, T. (Eds.). (1997). *Ethical dilemmas and nursing practice.* Stamford, CT: Appleton & Lange.

Desjarlais, R., Isenberg, L., Good, B., & Kleinman, A. (1995). *World mental health: Problems and priorities in low-income countries.* Oxford, UK: Oxford University Press.

Dodd, S. J., Jansson, B., Brown-Saltzman, K., Shirk, M., & Wunch, K. (2004). Expanding nurses' participation in ethics: An empirical examination of ethical activism and ethical assertiveness. *Nursing Ethics, 11*(1), 15–27.

DuVal, G. (2004). Ethics in psychiatric research: Study design issues. *Canadian Journal of Psychiatry, 49*(1), 55–59.

Dwyer, J. (1994). Primum non tacere: An ethics of speaking up. *Hastings Center Report, 24*(1), 13–18.

Epp, J. (1988). *Mental health for Canadians: Striking a balance* (Cat. H39–128/1988E). Ottawa, ON: Supply and Services Canada.

Epstein, R. (1994). *Keeping boundaries: Maintaining safety and integrity in the psychotherapeutic process.* Washington, DC: American Psychiatric Press.

Eriksson, K., & Kjellin, L. (1989). Study of psychiatric care, especially compulsory care, in two Swedish counties: The psychiatric personnel's attitudes and experience of compulsory care. *Nordic Journal of Psychiatry, 43,* 365–368.

Eriksson, K., & Westrin, C. (1995). Coercive measures in psychiatric care: Reports and reactions of patients and people involved. *Acta Psychiatrica Scandinavica, 92,* 225–230.

Fisher, A. (1995). The ethical problems encountered in psychiatric nursing practice with dangerous mentally ill persons. *Scholarly Inquiry for Nursing Practice: An International Journal, 9*(2), 193–208.

Forchuk, C. (1991). Ethical problems encountered by mental health nurses. *Issues in Mental Health Nursing, 12,* 375–383.

Fowler, M. (1997). Nursing's ethics. In A. Davis, J. Liaschenko, M. Aroskar, & T. Drought (Eds.), *Ethical dilemmas and nursing practice* (pp. 17–34). Stamford, CT: Appleton & Lange.

Fry, S., Harvey, R., Hurley, A., & Foley, B. (2002). Development of a model of moral distress in the military. *Nursing Ethics, 9*(4), 373–387.

Gallop, R. (1993). Balance of power in the provider/client relationship. *College Communiqué, 18*(3), 9–12.

Gallop, R. (1997). Caring about the client: The role of gender, empathy and power in the therapeutic process. In S. Tilley (Ed.), *The mental health nurse: Views from practice and education* (pp. 28–42). Oxford, UK: Blackwell Science.

Gallop, R., McCay, E., Guha, M., & Khan, P. (1999). The experience of hospitalization and restraint of women who have a history of childhood sexual abuse. *Health Care for Women International, 20*(4), 401–416.

Gallup (2005, December). Nurses remain atop honesty and ethics list. Retrieved October 29, 2009, from http://www.gallup.com/poll/20254/Nurses-Remain-Atop-Honesty-Ethic

Garritson, S. (1988). Ethical decision making. *Journal of Psychosocial Nursing and Mental Health Services, 26*(4), 22–29, 35.

Gilligan, C. (1982). *In a different voice: Psychological theory and women's development.* Cambridge, MA: Harvard University Press.

Gostin, L. (2001). Beyond moral claims: A human rights approach in mental health. *Cambridge Quarterly of Healthcare Ethics, 10,* 264–274.

Griener, G. (2005). Electronic health records as a threat to privacy. *Health Law Review, 14*(1), 14–17.

Holmes, D. (2001). From iron gaze to nursing care: Mental health nursing in the era of panopticism. *Journal of Psychiatric and Mental Health Nursing, 8,* 7–15.

Holmes, D., & Jacob, J. (2007). Seclusion practice: A critical examination of the nurses" decision-making process. *BioMedCentrel Psychiatry, 7*(Suppl. 1), S147. Available at: www.biomedcentral.com/147–244X/7/S1/S147

Holmes, D., Kennedy, S., & Perron, A. (2004). The mentally ill and social exclusion: A critical examination of the use of seclusion from the patient's perspective. *Issues of Mental Health Nursing, 25*(6), 559–578.

Hoop, J. (2008). Ethical considerations in psychiatric genetics. *Harvard Review of Psychiatry, 16*(6), 322–336.

Illes, J., & Racine, E. (2005). Imaging or imagining? A neuroethics challenge informed by genetics. *American Journal of Bioethics, 5*(2), 5–18.

Ipperciel, D. (2003). Dialogue and discussion in a moral context. *Nursing Philosophy, 4,* 211–224.

Jameton, A. (1993). Dilemmas of moral distress: Moral responsibility and nursing practice. *AWONN's Clinical Issues in Perinatal and Women's Health Nursing, 4*(4), 542–551.

Jonsen, A. (1991). Casuistry as methodology in clinical ethics. *Theoretical Medicine, 12,* 295–307.

Jonsen, A., & Toulmin, S. (1988). *The abuse of casuistry: A history of moral reasoning.* Berkeley, CA: University of California Press.

Kant, I. (1996). *Practical philosophy.* M. Gregor, (Trans.). Cambridge, UK: Cambridge University Press.

Kaplan, B., & Litewka, S. (2008). Ethical challenges of telemedicine and telehealth. *Cambridge Quarterly of Healthcare Ethics, 17,* 401–416.

Kirby, M. (2004, November). *Interim report on mental health, mental illness and addiction of the Standing Senate Committee on Social Affairs, Science and Technology.* Retrieved February 20, 2006, from http://www.parl.gc.ca/38/1/parlbus/commbus/senate/com-e/soci-e/rep-e/repintnov04-e.htm

Kjellin, L., Westrin, C-G., Eriksson, K., Axelsson, M., Candefjord, I. L., Ekblom, B., et al. (1993). Coercion in psychiatric care: Problems of medical ethics in a comprehensive-empirical study. *Behavioral Sciences and the Law, 11,* 323–334.

Larue, C., Dumais, A., Ahern, E., Bernheim, E., & Mailhot, M-P. (2009). Factors Influencing Decisions on Seclusion and Restraint. *Journal of Psychiatric and Mental Health Nursing, 16,* 440–446.

Leary, V. (1994). The right to health in international human rights law. *Health and Human Rights, 1*(1), 25–57.

Levine, M. (1977). Nursing ethics and the ethical nurse. *American Journal of Nursing, 77*(5), 845–849.

Liaschenko, J. (1994). Making a bridge: The moral work with patients we do not like. *Journal of Palliative Care, 10*(3), 83–89.

Liaschenko, J., & Peter, E. (2003). Feminist ethics. In V. Tschudin (Ed.), *Approaches to ethics: Nursing beyond boundaries.* Edinburgh, UK: Butterworth/Heinemann.

Loughrey, L., Jackson, J., Molla, P., & Wobbleton, J. (1997). Patient self-mutilation: When nursing becomes a nightmare. *Journal of Psychosocial Nursing, 35*(4), 30–34.

Lützen, K., & da Silva, A. B. (1996). The role of virtue ethics in psychiatric nursing. *Nursing Ethics, 3*(3), 202–211.

MacIntyre, A. (1984). *After virtue* (2nd ed.). Notre Dame, IN: University of Notre Dame.

Magnusson, A., & Lützén, K. (1999). Intrusion into patient privacy: A moral concern in the home care of persons with chronic mental illness. *Nursing Ethics, 6*(5), 399–410.

Mann, J., Gostin, L., Gruskin, S., Brennan, T., Lazzarini, Z., & Fineberg, H. (1999). Health and human rights. In J. Mann, S. Gruskin, M. Grodin, & G. Annas (Eds.). *Health and human rights: A reader* (pp. 7–20). New York, NY: Routledge.

Marangos-Frost, S., & Wells, D. (2000). Psychiatric nurses' thoughts and feelings about restraint use: a decision dilemma. *Journal of Advanced Nursing, 31*(2), 362–369.

Martin, N. (2001). Feminist bioethics and psychiatry. *Journal of Medicine and Philosophy, 26*(4), 431–441.

McCain, M., & Kornegay, K. (2005). Behavioral health restraint: The experience and beliefs of seasoned psychiatric nurses. *Journal for Nurses in Staff Development, 21*(5), 236–242.

McDaniel, C. (1997). Development and psychometric properties of the Ethics Environment Questionnaire. *Medical Care, 35,* 901–914.

McFarland-Icke, B. R. (1999). *Nurses in Nazi Germany: Moral choice in history.* Princeton, NJ: Princeton University Press.

McLaughlin, C. (1999). An exploration of psychiatric nurses' and patients' opinions regarding in-patient care for suicidal patients. *Journal of Advanced Nursing, 29*(5), 1042–1051.

Medical Research Council of Canada, Natural Sciences and Engineering Research Council of Canada, & Social Sciences and Humanities Council of Canada. (1998). *Tri-council policy statement: Ethical conduct for research involving humans.* Ottawa, ON: Authors.

Mental Disability Rights International. (2002). Not on the agenda: Human rights of people with mental disabilities in Kosovo. Retrieved February 19, 2006, from http://www.mdri.org/pdf/KosovoReport.pdf

Midence, G., Gregory, S., & Stanley, R. (1996). The effects of a patient suicide on nursing staff. *Journal of Clinical Nursing, 5,* 15–20.

Mill, J. S. (2002). *The basic writings of John Stuart Mill: On liberty, the subjection of women and utilitarianism.* New York, NY: Modern Library.

Moore, D. (1999, August 20). Actor urges people to take control of their mental health. *Edmonton Journal,* A12.

Muller, A., & Poggenpoel, M. (1996). Patients' internal world experience of interacting with psychiatric nurses. *Archives of Psychiatric Nursing, 10*(3), 143–150.

Nathaniel, A. (2002). Ethics and human rights. *American Nurses Association Issues Update, 1*(2), 3–8.

Niebuhr, R. (1963). *The responsible self.* San Francisco, CA: Harper.

Nietzsche, F. (2000). *Basic writings of Nietzsche.* New York, NY: The Modern Library.

Noddings, N. (1984). *Caring: A feminine approach to ethics and moral education.* Berkeley, CA: University of California Press.

Oberle, K., & Bouchal, S. R. (2009). *Ethics in Canadian nursing practice: Navigating the journey.* Toronto, ON: Pearson Education.

Olofsson, B., Gilje, F., Jacobsson, L., & Norberg, A. (1998). Nurses' narratives about using coercion in psychiatric care. *Journal of Advanced Nursing, 28*(1), 45–53.

Olson, L. (1998). Hospital nurses' perceptions of the ethical climate of their work setting. *Image, the Journal of Nursing Science, 30,* 345–349.

Ormrod, J., & Ambrose, L. (1999). Public perceptions about confidentiality in mental health services. *Journal of Mental Health, 8*(4), 413–421.

Paine, T. (1996). *Rights of man.* Ware, UK: Wordsworth Editions.

Peter, E., & Morgan, K. P. (2001). Explorations of a trust approach for nursing ethics. *Nursing Inquiry, 8*(3), 3–10.

Peternelj-Taylor, C. (2003). Whistleblowing and boundary violations: Exposing a colleague in the forensic milieu. *Nursing Ethics, 10*(5), 526–537.

Radden, J., & Sadler, J. (2008). Character virtues in psychiatric practice. *Harvard Review of Psychiatry, 16*(6), 373–380.

Ricouer, P. (1992). *Oneself as another.* K. Blamey, (Trans.). Chicago, IL: University of Chicago Press. (Original work published 1990)

Robertson, M., Morris, K., & Walter, G. (2007). Overview of psychiatric ethics V: Utilitarianism and the ethics of duty. *Australasian Psychiatry, 15*(5), 402–410.

Rodgers, S. (2004). Sexual abuse by health care professionals: The failure of reform in Ontario. *Health Law Journal, 12,* 71–102.

Roper, C. (Ed.). (2003). *Conversations between service receivers: On mental health nursing and the psychiatric service system.* Melbourne, Australia: Centre for Psychiatric Research and Practice.

Rowlands, M. (2004). *The philosopher at the end of the universe: Philosophy explained through science fiction films.* New York, NY: St. Martin's Press.

Ryan, C., & Bowers, L. (2005). Coercive measures in a psychiatric intensive care unit. *Journal of Psychiatric and Mental Health Nursing, 12,* 695–702.

Saul, J. R. (2001). *On equilibrium.* Toronto, ON: Penguin/Viking.

Scott, A. (2003). Virtue, nursing and the moral domain of practice. In V. Tschudin (Ed.), *Approaches to ethics: Nursing beyond boundaries* (pp. 25–32). Edinburgh, UK: Butterworth/Heinemann.

Scott, A. (1998). Professional ethics: Are we on the right track? *Nursing Ethics, 5*(6), 477–496.

Sherwin, S. (1992). *No longer patient: Feminist ethics and health care.* Philadelphia, PA: Temple University Press.

Sibbald, B. (2005) Nurse to know: Ethics in action. *Canadian Nurse, 101*(5), 44.

Singer, P., & Singer, R. (Eds.). (2005). *The moral of the story: An anthology of ethics through literature.* Oxford, UK: Blackwell.

Sjöstedt, E., Dahlstrand, A., Severinsson, E., & Lützén, K. (2001). The first nurse-patient encounter in a psychiatric setting: Discovering a moral commitment in nursing. *Nursing Ethics, 8*(4), 313–327.

Slomka, J., Agich, G., Stagno, S., & Smith, M. (1998). Physical restraint elimination in the acute care setting: Ethical considerations. *HEC Forum, 10*(3–4), 244–262.

Somerville, M. (2000). *The ethical canary: Science, society and the human spirit.* Toronto, ON: Penguin Books.

Strong, C. (2000). Specified principlism: What is it, and does it really resolve cases better than casuistry? *Journal of Medicine and Philosophy, 25*(3), 323–341.

Sumner, L. (2000). Rights. In H. LaFollette (Ed.), *The Blackwell guide to ethical theory* (pp. 288–305). Oxford, UK: Blackwell.

Szasz, T. (1961). The myth of mental illness: Foundations of a theory of personal conduct. New York, NY: Harper & Row.

Szasz, T. (1993). *A lexicon of lunacy: Metaphoric madness, moral responsibility and psychiatry.* New Brunswick, NJ: Transaction Publishing.

Szasz, T. (2005). "Idiots, infants, and the insane": Mental illness and legal incompetence. *Journal of the Institute of Medical Ethics, 31*(2), 78–81.

Tschudin, V. (2003). Preface. In V. Tschudin (Ed.), *Approaches to ethics: Nursing beyond boundaries.* Edinburgh, UK: Butterworth/Heinemann.

Usher, K., & Holmes, C. (1997). Ethical aspects of phenomenological research with mentally ill people. *Nursing Ethics, 4*(1), 49–56.

Van der Merwe, Bowers, L., Jones, J., Simpson, A., Haglund, K. (2009). Locked doors in acute inpatient psychiatry: a literature review. *Journal of Psychiatric & Mental Health Nursing, 16*(3):293–299.

Vuckovich, P., & Artinian, B. (2005). Justifying coercion. *Nursing Ethics, 12*(4), 370–380.

Waldron, J. (1987). *"Nonsense upon stilts": Bentham, Burke and Marx on the rights of man.* London, UK: Methuen.

Walker, T. (2009). What principlism misses. *Jornal of Medical Ethics, 35*(4), 229–231.

Webster, G., & Baylis, F. (2000). Moral residue. In S. Rubin & L. Zoloth (Eds.), *Margin of error: The ethics of mistakes in the practice of medicine* (pp. 217–232). Hagerstown, MD: University Publishing Group.

Wong, J., Poon, Y., & Hui, E. (2005). I can put the medicine in his soup. *Journal of Medical Ethics, 31,* 262–265.

World Health Organization. (2001). *World Health Report 2001: Mental health: New understandings, new hope.* Geneva, Switzerland: Author.

World Health Organization. (2005). *Glaring inequalities for people with mental disorders addressed in new WHO effort.* Retrieved February 20, 2006, from http://www.who.int/mediacentre/news/notes/2005/np14/en/print.html

World Psychiatric Association. (1996). Madrid declaration of ethical standards for psychiatric practice. Retrieved February 20, 2006, from http://www.wpanet.org/generalinfo/ethic1.html

CHAPTER 8

Theoretic Basis of Psychiatric and Mental Health Nursing

Ginette Pagé

Adapted from the chapter "Theoretic Basis of Psychiatric and Mental Health Nursing" by Mary Ann Boyd

LEARNING OBJECTIVES

After studying this chapter, you will be able to:

- Discuss the need for theory-based psychiatric and mental health (PMH) nursing practice.
- Compare the key elements of theories that provide a basis for such practice.
- Describe the common nursing models used in PMH nursing.
- Identify theories that contribute to our understanding of human beings and their behaviours.

KEY CONCEPT

- theory

KEY TERMS

• anima • animus • archetype • behaviourism • classical conditioning • cognition • collective unconscious • conscious • countertransference • diathesis-stress model • disinhibition • ego • elicitation • empathy • extrovert • formal support systems • genetics • genomics • id • informal support systems • interpersonal relations • introvert • modelling • object relations • operant behaviour • preconscious • persona • role • self-actualization • self-efficacy • self-system • shadow • social distance • superego • transaction • transference • unconditional positive regard • unconscious

This chapter presents an overview of some of the nursing and other theories that serve as the knowledge base for PMH nursing practice. Many of the theories underlying this practice are evolving, and only some have research support to date. As acknowledged in the *Canadian Standards of Psychiatric-Mental Health Nursing*, PMH nurses use knowledge from nursing, the health sciences, and related mental health disciplines in their practice. The chapter begins, then, with selected nursing theories and moves to some of the many theories that underlie our understanding of the biologic,

psychological, social, and spiritual aspects of human knowledge and experience.

NURSING THEORIES

Nursing **theories** are essential in conceptualizing nursing practice. Some theories described here are commonly referred to as models, not as theories, and we have followed common practice. We are not, however, differentiating between a model and a theory, as this remains an area of some debate within nursing.

KEY CONCEPT A "**theory** is an imaginative grouping of knowledge, ideas, and experience that are represented symbolically and seek to illuminate a given phenomenon" (Watson, 1988, p. 1).

A nurse may choose to base his or her practice consistently on one nursing theory or may choose to use a specific theory depending on the care situation. For example, in nursing a person with schizophrenia who has problems related to maintaining self-care, Dorothea Orem's deficit theory (1991) may be particularly useful. Peplau's model (1952) may be more helpful in addressing relationship issues. The theory or theories used by a nurse reveal the way that nurse conceives his or her practice.

Nightingale: The Visionary

Florence Nightingale (1820–1910), the founder of modern nursing, is recognized as the first nurse researcher and the pioneer of theory development in nursing. Many nurses believe that "if her model for nursing had been followed, the nursing profession would be in a much more advantageous position in society today" (MacPhail, 1988, p. 49). The respect for her legacy is apparent: International Nurses Day is celebrated on her birthday, May 12, and Canada's National Nursing Week occurs the second week of May. Nightingale's model, developed in the mid-1800s, emerged from her work in hospitals and in the Crimean War, where unhealthy physical environments for the sick prevailed (Nightingale, 1859). This is the reason that the primary focus of her model, although not neglecting psychosocial and spiritual needs, is on improving environmental conditions. Nightingale's intent was to create healthy surroundings that help alleviate suffering and promote well-being. Health, for her, included the ability to use "every power we have." For example, she considered that giving false reassurance to sick people was unacceptable behaviour. For Nightingale, the curative process was accomplished by nature alone: medicine and nursing do not cure. Nursing activities, therefore, were to "put the patient in the best condition for nature to act upon [him or her]" (p. 75).

Interpersonal Relations Models

Hildegard Peplau: Interpersonal Relations

Hildegard Peplau's (1909–1999) perspective continues to be an important base for the practice of PMH nursing. Influenced by Harry Stack Sullivan (discussed later in this chapter), Peplau (1952) introduced the first systematic framework for PMH nursing in her book *Interpersonal Relations in Nursing*. One of her major contributions was the introduction of the nurse–patient relationship,

including a conceptualization of its phases (see Chapter 9). Although her work continues to stimulate debate, she led PMH nursing out of the confinement of custodial care into a unique PMH nursing model for practice.

Peplau (1992) believed in the importance of the interpersonal environment, which included interactions between person and family, parent and child, or patient and nurse. She emphasized empathic linkage, the ability to feel in oneself the feelings experienced by another person or people. The interpersonal transmission of anxiety or panic is the most common empathic linkage, but other feelings, such as anger, disgust, and envy, can also be communicated nonverbally to others. Peplau believed that if nurses pay attention to what they feel during a relationship with a patient, they can gain invaluable observations of feelings a patient is experiencing, even those the patient has not yet recognized or spoken about.

CRNENOTE

In being empathic as a nurse, one should know that it is not enough to attempt to understand the patient's experience. Nurses need to communicate to their patients that they are attempting to understand.

The **self-system** is an important concept in Peplau's model. Drawing from Sullivan (1953), Peplau defined the self as an "antianxiety system" and a product of socialization. The self proceeds through personal development that is always open to revision but tends toward stability. For example, in parent–child relationships, patterns of approval, disapproval, and indifference are used by children to define themselves. If the verbal and nonverbal messages have been derogatory, children incorporate these messages and also view themselves negatively. The concept of need is also important to Peplau's model. Needs are primarily of biologic origin but are met within a sociocultural environment. When a biologic need is present, it gives rise to tension that is reduced and relieved by behaviours meeting that need. According to Peplau, nurses are not concerned about needs per se but recognize the patients' patterns and style of meeting their needs in relation to their health status. Nurses interact with patients to identify available resources, such as food, interpersonal support, and support for interaction patterns that help patients obtain what is required to satisfy their needs.

Anxiety is another key concept for Peplau, who contended that professional practice is unsafe if anxiety is not understood. If anxiety is not recognized, it continues to rise and escalates toward panic. There are various levels of anxiety (mild, moderate, severe, and panic levels), each having observable behavioural cues. These cues are sometimes called *defensive*, but Peplau argues that they are often "relief behaviours." For example, some people

Hildegard Peplau (1909–1999)
Psychiatric Nurse of the Century

Peplau, born in 1909, became a nurse in 1931 in Pennsylvania. During World War II she joined the Army Nurse Corps and worked in a neuropsychiatric clinic in London. She obtained a Master's Degree (1947) and a PhD (1953) from Columbia University. Peplau took the lead in the development of psychiatric nursing as a specialty at the Master's level and developed the theory of psychodynamic nursing. Peplau has numerous publications, with her most influential works being *Interpersonal Relations in Nursing* (1952), *Aspects of Psychiatric Nursing* (1957), and *Principles of Patient Counselling* (1964).

Her ideas regarding the centrality of relationship to nursing practice and the efficacy of the use of self as a nursing tool have had far reaching effects. She envisioned nursing as an independent discipline from medicine and worked to ensure that this was so. Drawing on interdisciplinary knowledge from psychology, education, and pragmatic educational philosophy, she deeply influenced the professional and scientific development of nursing. Her achievements occurred during a time when strong leadership from women was frowned upon, and she faced many conflicts and controversies throughout a 50-year career that included being President of the American Nurses Association and consultant to the World Health Organization in psychiatric nursing. She was named as one of 50 Great Americans by Marquis' *Who's Who*. Hildegard Peplau was an honorary member of the Canadian Federation of Mental Health Nurses.

Source: Calaway, B. J. (2002). *Hildegard Peplau: Psychiatric nurse of the century*. New York, NY: Springer.

may relieve their anxiety by yelling and swearing, whereas others seek relief by withdrawing. In both instances, anxiety, according to Peplau, is generated by an unmet self-system security need.

Ida Jean Orlando: The Dynamic Nurse–Patient Relationship

In 1954, Ida Jean Orlando (b. 1926) studied the factors that enhanced or impeded the integration of mental health principles in the basic nursing curriculum. From this study, she published *The Dynamic Nurse–Patient Relationship* (1961). In this work, Orlando identified three areas of nursing concern: the nurse–patient relationship, the nurse's professional role, and the identity and development of knowledge that is distinctly nursing. A nursing situation involves the behaviour of the patient, the reaction of the nurse, and anything that does not relieve the distress of the patient. According to Orlando (1961, 1972), patient distress is related to the inability of the individual to meet or communicate his or her own needs.

Orlando's contribution to nursing practice focuses on the whole patient, rather than on disease or institutional demands. Her ideas continue to be useful today, and current research supports her model (Olson & Hanchett, 1997).

A small nursing study investigated whether Orlando's theory-based practice had a measurable impact on patients' immediate distress when compared with non-specified nursing interventions (Potter & Bockenhauer, 2000). Orlando's approach consisted of the nurse validating the patient's distress before taking any action to reduce it. Patients being cared for by the Orlando group (*n* = 19) experienced significantly less stress than those being cared for with traditional nursing care (*n* = 11).

Existential and Humanistic Theoretic Perspectives

Joyce Travelbee: Seeking Life Meaning

As well as being influenced by Peplau and Orlando, Joyce Travelbee (1926–1973) provided an existential perspective to nursing based on the works of Viktor Frankl, an existential philosopher (see Spiritual Theories section later in this chapter). Existentialists believe that humans seek meaning in their life and experiences. "Suffering" is a feeling of displeasure ranging from simple and transitory mental, physical, or spiritual discomfort to extreme anguish and to those phases beyond anguish, namely, the malignant phase of despair. Despair can be experienced as "not caring"; the terminal phase that follows is apathetic indifference (Travelbee, 1971). Travelbee also applied the concept of hope and defined it as a mental state characterized by the desire to gain an end or accomplish a goal combined with some degree of expectation that what is desired or sought is attainable.

Travelbee expanded the area of concern of mental illness to include long-term physical illnesses. Focusing her attention on individuals who must learn to live with chronic illness, she believed that the nurse's spiritual values and philosophical beliefs about suffering would determine the extent to which the nurse could help ill people find meaning in these situations.

Travelbee's model was never subjected to empiric testing, but it was influential to Paterson and Zderad's work in *Humanist Nursing* (1976) and is congruent with their phenomenological approach. Overall, her use of the interpersonal process as a nursing intervention (Travelbee, 1969) and her focus on suffering and illness helped to define areas of concern for nursing.

Patricia Benner: Primacy of Caring

Patricia Benner (b. 1934) derived her notion of nursing as a caring relationship. As a caring profession, nursing "is guided by the moral art and ethics of care and responsibility" (Benner & Wrubel, 1989, p. xi), and nursing practice is based upon "the lived experience of health and illness" (p. 8). Based upon Heidegger's phenomenological philosophy, Benner describes the person as "a self interpreting being … [who] gets defined in the course of a life … [and] has an effortless and nonreflective understanding of the self in the world" (p. 41). Well-being (the human experience of health or wholeness) is, as is being ill, a distinct way of being in the world. With a phenomenological view, Benner believes the environment situates meaning. People enter situations with their own sets of meanings, habits, and perspectives, and their personal interpretations affect the way they respond in those situations. Within this perspective, Chesla (1994) examined parents who cared for offspring with schizophrenia.

Jean Watson: Caring

The science of caring was initiated by Jean Watson (b. 1940). Watson (1979) believes that caring is the foundation of nursing and recommends that specific theories of caring be developed in relation to specific human conditions and health and illness experiences. She distinguishes between caring and curing, which is considered the work of medicine. The science of caring is based on 7 assumptions and 10 "carative" factors (Barnhart, Bennett, Porter, & Sloan, 1994). One of her assumptions is that "effective caring promotes health and individual or family growth" (p. 153), and one of her carative factors is that "a trusting relationship … involves congruence, **empathy**, nonpossessive warmth, and effective communication" (p. 152). The model has evolved to address, more specifically, the spiritual dimension of the nurse's role, including helping the patient to grow spiritually (Watson, 1988). For Watson, spiritual well-being is the foundation of human health, and she suggests that a troubled soul can lead to illness and disease.

Watson's view is applicable to the care of those who seek help for mental illness. This model emphasizes the importance of sensitivity to self and others; the development of helping and trusting relations; the promotion of interpersonal teaching and learning; and provision for a supportive, protective, and corrective mental, physical, sociocultural, and spiritual environment. Research studies supporting the model use qualitative approaches (Baldursdottir & Jonsdottir, 2002).

Philip Barker: The Tidal Model

Philip Barker's Tidal Model (Barker, 1998; Barker & Buchanan-Barker, 2005), which emerged from the Newcastle University study of the need for nursing (Barker, Jackson & Stevenson, 1998), incorporates Barker's (b. 1946) and his colleagues' Model for Empowering Interactions. It emphasizes the centrality of the lived experience of the person-in-care and is based on the assumption that people are their life stories and that they generate meaning through such stories (Barker, 2001b). The interpersonal nurse–client relationship is

important and envisioned as a respectful collaboration with the person seeking care. The nursing assessment of the person is to be holistic, with the aim of discovering whom the person is through his or her story and his or her perspectives on what is happening during the "current episode of care" (Barker, 2004, p. 341). This assessment is not considered a clinical or therapeutic assessment; it is, rather, the basis for a conversation between the nurse and the person seeking care. As change is a core element in this model (hence the metaphor of the tide), the nurse's role is focused on and shaped by the changing needs of clients across the continuum of care (e.g., critical, transitional, or developmental care). The need for services to be interdependent is argued (Barker, 2001a). Box 8-1 outlines the Tidal Model's "ten commitments" of care.

Systems Models

The McGill Model of Nursing: Health Promotion

Under the guidance of Dr. Moyra Allen, the McGill Model of Nursing was developed by the students and faculty of McGill University School of Nursing. It distinguishes nursing from other health disciplines but also identifies the complementary relationship that exists with them (Allen, 1977). The four major concepts of the model are health, family (person), collaboration, and learning (Gottlieb & Rowat, 1987). Health is considered the focus of the practice of nursing and is seen as coexisting with illness. Coping and development are health processes that facilitate functioning and satisfaction with life; family (person) is viewed as the unit of concern. The person is perceived through his or her web of significant relationships. Family and person are considered open systems in constant interaction with their environment. The environment is viewed "as the context within which health and healthy ways of living are learned" (p. 56). Collaboration and learning are essentials for the nurse to structure a learning environment to meet "the needs, goals, and problem-solving styles of the family (person) … based upon the family [person's] strengths and resources"(p. 51).

Imogene M. King: Goal Attainment

The theory of goal attainment developed by Imogene M. King (1923–2007) is based on a systems model that includes three interacting systems: personal, interpersonal, and social (King, 1971). She believes that human beings interact with the environment and that the individual's perceptions influence reactions and interactions. For King, nursing involves caring for the human being, with the goal of health defined as adjusting to the stressors in both internal and external environments. She defines

BOX 8.1

Ten Commitments of the Tidal Model

1. **Value the voice:** The person's story is the beginning and endpoint of the helping encounter. All nursing care plans and documents should be written in the person's own voice.
2. **Respect the language:** Each person has developed his or her own unique way of telling his or her story. It is not necessary to use the language of psychiatry and psychiatric nursing.
3. **Develop genuine curiosity:** Those who seek to be of assistance to the person need to develop ways of expressing genuine interest in the person's story so that they might better understand it and the storyteller.
4. **Become the apprentice:** The person is the expert/authority on his or her life story.
5. **Reveal personal wisdom:** One of the key tasks for the helper is to assist in revealing the person's life wisdom that will sustain and guide his or her recovery.
6. **Be transparent:** Both the person and the professional embody the opportunity to become a team. The professional can support this by being transparent at all times, helping the person understand *what* is being done and *why*.
7. **Use the available toolkit:** The person's story contains numerous examples of "what has worked" or "what might work" for this person.
8. **Craft the step beyond:** The helper and the person work together to construct an appreciation of what needs to be done now. The first step is the crucial step, revealing the power of change and pointing toward the ultimate goal of recovery.
9. **Give the gift of time:** There is no value in asking "how much time do we have?" The question is, "how do we use this time?"
10. **Know that change is constant:** The professional helper needs to become aware of how change is happening and discover the way that knowledge may steer the person out of danger and distress and help remain on to the journey to recovery.

Available at: http://www.tidal-model.com/Ten%20Commitments.htm

---

nursing as a "process of human interactions between nurse and patient whereby each perceives the other and the situation; and through communication, they set goals, explore means, and agree on means to achieve goals" (King, 1981, p. 144). The process is initiated to help the patient cope with a health problem that compromises the ability to maintain social roles, functions, and activities of daily living (King, 1992).

In this theory, the person is goal oriented and purposeful, is reacting to stressors, and is viewed as an open system interacting with the environment. One of the variables in the nursing situation is the perceptions of the nurse and the client. The derived proposition is that "if perceptual accuracy (PA) is present in nurse-client interactions (I), transactions (T) will occur" (Sieloff-Evans, 1991, p. 30). The quality of nurse–patient interactions may have positive or negative influences on the promotion of health in any nursing situation. It is within this interpersonal system of nurse and client that the healing process is performed. Interaction is depicted in which the outcome is a **transaction**, defined as the transfer of value between two or more people. This behaviour is unique, is based on experience, and is goal directed.

King's work reflects her understanding of the systematic process of theory development, and her theory continues to be developed and applied in different settings, including PMH care. The King theory has been applied to group therapy for inpatient juvenile offenders, maximum security state offenders, and community parolees (Laben, Dodd, & Snead, 1991). King's theory has also been used as a nursing framework for individual psychotherapy (DeHowitt, 1992).

Betty Neuman: Systems and Stress

Betty Neuman (b. 1924) also used a systems approach as a model of nursing care. Neuman wanted to extend care beyond an illness model, incorporating concepts of problem finding and prevention and the newer behavioural science concepts and environmental approaches into wellness. Neuman developed her framework in the late 1960s as chair of the University of California at Los Angeles graduate nursing program. The purpose of Neuman's systems model (1989) is to guide the actions of the professional caregiver through the assessment and intervention processes by focusing on two major components: the nature of the relationship between the nurse and patient and the patient's response to stressors. The patient may be an individual, group (e.g., a family), or community. The nurse is an "intervener" who attempts to reduce an individual's encounter with stress and to strengthen the person's ability to deal with stressors. The patient is viewed as a collaborator in setting health care goals and determining interventions. Neuman was one of the first PMH nurses to include the concept of stressors in understanding nursing care.

The model continues to be developed and applied. For example, the latest edition of the Neuman's systems model is applied to a diversity of settings, including community health, family therapy, renal nursing, perinatal nursing, and mental health nursing of older adults (Neuman,

Newman, & Holder, 2000). The model has also been applied to nursing care of patients with multiple sclerosis (Knight, 1990) and quality-of-life indicators defined as a perception of good physical health, being comfortable with socioeconomic status, and developing a psychospiritual self (Hinds, 1990). The Neuman Systems Model Trustee Group, Inc. was established in 1988 to preserve, protect, and perpetuate the integrity of the model for the future of nursing.

Dorothea Orem: Self-Care

Self-care is the focus of the general theory of nursing initiated by Dorothea Orem (1914–2007) in the early 1960s. The theory has three main focuses: self-care, self-care deficit, and a theory of nursing systems (Orem, 1991). Self-care is defined as those activities performed independently by an individual to promote and maintain personal well-being throughout life. Self-care deficits occur when an individual has a deficit in attitude (motivation), knowledge, or skill that impedes the meeting of self-care needs. Nurses can help individuals meet self-care requisites through five approaches: acting or doing for, guiding, teaching, supporting, and providing an environment to promote the patient's ability to meet current or future demands. The nursing systems theory refers to a series of actions a nurse takes to meet the patient's self-care requisites, varying from the individual being totally dependent on the nurse for care to needing only some education and support. Orem's model is used extensively in PMH nursing because of its emphasis on promoting independence of the individual and on self-care activities (Campbell & Soeken, 1999).

Callista Roy: Adaptation

Callista Roy's (b. 1939) nursing model is often selected by nurses working in inpatient psychiatric units because they find its concepts particularly relevant to their practice. Roy's adaptation model (1974), originating in 1964, describes humans as living adaptive systems with two coping mechanisms: the regulator and the cognator. The regulator copes with physiologic stimuli and the cognator with psychosociocultural stimuli. Manifestations of the coping mechanisms can be assessed by four adaptive modes: physiologic needs, self-concept, role function, and interdependence. In this model, the nursing process has six steps: "assessment of behaviour, assessment of stimuli (focal, contextual, and residual), nursing diagnosis, goal setting, intervention, and evaluation" (Lutjens, 1991a, p.10).

Martha Rogers: Unitary Human Beings

The key concept of nursing for Martha Rogers (1914–1994) is energy fields, which are open systems (Rogers, 1970). With its principles of homeodynamics—integrality, resonancy, and helicy—her abstract system offers a perspective of change as continuous and evolutionary (Rogers, 1994). Health and nonhealth are considered value laden, with the purpose of nursing being the promotion of human betterment. Important concepts are accelerating change, paranormal phenomena, and rhythmic manifestation of change. Rogers' science enables us to see human phenomena differently (Lutjens, 1991b), including a psychiatric disorder (Thompson, 1990). Her influence on other nursing perspectives, such as Margaret Newman's health as synthesis of disease and nondisease and Rosemarie Parse's health as human becoming, is evident. According to Lego (1973), the holistic, unitary human beings approach differentiates a nurse psychotherapist from other psychotherapists.

Margaret Newman: Health as Expanding Consciousness

Health in Newman's (b. 1933) perspective, an open system model, is conceived as the pattern of the whole of the unitary human being in interaction with the environment (Newman, 1986; Rogers, 1970). "Consciousness is defined as the informational capacity of the system" (p. 33). The evolving patterning of consciousness can be explained by the integration of the three concepts of movement, time, and space. "Movement is the natural condition of life… It is the fullest expression of consciousness in matter" (p. 58) and the means to reality. "Rhythm is basic to movement" (p. 59). To be a nurse is not to react to a client but to be "with" him or her in a sharing rhythmic relationship that is intrinsically related to the concepts of time and space. Expansion of consciousness, or change in perspective, comes from the recognition of the life pattern of the person and acceptance of what it means to that person. A PMH nurse utilizing Newman's view would consider the person's behaviour as a manifestation of his or her pattern. A means to assess and understand a person's behaviour in this manner is the "Auto-patterning Index" (Pagé, 1988). The rhythmic patterns of activities reveal the person's life pace and space at a given time. Psychiatric pathology can be considered as a pattern manifestation and "if becoming ill is the only way an individual's pattern can manifest itself, then that is health for that person" (Newman, 1979, p.58). Removal of the pathology will not change the person's pattern.

■ BIOLOGIC THEORIES

Biologic theories are clearly important in understanding the manifestations of mental disorders and caring for people with these illnesses. Chapter 10 explains many of the important neurobiologic theories, and Chapter 14 focuses on psychopharmacology. Many of the biologically focused interventions explained in Chapter 13 have their theoretic roots in basic nursing knowledge. This chapter describes two biologic approaches used to understand the expression of mental disorders.

Psychiatric Genetics

It has been noted for many decades that some families seem to have a susceptibility to a particular psychiatric illness. In fact, the 1823 archives of London's Bethlehem Royal Hospital ("Bedlam") indicate that the coversheet of case notes required the physician to answer "whether heredity?" (McGuffin & Southwick, 2003, p. 658). Paradoxically, recent discoveries in **genetics** (the study of specific DNA sequences or gene) and **genomics** (the study of the complete DNA structure or genome) make the answer to that question a more difficult and complex one while, at the same time, providing evidence for the role of genes in psychopathology. The understanding of single gene disorders, such as Huntington's disease and early onset familial Alzheimer's disease, has advanced with research but the pattern of inheritance of schizophrenia or bipolar disorders is more complex and involves multiple genes and environmental factors. For instance, there is some evidence of contributions to schizophrenia in linkage regions on chromosomes 8p, 13Q, and 22q and to bipolar disorder on chromosomes 13q and 22q regions, suggesting a genetic overlap (McGuffin & Southwick). The identifying role, if any, of genetics in some forms of addiction and in suicidal behaviour is also at an early stage (Courtet, 2005).

We do know, however, that genetics is not fate: nurture plays a role as well as nature. Environmental factors coact or interact with genes to increase (or to reduce) vulnerability to psychopathology (McGuffin & Southwick, 2003). The **diathesis-stress model** holds that certain genes or genetic combinations produce a diathesis, or constitutional predisposition or vulnerability to a disorder. When diathesis is combined with environmental stressors, abnormal behaviour results. According to this model, for a mental disorder to develop, there must be an interaction between diathesis and stress. Deciphering complicated gene–environment interaction in psychopathology is an exciting research area. Examples of relevant research include a study that shows how attribution of negative life events predicts alcohol use in undergraduate college students (Goldstein, Abela, Buchanan, & Buchanan, 2001) and one that reveals that maltreated children, with genotypes conferring low levels of monoamine oxidase A expression, developed conduct disorder, antisocial personality, and adult violent crime more often than children with high-activity genotypes (Moffitt, Caspi, & Rutter, 2005).

Studies in psychiatric genetics include twin and adoption studies (attempting to determine the role of heredity versus environment), linkage studies (finding the region of the genome that is inherited by affected people and not by unaffected people), and association studies (determining if an identified gene looks different in people with a disorder than in matched controls; Conley, Steele, & Puskar, 2004). The ethical concerns related to psychiatric genetics must be addressed alongside the progress of this research. Atrocities have been committed in the name of "eugenics" (e.g., the Nazi "extermination" of people with psychiatric illness), and information on an individual's genetic inheritance may lead to discrimination. Certainly, future findings in genetics will change the way mental disorders are understood and may affect the way individual responsibility is viewed (Corvin & Gill, 2003; Propping, 2005). Nurses need to keep abreast of the advances in genetic theory, testing, and intervention (Horner, 2004).

General Adaptation Syndrome

Hans Selye's (1907–1982) landmark studies on stress described the interaction of environmental events and biologic responses (Selye, 1956). Selye looked for a link between illness and stressful events and identified the *general adaptation syndrome* (GAS), describing a three-stage process:

- Alarm reaction
- Resistance
- Exhaustion

He hypothesized that during the alarm stage, patients exhibit an adrenocortical response associated with "fight-or-flight" behaviour. During the resistance phase, the body adapts to stress but functions at a lower than optimal level. If the adaptive mechanisms fail or wear out, the individual enters the third stage, exhaustion. At this point, the negative effects of the stressor spread to the entire organism, and Selye believed that ensuing illnesses could ultimately lead to death. Current research supports the relationship between illness and stressful events as argued by Selye, but new understandings about the specificity of responses, such as those within the neuroendocrine system, raise new questions about a general physical adaptation response.

Applicability of Biologic Theories to Psychiatric and Mental Health Nursing

Both Selye's biophysical model and the diathesis-stress model are addressed by nurse theorists. Neuman's systems and stress model (1989) borrows Selye's definition of stress and includes a component guiding the actions of the caregiver, which implies the client's response to stressors. Roy's adaptation model (1974) is linked to Selye's model by its physiologic mode of nursing assessment. Any holistic approach to care must acknowledge that humans are embodied beings with a genetic inheritance that shapes their responses to their environment and experiences.

PSYCHOLOGICAL THEORIES

Psychodynamic Theories

Psychodynamic theories explain human development processes, especially in early childhood, and their effects on thought and behaviour. The study of the unconscious is a key aspect of psychodynamic theory (Ellenberger, 1970). Many important concepts in PMH nursing began with the Austrian physician Sigmund Freud (1856–1939). Psychodynamic theories initially attempted to explain the cause of mental disorders, but etiologic explanations have not been consistently supported by empiric research. These theories, however, proved to be especially important in the development of therapeutic relationships, techniques, and interventions (Table 8-1).

Psychoanalytic Theory

Study of the Unconscious

In Freud's psychoanalytic model, the human mind was conceptualized in terms of **conscious** mental processes (an awareness of events, thoughts, and feelings with the ability to recall them) and **unconscious** mental processes (thoughts and feelings that are outside awareness and are not remembered). Freud believed that the unconscious part of the human mind is only rarely recognized by the conscious part, as in remembered dreams. The term **preconscious** was used to describe unconscious material that is capable of entering consciousness. Uncovering unconscious material to help patients gain insight into unresolved issues was basic to the psychotherapy Freud developed.

Personality and Its Development

Freud's personality structure consists of three parts: the id, ego, and superego (Freud, 1927). According to Freud, the **id** is formed by unconscious desires, primitive instincts, and unstructured drives, including sexual and aggressive tendencies that arise from the body. The **ego** consists of the sum of certain mental mechanisms, such as perception, memory, and motor control, as well as specific defence mechanisms. The ego controls movement, perception, and contact with reality. The capacity to form mutually satisfying relationships is a fundamental function of the ego, which is not present at birth but is formed throughout a child's development. The **superego** is that part of the personality structure associated with ethics, standards, and self-criticism. A child's identification with important and esteemed people in early life, particularly parents, helps form the superego.

Object Relations and Identification

Freud introduced the concept of **object relations,** the psychological attachment to another person or object.

He believed that the choice of a love object in adulthood and the nature of the relationship depend on the nature and quality of the child's object relationships during the early formative years. A child's first love object is the mother, who is the source of nourishment and the provider of pleasure. Gradually, as the child separates from the mother, the nature of this initial attachment influences any future relationships. The development of the child's capacity for relationships with others progresses from a state of narcissism to social relationships, first within the family and then within the larger community. Although the concept of object relations is fairly abstract, it can be understood in terms of a child who imitates her mother and then becomes like her mother in adulthood. This child has incorporated her mother as a love object, identifies with her, and becomes like her as an adult. This process becomes especially important in understanding an abused child who, under certain circumstances, becomes the adult abuser.

Anxiety and Defence Mechanisms

For Freud, anxiety was a specific state of unpleasantness accompanied by motor discharge along definite pathways, the reaction to danger of object loss. Defence mechanisms protected a person from unwanted anxiety. Although they are defined differently than in Freud's day, defence mechanisms still play an explanatory role in contemporary PMH practice. Defence mechanisms are discussed in Chapter 9; they are listed in Appendix H.

Sexuality

According to Freud, the energy or psychic drive associated with the sexual instinct, called the *libido,* literally translated from Latin to mean "pleasure" or "lust," resides in the id. When sexual desire is controlled and not expressed, tension results and is transformed into anxiety (Freud, 1905). Freud believed that adult sexuality is an end product of a complex process of development that begins in early childhood and involves a variety of body functions or areas (oral, anal, and genital zones) that correspond to stages of relationships, especially with parents.

Psychoanalysis

Freud (1949) developed *psychoanalysis,* a therapeutic process of accessing the unconscious and resolving the conflicts that originated in childhood with a mature adult mind. As a system of psychotherapy, psychoanalysis attempted to reconstruct the personality by examining free associations (spontaneous, uncensored verbalizations of whatever comes to mind) and the interpretation of dreams (Freud, 1955). Freud believed that therapeutic relationships had their beginnings within the psychoanalytic framework.

Table 8.1	Psychodynamic Models		
Theorist	**Overview**	**Major Concepts**	**Applicability**
Psychoanalytic Models			
Sigmund Freud (1856–1939)	Founder of psychoanalysis. Believed that the unconscious could be accessed through dreams and free association. Developed a personality theory and theory of infantile sexuality.	Id, ego, superego Consciousness Unconscious mental processes Libido Object relations Anxiety and defence mechanisms Free associations, transference, and countertransference	Individual therapy approach used for enhancement of personal maturity and personal growth
Anna Freud (1895–1982)	Application of ego psychology to psychoanalytic treatment and child analysis with emphasis on the adaptive function of defence mechanisms.	Refinement of concepts of anxiety, defence mechanisms	Individual therapy, childhood psychoanalysis
Neo-Freudian Models			
Alfred Adler (1870–1937)	First defected from Freud. Founded the school of individual psychology.	Inferiority	Added to the understanding of human motivation
Carl Gustav Jung (1875–1961)	After separating from Freud, founded the school of psychoanalytic psychology. Developed new therapeutic approaches.	Redefined libido Introversion Extroversion Persona	Personalities are often assessed on the introversion and extroversion dimensions
Karen Horney (1885–1952)	Opposed Freud's theory of castration complex in women and his emphasis on the Oedipus complex. Argued that neurosis was influenced by the society in which one lived.	Situational neurosis Character	Beginning of feminist analysis of psychoanalytic thought
Interpersonal Relations			
Harry Stack Sullivan (1892–1949)	Impulses and striving need to be understood in terms of interpersonal situations.	Participant observer Parataxic distortion Consensual validation	Provided the framework for the introduction of the interpersonal theories in nursing
Humanist Theories			
Abraham Maslow (1921–1970)	Concerned himself with healthy rather than sick people. Approached individuals from a holistic-dynamic viewpoint.	Needs Motivation	Used as a model to understand how people are motivated and needs that should be met
Frederick S. Perls (1893–1970)	Awareness of emotion, physical state, and repressed needs would enhance the ability to deal with emotional problems.	Reality Here-and-now	Used as a therapeutic approach to resolve current life problems that are influenced by old, unresolved emotional problems
Carl Rogers (1902–1987)	Based theory on the view of human potential for goodness. Used the term *client* rather than *patient*. Stressed the relationship between the therapist and the client.	Empathy Positive regard	Individual therapy approach that involves never giving advice and always clarifying client's feelings

Transference and Countertransference

Transference is the displacement of thoughts, feelings, and behaviours originally associated with significant others from childhood onto a person in a current therapeutic relationship (Moore & Fine, 1990). For example, a woman's feelings toward her parents as a child may be directed toward the therapist. If a woman were unconsciously angry with her parents, she may feel unexplainable anger and hostility toward her therapist. In psychoanalysis, the therapist uses transference as a therapeutic tool to help the patient understand emotional problems and their origin. It is considered an essential aspect to therapy. **Countertransference**, on the other hand, is defined as the direction of all the therapist's feelings and attitudes toward the patient. Feelings and perceptions caused by countertransference may interfere with the therapist's ability to understand the patient.

Neo-Freudian Models

Many of Freud's followers ultimately established their own forms of psychoanalysis. The various psychoanalytic schools have adopted other names because their doctrines deviated from Freudian theory.

Adler's Foundation for Individual Psychology

Alfred Adler (1870–1937), a Viennese psychiatrist and founder of the school of individual psychology, was an early colleague of Freud. He disagreed with Freud's focus on instinctual determination and focused instead on the social aspects of human existence. Adler believed mental health involves love, work, and community. For Adler (1963), life goals are important, and the motivating force in human life is a striving for superiority. Seeking perfection and security while trying to avoid feelings of inferiority can lead the individual to adopt a life goal that is unrealistic and frequently expressed as an unreasoning desire for power and dominance (i.e., *inferiority complex*). Because inferiority is intolerable, the compensatory mechanisms set up by the mind may get out of hand, resulting in self-centred neurotic attitudes, overcompensation, and a retreat from the real world and its problems.

Adler focused on growth, lifestyle, and becoming: Humans are looking to realize their potential, to flourish within their community. Adlerian theory is based on principles of mutual respect, choice, responsibility, consequences, and belonging. Today, his theory and principles are applied to both psychotherapy (including family therapy) as well as education and exert a strong influence on the development of such psychotherapeutic approaches as Ellis's (1973) Rational Emotive Therapy, in which people look to take risks and to become more responsible for their behaviour.

Jung's Analytical Psychology

One of Freud's earliest colleagues, Carl Gustav Jung (1875–1961), a Swiss psychoanalyst, created a model called *analytical psychology*. For Jung, humans were influenced not only by their past but also by what they were hoping for in the future. He supported the idea, not only of a personal unconscious, but of a second psychic system called the **collective unconscious.** The collective unconscious is universal, shared by all humans, and inherited rather than individually developed. Within the collective unconscious are **archetypes**, forms or symbols common to all cultures. The image of "mother" or "hero" or "trickster," for instance, have similar forms in every society and are important commonalities for humans (Jung, 1959). Jung described humans as having both feminine and masculine characteristics and thought that therapy may be directed at helping an individual develop more fully as a person by embracing both aspects of himself or herself. The feminine side of men is the **anima**; the masculine side of women is the **animus**. His concept of **persona** (the mask one wears in society, one's public self) is similar to Freud's superego (Jung, 1966). The **shadow** is Jung's image for the dark side of every person, the side we do not like to recognize or show to others. For people to evolve as individuals, they need to become aware of and integrate their shadow into their personality not attempt to extinguish it.

Jung believed in the existence of two psychological types: the **extrovert** (who finds meaning in the world) and the **introvert** (who finds meaning within). He also described four primary modes of orientation to the world: *thinking, feeling, intuition,* and *sensation*. Although he argued that each of these functions exists in an individual, certain preferences will dominate. Our unconscious is revealed often through our least developed mode. The Myers-Briggs Type Indicator test is based on Jung's personality theory.

Horney's Feminine Psychology

Karen Horney (1885–1952), a German-American psychiatrist, challenged many of Freud's basic concepts and introduced principles of feminine psychology. Recognizing a male bias in psychoanalysis, Horney questioned the traditional psychoanalytic belief that women felt disadvantaged because of their genital organs. Freud believed that women felt inferior to men because their bodies were less completely equipped, a theory he described as "penis envy." Horney rejected this concept, as well as the Oedipus complex, arguing that there are significant cultural reasons why women may strive to obtain qualities or privileges that are defined by a society as being masculine. She argued that women truly were at a disadvantage because of the authoritarian culture in which they lived (Horney, 1939). Her primary concept was that of basic anxiety: early (childhood) feelings of helplessness and isolation with which one strives to cope and resolve. According to Horney, this anxiety underlies all of an individual's relationships. Behaviour can be understood as a reaction to basic anxiety. Horney (1950) named the unrealistic expectations that one puts on oneself "tyranny of the should." Along with other Neo-Freudians, such as Eric Fromm, she introduced sociocultural dimensions of human behaviour into the psychoanalytical model.

Interpersonal Theories: Sullivan's Interpersonal Relations

Interpersonal theories were developed as an alternative explanation for human development and behaviour. Although there are similarities between psychoanalytic and interpersonal theories, the major difference is that interpersonal theories give priority to relationships in personality development, with instincts and drives being less important. Childhood relationships with parenting figures are seen as especially significant and believed to influence important adult relationships, such as the choice of a mate.

Harry Stack Sullivan (1892–1949), an American psychiatrist, extended the concept of **interpersonal relations** to include characteristic interaction patterns. Sullivan studied personality characteristics that could be directly observed, heard, and felt. He believed that the health or sickness of one's personality was determined by the characteristic ways in which one dealt with other people. Health also depended on the constantly changing physical, social, and interpersonal environment as well as past and current life experiences (Sullivan, 1953).

Humanistic Theories

Humanistic theories were generated as a reaction against psychoanalytic premises of instinctual drives. Humanistic theories are based on the views of human potential for goodness. Instead of focusing on instinctual drives, humanist therapists focus on one's ability to learn about oneself, acceptance of self, and exploration of personal capabilities. Within the therapeutic relationship, the patient begins to develop positive attitudes and views himself or herself as a person of worth. The focus is not on investigation of repressed memories but on learning to experience the world in a different way.

Rogers' Client-Centred Therapy

Carl Rogers (1902–1987), an American psychologist, developed new methods of client-centred therapy. Rogers (1980) defined empathy as the capacity to assume the internal reference of the client in order to perceive the world in the same way as the client. To use empathy in the therapeutic process, the counsellor must be nondirective but not passive. Thus, the counsellor's attitude and nonverbal communication are crucial. He advocated that

the therapist develops **unconditional positive regard**, a nonjudgmental caring, for the client (Rogers, 1980) and believed that the therapist's emotional investment (i.e., true caring) in the client is essential to the therapeutic process. Genuineness on the part of the therapist, in contrast with the passivity of the psychoanalyst, is seen as key.

Gestalt Therapy

Another humanistic approach created as a response to the psychoanalytic model was Gestalt therapy, developed by Frederick S. (Fritz) Perls (1893–1970), a German-born former psychoanalyst who immigrated to the United States. Perls believed that modern civilization inevitably produces neurotic anxiety because it forces people to repress natural desires and frustrates an inherent human tendency to adjust biologically and psychologically to the environment. For a person to be cured, unmet needs must be brought back to awareness. Perls did not believe that the intellectual insight gained through psychoanalysis enabled people to change. Instead, he devised individual and group exercises that enhanced a person's awareness of emotions, physical state, and repressed needs as well as physical and psychological stimuli in the here-and-now environment (Perls, 1969).

Maslow's Hierarchy of Needs

Abraham Maslow (1921–1970) developed a humanistic model that is used in PMH nursing today (Maslow, 1998). His major contributions were to the understanding of needs and motivation (Maslow, 1970). He studied exemplary healthy individuals (e.g., Albert Einstein) whom he saw as self-actualizing and described their characteristics. For instance, he noted that they were creative and had a deep sense of kinship with others and a strong sense of ethics. People are self-actualized when they are making the most of their unique human potential. Maslow's view of human motivation was based on a hierarchy of needs, ranging from lower-level survival needs, such as air, water, basic food, and shelter, to higher-level needs, such as those for belonging and esteem and, finally, for **self-actualization.** One must meet lower-level needs before moving to the higher-level ones. According to Maslow's model, values such as truth, beauty, and justice are aspects of our metaneeds, and their persistent deprivation can lead to spiritual-existential ailments often expressed as apathy, boredom, hopelessness, and powerlessness (Hoffman, 1996). Maslow's model offers a framework for assessment.

Applicability of Psychodynamic Theories to Psychiatric and Mental Health Nursing

Several concepts in psychodynamic models are core elements in PMH nursing practice, such as interpersonal relationships, needs, anxiety, defence mechanisms, transference, and countertransference. Many of these concepts are further developed within nursing theories. For instance, Freud's concept of anxiety contrasts with Peplau's (1952) levels of anxiety, and Frankl's logotherapy has commonalities with Travelbee's human-to-human relationship model. A key psychodynamic concept, the therapeutic relationship, is recognized as a core of PMH nursing intervention.

Behavioural Theories

Behavioural theories, with roots in the discipline of psychology, offer important explanatory models for PMH nursing in terms of the way in which people act and learn (Table 8-2).

Early Stimulus-Response Theories

Pavlovian Theory

One of the earliest behavioural theorists was Ivan P. Pavlov (1849–1936), who was studying the gastric functioning of dogs when he noticed that stomach secretions of dogs were stimulated by triggers other than food, such as the sight and smell of food. He became interested in this anticipatory secretion. Through his experiments, he was able to stimulate secretions with a variety of other laboratory nonphysiologic stimuli. Thus, a clear connection was made between thought processes and physiologic responses.

In Pavlov's model, there is an unconditioned stimulus (not dependent on previous training) that elicits an unconditioned (i.e., specific) response. In his experiments, meat was the unconditioned stimulus, and salivation was the unconditioned response. Pavlov would then select other stimuli, such as a bell, a ticking metronome, and a triangle drawn on a large cue card, presenting this conditioned stimulus just before the meat, the unconditioned stimulus. If the conditioned stimulus was repeatedly presented before the meat, eventually salivation was elicited by the conditioned stimulus. This phenomenon was called **classical** (Pavlovian) **conditioning** (Pavlov, 1927/1960).

Table 8.2	Behavioural Theorists		
Theorist	**Overview**	**Major Concepts**	**Applicability**
Stimulus-Response Theories			
Ivan P. Pavlov (1849–1936)	Classical conditioning	Unconditioned stimuli Unconditioned response Conditioned stimuli	Important in understanding learning of automatic responses such as habitual behaviours
John B. Watson (1878–1958)	Introduced behaviourism, believed that learning was classical conditioning called *reflexes*; rejected distinction between the mind and the body.	Principle of frequency Principle of recency	Focuses on the relationship between the mind and the body
Reinforcement Theories			
B. F. Skinner (1904–1990)	Developed an understanding of the importance of reinforcement and differentiated types and schedules.	Operant behaviour Respondent behaviour Continuous reinforcement Intermittent reinforcement	Important in behaviour modification
Edward L. Thorndike (1874–1949)	Believed in the importance of effects that followed behaviour.	Reinforcement	Important in behaviour modification programs
Cognitive Theories			
Albert Bandura (b. 1925)	Developed social cognitive theory, a model for understanding how behaviour is learned from others.	Modelling Disinhibition Elicitation Self-efficacy	Important in helping patients learn appropriate behaviours
Aaron Beck (b. 1921)	Conceptualized distorted cognitions as a basis for depression.	Cognitions Beliefs	Important in cognitive therapy
Kurt Lewin (1890–1947)	Developed field theory, a system for understanding learning, motivation, personality, and social behaviour.	Life space Positive valences Negative valences	Important in understanding motivation for changing behaviour
Edward Chace Tolman (1886–1959)	Introduced the concept of cognitions; believed that human beings act on beliefs and attitudes and strive toward goals.	Cognition	Important in identifying the person's beliefs

John B. Watson and the Behaviourist Revolution

At about the same time Pavlov was working in Russia, John B. Watson (1878–1958) initiated the psychological revolution known as **behaviourism** in the United States. He developed two principles: frequency and recency. The principle of frequency states that the more often a given response is made to a given stimulus, the more likely the response to that stimulus will be repeated. The principle of recency states that the more recently a given response to a particular stimulus is made, the more likely it will be repeated. Watson's major contribution was the rejection of the distinction between body and mind and his emphasis on the study of objective behaviour (Watson & Rayner, 1917).

Reinforcement Theories

Edward L. Thorndike

A pioneer in experimental animal psychology, Edwin L. Thorndike (1874–1949) studied the problem-solving behaviour of cats to determine whether animals solved problems by reasoning or instinct. He found that neither choice was completely correct; animals gradually learn the correct response by "stamping in" the stimulus-response connection. The major difference between Thorndike and behaviourists such as Watson was that Thorndike believed in the importance of the effects that followed the response or the reinforcement of the behaviour. He was the first reinforcement theorist, and his view of learning became the dominant view in learning theory (Thorndike, 1916).

B. F. Skinner

One of the most influential behaviourists, B. F. Skinner (1904–1990) recognized two different kinds of learning, each involving a separate kind of behaviour. *Respondent behaviour*, or the end result of classical conditioning, is elicited by specific stimuli. Given the stimulus, the response occurs automatically. The other kind of learning is referred to as **operant behaviour**. In this type of learning, the distinctive characteristic is the consequence of a particular behavioural response not a specific stimulus. The learning of operant behaviour is also known as *conditioning*, but it is different from the conditioning of reflexes. If a behaviour occurs and is followed by reinforcement, it is probable that the behaviour will recur. For example, if a child climbs on a chair, reaches the faucet, and is able to get a drink of water successfully, it is more likely that the child will repeat the behaviour (Skinner, 1935). Skinner wrote a book about a utopian community based on the principles of behaviourism that he titled *Walden II* (Skinner, 1976).

Cognitive Theories

The initial behavioural studies focused attention on human actions without attention to the internal thinking process. As complex behaviour was examined and could not be accounted for by strictly behavioural explanations, thought processes became new subjects for study. Cognitive theories, an outgrowth of different theoretic perspectives including the behavioural and the psychodynamic, attempted to link internal thought processes with human behaviour.

Albert Bandura's Social Cognitive Theory

Acquiring behaviours by learning from other people is the basis of social cognitive theory developed by the psychologist Albert Bandura, who was born in Mundare, Alberta (b. 1925). Bandura developed his ideas after being concerned about violence on television contributing to aggression in children. He believes that important behaviours are learned by internalizing behaviours of others. His initial contribution was identifying the process of **modelling**: pervasive imitation or one person trying to be like another. According to Bandura, the model may not need to be a real person but could be a character in history or generalized to an ideal person (Bandura, 1977).

The concept of **disinhibition** is important to Bandura's model and refers to the situation in which someone has learned not to make a response; then, in a given situation, when another is making the inhibited response, the individual becomes disinhibited and also makes the response. Thus, the response that was "inhibited" now becomes disinhibited through a process of imitation. For example, during severe dieting, an individual may have learned to resist eating large amounts of food. However, when at a party with a friend who eagerly fills a plate at a buffet, the person also eats large amounts of food.

In the instance of disinhibition, the desire to eat is already there, and the individual indulges that desire. However, in another instance called **elicitation**, there is no desire present but when one person starts an activity, others want to do the same. An example of this occurs when a child is playing with a toy and the other children now want to play with the same toy even though they showed no interest in it before that time.

An important concept of Bandura's is **self-efficacy**, a person's sense of his or her ability to deal effectively with the environment (Bandura, 1993). Efficacy beliefs influence how people feel, think, motivate themselves, and behave. The stronger the self-efficacy, the higher the goals people set for themselves and the firmer their commitment to them.

Aaron T. Beck: Thinking and Feeling

American psychiatrist Aaron T. Beck (b. 1921) of the University of Pennsylvania devoted his career to understanding the relationship between **cognition** and mental health. For Beck, cognitions are verbal or pictorial events in the stream of consciousness. He realized the importance of cognitions when treating people with depression, finding that the depression improved when patients began thinking differently.

He believed that people with depression had faulty information-processing systems that led to biased cognitions. These faulty beliefs cause errors in judgment that become habitual errors in thinking. These individuals incorrectly interpret life situations, judge themselves too harshly, and jump to inaccurate conclusions. A person may, for example, truly believe that he or she has no friends and therefore no one cares. On examination, the evidence for the beliefs is based on the fact that there has been no contact with anyone because of moving from one city to another. Thus, a distorted belief is the basis of the cognition. Beck, Thase, & Wright (2003) developed cognitive therapy, a successful approach for the treatment of depression (see Chapter 20). See Chapter 15 for an overview of Cognitive-Behavioural Therapy.

Applicability of Behavioural Theories to Psychiatric and Mental Health Nursing

Interventions based on behavioural theories are important in PMH nursing. For example, patient education interventions are usually based on learning principles derived from any number of the behavioural theories, and the teaching of new coping skills for patients regarding their symptoms of mental illnesses is usually based on behavioural theories. Changing an entrenched habit involves helping people to identify what motivates them and how new lifestyle habits can become permanent. Examples of behavioural interventions used on inpatient hospital units include the privilege systems and token economies.

Developmental Theories

Developmental theories explain normal human growth and development and focus on change over time. Many developmental theories are presented in terms of stages based on the assumption that normal development proceeds longitudinally from the beginning to the ending stage. Although this approach is useful, unless a stage model is truly supported by evidence, the model does not represent reality.

Erik Erikson: Psychosocial Development

Freud and Sullivan both published treatises on stages of human development, but Erik Erikson (1902–1994) outlined the psychosocial developmental model that is most often used in nursing. Erikson's model was an expansion of Freud's psychosexual development theory. Whereas Freud emphasized intrapsychic experiences, Erikson recognized the importance of culture. He believed that similar events may be experienced differently depending on a person's reaction, family background, and cultural situation.

Each of Erikson's eight stages is associated with a specific task that can be successfully or unsuccessfully resolved. The model is organized according to developmental conflicts by age: basic trust versus mistrust, autonomy versus shame and doubt, initiative versus guilt, industry versus inferiority, identity versus role diffusion, intimacy versus isolation, generativity versus stagnation, and ego integrity versus despair. Erikson's wife, Joan Serson Erikson, extended his theory to include old age as a ninth stage, gerotranscendence (Erikson & Erikson, 1997). Gerotranscendence theory focused on the continued growth in dimensions such as spirituality and inner strength (see Chapter 29).

Within Erikson's theory, successful resolution of a crisis leads to essential strength and virtues. For example, a positive outcome of the trust versus mistrust crisis is the development of a basic sense of trust. If the crisis is unsuccessfully resolved, the infant moves into the next stage without a sense of trust. According to this model, a child who is mistrustful will have difficulty completing the next crisis successfully and, instead of developing a sense of autonomy, will more likely be full of shame and doubt (Erikson, 1963).

Identity and Adolescence

One of Erikson's major contributions was the recognition of the turbulence of adolescent development. Erikson wrote extensively about adolescence, youth, and identity formation. When adolescence begins, childhood ways must be given up, and body changes must be reconciled with the individual's social position, previous history, and identifications. An identity is formed. This task of reconciling how young people see themselves and how society perceives them can become overwhelming and lead to role confusion and alienation (Erikson, 1968).

Research Evidence for Erikson's Models

Two major areas of study support Erikson's models. One area of research focuses on the developmental stages and the second on gender differences. In one early study, male college students who measured low on identity also scored low on intimacy ratings (Orlofsky, Marcia, & Lesser, 1973). These results lend support to the idea that identity precedes intimacy. In still another study, intimacy was found to begin developing early in adolescence, before the development of identity (Ochse & Plug, 1986). Studying fathers with young children, Christiansen and

Palkovitz (1998) found that generativity was associated with a paternal identity, psychosocial identity, and psychosocial intimacy. In addition, fathers who had a religious identification also had higher generativity scores than did others. These studies suggest that these well-known stages may be neither fixed nor sequential.

Evidence also suggests that girls' development is different than boys. One study shows that *generativity* (defined as the need or drive to produce, create, or effect a change) is associated with well-being in both males and females, but in males, generativity is related to the urge for self-protection, self-assertion, self-expansion, and mastery. In women, the antecedents may be the desire for contact, connection, and union (Ackerman, Zuroff, & Moskowitz, 2000).

Jean Piaget: Learning in Children

One of the most influential people in child psychology was Jean Piaget (1896–1980), who contributed more than 40 books and 100 articles on child psychology alone. Piaget viewed intelligence as an adaptation to the environment. He proposed that cognitive growth is like embryologic growth: An organized structure becomes more and more differentiated over time. Piaget developed a system that explains how knowledge develops and changes. Each stage of cognitive development represents a particular structure with major characteristics. Piaget's theory was developed through observation of his own children and therefore never received formal testing.

The major strength of his model was its recognition of the central role of cognition in development and the discovery of surprising features of young children's thinking. For PMH nursing, Piaget's model provides a framework on which to define different levels of thinking and use the data in the assessment and intervention processes. For example, the assessment of concrete thinking would be typical of people with schizophrenia who are unable to perform abstract thinking.

Carol Gilligan: Gender Differentiation

Carol Gilligan (b. 1936) argues that most development models are male centred and therefore inappropriate for girls and women (Gilligan, 1994). For Gilligan, attachment within relationships is the important factor for successful female development. After comparing male and female personality development, she highlighted the differences (Gilligan, 1982). Although the first primary relationship of both boys and girls is with the mother, in developing identity, boys separate from their mother and girls attach. Thus, girls probably learn to value relationships and become interdependent at an earlier age. They learn to value the ideal of care, begin to respond to human need, and want to take care of the world by sustaining attachments so that no one is left alone. According to Gilligan, female development does not follow a progression of stages but is based on experiences within relationships. However, some researchers suggest that relationships may also be equally important for boys in their development of a strong sense of self (Nelson, 1996).

Gilligan's conclusion that female development depends on relationships has implications for everyone who provides care to women. Traditional models that advocate separation as the primary goal of human development immediately place women at a disadvantage. By negating the value and importance of attachments within relationships, the natural development of women is impaired. If Erikson's model is applied to women, their failure to separate then becomes defined as a developmental failure (Gilligan, 1982). Currently, there is considerable debate about whether Erikson's developmental model is applicable to women.

Applicability of Developmental Theories to Psychiatric and Mental Health Nursing

Developmental theories are used in understanding childhood and adolescent experiences and their manifestations as adult problems. When working with children, nurses can use developmental models to help gauge development and mood. However, because most of the models are based on the assumptions of the linear progression of stages and have not been adequately tested, applicability has limitations. In addition, these models were based on a relatively small number of children who typically were raised in a Western middle-class environment. Most do not account for gender differences and diversity in lifestyles and cultures.

SOCIAL THEORIES

Numerous social theories underlie PMH nursing practice, and the nursing profession itself serves a specific societal function. This section represents a sampling of important social theories that nurses may use. This discussion is not exhaustive and should be viewed by the student as including only some of the theoretic perspectives that may be applicable.

Family Dynamics

Family dynamics are the patterned interpersonal and social interactions that occur within the family structure over the life of a family. Family dynamics models are based on systems theory describing a phenomenon in terms of a set of interrelated parts, in which the change of one part affects the total functioning of the system. A system can be "open" and interacting in the environment or "closed," completely self-contained, and not influenced by the environment. The family is viewed organizationally as an open system in which one member's actions influence the functioning of the total system. Most of the theoretic explanations have emerged from treatment case studies, rather than from systematic development of theory based on generalizable research. Consequently, the limitation of available research should be considered when these models are used to understand family interactions and plan patient care (see Chapter 17).

Applicability of Family Theories to Psychiatric and Mental Health Nursing

Family theories are especially useful to nurses who are assessing family dynamics and planning interventions (Wright & Leathy, 2005). Family systems models are used to help nurses form collaborative relationships with patients and families dealing with health problems. Generalist PMH nurses will not be engaged in family therapy. However, they will be caring for individuals and families. Understanding family dynamics is important in every nurse's practice. Many family interventions are consistent with these theories (see Chapter 17). Many of the symptoms of mental disorders, such as hallucinations or delusions, have implications for the total family and its interactions.

Balance Theory and Social Distance

A useful theory for understanding caregiving activities within a community is balance theory, proposed in 1966 by sociologist Eugene Litwak (b. 1925). This theory explains the importance of informal and formal support systems in the delivery of health care.

Formal support systems are large organizations, such as hospitals and nursing homes, which provide care to individuals. **Informal support systems** are family, friends, and neighbours. Litwak found that individuals with strong informal support networks actually live longer than those without this type of support. In addition, those without informal support have significantly higher mortality rates when the causes of death are accidents (e.g., smoking in bed) or suicides (Litwak, 1985).

A key concept in balance theory is **social distance,** the degree to which the values of the formal organization and primary group members differ. The formal and informal groups are considered to be balanced when they are at a midpoint of social distance, that is, close enough to communicate but not so close to destroy each other—neither enmeshment nor isolation (Litwak, Messeri, & Silverstein, 1990; Messeri, Silverstein, & Litwak, 1993). If the primary groups and the formal care system begin performing similar caregiving services, the formal system increases the social distance by developing linkages with the primary group. Thus, a balance is maintained between the two systems. For example, if a patient relies only on the health care provider for care and support (e.g., calls the nurse every day, visits the physician weekly, refuses any help from family), the individual will be linked with an informal support system for help with some of the caregiving tasks. If the individual refuses any health promotion interventions from providers, the patient will be directly approached by the health care team.

Applicability of Balance Theory to Psychiatric and Mental Health Nursing

Balance theory is a practical model for conceptualizing delivery of mental health care in the community, particularly in rural areas where resources are limited. By using the framework of formal and informal support systems and social distance, mental health services can be developed and evaluated from this perspective. Nurse researchers at the Southeastern Rural Mental Health Research Center at the University of Virginia developed a model for establishing linkages of formal and informal caregivers for mental health service for those with serious mental illnesses in rural areas (Fox, Blank, Kane, Hargrove, & David, 1994). In this model, case managers adjust the social distance between the formal and informal systems by identifying communication barriers and helping the two groups work together. For example, a patient misses an appointment because of a lack of transportation. The case manager helps the patient communicate the problem to the system to obtain another appointment. Informal caregivers are valued by the case manager, who recognizes the important services performed by family and friends. Thus, linkages between mental health providers (formal support) and the consumer network (informal support) are reinforced.

Role Theories

A **role** describes an individual's social position and function within an environment. Anthropologic theories explain members' roles that relate to a specific society. For example, the universal roles of healer may be assumed by a nurse in one culture and a spiritual leader in another. Societal expectations, social status, and rights are attached to these roles. Psychological theories, which are concerned about roles from a different perspective, focus on the relationship of an individual's role: the self. The responsibilities of a parent are often in conflict with the personal needs for time alone. All of the Neo-Freudian and humanist models that have been discussed focus on reciprocal social relationships or interactions that determine how the mind develops.

Applicability of Role Theories to Psychiatric and Mental Health Nursing

Role theories emphasize the importance of social interaction in either the individual's choice of a particular role or society's recognition of it. Several nursing models have role as a major concept, including King (1971), Roy (1974), and Peplau (1952). PMH nursing uses role concepts in understanding group interaction and the role of the patient in the family and community (see Chapters 16 and 17). In addition, milieu therapy approaches discussed in later chapters are based on the patient's assumption of a role within the psychiatric care environment.

Sociocultural Perspectives

Theories of Gender and Culture

In the 20th century, gender and culture came to be recognized as playing a significant part in determining human behaviours, including the manifestation of illness, as well as influencing our understandings of mental health and mental illness. (See Box 2-3 in Chapter 2 for examples of culturally specific illnesses.) Coinciding with this recognition was the development of a critical and emancipatory scholarship calling not only for the study of the influence of culture and gender on mental illness but also for a critique of how power differences can result in psychiatric care that can stigmatize and marginalize minority groups. Feminist theories have been applied to reintroduce validity to concepts such as emotions and embodied knowledge that were previously deemed irrational. Likewise, postcolonial theories and Marxist approaches have been introduced and call on nurses to attend to the ways that the various notions of race and class function in our understanding of psychiatric illness and mental health, respectively. "The social and moral mandate of nursing is now seen to include illumination of the experiences of those marginalized within society and within health care" (Reimer, Kirkham, & Anderson, 2002, p. 2).

Madeleine Leininger: Transcultural Health Care

Concern about the impact of culture on the treatment of children with psychiatric and emotional problems led Madeleine Leininger (b. 1924), a nurse anthropologist, to develop a new field called transcultural nursing, which is directed toward holistic, congruent, and beneficent care. She used concepts from anthropology and nursing (from such theorists as Henderson [1966], Rogers [1970], and Watson [1979]) to depict universal and diverse dimensions of human caring. Because caring is an integral part of being human, as well as a learned behaviour, caring is culturally based (Leininger, 1991, 1999). Care is considered the essence of nursing, and caring manifestations include compassion, presence, and enabling (Leininger, 1993). Nursing care in one culture is different from that in another because definitions are different. Leininger developed a model to depict her theory symbolically. The model depicts the "world view, religion, kinship, cultural values, economics, technology, language, ethnohistory, and environmental factors that are predicted to explain and influence culture care" (p. 27).

Applicability of Sociocultural Theories to Psychiatric and Mental Health Nursing

The use of sociocultural theories is especially important for PMH nurses. In any individual or family assessment, the sociocultural aspect is integral to mental health. It would be impossible to complete an adequate assessment without considering the role of the individual within the family and within society. Interventions are based on the understanding and significance of familial and cultural norms. It would be impossible to interact with a family in a meaningful way without an understanding of the family's cultural values. In the inpatient setting, the nurse is responsible for designing the social environment of the unit as well as ensuring that the patient is safe from harm. To accomplish this complex task, an understanding of the unit as a small social community helps the nurse use the environment in patient treatment (see Chapter 13). In addition, many group interventions are based on sociocultural theories (see Chapter 16).

■■■ SPIRITUAL THEORIES

Frankl's Logotherapy

Viktor Frankl (1905–1997) is considered a humanist and an existentialist. His perspective comes from his clinical background and his personal experiences as a prisoner in Nazi concentration camps during World War II. Logotherapy is concerned with meaning. It is based on three assumptions: freedom of will, will to meaning, and meaning of life. Without meaning, life is empty. The goal of logotherapy is to help the person find meaning (Frankl, 1992).

Yalom's Existential Psychotherapy

Irving Yalom (b. 1931) grounds his existential psychotherapy upon what he considers central or ultimate life concerns: death, freedom, isolation, and meaningless. As each person attempts to confront these concerns, conflicts may arise. In his theory, Yalom (1980) describes how life concerns play a role in psychopathology and psychotherapy. For instance, "fear of death plays a major role in our internal experience; it haunts as does nothing else" (p. 27). A childhood developmental task is to deal with this fear. Often, however, we use denial to keep awareness of death at bay. Ineffective modes of facing our mortality can result in psychopathology; psychotherapy, therefore, may need to be aimed at death awareness. Yalom does not claim the existential orientation is *the* paradigm from which to understand all behaviour: the human being is too complex for this to be possible. However, existential psychotherapy is a useful, systematic approach for addressing many people's clinical situation or symptoms.

Applicability of Spiritual Theories to Psychiatric and Mental Health Nursing

As well as directly influencing nurse theorists such as Travelbee, these theoretic perspectives allow nurses to explore the way the search for meaning in life and death shapes human development, experience, and understanding.

SUMMARY OF KEY POINTS

- ☐ Nursing theories form the conceptual basis for nursing practice and are useful in a variety of PMH settings.
- ☐ The biologic framework forms a basis for nursing considerations based on such models as psychiatric genetics and the interaction of nature and nurture.
- ☐ The traditional psychodynamic framework helped form the basis of early nursing interpersonal interventions, including the development of therapeutic relationships and the use of such concepts as transference, countertransference, empathy, and object relations.
- ☐ The cognitive and behavioural theories are often used in strategies that help patients change behaviour and thinking.
- ☐ Sociocultural theories remain important in understanding and interacting with patients as members of families, cultures, and society.
- ☐ Spiritual theories offer a way to consider the human search for meaning in life and how a patient's view of life can affect his or her health and well-being.

CRITICAL THINKING CHALLENGES

1 Compare and contrast the basic ideas of the nursing theorists.

2 Discuss the importance of the biologic theories in mental health practice. Compare Selye's model with the diathesis-stress model.

3 Discuss the similarities and differences between Freud's ideas and the Neo-Freudians, including Jung, Adler, Horney, and Sullivan.

4 Compare and contrast the basic ideas of psychodynamic and behavioural theories.

5 Compare and differentiate classical conditioning from operant conditioning.

6 Define the following terms and discuss their applicability to PMH nursing: *classical conditioning, operant conditioning, positive reinforcement,* and *negative reinforcement.*

7 List the major developmental theorists and their main ideas.

8 Discuss the way in which cognitive therapy approaches can be used in PMH nursing practice.

9 How might a nurse's own death awareness affect his or her ability to help patients deal with a fear of death?

WEB LINKS

www.florence-nightingale.co.uk   This is the site of the Florence Nightingale Museum.

www.freud.org.uk   This is the website of the Freud Museum in London. It has pictures, publications, and links to other relevant sites.

www.jungianstudies.org   This is the site of the International Association of Jungian Studies, which should be of interest to anyone interested in Jung's work.

www.kumc.edu/gec/geneinfo.html   This site, created for genetic professionals by University of Kansas, provides clinical information regarding genetic disorders, tests, and links to other sites.

publish.uwo.ca/~cforchuk/peplau/hpcb.html   This is the site of Hildegard Peplau's home page.

www.sandiego.edu/ACADEMICS/nursing/theory   This site on nursing theory was developed by the Hahn School of Nursing and Health Sciences.

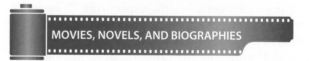

MOVIES, NOVELS, AND BIOGRAPHIES

Florence Nightingale: 1985. This made-for-TV movie, starring Jaclyn Smith as Florence Nightingale, shows how the aristocratic Nightingale defied Victorian convention as a nurse in London and during the Crimean War. It is the fact-based story of "the Lady with the Lamp" and her efforts to reform health care (e.g., hospital sanitation) that lead to the establishment of modern nursing.

VIEWING POINTS: Consider the opposition that Florence Nightingale faced in changing the thinking of her contemporaries. What qualities did she bring to this challenge and what strategies did she use that made her so successful?

Freud: 1962. This video depicts Sigmund Freud as a young physician, focusing on his early psychiatric theories and treatments. His struggles for acceptance of his ideas among the Viennese medical community are depicted. This film provides an interesting overview of the impact of psychoanalysis.

VIEWING POINTS: Watch for the influence of political thinking on the gradual acceptance of Freud's ideas. Discuss the "dream sequence" and its impact on the development of psychoanalysis as a therapeutic technique.

When Nietzsche Wept: 1992. This award-winning novel, written by Irving Yalom, the author of *Existential Therapy* (and also referred to previously in this chapter), is set in 19th century Vienna and features an imagined therapist–patient relationship between Josef Breuer, a founding father of psychoanalysis, and Friedrich Nietzsche, the great philosopher.

READING POINTS: Consider how psychoanalysis evolved from the early days of the "talking cure" as depicted in this work.

REFERENCES

Ackerman, S., Zuroff, D. C., & Moskowitz, D. S. (2000). Generativity in midlife and young adults: Links to agency, communion, and subjective well-being. *International Journal of Aging and Human Development, 5*(1), 17–41.

Adler, A. (1963). *The practice and theory of individual psychotherapy.* Paterson, NJ: Littlefield, Adams.

Allen, M. (1977). Comparative theories of the expanded role in nursing and its implications for nursing practice: A working paper. *Nursing Papers/Perspectives en Nursing, 9,* 38–45.

Baldursdottir, G., & Jonsdottir, H. (2002). The importance of nurse caring behaviours as perceived by patients receiving care at an emergency department. *Heart & Lung, 31*(1), 67–75.

Bandura, A. (1977). *Social learning theory.* Englewood Cliffs, NJ: Prentice-Hall.

Bandura, A. (1993). Perceived self-efficacy in cognitive development and function: American Educational Research Association Annual Meeting. *Educational Psychologist, 28*(2), 117–148.

Barker, P. (1998). It's time to turn the tide. *Nursing Times, 94*(46), 70–72.

Barker, P. (2001a). The Tidal Model: Developing a person-centred approach to psychiatric and mental health nursing. *Perspectives in Psychiatric Care, 37,* 79–87.

Barker, P. (2001b). The Tidal Model: The lived-experience in person-centred mental health nursing care. *Nursing Philosophy, 2,* 213–223.

Barker, P. J. (2004). *Assessment in psychiatric and mental health nursing: In search of the whole person* (2nd ed., pp. 337–346). Cheltenham, UK: Nelson Thornes Ltd.

Barker P., & Buchanan-Barker, P. (2005). *The Tidal Model: A guide for mental health professionals.* London and New York: Brunner-Routledge.

Barnhart, D. A., Bennett, P. M., Porter, B. D., & Sloan, R. S. (1994). Jean Watson: Philosophy and science of caring. In A. Marriner-Tomey (Ed.), *Nursing theorists and their work* (3rd ed., pp. 148–162). St. Louis, MO: Mosby.

Beck, A. T., Thase, M. D., & Wright, J. H. (2003). Cognitive therapy. In R. E. Hales & S. C. Ydofsky (Eds.), *Textbook of clinical psychiatry* (4th ed., pp. 1245–1283). Washington, DC: American Psychiatric Publishers, Inc.

Benner, P., & Wrubel, J. (1989). *The primacy of caring: Stress and coping in health and illness.* Menlo Park, CA: Addison-Wesley.

Calaway, B. J. (2002). *Hildegard Peplau: Psychiatric nurse of the century.* New York, NY: Springer.

Campbell, J. C., & Soeken, K. L. (1999). Women's responses to battering: A test of the model. *Research in Nursing and Health, 22*(1), 49–58.

Chesla, C. (1994). Parents' caring practices with schizophrenic offspring. In P. Benner (Ed.), *Interpretive phenomenology: Embodiment, caring and ethics in health and illness* (pp. 167–184). Newbury Park CA: Sage Publications, Inc.

Christiansen, S. L., & Palkovitz, R. (1998). Exploring Erikson's psychosocial theory and development: Generativity and its relationship to paternal identity, intimacy, and involvement in childcare. *Journal of Men's Studies, 7*(1), 133–156.

Conley, Y. P., Steele, A. M., & Puskar, K. R. (2004). Genetic susceptibility to psychiatric disorders. *MEDSURG Nursing, 13*(5), 319–325.

Corvin, A., & Gill, M. (2003). Psychiatric genetics in the post-genome age. *British Journal of Psychiatry, 182,* 95–96.

Courtet, P. (2005). The genetic basis of suicidal behavior. *Psychiatric Times, 22*(9), 26-28.

DeHowitt, M. (1992). King's conceptual model and individual psychotherapy. *Perspectives in Psychiatric Care, 28*(4), 11–14.

Ellenberger, H. (1970). *The discovery of the unconscious: The history and evolution of dynamic psychiatry.* London, UK: Allen Lane, Penguin Press.

Ellis, A. (1973). *Humanistic psychotherapy: The rational-emotive approach.* New York, NY: McGraw-Hill.

Erikson, E. (1963). *Childhood and society* (2nd ed.). New York, NY: Norton.

Erikson, E. (1968). *Identity: Youth and crisis.* New York, NY: Norton.

Erickson, E., & Erikson, J., (1997). *The lifecycle completed, extended version.* New York, NY: Norton.

Fox, J., Blank, M., Kane, C., Hargrove, C. F., & David, S. (1994). Balance theory as a model for coordinating delivery of rural mental health services. *Applied and Preventive Psychology, 3*(2), 121–129.

Frankl, V. (1992). *Man's search for meaning: An introduction to logotherapy* (4th ed.). Boston, MA: Beacon Press.

Freud, S. (1905). Three essays on the theory of sexuality. In J. Strachey, A. Freud, A. Strachey, & A. Tyson (Eds.). (1953). *The standard edition of the complete psychological works of Sigmund Freud* (pp. 135–248). London, UK: Hogarth Press.

Freud, S. (1927). The ego and the id. In E. Jones (Ed.), 1957), *The international psycho-analytical library* (No. 12). London, UK: Hogarth Press.

Freud, S. (1949). *An outline of psychoanalysis.* New York, NY: Norton.

Freud, S. (1955). *An interpretation of dreams.* London, UK: Hogarth Press.

Gilligan, C. (1982). *In a different voice.* Cambridge, MA: Harvard University Press.

Gilligan, C. (1994). Joining the resistance: Psychology, politics, girls and women. In M. Berger (Ed.), *Women beyond Freud: New concepts of feminine psychology* (pp. 99–145). New York, NY: Brunner Mazel.

Goldstein, B., Abela, J. R., Buchanan, G. M., & Buchanan, M. E. (2001). Attributional styles and life events: A diathesis-stress theory of alcohol consumption. *Psychological Reports, 87*(3 Pt. 1), 949–955.

Gottlieb, L., & Rowat, K. (1987). The McGill model of nursing: A practice-derived model. *Advances in Nursing Science, 9*(4), 51–61.

Henderson, V. (1966). *The nature of nursing: A definition and its implications for practice, research, and education.* New York, NY: Macmillan.

Hinds, C. (1990). Personal and contextual factors predicting patients' reported quality of life: Exploring congruency with Betty Neuman's assumptions. *Journal of Advanced Nursing, 15,* 456–462.

Hoffman, E. (Ed.). (1996). *Future visions: The unpublished papers of Abraham Maslow.* Newbury Park, CA: Sage Publications, Inc.

Horner, K. (2004). Ethics and genetics: Implications for CNS practice. *Clinical Nurse Specialist, 18*(5), 228–231.

Horney, K. (1939). *New ways in psychoanalysis.* New York, NY: Norton.

Horney, K. (1950). *Neurosis and human growth.* New York, NY: Norton.

Jackson, S., & Stevenson, C. (1998). The gift of time from the friendly professional. *Nursing Standard, 12,* 31–33.

Jung, C. G. (1959). *The basic writings of C. G. Jung.* New York, NY: Modern Library.

Jung, C. (1966). On the psychology of the unconscious. V. The personal and the collective unconscious. In C. Jung (Ed.), *Collected works of C. G. Jung* (2nd ed., Vol. 7, pp. 64–79). Princeton, NJ: Princeton University Press.

King, I. (1971). *Toward a theory for nursing: General concepts of human behavior.* New York, NY: John Wiley and Sons.

King, I. (1981). *A theory for nursing: Systems, concepts, process.* New York, NY: John Wiley and Sons.

King, I. (1992). King's theory of goal attainment. *Nursing Science Quarterly, 5*(1), 19–26.

Knight, J. (1990). The Betty Neuman systems model applied to practice: A client with multiple sclerosis. *Journal of Advanced Nursing, 15,* 447–455.

Laben, J., Dodd, D., & Snead, L. (1991). King's theory of goal attainment applied in group therapy for inpatient juvenile sexual offenders, maximum security state offenders, and community parolees, using visual aids. *Issues in Mental Health Nursing, 12*(1), 51–64.

Lego, S. (1973). Nurse psychotherapists: How are we different? *Perspectives in Psychiatric Care, 11,* 144–147.

Leininger, M. (1991). *Culture care diversity and universality: A theory of nursing.* New York, NY: National League for Nursing.

Leininger, M. (1993). Assumptive premises of the theory. In C. Reynolds & M. Leininger (Eds.), *Madeleine Leininger: Cultural care diversity and universality theory. Notes on nursing theories* (Vol. 8, pp. 15–30). Newbury Park, CA: Sage Publications, Inc.

Leininger, M. (1999). What is transcultural nursing and culturally competent care? *Journal of Transcultural Nursing, 10*(1), 9.

Litwak, E. (1985). Complementary roles for formal and informal support groups: A study of nursing homes and mortality rates. *Journal of Applied Behavioural Science, 21*(4), 407–425.

Litwak, E., Messeri, P., & Silverstein, M. (1990). The role of formal and informal groups in providing help to older people. *Marriage and Family Review, 15*(1–2), 171–193.

Lutjens, L. R., (1991a). *Callista Roy: An adaptation model.* Newbury Park, CA: Sage Publications, Inc.

Lutjens, L. R., (1991b). *Martha Rogers: The science of unatary human beings.* Newbury Park, CA: Sage Publications, Inc.

MacPhail, J., (1988). The professional image: Impact and strategies for change. In *Canadian Nursing: Issues and perspectives* (pp. 47–58). Toronto, ON: McGraw-Hill Ryerson.

Maslow, A. (1970). *Motivation and personality* (rev. ed.). New York, NY: Harper & Brothers.

Maslow, A. (1998). *Toward a psychology of being* (3rd ed.). New York, NY: John Wiley & Sons.

McGuffin, P., & Southwick, L. (2003). Fifty years of the double helix and its impact on psychiatry. *Australian and New Zealand Journal of Psychiatry, 37,* 657–661.

Messeri, P., Silverstein, M., & Litwak, E. (1993). Choosing optimal support groups: A review and reformulation. *Journal of Health and Social Behaviour, 34*(6), 122–137.

Moffitt, T., Caspi, A., & Rutter, M. (2005). Strategy for investigating interactions between measured genes and measured environments. *Archives of General Psychiatry, 62,* 473–481.

Moore, B., & Fine, B. (Eds.). (1990). *Psychoanalytic terms and concepts.* New Haven, CT: American Psychoanalytic Association and Yale University Press.

Nelson, M. (1996). Separation versus connection, the gender controversy: Implications for counseling women. *Journal of Counseling and Development, 74*(4), 339–344.

Neuman, B. (1989). *The Neuman systems model* (2nd ed.). East Norwalk, CT: Appleton & Lange.

Neuman, B., Newman, D. M. L., & Holder, P. (2000). Leadership and scholarship integration: Using the Neuman system model for 21st century professional nursing practice. *Nursing Science Quarterly, 13*(1), 60–63.

Newman, M. A. (1979). *Theory development in nursing.* Philadelphia, PA: F.A. Davis Company.

Newman, M. A. (1986). *Health as expanding consciousness.* St. Louis, MO: Mosby-Year Book.

Nightingale, F. (1859). *Notes on nursing: What it is and what it is not.* London, UK: Harrison, Bookseller to the Queen.

Ochse, R., & Plug, C. (1986). Cross-cultural investigation of the validity of Erikson's theory of personality development. *Journal of Personality and Social Psychology, 50*(6), 1240–1252.

Olson, J., & Hanchett, E. (1997). Nurse-expressed empathy, patient outcomes, and the development of a middle-range theory. *Image: The Journal of Nursing Scholarship, 29*(1), 71–76.

Orem, D. (1991). *Nursing concepts of practice* (4th ed.). St. Louis, MO: Mosby–Year Book.

Orlando, I. J. (1961). *The dynamic nurse–patient relationship.* New York, NY: G. P. Putnam's Sons.

Orlando, I. J. (1972). *The discipline and teaching of nursing process.* New York, NY: G. P. Putnam's Sons.

Orlofsky, J., Marcia, J., & Lesser, I. (1973). Ego identity status and the intimacy versus isolation crisis of young adulthood. *Journal of Personality and Social Psychology, 27*(2), 211–219.

Pagé, G. (1988). *An exploration of the relationship between daily patterning and weight loss.* (Doctoral dissertation, Wayne State University). *Dissertation Abstracts Int.,* 50, 497b.

Paterson, J. G., & Zderad, L. T. (1976). *Humanistic nursing.* New York, NY: John Wiley & Sons.

Pavlov, I. P. (1927/1960). *Conditioned reflexes.* New York, NY: Dover Publications.

Peplau, H. (1952). *Interpersonal relations in nursing.* New York, NY: G. P. Putnam & Sons.

Peplau, H. (1992). Interpersonal relations: A theoretical framework for application in nursing practice. *Nursing Science Quarterly, 5*(1), 13–18.

Perls, F. (1969). *In and out of the garbage pail.* Lafayette, CA: Real People Press.

Potter, M. L., & Bockenhauer, B. J. (2000). Implementing Orlando's nursing theory. *Journal of Psychosocial Nursing and Mental Health Services, 3813,* 14–21.

Propping, P. (2005). The biography of psychiatric genetics: From early achievements to historical burden, from an anxious society to critical geneticists. *American Journal of Medical Genetics: Neuropsychiatric Genetics, 136*(1), 2–7.

Reimer Kirkham, S., & Anderson, J. M. (2002). Postcolonial nursing scholarship: From epistemology to method. *Advances in Nursing Science, 25*(1), 1–17.

Rogers, C. (1980). *A way of being.* Boston, MA: Houghton Mifflin.

Rogers, M. E. (1970). *An introduction to the theoretical basis of nursing.* Philadelphia, PA: F.A. Davis.

Rogers, M. E. (1994). The science of unitary human being: Current perspectives. *Nursing Science Quarterly, 7*(1), 33–35.

Roy, C. (1974). The Roy adaptation model. In J. P. Riehl & C. Roy, (Eds.), *Conceptual models for nursing practice* (pp. 135–144). New York, NY: Appleton-Century-Crofts.

Selye, H. (1956). *The stress of life.* New York, NY: McGraw-Hill.

Sieloff-Evans, C. (1991). *Imogene King: A conceptual framework for nursing.* CA: Sage Publications, Inc.

Skinner, B. F. (1935). The generic nature of the concepts of stimulus and response. *Journal of General Psychology, 12,* 40–65.

Skinner, B. F. (1976). *Walden II.* New York, NY: Macmillan.

Sullivan, H. (1953). *The interpersonal theory of psychiatry.* New York, NY: Norton.

Thompson, J. E. (1990). Findings the borderline's border: Can Martha Rogers help? *Perspectives in Psychiatric Care, 26*(4), 7–10.

Thorndike, E. L. (1916, c1906). *The principles of teaching, based on psychology.* New York, NY: A. G. Seiler.

Travelbee, J. (1969). *Intervention in psychiatric nursing: Process in the one-to-one relationship.* Philadelphia, PA: F.A. Davis.

Travelbee, J. (1971). *Interpersonal aspects of nursing* (2nd ed.). Philadelphia, PA: F. A. Davis.

Watson, J. (1979). *Nursing: The philosophy and science of caring* (2nd ed.). Boston, MA: Little, Brown.

Watson, J. (1988). *Nursing: Human science and human care: A theory of nursing.* New York, NY: National League for Nursing.

Watson, J. B., & Rayner, R. (1917). Emotional reactions and psychological experimentation. *American Journal of Psychology, 28,* 163–174.

Wright, L., & Leahy, M. (2005). *Nurses and families: A guide to family assessment and intervention* (3rd ed.). Philadelphia, PA: FA Davis.

Yalom, I. D. (1980). *Existential psychotherapy.* New York, NY: Basic Books.

Communication and the Therapeutic Relationship

Cheryl Forchuk

LEARNING OBJECTIVES

After studying this chapter, you will be able to:

- Identify the importance of self-awareness in nursing practice.
- Develop a repertoire of verbal and nonverbal communication skills.
- Develop a process for selecting effective communication techniques.
- Explain how the nurse can establish a therapeutic relationship with clients by using rapport and empathy.
- Explain the physical, emotional, social, and spiritual boundaries of the nurse–client relationship.
- Discuss the significance of defence mechanisms.
- Explain what occurs in each of the three phases of the nurse–client relationship: orientation, working, and resolution.

KEY CONCEPTS

- nurse–client relationship
- self-awareness
- therapeutic communication

KEY TERMS

• active listening • boundaries • communication blocks • content themes • countertransference • defence mechanisms • empathic linkages • empathy • nontherapeutic • nonverbal communication • orientation phase • passive listening • process recording • rapport • resolution phase • self-disclosure • symbolism • transference • verbal communication • working phase

*C*lients with psychiatric disorders have special communication and relationship needs that require advanced therapeutic communication skills. In psychiatric and mental health (PMH) nursing, the nurse–client relationship is an important intervention tool that is used to reach treatment goals. The purposes of this chapter are to (1) help the nurse develop self-awareness and communication techniques needed for a therapeutic nurse–client relationship, (2) examine the specific stages or steps involved in establishing the relationship, (3) explore the specific factors that make a nurse–client relationship successful and therapeutic, and (4) differentiate therapeutic from **nontherapeutic** relationships.

Self-Awareness

Self-awareness is the process of understanding one's own beliefs, thoughts, motivations, biases, and limitations and recognizing how they affect others. Without self-awareness, nurses will find it impossible to establish and maintain therapeutic relationships with clients. "Know thyself" is a basic tenet of PMH nursing (see Box 9-1).

To come to self-awareness, nurses can carry out self-examination. Self-examination involves reflecting on the personal meaning of the current nursing situation. This reflection can relate to similar past situations and issues related to personal values. Self-examination can provoke

BOX 9.1

"Know Thyself"

- Do you have any physical problems or illnesses?
- Have you had significant traumatic life events (e.g. divorce, death of a significant person, abuse, disaster)?
- Do your family or significant others have prejudiced or embarrassing beliefs and attitudes about groups different than yours?
- Would sociocultural factors in your background contribute to being rejected by members of other cultures?
- Do you have strong religious beliefs that shape your daily life?
- If you answer "yes" to any of these questions, how would these experiences and beliefs affect your ability to care for clients with these characteristics?

anxiety and is rarely comfortable, either alone or with help from others. Self-examination without the benefit of another's perspective can lead to a biased view of self. Conducting self-examinations with a trusted individual who can give objective but realistic feedback is best. The development of self-awareness requires a willingness to be introspective and to examine personal beliefs, attitudes, and motivations.

KEY CONCEPT **Self-awareness** is the process of understanding one's own beliefs, thoughts, motivations, biases, and limitations and recognizing how they affect others.

THE BIO/PSYCHO/SOCIAL/ SPIRITUAL SELF

Each nurse brings a bio/psycho/social/spiritual self to nursing practice. The client perceives the biologic dimension of the nurse in terms of physical characteristics: age, gender, body weight, height, ethnic or racial background, and any other observed physical characteristics. The nurse, too, can have a certain genetic composition, chronic illness, or unobservable physical disability that may influence the quality or delivery of nursing care. The nurse's psychological state also influences how he or she analyzes client information and selects treatment interventions. An emotional state or behaviour can inadvertently influence the therapeutic relationship. For example, a nurse who has just learned that her child is using illegal drugs and who has a client with a history of drug use may inadvertently project a judgmental attitude toward her client, which would interfere with the formation of a therapeutic relationship. The nurse needs to examine underlying emotions, motivations, and beliefs and determine how these factors shape behaviour.

The nurse's social biases can be particularly problematic for the nurse–client relationship. Although the nurse may not verbalize these values to clients, some are readily evident in the nurse's behaviour and appearance, such as how the nurse acts or appears at work. The nurse's spiritual beliefs or feelings can also affect nurse–client interactions. For instance, beliefs about divorce, abortion, or homosexuality can affect how the nurse interacts with a client who is dealing with such issues.

UNDERSTANDING PERSONAL FEELINGS AND BELIEFS AND CHANGING BEHAVIOUR

Nurses must understand their own personal feelings and beliefs and try to avoid projecting them onto clients. This is not an easy task. For instance, due to ethnocentrism, our own sociocultural values may not be readily apparent. It takes effort to develop self-awareness, but it will enhance the nurse's objectivity and foster a nonjudgmental attitude, which is so important in building and maintaining trust throughout the nurse–client relationship. Soliciting feedback from colleagues and supervisors about how personal beliefs or thoughts are being projected onto others is a useful self-assessment technique. One of the reasons that ongoing clinical supervision is so important is that the supervisor really knows the nurse and can continually observe for inappropriate communication and question assumptions that the nurse may hold, as well as reinforce helpful behaviour.

Once a nurse has identified and analyzed personal beliefs and attitudes, behaviours that were driven by prejudicial ideas may change. The change process requires introspective analysis that may result in viewing the world differently. Through self-awareness and conscious effort, the nurse can change learned behaviours to engage effectively in therapeutic relationships with clients. Nevertheless, sometimes a nurse realizes that some attitudes are too ingrained to support a therapeutic relationship with a client with different beliefs. In such cases, the nurse should refer the client to someone who can be therapeutically helpful.

Communication

Effective communication skills, including verbal and nonverbal techniques, are the building blocks for all successful relationships. The nurse–client relationship is built on therapeutic communication, the ongoing process of interaction through which meaning emerges (see Box 9-2). **Verbal communication**, which is principally achieved by spoken words, includes the underlying emotion, context,

Principles of Therapeutic Communication

1. The client should be the primary focus of the interaction.
2. A professional attitude sets the tone of the therapeutic relationship.
3. Use self-disclosure cautiously and only when the disclosure has a therapeutic purpose.
4. Avoid social relationships with clients.
5. Maintain client confidentiality.
6. Assess the client's intellectual competence to determine the level of understanding.
7. Implement interventions from a theoretic base.
8. Maintain a nonjudgmental attitude. Avoid making judgments about the client's behaviour and giving advice. By the time the client sees the nurse, he or she has had plenty of advice.
9. Guide the client to reinterpret his or her experiences rationally.
10. Track the client's verbal interaction through the use of clarifying statements. Avoid changing the subject unless the content change is in the client's best interest.

and connotation of what is actually said. **Nonverbal communication** includes gestures, expressions, and body language. Both the client and the nurse use verbal and nonverbal communication. **Empathic linkages** are the direct communication of feelings. To respond therapeutically in a nurse–client relationship, the nurse is responsible for assessing and interpreting all forms of client communication.

• CRNENOTE

In analyzing client–nurse communication, nonverbal behaviours and gestures are communicated first. If a client's verbal and nonverbal communication are contradictory, priority should be given to the nonverbal behaviours and gestures since they operate on a more basic and less conscious level and are therefore harder to mask.

KEY CONCEPT **Therapeutic communication** is the ongoing process of interaction through which meaning emerges.

Therapeutic and social relationships are very different. In a therapeutic relationship, the nurse focuses on the client and client-related issues, even when engaging in social activities with that client. For example, a nurse may take a client shopping and out for lunch. Even though the nurse is engaged in a social activity, that trip should have a definite purpose, and conversation should focus only on the client. The nurse must not attempt to meet his or her own social or other needs during the activity.

■ USING VERBAL COMMUNICATION

The process of verbal communication involves a sender, a message, and a receiver. The client is often the sender, and the nurse is often the receiver (Fig. 9-1), but communication always works two ways. The client formulates an idea, encodes a message (puts ideas into words), and then transmits the message with emotion. The client's words and their underlying emotional tone and connotation communicate his or her needs and emotional problems. The nurse receives the message, decodes it (interprets the message, including its feelings, connotation, and context), and then responds to the client. On the surface, this interaction is deceptively simple; unseen complexities, however, lie beneath. Is the message that the nurse receives consistent with the client's original idea? Did the nurse interpret the message as the client intended? Is the verbal message consistent with the nonverbal flourishes that accompany it? Validation is essential to ensure that the nurse has received the information accurately. (See section "Validation" later in this chapter for further discussion.)

Self-Disclosure

One of the most important principles of therapeutic communication for the nurse to follow is to focus the interaction on the client's concerns. **Self-disclosure**, telling the client personal information, generally is not a good idea since the conversation should focus on the client, not the nurse. If a client asks the nurse personal

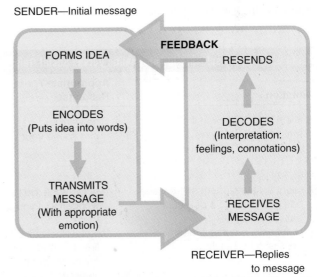

FIGURE 9.1 The communication process. (Adapted from Boyd, M. [1995]. Communication with clients, families, healthcare providers, and diverse cultures. In M. Strader & P. Decker [Eds.], *Role transition to client care management* [p. 431]. Norwalk, CT: Appleton & Lange.)

questions, the nurse should elicit the underlying reason for the request. The nurse can then determine how much personal information to disclose, if any. In revealing personal information, the nurse should be purposeful and have identified therapeutic outcomes. For example, a male client who was struggling with the implications of marriage and fidelity asked a male nurse if he had ever had an extramarital affair. The nurse interpreted the client's statement as seeking role-modelling behaviour for an adult man and judged self-disclosure in this instance to be therapeutic. He responded honestly that he did not engage in affairs and redirected the discussion back to the client's concerns.

Nurses sometimes may feel uncomfortable avoiding clients' questions for fear of seeming rude. Sometimes they disclose too much personal information because they are trying to be nice. However, being nice is not necessarily therapeutic. As appropriate, redirecting the client, giving a neutral or vague answer, or saying "Let's talk about you" may be all that is necessary to limit self-disclosure. In some instances, nurses may need to tell the client directly that they will not share personal information (Table 9-1).

Verbal Communication Techniques

PMH nurses use many verbal techniques in establishing relationships and helping clients focus on their problems. Asking a question, restating, and reflecting are examples of such techniques. These techniques may at first seem artificial, but with practice, they can be useful.

One of the most difficult but often most effective techniques is the use of silence during verbal interactions.

By maintaining silence, the nurse allows the client to gather thoughts and to proceed at his or her own pace.

Listening is another valuable tool. Silence and listening differ in that silence consists of deliberate pauses to encourage the client to reflect and eventually respond. Listening is an ongoing activity by which the nurse attends to the client's verbal and nonverbal communication. The art of listening is developed through careful attention to the content and meaning of the client's speech. There are two types of listening: passive and active. **Passive listening** involves sitting quietly and letting the client talk. A passive listener allows the client to ramble and does not focus or guide the thought process. Passive listening does not foster a therapeutic relationship.

Through **active listening,** the nurse focuses on what the client is saying to interpret and respond to the message objectively. While listening, the nurse concentrates only on what the client says and the underlying meaning. The nurse's verbal and nonverbal behaviours indicate active listening. The nurse usually responds indirectly, using techniques such as open-ended statements, reflection (Table 9-2), and questions that elicit additional responses from the client. In active listening, the nurse should avoid changing the subject and instead follow the client's lead, although at times, it is necessary to respond directly to help a client focus on a specific topic or to clarify thoughts and beliefs.

CRNENOTE

Self-disclosure can be used in very specific situations, but self-disclosure is not the first intervention to consider. In prioritizing interventions, active listening is one of the first methods to be used.

Table 9.1 Self-Disclosure in Therapeutic Versus Social Relationships		
Situation	**Appropriate Therapeutic Response**	**Inappropriate Social Response With Rationale**
A client asks the nurse if she had fun over the weekend.	"The weekend was fine. How did you spend your weekend?"	"It was great. My boyfriend and I went to dinner and a movie." (This self-disclosure has no therapeutic purpose. The response focuses the conversation on the nurse, not on the client.)
A client asks a student nurse if she has ever been to a particular bar.	"Many people go there. I'm wondering if you have ever been there."	"Oh yes—all the time. It's a lot of fun." (Sharing information about outside activities is inappropriate.)
A client asks a nurse if mental illness is in his family.	"Mental illnesses do run in families. I've had a lot of experience caring for people with mental illnesses."	"My sister is being treated for depression." (This self-disclosure has no purpose, and the nurse is missing the meaning of the question.)
While shopping with a client, the nurse sees a friend, who approaches them.	To her friend: "I know it looks like I'm not working, but I really am. I'll see you later."	"Hi, Bob. This is Jane Doe, a client." (Introducing the client to the friend is very inappropriate and violates client confidentiality.)

Table 9.2	Verbal Communication Techniques		
Technique	**Definition**	**Example**	**Use**
Acceptance	Encouraging and receiving information in a nonjudgmental and interested manner	*Client*: I have done something terrible. *Nurse*: I would like to hear about it. It's OK to discuss it with me.	Used in establishing trust and developing empathy.
Confrontation	Presenting the client with a different reality of the situation	*Client*: My best friend never calls me. She hates me. *Nurse*: I was in the room yesterday when she called.	Used cautiously to immediately redefine the client's reality. However, it can alienate the client if used inappropriately. A nonjudgmental attitude is critical for confrontation to be effective.
Doubt	Expressing or voicing doubt when a client relates a situation	*Client*: My best friend hates me. She never calls me. *Nurse*: From what you have told me, that does not sound like her. When did she call you last?	Used carefully and only when the nurse feels confident about the details. It is used when the nurse wants to guide the client toward other explanations.
Interpretation	Putting into words what the client is implying or feeling	*Client*: I could not sleep because someone would come in my room and rape me. *Nurse*: It sounds like you were scared last night.	Used in helping the client identify underlying thoughts or feelings.
Observation	Stating to the client what the nurse is observing	*Nurse*: You are trembling and perspiring. When did this start?	Used when a client's behaviours (verbal or nonverbal) are obvious and unusual for that client.
Open-ended statements	Introducing an idea and letting the client respond	*Nurse*: Trust means.... *Client*: That someone will keep you safe.	Used when helping the client explore feelings or gain insight.
Reflection	Redirecting the idea back to the client	*Client*: Should I go home for the weekend? *Nurse*: Should you go home for the weekend?	Used when the client is asking for the nurse's approval or judgment. Use of reflection helps the nurse maintain a nonjudgmental approach.
Restatement	Repeating the main idea expressed; lets the client know what was heard	*Client*: I hate this place. I don't belong here. *Nurse*: You don't want to be here.	Used when trying to clarify what the client has said.
Silence	Remaining quiet, but nonverbally expressing interest during an interaction	*Client*: I am angry!! *Nurse*: (Silence) *Client*: My wife had an affair.	Used when the client needs to express ideas but may not know quite how to do it. With silence, the client can focus on putting thoughts together.
Validation	Clarifying the nurse's understanding of the situation	*Nurse*: Let me see if I understand.	Used when the nurse is trying to understand a situation the client is trying to describe.

Some verbal techniques, however, block interactions and inhibit therapeutic communication (Table 9-3). One of the biggest blocks to communication is giving advice, particularly that which others have already given. Giving advice is different from supporting a client through decision making. The therapeutic dialogue presented in Box 9-3 differentiates between advice (telling the client what to do or how to act) and therapeutic communication, by which the nurse and the client explore alternative ways of viewing the client's world. The client then can reach his or her own conclusions about the best approaches to use. Refer to Box 9-4 for a summary of a research study on boundaries between clients and PMH nurses.

Table 9.3	Techniques That Inhibit Communication		
Technique	**Definition**	**Example**	**Problem**
Advice	Telling a client what to do	*Client*: I can't sleep. It is too noisy. *Nurse*: Turn off the light and shut your door.	The nurse solves the client's problem, which may not be the appropriate solution and encourages dependency on the nurse.
Agreement	Agreeing with a particular viewpoint of a client	*Client*: Abortions are sinful. *Nurse*: I agree.	The client is denied an opportunity to change his or her view now that the nurse agrees.
Challenges	Disputing a client's beliefs with arguments, logical thinking, or direct order	*Client*: I'm a cowboy. *Nurse*: If you are a cowboy, what are you doing in the hospital?	The nurse belittles the client and decreases self-esteem. The client will avoid relating to the nurse who challenges.
Disapproval	Judging a client's situation and behaviour	*Client*: I'm so sorry. I did not mean to kill my mother. *Nurse*: You should be. How could anyone kill their mother?	The nurse belittles the client. The client will avoid the nurse.
Reassurance	Telling a client that everything will be OK	*Client*: Everyone thinks I'm bad. *Nurse*: You are a good person.	The nurse makes a statement that may not be true. The client is blocked from exploring feelings.

BOX 9.3

Therapeutic Dialogue: *Giving Advice Versus Recommendations*

Ms. J has just received a diagnosis of phobic disorder and been given a prescription for fluoxetine. She was referred to the home care agency because she does not want to take her medication. She is fearful of becoming suicidal. Two approaches are given below.

INEFFECTIVE COMMUNICATION (ADVICE)

Nurse: Ms. J, the doctor has ordered the medication because it will help you.

Ms. J: I don't want to take the medication because I am afraid of becoming suicidal. I heard that some of this psychiatric medication does that. I haven't had any attacks for 2 weeks.

Nurse: This medication has rarely had that side effect. You should try it and see if you have any suicidal thoughts.

Ms. J: OK. (The nurse leaves and Ms. J does not take the medication. Within a week, Ms. J is taken to the emergency room with a panic attack.)

EFFECTIVE COMMUNICATION (RECOMMENDATIONS)

Nurse: Ms. J, how have you been doing?

Ms. J: So far, so good. I haven't had any attacks for 2 weeks.

Nurse: I understand that the doctor gave you a prescription for medication that may help with the panic attacks.

Ms. J: Yes, but I don't want to take it because I am afraid of becoming suicidal. I heard that some of this psychiatric medication does that.

Nurse: Have you ever had feelings of hurting yourself?

Ms. J: Not really.

Nurse: If you took the medication and had thoughts like that, what would you do?

Ms. J: I don't know.

Nurse: I think I see your dilemma. This medication may help your panic attacks, but the suicidal thoughts are a real fear. Is that it?

Ms. J: Yeah, that's it.

Nurse: Are there any circumstances under which you would be able to try the medication?

Ms. J: If I knew that I would not have suicidal thoughts.

Nurse: I can't guarantee that, but I could call you every few days to see if you are having any of these thoughts and help you deal with them.

Ms. J: Oh, that will be OK.

(Ms. J successfully took the medication.)

CRITICAL THINKING CHALLENGE

- Contrast the communication in the first scenario with that in the second.
- What therapeutic communication techniques did the second nurse employ that may have contributed to a better outcome?
- Are there any cues in the first scenario that indicate that the client will not follow the nurse's advice? Explain.

BOX 9.4

Research for Best Practice: Boundaries Between Clients and Mental Health Nurses

Campbell, R. J., Yonge, O., & Austin, W. (2005). Intimacy boundaries between mental health nurses and psychiatric patients. Journal of Psychosocial Nursing and Mental Health Services, 43(5), 33–41.

THE QUESTION: What are the attitudes and behaviours of mental health nurses toward clients in the areas of attraction, dating, and sexual relationships?

METHODS: A self-administered survey with a majority of forced-choice, refined-response items was sent by mail to 2,009 nurses (896 registered nurses and 1,113 registered psychiatric nurses) in Alberta. The response rate was 45.9%. The questionnaire was composed of 37 questions with 171 variables and took approximately 15–30 minutes to complete. Analysis involved examination of basic frequency distributions, percentage distributions, and cross-tabulations.

FINDINGS: Almost all respondents strongly agreed that it was inappropriate to go on a date with a current client (98.9%) or to have a sexual relationship with a current client (99.3%). Only one respondent reported having dated a current client (rarely), and nine respondents reported having dated a discharged client (rarely or sometimes). Six nurses reported that they had had a sexual relationship with a discharged client in the past.

IMPLICATIONS FOR PRACTICE: Nurses need to recognize that the potential for intimacy boundary violations with clients exists. Although most nurses in the study reported never dating or having sexual relationships with current or discharged clients, a few respondents reported having done so. Nurses who do engage in such inappropriate behaviours can face disciplinary action and lawsuits.

USING NONVERBAL COMMUNICATION

Gestures, facial expressions, and body language actually communicate more than verbal messages. Under the best circumstances, body language mirrors or enhances what is verbally communicated. However, if verbal and nonverbal messages are conflicting, the listener will most likely believe the nonverbal message since it functions on a more basic level. For example, if a client says that he feels fine but has a sad facial expression and is slumped in a chair away from others, the message of sadness and depression likely will be accepted, rather than the client's words. The same is true of a nurse's behaviour. If a nurse tells a client that she is happy to see him, but her facial expression communicates indifference, the client will receive the message that the nurse is bored.

Because people with psychiatric problems often have difficulty verbally expressing themselves and interpreting the emotions of others, nurses need to assess continually the nonverbal communication needs of clients. Eye contact (or lack thereof), posture, movement (e.g., shifting in chair, pacing), facial expressions, and gestures are nonverbal behaviours that communicate thoughts and feelings. A client with low self-esteem may be unable to maintain eye contact and thus may spend a great deal of time looking toward the floor. A client who is pacing and restless may be upset or having a reaction to medication. A clenched fist usually indicates that a person feels angry or hostile.

Nonverbal behaviour is culturally specific. The nurse must therefore be careful to understand his or her own cultural context as well as that of the client. For example, in some cultures (e.g., Canadian Aboriginal nations), it is

| Closed body and closed attitude | Open body and open attitude |

FIGURE 9.2 Open and closed body language.

considered disrespectful to look a person straight in the eye. In other cultures, not looking a person in the eye may be interpreted as "hiding something" or low self-esteem. Whether one points with the finger, nose, or eyes and how much hand gesturing one uses are other examples of nonverbal communication that may vary considerably among cultures.

Nurses should use positive body language, such as sitting at the same eye level as the client with a relaxed posture that projects interest and attention. Leaning slightly forward helps engage the client. Generally, the nurse should not cross his or her arms or legs during therapeutic communication because such postures erect barriers to interaction. Uncrossed arms and legs project openness and a willingness to engage in conversation (Fig. 9-2). Any verbal response should be consistent with nonverbal messages.

RECOGNIZING EMPATHIC LINKAGES

Empathic linkages are the communication of feelings (Peplau, 1952). This commonly occurs with anxiety. For example, a nurse may be speaking with a client who is highly anxious, and the nurse may notice his or her own speech becoming more rapid in tandem with the client's. The nurse may also become aware of subjective feelings of anxiety. It may be difficult for the nurse to determine whether the anxiety was communicated interpersonally, or whether the nurse is personally reacting to some of the content of what the client is communicating. However, being aware of one's own feelings and analyzing them is crucial to determining the source of the feeling.

SELECTING COMMUNICATION TECHNIQUES

In therapeutic communication, the nurse chooses the best words to say and uses nonverbal behaviours that are consistent with these words. If a client is angry and upset, should the nurse invite the client to sit down and discuss the problem, walk quietly with the client, or simply observe the client from a distance and not initiate conversation? Choosing the best response begins with assessing and interpreting the meaning of the client's communication—both verbal and nonverbal.

> **• CRNENOTE**
>
> Applying communication techniques requires consideration of the ultimate goal and the ability of the client to benefit from the intervention. Giving advice rarely works.

Nurses should not necessarily take verbal messages literally, especially when a client is upset or angry. For example, one nurse walked into the room of a newly admitted client who accused, "You locked me up and threw away the key." The nurse could have responded defensively that she had nothing to do with the client being admitted; however, that response would have ended in an argument, and communication would have been blocked. Fortunately, the nurse recognized that the client was communicating frustration at being in a locked psychiatric unit and did not take the accusation personally.

The nurse also needs to identify the desired client outcome. To do so, the nurse should engage the client with eye contact (if culturally appropriate) and quietly try to interpret the client's feelings. In the example just discussed, the desired outcome was for the client to clarify the hospitalization experience. The nurse responded by saying, "It must be frustrating to feel locked up." The nurse focused on the client's feelings, rather than the accusations, which reflected an understanding of the client's feelings. The

client knew that the nurse accepted these feelings, which led to further discussion. It may seem impossible to plan reactions for each situation, but with practice, the nurse will begin to respond consistently in a therapeutic way.

APPLYING COMMUNICATION CONCEPTS

When the nurse is interacting with clients, additional considerations can enhance the quality of communication. This section describes the importance of rapport, validation, empathy, and the role of boundaries and body space in nurse–client interactions.

Rapport

Rapport, interpersonal harmony characterized by understanding and respect, is important in developing a trusting, therapeutic relationship. Nurses establish rapport through interpersonal warmth, a nonjudgmental attitude, and a demonstration of understanding. A skilled nurse will establish rapport that will alleviate the client's anxiety in discussing personal problems.

People with psychiatric problems often feel alone and isolated. Establishing rapport helps lessen the feelings of being alone. When rapport develops, a client feels comfortable with the nurse and finds self-disclosure easier. The nurse also feels comfortable and recognizes that an interpersonal bond or alliance is developing. All these factors—comfort, sense of sharing, and decreased anxiety—are important in establishing and building the nurse–client relationship.

Validation

Validation is explicitly checking out one's own thoughts or feelings with another person. To do so, the nurse must own his or her own thought or feeling by using "I" statements. The validation generally refers to observations, thoughts, or feelings and seeks explicit feedback. For example, a nurse who sees a client pacing the hallway before a planned family visit may conclude that the client is anxious. Validation may occur with a statement such as, "I notice you pacing the hallway. I wonder if you are feeling anxious about the family visit?" The client may agree, "Yes. I keep worrying about what is going to happen!" or disagree, "No. I have been trying to get into the bathroom for the last 30 minutes, but my roommate is still in there!"

Empathy

The use of empathy in a therapeutic relationship is central to PMH nursing. **Empathy** is the ability to experience, in the present, a situation as another did at some time in the past. It is the ability to put oneself in another person's circumstances and feelings. The nurse does not actually have to have had the experience but has to be able to imagine the feelings associated with it. For empathy to develop, there must be a giving of self to the other individual and a reciprocal desire to know each other personally. The process involves the nurse receiving information from the client with open, nonjudgmental acceptance and communicating this understanding of the experience and feelings so that the client feels understood.

Bio/psycho/social/spiritual Boundaries and Body Space Zones

Boundaries are the defining limits of individuals, objects, or relationships. Boundaries mark territory or what is "mine" or "not mine." Human beings have many different types of boundaries. Material boundaries, such as fences around property, artificially imposed territorial lines, and bodies of water can define territory as well as provide security and order. Personal boundaries can be conceptualized within the bio/psycho/social/spiritual model as including physical, psychological, social, and spiritual dimensions. Physical boundaries are those established in terms of physical closeness to others—whom we allow to touch us or how close we want others to stand near us. Psychological boundaries are established in terms of emotional distance from others—how much of our innermost feelings and thoughts we want to share. Social boundaries, such as norms, customs, and roles, help us establish our closeness and place within the family, culture, and community. Spiritual boundaries, related to such things as our understanding of the meaning of life, our religious values, and/or our sense of relationship with a greater power, shape our way of being in the world. Boundaries are not fixed, but dynamic. When boundaries are involuntarily transgressed, the individual feels threatened and responds to the perceived threat. The nurse must elicit permission before implementing interventions that invade personal space and boundaries.

Personal Boundaries

Every individual is surrounded by four different body zones. These were identified by Hall (1990) as the intimate zone (e.g., whispering and embracing), the personal zone (e.g., for close friends), the social zone (e.g., for acquaintances), and the public zone (usually for interacting with strangers). These zones provide varying degrees of protection against unwanted physical closeness during interactions. The actual sizes of the different zones vary according to culture. Some cultures define the intimate zone narrowly and the personal zones widely. Thus, friends in these cultures stand and sit close while interacting. People of other cultures define the intimate zone widely and are uncomfortable when others stand close to them. The variability of intimate and personal zones has implications for nursing. For a client to be

comfortable with a nurse, the nurse needs to protect the intimate zone of that individual. The client usually will allow the nurse to enter the personal zone but will express discomfort if the nurse breaches the intimate zone. For the nurse, the difficulty lies in differentiating the personal zone from the intimate zone for each client.

The nurse's awareness of his or her own need for intimate and personal space is another prerequisite for therapeutic interactions with the client. It is important that a nurse feels comfortable while interacting with clients. Establishing a comfort zone may well entail fine-tuning the size of body zones. Recognizing this will help the nurse understand occasional inexplicable reactions to the proximity of clients.

Professional Boundaries

For nurses, professional boundaries are also essential to consider in the context of the nurse–client relationship. Clients often enter such relationships at a very vulnerable point, and nurses need to be aware of professional boundaries to avoid exploitation of the client. For example, in a friendship, there is a two-way sharing of personal information and feelings, but as mentioned previously, the focus is on the client's needs, and the nurse generally does not share personal information or attempt to meet his or her own needs through the relationship. The client may seek a friendship or sexual relationship with the nurse (or vice versa), which would be inconsistent with the professional role. Although professional boundaries are about power, influence, and control, they are not clear and precise. Professional boundaries can become blurred and ambiguous, given the familiarity, trust, and emotional intensity that are often involved in therapeutic relationships. It is important to be vigilant about the potential abuse of power that is present in all such relationships (Austin, Bergum, Nuttgens, & Peternelj-Taylor, 2006).

Indicators that the relationship may be moving outside the professional boundaries are gift giving on either party's part, spending more time than usual with a particular client, strenuously defending or explaining the client's behaviour in team meetings, the nurse feeling that he or she is the only one who truly understands the client, keeping secrets, and frequently thinking about the client outside of the work situation (Forchuk et al., 2006; Gallop et al., 2002). Provincial regulatory bodies may have guidelines or firm rules, such as how long after a therapeutic relationship must be terminated before engaging in a romantic or sexual relationship. Within psychiatric disciplines, a romantic or sexual relationship with a former client can be considered as always inappropriate, regardless of the length of time that the professional relationship has been terminated. In nursing, the guidelines are generic and do not identify differences between specialties. Nevertheless, the professional implications of a personal relationship following a nursing relationship that involved psychotherapy are serious and must be carefully considered.

Guidelines are generally more vague about when a friendship would be appropriate, but such relationships are not appropriate when the nurse is actively providing care to the client. Exceptions may be when a relationship preceded the nursing context and another nurse is unavailable to provide care, such as in a nursing outpost (College of Nurses of Ontario, 2006). Similarly, relationships to meet the nurse's needs that are acquired through the nursing context, such as a relationship with a family member of the client, also breach professional boundaries. It is important for the nurse to be familiar with the specific standards of practice related to boundaries and therapeutic relationships of his or her provincial regulatory and professional associations. Table 9-4 summarizes some of these standards. When concerns arise related to therapeutic boundaries, the nurse must seek clinical supervision or transfer the care of the client immediately.

Defence Mechanisms

Defence mechanisms (or coping mechanisms) are the automatic psychological processes protecting the individual against anxiety and from the awareness of internal or external dangers or stressors (Table 9-5). Individuals often are unaware of these processes, although they mediate reactions to emotional conflicts and to internal and external stressors (American Psychiatric Association, 2000). The concept of defence mechanisms originated with Freud's psychoanalytic theory and was conceived as the way the ego protected the individual from overwhelming anxiety (see Chapter 8). All healthy individuals use various defence mechanisms throughout their lives. A defence mechanism becomes pathological when it is used so persistently that it becomes maladaptive. Suppression or denial, for instance, involves a process where anxiety-provoking information is not accepted (for suppression, this is conscious and for denial, this is unconscious). This may be either maladaptive or adaptive, depending on its severity and the context in which it occurs. Other defence mechanisms such as projection (attributing one's own feelings onto another), splitting (self or others viewed as all bad or all good), and acting out (expressing unconscious feelings in actions rather than words), however, are almost invariably maladaptive.

As nurses develop therapeutic relationships, they will recognize their clients, and perhaps themselves, using defence mechanisms. (As defence mechanisms are almost always used unconsciously, it will be difficult for a nurse to readily identify his or her own.) With experience, the nurse will evaluate the purpose of a defence mechanism and then determine whether or not it should be discussed with the client. For example, if a client is using humour to alleviate an emotionally intense situation, that may be very appropriate. On the other hand, if someone continually rationalizes antisocial behaviour, the use of the defence mechanism should be discussed.

CRNENOTE

When studying defence mechanisms, focus on those mechanisms and coping styles that are similar. For example, displacement, repression, and projection should be differentiated. Use these concepts in clinical assignments.

Table 9.4	**Canadian Provincial Standards of Practice Regarding Therapeutic Nurse–Client Relationships**	
Province Territory	**Standards of Practice/Best Practice Guidelines**	**Web site**
Alberta	College and Association of Registered Nurses of Alberta:	
	Nursing Practice Standards with CNA Code of Ethics for Registered Nurses (2008)	http://www.nurses.ab.ca/Carna-Admin/Uploads/new_nps_with_ethics.pdf
	Professional Boundaries for Registered Nurses: Guidelines for the Nurse–Client Relationship	http://www.nurses.ab.ca/Carna-Admin/Uploads/Professional%20Boundaries%20Guidelines.pdf
	College of Registered Psychiatric Nurses of Alberta:	
	Competency Profile (2001)	http://www.crpna.ab.ca/RPN%20Competency%20Profile%20REVISED%202007.pdf
British Columbia	College of Registered Nurses of British Columbia:	
	Professional Standards for Registered Nurses and Nurse Practitioners	http://www.crnbc.ca/downloads/128_Prof%20Standards%202005.pdf
	Nurse–Client Relationships	http://www.crnbc.ca/downloads/432.pdf
	College of Registered Psychiatric Nurses of British Columbia:	
	Standards of Psychiatric Nurses in British Columbia	http://www.crpnbc.ca/standards_ethics.pdf

Continued

Table 9.4   Canadian Provincial Standards of Practice Regarding Therapeutic Nurse–Client Relationships (*Continued*)

Province Territory	Standards of Practice/Best Practice Guidelines	Web site
Manitoba	College of Registered Nurses of Manitoba: Standards of Practice for Registered Nurses	http://cms.tng-secure.com/file_download.php?fFile_id = 140
	Professional Boundaries for Therapeutic Relationships	http://cms.tng-secure.com/file_download.php?fFile_id = 144
	College of Registered Psychiatric Nurses of Manitoba: Standards of Psychiatric Nursing Practice	http://crpnm.mb.ca/CRPNM_v0/standards/standards.pdf
New Brunswick	Nurses Association of New Brunswick: Standards of Practice for Registered Nurses	http://www.nanb.nb.ca/pdf_e/Publications/General_Publications/StandardsofRegistered-NursesE.pdf
	Standards for the Therapeutic Nurse–Client Relationship	http://www.nanb.nb.ca/pdf_e/Publications/General_Publications/Standards_for_the_therapeutic_Nurse-Client_Relationship_English.pdf
Newfoundland and Labrador	Association of Registered Nurses of Newfoundland and Labrador: Standards for Nursing Practice	http://www.arnnl.nf.ca/PDF/Standards_for_Nursing_Practice_April_07.pdf
Northwest Territories	Registered Nurses Association of the Northwest Territories and Nunavut: Standards of Nursing Practice for Registered Nurses	http://www.rnantnu.ca/Portals/0/Documents/Standards_Nrsing_Prac_2006.pdf
Nova Scotia	College of Registered Nurses of Nova Scotia: Standards for Nursing Practice	http://www.crnns.ca/documents/standards2004.pdf
	Professional Boundaries and Expectations for Nurse–Client Relationships	http://www.crnns.ca/documents/professional-boundaries.pdf
Ontario	College of Nurses of Ontario: Professional Standards	http://www.cno.org/docs/prac/41006_ProfStds.pdf
	Therapeutic Nurse–Client Relationships	http://www.cno.org/docs/prac/41033_Therapeutic.pdf
	Registered Nurses' Association of Ontario: Establishing Therapeutic Relationships	http://www.rnao.org/Page.asp?PageID = 828&ContentID = 801
Prince Edward Island	The Association of Registered Nurses of Prince Edward Island: Standards for Nursing Practice	http://www.arnpei.ca/default.asp?id = 190&sfield = content.id&search = 72&mn = 1.25.30
Quebec	Ordre des infirmières et infirmiers du Québec: Le Plan Thérapeutique Infirmier	http://www.oiiq.org/infirmieres/plan/index.asp
Saskatchewan	Saskatchewan Registered Nurses' Association: Standards and Foundation Competencies for the Practice of Registered Nurses	http://www.srna.org/nurse_resources/standards_competencies.pdf
	Registered Psychiatric Nurses Association of Saskatchewan: Standards for Psychiatric Nursing Practice	http://www.rpnas.com/public/jsp/content/documentation/standards.jsp
Yukon	Yukon Registered Nurses Association: Standards for Registered Nursing Practice in the Yukon	http://www.yrna.ca/pdf/Standards2005.pdf
National	Canadian Federation of Mental Health Nurses: The Canadian Standards of Psychiatric-Mental Health Nursing Practice	http://www.cfmhn.ca/standards.html

Table 9.5   Specific Defence Mechanisms and Coping Styles*

Defence Mechanism	Definition	Example
Denial	Refusing to acknowledge some painful aspect of external reality or subjective experience that would be apparent to others (psychotic denial is used when there is gross impairment in reality testing)	A teenager's best friend moves away, but the adolescent says that he does not feel sad.
Displacement	Transferring a feeling about, or a response to, one object onto another (usually less threatening) substitute object	A child is mad at her mother for leaving for the day but says that she is really mad at the sitter for serving her food she does not like.
Dissociation	Experiencing a breakdown in the usually integrated functions of consciousness, memory, perception of self or the environment, or sensory and motor behaviour	An adult relates severe sexual abuse experienced as a child, but she does it without feeling. She says that the experience was as if she were outside her body watching the abuse.
Idealization	Attributing exaggerated positive qualities to others	An adult falls in love and fails to see the negative qualities in the other person.
Projection	Falsely attributing to another one's own unacceptable feelings, impulses, or thoughts	A child is very angry at a parent, but accuses the parent of being angry.
Rationalization	Concealing the true motivations for one's own thoughts, actions, or feelings through the elaboration of reassuring or self-serving but incorrect explanations	A man is rejected by his girlfriend, but he explains to his friends that her leaving was best because she was beneath him socially and would not be liked by his family.
Reaction formation	Substituting behaviours, thoughts, or feelings that are diametrically opposed to one's own unacceptable thoughts or feelings (this usually occurs in conjunction with their repression)	A wife finds out about her husband's extramarital affairs and tells her friends that she thinks his affairs are perfectly appropriate. She truly does not feel, on a conscious level, any anger or hurt.
Repression	Expelling disturbing wishes, thoughts, or experiences from conscious awareness (the feeling component may remain conscious, detached from its associated ideas)	A woman does not remember the experience of being raped in the basement, but she does feel anxious when going into the house.
Undoing	Words or behaviours designed to negate or to make amends symbolically for unacceptable thoughts, feelings, or actions	A man has sexual fantasies about his wife's sister. He takes his wife away for a romantic weekend.

*The following defence mechanisms and coping styles are identified in the DSM-IV as being used when the individual deals with emotional conflicts or stressors (either internal or external).

Adapted from American Psychiatric Association. (2000). Diagnostic and statistical manual of mental disorders (4th ed., Text revision, pp. 811–814). Washington, DC: Author.

■ ANALYZING INTERACTIONS

Many people with psychiatric disorders have difficulty communicating. For example, perceptual, cognitive, and information-processing deficits, typical of people with schizophrenia, can interfere with the person's ability to express ideas, understand concepts, and accurately perceive the environment. Because of the complexity of communication, mental health professionals monitor their interactions with clients using various methods, including audio recording, video recording, and **process recording** (writing a verbatim transcript of the interaction). A video or audio recording of an interaction provides the most accurate monitoring but is cumbersome to use. Process recording, one of the easiest methods to use, is adequate in most situations. Nurses should use it when first learning therapeutic communication and during times when communication becomes a problem.

In a process recording, the nurse records, from memory, the verbatim interaction immediately after the communication (Box 9-5). The nurse then analyzes the content of the interaction in terms of the words and their meaning for both the client and the nurse. The analysis is especially important because the ability to communicate verbally is often compromised in people with mental disorders. Words may not have the same meaning for the client as they do for the nurse. Clarification of meaning becomes especially important. The analysis can identify symbolic meanings, themes, and blocks in communication. **Symbolism**, the use of a word or phrase to represent an object, event, or feeling, is used universally. For example, automobiles are named for wild animals that represent speed, prowess, and beauty. In people with mental disorders, the use of words to symbolize events, objects, or feelings is often idiosyncratic, and they cannot explain their choices. For

---

BOX 9.5

Process Recording

Setting: The living room of Mr. S's home. His parents are in the room but cannot hear the conversation. Mr. S is sitting on the couch and the nurse is sitting on a chair. This is the nurse's first visit after Mr. S's discharge from the hospital.

Client	Nurse	Comments/Interpretation
	How are you doing, Mr. S?	*Plan:* Initially develop a sense of trust and initiate a therapeutic relationship.
I'm fine. It's good to be home. I really don't like the hospital.	You didn't like the hospital?	*Interpretation:* Mr. S does not want to return to the hospital. Use reflection to begin to understand his experience.
NO. The nurses lock you up. Are you a nurse?	Yes. I'm a nurse. I'm wondering if you think that I will lock you up?	*Interpretation:* Mr. S is wondering what my role is and whether I will put him back in the hospital.
You could tell my mom to put me back in the hospital.	Any treatment that I recommend will be thoroughly discussed with you first. I am here to help you stay out of the hospital. I will not discuss anything with your mother unless you give me the permission to do so.	Use interpretation to clarify Mr. S's thinking. Mr. S is wondering about my relationship with his mother. Explain my role.

---

example, a person who is feeling scared and anxious may tell the nurse that bombs and guns are exploding. It is up to the nurse to make the connection between the bombs and guns and the client's feelings and then validate this with the client. Because of the client's cognitive limitations, the individual may express feelings only symbolically.

Some clients, for example, those with developmental handicaps or organic brain difficulties, may have difficulty with abstract thinking and symbolism. Conversations may be interpreted literally. For example, in response to the question "What brings you to the hospital?" a client might reply, "the ambulance." In these situations, the nurse must be cautious to avoid using symbols or metaphors. Concrete language, that is, language reflecting what can be observed through the senses, will be more easily understood.

Verbal behaviour is also interpreted by analyzing **content themes**. Clients often express concerns or feelings repeatedly in several different ways. After a few sessions, a common theme emerges. Themes may emerge symbolically, as in the case with the client who constantly talks about the "guns and bombs." Alternatively, a theme may simply be identified as a recurrent thread of a story that a client retells at each session. For example, one client always explained his early abandonment by his family. This led the nurse to hypothesize that he had an underlying fear of rejection. The nurse was then able to test whether there was an underlying fear and to develop strategies to help the client explore the fear (Box 9-6). It is important to involve clients in analyzing themes so that they may learn this skill. Within the therapeutic relationship, the person who does the work is the one who develops the competencies, so the nurse

BOX 9.6

Themes and Interactions

Session 1	Client discusses the death of his mother at a young age.
Session 2	Client explains that his sister is now married and never visits him.
Session 3	Client says that his best friend in the hospital was discharged and he really misses her.
Session 4	Client cries about a lost kitten.

Interpretation: Theme of loss is pervasive in several sessions.

---

must be careful to share this opportunity with the client (Peplau, 1952).

Communication blocks are identified by topic changes that either the nurse or the client makes. Topics are changed for various reasons. A client may change the topic from one that does not interest him or her to one that he or she finds more meaningful. However, an individual often changes the topic because he or she is uncomfortable with a particular subject. Once a topic change is identified, the nurse or client hypothesizes the reason for it. If the nurse changes the topic, he or she needs to determine why. The nurse may find that he or she is uncomfortable with the topic or may not be listening to the client. Beginning mental health nurses who are uncomfortable with silences or trying to elicit specific information from the client often change topics.

The nurse must also record and interpret the client's nonverbal behaviour in light of the verbal behaviour. Is the client saying one thing verbally and another nonverbally? The nurse must consider the client's cultural background. Is the behaviour consistent with cultural norms? For example, if a client denies any problems but is affectionate and physically demonstrative (which is antithetical to his or her naturally stoic cultural beliefs and behaviours), the nonverbal behaviour is inconsistent with what is normal behaviour for that person. Further exploration is needed to determine the meaning of the culturally atypical behaviour.

The Nurse–Client Relationship

The nurse–client relationship is a dynamic process that changes with time. It can be viewed in steps or phases with characteristic behaviours for both the client and the nurse. This text uses an adaptation of Hildegard Peplau's model that she introduced in her seminal work, *Interpersonal Relations in Nursing* (1952, 1988). The nurse–client relationship is conceptualized in three overlapping phases that evolve with time: orientation phase, working phase, and resolution phase. Box 9-7 gives a recent research example testing an intervention based on this approach.

The **orientation phase** is the phase during which the nurse and client get to know each other. During this phase, which can last from a few minutes to several months, the client develops a sense of trust in the nurse. The second phase is the **working phase**, in which the client uses the relationship to examine specific problems and learn new ways of approaching them. The final stage, the **resolution phase**, is the termination stage of the relationship and lasts from the time the problems are actually resolved to the close of the relationship. The relationship does not evolve as a simple linear relationship. Instead, the relationship may be predominantly in one phase, but reflections of all phases can be seen in each interaction.

KEY CONCEPT The **nurse–client relationship** is a dynamic process that changes with time. It can be viewed in steps or phases with characteristic behaviours for both the client and the nurse.

ORIENTATION PHASE

The orientation phase begins when the nurse and client meet and ends when the client begins to identify problems to be examined. During the orientation phase, the nurse discusses the client's expectations, explains the purpose of the relationship and its boundaries, and facilitates the development of the relationship. It is natural for the nurse and client to be more nervous during the first few sessions. The goal of the orientation phase is to develop trust and security within the nurse–client relationship. During this initial phase, the nurse listens intently to the client's history and perception of problems and begins to understand the client and identify themes. The use of empathy facilitates the development of a positive therapeutic relationship.

First Meeting

During the first meeting, outlining both nursing and client responsibilities is important. The nurse is responsible for providing guidance throughout the therapeutic relationship, protecting confidential information, and maintaining professional boundaries. The client is responsible for attending agreed-upon sessions, interacting during the sessions, and participating in the nurse–client relationship. The nurse should also explain clearly to the client meeting times, handling of missed sessions, and the estimated length of the relationship. Issues related to recording information and how the nurse will work within the interdisciplinary team should also be made explicit.

BOX 9.7

Research for Best Practice: Therapeutic Relationships—From Psychiatric Hospital to Community

Forchuk, C., Martin, M. L., Chan, Y-C., & Jensen, E. (2005). Therapeutic relationships: From psychiatric hospital to community. Journal of Psychiatric and Mental Health Nursing, 12, 556–564.

THE QUESTION: This study tested the effectiveness of a transitional discharge model (TDM) based on sustaining therapeutic relationships over the discharge process. The therapeutic relationships included staff and peer relationships.

METHODS: The authors provided a history and overview of TDM. The current study included 26 tertiary care psychiatric wards that were matched into 13 pairs of similar wards. Of these, one half implemented TDM (intervention group), and the other half continued with the usual care (control group).

There were 390 research subjects who were followed up for 1 year after discharge. Comparisons of quality of life and use of services (costs) were made between the intervention and the control groups.

FINDINGS: The quality of life and postdischarge costs were not significantly different between the intervention and control groups. However, the intervention group subjects were able to leave the hospital an average of 116 days sooner than the control group subjects. This is equal to a savings of more than $12 million Canadian.

IMPLICATIONS FOR PRACTICE: Strategies focusing on developing and sustaining therapeutic relationships have the potential for significant health cost savings.

Usually, both the nurse and the client feel anxious at the first meeting. The nurse should recognize the anxieties and attempt to alleviate them before the meeting. The client's behaviour during this first meeting may indicate to the nurse some of the client's problems in interpersonal relationships. For example, a client may talk nonstop for 15 minutes or may brag of sexual conquests. What the client chooses to tell or not to tell is significant. What a client first does or says may not accurately indicate his or her true feelings or the situation. In the beginning, clients may deny problems or choose not to discuss them as defence mechanisms or to prevent the nurse from getting to know them. The client is usually nervous and insecure during the first few sessions and may exhibit behaviour reflective of these emotions, such as rambling. Usually, by the third session, the client can focus on a topic.

Confidentiality in Treatment

Ideally, nurses include people who are important to the client in planning and implementing care. The nurse and client should discuss the issue of confidentiality in the first session. The nurse should be clear about any information that is to be shared with anyone else. Usually, the nurse shares significant assessment data and client progress with a supervisor and a physician. Most clients expect the nurse to communicate with other mental health professionals and are comfortable with this arrangement. Boundaries around what information can be shared with whom and under what circumstances are covered under provincial/territorial legislation such as mental health acts and health information acts. It is therefore important that each nurse be aware of the legislation in the province or territory in which he or she is practising.

Testing the Relationship

This first part of the orientation phase, called the "honeymoon phase," is usually pleasant. However, the therapeutic team typically hits rough spots before completing this phase. The client begins to test the relationship to become convinced that the nurse will really accept him or her. Typical testing behaviours include forgetting a scheduled session or being late. Clients may also express anger at something a nurse says or accuse the nurse of breaking confidentiality. Another common pattern is for the client to first introduce a relatively superficial issue as if it is the major problem. The nurse must recognize that these behaviours are designed to test the relationship and establish its parameters, not to express rejection or dissatisfaction with the nurse. The student nurse often feels personally rejected during the client's testing and may even become angry with the client. If the nurse simply accepts the behaviour as testing and continues to be available to the client and consistent in responses, these behaviours usually subside. Testing needs to be understood as a normal way that human beings develop trust.

Some issues specific to psychiatric clients can occur. For example, a client experiencing paranoia, by definition, is going to have difficulty establishing trust and may require a longer orientation phase. A client who is depressed may have difficulty expressing needs and may require periods of silence to feel comfortable in moving forward in the relationship.

WORKING PHASE

When the client begins identifying problems to work on, the working phase of the relationship has started. Problem identification can yield a wide range of issues, such as managing symptoms of a mental disorder, coping with chronic pain, examining issues related to sexual abuse, and dealing with problematic interpersonal relationships. Through the relationship, the client begins to explore the identified problems and develop strategies to resolve them. By the time the working phase is reached, the client has developed enough trust that he or she can examine the identified problems within the security of the therapeutic relationship. In the working phase, the nurse can use various verbal and nonverbal techniques to help the client examine problems.

Transference (unconscious assignment to others of the feelings and attitudes that the client originally associated with important figures) and **countertransference** (the provider's emotional reaction to the client based on personal unconscious needs and conflicts) become important issues in the working phase. For example, a client could be hostile to a nurse because of the underlying resentment of authority figures; the nurse, in turn, could respond defensively because of earlier experiences of anger. The client uses transference to examine problems. During this phase, the client is psychologically vulnerable and emotionally dependent on the nurse. The nurse needs to recognize countertransference and prevent it from eroding professional boundaries.

Many times, nurses are eager to implement rehabilitation plans. However, this cannot be done until the client trusts the nurse and identifies what issues he or she wishes to work on in the context of the relationship.

RESOLUTION PHASE

The final stage of the nurse–client relationship is the resolution phase, which begins when the actual problems are resolved and ends with the termination of the relationship. During this phase, the client is redirected toward a life without this specific therapeutic relationship. The client connects with community resources, solidifies a newly found understanding, and practices new behaviours. The client takes responsibility for follow-up appointments and interacts with significant others in new ways. New problems are not addressed during this phase, except in terms of what was learned during the working stage. The nurse assists the client in strengthening relationships, making referrals, and recognizing and understanding signs of future relapse.

Termination begins the first day of the relationship, when the nurse explains that this relationship is time limited and was established to resolve the client's problems and help him or her handle them. Because a therapeutic relationship is dependent, the nurse must constantly evaluate the client's level of dependence and continually support the client's move toward independence. Termination is usually stressful for the client, who must sever ties with the nurse who has shared thoughts and feelings and given guidance and support over many sessions. Depending on previous experiences with terminating relationships, some clients may not handle their emotions well during termination. Some may not show up for the last session at all to avoid their feelings of sadness and separation. Many clients display anger about the relationship ending. Clients may express anger toward the nurse or displace it onto others. For example, a client may shout obscenities at another client after being told that his or her therapeutic relationship

with the nurse will end in a few weeks. One of the best ways to handle the anger is to help the client acknowledge it, to explain that anger is a normal emotion when a relationship is ending, and to reassure the client that it is acceptable to feel angry. The nurse should also reassure the client that anger subsides once the relationship is over.

Another typical termination behaviour is raising old problems that have already been resolved. The nurse may feel frustrated if clients in the termination phase present resolved problems as if they were new. The nurse may feel that the sessions were unsuccessful. In reality, clients are unconsciously attempting to prolong the relationship and avoid its ending. Nurses should avoid addressing these problems. Instead, they should reassure clients that they already covered those issues and learned methods to control them. They should explain that the client may be feeling anxious about the relationship ending and redirect the client to newly found skills and abilities in forming new relationships, including support groups and social groups. The final meeting should focus on the future (see Box 9-8). The nurse can reassure the client that the nurse will remember him or her, but the nurse should not agree to see the client outside the relationship. Many clients who have difficulty establishing relationships may similarly have difficulty letting go of supportive relationships. The ending of the therapeutic relationship is a significant opportunity for client learning, including the opportunity for a healthy

---

BOX 9.8

Therapeutic Dialogue: **The Last Meeting**

INEFFECTIVE APPROACH

Nurse: Today is my last day.

Client: I need to talk to you about something important.

Nurse: What is it?

Client: I have been hearing voices again.

Nurse: Oh, how often?

Client: Every night. You are the only one I'm going to tell.

Nurse: I think you should tell the new nurse.

Client: She is too new. She won't understand. I feel so bad about your leaving. Is there any way you can stay?

Nurse: Well, I could check on you tomorrow.

Client: Oh, would you? I would really appreciate it if you would give me your new telephone number.

Nurse: I don't know what the number will be, but it will be listed in the telephone book.

EFFECTIVE APPROACH

Nurse: Today is my last day.

Client: I need to talk to you about something important.

Nurse: We talked about that. Anything "important" needs to be shared with the new nurse.

Client: But, I want to tell you.

Nurse: Saying good-bye can be very hard.

Client: I will miss you.

Nurse: Your feelings are very normal when relationships are ending. I will remember you in a very special way.

Client: Can I please have your telephone number?

Nurse: No, I can't give that to you. It is important that we say good-bye today.

Client: OK. Good-bye. Good luck.

Nurse: Good-bye.

CRITICAL THINKING CHALLENGE

• What were some of the mistakes the nurse in the first scenario made?

• In the second scenario, how does therapeutic communication in the termination phase differ from effective communication in the working phase?

good-bye. The nurse needs to plan for and to support this learning.

NONTHERAPEUTIC RELATIONSHIPS

Although it is hoped that all nurse–client relationships will go through the phases described in the previous section, this is not always the case. Nontherapeutic relationships also go through predictable phases (Forchuk et al., 2000). These relationships also start in the orientation phase. However, trust is not established, and the relationship moves to a *phase of grappling and struggling*. The nurse and client both feel very frustrated and keep varying their approach with each other in an attempt to establish a meaningful relationship. This is different from a prolonged orientation phase in that the efforts are not sustained; they vary constantly. The nurse may try longer meetings, shorter meetings, being more or less directive, and varying the therapeutic stance from warm and friendly to aloof. Clients in this phase may try to talk about the past but then change to discussions of the here and now. They may try talking about their family and in the next meeting talk about their work goals. Both the client and the nurse grapple and struggle to come to a common ground, and both become increasingly frustrated with each other. Eventually, the frustration becomes so great that the pair gives up on each other and moves to a *phase of mutual withdrawal*. The nurse may schedule seeing this client at the end of the shift and "run out of time" so that the meeting never happens. The client will leave the unit or otherwise be unavailable during scheduled meeting times. If a meeting does occur, the nurse will try to keep it short. "What's the point—we just cover the same old ground anyway." The client will attempt to keep it superficial and stay on safe topics. "You can always ask about your medications—nurses love to health teach, you know." Obviously, no therapeutic progress can be made in such a relationship. The nurse may be hesitant to ask for a therapeutic transfer, assuming that a relationship would similarly fail with another nurse. However, each relationship is unique, and difficulties in one relationship do not predict difficulties in the next. Clinical supervision early on may assist the development of the relationship, but often a therapeutic transfer to another nurse is required.

SUMMARY OF KEY POINTS

◻ To deal therapeutically with the emotions, feelings, and problems of clients, nurses must understand their own cultural values and beliefs and interpersonal strengths and limitations.

◻ The nurse–client relationship is built on therapeutic communication, including verbal and nonverbal interactions between the nurse and the client. Some communication skills include active listening, positive body language, appropriate verbal responses, and the ability of the nurse to interpret appropriately and analyze the client's verbal and nonverbal behaviours.

◻ Two of the most important communication concepts are empathy and rapport.

◻ In the nurse–client relationship, as in all types of relationships, certain physical, psychological, social, and spiritual boundaries and limitations need to be observed.

◻ The therapeutic nurse–client relationship consists of three major and overlapping stages or phases: the orientation phase, in which the client and nurse meet and establish the parameters of the relationship; the working phase, in which the client identifies and explores problems; and the resolution phase, in which the client learns to manage the problems and the relationship is terminated.

◻ The nontherapeutic relationship also consists of three major and overlapping phases: the orientation phase, the grappling and struggling phase, and the phase of mutual withdrawal.

CRITICAL THINKING CHALLENGES

1 Describe how you would communicate with a client who is concerned that a psychiatric diagnosis will negatively affect his or her social and work relationships.

2 Your client does not seem inclined to talk about his or her illness. Describe the measures you would take to initiate a therapeutic relationship with him or her. Who chooses the content to be discussed?

3 Your client does not appear for the last scheduled meeting. What will you do?

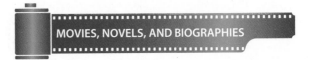

MOVIES, NOVELS, AND BIOGRAPHIES

In Treatment: 2008. This American television show is about a Washington-based psychotherapist, Paul Weston, played by Gabriel Byrne. We see him doing therapy with his clients Monday to Thursday, and on Friday, we get to watch his visit with his own therapist. [Being analyzed yourself is an expectation for psychoanalysts.]

VIEWING POINTS: What aspects of therapeutic relationships can you identify in Dr. Weston's session? Look for ways in which transference and countertransference are portrayed.

Analyze This: 1999. In this comedy, Billy Crystal plays psychiatrist Dr. Ben Sobel. His client is Paul Vitti (Robert De Niro), a mobster who is having panic attacks. Dr. Sobel is intimidated into seeing his new client at all hours and places and into accepting expensive (stolen?) gifts from him. Power issues become very interesting in this unusual therapeutic relationship.

VIEWING POINTS: The issue of therapeutic boundaries is a source of comedy in this film. What normal therapeutic boundaries are being violated? Whose needs are being met throughout the film? What would be appropriate if a client evoked personal unresolved issues for the therapist?

Good Will Hunting: 1997. Robin Williams plays a therapist to Will Hunting, a janitor identified as a mathematical genius, played by Matt Damon. Through a strong relationship, Will begins to realize his potential.

VIEWING POINTS: Watch closely how the relationship develops between the characters played by Williams and Damon. How does the relationship change as the characters move through different stages of their relationship?

REFERENCES

American Psychiatric Association. (2000). *Diagnostic and statistical manual of mental disorders* (4th ed., Text Revision). Washington, DC: Author.

Austin, W., Bergum, V., Nuttgens, S., & Peternelj-Taylor, C. (2006). A re-visioning of boundaries in professional helping relationships: Exploring other metaphors. *Ethics & Behavior, 16*(2), 77–94.

Boyd, M. (1995). Communication with clients, families, healthcare providers, and diverse cultures. In M. Strader & P. Decker (Eds.), *Role transition to client care management* (p. 431). Norwalk, CT: Appleton & Lange.

Campbell, R. J., Yonge, O., & Austin, W. (2005). Intimacy boundaries between mental health nurses and psychiatric patients. *Journal of Psychosocial Nursing and Mental Health Services, 43*(5), 33–41.

College of Nurses of Ontario. (2006). *Practice standard: Therapeutic nurse-client relationship* (Rev. ed.). Toronto, ON: Author.

Forchuk, C., Carmichael, C., Golea, G., Johnston, N., Martin, M. L., Patterson, P., et al. (2006). *Nursing best practice guideline: Establishing therapeutic relationships* (Rev. ed.). Toronto, ON: Registered Nurses Association of Ontario.

Forchuk, C., Martin, M. L., Chan, Y-C., & Jensen, E. (2005). Therapeutic relationships: From psychiatric hospital to community. *Journal of Psychiatric and Mental Health Nursing, 12*, 556–564.

Forchuk, C., Westwell, J., Martin, M. L., Bamber-Azzapardi, W., Kosterewa-Tolman, D., & Hux, M. (2000). The developing nurse–client relationship: Nurses = perspectives. *Journal of the American Psychiatric Nurses Association, 6*(1), 3–10.

Gallop, R., Choiniere, J., Forchuk, C., Golea, G., Jonston, N., Levac, A. M., et al. (2002). *Nursing best practice guideline: Establishing therapeutic relationships*. Toronto, ON: Registered Nurses Association of Ontario.

Hall, E. T. (1990). *The hidden dimension*, New York, NY: Anchor Books.

Peplau, H. E. (1952/1988 reissued). *Interpersonal relations in nursing*. London, UK: MacMillan.

CHAPTER 10

Biological Foundations of Psychiatric and Mental Health Nursing Practice

Anne Marie Creamer

Adapted from the chapter "The Biologic Foundations of Psychiatric Nursing" by Susan McCabe and Mary Ann Boyd

KEY CONCEPTS

- neurotransmitters
- plasticity

LEARNING OBJECTIVES

After studying this chapter, you will be able to:

- Describe the association between biologic functioning and symptoms of psychiatric disorders.
- Describe the approaches researchers have used to study the central nervous system and the significance of each approach.
- Locate the brain structures primarily involved in psychiatric disorders and describe the primary functions of these structures.
- Assess symptoms of common psychiatric disorders in terms of central nervous system functioning.
- Describe the mechanisms of neuronal transmission.
- Identify the location and function of neurotransmitters significant to hypotheses regarding major mental disorders.
- Discuss the basic utilization of new knowledge gained from fields of study, including psychoendocrinology, psychoimmunology, and chronobiology.
- Discuss the role of genetics in the development of psychiatric disorders.

KEY TERMS

- amino acids • animal model • autonomic nervous system • basal ganglia
- biogenic amines • biologic markers • chronobiology • circadian cycle • cortex
- frontal, parietal, temporal, and occipital lobes • genome • hippocampus
- limbic system • neurohormones • neuropeptides • psychoendocrinology
- psychoimmunology • receptors • risk factors • symptom expression
- synapse • zeitgebers

All behaviours recognized as human result from actions that originate in the brain and its amazing interconnection of neural networks. Modern research has increased understanding of how the complex circuitry of the brain interacts with the external environment, memories, and experiences. Through the spinal column and peripheral nerves, along with other systems, such as the endocrine and immune systems, the brain constantly receives and processes information. As the brain shifts and sorts through the amazing amount of information it processes every hour, it decides on actions and initiates behaviours that allow each person to act in entirely unique and very human ways.

Foundational Concepts

This chapter is a review of the basic information necessary for understanding neuroscience as it relates to the role of the psychiatric and mental health (PMH) nurse. The review includes basic central nervous system (CNS) structures and functions, basic mechanisms of neurotransmission, general functions of the major neurotransmitters, basic structure and function of the endocrine system, genetic research, circadian rhythms, neuroimaging techniques, and biologic tests. This chapter was written with the assumption that the reader has a basic knowledge of human biology, anatomy, and pathophysiology. The chapter is not intended as a full presentation of neuroanatomy and physiology but rather as an overview of the structures and functions most critical to the role of the PMH nurse.

■■■ THE BIOLOGIC BASIS OF BEHAVIOUR

As our understanding of the brain grows, evidence accumulates that most human behaviours have a biologic basis. Whether it is responding angrily to someone, impulsively making a purchase, or struggling to make a decision, behaviours are in large part rooted in the neurocircuitry of the brain. So when common psychiatric symptoms manifest as abnormal behaviours (e.g., seeing things that are not there, attempting suicide, talking in odd or unusual ways), we look to the brain. **Symptom expression** is a term referring to the behavioural symptoms seen in mental illness and the link to the neurobiologic basis of the symptom. Because symptoms of psychiatric illness are expressed mainly as behavioural disturbance and because behavioural symptoms are linked to anomalies in brain functioning, PMH nurses need to understand disease symptoms in relation to brain function.

Just as a breathing problem is often a symptom of a respiratory disorder, psychiatric symptoms are often indicators of CNS problems. Understanding this fundamental concept makes it much easier to understand the scientific rationale for many of the nursing care and treatment decisions presented in this book.

As you read this chapter, think about what you know about the symptoms of mental illness. PMH nurses must be able to make the connection among (1) patients' psychiatric symptoms, (2) the probable alterations in brain functioning linked to those symptoms, and (3) the rationale

---

IN A LIFE

King George III (1739–1820)

Bipolar Illness Misdiagnosed

Public Persona

Crowned King of England at age 22, George III headed the most influential colonial power in the world at that time. England thrived in the peacetime after the Seven Years' War with France but simultaneously taxed its American colonies so heavily and resolutely that the colonies rebelled. Could the American Revolution be blamed on King George III's state of mind?

Personal Realities

At age 50, the king first experienced abdominal pain and constipation, followed by weak limbs, fever, tachycardia, hoarseness, and dark red urine. Later, he experienced confusion, racing thoughts, visual problems, restlessness, delirium, convulsions, and stupor. His strange behaviour included ripping off his wig and running about naked. Although he recovered and did not have a relapse for 13 years, he was considered to be mad. Relapses after the first relapse became more frequent, and the king was eventually dethroned by the Prince of Wales. It was believed that King George III suffered bipolar disorder.

However, was George's madness in reality a genetically transmitted blood disease that caused thought disturbances, delirium, and stupor? The genetic disease porphyria is caused by defects in the body's ability to make haem. The diseases are generally inherited in an autosomal dominant fashion. The retrospective diagnosis was not made until 1966 (Macalpine & Hunter, 1966).

Other members of the royal family who suffered from this hereditary disease were Queen Anne of Great Britain; Frederic the Great of Germany; George IV of Great Britain (son of George III); and George IV's daughter, Princess Charlotte, who died during childbirth from complications of the disease. After Charlotte's death, Victoria became Queen.

Macalpine, I., & Hunter, R. (1966). The insanity of King George 3d: A classic case of porphyria. *British Medical Journal, 5479*(1), 65–71.

---

for treatment and care practices. Knowledge of the CNS is an inescapable aspect of modern PMH nursing.

Animal Modelling

How do scientists come to know about the workings of the brain? Animal modelling is the most common research method for studying the CNS. It involves using nonhuman organisms (animals such as rats and mice) to study biologic processes and how certain diseases affect those processes. **Animal models** resemble humans in anatomical structure, function, and genetics, allowing for research and learning that would not be possible to do with humans. Using animals, scientists can induce disease that occurs in humans and test treatments before attempting to treat humans who have that disease. Common examples of using animals to study human illness include studying cancer in mice, studying tissue reactions to transplanted cells in pigs, and analyzing DNA from a fly to study the genetic links of a disease. Animal models allow researchers to examine diseases such as high blood pressure, Parkinson's, depression, and Alzheimer's, as well as the neurobiology of normal behaviours, such as eating, mating, and learning. Researchers can then use the animal model to study what controls a behaviour or the way a disease progresses and how symptom expression occurs. Animal models are increasingly being used to explore psychiatric illnesses, such as schizophrenia, bipolar disorder, and anxiety disorders, and to expand our knowledge of the illnesses, including the genetic basis for common psychiatric disorders. Every drug used to treat psychiatric disorders was first researched and tested in animal models. However, it should be noted that the use of animals for medical research is a subject of ethical debate, focused especially around concepts such as the moral status of humans and animals and the underlying assumptions made about animal research (Hale, 2008; Walker, 2006).

Genetics

Family members of individuals who have one of the major mental disorders, such as schizophrenia, bipolar disorder, or panic disorder, have an increased risk for the same disorder. Animal models have greatly increased the ability of researchers to understand the influence of genetics on symptom expression in psychiatric disorders, and many of the common psychiatric disorders that nurses encounter have a known genetic component. As genetic knowledge increases, treatments that work at the genetic level are rapidly being developed (Kendler & Greenspan, 2006).

Genetic *processes* control how humans develop from a single-cell egg into an adult human. Genes control the regrowth of hair and skin cells, the growth and connection of nervous system cells, and our biologic reaction to stress, among other processes. Genes make humans dynamic organisms, capable of growth, change, and development. The Human Genome Project, which started in 1990, mapped the complete set of human genes, or **genome**, carried by all of us and transmitted to our offsprings. There are about 30,000 genes in the human genome, with the brain accounting for only about 1% of the body's DNA. The completed human genome provided researchers with a road map of the exact sequence of the 3 billion nucleotide bases that make up human organisms. If printed out, the entire human genome sequence would fill one thousand 1,000-page telephone books. Now that it is completed, the genome map can be used for studying the function of each gene and the disease-inducing capacity of those genes when they malfunction.

A gene comprises short segments of DNA and is packed with the instructions for making proteins that have a specific function. When genes are absent or malfunction, protein production is altered, and bodily functions are disrupted. In this fashion, genes play a role in cancer, heart disease, diabetes, and many psychiatric disorders. For example, recent research has demonstrated that approximately 1% of individuals with schizophrenia have 22q11.2 deletion syndrome, a genetic subtype of schizophrenia in which there is a deletion on part of chromosome 22. In most newly diagnosed cases of this syndrome, the patient has the genetic mutation while the parents are unaffected (Kapadia & Bassett, 2008).

Gene expression is the result of the genes' direction or the production of these proteins. It is not a static condition fixed at some point in neuronal development. Individual nerve cells may respond to neurochemical changes outside the cell, producing different proteins for adaptation to the new environment. This dynamic nature of gene function highlights the manner in which the body and the environment interact and how environmental factors influence gene expression.

Population Genetics

The study of molecular genetics in psychiatric disorders is in its infancy. Because the exact genetic basis of psychiatric disorder remains unclear and animal models are hard to produce for some disorders, much of what we know about the genetics of psychiatric disorders comes from studies that trace given disorders within groups of people. This technique, called *population genetics*, involves the analysis of genetic transmission of a trait within families and populations to determine risks and patterns of transmission. The risk for a given disorder occurring in the general population can then be compared with the risk within families and between groups of relatives. These studies rely on the initial identification of an individual who has the disorder and include the following principal methods:

- Family studies, which analyze the occurrence of a disorder in first-degree relatives (biologic parents, siblings, and children), second-degree relatives (grandparents, uncles, aunts, nieces, nephews, and grandchildren), and so on.
- Twin studies, which analyze the presence or absence of the disorder in pairs of twins. The *concordance rate* is the measure of similarity of occurrence in individuals with similar genetic makeup.
- Adoption studies, which compare the risk for the illness developing in offsprings raised in different environments. The strongest inferences may be drawn from studies that involve children separated from their parents at birth.

Few traits are completely heritable. Colour blindness and blood type are examples of traits that exist because of heredity alone. Monozygotic twins have identical genetic contributions; therefore, both would have colour blindness or the same blood type if they expressed that gene.

This is 100% concordance. If a disorder were completely unrelated to genetics, then monozygotic twins would have the same concordance rates as dizygotic (fraternal) twins, who share roughly the same proportion of genes that ordinary siblings do—50%. If there is a genetic contribution with environmental influence, the concordance rates would be less than 100% for monozygotic twins but significantly greater than for dizygotic twins. Such is the case with several psychiatric disorders. Although no conclusive evidence exists for a complete genetic cause of most psychiatric disorders, significant evidence suggests that strong genetic contributions exist for most (Green et al., 2003; Harrison & Owen, 2003; Lea, 2000; McGuffin et al., 2003; Merikangas & Avenevoli, 2000). It is likely that psychiatric disorders are *polygenic*. This means that more than one gene is involved in producing a psychiatric disorder and that the disorder develops from genes interacting, which produces a risk factor, and environmental influences that lead to the expression of the illness. The environmental factors may include stress, infections, poor nutrition, catastrophic loss, complications during pregnancy, and exposure to toxins, for example. Thus, genetic compositions convey vulnerability, or a risk for the illness, but the right set of environmental factors must be present for the disease to develop in the at-risk individual. Additionally, specific genes may convey risk for more than one disorder (Kendler & Greenspan, 2006).

When considering information regarding risks for genetic transmission of psychiatric disorders, it is important to remember several key points:

- Psychiatric disorders have been described and labelled quite differently across generations, and errors in diagnosis may occur.
- Similar psychiatric symptoms may have considerably different causes, just as symptoms such as chest pain may occur in relation to many different causes.
- Genes that are present may not always cause the appearance of the trait.
- Several genes work together in an individual to produce a given trait or disorder.
- A biologic cause is not necessarily solely genetic in origin. Environmental influences alter the body's functioning and often mediate or worsen genetic **risk factors**.

As public awareness of genetic evidence grows, it is likely that a PMH nurse will be faced with patients or family members requesting genetic testing or needing information regarding their likelihood of risk for a psychiatric disorder. As a result, PMH nurses increasingly will need greater understanding of the role genetics play in mental illness.

Risk Factors

The concept of genetic susceptibility suggests that an individual may be at increased risk for a psychiatric disorder. Research into *risk factors* is an important avenue of study. Just as knowledge of risk factors for diabetes and heart disease led to the development of preventive interventions, learning more about risk factors for psychiatric disorders will lead to preventive care practices. Specific risk factors for psychiatric disorders are just beginning to be understood, and some of the environmental influences listed previously may be examples of risk factors. These events, circumstances, or demographic features are more likely to occur in individuals who experience a particular psychiatric disorder. In the absence of one specific gene for major psychiatric disorders, risk factor assessment may be a logical alternative for predicting who is more likely than others to experience psychiatric disorders or certain conditions, such as aggression or suicidality. This is a growing area of psychiatric nursing.

Current Approaches and Technologic Advances

Neuroscience researchers have applied several approaches to the study of the CNS structure and function. These approaches occur with both human research and animal models. The approaches, highlighted in Table 10-1, include the following:

- Comparative
- Developmental
- Chemoarchitectural
- Cytoarchitectural
- Functional

These different approaches to studying the CNS have significantly increased our understanding of normal CNS functioning and how a disease affects behaviour and contributes to the development of psychiatric disorders. Research shows that areas of the brain, and the groups of nerve cells that constitute that area, often work together as functional units. A hierarchy of function exists in which primary sensory input is used in an increasingly more complex and integrated manner across areas of the brain. In addition, some areas of the brain, such as those that control basic levels of alertness and attention, must work correctly for information to be received, understood, and used by higher levels of the brain to organize a response. The brain's functional units work together to control or contribute to specific behaviours or emotions.

The *integrated approach* to brain development is the term used to describe the interactive working of brain areas and function. Understanding the work as an integration of parts allows us to understand that specific areas of the brain control specific functions. For example, there is a speech area in the brain, a mood area, an appetite area, and so on. Understanding the functions of areas of the brain

Table 10.1	Approaches to the Study of Neuroanatomy	
Approach	**Purpose**	**Potential Limitations**
Comparative	Explores and compares behaviour across animal nervous systems, from a simple primitive cordlike structure in some species to the large complex structure of the human brain	Difficult to correlate animal behaviour to human, especially emotional New brain structures do not necessarily correlate to new behaviour
Developmental	Studies nervous system structure within an individual or species of animal across different stages of development	Impossible to follow one human being's neuronal development Individual variation in development complicates comparisons of individuals across a specific point of time in development
Chemoarchitectural	Identifies differences in location of neurochemicals such as neurotransmitters throughout the brain	Boundaries between regional changes are subtle and may vary across individuals
Cytoarchitectural	Identifies differences or variations in cell type, structure, and density throughout the brain, mapping these variations by location	Boundaries between regional changes are subtle and may vary across individuals
Functional	Identifies location of predominant control over various behavioural functions within the brain Studies often conducted on the basis of dysfunction from a localized injury to the brain	Several regions or structures within the brain may contribute to one behaviour, making predominant control difficult to assign Controversy exists in correlating normal brain function to damaged brain tissue

allows nurses to assess a patient's symptoms as, in large part, an expression of a problem with a specific brain area. Just as a person with an irregular heart beat is experiencing disruption in normal cardiac function, a person who fails to eat because of depression is experiencing a disruption in the brain's normal appetite and mood function.

> **KEY CONCEPT** **Plasticity** is the ability of the brain to change its structure and function in response to internal and external pressures (Kleim & Jones, 2008).

Neuroplasticity is an increasingly important concept when describing brain function. The changes in neural environment can come from internal sources, such as a change in electrolytes, or from external sources, such as a virus or toxin. External pressures to the neural environment also include behavioural, sensory, and cognitive experiences. With neuroplasticity, nerve signals may be rerouted, cells may learn new functions, sensitivity or number of cells may increase or decrease, or some nerve tissue may be regenerated in a limited way. Brains are most plastic during infancy and young childhood, when large adaptive learning tasks should normally occur. With age, brains become less plastic, which explains why it is easier to learn a second language at the age of 5 years than 55 years. Neuroplasticity contributes to understanding how function may be restored over time after brain damage occurs or how an individual may react over time to continuous pharmacotherapy regimens.

NEUROIMAGING

Since the 1980s, technologic advances in neuroimaging techniques have been a major aid to the current understanding of how the human brain functions. As knowledge grows, neuroimaging techniques are moving from research to routine clinical use, requiring PMH nurses to understand this technology. Two basic neuroimaging methods are structural and functional neuroimaging.

Structural Neuroimaging

Structural neuroimaging techniques were the first form of neuroimaging that allowed visualization of brain structures. Structural images show what normal structures of the brain look like and allow clinicians to identify tissue abnormalities, changes, or damage. Commonly used structural neuroimaging techniques include computed axial tomography (CT) scanning and magnetic resonance imaging (MRI). Although these techniques are useful in identifying what the brain looks like, they do not reveal anything about how the brain works.

Computed Axial Tomography

CT scanning first allowed scientists and clinicians to see structures inside the brain without more invasive and potentially dangerous methods. CT scans still use an x-ray beam passed through the head in serial slices. High-speed computers measure the decreased strength in the x-ray beam that results from absorption, and the computer assigns a shade of gray that reflects that change. The degree of energy absorbed by a tissue is proportionally related to its density. For example, cerebrospinal fluid (CSF) decreases the least, so it appears the darkest, whereas bone absorbs the most and appears light. White matter and gray matter are more difficult to discriminate with CT technology.

CT scans can be done with or without contrast material. Contrast materials are used to increase the visibility of certain tissues or blood vessels. If a contrast agent is used, an iodinated or other material is intravenously administered to enhance the CT image. Although CT scanning is a relatively safe, noninvasive procedure, the contrast material may have some adverse effects in some patients. Some patients receiving contrast materials report a metallic taste in the mouth, and some experience mild nausea, rashes, or joint pain. In rare instances, severe allergic responses, including anaphylaxis, may develop, so nurses must closely monitor patients who have received contrast materials. In addition, because the CT equipment itself may frighten the patient, the nurse should educate the patient about the scan. Some patients may need to be accompanied by a nurse during the procedure for ongoing reassurance.

Magnetic Resonance Imaging

MRI is performed by placing a patient into a long tube that contains powerful magnets. The magnetic field causes hydrogen-containing molecules (primarily water) to line up and move in symmetric ways around their axes. The magnetic field is then interrupted in pulses, causing the molecules to turn 90 or 180 degrees. Electromagnetic energy is released when the molecules return to their original position. The energy released is related to the density of the tissue and is detected by the MRI device, resulting in a scan measurement of the density of the examined tissue. The CT scan is limited to one-dimensional images, but the MRI can produce three-dimensional images extremely clearly, allowing for discrimination of white and gray matters and other subtle changes in the tissue.

MRI scans produce more information than CT images, but MRI scans also are more complicated and costly. In addition, MRI scans cannot be used for all patients. Because MRI uses magnet energy, individuals with pacemakers, metal plates, bone replacements, aneurysm clips, or other metal in their body cannot undergo the procedure; pregnant women also cannot have MRI scans. The loud noise of the equipment and the very narrow tube in which the patient must lie still can trigger claustrophobic responses in some people. Adequate preparation of the patient by the nurse should eliminate any surprises. Assistance with shallow breathing techniques, mental

distractions, or other anxiety-reducing strategies may help. Many MRI facilities are equipped with music to mask the whirring of the equipment and provide a distraction through the long testing period. Some tubes are now being made of clear plastic to decrease the claustrophobic sensation.

Functional Neuroimaging

Although structural imaging identifies what the brain looks like, the scans do not show how the brain is working. Functional neuroimaging techniques measure physiologic activities, providing insight into how the brain works. These methods let researchers study such activities as cerebral blood flow, neuroreceptor location and function, and distribution patterns of specific chemicals within the brain. Single photon emission computed tomography (SPECT) and positron emission tomography (PET) are the primary methods used to observe metabolic functioning. Both procedures require administering radioactive substances that emit charged particles, which are then measured by scanning equipment. Because these procedures measure function, the patient is usually asked to perform specific tasks during the test. The Wisconsin Card Sorting Test (WCST), which is commonly used, requires the individual to sort cards with different numbers, colours, and shapes into piles based on specified rules. This task requires the use of the brain's frontal lobe, an important area for concept formation and decision making and an area that often is disrupted in many psychiatric disorders. Figure 10-1 illustrates the differences between the frontal lobe activity of a pair of twins, one with schizophrenia and one without.

Single Photon Emission Computed Tomography

SPECT is helpful in measuring regional cerebral blood flow. Evidence documents the use of SPECT scans in differentiating depression from dementia (Cho et al., 2002). Well documented in Alzheimer's disease (Vercelletto et al., 2002), decreased cerebral blood flow in specific areas of the brain is not found in depression. SPECT scans are also used to confirm changes in cerebral blood flow caused by certain drugs. For example, caffeine and nicotine cause a generalized decrease in cerebral blood flow. New compounds have been developed recently to visualize the numbers or density of **receptors** in various areas of the brain, which may assist in understanding the effects of psychopharmacologic medications and neuroplastic changes in brain tissue over time.

Positron Emission Tomography

PET measures glucose consumption in various brain regions. Because cells use glucose as fuel for cellular

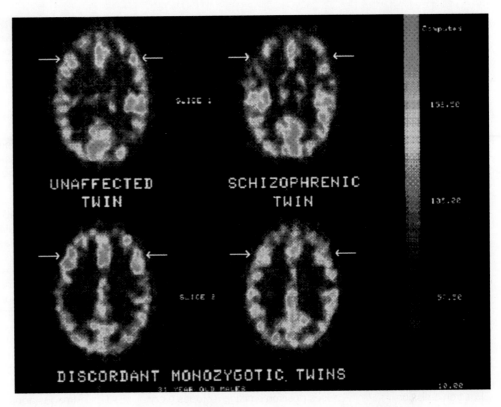

FIGURE 10.1 Differences in the frontal lobe activity of a pair of twins, one with the mental disorder of schizophrenia and one who does not have the disorder. Figure courtesy of Dr. K. F. Berman and Dr. D. R. Weinberger, Clinical Brain Disorders Branch, National Institute of Mental Health.

action, the higher the rate of glucose use detected by the PET scan, the higher the rate of metabolic activity in different areas of the brain. Abnormalities in glucose consumption, indicating more or less cellular activity, are found in Alzheimer's disease, seizures, strokes, tumours, and a number of psychiatric disorders. Scanning may be performed while the individual is at rest or performing a cognitive task. PET scans are often used to measure regional cerebral blood flow and neurotransmitter system functions.

Bridging the Structure-Function Gap

As structural and functional neuroimaging techniques advance, attempts are being made to develop imaging procedures that detail structure and function at the same time. Magnetic resonance spectroscopy (MRS) and functional magnetic resonance imaging (fMRI) are examples. The fMRI is useful for showing structure while localizing function and providing clear, high-resolution images. Like other forms of neuroimaging, the fMRI is noninvasive, but it requires no radioactive agent, making it economical and safer than PET and SPECT (Hennig, Speck, Koch, & Weiller, 2003).

MRS uses the same machinery as fMRI and provides precise and clear images of neuronal membranes as well as measures of metabolic cellular function (Heerschap, Kok, & Van De, 2003). In addition to these procedures, electromagnet encephalography (EEG/MEG) is being

used. This procedure combines traditional EEG measurement (discussed later in this chapter) with imaging to visualize cellular electrical activity in the brain. Table 10-2 summarizes these neuroimaging methods. Although these neuroimaging procedures are used primarily as research tools, they also are becoming useful in clinical practice.

Neuroanatomy of the Central Nervous System

With advances in brain science comes greater understanding of the biologic basis of mental illnesses. Therefore, PMH nurses must increasingly be aware of the anatomic intricacy of the CNS as a foundation for modern psychiatric nursing assessments and interventions.

Although this section discusses each functioning area of the brain separately, each area is intricately connected with the others, and each functions interactively. The CNS contains the brain, brain stem, and spinal cord, whereas the total human nervous system includes the peripheral nervous system (PNS) as well. The PNS consists of the neurons that connect the CNS to the muscles, organs, and other systems in the periphery of the body. Whatever affects the CNS may also affect the PNS, and vice versa.

Table 10.2	Methods of Neuroimaging	
Method	**Description**	**Considerations**
Structural Imaging		
Computed tomography (CT), also called computed axial tomography (CAT)	Uses x-ray technology to measure tissue density; is readily available; can be completed quickly, and less costly; may be used for screening, but many disease states are not clearly seen; use of contrast medium improves resolution	Contrast medium may produce allergic reactions; individuals with increased risk for contrast media complications include those with History of previous reactions Cardiac disease Hypertension Diabetes Sickle cell disease Contraindications for use of contrast: Iodine/shellfish allergies Renal disease Pregnancy
Magnetic resonance imaging (MRI)	Uses a magnetic field to magnetize hydrogen atoms in soft tissue, changing their alignment—this creates a tiny electric signal, which can be received to produce an image; produces greater resolution than a CT, diagnosing more subtle pathologic changes	Patients may experience headaches, dizziness, and nausea; symptoms of anxiety, claustrophobia, or psychosis can increase; contraindicated when patients have aneurysm clips, internal electrical, magnetic, or mechanical devices such as pacemakers, metallic surgical clips, sutures, or dental work, which distort the image; claustrophobia
Functional Neuroimaging		
Positron emission tomography (PET)	Uses positron emitting isotopes (very short-lived radioactive entities such as oxygen-15) to image brain functioning; isotopes are incorporated into specific molecules to study cerebral metabolism, cerebral blood flow, and specific neurochemicals	Images appear blurry, lacking anatomic detail, but have been extremely useful in research to study distribution of neuroreceptors and the action of pharmacologic agents; invasive procedure, use of radioactivity limits the number of scans done with a single individual
Single photon emission computed tomography (SPECT)	Like PET, SPECT uses radioisotopes that produce only one photon; data are collected as a three-dimensional volume, and two-dimensional images can be constructed on any plane; cheaper than PET technology	Less resolution and sensitivity than the PET, but inhalation methods may be used, allowing for some repeated studies; useful in drug dependency research
Functional magnetic resonance imaging (fMRI)	Combines spatial resolution of MRI with the ability to image neural activity; is able to show sequential, movie-type images of blood flow in the brain as it is happening; shows whether brain activity occurs simultaneously or sequentially in different areas of the brain while engaged in selected activities	Requires no radiation and can be completely noninvasive; individual can be imaged many times, in different clinical states, before or after treatments; removes many of the ethical constraints when studying children and adolescents with psychiatric disorders
Magnetic resonance spectroscopy (MRS)	Uses the same imaging equipment of the fMRI; by altering scanning parameters, signals represent specific chemicals in the brain	Noninvasive, repeatable, may be ideal for longitudinal studies, but has limited spatial resolution, especially with molecules that occur in low concentrations

■ CEREBRUM

The largest part of the human brain, the cerebrum, fills the entire upper portion of the cranium. The **cortex**, or outermost surface of the cerebrum, makes up about 80% of the human brain. The cortex is several millimeters thick and is composed of cell bodies mixed with capillary blood vessels. This mixture makes the cortex grey brown, thus the term *grey matter*. The cortex contains a number of bumps and grooves in a fully developed adult brain, as

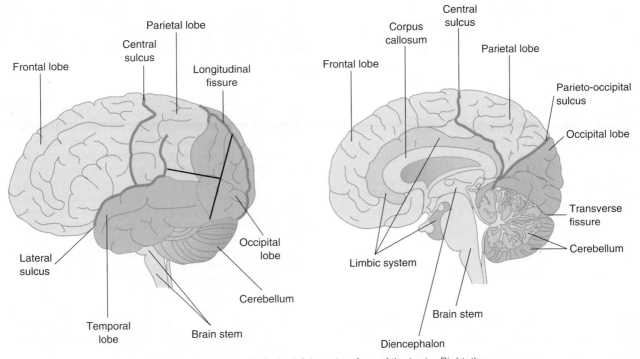

FIGURE 10.2 Lateral and medial surfaces of the brain. *Left*: the left lateral surface of the brain. *Right*: the medial surface of the right half of a sagittally hemisected brain.

shown in Figure 10-2. This "wrinkling" allows for a large amount of surface area to be confined in the limited space of the skull. The increased surface area allows for more potential connections between cells within the cortex. The grooves are called *fissures* if they extend deep into the brain and *sulci* if they are shallower. The bumps or convolutions are called *gyri*. Together, they provide many of the landmarks for the subdivisions of the cortex. The longest and deepest groove, the longitudinal fissure, separates the cerebrum into left and right hemispheres. Although these two divisions are nearly symmetric, there is some variation in the location and size of the sulci and gyri in each hemisphere. Substantial variation in these convolutions is found in the cortex of different individuals.

Left and Right Hemispheres

The cerebrum can be roughly divided into two halves, or hemispheres. Each hemisphere controls functioning mainly on the opposite side of the body. For about 95% of people, the left hemisphere is dominant, whereas about 5% of individuals have mixed dominance. The right hemisphere provides input into receptive nonverbal communication, spatial orientation, and recognition; intonation of speech and aspects of music; facial recognition and facial expression of emotion; and nonverbal learning and memory. In general, the left hemisphere is more involved with verbal language function, including areas for both receptive and expressive speech control. In addition, the left hemisphere provides strong contributions to temporal order and sequencing, numeric symbols, and verbal learning and memory. However, it is important to note that the intact brain may not be neatly organized with one side being the dominant because the degree of lateralization differs across individuals (Papousek & Schulter, 2006).

The two hemispheres are connected by the corpus callosum, a bundle of neuronal tissue that allows information to be exchanged quickly between the right and left hemispheres. An intact corpus callosum is required for the hemispheres to function in a smooth and coordinated manner.

Lobes of the Brain

The lateral surface of each hemisphere is further divided into four lobes: the **frontal**, **parietal**, **temporal**, **and occipital lobes** (Fig. 10-3). The lobes work in coordinated ways, but each is responsible for specific functions. Knowledge of these unique functions is helpful for understanding how damage to these areas produces the symptoms of mental illness and how medications that affect the functioning of these lobes can produce certain effects.

Frontal Lobes

The right and left frontal lobes make up about one fourth of the entire cerebral cortex and are proportionately larger in humans than in any other mammal. The precentral

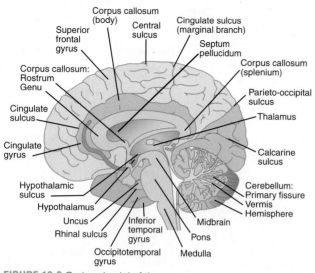

FIGURE 10.3 Gyri and sulci of the cortex.

Frontal Lobe Syndrome

In the 1860s, Phineas Gage became a famous example of frontal lobe dysfunction. Mr. Gage was a New England railroad worker who had a thick iron-tamping rod propelled through his frontal lobes by an explosion. He survived, but suffered significant changes in his personality. Mr. Gage, who had previously been a capable and calm supervisor, began to show impatience, labile mood, disrespect for others, and frequent use of profanity after his injury (Harlow, 1868). Similar conditions are often called *frontal lobe syndrome*. Symptoms vary widely from individual to individual. In general, after damage to the dorsolateral (upper and outer) areas of the frontal lobes, the symptoms include a lack of drive and spontaneity. With damage to the most anterior aspects of the frontal lobes, the symptoms tend to involve more changes in mood and affect, such as impulsive and inappropriate behaviour.

The rendering shows the route the tamping rod took through Phineas Gage's skull. The angle of entry of the rod shot it behind the left eye and through the front part of the brain, sparing regions that are directly concerned with vital functions like breathing and heartbeat.

gyrus, the gyrus immediately anterior to the central sulcus, contains the primary motor area, or homunculi. Damage to this gyrus, or to the anterior neighbouring gyri, causes spastic paralysis in the opposite side of the body. The frontal lobe also contains Broca's area, which controls the motor function of speech. Damage to Broca's area produces expressive aphasia, or difficulty with the motor movements of speech. The frontal lobes are also thought to contain the highest or most complex aspects of cortical functioning, which collectively make up a large part of what we call personality. Working memory is an important aspect of frontal lobe function, including the ability to plan and initiate activity with future goals in mind. Insight, judgment, reasoning, concept formation, problem-solving skills, abstraction, and self-evaluation are all abilities that are modulated and affected by the action of the frontal lobes. These skills are often referred to as *executive functions* because they modulate more primitive impulses through numerous connections to other areas of the cerebrum.

When normal frontal lobe functioning is altered, executive functioning is decreased, and modulation of impulses can be lost, leading to changes in mood and personality. The importance of the frontal lobe and its role in the development of symptoms common to psychiatric disorders are emphasized in later chapters that discuss disorders such as schizophrenia, attention-deficit hyperactivity disorder, and dementia. Box 10-1 describes how altered frontal lobe function can affect mood and personality.

Parietal Lobes

The postcentral gyrus, immediately behind the central sulcus, contains the primary somatosensory area (Fig. 10-3). Damage to this area and neighbouring gyri results in deficits in discriminative sensory function but not in the ability to perceive sensory input. The posterior areas of the parietal lobe appear to coordinate visual and somatosensory information. Damage to this area produces complex sensory deficits, including neglect of contralateral sensory stimuli and spatial relationships. The parietal lobes contribute to the ability to recognize objects by touch; calculate; write; recognize fingers of the opposite hands; draw; and organize spatial directions, such as how to travel to familiar places.

Temporal Lobes

The temporal lobes contain the primary auditory and olfactory areas. Wernicke's area, located at the posterior aspect of the superior temporal gyrus, is primarily responsible for receptive speech. The temporal lobes also integrate sensory and visual information involved in the control of written and verbal language skills, as well as visual recognition. The hippocampus, an important structure discussed in its own section later in this chapter, lies in the internal aspects of each temporal lobe and contributes to memory. Other internal structures of this lobe are involved in the modulation of mood and emotion.

Occipital Lobes

The primary visual area is located in the most posterior aspect of the occipital lobes. Damage to this area results in a condition called *cortical blindness*. In other words, the retina and optic nerve remain intact, but the individual cannot see. The occipital lobes are involved in many aspects of visual integration of information, including colour vision, object and facial recognition, and the ability to perceive objects in motion.

Association Cortex

Although not a lobe, the association cortex is an important area that allows the lobes to work in an integrated manner. Areas of one lobe of the cortex often share functions with an area of the adjacent lobe. When these neighbouring nerve fibers are related to the same sensory modality, they are often referred to as *association* areas. For example, an area in the inferior parietal, posterior temporal, and anterior occipital lobes integrates visual, somatosensory, and auditory information to provide the abilities required for basic academic skills. These areas, along with numerous connections beneath the cortex, are part of the mechanisms that allow the human brain to work as an integrated whole.

Subcortical Structures

Beneath the cortex are layers of tissue composed of the axons of cell bodies. The axonal tissue forms pathways that are surrounded by glia, a fatty or lipid substance, which has a white appearance and gives these layers of neuron axons their name—*white matter*. Structures inside the hemispheres, beneath the cortex, are considered subcortical. Many of these structures, essential in the regulation of emotions and behaviours, play important roles in our understanding of mental disorders. Figure 10-4 provides a coronal section view of the grey matter, white matter, and important subcortical structures.

Basal Ganglia

The **basal ganglia** are subcortical grey matter areas in both the right and left hemispheres that contain many cell bodies or nuclei. The basal ganglia are involved with motor functions and in association with both the learning and the programming of behaviours or activities that are repetitive and, done over time, become automatic. The basal ganglia have many connections with the cerebral

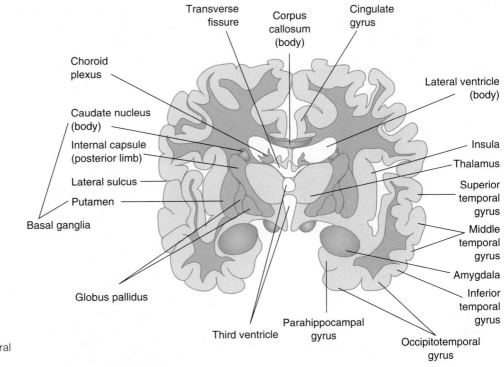

FIGURE 10.4 Coronal section of the brain, illustrating the corpus callosum, basal ganglia, and lateral ventricles.

cortex, thalamus, midbrain structures, and spinal cord. Damage to portions of these nuclei may produce changes in posture or muscle tone. In addition, damage may produce abnormal movements, such as twitches or tremors. The basal ganglia can be adversely affected by some of the medications used to treat psychiatric disorders, leading to side effects and other motor-related problems. The primary subdivisions of the basal ganglia are the putamen, globus pallidus, and caudate.

Limbic System

The **limbic system** is essential to understanding the many hypotheses related to psychiatric disorders and emotional behaviour in general. Basic emotions, needs, drives, and instinct begin and are modulated in the limbic system. Hate, love, anger, aggression, and caring are basic emotions that originate within the limbic system. Not only does the limbic system function as the seat of emotions, but also, because emotions are often generated based on our personal experiences, the limbic system is involved with aspects of memory. Hypothesized changes in the limbic system play a significant role in many theories of major mental disorders, including schizophrenia, depression, and anxiety disorders (discussed in later chapters). The limbic system is called a "system" because it comprises several small structures that work in a highly organized way. These structures include the hippocampus, thalamus, hypothalamus, amygdala, and limbic midbrain nuclei. See Figure 10-5 for identification and location of the structures within the limbic system and their relationship to other common CNS structures.

Hippocampus

The **hippocampus** is involved in storing information, especially the emotions attached to a memory. Our emotional response to memories and our association with other related memories are functions of how information

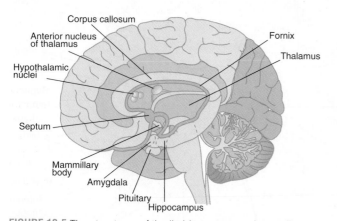

FIGURE 10.5 The structures of the limbic system are integrally involved in memory and emotional behaviour. Theories link changes in the limbic system to many major mental disorders, including schizophrenia, depression, and anxiety disorders.

is stored within the hippocampus. Although memory storage is not limited to one area of the brain, destruction of the left hippocampus impairs verbal memory, and damage to the right hippocampus results in difficulty with recognition and recall of complex visual and auditory patterns. Deterioration of the nerves of the hippocampus and other related temporal lobe structures found in Alzheimer's disease produces the disorder's hallmark symptoms of memory dysfunction.

Thalamus

The thalamus is composed of several distinct subnuclei, each with its own specialized connections to many regions in the cerebral cortex. Sometimes called the "relay-switching centre of the brain," the thalamus functions as a regulatory structure to relay all sensory information, except smell, sent to the CNS from the PNS. The thalamus relays and regulates by filtering incoming information and determining what to pass on or what not to pass on to the cortex. In this fashion, the thalamus prevents the cortex from becoming overloaded with sensory stimulus. The thalamus is thought to play a part in controlling electrical activity in the cortex. The thalamus is of special interest in schizophrenia because it may play a role in the development of several cognitive disturbances, such as memory tasks.

Hypothalamus

Basic human activities, such as sleep-rest patterns, body temperature, and physical drives (e.g., hunger and sex), are regulated by the hypothalamus, which rests deep within the brain. Dysfunction of this structure, whether from disorders or as a consequence of the adverse effects of drugs used to treat mental illness, produces common psychiatric symptoms, such as appetite and sleep problems.

Nerve cells within the hypothalamus secrete hormones: for example, antidiuretic hormone, which when sent to the kidneys, accelerates the reabsorption of water, and oxytocin, which acts on smooth muscles to promote contractions, particularly within the walls of the uterus. Because cells within the nervous system produce these hormones, they are often referred to as **neurohormones** and form a communication mechanism through the bloodstream to control organs that are not directly connected to nervous system structures.

Deregulation of the hypothalamus can be manifested in symptoms of certain psychiatric disorders. For example, patients with schizophrenia often wear heavy coats during the hot summer months and do not appear hot. Before the role of the hypothalamus in schizophrenia was understood, psychological reasons were used to explain such symptoms. It is increasingly clear that such a symptom relates to deregulation of the hypothalamus's normal role in temperature regulation and is biologically based (Shiloh et al., 2001).

Pituitary

The pituitary gland, often called the *master gland*, has two distinct parts, the anterior pituitary and the posterior pituitary. Located just below the hypothalamus, the anterior pituitary consists of glandular epithelial tissue and is connected to the hypothalamus by a vascular link. In contrast, the posterior pituitary is composed of neural tissue and is connected to the hypothalamus by a neural pathway. When stimulated, the posterior pituitary releases oxytocin or vasopressin, two small peptide hormones that are produced in the hypothalamus. The anterior pituitary produces and releases six different hormones—growth hormone (GH), thyroid-stimulating hormone (TSH), adrenocorticotropin hormone (ACTH), follicle-stimulating hormone (FSH), luteinizing hormone (LH), and prolactin—when stimulated by a corresponding hormone from the hypothalamus (e.g., corticotrophin-releasing hormone stimulates secretion of ACTH). Together with the pituitary gland, the hypothalamus functions as one of the primary regulators of many aspects of the endocrine system. Its functions are involved in the control of visceral activities, such as body temperature, arterial blood pressure, hunger, thirst, fluid balance, gastric motility, and gastric secretions.

Of note, increased release of prolactin can result from blockade of naturally occurring dopamine by various medications including antipsychotics, antidepressants, opiates, and cocaine (Molitch, 2005). This can result in galactorrhea, menstrual irregularities in women, erectile dysfunction in men, and loss of libido and infertility in both men and women.

Amygdala

The amygdala is directly connected to more primitive centres of the brain involving the sense of smell. It has numerous connections to the hypothalamus and lies adjacent to the hippocampus. The amygdala provides an emotional component to memory and is involved in modulating aggression and sexuality. Impulsive acts of aggression and violence have been linked to dysregulation of the amygdala, and erratic firing of the nerve cells in the amygdala is a focus of investigation in bipolar mood disorders (see Chapter 20). The amygdala is also part of the brain most affected by psychoactive drugs.

Limbic Midbrain Nuclei

The limbic midbrain nuclei are a collection of neurons (including the ventral tegmental area and the locus caeruleus) that appear to play a role in the biologic basis of addiction. Sometimes referred to as the pleasure centre or reward centre of the brain, the limbic midbrain nuclei function to reinforce chemically certain behaviours, ensuring their repetition. Emotions such as feeling satisfied with good food, the pleasure of nurturing, and the enjoyment of sexual activity originate in the limbic midbrain nuclei. The reinforcement of activities such as nutrition, procreation, and nurturing young are all primitive aspects of ensuring the survival of a species. When functioning in abnormal ways, the limbic midbrain nuclei can begin to reinforce unhealthy or risky behaviours, such as drug abuse. Exploration of this area of the brain is in its infancy but offers potential insight into addictions and their treatment.

■ OTHER CENTRAL NERVOUS SYSTEM STRUCTURES

The *extrapyramidal motor system* is a bundle of nerve fibers connecting the thalamus to the basal ganglia and cerebral cortex. Muscle tone, common reflexes, and automatic voluntary motor functioning, such as walking, are controlled by this nerve track. Dysfunction of this motor track can produce hypertonicity in muscle groups. In Parkinson's disease, the cells that compose the extrapyramidal motor system are severely affected, producing many involuntary motor movements. A number of medications, which are discussed in Chapter 14, also affect this system.

The *pineal body* is located above and medial to the thalamus. Because the pineal gland easily calcifies, it can be visualized by neuroimaging and often is a medial landmark. Its functions remain somewhat of a mystery, despite long knowledge of its existence. It contains secretory cells that emit the neurohormone melatonin and other substances. These hormones are thought to have a number of regulatory functions within the endocrine system. Information received from light-dark sources controls release of melatonin, which has been associated with sleep and emotional disorders. In addition, a modulation of immune function has been postulated for melatonin from the pineal gland.

The *locus caeruleus* is a tiny cluster of neurons that fan out and innervate almost every part of the brain, including most of the cortex, the thalamus and hypothalamus, the cerebellum, and the spinal cord. Just one neuron from the caeruleus can connect to more than 250,000 other neurons. Although it is very small, because of its wide-ranging neuronal connections, this tiny structure has influence in the regulation of attention, time perception, sleep-rest cycles, arousal, learning, pain, and mood, and it seems most involved with information processing of new, unexpected, and novel experiences. Some think its function/dysfunction may explain why individuals become addicted to substances and seek risky behaviours, despite awareness of negative consequences.

The *brain stem*, located beneath the thalamus, is composed of the midbrain, pons, and medulla and has important life-sustaining functions. Nuclei of numerous neural pathways to the cerebrum are located in the brain stem.

Table 10.3   Classic and Putative Neurotransmitters, Their Distribution and Proposed Functions

Neurotransmitter	Cell Bodies	Projections	Proposed Function
Acetylcholine			
Dietary precursor: choline	Basal forebrain Pons Other areas	Diffuse throughout the cortex, hippocampus Peripheral nervous system	Important role in learning and memory Some role in wakefulness and basic attention Peripherally activates muscles and is the major neurochemical in the autonomic system
Monoamines			
Dopamine Dietary precursor: tyrosine	Substantia nigra Ventral tegmental area Arcuate nucleus Retina olfactory bulb	Striatum (basal ganglia) Limbic system and cerebral cortex Pituitary	Involved in involuntary motor movements Some role in mood states, pleasure components in reward systems, and complex behaviour such as judgment, reasoning, and insight
Norepinephrine Dietary precursor: tyrosine	Locus caeruleus Lateral tegmental area and others throughout the pons and medulla	Very widespread throughout the cortex, thalamus, cerebellum, brain stem, and spinal cord Basal forebrain, thalamus, hypothalamus	Proposed role in learning and memory, attributing value in reward systems; fluctuates in sleep and wakefulness Major component of the sympathetic nervous system responses, including "fight-or-flight"
Serotonin Dietary precursor: tryptophan	Raphe nuclei Others in the pons and medulla	Very widespread throughout the cortex, thalamus, cerebellum, brain stem, and spinal cord	Proposed role in the control of appetite, sleep, mood states, hallucinations, pain perception, and vomiting
Histamine Dietary Precursor: histidine	Hypothalamus	Cerebral cortex Limbic system Hypothalamus Found in all mast cells	Control of gastric secretions, smooth muscle control, cardiac stimulation, stimulation of sensory nerve endings, and alertness
Amino Acids			
GABA	Derived from glutamate without localized cell bodies	Found in cells and projections throughout the CNS, especially in intrinsic feedback loops and interneurons of the cerebrum Also in the extrapyramidal motor system and cerebellum	Fast inhibitory response postsynaptically, inhibits the excitability of the neurons and therefore contributes to seizure, agitation, and anxiety control
Glycine	Primarily the spinal cord and brain stem	Limited projection, but especially in the auditory system and olfactory bulb Also found in the spinal cord, medulla, midbrain, cerebellum, and cortex	Inhibitory Decreases the excitability of spinal motor neurons but not cortical
Glutamate	Diffuse	Diffuse, but especially in the sensory organs	Excitatory Responsible for the bulk of information flow
Neuropeptides			
Endogenous opioids, (e.g., endorphins, enkephalins)	A large family of neuropeptides, which has three distinct subgroups, all of which are manufactured widely throughout the CNS	Widely distributed within and outside the CNS	Suppresses pain, modulates mood and stress Likely involvement in reward systems and addiction Also may regulate pituitary hormone release Implicated in the pathophysiology of diseases of the basal ganglia
Melatonin One of its precursors serotonin	Pineal body	Widely distributed within and outside the CNS	Secreted in dark and suppressed light, helps regulate the sleep-wake cycle as well as other biologic rhythms

Continued

Table 10.3	Classic and Putative Neurotransmitters, Their Distribution and Proposed Functions (*Continued*)		
Neurotransmitter	**Cell Bodies**	**Projections**	**Proposed Function**
Substance P	Widespread, significant in the raphe system and spinal cord	Spinal cord, cortex, brain stem, and especially sensory neurons associated with pain perception	Involved in pain transmission, movement, and mood regulation
Cholecystokinin	Predominates in the ventral tegmental area of the midbrain	Frontal cortex where it is often colocalized with dopamine Widely distributed within and outside the CNS	Primary intestinal hormone involved in satiety, also has some involvement in the control of anxiety and panic

They are significantly involved in mediating symptoms of emotional dysfunction. These nuclei are also the primary source of several neurochemicals, such as serotonin, that are commonly associated with psychiatric disorders. Table 10-3 summarizes some of the key related nuclei.

The *cerebellum* is in the posterior aspect of the skull, beneath the cerebral hemispheres. This large structure controls movements and postural adjustments. To regulate postural balance and positioning, the cerebellum receives information from all parts of the body, including muscles, joints, skin, and visceral organs, as well as from many parts of the CNS.

Closely associated with the spinal cord, but not lying entirely within its column, is the **autonomic nervous system**, a subdivision of the PNS. It was originally given this name for being independent of conscious thought, that is, automatic. However, it does not necessarily function as autonomously as the name indicates. This system contains efferent (nerves moving away from the CNS) or motor system neurons, which affect target tissues such as cardiac muscle, smooth muscle, and the glands. It also contains afferent nerves, which are sensory and conduct information from these organs back to the CNS.

The autonomic nervous system is further divided into the sympathetic and parasympathetic nervous systems. These systems, although peripheral, are included here because they are involved in the emergency, or "fight-or-flight," response as well as the peripheral actions of many medications (see Chapter 14). Figure 10-6 illustrates the innervations of various target organs by the autonomic nervous system. Table 10-4 identifies the actions of the sympathetic and parasympathetic nervous systems on various target organs.

Neurophysiology of the Central Nervous System

At their most basic level, the human brain and connecting nervous system are composed of billions of cells (Fig. 10-7). Most are connective and supportive glial cells with ancillary functions in the nervous system.

◼◼ NEURONS AND NERVE IMPULSES

About 10 billion cells are nerve cells, or neurons, responsible for receiving, organizing, and transmitting information. Each neuron has a cell body, or soma, which holds the nucleus containing most of the cell's genetic information. The soma also includes other organelles, such as ribosomes and endoplasmic reticulum, both of which carry out protein synthesis; the Golgi apparatus, which contains enzymes to modify the proteins for specific functions; vesicles, which transport and store proteins; and lysosomes, responsible for degradation of these proteins. Located throughout the neuron, mitochondria, containing enzymes and often called the "cell's engine," are the site of many energy-producing chemical reactions. These cell structures provide the basis for secreting numerous chemicals by which neurons communicate.

It is not just the vast number of neurons that accounts for the complexities of the brain but also the enormous number of neurochemical interconnections and interactions between neurons. A single motor neuron in the spinal cord may receive signals from more than 10,000 sources of interconnections with other nerves. Although most neurons have only one axon, which varies in length and conducts impulses away from the soma, each has numerous dendrites, receiving signals from other neurons. Because axons may branch as they terminate, they also have multiple contacts with other neurons.

Nerve signals are prompted to fire by a variety of chemical or physical stimuli. This firing produces an electrical impulse. The cell's membrane is a double layer of phospholipid molecules with embedded proteins. Some of these proteins provide water-filled channels through which inorganic ions may pass (Fig. 10-8). Each of the common ions—sodium, potassium, calcium, and chloride—has its own specific molecular channel. These channels are voltage gated and thus open or close in response to changes in the electrical potential across the membrane. At rest, the cell membrane is polarized with a positive charge on the outside and about a 270-mV charge on the inside, owing to the resting distribution of sodium and potassium ions. As potassium passively diffuses across the membrane, the sodium pump uses energy to move sodium from the inside

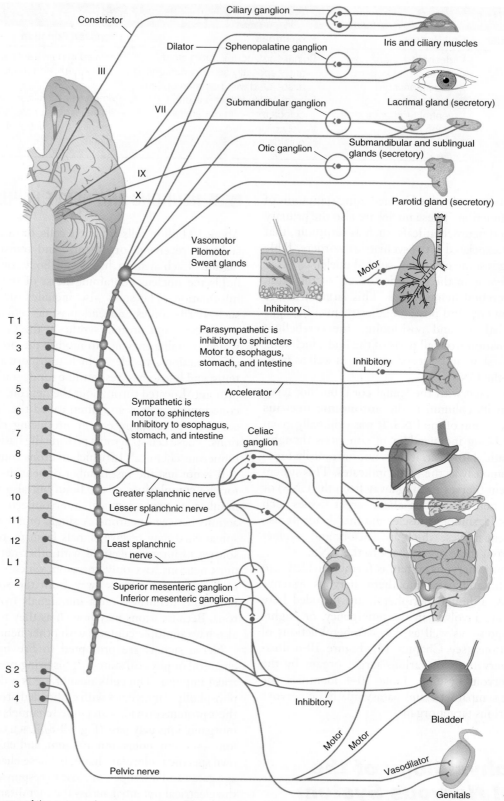

FIGURE 10.6 Diagram of the autonomic nervous system. Note that many organs are innervated by both sympathetic and parasympathetic nerves. (Adapted from Schaffe, E. E., & Lytle, I. M. [1980]. *Basic physiology and anatomy*. Philadelphia, PA: J. B. Lippincott.)

Table 10.4	Peripheral Organ Response in the Autonomic Nervous System	
Effector Organ	**Sympathetic Response**	**Parasympathetic Response (Acetylcholine)**
Eye • Iris sphincter muscle • Ciliary muscle	Preganglionic neurons—acetylcholine Postganglionic neurons—mostly norepinephrine Dilation Relaxation	Constriction to normal Accommodation for near vision
Heart • Sinoatrial node • Atria • Atrioventricular node	Increased rate Increased contractility Increased contractility	Decrease rate to normal Decrease in contractility Decrease in conduction velocity
Blood vessels	Depending on type of sympathetic receptor, stimulation can cause constriction or dilation	Dilation of vessels supplying penis and clitoris only
Lungs • Bronchial muscles • Bronchial glands	Relaxation	Constriction to normal Secretion
Gastrointestinal Tract • Motility and tone • Sphincters • Secretion glands	Relaxation (decrease peristalsis) Contraction Decrease secretion	Increased (for normal peristalsis) Relaxation Stimulation
Urinary Bladder • Detrusor muscle • Trigone and sphincter	Relaxation Contraction	Contraction Relaxation
Uterus	Contraction (pregnant) Relaxation (nonpregnant)	Variable
Skin • Pilomotor muscles • Sweat glands	Contraction Increased secretion	No effect No effect
Glands • Salivary • Sweat • Adrenal medulla • Endocrine pancreas	Stimulation of small volume of thick saliva Increased secretion Stimulation of epinephrine and norepinephrine secretion Inhibition of insulin secretion; stimulation of glucagon secretion	Stimulation of large volume of watery saliva None None Stimulation of insulin and glucagon secretion

of the cell against a concentration gradient to maintain this distribution. An action potential, or nerve impulse, is generated as the membrane is depolarized and a threshold value is reached, which triggers the opening of the voltage-gated sodium channels, allowing sodium to surge into the cell. The inside of the cell briefly becomes positively charged and the outside negatively charged. Once initiated, the action potential becomes self-propagating, opening nearby sodium channels. This electrical communication moves into the soma from the dendrites or down the axon by this mechanism.

SYNAPTIC TRANSMISSION

For one neuron to communicate with another, the electrical process must change to a chemical communication. The synaptic cleft, a junction between one nerve and another, is the space where the electrical intracellular signal becomes a chemical extracellular signal. Various substances are recognized as the chemical messengers between neurons.

KEY CONCEPT **Neurotransmitters** are small molecules that directly and indirectly control the opening or closing of ion channels.

Neurotransmitters are small molecules that directly and indirectly control the opening or closing of ion channels. Neuromodulators are chemical messengers that make the target cell membrane or postsynaptic membrane more or less susceptible to the effects of the primary neurotransmitter. Some of these neurochemicals are synthesized quickly from dietary precursors, such as tyrosine or tryptophan, or enzymes inside the cytoplasm of the neuron, but most synthesis occurs in the ends of the axons, called *terminals*, or the neuron itself. Some

FIGURE 10.7 Cell body and organelles of an axon.

FIGURE 10.8 Initiation of a nerve impulse. The initiation of an action potential, or nerve impulse, involves the opening and closing of the voltage-gated channels on the cell membrane and the passage of ions into the cell. The resulting electrical activity sends communication impulses from the dendrites or axon into the body.

neurochemicals can reduce the membrane potential and enhance the transmission of the signal between neurons. These chemicals are called *excitatory neurotransmitters*. Other neurochemicals have the opposite effect, slowing down nerve impulses, and these substances are called *inhibitory neurotransmitters*.

As the electrical action potential reaches the terminals, calcium ion channels are opened, causing an influx of Ca⁺⁺ ions into the neuron. This increase in calcium stimulates the release of neurotransmitters into the **synapse.** Rapid signaling between neurons requires a ready supply of neurotransmitters. These neurotransmitters are

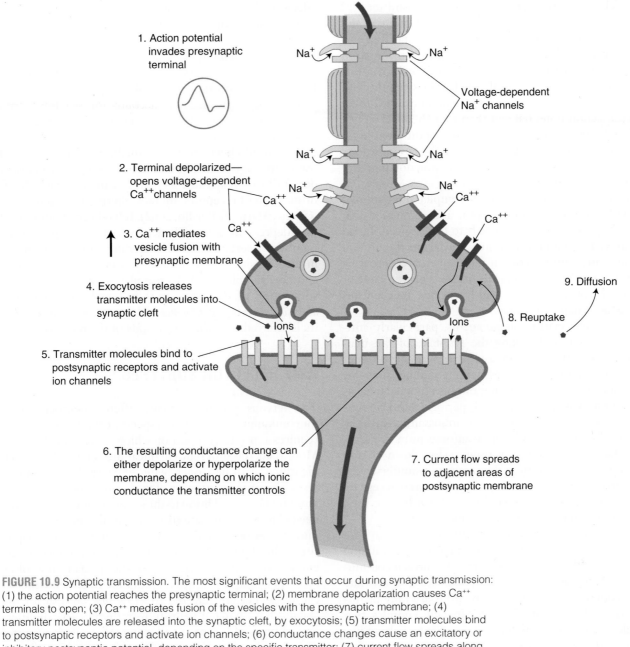

1. Action potential invades presynaptic terminal

Voltage-dependent Na⁺ channels

2. Terminal depolarized— opens voltage-dependent Ca⁺⁺ channels

3. Ca⁺⁺ mediates vesicle fusion with presynaptic membrane

4. Exocytosis releases transmitter molecules into synaptic cleft

5. Transmitter molecules bind to postsynaptic receptors and activate ion channels

6. The resulting conductance change can either depolarize or hyperpolarize the membrane, depending on which ionic conductance the transmitter controls

7. Current flow spreads to adjacent areas of postsynaptic membrane

8. Reuptake

9. Diffusion

Ions

FIGURE 10.9 Synaptic transmission. The most significant events that occur during synaptic transmission: (1) the action potential reaches the presynaptic terminal; (2) membrane depolarization causes Ca⁺⁺ terminals to open; (3) Ca⁺⁺ mediates fusion of the vesicles with the presynaptic membrane; (4) transmitter molecules are released into the synaptic cleft, by exocytosis; (5) transmitter molecules bind to postsynaptic receptors and activate ion channels; (6) conductance changes cause an excitatory or inhibitory postsynaptic potential, depending on the specific transmitter; (7) current flow spreads along the postsynaptic membrane; and (8) transmitter remaining in the synaptic cleft returns to the presynaptic terminal by reuptake or (9) diffuses into the extracellular fluid. (Adapted and reproduced with permission from Schauf, C., Moffett, D., & Moffett, S. (1990). *Human physiology*. St. Louis, MO: Times Mirror/Mosby.)

stored in small vesicles grouped near the cell membrane at the terminals. Because nerve terminals do not have the ability to manufacture proteins, the transmitters that fill these vesicles are small molecules, such as the bioamines (dopamine and norepinephrine) or the amino acids (glutamate or γ-aminobutyric acid [GABA]). Actions of these small molecules are discussed in the Neurotransmitters section later in this chapter. When stimulated, the vesicles containing the neurotransmitter fuse with the cell membrane, and the neurotransmitter is released into the

synapse (Fig. 10-9). The neurotransmitter then crosses the synaptic cleft to a receptor site on the postsynaptic neuron and stimulates adjacent neurons. This is the process of neuronal communication.

Embedded in the postsynaptic membrane are a number of proteins that act as receptors for the released neurotransmitters. The "lock-and-key" analogy has often been used to describe the fit of a given neurotransmitter to its receptor site. Each neurotransmitter has a specific receptor, or protein, for which it and only it will fit. The target cell, when stimulated by the neurotransmitter, will then respond by evoking its own action potential and either producing some action common to that cell or acting as a relay to keep the messages moving throughout the CNS. This pattern of the electrical signal from one neuron, converted to chemical signal at the synaptic cleft, picked up by an adjacent neuron, again converted to an electrical action potential and then to a chemical signal, occurs billions of times a day in billions of different brain cells. It is this electrical-chemical communication process that allows the structures of the brain to function together in a coordinated and organized manner.

When the neurotransmitter has completed its interaction with the postsynaptic receptor and stimulated that cell, its work is done, and it needs to be removed. It can be removed by natural diffusion away from the area of high neurotransmitter concentration at the receptors by being broken down by enzymes in the synaptic cleft or through reuptake through highly specific mechanisms into the presynaptic terminal.

Many psychopharmacologic agents, particularly antidepressants, act by blocking the reuptake of the neurotransmitters, thereby increasing the available amount of chemical messenger. Presynaptic binding sites for neurotransmitters may serve not only as reuptake mechanisms but also as autoreceptors to perform various regulatory functions on the flow of neurotransmitters into the synapse. When these presynaptic autoreceptors are saturated, the neuron knows it is time to slow down or stop releasing neurotransmitters. The neurotransmitters taken back into the presynaptic neuron may be stored in vesicles for rerelease, or they may be broken down by enzymes, such as monoamine oxidase, and removed entirely.

The primary steps in synaptic transmission are summarized in Figure 10-9. The preceding discussion contains only the basic mechanisms of neuronal communication. Many other factors that modulate or contribute to the communication between neurons are only beginning to be discovered. Examples include peptides that are released into the synapse and thought to behave like neurotransmitters or that also can appear in combination with another neurotransmitter. These peptides, known as *co-transmitters*, are believed to have a modulatory effect on the primary neurotransmitter.

RECEPTOR ACTIVITY

Both presynaptic and postsynaptic receptors have the capacity to change, developing either a greater-than-usual response to the neurotransmitter, known as *supersensitivity*, or a less-than-usual response, called *subsensitivity*. These changes represent the concept of neuroplasticity of brain tissue, which was discussed earlier in the chapter. The change in sensitivity of the receptor is most commonly caused by the effect of a drug on a receptor site or by disease that affects the normal functioning of a receptor site. Drugs can affect the sensitivity of the receptor by altering the strength of attraction or affinity of a receptor for the neurotransmitter, by changing the efficiency with which the receptor activity translates the message inside the receiving cell, or by decreasing over time the number of receptors.

These mechanisms may account for the long-term, sometimes severely adverse, effects of psychopharmacologic drugs, the loss of effectiveness of a given medication, or the loss of effectiveness of a medication after repeated use in treating recurring episodes of a psychiatric disorder. A disease may cause a change in the normal number or function of receptors, thereby altering their sensitivity (Garcia, Marin, & Perillo, 2002). It has been hypothesized that depression is caused by a reduction in the normal number of certain receptors, leading to an abnormality in their sensitivity to neurotransmitters such as serotonin and norepinephrine. A decreased response to continued stimulation of these receptors is usually referred to as *desensitization* or *refractoriness*. This suspected subsensitivity is referred to as *down-regulation* of the receptors.

RECEPTOR SUBTYPES

The nervous system uses many different neurochemicals for communication, and each specific chemical messenger requires a specific receptor on which the chemical can act. More than 100 different chemical messengers have been identified, with new ones being uncovered frequently as research on the functioning of the brain becomes more and more precise. In addition to the sheer number of receptors needed to accommodate these chemicals, the neurotransmitters may produce different effects at different synaptic sites. The ability of a neurotransmitter to produce different actions is, in part, because of the specialization of its receptors. The different receptors for each neurochemical messenger are referred to as *receptor subtypes* for the chemical. Each major neurotransmitter has several different subtypes of receptors, allowing the neurotransmitter to have different effects in different areas of the brain. For example, dopamine, a common neurotransmitter discussed in the next section, has five different subtypes of receptors that have been identified. Numbers usually name the receptor subtypes. In the example of dopamine, the various subtypes of receptors are called D_1, D_2, D_3, and so on. Knowledge of the different subtypes helps in understanding both the effects and side effects of medications used to treat mental disorders.

NEUROTRANSMITTERS

Many substances have been identified as possible chemical messengers, but not all chemical messengers are neurotransmitters. Classic neurotransmitters are those that meet certain criteria agreed on by neuroscientists. The traditional criteria include the following:

- The chemical is synthesized inside the neuron.
- The chemical is present in the presynaptic terminals.
- The chemical is released into the synaptic cleft and causes a particular effect on the postsynaptic receptors.
- An exogenous form of the chemical administered as a drug causes identical action.
- The chemical is removed from the synaptic cleft by a specific mechanism.

Neurotransmitters can be grouped into categories that reflect chemical similarities of the neurotransmitter. Common practice classifies certain chemicals as neurotransmitters even though their ability to meet the strict traditional definition may be incomplete. For the purposes of this section, the classification of neurotransmitters will use this common system of classifying neurotransmitters. Common categories of neurotransmitters include

- Cholinergic neurotransmitters
- Biogenic amine neurotransmitters (sometimes called *monoamines* or *bioamines*)
- Amino acid neurotransmitters
- Neuropeptide neurotransmitters

Neurotransmitters are also classified by whether their action causes physiologic activity to occur or to stop occurring. All of the neurotransmitters commonly involved in the development of mental illness or affected by the drugs used to treat these illnesses are excitatory except one, GABA, which is inhibitory. The significance of this concept is discussed in the section about amino acids. Neurotransmitters are found wherever there are neurons, and neurons are contained in both the CNS and PNS. Because psychiatric mental disorders occur in the CNS, the following sections discuss neurotransmitters from the perspective of the CNS.

Cholinergic

Acetylcholine (ACh) is a primary cholinergic neurotransmitter. Found in the greatest concentration in the PNS, ACh provides the basic synaptic communication for the parasympathetic neurons and part of the sympathetic neurons, which send information to the CNS. Understanding both the action of ACh and the receptor subtypes for this neurotransmitter assists PMH nurses in understanding the complex side effects of common medications used to treat mental disorders.

Cholinergic neurons, so named because they contain ACh, follow diffuse projections throughout the cerebral cortex and limbic system, arising primarily from cell bodies in the base of the frontal lobes. Pathways from this region also project throughout the hippocampus (Fig. 10-10). These connections suggest that ACh is involved in higher intellectual functioning and memory. Individuals who have Alzheimer's disease or Down

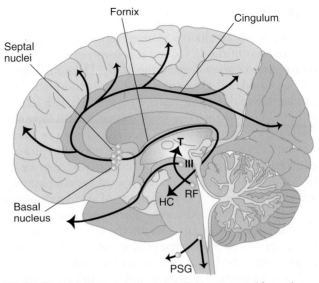

FIGURE 10.10 Cholinergic pathways. HC, hippocampal formation; PSG, parasympathetic ganglion cell; RF, reticular formation; T, thalamus. (Adapted from Nolte, J., & Angevine, J. (1995). *The human brain: In photographs and diagrams.* St. Louis, MO: Mosby.)

syndrome often exhibit patterns of cholinergic neuron loss in regions innervated by these pathways (such as the hippocampus), which may contribute to their memory difficulties and other cognitive deficits. Some cholinergic neurons are afferent to these areas bringing information from the limbic system, highlighting the role that ACh plays in communicating emotional state to the cerebral cortex. ACh is an excitatory neurotransmitter, meaning that when released into a synapse, it causes the postsynaptic neuron to initiate some action.

The subtypes of ACh receptors are divided into two groups: the muscarinic receptors and the nicotinic receptors. Many psychiatric medications are anticholinergic agents, which block the effects of the muscarinic ACh receptors. This blocking effect of ACh causes common side effects, such as dry mouth, blurred vision, constipation, urinary retention, and tachycardia, which are seen in many psychotropic medications. Excessive blockade of ACh can cause confusion and delirium, especially in elderly patients, as discussed in Chapter 31. Table 10-4 lists the effects of ACh on various organs in the parasympathetic system.

Biogenic Amines

The **biogenic amines** (bioamines) consist of small molecules manufactured in the neuron that contain an amine group, thus the name. These include dopamine, norepinephrine, and epinephrine, which are all synthesized from the amino acid tyrosine; serotonin, which is synthesized from tryptophan; and histamine, manufactured from histidine. Of all the neurotransmitters, the biogenic amines are most central to current hypotheses of psychiatric disorders and thus are described individually in more detail.

Dopamine

Dopamine is an excitatory neurotransmitter found in distinct regions of the CNS, and it is involved in cognitive, motor, and neuroendocrine functions. Dopamine levels are decreased in Parkinson's disease, and abnormally high production of dopamine has been associated with schizophrenia, discussed in more detail in Chapter 18. Dopamine is also the neurotransmitter that stimulates the body's natural "feel good" reward pathways, producing pleasant euphoric sensation under certain conditions. Abnormalities of dopamine use within the reward system pathways are suspected to be a critical aspect of the development of drug and other addictions. The dopamine pathways are distinct neuronal areas within the CNS in which the neurotransmitter dopamine predominates. Three major dopaminergic pathways have been identified.

The mesocortical and mesolimbic pathways originate in the ventral tegmental area and project into the medial aspects of the cortex (mesocortical) and the medial aspects of the limbic system inside the temporal lobes, including the hippocampus and amygdala (mesolimbic). Sometimes they are considered to be one pathway and at other times two separate pathways. The mesocortical pathway has major effects on cognition, including such functions as judgment, reasoning, insight, social conscience, motivation, the ability to generalize learning, and reward systems in the human brain. It contributes to some of the highest seats of cortical functioning. The mesocortical system may be linked to the positive symptoms of schizophrenia. The mesolimbic pathway also strongly influences emotions and has projections that affect memory and auditory reception. Abnormalities in the mesolimbic system may be linked with negative symptoms of schizophrenia.

Another major dopaminergic pathway begins in the substantia nigra and projects into the basal ganglia, parts of which are known as the *striatum*. Therefore, this pathway is called the *nigrostriatal pathway*. This influences the extrapyramidal motor system, which serves the voluntary motor system and allows involuntary motor movements. Destruction of dopaminergic neurons in this pathway has been associated with Parkinson's disease.

The last dopamine pathway originates from projections of the mesolimbic pathway and continues into the hypothalamus, which then projects into the pituitary gland. Therefore, this pathway, called the *tuberoinfundibular pathway*, has an impact on endocrine function and other functions, such as metabolism, hunger, thirst, sexual function, circadian rhythms, digestion, and temperature control. Figure 10-11 illustrates the dopaminergic pathways.

As noted previously, scientists have identified at least five subtypes of dopamine receptors in the CNS. These subtypes are distributed differently throughout the brain. For example, the D_1 subtype receptor and its related receptor subtype, D_5, predominate in areas that affect

FIGURE 10.11 Dopaminergic pathways. C, caudate nucleus; H, hypothalamus; HC, hippocampal formation; P, putamen; V, ventral striatum. (Adapted from Nolte, J., & Angevine, J. (1995). *The human brain: In photographs and diagrams*. St. Louis, MO: Mosby.)

memory and emotions, such as the cortex, hippocampus, and amygdala. They have not been detected in the substantia nigra. D_2 receptors are richly distributed throughout the neurons in the extrapyramidal motor system, whereas D_4 receptors are richly distributed in the frontal cortex, with few in the nigrostriatal system. Antipsychotic medications, discussed in Chapter 14, act by blocking the effects of dopamine at the receptor sites.

Many of the medications that are most effective on the acute symptoms of psychosis have a strong attraction or affinity for D_2 receptors and a weaker but modest correlation with D_1 receptors. Because D_2 receptors predominate in the nigrostriatal pathway, medications that have a weaker blockade of D_2 will have fewer extrapyramidal motor system effects. Side effects and adverse effects from the involuntary motor system are at times extremely debilitating to individuals. Based on the assumption that these dopamine receptor subtypes have different functions in the CNS, new medications are being designed to affect more predominantly one subtype than another, presumably avoiding effects on systems containing other subtypes and thus avoiding potential side effects of the medication. Researchers are attempting to develop new antipsychotic medications that avoid or minimize the effects on D_2 and therefore diminish the occurrence of extrapyramidal effects.

Norepinephrine

Norepinephrine was first demonstrated to be the primary neurotransmitter of the PNS in 1946. Whereas it is commonly found in the PNS, norepinephrine is critical to CNS functioning as well. Norepinephrine is an excitatory neurochemical that plays a major role in generating and maintaining mood states. Decreased norepinephrine has been associated with depression, and excessive norepinephrine has been associated with manic symptoms (Montgomery, 2000). Because norepinephrine is so heavily concentrated in the terminal sites of sympathetic nerves, it can be released quickly to ready the individual for a fight-or-flight response to threats in the environment. For this reason, norepinephrine is thought to play a role in the physical symptoms of anxiety.

Nerve tracts and pathways containing predominantly norepinephrine are called *noradrenergic* and are less clearly delineated than the dopamine pathways. In the CNS, noradrenergic neurons originate in the locus caeruleus, where more than half of the noradrenergic cell bodies are located. Because the locus caeruleus is one of the major timekeepers of the human body, norepinephrine is involved in sleep and wakefulness. From the locus caeruleus, noradrenergic pathways ascend into the neocortex, spread diffusely (Fig. 10-12), and enhance the ability of neurons to respond to whatever input they may be receiving. In addition, norepinephrine appears to be involved in the process of reinforcement, which facilitates learning. Noradrenergic pathways innervate the hypothalamus and thus are involved to some degree in endocrine function. Anxiety disorders and depression are examples of psychiatric illnesses in which dysfunction of the noradrenergic neurons may be involved.

Epinephrine

Epinephrine is very similar to norepinephrine chemically; however, in contrast to norepinephrine, only very small amounts of epinephrine are produced and released in the brain. Relatively few neurons in the brain use epinephrine as a neurotransmitter and those are located in the caudal pons and the medulla. Epinephrine is found in much higher concentrations in the rest of the body, where it is secreted directly from the adrenal gland into the blood circulation. Little discussion of the role of epinephrine in mental illness is found in the literature.

Serotonin

Serotonin (also called 5-hydroxytryptamine or 5-HT) is primarily an excitatory neurotransmitter that is diffusely distributed within the cerebral cortex, limbic system, and basal ganglia of the CNS. Serotonergic neurons also project into the hypothalamus and cerebellum. Figure 10-13 illustrates serotonergic pathways. Serotonin plays a role in emotions, cognition, sensory perceptions, and essential biologic functions, such as sleep and appetite. During the rapid-eye-movement (REM) phase of sleep, or the dream

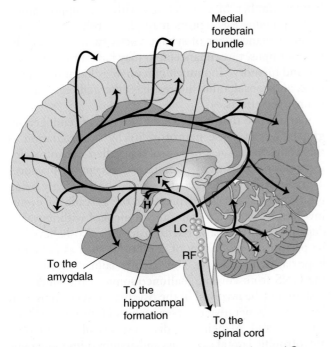

FIGURE 10.12 Noradrenergic pathways. H, hypothalamus; LC, locus caeruleus; RF, reticular formation; T, thalamus. (Adapted from Nolte, J., & Angevine, J. (1995). *The human brain: In photographs and diagrams*. St. Louis, MO: Mosby.)

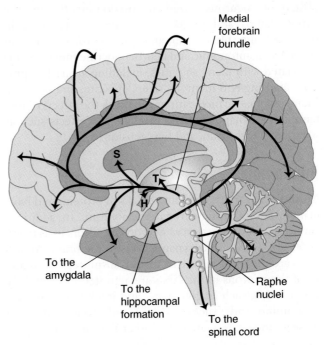

FIGURE 10.13 Serotonergic pathways. H, hypothalamus; S, septal nuclei; T, thalamus. (Adapted from Nolte, J., & Angevine, J. (1995). *The human brain: In photographs and diagrams*. St. Louis, MO: Mosby.)

state, serotonin concentrations decrease, and muscles subsequently relax. Serotonin is also involved in the control of food intake, hormone secretion, sexual behaviour, thermoregulation, and cardiovascular regulation. Some serotonergic fibres reach the cranial blood vessels within the brain and the pia mater, where they have a vasoconstrictive effect. The potency of some new medications for migraine headaches is related to their ability to block serotonin transmission in the cranial blood vessels. Descending serotonergic pathways are important in central pain control. Depression and insomnia have been associated with decreased levels of serotonin, whereas mania has been associated with increased serotonin. Some of the most well-known antidepressant medications, such as Prozac and Zoloft, which are discussed in more depth in Chapter 14, function by raising serotonin levels within certain areas of the CNS (Harmer, Hill, Taylor, Cowen, & Goodwin, 2003). Obsessive-compulsive disorder, panic disorder, and other anxiety disorders are believed to be associated with dysfunction of the serotonin pathways, explaining why antidepressant medications have several uses in treating mental disorders (Kapczinski, Lima, Souza, Cunha, & Schmitt, 2003).

Numerous subtypes of serotonin receptors also exist, and each of these appears to have a distinct function. $5\text{-}HT_{1a}$ is involved in the control of anxiety, aggression, and depression. Drugs such as lysergic acid diethylamide (LSD) affect $5\text{-}HT_2$ and produce hallucinatory effects.

Histamine

Histamine neurons originate predominantly in the hypothalamus and project to all major structures in the cerebrum, brain stem, and spinal cord. Exerting an influence in autonomic and neuroendocrine function, it is associated with many activities, including arousal, cognition, learning and memory, sleep, appetite, and seizures. Many psychiatric medications can block the effects of histamine postsynaptically and produce side effects such as sedation, weight gain, and hypotension.

Amino Acids

Amino acids are the building blocks of proteins and have many roles in intraneuronal metabolism. In addition, amino acids can function as neurotransmitters in as many as 60% to 70% of the synaptic sites in the brain. Amino acids are the most prevalent neurotransmitters. Virtually all of the neurons in the CNS are activated by excitatory amino acids, such as glutamate, and inhibited by inhibitory amino acids, such as GABA and glycine. Many of these amino acids coexist with other neurotransmitters.

γ-Aminobutyric Acid

GABA is the primary inhibitory neurotransmitter for the CNS. The pathways of GABA exist almost exclusively in the CNS, with the largest GABA concentrations in the hypothalamus, hippocampus, basal ganglia, spinal cord, and cerebellum. GABA functions in an inhibitory role in control of spinal reflexes and cerebellar reflexes. It has a major role in the control of neuronal excitability through the brain. In addition, GABA has an inhibitory influence on the activity of the dopaminergic nigrostriatal projections. GABA also has interconnections with other neurotransmitters. For example, dopamine inhibits cholinergic neurons, and GABA provides feedback and balance. Dysregulation of GABA and GABA receptors has been associated with anxiety disorders, and decreased GABA activity is involved in the development of seizure disorders.

Two specific subtype receptors have been identified for GABA: A and B. Two classes of medication, benzodiazepine antianxiety drugs and sedative-hypnotic barbiturate drugs, work because of their affinity for GABA receptor sites. Interest in the beneficial effects of these drugs has led to increased interest in GABA receptor sites. Researchers are finding endogenous chemicals that bind to the same receptor sites as benzodiazepines and serve as natural inhibitory regulators (Fritschy & Brunig, 2003).

Glutamate

Glutamate, the most widely distributed excitatory neurotransmitter, is the main transmitter in the associational areas of the cortex. Glutamate can be found in a number of pathways from the cortex to the thalamus, pons, striatum, and spinal cord. In addition, glutamate pathways have a number of connections with the hippocampus. Some glutamate receptors may play a role in the long-lasting enhancement of synaptic activity. In turn, in the hippocampus, this enhancement may have a role in learning and memory. Too much glutamate is harmful to neurons, and considerable interest has emerged regarding its neurotoxic effects.

Conditions that produce an excess of endogenous glutamate can cause neurotoxicity by overexcitation of the neuronal tissue. This process, called excitotoxicity, increases the sensitivity of glutamate receptors, produces overactivation of the receptors, and is increasingly being understood as a critical piece of the cascade of events involved in physical symptoms of alcohol withdrawal in dependent individuals. Excitotoxicity is also believed to be part of the pathology of conditions such as ischemia, hypoxia, hypoglycemia, and hepatic failure. Damage to the CNS from chronic malfunctioning of the glutamate system may be involved in the psychiatric symptoms seen in neurodegenerative diseases such as Huntington's, Parkinson's, and Alzheimer's diseases; vascular dementia; amyotrophic lateral sclerosis; and acquired immune deficiency syndrome (AIDS)-related dementia (MacGregor, Avshalumov, & Rice, 2003). Degeneration of glutamate neurons has more recently been implicated in the development of schizophrenia (Kurup & Kurup, 2003).

Neuropeptides

Peptides are short chains of amino acids. **Neuropeptides** exist in the CNS and have a number of important roles as neurotransmitters, neuromodulators, or neurohormones. Neuropeptides were first thought to be pituitary hormones, such as adrenocorticotropin, oxytocin, and vasopressin, or hypothalamic-releasing hormones, such as corticotropin-releasing hormone and thyrotropin-releasing hormone (TRH). However, when an endogenous morphine-like substance was discovered in the 1970s, the term *endorphin*, or endogenous morphine, was introduced. Although amino acids and monoamine neurotransmitters can be produced directly from dietary precursors in any part of the neuron, neuropeptides are, almost without exception, synthesized from messenger RNA in the cell body. To date, two types of neuropeptides have been identified: opioid and nonopioid. Opioid neuropeptides, such as endorphins, enkephalins, and dynorphins, act in endocrine functioning and pain suppression. Nonopioid neuropeptides, such as substance P and somatostatin, play roles in pain transmission and endocrine functioning.

There are considerable variations in the distribution of individual neuropeptides, but some areas are especially rich in cell bodies containing neuropeptides. These areas include the amygdala, striatum, hypothalamus, raphe nuclei, brain stem, and spinal cord. Many of the interneurons of the cerebral cortex contain neuropeptides, but there are considerably fewer in the thalamus and almost none in the cerebellum.

The complexities of neuronal transmission are enormous. PMH nurses have a significant role in assessing symptoms and administering and monitoring medications for patients with psychiatric disorders. Knowledge of neurotransmitters is essential because even a single dose of a drug affecting this system may cause relief of symptoms or have adverse effects. The actions of psychopharmacologic agents and related nursing responsibilities are discussed more fully in Chapter 14. In addition, many nursing interventions designed to effect changes in such functions as sleep, diet, stress management, exercise, and mood modulation affect these neurotransmitters and neuropeptides, directly or indirectly. More research is needed to understand the bio/psycho/social/spiritual aspects of nursing care.

New Fields of Study

As the complexity of the nervous system and its interrelationship with other body systems and the environment have become more fully understood, new fields of study have emerged. From the discussion of neuroanatomy and neurotransmitters, it is logical to deduce that understanding the endocrine system and its interrelationship with the nervous system is essential. Although it has long been observed that individuals under stress have compromised immune systems and are more likely to acquire common diseases, only recently have changes in the immune system been linked to some psychiatric illnesses (Sperner-Unterweger, 2005; Fetissov & Déchelotte, 2008). In addition, as biologic rhythms have become more fully understood and defined, new information suggests that dysfunction of these rhythms may not only result from a psychiatric illness but also contribute to its development. Therefore, the following sections provide a brief overview of psychoendocrinology, psychoimmunology, and chronobiology.

■■■◗ PSYCHOENDOCRINOLOGY

Psychoendocrinology examines the relationships among the nervous system, endocrine system, and behaviour. Messages are conveyed within the endocrine system mainly by hormones, and neurohormones are those substances excreted by special neurons within the nervous system. Neurohormones are cellular substances and are secreted into the bloodstream and transported to a site where they exert their effect. Of the several types of hormones, peptides are the most common hormones in the CNS.

The hypothalamus sends and receives information through the pituitary, which then communicates with structures in the peripheral aspects of the body. Figure 10-14 presents an example of the communication

FIGURE 10.14 Hypothalamic and pituitary communication system. The neurohormonal communication system between the hypothalamus and the pituitary exerts effects on many organs and systems.

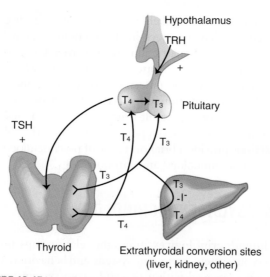

FIGURE 10.15 Hypothalamic–pituitary–thyroid axis. The regulation of thyroid-stimulating hormone (TSH or thyrotropin) secretion by the anterior pituitary. Positive effects of thyrotropin-releasing hormone (TRH) from the hypothalamus and negative effects of circulating triiodothyronine (T_3) and T_3 from intrapituitary conversion of thyroxine (T_4).

of the anterior pituitary with a number of organs and structures. Axes, the structures within which the neurohormones are providing messages, are the most often studied aspect of the neuroendocrine system. These axes always involve a feedback mechanism. For example, the hypothalamic–pituitary–thyroid axis regulates the release of thyroid hormone by the thyroid gland using TRH hormone from the hypothalamus to the pituitary and TSH from the pituitary to the thyroid. Figure 10-15 illustrates the hypothalamic–pituitary–thyroid axis. The hypothalamic–pituitary–gonadal axis regulates estrogen and testosterone secretion through LH and FSH.

Interest in psychoendocrinology is heightened by various endocrine disorders that produce psychiatric symptoms. Addison's disease (hypoadrenalism) produces depression, apathy, fatigue, and occasionally psychosis. Hypothyroidism produces depression and some anxiety. Administration of steroids can cause depression, hypomania, irritability, and in some cases, psychosis. Some psychiatric disorders have been associated with endocrine system dysfunction. For example, some individuals with mood disorders show evidence of dysregulation in adrenal, thyroid, and growth hormone axes.

■ PSYCHOIMMUNOLOGY

Psychoimmunology is the study of immunology as it relates to emotions and behaviour. The immune system protects the body from foreign pathogens. Overactivity of the immune system can occur in autoimmune diseases such as systemic lupus erythematosus (SLE), allergies, or anaphylaxis. Too little activity may result from cancer and serious infections, as is the case with AIDS. Evidence suggests that communication between the nervous system and the immune system is bidirectional. Specific immune system dysfunctions may result from damage to the hypothalamus, hippocampus, or pituitary and may produce symptoms of psychiatric disorders. Negative events and emotions influence catecholamines (norepinephrine and epinephrine), adrenocorticotropic hormone (ACTH), cortisol, growth hormone, and prolactin (Glazer & Kiecolt-Glazer, 2005). Each of these hormones can affect the immune function. Figure 10-16 illustrates the interaction between stress and the immune system. This figure also demonstrates the true bio/psycho/social/spiritual nature of the complex interrelationship of the nervous system, the endocrine system, the immune system, and environmental or emotional stress.

Immune dysregulation may also be involved in the development of psychiatric disorders. This can occur by allowing neurotoxins to affect the brain, damaging the neuroendocrine tissue or damaging tissues in the brain at locations such as the receptor sites. Some antidepressants have been thought to have antiviral effects. Symptoms of diseases such as depression may follow an occurrence of serious infection, and prenatal exposure to infectious organisms may be associated with the development of schizophrenia. Stress and conditioning have specific effects on the suppression of immune function (Ekman, Persson, & Nilsson, 2002; Friedman, 2000; Ishihara, Makita, Imai, Hashimoto, & Nohara, 2003). In many cases, individuals with SLE experience symptoms of depression, insomnia, nervousness, and confusion. Although there is still much to learn about the relationship of psychiatric disorders and the immune system, it is clear that PMH nurses must develop and implement interventions designed to enhance immune function in psychiatric patients.

■ CHRONOBIOLOGY

Chronobiology involves the study and measure of time structures or biologic rhythms. Some rhythms have a **circadian cycle**, or 24-hour cycle, whereas others, such as the menstrual cycle, operate in different periods. Rhythms exist in the human body to control endocrine secretions, sleep-wake cycles, body temperature, neurotransmitter synthesis, and more. These cycles may become deregulated and may begin earlier than usual, known as a phase advance, or later than usual, known as a phase delay.

Zeitgebers are specific events that function as time givers or synchronizers and that set biologic rhythms. Light is the most common example of an external zeitgeber. The suprachiasmatic nucleus of the hypothalamus is an example of an internal zeitgeber. Some theorists think that psychiatric disorders may result from one or more biologic rhythm dysfunctions. For example, depression may be, in

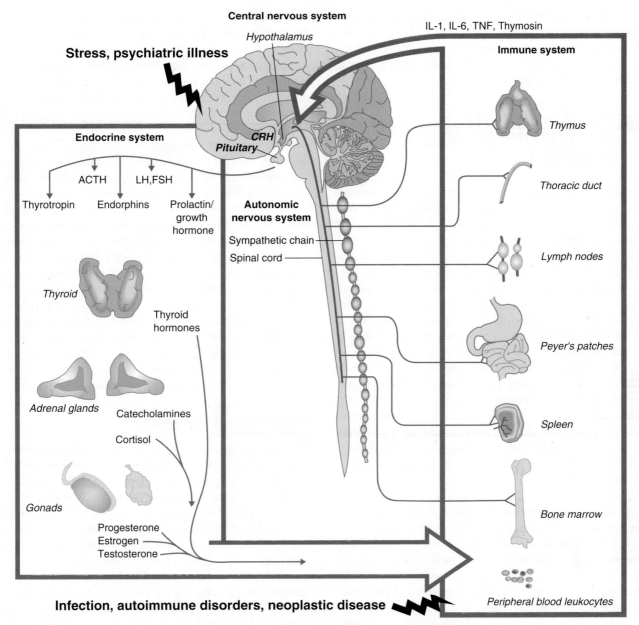

FIGURE 10.16 Examples of the interaction between stress or psychiatric illness and the immune system through the endocrine system. ACTH, adrenocorticotropic hormone; CRH, corticotropin-releasing hormone; FSH, follicle-stimulating hormone IL, interleukin; LH, luteinizing hormone; TNF, tumour necrosis factor.

part, a phase advance disorder, including early morning awakening and decreased time of onset of REM sleep. Seasonal affective disorder may be the result of shortened exposure to light during the winter months. Exposure to specific artificial light often relieves symptoms of fatigue, overeating, hypersomnia, and depression.

Diagnostic Approaches

Now that researchers understand more about neural transmission, brain functioning, and psychopharmacology, focus is shifting to applying the knowledge in order to find biologic markers for the psychiatric disorders previously thought to have only a psychological component. **Biologic markers** are diagnostic test findings that occur only in the presence of the psychiatric disorder and include such findings as laboratory and other diagnostic test results and neuropathologic changes noticeable in assessment. These markers increase diagnostic certainty and reliability and may have predictive value, allowing for the possibility of preventive interventions to forestall or avoid the onset of illness.

In addition, biologic markers could assist in developing evidence-based care practices. If markers can be used reliably, it would be much easier to identify the most effective treatments and to determine the expected prognosis for given conditions. The PMH nurse should be aware of the most current information on biologic markers so that information, limitations, and results can be discussed knowledgeably with the patient.

LABORATORY TESTS AND NEUROPHYSIOLOGIC PROCEDURES

For many years, laboratory tests have attempted to measure levels of neurotransmitters and other CNS substances in the bloodstream. Many of the metabolites of neurotransmitters can be found in the urine and CSF as well. However, these measures have had only limited utility in elucidating what is happening in the brain. Levels of neurotransmitters and metabolites in the bloodstream or urine do not necessarily equate with levels in the CNS. In addition, availability of the neurotransmitter or metabolite does not predict the availability of the neurotransmitter in the synapse, where it must act or directly relate to the receptor sensitivity. However, in addition to neuroimaging procedures like MRIs, studies of fresh brain tissue removed in neurosurgery and postmortem studies have helped localize neurotransmitters, their function, and pharmacological properties (Raiteri, 2006). These studies have provided clues but remain without conclusive predictive value and therefore are not routinely used.

Another laboratory approach to the study of some of the psychiatric disorders is the challenge test. A challenge test has been most often used in the study of panic disorders. These tests are usually conducted by intravenously administering a chemical known to produce a specific set of psychiatric symptoms. For example, lactate or caffeine may be used to induce the symptoms of panic in a person who has panic disorder. The biologic response of the individual is then monitored. These tests have been developed primarily for research purposes.

Endocrine stimulation tests, such as the TRH stimulation test, dexamethasone suppression test (DST), and corticotrophin-releasing hormone (CRH) test, have some limited clinical utility. In the TRH stimulation test, TRH is administered, and the TSH blood level is measured over time, usually at intervals during a period of 3 to 4 hours. The patient with hypothyroidism has an elevated TSH level. A blunted TRH stimulation test has been proposed as a biologic marker for major depression; however, only about 30% of individuals with major depression show the response.

The DST and CRH test are used to assess the function of the hypothalamic–pituitary–adrenocorticotropin system. The DST involves administering dexamethasone at 11 PM. Cortisol blood levels are then measured at one

or more points the next day. In the healthy individual, dexamethasone suppresses cortisol levels, but results of numerous studies suggest that there is nonsuppression in certain types of depression. Many medical conditions, such as diabetes mellitus; obesity; infection; pregnancy; recent surgery; and use of medications, such as carbamazepine or high doses of estrogen, may alter the test results, producing false-positive results. Overall, a positive result, or abnormal nonsuppression, appears to indicate major depression, but a negative result does not rule out depression. Considerable controversy, therefore, exists regarding the clinical usefulness of this test.

Although no commonly used laboratory tests exist that directly confirm a mental disorder, laboratory tests are still an active part of care and assessment of psychiatric patients. Many physical conditions mimic the symptoms of mental illness, and many of the medications used to treat psychiatric illness can produce health problems. For these reasons, the routine care of patients with psychiatric disorders includes the use of laboratory tests such as complete blood counts, thyroid studies, electrolytes, hepatic enzymes, and other evaluative tests. PMH nurses need to be familiar with these procedures and assist patients in understanding the use and implications of such tests.

Electroencephalography

EEG is a tried and true method for investigating what is happening inside the living brain. Developed in the 1920s by Hans Berger, an EEG measures electrical activity in the uppermost nerve layers of the cortex. Usually, 16 electrodes are placed on the patient's scalp. The EEG machine, equipped with graph paper and recording pens, is turned on, and the pens then trace the electrical impulses generated over each electrode. Until the use of CT in the 1970s, the EEG was the only method for identifying brain abnormalities. It remains the simplest and most noninvasive method for identifying some disorders. It is increasingly being used to identify individual neuronal differences and most recently to predict a person's response to common antidepressant medication (Cook et al., 2002).

An EEG may be used in psychiatry to differentiate possible causes of the patient's symptoms. For example, some types of seizure disorders, such as temporal lobe epilepsy, head injuries, or tumours, may present with predominantly psychiatric symptoms. In addition, metabolic dysfunction, delirium, dementia, altered levels of consciousness, hallucinations, and dissociative states may require EEG evaluation.

Spikes and wave-pattern changes are indications of brain abnormalities. Spikes may be the focal point from which a seizure occurs. However, abnormal activity often is not discovered on a routine EEG while the individual is awake. For this reason, additional methods are sometimes used. Nasopharyngeal leads may be used to get physically closer to the limbic regions. The patient may be exposed to a flashing strobe light while the examiner looks for activity that is not in phase with the flashing light or may be asked to hyperventilate for 3 minutes to induce abnormal activity if it exists. Sleep deprivation may also be used. This involves keeping the patient awake throughout the night before the EEG evaluation. The patient may then be drowsy and fall asleep during the procedure. Abnormalities are more likely to occur when the patient is asleep. Sleep may also be induced using medication; however, many medications change the wave patterns on an EEG. For example, the benzodiazepine class of drugs increases the rapid and fast beta activity. Many other prescribed and illicit drugs, such as lithium, which increases theta activity, can cause EEG alterations. In addition to reassuring, preparing, and educating the patient for the examination, the nurse should carefully assess the history of substance use and report this information to the examiner. If a sleep deprivation EEG is to be done, caffeine or other stimulants that might assist the patient in staying awake should be withheld because they may change the EEG patterns.

Polysomnography

Polysomnography is a special procedure that involves recording the EEG throughout a night of sleep. This test is usually conducted in a sleep laboratory. Other tests are usually performed at the same time, including electrocardiography and electromyography. Blood oxygenation, body movement, body temperature, and other data may be collected as well, especially in research settings. This procedure is usually conducted for evaluating sleep disorders, such as sleep apnea, enuresis, or somnambulism. However, sleep pattern changes are frequently researched in mental disorders as well.

Researchers have found that normal sleep divisions and stages are affected by many factors, including drugs, alcohol, general medical conditions, and psychiatric disorders (Holcomb, 2006). For example, REM latency, the length of time it takes for an individual to enter the first REM episode, is shortened in depression. Reduced delta sleep is also observed. These findings have been replicated so frequently that some researchers consider them biologic markers for depression.

Other Neurophysiologic Methods

Evoked potentials (EPs), also called event-related potentials, use the same basic principles as an EEG. They measure changes in electrical activity of the brain in specific regions as a response to a given stimulus. Electrodes placed on the scalp measure a large waveform that stands out after the administration of repetitive stimuli, such as a click or flash of light. There are several different types of EPs to be measured, depending on the sensory area affected by the stimulus, the cognitive task required, or the region monitored, any of which can change the length of time until the wave occurrence. EPs are used extensively in psychiatric research. In clinical practice, EPs are used primarily in the assessment of demyelinating disorders, such as multiple sclerosis.

However, brain electrical activity mapping (BEAM) studies, which involve a 20-electrode EEG that generates computerized maps of the brain's electrical activity, have found a slowing of electrical activity in the frontal lobes of individuals who have schizophrenia. These findings initially suggested a "hypofrontality" in schizophrenia; however, later research found that this was an inconsistent finding (McGuire, Howes, Stone, & Fusar-Poli, 2008; see Chapter 18). Nonetheless, neurophysiologic methods provide only rough approximations compared with current structural and functional neuroimaging techniques.

• CRNENOTE

CRNENOTE The direct influence of biologic factors can be overlooked by a nurse who assumes mental health problems (e.g., difficulty managing anger) are primarily psychosocial in nature.

Integration of the Biologic, Psychological, Social, and Spiritual Domains

Basic knowledge in the neurosciences has become essential content for the practicing PMH nurse. In a truly holistic bio/psycho/social/spiritual model, all psychological and social influences are seen as interacting with the complex human biologic system. For example, treatment of generalized anxiety disorder would involve addressing etiologies in each of these areas (see Fig. 10-17). As research continues to increase our understanding of the biologic dimension of psychiatric disorders and mental health, nursing care will focus on human biology in increasingly sophisticated ways. PMH nurses must integrate this information into all aspects of nursing management, including

- *Assessment*—genetic, physical, and environmental factors that contribute to the symptoms of psychiatric disorders; biologic rhythm changes; cognitive abilities that may affect or complicate interventions; and risk factors that may predict development of psychiatric symptoms or disorders
- *Diagnosis*—difficulties related to diet, exercise, or sleep that may change the individual's biology; quality-of-life

Spiritual

1. Spiritual distress
2. Fear of death
3. Fear life has no meaning

Biologic

1. Possible dysregulation of SNS
2. Serotonin dysfunction
3. GABA and benzodiazepine receptor dysfunction
4. Genetic factors
5. Increased consumption of anxiety provoking substances
6. Endocrine dysfunction, e.g., hypothyroidism

Social

1. High-stress lifestyle
2. Multiple life stresses

Psychological

1. Inaccurate assessment of perceived environmental dangers
2. Unresolved unconscious conflicts
3. Hypersensitivity to stress and anxiety-provoking events

FIGURE 10.17 Bio/psycho/social/spiritual etiologies for patients with generalized anxiety disorders. GABA, γ-aminobutyric acid; SNS, sympathetic nervous system.

difficulties based on biologic changes; and knowledge deficits concerning the biologic basis of psychiatric disorders or treatment

- *Interventions*—designed to modify biologic changes and physical functioning; designed to enhance biologic treatments; or modified to consider cognitive dysfunction related to psychiatric disorders

SUMMARY OF KEY POINTS

☐ Neuroscientists now view behaviour and cognitive function as a result of complex interactions within the central nervous system and its plasticity or its ability to adapt and change in both structure and function.

☐ Each hemisphere of the brain is divided into four lobes: the frontal lobe, which controls motor speech function, personality, and working memory—often called the executive functions that govern one's ability to plan and initiate action; the parietal lobe, which controls the sensory functions; the temporal lobe, which contains the primary auditory and olfactory areas; and the occipital lobe, which controls visual integration of information.

☐ The structures of the limbic system are integrally involved in memory and emotional behaviour. Dysfunction of the limbic system has been linked with major mental disorders, including schizophrenia, depression, and anxiety disorders.

☐ Neurons communicate with each other through synaptic transmission. Neurotransmitters excite or inhibit a response at the receptor sites and have been linked to certain mental disorders. These neurotransmitters include acetylcholine, dopamine, norepinephrine, serotonin, g-aminobutyric acid, and glutamate.

☐ Psychoendocrinology examines the relationship between the nervous system and endocrine system and the effects of neurohormones excreted by special neurons to communicate with the endocrine system in effecting behaviour. Psychoimmunology focuses on the nervous system as regulating immune function, which may play a significant role in effecting psychological states and psychiatric disorders. Chronobiology focuses on the study and measure of time structures or biologic rhythms occurring in the body and associates dysregulation of these cycles as contributing factors to the development of psychiatric disorders.

◻ Biologic markers are physical indicators of disturbances within the central nervous system that differentiate one disease process from another, such as biochemical changes or neuropathologic changes. These biologic markers can be measured by several methods of testing, including challenge tests, electroencephalography, polysomnography, evoked potentials, CT scanning, magnetic resonance imaging, positron emission tomography, and single photon emission computed tomography, all of which the PMH nurse must be familiar with.

CRITICAL THINKING CHALLENGES

1 Explain the significance of mental disorders being described as *polygenetic*.

2 A patient who is scheduled for magnetic resonance imaging asks how this test can possibly help explain why he is "all nerved up." He states that his friend had a CT scan, and he wants that instead. What would you say to assist this patient in understanding the difference between the two tests?

3 Define the five different approaches to the study of neuroanatomy and discuss their utility in understanding mental disorders.

4 A woman who has experienced a "ministroke" continues to regain lost cognitive function months after the stroke. Her husband takes this as evidence that she never had a stroke. How would you approach patient teaching and counselling for this couple to help them understand this occurrence if the stroke did damage to her brain?

5 Choose a patient for whom you are caring. Review his or her psychotropic medications and discuss their impact on the patient's CNS. Discuss what side effects might be seen and why.

6 Mr. S is unable to sleep after watching an upsetting documentary. Identify the neurotransmitter activity that may be interfering with his sleep. (Hint: fight-or-flight.)

7 Describe what behavioural symptoms or problems may be present in a patient with dysfunction of the following brain areas:
 a. Basal ganglia
 b. Hippocampus
 c. Limbic system
 d. Thalamus
 e. Hypothalamus
 f. Frontal lobe

8 Compare and contrast the functions of the sympathetic and parasympathetic nervous systems.

9 Discuss the steps in synaptic transmission, beginning with the action potential and ending with how the neurotransmitter no longer communicates its message to the receiving neuron.

10 Examine how a receptor's usual response to a neurotransmitter might change.

11 Compare the role of dopamine and acetylcholine in the CNS.

12 Explain how dopamine, norepinephrine, and serotonin all contribute to endocrine system regulation. Suggest some other transmitters that may affect endocrine function.

13 Discuss how the fields of psychoendocrinology, psychoimmunology, and chronobiology overlap.

14 Compare the methods used to find biologic markers of psychiatric disorders reviewed in this chapter. Consider the potential risks and benefits to the patient.

15 Determine the actions you would take in preparing a patient for an MRI scan.

16 Ask a psychiatric clinician, "What is the greatest diagnostic mystery you've encountered?"

WEB LINKS

www.loni.ucla.edu   This is the site of the Laboratory of Neuro Imaging (LONI) at the University of California at Los Angeles. LONI is dedicated to the development of comprehensive brain mapping as a means to improve understanding of the brain.

www.med.harvard.edu/AANLIB/home.html   This is the site of the Whole Brain Atlas, which provides images of brain structures.

MOVIES, NOVELS, AND BIOGRAPHIES

The Madness of King George: 1994. This movie depicts the experience of King George III as his mental health deteriorates and he loses much of his autonomy to his physicians, despite his royal status.

 VIEWING POINTS: Identify the suppositions (hypotheses) of the physicians as they attempt to understand the way the human body functions. Were their actions in the treatment of King George based solely on these suppositions?

REFERENCES

Cho, M. J., Lyoo, I. K., Lee, D. W., Kwon, J. S., Lee, J. S., Lee, D. S., et al. (2002). Brain single photon emission computed tomography findings in depressive pseudodementia patients. *Journal of Affective Disorders, 69*(1–3), 159–166.

Cook, I.A., Leuchter, A.F., Morgan, M., Witte, E., Stubbeman, W.F., Abrams, M., et al. (2002). Early changes in prefrontal activity characterize clinical responders to antidepressants. *Neuropsychopharmacology, 27*(1), 120–31.

Ekman, R., Persson, R., & Nilsson, C. L. (2002). Neurodevelopmental influences on the immune system reflecting brain pathology. *Neurotoxic Research, 4*(5–6), 565–572.

Fetissov, S., & Déchelotte, R. (2008). The putative role of neuropeptide autoantibodies in anorexia nervosa. *Current Opinion in Clinical Nutrition and Metabolic Care, 11*, 428–434.

Friedman, M. J. (2000). What might the psychobiology of posttraumatic stress disorder teach us about the future approaches to pharmacotherapy? *Journal of Clinical Psychiatry, 61*(7), 44–51.

Fritschy, J. M., & Brunig, I. (2003). Formation and plasticity of GABAergic synapses: Physiological mechanisms and pathophysiological implications. *Pharmacologic Therapy, 98*(3), 299–323.

Garcia, D. A., Marin, R. H., & Perillo, M. A. (2002). Stress-induced decrement in the plasticity of the physical properties of chick brain membranes. *Molecular Membrane Biology, 19*(3), 221–230.

Glazer, R., & Kiecolt-Glazer, J. K. (2005). Stress-induced immune dysfunction: Implications for health. *Nature Reviews Immunology, 5*, 243–251.

Green, R. C., Cupples, L. A., Kurz, A., Auerbach, S., Go, R., Sadovnick, D., et al. (2003). Depression as a risk factor for Alzheimer disease: The MIRAGE Study. *Archives of Neurology, 60*(5), 753–759.

Hale, B. (2008). Open to debate: Moral considerations and the lab monkey. *American Journal of Bioethics, 8*(6), 53–54.

Harlow, J. M. (1868). Recovery after severe injury to the head. *Publication of the Massachusetts Medical Society, 2*, 327.

Harmer, C. J., Hill, S. A., Taylor, M. J., Cowen, P. J., & Goodwin, G. M. (2003). Toward a neuropsychological theory of antidepressant drug action: Increase in positive emotional bias after potentiation of norepinephrine activity. *American Journal of Psychiatry, 160*, 990–992.

Harrison, P. J., & Owen, M. S. (2003). Genes for schizophrenia? Recent findings and their pathophysiological implications. *Lancet, 361*(9355), 417–419.

Heerschap, A., Kok, R. D., & Van De, W. (2003). Antenatal proton MR spectroscopy of the human brain in vivo. *Childrens Nervous System, 17*, 44–46.

Hennig, J., Speck, O., Koch, M. A., & Weiller, C. (2003). Functional magnetic resonance imaging: A review of methodological aspects and clinical applications. *Journal of Magnetic Resonance Imaging, 18*(1), 1–15.

Holcomb, S. (2006). Recommendations for assessing insomnia. *Nurse Practitioner, 31*(2), 55–60.

Ishihara, S., Makita, S., Imai, M., Hashimoto, T., & Nohara, R. (2003). Relationship between natural killer activity and anger expression in patients with coronary heart disease. *Heart Vessels, 18*(2), 85–92.

Kapadia, R. K., & Bassett, A. S. (2008). Recognizing a common genetic syndrome: 22q11.2 deletion syndrome. *Canadian Medical Association Journal, 178*, 391–393.

Kapczinski, F., Lima, M. S., Souza, J. S., Cunha, A., & Schmitt, R. (2003). Antidepressants for generalized anxiety disorder (Cochrane Review). *Cochrane Database System Review, 2*, CD003592.

Kendler, K. S., & Greenspan, R. J. (2006). The nature of genetic influences on behavior: Lessons from "simpler" organisms. *American Journal of Psychiatry, 163*, 1683–1694.

Kleim, J., & Jones, T. A. (2008). Principles of experience–dependent neuroplasticity: Implications for rehabilitation after brain damage. *Journal of Speech, Language, and Hearing Research, 51*, S225–S239.

Kurup, R. K., & Kurup, P. A. (2003). Hypothalamic digoxin: Central role in conscious perception, neuroimmunoendocrine integration and coordination of cellular function—relation to hemispheric dominance. *Medical Hypotheses, 60*(2), 243–257.

Lea, D. H. (2000). A clinician's primer in human genetics: What nurses need to know. *Nursing Clinics of North America, 35*(3), 583–614.

Macalpine, I., & Hunter, R. (1966). The insanity of King George 3d: A classic case of porphyria. *British Medical Journal, 5479*(1), 65–71.

MacGregor, D. G., Avshalumov, M. V., & Rice, M. E. (2003). Brain edema induced by in vitro ischemia: Causal factors and neuroprotection. *Journal of Neurochemistry, 85*(6), 1402–1411.

McGuffin, P., Rijsdijk, F., Andrew, M., Sham, P., Katz, R., & Cardno, A. (2003). The heritability of bipolar affective disorder and the genetic relationship to unipolar depression. *Archives of General Psychiatry, 60*, 497–502.

McGuire, P., Howes, O., Stone, J., & Fusar-Poli, P. (2008). Functional neuroimaging in schizophrenia: Diagnosis and drug discovery. *Trends in Pharmacological Sciences, 29*, 91–98.

Merikangas, K. R., & Avenevoli, S. (2000). Implications of genetic epidemiology for the prevention of substance use disorders. *Addictive Behaviors, 25*, 807–820.

Montgomery, S. A. (2000). Understanding depression and its treatment: Restoration of chemical balance or creation of conditions promoting recovery. *Journal of Clinical Psychiatry, 61*(6), 3–6.

Nolte, J., & Angevine, J. (1995). *The human brain: In photographs and diagrams.* St. Louis, MO: Mosby.

Papousek, I., & Schulter, G. (2006). Individual differences in functional asymmetries of the cortical hemispheres. Revival of laterality research in emotion and psychopathology. *Cognitie, Creier, Comportament /Cognition, Brain, Behavior, 10*, 269–298.

Raiteri, M. (2006). Functional pharmacology in human brain. *Pharmacological Reviews, 58*, 162–193.

Schauf, C., Moffett, D., & Moffett, S. (1990). *Human physiology.* St. Louis, MO: Times Mirror/Mosby.

Shiloh, R., Weizman, A., Epstein, Y., Rosenberg, S. L., Valevski, A., Dorfman-Etrog, P., et al. (2001). Abnormal thermoregulation in drug-free male schizophrenia patients. *European Neuropsychopharmacology, 11*(4), 285–288.

Siegel, J., Badr, S., & Krieger, A. (2005). When sleep is the enemy. *Patient Care, 39*(1), 30–39.

Sperner-Unterweger, B. (2005). Immunological aetiology of major psychiatric disorders: Evidence and therapeutic implications. *Drugs, 65*, 1493–1520.

Vercelletto, M., Martinez, F., Lanier, S., Magne, C., Jaulin, P., & Bourin, M. (2002). Negative symptoms, depression and Alzheimer's disease. *International Journal of Geriatric Psychiatry, 17*(4), 383–387.

Walker, R. (2006). Human and animal subjects of research: The moral significance of respect versus welfare. *Theoretical Medicine & Bioethics, 27*, 305–331.

UNIT *III*

Interventions in Psychiatric and Mental Health Nursing Practice

The Assessment Process

Gerri Lasiuk

Adapted from the chapter "The Assessment Process"
by Mary Ann Boyd

*T*he **nursing process** is a problem-solving method by which nurses can translate value into practice. The four essential components of the nursing process are assessment, planning, implementation, and evaluation. This chapter deals with **assessment**—activities involved with the collection, validation, analysis, synthesis, and documentation of information concerning clients' responses to health and illness.

ASSESSMENT AS A PROCESS

Standard II of the *Canadian Standards of Psychiatric and Mental Health Nursing* states:

Effective assessment, diagnosis and monitoring is central to the nurse's role and is dependent upon theory, as well as upon understanding the meaning of the health or illness experience from the perspective of the client. The nurse explains to the client the assessment process and content and provides feedback. Knowledge is integrated with the nurse's conceptual model of nursing practice, provides a framework for processing client data and for developing client-focused plans of care. The nurse makes professional judgments regarding the relevance and importance of the data, recognizing and including the client as a valued partner. (Canadian Federation of Mental Health Nurses, 2006, p. 11)

This statement underscores the importance of assessment as the basis for developing a plan of care.

Assessment is not a one-time activity. Rather, it is a purposeful, systematic, and dynamic process that is ongoing throughout the nurse's relationship with individuals in his or her care. Effective assessment involves

1. Collaborating with clients and with other members of the health care team to gather holistic assessments through observation, examination, interview, and consultation, while being attentive to issues of confidentiality and pertinent legal statutes.

2. Documenting and analyzing baseline data to identify health status, potential for wellness, health care deficits, potential for danger to self and others; alterations in thought content and/or process, affect behaviour, communication, and decision-making abilities; substance use and dependency; and history of trauma and/or abuse (emotional, physical, neglect, sexual, or verbal).

3. Formulating and documenting a plan of care in collaboration with the client and with the mental health care team and recognizing variability in the client's ability to participate in the process.

4. Refining and expanding client assessment information by assessing and documenting significant change(s) in the client's status and by comparing new data with the baseline assessment and client goals.

5. Continuously assessing and anticipating potential needs and risks. Collaborating with the client to examine his/her environment for risk factors—self-care, housing, nutrition, economic, psychological, and social.

6. Determining most appropriate and available therapeutic modality that meets client's needs, and assisting the client to access these resources (Canadian Federation of Mental Health Nurses, 2006, p. 11).

KEY CONCEPT **Assessment** is a purposeful, systematic, and dynamic process that is ongoing throughout the nurse's relationship with individuals in his or her care. It involves the collection, validation, analysis, synthesis, organization, and documentation of client health–illness information.

Types of Assessment

Depending on the client's needs and the context of care, an assessment may be comprehensive or focused. A **comprehensive assessment** includes a health history and physical examination; considers the psychological, emotional, social, spiritual, ethnic, and cultural dimensions of health; attends to the meaning of the client's health–illness experience; and evaluates how all of this affects the individual's daily living (Fig. 11-1). It is typically done in collaboration with other members of the health care team. The purpose of a comprehensive assessment is to develop a holistic understanding of the individual's problems and needs as well as his or her strengths and resources. With this, the treatment team collaborates with the client to establish a diagnosis, identify treatment goals, and develop a plan of care.

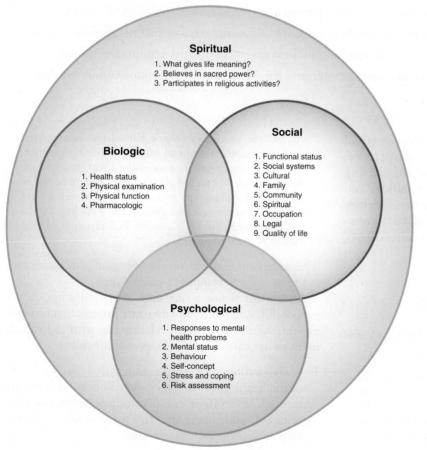

FIGURE 11.1 Bio/psycho/social/spiritual nursing assessment.

Because of its broad scope and the time it takes to develop rapport, a comprehensive assessment may take days or even weeks to complete. Members of the health care team collect information from several sources, including the individual and his or her family, other health care providers, social service and justice personnel, educators, employers, and existing client records. All this is done while attending to issues of confidentiality and pertinent legal statutes.

A **focused assessment** is the collection of specific information about a particular need, problem, or situation and may involve evaluation of such things as medication effects, risk for self-harm, knowledge deficits, or the adequacy of supports and resources. As the name suggests, focused assessments are briefer, narrower in scope, and more present oriented than are comprehensive assessments. Focused assessments are also used to screen individuals who are at high risk for particular problems or disorders. In these instances, nurses often employ standardized assessment tools (e.g., Glasgow Coma Scale, Mini-Mental Status Examination, or Hamilton Depression Inventory).

> ### • CRNENOTE
> Assessment is a part of all nurse–client interactions. It requires a broad theoretical knowledge of human, social, and health sciences; the ability to think critically; and psychomotor and interpersonal skills. Assessment activities include observation, examination, interview, and consultation.

The type of assessment most appropriate for a given situation rests on two key factors: the immediate needs of the client and the practice setting. Efforts to perform a comprehensive assessment during a psychiatric emergency (e.g., when an individual is floridly psychotic or actively suicidal) can be both dangerous and futile. The quality and trustworthiness of the information collected in these circumstances are biased by the client's symptoms and by the high emotionality of the situation. The priority in such situations is to perform a focused assessment that provides the treatment team with sufficient information to treat the client's symptoms and to ensure the safety of all involved.

The type of assessment a nurse performs is also largely determined by the setting in which he or she works. The mandate of a psychiatric and mental health (PMH) facility or program will determine the type of service it offers, which in turn dictates the nature of the assessment required. During the course of a first admission to a psychiatric unit, for example, an individual is likely to undergo a comprehensive assessment. In contrast, nurses working with a telehealth line or with a mobile mental health crisis team will collect only the information required to address the immediate problem or crisis.

Assessment Techniques

Psychiatric and mental health assessments involve observation of the individual at different times of the day and in different circumstances, interviews with the individual and family members, analyses and synthesis of findings from physical and mental examinations into a care plan, and consultation with other health care providers.

Observation

Although verbal communication is vital to the assessment process, nonverbal cues also communicate important information about the client's health–illness experience (see Chapter 9). Nurses learn to engage all of their senses and to seamlessly integrate assessment into all their encounters with clients. Close attention to nuances of dress, manner, facial expression, gestures, and interactions with others (particularly when the individual is not aware of being observed) provide important information that may not otherwise be revealed through conversation. For example, as well as observing hygiene and personal grooming, the nurse considers whether the client's dress is appropriate to the season and situation. Other important observations include behavioural evidence of perceptual disturbances or disordered thoughts (e.g., listening or talking to unseen others) and apparent inconsistencies between what an individual reports and what the nurse observes.

Examination

A comprehensive health assessment includes a health history, a physical examination, and diagnostic testing. This is particularly important in the provision of holistic PMH care because individuals with mental illness are at high risk for a range of physical problems and are less likely than those in the general population to seek regular medical care (Cormac, Ferriter, Benning, & Saul, 2005; Hahm & Segal, 2005; Maj, 2009). Common risk factors in this group include smoking, alcohol and drug use, obesity, poverty, and self-care deficits. It is also important to remain cognizant that medical conditions can mask, imitate, or exacerbate psychiatric symptoms and that psychiatric medications have significant short-term and long-term side effects. The situation is further complicated because some mental illnesses cause an individual to misattribute physical sensations, making it difficult to recognize and describe his or her symptoms.

The **mental status examination** (MSE) is a structured approach to assessing an individual's psychological, emotional, social, and neurologic functioning. Although the components of the MSE are standard across clinical settings, the findings are highly subjective and rely heavily on the clinician's knowledge, communication skills, interpretation, and judgment. For this reason, it is important for clinicians to be self-reflective and to collaborate with colleagues to develop an unbiased understanding of the client's experience.

Interview

An assessment interview is a semistructured conversation aimed at building rapport, obtaining facts, clarifying perceptions and meanings, validating observations, and comparing understandings. Skillful interviewing is much more than peppering an individual with questions about signs and symptoms; it is both an art and a science and takes years of practice to develop (Box 11-1). Effective interviewers train themselves to be fully present to the individual before them, no matter how brief the encounter. They are genuinely warm and respectful and approach individuals in their care as collaborators working toward the same ends. Above all, competent interviewers engage in what Rogers (1975) referred to as empathic listening,

which he describes as:

> entering the private perceptual world of the other and becoming thoroughly at home in it. [Empathic listening] involves being sensitive, moment by moment, to the changing felt meanings which flow in the other person and to the fear or rage or tenderness or confusion or whatever he or she is experiencing. It means temporarily living in the other's life, moving about in it delicately without making judgments (p. 4).

Because many psychiatric symptoms are beyond an individual's awareness, sometimes only those around them are aware of them. For that reason, nurses may also interview family and friends to obtain client-related information. That being said, the Canadian *Privacy Act* imposes obligations on government departments and public agencies, including health-serving facilities, to respect privacy rights and to limit the collection, use, and disclosure of personal information. Today, every province and territory has privacy laws, and it is the responsibility of every nurse to know the limits of information sharing under that legislation.

It is often the case that novice interviewers are so overwhelmed by their own anxieties about interviewing that they become unduly focused on their own experience and on asking questions to elicit needed information. When this happens, the interpersonal nature of the interaction is forgotten. Box 11-2 identifies some interviewer behaviours that are barriers to effective interviewing.

Collaboration

Although nurses have long been vital contributors to interdisciplinary teams, recent health care reforms reiterate the importance of interdisciplinary collaboration. In large part, this is a response to concerns expressed both in the Romanow report (2002) and by the Health Council of Canada about the lack of continuity among health care providers and the institutions in which they work. The shift toward primary health care brings with it an emphasis on teams of health professionals who are accountable for providing comprehensive services to clients. There is a clear consensus that working partnerships among nurses, physicians, and other practitioners result in better health, improved access to services, more efficient use of resources, and higher levels of satisfaction for both consumers and health professionals.

PMH teams typically include the client and his or her family, nurses, physicians, psychologists, social workers, pharmacists, occupational therapists, and recreational therapists. Depending on the treatment setting and the client's particular needs, however, other professionals (e.g., teachers, clergy or spiritual leaders, other medical specialists) may be regular contributors to the team or participate on an *ad hoc* basis. One member of the team is usually assigned to be the client's primary therapist and takes on the role of coordinating team activities to

---

BOX 11.1

Factors That Facilitate Effective Interviewing

- As much as possible, **negotiate the terms of the interview with all the participants** (e.g., choose a mutually agreeable time and place; clearly state your intent; and continually create opportunities for participants to express their thoughts, feelings, wants, and needs). This conveys respect, establishes a human connection, and fosters rapport.
- **The environment.** Choose a private and comfortable setting that is free from interruption.
- **Realistic time management.** Be clear at the outset how much time you have available for an interview and make a realistic plan about what you can achieve. Communicate that to participants.
- **Be attentive to your nonverbal communication.** Sit at the same level of other participants. Maintain an open body posture and actively attend to the encounter. If you intend to make notes, inform others of this at the beginning of the interview. Keep your notes brief; most of your attentional resources should be focused on the interaction.
- **Avoid jargon** and choose language that is clear, simple, and developmentally and culturally appropriate to all participants. Repeatedly check with participants to ensure that they understand what you are saying.
- **Begin with a less sensitive topic and move toward sensitive issues as rapport develops.**
- Leave some time at the end of the encounter for **closure and future planning.** The interviewer is responsible for timekeeping. This involves monitoring the available time and notifying other participants when the interview is coming to an end. Closure activities help participants to disengage from the encounter and orient themselves to the future.

BOX 11.2

Barriers to Effective Interviewing

- **Having a lack of clarity about the purpose and parameters of the interview** is like embarking on a journey without a clear idea of where you are going, your means of travel, and the time you have allotted for the trip. Although you may have some interesting experiences, you also risk missing some important things. A statement such as, "Mrs. Woods, my name is Kate Donovan. I am a nurse on this unit, and I would like to spend the next hour or so getting to know more about you and completing your admission assessment. Is that okay with you?" conveys respect, informs the client of your intent, and begins the process of negotiating a contract for the encounter.

- **Asking too many closed-ended questions**. Closed-ended questions invite brief responses and are most useful for eliciting specific facts, like those needed in a focused assessment. Heavy reliance on them tends to orient the interview around the interviewer's desire for information and prevents clients from introducing or expanding on topics of importance to them.

- **Avoiding silence**. Often in response to their own discomfort or anxiety, interviewers rush to fill all silences with words. Pauses in the conversation allow both the client and the interviewer time to reflect on their experience in the moment, to formulate or elaborate on their responses,

to switch speakers, or to turn the conversation to a new topic.

- **Asking complex questions**. A complex question is really several questions presented as one, as in, "Why did you come to the hospital today, who brought you, and how did you get here?" These types of questions are confusing to the respondent, who often does not know which to answer first. Successful interviewers ask one question at a time, listen carefully to the answer, and probe for more detail if it is not clear.

- **Making assumptions**. Effective interviewers are those who understand that each individual experiences and understands the world in their own unique way. The failure to clarify and validate what the client means results in misunderstanding and inaccuracies.

- **Avoiding or ignoring expressions of emotion**. Emotions are rich communications. They provide insight into the meaning an individual assigns to an experience or event. Minimizing or ignoring an expression of emotion sends a powerful message. For example, "There are parts of you that I do not acknowledge," or "Your emotions are frightening or unimportant," Competent practitioners need to maintain a high level of self-awareness in order to remain grounded in their own experience so that they can bear witness to others.

---

address the client's needs. Teams meet together frequently to share information, to develop and evaluate treatment goals, and to provide ongoing support.

In most PMH treatment facilities, the interdisciplinary team works to develop a psychiatric diagnosis based on the *Diagnostic and Statistical Manual of Mental Health Disorders*, 4th ed., Text revision (*DSM-IV-TR*; American Psychiatric Association, 2000). This diagnosis provides a framework for understanding clients' responses to mental illness.

BIO/PSYCHO/SOCIAL/SPIRITUAL PSYCHIATRIC AND MENTAL HEALTH NURSING ASSESSMENT

A bio/psycho/social/spiritual psychiatric and mental health nursing assessment rests on the assumption that humans are whole, integrated beings who live in constant and reciprocal relationship with their physical and social environments. One's state of health–illness reflects "the extent to which an individual or group is able to realize aspirations and satisfy needs and to change or cope with the environment" (Canadian Nurses Association, 2005). The bio/psycho/social/spiritual model presented in Chapter 6 provides a framework for assessing the physical, psychological, emotional, social, spiritual, ethnic, and cultural dimensions of health. Whereas the goal of medical assessment is the diagnosis and treatment of disease

and illness, nursing assessment aims to develop a holistic understanding of the individual's health–illness experience. Besides identifying health problems and deficits, it attends to strengths and resources and evaluates how these affect the individual's daily living.

Types and Sources of Information

Client information or data fall into two broad categories: *objective* and *subjective*. **Objective data** (also called *signs*) are directly observable and measurable. The physical examination, vital signs, and diagnostic tests all yield objective data. In contrast, subjective data (*symptoms*) are neither directly observable nor measurable. Subjective data are what the client and others report about their thoughts, attitudes, beliefs, emotions, perceptions, experiences, and motivations. A health history provides this type of data. Subjective information provides a window into an individual's inner experience. This experience is influenced by personal history, learning, ethnicity, culture, and spirituality and offers insight into the sense an individual makes of the world. It is critical for nurses to remember that individuals act and react to the *meanings they assign* to events and experiences, rather than to the events or experiences themselves.

Both objective and subjective data are generated from *primary* or *secondary* sources. The individual or client is the primary source of information about himself or herself. Secondary data, on the other hand, come from all other sources, including family, other health care providers, written reports, and client records.

Documentation

Health care records are important vehicles for communication as well as being legal documents. The type of information collected and how it is documented are regulated by the program or facility in which the nurse practices. In turn, programs and facilities develop documentation policies and procedures to comply with provincial and territorial legislation.

Generally speaking, there are two common approaches to documentation: *source-oriented* and *problem-oriented* documentations. In source-oriented documentation, each discipline is assigned a section of the client record (e.g., nurse's notes or physician's notes). Although this approach clearly identifies the discipline of the person making the entry, it tends to fragment the data, which is antithetical to holistic care. In problem-oriented documentation, everyone involved with the care of an individual makes entries in the same section of the record. This not only facilitates interdisciplinary collaboration but also keeps team members oriented toward the client's identified goals, needs, and problems.

Information may be entered in the client record in several ways, including fill-in forms, flow sheets, checklists, and narrative notes. Computerized documentation is becoming more common because it is efficient, saves time, and facilitates electronic sharing of client information. In many settings, practitioners use the SOAP, DAR, or PIE methods to organize their notes (Box 11-3). Another approach to documentation is *charting by exception*, which involves documenting only those client health–illness responses that deviated from well-articulated standards.

BOX 11.3

Methods of Documentation

SOAP METHOD
S = Subjective data
O = Objective data
A = Assessment/clinical judgment
P = Plan/implementation/evaluation

DAR METHOD
D = Data
A = Action
P = Plan

PIE METHOD
P = Problem
I = Implementation
E = Evaluation

Biologic Domain

Health History

The health history (Table 11-1) establishes a subjective database about the client's current and past health–illness experience, identifies strengths and resources, identifies actual and potential health problems and deficits, and is an opportunity to build rapport. Depending on the practice setting, different members of the health care team may take responsibility for sections of the health history. For example, the social worker may perform the family and social assessments, the occupational therapist undertakes the occupational assessment, and the recreational therapist often assesses the individual's exercise and leisure activities. Box 11-4 outlines the components of a health history and relates the significance of important findings to mental health and illness.

Physical Examination

Physical examination is a process by which a clinician collects objective information about the client's health. Components include anthropomorphic measurements

---

BOX 11.4

PQRST Method of Symptom Analysis

Many practitioners use the PQRST acronym to guide their analysis of the nature and characteristics of reported symptoms.

P = Precipitating/ palliative factors	**Ask:** What were you doing when you first noticed it? What makes it better? Worse?
Q = Quality/quantity	**Ask:** Describe the symptom in your own words. What does it feel/look/sound like? Has it changed during this episode? If yes, how? How often do you experience it? How does it affect your day-to-day life?
R = Region/radiation/ related symptoms	**Ask:** Point to where it is. Does it occur or spread anywhere else? What else have you noticed about it?
S = Severity	**Ask:** One a scale of 0 to 10, with 10 being the most severe that this symptom has ever been, where do you rate it at this moment? Using the same scale, what is the usual severity of this symptom?
T = Time	**Ask:** When was the first time you ever experienced it? How often does it occur? How long does it usually last? When did this episode begin?

Table 11.1	Health History and Significance to Psychiatric and Mental Health Problems
Data	**Considerations/Significance**
Source of Information	Ideally, the client is the primary source of information; consultation with secondary sources is necessary with minors or when the client is unable to do so.
	Note the apparent reliability and consistency of the information provided.
Identification/Biographic Information	Legal name/nicknames/aliases; date and place of birth; gender; address; telephone numbers; relationship status; next of kin; ethnicity; religious/spiritual affiliation; employer; education; provincial/territorial health insurance number.
	Because this information is relatively nonthreatening, it is a safe place to begin an assessment. It also provides important clues about an individual's current living situation.
Primary Reason for Seeking Care	Record this verbatim because it speaks to the client's and family's perception of and insight into existing problems; its judgment; and goals for treatment.
Past Health	
Past illness, injury, and/or hospitalization	Note positive history of childhood diseases, especially viral infection, which have been linked to some psychiatric disorders (e.g., schizophrenia).
	Inquire about surgeries and trauma, particularly those resulting in concussion or loss of consciousness.
	Ask about parental alcohol and drug use (especially during pregnancy); birth trauma; lengthy/repeated separation from parents/caregivers because of hospitalization; a pattern of injury suggestive of childhood abuse/neglect; and surgeries.
Chronic illnesses	Chronic illnesses (e.g., diabetes and thyroid dysfunction), even when well-controlled, may affect mental status.
	Highlight known allergies, type of reaction, usual treatment, and effectiveness of treatment.
Family Health History	Record the name, age, and current health status of close relatives (spouse/partner, children, parents, siblings, grandparents, and aunts/uncles). If a family member is deceased, note the date and cause of death and indications of unresolved grief/loss.
	Inquire specifically about diseases/disorders that "run in the family," particularly psychiatric disorders and addictions. A genogram is a useful tool for recording this information.
	Many psychiatric disorders are genetically linked, so a family health history provides information about the client's risk factors. It also provides clues about social roles, the availability of social support, and family resources/stressors.
	Coping strategies, both effective and ineffective, are learned early in life from our family of origin. A family health history can help to identify these.
Developmental Considerations	Note social and educational difficulties, as well as failure to achieve expected developmental milestones. These may be indicative of attentional or interpersonal deficits; behavioural problems; a chaotic family environment; acquired brain injury; or childhood mental illness.
	Ask about early parental death or separation because these may be associated with alterations in attachment and later relationship difficulties.
	The Canadian Government's practice of removing aboriginal children to residential schools traumatized children, fragmented families, decimated cultures/languages, and contributed to serious social and psychological problems that still reverberate among First Nations people.
Immunization/HIV/Hepatitis Status	Individuals with severe and persistent mental illness often live in severe poverty and lack knowledge and resources for health promotion. In addition, many have lifestyles that put them at risk for serious communicable diseases.
Psychological Trauma	Ask: "Have you ever experienced or witnessed anything that threatened your life or safety or the life or safety of a loved one?" If yes, probe for details.
	Psychological trauma associated with natural disasters, motor vehicle crashes, combat, abuse/assault (physical or sexual), and childhood neglect is associated with a number of PMH problems (e.g., particularly posttraumatic stress disorder, other anxiety disorders, and depression).
Current Health Status	Provides information about medical conditions that affect mental status, global functioning, and quality of life.
	A systematic approach to performing a health history ensures thoroughness, helps the clinician to organize/cluster the data, and cues the informant's memory.
	Analyze significant symptoms (see Box 11-4).
Integumentary	Ask about problems/changes in the skin, hair, and nails. Note the presences of scars; piercings/body art; lesions/sores; rashes; discolouration; itching; or unusual sensations.
	Piercings and body art are expressions of one's personal aesthetic, which is part of self-concept. They may also indicate identification with particular social groups.

Continued

Table 11.1	Health History and Significance to Psychiatric and Mental Health Problems *(Continued)*
Data	**Considerations/Significance**
Sensory systems	Note sensory deficits and the use of eye glasses, contact lenses, hearing aids, and dentures. Uncorrected sensory deficits can affect an individual's day-to-day function and ability to communicate. Record the report of unusual perceptions or sensations because these may be related to perceptual or thought disturbances.
Respiratory	Note problems/disease, recurrent infections, cough, sputum, shortness of breath, noisy respirations, and smoking history.
Cardiovascular/ hematologic	Inquire about history of cardiac disease/problems; palpitations; arrhythmias; murmurs; dizzy spells; coldness/blueness/swelling of extremities; leg pain while walking. Individuals who experience panic episodes often present at emergency departments because their signs and symptoms mimic heart attack. Inquire about anemia, bleeding disorders, fatigue, blood transfusions, bruising, and cancers. Monitoring of some long-term neuroleptic medication use (e.g., lithium and clozapine) requires regular blood tests.
Gastrointestinal	Ask about changes in appetite, weight, and bowel patterns; nausea, vomiting, indigestion, gastroesophageal reflux disease; antacid and laxative use; history of disease (e.g., ulcers, irritable bowel syndrome, and cancer); and rectal discharge/bleeding. Alterations in gastrointestinal function are implicated in many psychiatric disorders. An individual may not notice hunger or have the energy to prepare food. Others may handle distressing emotions by eating more than usual. Anticholinergic effects of antipsychotic medication can cause constipation, whereas lithium carbonate can cause diarrhea.
Genitourinary	Note pain/burning on urination, frequency, urgency, dribbling/incontinence, hesitancy, colour of urine, history of urinary tract infection/kidney disease, and frequent night-time urination. Anticholinergic effects of antipsychotic medication can cause urinary hesitancy and/or retention.
Reproductive/breasts	Ask females about menarche; usual pattern of menses (frequency, duration, colour/amount of bleeding, and recent changes); obstetrical history (pregnancies, live births, miscarriages, abortions); infertility; dysmenorrhoea (pain, excessive bleeding); past or current infection/disease (e.g., sexually transmitted infections, sores/lesions, and unusual discharge or odour); date of last Pap smear; sexual orientation; sexual activity (including level of sexual desire, change in frequency of sexual activity, satisfaction with sexual relationships, painful intercourse); and contraceptive use.
	Ask males about number of children; infertility; past or current infection/disease (e.g., sexually transmitted infections, sores/lesions, and penile/rectal discharge); date of last testicular and prostate examinations; sexual orientation; sexual activity (including level of sexual desire, change in frequency of sexual activity, satisfaction with sexual relationships, painful intercourse, erectile/ejaculatory problems); and contraceptive use.
	Ask both men and women about past disease; changes in breasts or nipples (e.g., masses/lumps, pain, and discharge); and breast self-examination. Note the date of female clients' last mammogram.
	Attitudes, beliefs, and expressions of sexuality provide important information about an individual's self-concept, gender identification, quality of relationships, and overall satisfaction with life.
	Changes in level of desire and frequency of sexual activity are common in many psychiatric disorders, including depression, anxiety, and mania.
	Side effects of selective serotonin reuptake inhibitors (SSRIs) are decreased sexual desire and erectile/ejaculatory dysfunction.
	Suicide rates among gay and lesbian youth are higher than the national average.
Musculoskeletal	Note problems with mobility; limited range of motion; pain or weakness; joint problems; disease/injury (e.g., osteoporosis); use of prosthetics; and impairments to activities of daily living.
Endocrine	Ask about disease/illness (e.g., diabetes, hypothyroidism/hyperthyroidism, and goitre); changes in height, weight, hair and skin, appetite, and energy level; excessive thirst; frequent urination; weakness; heat/cold intolerance; and current hormone therapy. Diseases of the endocrine system can imitate symptoms associated with psychiatric disorders (e.g., depression, anxiety, mania, eating disorders, and dementia).
Neurologic	Ask about head trauma; alterations in consciousness; seizures; headaches; changes in cognition and memory; sensory and motor disturbances (numbness, tingling, loss of sensation, tremors, lack of coordination, balance problems, and pain). As well, inquire about alterations in personality, speech, or ability to manage activities of daily living. Neurologic signs and symptoms are associated with many psychiatric disorders as well as with side effects/toxicity of some neuroleptic medications (e.g., neuroleptic malignant syndrome [NMS], serotonin syndrome, and lithium toxicity).

Continued

Table 11.1	Health History and Significance to Psychiatric and Mental Health Problems (*Continued*)
Data	**Considerations/Significance**
Current Medications (including over-the-counter preparations and herbal remedies)	Specify the name of the medication, purpose, usual dose, frequency, effectiveness, side effects, prescriber, and the length of time the client has been taking it. This information helps to assess the client's health-promoting behaviours and potential knowledge deficits. Individuals with serious and persistent mental illness often take several different medications, which puts them at risk for drug–drug and drug–food interactions.
Health/Lifestyle Health promotion/maintenance	Ask individuals to describe what they do on a daily, weekly, and yearly basis to promote and maintain their health. Note the dates of their last physical examination, visit to a dentist, and eye examination.
Nutritional patterns	Ask about usual eating patterns and whether there have been any recent changes. Changes in eating patterns are associated with many affective states and psychiatric disorders. Particularly note dissatisfaction with weight and shape as well as activities aimed at weight loss. Body dissatisfaction is a factor in eating disorders and contributes to self-concept. It is particularly common among girls/women, elite athletes, and those with occupations that emphasize physical appearance (e.g., modelling and dancing). Psychiatric symptoms, neuroleptic medication, and poverty can all affect nutritional status. The weight gain associated with many neuroleptic medications increases individuals' risk for type II diabetes.
Sleep/rest patterns	Changes in sleep patterns can be a response to stress or symptoms of a psychiatric disorder. Probe a positive response about alterations in usual sleep patterns. Ask about *sleep onset* (latency between going to bed and falling asleep); *sleep maintenance* (frequency of wakening during the night and ease of falling back to sleep); and *early morning wakening* (consistently waking up before one needs to be up). Also, ask about whether the individual generally feels rested/refreshed. Alterations in sleep patterns are common in many psychiatric disorders (e.g., depression, mania, and schizophrenia). For many individuals with serious and persistent mental illness, sleep disturbances are early signs of relapse.
Activity/exercise	Ask about usual activity level and type and amount of exercise. Involvement in social activities and hobbies enhances health and reduces stress. Withdrawal from these things may be early signs of illness. Two of the negative symptoms of schizophrenia are anhedonia (decreased ability to experience pleasure) and avolition (lack of motivational drive and energy). These explain why many individuals with schizophrenia sleep excessively. Alterations in usual activities are associated with many mental disorders including depression, mania, schizophrenia, and some eating disorders.
Tobacco, alcohol and nonprescription drug use, and problem gambling	*Tobacco.* Inquire about type (cigarettes, cigars, pipes, and chewing tobacco); age at first use; frequency; and efforts to stop use. *Alcohol.* Ask about age at first use; preferred type (beer, wine, or spirits); usual pattern of drinking; and any recent changes to that pattern. It is also important to explore whether the individual or those close to the individual believe that alcohol is a problem in the individual's life. If yes, probe for details. Many people use alcohol to self-medicate—that is, to cope with stress, unpleasant emotions, sleep disturbances, and so forth. *Nonprescription drugs.* Ask about the age of first use; drug(s) of choice; dose; route; and frequency of nonprescription drug use. Probe for information about the effects of drug use (physical, psychological, emotional, social, legal, and economic). *Problem gambling.* Ask at what age it began; game(s) of choice; frequency; and average amount of money lost per month. Probe for information about the consequences (physical, psychological, emotional, social, legal, and economic).

(e.g., height and weight), vital signs, an examination of all body systems, and diagnostic testing appropriate to the individual's age, level of risk, and sex. The physical examination aids in diagnosing disease or illness, establishes a baseline for evaluating change, and provides an opportunity to validate information provided in the health history. With respect to laboratory studies, particular attention is paid to any abnormalities of hepatic, renal, or urinary function because these systems metabolize or excrete many psychiatric medications. In addition, abnormal white blood cell (WBC) and electrolyte levels are noted. See Table 11-2 for selected hematologic measures and their relevance to psychiatric disorders.

Psychological Domain

The psychological domain encompasses responses to mental health problems, mental status, stress and coping, and risk assessment.

Table 11.2	Selected Hematologic Measures and Their Relevance to Psychiatric Disorders	
Test	**Result**	**Implications**
Complete Blood Count (CBC)		
Leukocyte count (WBC)	Leukopenia ($\downarrow$ WBC)	May be a side effect of phenothiazines, clozapine, carbamazepine
	Agranulocytosis ($\downarrow$ granulocytic WCB)	Lithium causes a benign mild to moderate increase (11,000–17,000/μL).
	Leukocytosis ($\uparrow$ WCB)	NMS can be associated with increases of 15,000–30,000/mm^3 in about 40% of cases.
WBC differential	"Shift to the left"—from segmented neutrophils to band forms	This shift suggests a bacterial infection but has been reported in about 40% of cases of NMS.
Red blood cell (RBC) count	Polycythemia ($\uparrow$ RBC)	Primary form (true polycythemia) is associated with several disease states; requires further evaluation.
		Secondary form is compensation for decreased oxygenation (e.g., chronic obstructive pulmonary disease [COPD]).
		Blood is more viscous, which is exacerbated by being dehydrated.
	$\downarrow$ RBCs	Associated with some types of anemia; requires further evaluation.
Hematocrit (Hct)	$\uparrow$ Hct	Associated with dehydration.
	$\downarrow$ Hct	Associated with anemia; may be related to alterations in mental status, including asthenia, depression, and psychosis.
		Twenty percent of women of childbearing age in North America have iron deficiency anemia.
Hemoglobin (Hgb)	$\downarrow$ Hgb	Indicative of anemia; evaluation of cause requires review of erythrocyte indices.
Erythrocyte indices, such as red cell distribution width (RDW)	$\uparrow$ RDW	Finding suggests a combined anemia resulting from both vitamin B$_{12}$ and folic acid deficiencies and iron deficiency, as found in chronic alcoholism.
		Oral contraceptives also decrease vitamin B$_{12}$.
Other Hematologic Measures		
Vitamin B$_{12}$	Deficiency	May be associated with neuropsychiatric symptoms such as psychosis, paranoia, fatigue, agitation, marked personality change, dementia, and delirium.
Folate	Deficiency	Associated with alcohol use and with medications such as phenytoin, oral contraceptives, and estrogens.
Platelet count	Thrombocytopenia ($\downarrow$ platelets)	Associated with use of some psychiatric medications, such as carbamazepine, phenothiazines, or clozapine and with other nonpsychiatric medications; may also cause thrombocytopenia.
		Also, associated with some disease states; requires further evaluation.
Serum Electrolytes		
Sodium	Hyponatremia (serum sodium)	Associated with significant alterations in mental status. May be related to Addison's disease; the syndrome of inappropriate secretion of antidiuretic hormone (SIADH); polydipsia; and carbamazepine use.
Potassium	Hypokalemia ($\downarrow$ serum potassium)	Associated with weakness, fatigue, electrocardiogram (ECG) changes, paralytic ileus, and muscle paresis.
		Common in individuals exhibiting bulimic behaviour, psychogenic vomiting, misuse of diuretics, and/or excessive laxative use. Hypokalemia may be life threatening.
Chloride	Elevation	Chloride tends to increase to compensate for lower bicarbonate.
	Decrease	Associated with binging and purging behaviour.

Continued

Table 11.2	Selected Hematologic Measures and Their Relevance to Psychiatric Disorders *(Continued)*	
Test	**Result**	**Implications**
Bicarbonate	Elevation	Associated with binging and purging, disordered eating, excessive laxative use, and/or psychogenic vomiting.
	Decrease	May develop in individuals who hyperventilate (e.g., panic disorder).
Renal Function Tests		
Blood urea nitrogen (BUN)	Elevation	Associated with alterations in mental status (e.g., lethargy and delirium), dehydration, and medications excreted by the kidney, such as lithium and amantadine.
Serum creatinine	Elevation	Indicative of decreased renal function; typically does elevate until 50% of nephrons in the kidney are damaged.
Serum Enzymes		
Amylase	Elevation	Associated with the binging and purging behaviour in eating disorders; tends to decline when these behaviours stop.
	Alanine aminotransferase (ALT) > Aspartate aminotransferase (AST)	This disparity is common in acute forms of viral and drug-induced hepatic dysfunction.
Alanine aminotransferase (ALT; formerly serum glutamic pyruvic transaminase, or SGPT)	Elevation	Mild elevations are common with use of sodium valproate.
Aspartate aminotransferase (AST; formerly serum glutamic oxaloacetic transaminase, or SGOT)	AST > ALT	Severe elevations are associated with chronic hepatic disease and myocardial infarction.
Creatine phosphokinase (CPK)	Elevations of the isoenzyme related to muscle tissue	Associated with muscle tissue injury. Level is elevated in NMS and by repeated intramuscular injections (e.g., depot antipsychotics).
Thyroid Function		
Serum triiodothyronine (T_3)	Decrease	Associated with hypothyroidism and other nonthyroid related diseases. Individuals with depression may convert less T_4 to T_3 peripherally, but not out of the normal range. Medications such as lithium and sodium valproate may suppress thyroid function, but clinical significance is unknown.
	Elevation	Indicative of hyperthyroidism; T_3 toxicosis is associated with alterations in mood, anxiety, and symptoms of mania.
Serum thyroxine (T_4)	Elevation	Indicative of hyperthyroidism.
Thyroid-stimulating hormone (TSH)	Elevation	Associated with hypothyroidism, which shares features of depression with the additional physical signs of cold intolerance, dry skin, hair loss, bradycardia, and so forth. Lithium may also cause elevations.
	Decrease	Considered nondiagnostic; may be associated with hyperthyroidism, pituitary hypothyroidism, or even euthyroid status.

Responses to Mental Health Problems

Psychiatric disorders are manifested as characteristic patterns of thoughts, behaviours, and affective states. Like other illnesses, these disorders affect individuals and their families in many different ways. An important part of assessing the psychological domain is to explore the individual's experience of illness. Many have specific fears about losing their job, about their family, or about their personal safety. It is also important to identify the person's strategies for managing the illness and the effectiveness of those strategies. A simple question such as "How do you deal with your voices when you are with other people?" may initiate a discussion about a particular experience or symptom.

Mental Status Examination

The MSE (Box 11-5) is a systematic assessment of an individual's appearance, affect, behaviour, and cognitive processes. It reflects the examiner's observations and impressions at the time of the interview and is used in a variety of clinical settings to evaluate developmental, neurologic, and psychiatric disorders.

KEY CONCEPT The **mental status examination** is a systematic assessment of an individual's appearance, affect, behaviour, and cognitive processes. It reflects the examiner's observations and impressions at the time of the interview and is used in a variety of clinical settings to evaluate developmental, neurologic, and psychiatric disorders.

General Observations

This section of the MSE provides a brief narrative summary of the examiner's observations and impressions of the individual at the time of the interview. Although an individual's health history remains relatively stable, his or her mental status is variable over time.

Appearance. Describe the individual's general appearance and presentation. Note manner and appropriateness of dress, personal hygiene, odours, pupil size, and obvious identifying characteristics, such as tattoos and piercings. Physical signs such as skin tone (e.g., duskiness, pallor,

---

BOX 11.5

Components of the Mental Status Examination

1. General observations
   a. Appearance
   b. Psychomotor behaviour
   c. Attitude toward interviewer
2. Mood
3. Affect
4. Speech characteristics
5. Perception
6. Thought
   a. Content
   b. Process/form
7. Sensorium
   a. Level of consciousness
   b. Orientation (person, place, time)
   c. Memory (immediate retention and recall; recent, short-term, and long-term)
   d. Attention and concentration
   e. Comprehension and abstract reasoning
8. Insight
9. Judgment

---

or flushing), nutritional status, and energy level (e.g., catatonia, lethargy, or restlessness) provide clues to the person's general level of health–illness.

Psychomotor Behaviour. Observe and note the individual's behaviour during the interview, including posture, gait, coordination, facial expression, mannerisms, gestures, and activity. Pay particular attention to cues to the person's emotional state (e.g., perspiration, clamminess, muscle tension, repetitive movements, general activity level).

Attitude Toward Interviewer. The individual's attitude toward the interviewer and the interview process may be described as accommodating, cooperative, open, friendly, apathetic, bored, guarded, suspicious, hostile, or evasive. The following is an example of how the interviewer may describe the individual:

> Mr. D. is a tall, thin, Caucasian man, who looks older than his stated age of 47 years. He is unshaven, his hair is uncombed, and he has a strong body odour. His clothing is stained and dishevelled but appropriate to the season. He reports feeling "jumpy," and he declined to sit during the interview, opting instead to pace around the interview room. His posture is erect and his movements are quick, purposeful, and well coordinated; he displays no unusual mannerisms. Mr. D. was cooperative to the interview process, although his verbal responses were brief, and he did not maintain eye contact.

Mood and Affect

In everyday usage, the terms *emotion*, *feelings*, and *mood* are used interchangeably. In the context of an MSE, however, these words refer to specific phenomena. *Emotion* is the individual's experience of a feeling state, whereas **mood** is "a pervasive and sustained emotion that colours the person's perception of the world" (Saddock & Saddock, 2003, p. 238). Mood is what the individual reports about his or her prevailing emotional state. Although mood does vary with internal and external changes, it tends to be stable over time and reflects the person's disposition or worldview. Mood can be assessed by asking a simple, open-ended question like, "How have you been feeling over the past while?" Whatever the person answers, the interviewer should probe to find whether this is typical or is a response to some recent life event. A person who is generally positive and content will remain so even when bad things happen. He or she will tend to view adversity as a temporary period of unpleasantness in a basically happy life. In contrast, an individual whose mood tends to be negative or depressed views life through dark-coloured glasses. He or she experiences life as difficult and sees happiness as fleeting.

Mood may be sustained for days or weeks, or it may fluctuate during the course of a day. For example, some depressed individuals have a diurnal variation in their mood; they experience their lowest mood in the morning, but as the day progresses, their mood lifts, and they feel somewhat better in the evening. Terms used to describe mood include **euthymic** (normal), **euphoric** (elated), and **dysphoric** (depressed, disquieted, restless).

Affect is the individual's emotional responsiveness during the interview and is inferred from facial expressions, vocalizations, and behaviour. During the assessment, an individual's affect may change as he or she talks about an immediate experience or recent life events. Affect is described in terms of its *range, intensity, appropriateness,* and *stability. Affective range* can be full or constricted. Individuals who express several emotions that are consistent with their stated feelings and the content of what they are saying are described as having a full range of affect that is congruent with the situation. On the other hand, a person who speaks of the recent, tragic death of a loved one in a monotone voice with little outward expression of his or her internal feeling state is described as having constricted affect. In evaluating the *appropriateness* of a particular response, the nurse must consider both the meaning of the event to the individual and cultural norms. Descriptions of *intensity* attempt to quantify an affective response. Intensity may be characterized as heightened, blunted, or flat. An example of heightened affect is the man who reacts to deaths of the victims of the September 11, 2001 attack as if they were all his personal friends. He states that his life stopped when the World Trade Center towers came down; he cried every day and could not eat or sleep for weeks afterward. The phrase *blunted affect* describes limited emotional expression, whereas *flat affect* is its near absence. The person whose affect is flat speaks in a monotone voice and has little or no facial expression. *Stability* of affect can be described as mobile (normal) or labile. If a person displays a wide range of strong emotions in a relatively short period of time, his or her affect is described as being labile.

Speech Characteristics

Patterns and characteristics of speech provide clues about the individual's thoughts, emotions, and cognitive organization. They also convey information about the person's understanding of the situation and ability to read and respond to social cues. Speech is described in terms vof its *quantity, rate and fluency of production,* and *quality.* In assessing speech *quantity,* the individual may be described as talkative, verbose, garrulous, subdued, reticent, or taciturn. *Rate of speech production* may be slow, hesitant, fast, or pressured, whereas *fluency* refers to the apparent ease with which speech is produced. *Pressured speech* is speech that is rapid and increased in amount and difficult to understand; it is often associated with mania. Aphasic disturbances are problems of speech output and may be neurologic, cognitive, or emotional in origin. *Speech quality* refers to its characteristics, such as monotone, whispered, slurred, mumbled, staccato, or loud. During conversation, the interviewer also notes speech impediments (e.g., stuttering), response latency (the length of time it takes for the individual to respond to a question or comment), and repetition, rhyming, or unusual use of words.

Perception

Perception is the complex series of mental events involved with taking in of sensory information from the environment and the processing of that information into mental representations. Two perceptual disturbances commonly associated with mental illness are hallucinations and illusions. **Hallucinations** are false sensory perceptions not associated with external stimuli and are not shared by others. Although auditory hallucinations are the most common type, they may occur in any of the five major sensory modalities: auditory, visual, tactile, olfactory, or gustatory. Most people are familiar with *hypnagogic hallucinations*—false sensory perceptions that occur while falling asleep; these are not associated with mental disorder. Of more concern are *command hallucinations,* the false perception of commands or orders that an individual feels obligated to obey. For example, a person may hear voices telling him or her to harm or kill oneself or someone else. *Illusions* are the misperception or misrepresentation of real sensory stimuli (e.g., misidentifying the wind as a voice calling one's name or thinking that a label on a piece of clothing is an insect).

Thought

Because thought is not directly observable, it is assessed through language in terms of its content and process (form). *Thought content* is what the person is thinking about (e.g., ideas, beliefs, preoccupations, and obsessions), and *thought process* is the manner in which thoughts are formed and expressed. Some individuals are very forthcoming about the content of their thoughts, whereas others are more reticent to talk about them. Assessing thought requires the clinician to carefully attend to and explore unusual or recurring themes in the individual's conversation. Box 11-6 lists some common disturbances of thought content.

Saddock and Saddock (2003) define thinking as "the goal-directed flow of ideas, symbols, and associations initiated by a problem or task and leading toward a reality-oriented conclusion" (p. 282). A number of mental disorders are characterized by disturbances in the form or process of normal thinking. Box 11-7 lists some common disturbances of thought process.

BOX 11.6

Common Disturbances of Thought Content

Delusion—a false, fixed belief, based on an incorrect inference about reality. It is not shared by others and is inconsistent with the individual's intelligence or cultural background and cannot be corrected by reasoning.

Delusions of control—the belief that one's thoughts, feelings, or will are being controlled by outside forces. The following are some specific examples of delusions of control:

- **Thought insertion**—the belief that thoughts or ideas are being inserted into one's mind by someone or something external to one's self

- **Thought broadcasting**—the belief that one's thoughts are obvious to others or are being broadcast to the world

- **Ideas of reference**—the belief that other people, objects, and events are related to or have a special significance for one's self (e.g., a person on television is talking to or about him or her)

Paranoid delusions—an irrational distrust of others and/or the belief that others are harassing, cheating, threatening, or intend one harm

Bizarre delusion—an absurd or totally implausible belief (e.g., light waves from space communicate special messages to an individual)

Somatic delusion—a false belief involving the body or bodily functions

Delusion of grandeur—an exaggerated belief of one's importance or power

Religious delusion—the belief that one is an agent of or specially favoured by a greater being

Depersonalization—the belief that one's self or one's body is strange or unreal

Magical thinking—the belief that one's thoughts, words, or actions have the power to cause or prevent things to happen; similar to Jean Piaget's notion of preoperational thinking in young children

Erotomania—the belief that someone (often a public figure) unknown to the individual is in love with them or involved in a relationship with them

Nihilism—the belief that one is dead or nonexistent

Obsession—a repetitive thought, emotion, or impulse

Phobia—a persistent, exaggerated, and irrational fear

BOX 11.7

Common Disturbances of Thought Process

Loosening of association—the lack of a logical relationship between thoughts and ideas; conversation shifts from one topic to another in a completely unrelated manner, making it confusing and difficult to follow

Circumstantiality—the individual takes a long time to make a point because his or her conversation is indirect and contains excessive and unnecessary detail

Tangentiality—similar to circumstantiality, except that the speaker does not return to a central point or answer the question posed

Thought blocking—an abrupt pause or interruption in one's train of thoughts, after which the individual cannot recall what he or she was saying

Neologisms—the creation of new words

Flight of ideas—rapid, continuous verbalization, with frequent shifting from one topic to another

Word salad—an incoherent mixture of words and phrases

Perseveration—a persisting response to a stimulus even after a new stimulus has been presented

Clang association—the use of words or phrases that have similar sounds but are not associated in meaning; may include rhyming or puns

Echolalia—the persistent echoing or repetition of words or phrases said by others

Verbigeration—the meaningless repetition of incoherent words or sentences; typically associated with psychotic states and cognitive impairment

Pressured speech—speech that is increased in rate and volume and is often emphatic and difficult to interrupt; typically associated with mania or hypomania

Sensorium

This portion of the MSE assesses brain function and cognitive abilities. The Mini-MSE (MMSE; Folstein, Folstein, & McHugh, 1975) is a valid and reliable instrument, widely used to screen for gross impairments in these areas. The MMSE evaluates orientation, memory, calculation, reading and writing, visuospatial ability, and language.

Level of Consciousness. Evaluating level of consciousness (LOC) assesses arousal or wakefulness. An altered LOC typically indicates organic brain impairment. If the individual is not conscious, the nurse applies increasing levels of stimulation (e.g., verbal, tactile, and painful) to elicit a response. Terms used to describe LOC include alert, awake, lethargic, somnolent, stuporous, or comatose.

Orientation. This reflects an individual's ability to perceive and grasp the significance of environmental information. The examiner determines **orientation** by asking questions about time, place, and person because impairments tend to exist in this order (i.e., a sense of time is impaired before a sense of place). The nurse begins with specific questions about the date, time of day, location of the interview, and name of the interviewer and moves to more general questions if necessary. For example, if the client knows the year, but not the exact date, the nurse can ask the season.

Memory. Memory function is traditionally divided into four spheres: *immediate retention and recall; recent memory; short-term memory;* and *remote or long-term memory.* To check immediate retention and recall, the nurse gives the person three unrelated words to remember and asks him or her to recite them immediately and at 5- and 15-minute intervals during the interview. To test recent memory, the nurse asks questions about events of the past few hours or days. Short-term memory involves things that occurred within the past few weeks or months. The nurse assesses remote or long-term memory by asking about events of years ago. If they are personal events and the answers seem incorrect, the nurse may check them with a family member.

Attention and Concentration. To test attention and concentration, the nurse asks the individual to count backward, aloud, from 100 by increments of 7 (e.g., 93, 86, 79, and so on) or to start with 20 and subtract 3. The nurse must decide which is most appropriate for the patient considering education and understanding; subtracting 3s from 20 is the easier of the two tasks. Another way to test these areas is to ask the person to spell a simple word, such as house, backward.

Comprehension and Abstract Reasoning. To test abstract reasoning and comprehension, the nurse asks the person to interpret a simple proverb. Examples include "people in glass houses shouldn't throw stones," "a rolling stone gathers no moss," and "a penny saved is a penny earned." The examiner should keep in mind that proverbs are highly culturally bound and may not be appropriate for persons whose first language is not English. An alternative is to ask the individual to explain the similarities between everyday objects (e.g., apple and orange) or concepts (e.g., truth and beauty).

Insight and Judgment

Insight and judgment are related concepts that involve the ability to examine ideas, conceptualize facts, solve problems, and think abstractly. **Insight** is understanding the reality of a set of circumstances. It reflects the person's awareness of his or her own thoughts and feelings and an ability to compare them with the thoughts and feelings of others. For example, individuals with impaired insight may not believe that they have mental illness. They may have delusions and hallucinations or be hospitalized for bizarre and sometimes dangerous behaviour but do not grasp that this is unusual or abnormal.

Judgment is the ability to reach a logical decision about a situation and to choose a course of action after examining and analyzing various possibilities. Throughout the interview, the nurse evaluates the person's problem-solving abilities and capacity to learn from past experience. For example, a nurse might conclude that an individual who repeatedly chooses partners who are abusive demonstrates poor judgment in selecting partners. Another way to assess judgment is to give a simple scenario and ask the person to identify the best response. An example of such a scenario is, "What would you do if you found a bag of money outside a bank on a busy street?" If the client responds, "run with it," his or her judgment is questionable.

Stress and Coping Patterns

Everyone lives with some degree of stress in their life (see Chapter 35 for a full discussion). For vulnerable individuals, however, stress may contribute to the development of mental disorders. Identification of major stressors in an individual's life helps the nurse to understand and support the use of successful coping behaviours in the future. The nurse should identify the individual's current stressors and coping strategies and evaluate the effectiveness of the latter. This information is vital to the overall plan of care because it highlights both problem areas and resources.

CRNENOTE

A comprehensive assessment should always identify stressors and coping patterns. Identifying how an individual copes with stress can be used as a basis of care in all nursing situations. Review content from Chapter 35 when studying these concepts.

Risk Assessment

Risk factors are those characteristics, conditions, situations, and events that increase the individual's vulnerability to threats to safety or well-being. Throughout this text, assessment of risk factors focuses on risks to safety, risks for developing PMH disorders, and risks for increasing, or exacerbating, symptoms and impairment in individuals with an existing psychiatric disorder.

Assessing safety is a priority and a part of every encounter with clients. Examples include the risk for self-harm or suicide, risk for violence toward others, and risk for adverse events, such as falls, seizures, allergic reactions, or elopement. Nurses must assess these risk factors on a priority basis. For example, they must assess the risk for violence or suicide and take measures to prevent injury, such as implementing environmental constraints, before addressing other assessment factors.

Suicide

A suicide risk assessment involves garnering specific details regarding:

Suicidal ideation—thoughts about self-harm or of self-inflicted death

Threats of suicide—a verbal or behavioural indication (direct or indirect) that an individual is planning to end his or her life

Suicide attempt—action taken to end one's life

To ascertain this information, the nurse asks specific questions about suicidal thoughts, previous suicide attempts (including dates and outcome), the existence and lethality of a suicide plan, access to means, and symptoms of hopelessness. See Chapter 38 for a full discussion.

- Do you currently think about harming or killing yourself? Have you in the past? If the answer to either of these questions is "yes," probe for details about when these thoughts occur and their frequency and intensity.
- Have you ever tried to harm or kill yourself? If the answer is "yes," probe for details about precipitating circumstances, means, and outcome. If the individual has thought about suicide but not acted on these thoughts, determine why not.
- Do you have a plan for how you might kill yourself? If the answer is "yes," ask for details (e.g., when and by what means).
- Do you have the things that you need to carry out this plan?
- Have you made preparations for your death (e.g., writing a good-bye note, putting finances in order, and/or giving away possessions)?
- Has something in your life happened to cause you to think this way? Probe for indications of hopelessness, a sense of helplessness, a loss of enjoyment in life, guilt or shame, anger, or impaired judgment.

From this assessment, the nurse and other members of the team determine the individual's level of risk for self-harm and intervene as necessary. Most PMH programs and facilities use rating scales to quantify an individual's risk for self-harm. Those deemed to be at high risk are usually hospitalized and constantly observed.

Assaultive or Homicidal Ideation

A safety assessment also includes an evaluation of the level of threat an individual poses to others. Of particular importance are delusions or hallucinations that involve harming or killing others. Questions to ask to ascertain assaultive or homicidal ideation are as follows:

- Do you intend to harm someone? If yes, whom?
- Do you have a plan for how you might do this? If yes, what are the details of the plan?
- Do you have the things that you need to carry out your plan? (If the plan requires a weapon, is it readily available?)

Social Domain

A comprehensive assessment also attends to social dimensions of an individual's life. Much of this information is elicited during the health history and the MSE, and it includes information about the individual's current living situation, the individual's family of origin, and the existence and quality of significant relationships (see Chapter 17). The treatment team also assesses work, education, and social and leisure activities. As well, the team observes the individual's interactions with those around him or her. This component of the assessment helps to identify important strengths and resources as well as problems and deficits.

Functional Status

Understanding how an individual functions in his or her day-to-day life is a vital part of assessment. Many mental health teams use the Global Assessment of Functioning (GAF) Scale (discussed in Chapter 2) as a single measure of functioning.

Ethnic and Cultural Assessment

Ethnicity and culture profoundly affect an individual's worldview and frame the person's beliefs about life, death, health and illness, and roles and relationships. As part of a comprehensive assessment, the nurse must consider ethnic and cultural factors that influence health and illness (see Chapter 3). To understand these, the nurse should ask the following questions:

- Do you think of yourself as belonging to a particular ethnic or cultural group? If yes, which one(s)?
- What parts of your culture are most important to you? (Probe for details about values, beliefs, personal practices, social customs, behaviours, etc.)
- What does health mean to you?
- What does illness mean to you?
- How do you define good and evil?
- What things do you do to make yourself physically and mentally healthy?
- To whom do you turn when you feel physically or mentally ill?

Nurses must be clear about their own spirituality to ensure that it does not interfere with assessment of the client's spirituality.

Spiritual Assessment

See Chapter 6 for a definition of spirituality. Examples of questions that may foster an understanding of an individual's spirituality include

- What gives your life meaning?
- What brings joy to your life?
- Do you believe in God or a higher power?

- Do you participate in any religious activities? If yes, which ones?
- Do you feel connected with the world?

SUMMARY OF KEY POINTS

☐ **Assessment** is a purposeful, systematic, and dynamic process that is ongoing throughout the nurse's relationship with individuals in his or her care. It involves the collection, validation, analysis, synthesis, organization, and documentation of the client's health–illness information.

☐ A **comprehensive assessment** includes a health history and physical examination; considers the psychological, emotional, social, spiritual, ethnic, and cultural dimensions of health; attends to the meaning of the client's health–illness experience; and evaluates how all this affects the individual's daily living. A **focused assessment** is the collection of specific information about a particular need, problem, or situation. It is briefer, narrower in scope, and more present oriented than a comprehensive assessment.

☐ Techniques of data collection include observation, interview, physical and mental examinations, and collaboration.

☐ Biologic assessment includes health history, physical examination, and diagnostic testing.

☐ Assessment of the psychological domain includes understanding the individual's response to mental health problems, MSE, evaluation of stress and coping, and risk assessment.

☐ The MSE is a systematic assessment of an individual's appearance, affect, behaviour, and cognitive processes. It reflects the examiner's observations and impressions at the time of the interview and is used in a variety of clinical settings to evaluate developmental, neurologic, and psychiatric disorders.

☐ Risk factors are those characteristics, conditions, situations, or events that increase the individual's vulnerability to threats to safety or well-being. Examples include the risk for self-harm or suicide, violence toward others, and the risk for adverse events, such as falls, seizures, allergic reactions, or elopement.

☐ The social assessment involves a family and relationship assessment, evaluation of functional status, and information about the individual's ethnicity and culture.

☐ Nurses must be aware of their own spiritual beliefs and ensure that those beliefs do not affect their spiritual assessment of the client.

CRITICAL THINKING CHALLENGES

1 A 23-year-old Caucasian woman is admitted to an acute psychiatric setting because she has been depressed for most of the past month. Yesterday she was taken to the Emergency Department after she cut her wrists. Her admission form states that this is her first psychiatric admission, although she reports bouts of depression since early adolescence. She and her fiancé have just ended their engagement and moved into separate apartments. She has not yet told anyone that she is pregnant. She reports that her mother believes that she was "living in sin" and that she would "pay for it." From this scenario, develop three assessment questions for each domain: biologic, psychological, and social.

2 Reflect on the biologic, psychological, emotional, social, and spiritual factors that affect your own self-concept. How do your personal beliefs, values, and experiences affect your interactions with individuals with mental health/psychiatric problems? How might these things facilitate or hinder you?

WEB LINKS

www.cfmhn.ca/index.html Canadian Federation of Mental Health Nurses (CFMHN). This site provides the *Standards of Psychiatric-Mental Health Nursing* (2006), information about the CFMHN activities, and links to sites of interest to PMH nurses.

www.cna-nurses.ca Canadian Nurses Association. This website provides a copy of the *Code of Ethics for Registered Nurses* (2008), information about current issues of interest to nurses, position statements, and links to other Canadian nursing organizations.

www.healthcouncilcanada.ca/en/ This site describes the mission, mandate, and activities of the Health Council of Canada.

laws.justice.gc.ca/en/P-21/index.html This is the site maintained by the Department of Justice Canada and contains the *Privacy Act*.

psychcentral.com/ocdquiz.htm This is a public service site that has several self-report mental health screening tests.

library.med.utah.edu/neurologicexam/html/mentalstatus_normal.html This site describes a full neurological examination, including the video clips of various components of the mental health status examination.

REFERENCES

American Psychiatric Association. (2000). *Diagnostic and statistical manual of mental disorders* (4th ed., Text revision). Washington, DC: Author.

Canadian Federation of Mental Health Nurses. (2006). *Canadian standards of psychiatric and mental health nursing* (3rd ed.). Retrieved June 11, 2009, from http://www.cfmhn.org/Documents/Standards%20%20english%20doc.htm

Canadian Nurses Association. (2005). *Canadian nurse practitioner core competency framework*. Ottawa, ON: Author.

Cormac, I., Ferriter, M., Benning, R., & Saul, C. (2005). Physical health and health risk factors in a population of long-stay psychiatric patients. *Psychiatric Bulleting, 29*, 18–20.

Folstein, M. F., Folstein, S. E., & McHugh, P. R. (1975). Mini-mental state: A practical method for grading the cognitive state of patients for the clinician. *Journal of Psychiatric Research, 12*, 189–198.

Hahm, H. C., & Segal, S. P. (2005). Failure to seek health care among the mentally ill. *American Journal of Orthopsychiatry, 75*(1), 54–62.

Maj, M. (2009). Physical health care in persons with severe mental illness: A public health and ethical priority. *World Psychiatry, 8*(1), 1–2.

Rogers, C. R. (1975). Empathic: An unappreciated way of being. *The Counseling Psychologist, 5*(2), 2–10. Available at: http://tcp.sagepub.com/cgi/reprint/5/2/2-a

Romanow, R. J. (2002). *Building on values: The future of health care in Canada. Final Report.* Ottawa, ON: National Library of Canada. Retrieved June 11, 2005, from http://www.cbc.ca/healthcare/final_report.pdf

Saddock. J., & Saddock, V. A. (2003). *Kaplan's & Saddock's synopsis of psychiatry: Behavioral sciences and clinical psychiatry* (9th ed.). Philadelphia, PA: Lippincott Williams & Wilkins.

CHAPTER 12

Diagnosis and Outcomes Development

Christine Davis

Adapted from the chapter "Diagnosis and Outcomes Development" by Doris Bell and Lorraine D. Williams

LEARNING OBJECTIVES

After studying this chapter, you will be able to:

- Define components of nursing diagnoses.
- Discuss the use of nursing diagnoses in psychiatric and mental health care.
- Define and explore alternatives to nursing diagnosis, such as the Tidal Model or the Recovery Model.
- Explain the use of best practice guidelines.
- Discuss the relationship between client-centred care, patient outcomes, and quality care.
- Discuss the use of individual outcomes in psychiatric and mental health nursing.
- Describe the process of developing individual outcomes with clients.
- Write individual outcome statements for psychiatric and mental health nursing care.

KEY CONCEPTS

- best practice guidelines
- client-centred care
- defining characteristics
- nursing diagnosis
- outcomes

KEY TERMS

- defining characteristics • diagnosis-specific outcomes • discharge outcomes
- indicators • initial outcomes • revised outcomes

After completing an assessment of the individual who is to receive care, the nurse generates appropriate nursing diagnoses based on the assessment data. With experience, the nurse can easily cluster the assessment data to support one nursing diagnosis over another. Mutually agreed-on goals flow from the nursing diagnoses and provide guidance in determining appropriate interventions. Initial outcomes are determined and then are monitored and evaluated throughout the care process. Measuring outcomes not only demonstrates clinical effectiveness but also helps to promote rational clinical decision making and is reflective of the nursing interventions. This chapter describes the development of nursing diagnosis, client-centred care, and individual outcomes in psychiatric and mental health (PMH) nursing

within the context of the Canadian health care system. As the terms "patient" and "client" are used interchangeably in the nursing literature, both terms are used in this chapter according to common use.

EVOLUTION OF NURSING DIAGNOSIS AND INDIVIDUAL OUTCOMES

The concepts of nursing diagnosis and individual outcomes are not new ones. Florence Nightingale identified patient problems and analyzed patient outcomes during the Crimean War. As early as 1962, Mildred Aydelotte published one of the first nursing studies involving patient outcomes. In 1984, Lang and Clinton proposed these outcomes: physical health status, mental health status, social and physical functioning, health attitude, knowledge and behaviour, use of professional health resources, and patient perception of the quality of nursing care. In 1989, Marek identified 15 outcome categories: physiologic measures, symptom control, frequency of service, home maintenance, psychosocial measures, well-being, functional status, goal attainment, patient behaviours, patient satisfaction, patient knowledge, rehospitalization, safety, cost, and resolution of nursing diagnoses. In the 1990s, efforts focused on developing outcomes that could be used to evaluate nursing effectiveness.

In Canada, in the early 2000s, the Registered Nurses Association of Ontario (RNAO) was funded by the Ontario Ministry of Health and Long-Term Care to develop, implement, evaluate, and revise Best Practice Guidelines (BPGs) that would inform nursing practice in a number of areas. The Nursing Best Practice Guideline (BPG) Program connects research and practice to ensure that individuals and families participate in and receive the most up-to-date evidence-based care, ensuring better outcomes for individuals and thereby reducing costs (RNAO Best Practice Guidelines, 2005).

 KEY CONCEPT   Best practice guidelines (BPGs), also termed clinical practice guidelines (CPGs), are broad or specific recommendations for health care based on the best current evidence.

See Box 12-1 for examples of available RNAO guidelines. See Web Links for access information. BPGs support nurses in making good clinical decisions. They are to be used flexibly and in conjunction with knowledge of the preferences of the people seeking care.

BOX 12.1

Examples of RNAO Practice Guidelines

Caring strategies for older adults with delirium, dementia, and depression
Client-centred care
Crisis intervention
Enhancing healthy adolescent development
Establishing therapeutic relationships
Postpartum depression
Suicidal ideation and behaviour
Supporting clients on methadone maintenance treatment
Supporting and sustaining families through expected and unexpected life events
Women abuse: screening, identification, and initial response

CURRENT TRENDS IN CANADA

The current trend in nursing in Canada is away from the nurse as an expert about a patient's needs and toward a client-centred approach with the recognition that individuals, as whole and unique beings (RNAO, 2002b), make meaning of their own lived experiences and participate in all aspects of their care (Canadian Collaborative Mental Health Initiative [CCMHI], 2006).

KEY CONCEPT   Client-centred care is an approach to care in which the client is recognized as a whole person with the right to autonomy, self-determination, and participation in decision-making (RNAO, 2002a).

The CCMHI, a consortium of 12 national organizations, representing community services, consumer, family and self-help groups, dietitians, family physicians, nurses, occupational therapists, pharmacists, psychologists, psychiatrists, and social workers was established in 2004 to enhance mental health services in primary health care. At the core of CCMHI's work are the needs of consumers or individuals (Gagne, 2005). Consumer "centredness," or client-centred care, involves individuals, families, and caregivers in all areas of care from treatment choices to evaluation (Gagne).

Although the importance of identifying outcomes of nursing interventions has been the subject of several nursing research studies since the 1960s, escalating health care costs have forced the demonstration of measurable outcomes. Concerns about quality, cost, and use of limited resources have contributed to the current emphasis on both evidence-based practice and individual outcomes. With the expansion of nursing knowledge gained through measuring intervention effectiveness, the nursing discipline itself will continue to evolve.

DERIVING A NURSING DIAGNOSIS

KEY CONCEPT   A nursing diagnosis is a clinical judgment about an identified problem or need that requires nursing interventions and nursing management. It is based on data generated from a nursing assessment. A formal nursing diagnosis statement includes defining characteristics and related factors (Carpenito-Moyet, 2004).

Because nursing diagnoses provide the basis for planning nursing interventions, they are used in diverse practice settings in multiple individual populations to assist individuals to achieve positive health outcomes (Delaney, Herr, Maas, & Specht, 2000). For nurses to improve their ability to make sound nursing diagnoses, they must actively apply nursing principles, concepts, and theories to the care of the individual (Kleinpell, 2003). The 2009–2011 taxonomy of nursing diagnoses from the North American Nursing Diagnosis Association (NANDA) can be found on *thePoint*.

> **KEY CONCEPT** **Defining characteristics** are key signs and symptoms (clues) that relate to each other and that validate a nursing diagnosis. The nurse analyzes these characteristic clues to formulate a cluster of data, which helps in selecting an appropriate diagnosis or diagnoses reflecting the actual or potential health status or problems of the individual.

Clusters of data lead the nurse to choose certain diagnoses over others. For example, when assessing an individual, the nurse observes that the individual's responses are often self-negating (e.g., "I always mess things up," "I never get it right"). The nurse also observes that the individual shows indecisiveness and lacks problem-solving abilities (e.g., "I can never decide what the right thing to do is, and when I do finally choose, it is always wrong"). Nonverbal and verbal information should be used to identify **defining characteristics**. Observations of the individual sitting with her head down, making no eye contact, and dressed in dirty clothes are important data that should be considered in support of a nursing diagnosis. Such observations support the hypothesis that the individual has a disturbance in self-esteem. Further assessment will help the nurse determine whether the self-esteem disturbance is chronic or situational.

Related factors are those that influence or change the individual's health status and are associated with the nursing diagnosis. Related factors are grouped into four categories: pathophysiologic (biologic or psychological or spiritual), treatment-related (medications, diagnostic studies, surgeries), situational (environmental, home, community, person), and maturational (age-related influences) (Carpenito-Moyet, 2004). To continue with the assessment example, the nurse learns that the individual has lost three jobs within the past year, resulting in financial problems. These situation-related factors further support the nursing diagnosis of self-esteem disturbance.

In the real world, most PMH nurses practice in an interdisciplinary or multidisciplinary environment. Nursing diagnoses are dimensional, not categorical (as is the *Diagnostic and Statistical Manual of Mental Disorders*, 4th ed., Text revision [*DSM-IV-TR*] psychiatric disorder diagnoses [American Psychiatric Association, 2000]), so they may be helpful to other members of the team. Degrees of problems can be considered and measurable outcomes developed. Despite the use of nursing diagnosis by other disciplines, the nursing interventions need to be clearly specified.

■ DEVELOPING INDIVIDUAL OUTCOMES

> **KEY CONCEPT** **Outcomes** are the individual's response to nursing care at a given point in time. An outcome is concise, stated in few words and in neutral terms. Outcomes describe an individual's state, behaviour, or perception that is variable and can be measured (Table 12-1).

According to the *Canadian Standards of Psychiatric-Mental Health Nursing* and the *Scope and Standards of Psychiatric–Mental Health Nursing Practice*, outcomes are expected to be individualized to each person (American

Table 12.1	Example of Outcomes	
Diagnosis	**Outcome**	**Intervention**
Spiritual distress Related to conflict between religious or spiritual beliefs and prescribed health regime	Will express religious or spiritual satisfaction **Indicators** a. Express decreased feelings of guilt and fear. b. State that conflict has been eliminated.	Provide accurate information about treatment plan. Encourage the client and the physician to consider alternative methods of therapy. Support client making informed decisions—even if decision conflicts with own values.

From Carpenito-Moyet, L. J. (2010). *Nursing diagnosis: Application to clinical practice* (13th ed.). Philadelphia, PA: Lippincott Williams & Wilkins.

Table 12.2	Clinical Path: Depression			
Day	Assessment Parameters	Nursing Diagnosis	Nursing Interventions	Patient Outcomes
1	Individual admits to having a suicide plan.	Risk for Self-Directed Violence	Institute suicide precautions.	Suicide: self-restraint
2 3	Individual is apathetic, does not wash or dress self.	Ineffective Health Maintenance	Maintain suicide precautions. Help individual with personal hygiene, exhibit patience.	Suicide: self-restraint Self-care: dressing and bathing

Table 12.3	Results of Nursing Interventions	
Diagnosis	Patient Outcome	Nursing Intervention
Anticipatory Grieving	Grief resolution (adjusting to impending loss) **Indicators** a. Express feelings about loss. b. Express feelings about how life will change due to loss. c. Maintain relationships until death occurs. d. Maintain nutrition. e. Maintain social support. f. Practice skills and role function needed in the future.	Provide supportive feedback to verbal concerns and feelings.

Nurses Association, American Psychiatric Association, & International Society of Psychiatric–Mental Health Nurses, 2000; Canadian Federation of Mental Health Nurses, 2006) (Table 12-2). Individual outcomes are linked to nursing diagnoses through the nursing process. By linking outcomes to the nursing diagnosis, it is possible to monitor nursing practice and facilitate clinical decision-making and knowledge development (Table 12-3).

Outcomes can be defined as an individual's response to care. Outcome identification has moved away from the clinical symptoms and laboratory signs that medicine has traditionally used to describe individual knowledge, behaviours, and quality of life. Outcomes are the end result of a process, a treatment, or a nursing intervention and should be monitored and documented over time and across clinical settings. **Diagnosis-specific outcomes** show that the intervention resolved the problem or nursing diagnosis (Table 12-4). At other times, the outcome is nonspecific (i.e., not diagnosis-specific, meaning it does not show resolution of the diagnosis). In that case, the outcome is abstract or general (Table 12-5).

Indicators answer the question, "How close is the individual moving toward the outcome?" The indicator represents the dimensions of the outcome. Outcome indicators represent or describe individual status, behaviours, or perceptions evaluated during an individual's assessment. Indicators are a measurement of individual progress in relation to the individual outcomes and can serve as intermediate outcomes in a clinical pathway or standardized care plan. See Table 12-6 for examples of

Table 12.4	Example of Condition: Diagnosis-Specific Outcomes	
Diagnosis	Outcome
Anxiety	a. Anxiety control b. Aggression control

Table 12.5	Example of System-Specific Outcome	
Diagnosis	Outcome
Disturbed Sensory Perception (hallucination)	Movement disorder occurrence **Indicators** a. Initiation of antipsychotic drugs b. Demonstration of choreic movement c. Demonstration of pelvic gyrations d. Increase or decrease in dosage of antipsychotic drugs

outcomes linked to nursing diagnoses and Table 12-7 for examples of expected outcomes from nursing interventions.

In nursing care planning, outcomes can be **initial outcomes** (those written after the initial individual interview and assessment), **revised outcomes** (those written after each evaluation), or **discharge outcomes** (those outcomes to be met before discharge). Because of the decreased length of stay or days of service, discharge outcomes often are not met but are passed along to the

Table 12.6	Example—Linkage of Nursing Diagnosis and Outcomes
Diagnosis	**Outcome**
1. Disturbed Body Image	Self-mutilation restraint
2. Chronic Confusion	Improved thought control
3. Ineffective Denial	Anxiety control

From Johnson, M., Maas, M., & Moorhead, S. (2000). *Iowa outcomes project: Nursing outcomes classification (NOC)* (2nd ed.). St. Louis, MO: Mosby.

Table 12.7	Expected Outcomes From Nursing Interventions
Nursing Intervention	**Expected Outcome**
Provide educational information about mental illness	Knowledge: disease process
Educational group in caregiving	Caregiver: individual relationship
Group therapy	Improved thought control
Weight control counselling	Knowledge: diet
Health teaching	Knowledge: medication
Teaching limit setting	Coping
Reality orientation	Identity: self
Life review	Hope
Teaching anger management	Impulse control

Based on Johnson, M., Maas, M., & Moorhead, S. (2000). *Iowa outcomes project: Nursing outcomes classification (NOC)* (2nd ed.). St. Louis, MO: Mosby.

community nurse. If these discharge outcomes continue to be relevant, they become initial outcomes in community or home care.

Documentation of Outcomes

Nurses are accountable for documentation of individual outcomes, nursing interventions, and any changes in diagnosis, care plan, or both. Individual responses to care are documented as changes in behaviour or knowledge and can include the degree of satisfaction with the health care provided (Kleinpell, 2003). Outcomes can be expressed in terms of the individual's actual responses (e.g., no longer reports hearing voices) or the status of a nursing diagnosis at a point in time after implementation of nursing interventions, such as "caregiver role strain resolved." This documentation is important for further research and quality of care studies.

Purposes of Individual Outcomes

The primary purposes of developing individual outcomes are to ensure the needs of the individual are being met and to ensure quality care. They provide guidelines for what is expected of the individual and direction for continuity of care that reflects current knowledge in the field of PMH nursing. The measurement of individual outcomes helps to meet the goal of continuous quality improvement.

Accountability is an important concept in health care. Nursing and other disciplines are being pressured within health services systems to justify their practice, to demonstrate to consumers that they deliver quality care, and to control health care costs. Measurement of outcomes can be used to determine quality of care during a single episode of illness and across the continuum of care and can assist in discharge planning. Outcomes also can be used to determine quality of care in different systems and between systems. Evaluation of individual outcomes can help validate nursing interventions by identifying which interventions are effective. Outcomes can also be a communication tool when working with other nurses, case managers, caregivers, and policy makers and can be used to conduct program evaluations and develop research databases.

■ EVALUATION

Evaluation of individual outcomes involves answering the following questions:

- What were the benefits for the individual?
- What was the individual's level of satisfaction?
- Was the outcome diagnosis specific or nonspecific?
- What is the cost-effectiveness of the intervention?

When measuring outcomes, nurses must consider the time frame. Identifying the intermediate outcome indicators that may be achieved in one setting versus the indicators that can be achieved in a second setting provides for a measurement of progression and enhances continuity of care. Nevertheless, not until the individual is discharged or moved to a community setting can it be known if indicators such as demonstration of confidence when alone at home, demonstration of confidence in role skills (worker/mother), and demonstration of self-advocacy behaviour are achieved.

Outcomes can be measured immediately after the nursing intervention or after time passes. Remember that outcomes based on health prevention and health promotion diagnoses can occur after considerable time has passed.

Future Practice Considerations

In some Canadian mental health settings, the NANDA nursing diagnosis taxonomy is seen to be less client centred and therefore less meaningful to the individual's lived experience. The antithesis of NANDA nursing diagnosis is the Tidal Model, a theory-based approach to mental health nursing emphasizing the "need for nurses to collaborate closely with the people by developing a therapeutic user-empowering relationship" (see Chapter 8).

That change is life's only constant is a core element in this theory (hence the metaphor of the tide). Care is grounded on an understanding of the individual's present and future needs in the personal domains of world, self, and other (Barker, 2001).

The Recovery Model is another example of an alternative to the more traditional way of working with people living with mental illness. The Recovery Model comes out of the consumer of mental health services movement and the work of Dr. William Anthony (1993). It supports individual potential for recovery and focuses on the personal journey involved. A vision of recovery need not be grounded in the etiology of the illness, it is argued, but rather in the person's opportunity for empowerment and meaningful support. Recovery is not a linear experience and can be happening even if symptoms reoccur. The underlying message is one of hope and resumption of a meaningful life despite serious mental illness (Anthony). For this to occur, external conditions that facilitate recovery need to evolve the upholding of human rights, a positive culture of healing, and recovery-oriented services (Jacobson & Greenley, 2001). A criticism expressed toward this model is that recovery may seem a matter of will power, with an implicit message that those who are not recovering are lacking in this quality. It is integral to this model, however, that the social implications of living with a mental illness must be addressed and that recovery should be a guiding principle in mental health care systems (The Canadian Mental Health Association, Ontario Division, 2003).

SUMMARY OF KEY POINTS

☐ The Canadian Standards of Psychiatric-Mental Health Nursing (Canadian Federation of Mental Health Nurses, 2006) support the importance of outcome identification.

☐ Outcomes must be measurable and indicative of the individual's progress.

☐ More research is needed to identify individual outcomes as they relate to nursing interventions and nursing diagnosis.

☐ Nursing diagnoses, nursing interventions, and individual outcomes are initially derived from the assessment data.

☐ Initial, revised, and discharge outcomes can be included in a nursing care plan.

☐ Outcome statements can cover the bio/psycho/social/spiritual domains.

☐ Nursing care, from assessment to outcome measurement, needs to be client centred. This means more than a recognition of the client's right to participate in health care decisions. It means genuine respect of the client's life experience and hopes for recovery.

CRITICAL THINKING CHALLENGES

1 Create a nursing care plan with NANDA diagnoses for Ben, a 19-year-old man admitted to your unit. Ben is an engineering student who lives at home to avoid going into debt while at university. Until recently, Ben was a stellar student and quite an athlete, involved in hockey and lacrosse. Over the past couple of months, Ben has been struggling with exams and playoffs. He is not sleeping well at night but is staying up all night and sleeping most of the day. He wanders around his parents' home at night rummaging in the basement. He has not eaten with the family for awhile, stating that he doesn't like what his mother or father has made for the meal. Ben's grooming is poor; he seldom showers or changes his clothes. Ben refuses to let anyone into his bedroom, yelling at his parents to go away and leave him alone. Ben's parents can hear him inside his room talking angrily. Ben has no history of drug or alcohol use. He has never been in trouble with the law. Ben has lots of friends but now refuses to talk on the telephone with them or to go out with them. His parents are very concerned about him.

2 Explore what it is like to experience and to live with a psychiatric diagnosis. Read about Hayne's (2003) Canadian phenomenological study in which she points to the "particular kind of power" (p. 722) that medical diagnostic language has. Do you think nursing diagnostic language has a similar power?

3 In order to understand personal journeys of recovery, turn to autobiographies about such journeys. Two Canadian sources are Capponi, P. (1992). *Upstairs at the crazy house.* Toronto, ON: Viking and Nunes, J., & Simmie, S. (2002). *Beyond crazy: Journeys through mental illness.* Toronto, ON: McClelland and Stewart.

4 What might the potential barriers be to implementing either the Tidal Model or the Recovery Model in a PMH care setting?

WEB LINKS

www.carmha.ca   This website is the Centre for Applied Research in Mental Health and Addictions at Simon Fraser University that has a number of evidence-based documents available.

www.rnao.org/bestpractices/index.asp   This website offers RNAO Best Practice Guidelines.

www.mentalhealth.org.uk   This website of Britain's Mental Health Foundation provides a wealth of free resources on mental health issues for both clients and caregivers, including international awareness events and the latest news in mental health research.

www.mhrecovery.com   This is a recovery-based website, supported by an Ohio county board that has best practices and resources listed. Beware that some pages represent commercial enterprises.

www.camimh.ca This is the site for the Canadian Alliance of Mental Illness and Mental Health, an alliance of mental health organizations comprised of health care providers, as well as the mentally ill and their families.

www.psrrpscanada.ca Site for Psychosocial Rehabilitation Canada/Réadaptation Psychosociale Canada—an association of individuals and organizations committed to the provision of psychosocial rehabilitation services to support the recovery of persons with serious mental health issues.

www.tidal-model.co.uk This site has information regarding the Tidal Model.

REFERENCES

American Nurses Association, American Psychiatric Association, & International Society of Psychiatric–Mental Health Nurses. (2000). *Scope and standards of psychiatric–mental health nursing practice.* Washington, DC: American Nurses Publishing.

American Psychiatric Association. (2000). *Diagnostic and statistical manual of mental disorders* (4th ed., Text revision). Washington, DC: Author.

Anthony, W. A. (1993). Recovery from mental illness: The guiding vision of the mental health service system in the 1990's. *Psychosocial Rehabilitation Journal, 16,* 11–23.

Aydelotte, M. K. (1962). The use of individual welfare as a criterion measure. *Nursing Research, 11,* 10–14.

Barker, P. (2001). The Tidal Model: Developing a person-centred approach to psychiatric and mental health nursing. *Perspectives in Psychiatric Care, 37,* 79–87.

Canadian Collaborative Mental Health Initiative. (2006). *Canadian Collaborative Mental Health Charter.* Mississauga, ON: Author.

Canadian Federation of Mental Health Nurses. (2006). *Canadian standards of psychiatric and mental health nursing.* Available at: http://www.cfmhn.org

Carpenito-Moyet, L. J. (2004). *Nursing diagnosis: Application to clinical practice* (10th ed.). Philadelphia, PA: Lippincott Williams & Wilkins.

Carpenito-Moyet, L. J. (2010). *Nursing diagnosis: Application to clinical practice* (13th ed.) Philadelphia, PA: Lippincott Williams & Wilkins.

Delaney, C., Herr, K., Maas, M., & Specht, J. (2000). Reliability of nursing diagnoses documented in a computerized nursing information system. *Nursing Diagnosis, 11*(3), 121–135.

Gagne, M. A. (2005). What is collaborative mental health care? An introduction to the collaborative mental health care framework. Report prepared for the Canadian Mental Health Care Initiative. Mississauga, ON: Canadian Mental Health Care Initiative.

Hayne, Y. (2003). Experiencing psychiatric diagnosis: Client perspectives on being named mentally ill. *Journal of Psychiatric and Mental Health Services, 10,* 722–729.

Jacobson, N., & Greenley, D. (2001). What is recovery? A conceptual model and explication. *Psychiatric Services, 52*(4), 482–485.

Johnson, M., Maas, M., & Moorhead, S. (2000). *Iowa outcomes project: Nursing outcomes classification (NOC)* (2nd ed.). St. Louis, MO: Mosby.

Kleinpell, R. M. (2003). Measuring advanced practice nursing outcome, strategies and resources. *Critical Care Nurse, February*(Suppl.), 6–10.

Lang, N. M., & Clinton, J. F. (1984). Assessment of quality of nursing care. *Annual Review of Nursing Research, 2,* 135–163.

Marek, K. D. (1989). Outcome measurement in nursing. *Journal of Nursing Quality Assurance, 4*(1), 1–9.

Registered Nurses Association of Ontario. (2002a). *Client-centered care.* Toronto, ON: Author.

Registered Nurses Association of Ontario. (2002b). Establishing therapeutic relationships. Toronto, ON: Author.

Registered Nurses Association of Ontario Best Practice Guidelines. (2005). Available at: http://www.rnao.org/bestpractices/index.asp

The Canadian Mental Health Association, Ontario Division (2003). *Recovery rediscovered: Implications for the Ontario mental health system.* Available at: http://www.ontario.cmha.ca/policy_positions.asp

CHAPTER
13

Psychiatric and Mental Health Nursing Interventions

Nicole Snow

Adapted from the chapter by "Psychiatric and Mental Health Nursing Interventions" by Mary Ann Boyd and Janet Landeen

LEARNING OBJECTIVES

After studying this chapter, you will be able to:

- Discuss the way clinical knowledge and judgment and a commitment to collaboration with clients and families determine the selection of nursing interventions.
- Discuss the application of nursing interventions for the biologic domain.
- Discuss the application of nursing interventions for the psychological domain.
- Discuss the application of nursing interventions for the social domain.
- Discuss the application of nursing interventions for the spiritual domain.

KEY CONCEPTS

- collaboration
- nursing interventions

KEY TERMS

- automatic thinking • behaviour modification • behaviour therapy • chemical restraint • cognitive interventions • conflict resolution • counselling • cultural brokering • de-escalation • distraction • guided imagery • home visits • illogical thinking • milieu therapy • observation • open communication • physical restraint • psychoeducation • recovery • reminiscence • seclusion • simple relaxation techniques • spiritual care • structured interaction • token economy • validation

$\mathcal{P}$sychiatric and mental health (PMH) nursing interventions are nursing activities that promote mental health, prevent mental illness, assess dysfunction, assist clients to regain or improve their coping abilities, and/or prevent further disabilities (Canadian Federation of Mental Health Nurses [CFMHN], 2006). Based on clinical knowledge and judgment and a commitment to collaboration and partnership with clients and their families, nursing interventions include any treatment that a nurse performs to enhance client outcomes. These interventions are direct (performed through interaction with the client) or indirect (performed away from, but on behalf of, the client) (McCloskey & Bulechek, 2000). Interventions can be either nurse-initiated treatment, which is an autonomous action in response to a nursing diagnosis, or physician-initiated treatment, which is a response to a medical diagnosis as a result of a physician's order. In PMH nursing, the *Canadian Standards of Psychiatric-Mental Health Nursing* (CFMHN) describe the scope of practice, delineate nursing competencies, and guide the selection of interventions for implementation in the plan of care (see Chapter 6).

KEY CONCEPT **Nursing interventions** are "any treatment or activity, based upon clinical judgment and knowledge, that a nurse performs to enhance patient/client outcomes" (McCloskey & Bulechek, 2000, p. 3).

After many different factors are considered, including the self-care activities of the client, selecting nursing approaches involves integrating biologic, psychological, social, and spiritual interventions into a comprehensive plan of care with and for the client with a psychiatric disorder (Fig. 13-1). PMH nurses provide care in various roles. In some settings, such as an acute care hospital or the home, the nurse provides direct nursing care. In other settings, such as the community, the nurse may assume the role of a case manager, who primarily coordinates care for all disciplines, including nursing. In this instance, the nurse may be responsible for all or part of direct nursing care as well as for ensuring that agreed-on care is appropriate for the client, even if other providers deliver it. The nurse may also be the leader or manager of a nursing unit and thus responsible for delegating the care to paraprofessional and nonprofessional providers; however, he or she remains accountable for the client's care. In all of these instances, the nurse, working in partnership with the client and/or the client's family, plans and initiates safe and appropriate interventions.

A Commitment to Collaboration and Client Centredness

Nursing interventions need to be based on a client-centred approach. This means that interventions are provided with respect for the preferences, values, and particular needs of the client and implemented as much as possible in partnership with the client and his or her family. The nurse needs to be able to discuss with them the risks and benefits of proposed interventions. In the *Canadian Collaborative Mental Health Care Charter* (Canadian Collaborative Mental Health Initiative, 2006), which was developed by national organizations of consumers and providers of mental health services (including the Canadian Nurses Association, the Registered Psychiatric Nurses of Canada, and the Canadian Federation of Mental Health Nurses), seven principles are identified regarding aspects of

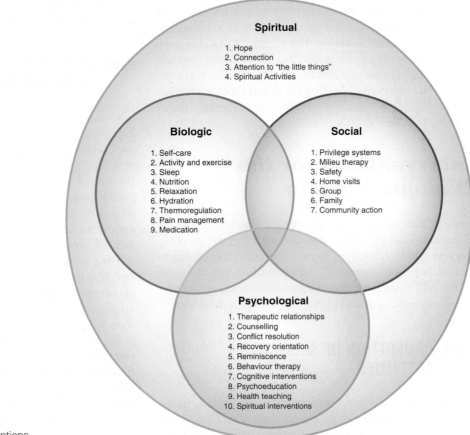

FIGURE 13.1 PMH nursing interventions.

collaborative clinical decisions and interventions: health promotion and prevention of mental health problems, holistic promotion, collaboration, partnership, respect for diversity, information exchange, and resources. Canadian nurses are committed to working together with clients and families.

⊕ **KEY CONCEPT Collaboration** is the process of working together toward common goals. Sharing knowledge and information can be an important aspect of the process.

Nursing Interventions and PMH Nursing

The *Nursing Interventions Classification* (NIC) (McCloskey & Bulechek, 2000) is an extensive system of specific interventions, with discrete activities for each. The NIC system is based on data collected from surveys of practicing nurses, who identified the interventions that were ultimately classified. The NIC taxonomy includes classes or groups of interventions categorized according to seven domains: physiologic basic, physiologic complex, behavioural, safety, family, health system, and community. The NIC taxonomy represents both basic and specialty advanced nursing practices. For example, both basic and specialist nurses use interventions such as reinforcing positive behaviour; however, the advanced practice psychiatric nurse may actually develop the plan and also use it as part of psychotherapy with the client. This text uses many NIC interventions (Box 13-1) and those identified in the *Canadian Standards of Psychiatric-Mental Health Nursing* (CFMHN, 2006; see Chapter 6).

Interventions for the Biologic Domain

Biologic interventions focus on physical functioning and are directed toward the client's self-care, activities and exercise, sleep, nutrition, relaxation, hydration, and thermoregulation as well as pain management and medication management. In the NIC taxonomy, these interventions are found within the physiologic basic and physiologic complex domains.

■■ PROMOTION OF SELF-CARE ACTIVITIES

Self-care is the ability to perform activities of daily living (ADLs) successfully. Many clients with PMH problems can manage self-care activities such as bathing, dressing appropriately, selecting adequate nutrition, and sleeping

regularly. (Although maintaining adequate nutrition and promoting normal sleep hygiene are considered self-care activities, they are discussed in separate sections because of their significance in mental health care.) Others, however, cannot manage such self-care activities, either because of their symptoms or as a result of the side effects of medications. Because nursing is concerned with maintaining the client's health and well-being, a focus on ADLs can become a nursing priority.

Dorothea Orem's (1991) nursing model is based on the concept of self-care deficit (see Chapter 8). Deficits in self-care may be related to attitude (motivation), knowledge, or skill. The model identifies five nursing approaches to deficits in a client's self-care: acting or doing for, guiding, teaching, supporting, and providing an environment to promote the client's ability to meet current or future demands. The emphasis is on helping the individual develop independence. In the inpatient setting, the PMH nurse works with the client so that basic self-care activities are completed. During acute phases of psychiatric disorders, the inability to attend to basic self-care tasks (e.g., getting dressed) is very common. Thus, the ability to complete personal hygiene activities (e.g., dental care, grooming) is monitored, and clients are assisted in completing such activities. In a psychiatric facility, clients are encouraged and expected to develop independence in completing these basic self-care activities. In the community, monitoring these basic self-care activities is always a part of the nursing visit or clinic appointment.

■■ ACTIVITY AND EXERCISE INTERVENTIONS

The nurse must attend to the client's level of activity. Encouraging regular activity and exercise can improve general well-being and physical health. A healthy lifestyle that includes daily exercise can help clients deal with the weight gain and type II diabetes associated with many psychotropic medications. In some psychiatric disorders (e.g., schizophrenia), people become sedentary and appear to lack the motivation to complete ADLs. This lack of motivation is part of the disorder and requires nursing intervention. In addition, side effects of medication that include sedation and lethargy can compound the problem. It is possible for exercise behaviour to become an abnormal focus of attention, such as for some clients with anorexia nervosa.

When assuming the responsibility of a direct care provider, the nurse can help clients identify realistic activities and exercise goals. Some institutions have other professionals (e.g., recreational therapists) available for the implementation of exercise programs. As a case manager, the nurse should consider the activity needs of individuals when jointly setting goals. As a leader or manager of a psychiatric unit, the nurse can influence ward routine.

BOX 13.1

Nursing Intervention Classification Taxonomy

1. Physiologic: Basic—Care That Supports Physical Functioning
   A. Activity and exercise management: Interventions to organize or assist with physical activity and energy conservation and expenditure
   B. Elimination management: Interventions to establish and maintain regular bowel and urinary elimination patterns and manage complications due to altered patterns
   C. Immobility management: Interventions to manage restricted body movement and the sequelae
   D. Nutrition support: Interventions to modify or maintain nutritional status
   E. Physical comfort promotion: Interventions to promote comfort using physical techniques
   F. Self-care facilitation: Interventions to provide or assist with routine ADLs
2. Physiologic: Complex—Care That Supports Homeostatic Regulation
   G. Electrolyte and acid–base management: Interventions to regulate electrolyte/acid–base balance and prevent complications
   H. Drug management: Interventions to facilitate the desired effects of pharmacologic agents
   I. Neurologic management: Interventions to optimize neurologic functions
   J. Perioperative care: Interventions to provide care before, during, and immediately after procedures (e.g., psychosurgery, electroconvulsive therapy)
   K. Respiratory management: Interventions to promote airway patency and gas exchange
   L. Skin/wound management: Interventions to maintain or restore tissue integrity
   M. Thermoregulation: Interventions to maintain body temperature within a normal range
   N. Tissue perfusion management: Interventions to optimize the circulation of blood and fluids to the tissues
3. Behavioural—Care That Supports Psychosocial Functioning and Facilitates Lifestyle Changes
   O. Behavioural therapy: Interventions to reinforce or promote desirable behaviours or alter undesirable behaviours

   P. Cognitive therapy: Interventions to reinforce or promote desirable cognitive functioning or alter undesirable cognitive functioning
   Q. Communication enhancement: Interventions to facilitate delivering and receiving verbal and nonverbal messages
   R. Coping assistance: Interventions to assist another to build on own strengths, adapt to a change in function, or achieve a higher level of function
   S. Client education: Interventions to facilitate learning
   T. Psychological comfort promotion: Interventions to promote comfort using psychological techniques
4. Safety—Care That Supports Protection Against Harm
   U. Crisis management: Interventions to provide immediate, short-term help in both psychological and physiologic crises
   V. Risk management: Interventions to initiate risk reduction activities and continue monitoring risks over time
5. Family—Care That Supports the Family Unit
   W. Childbearing care: Interventions to assist in understanding and coping with the psychological and physiologic changes during the childbearing period
   X. Life span care: Interventions to facilitate family unit functioning and promote the health and welfare of family members throughout the life span
6. Health System—Care That Supports Effective Use of the Health Care Delivery System
   Y. Health system mediation: Interventions to facilitate the interface between the client/family and the health care system
      a. Health system management: Interventions to provide and enhance support services for the delivery of care
      b. Information management: Interventions to facilitate communication among health care providers
7. Community—Care That Supports the Health of the Community
      a. Community health promotion: Interventions that promote health of the community
      b. Community risk management: Interventions that assist in detecting or preventing health risk to the whole community

Source: McCloskey, J., & Bulechek, G. (2000). *Nursing interventions classification (NIC)* (3rd ed.) St. Louis, MO: Mosby, with permission.

■ SLEEP INTERVENTIONS

Many psychiatric disorders and medications are associated with sleep disturbances. Sleep is also disrupted in clients with dementia; such clients may have difficulty falling asleep or may frequently awaken during the night. In dementia of the Alzheimer type, individuals may reverse their sleeping patterns by napping during the day and staying awake at night.

Nonpharmacologic interventions are always used first for sleep disturbances because of the side-effect risks associated with the use of sedatives and hypnotics (see Chapter 14). Sleep interventions to communicate to clients include the following:

- Go to bed only when tired or sleepy
- Establish a consistent bedtime routine
- Avoid stimulating foods, beverages, or medications
- Avoid naps in the late afternoon or evening
- Eat lightly before retiring and limit fluid intake
- Use bed only for sleep or intimacy
- Avoid emotional stimulation before bedtime
- Use behavioural and relaxation techniques
- Limit distractions

NUTRITION INTERVENTIONS

Psychiatric disorders and medication side effects can affect eating behaviours. For varying reasons, some clients eat too little, whereas others eat too much. For instance, homeless clients with mental illness have difficulty maintaining adequate nutrition because of their deprived lifestyle. Substance abuse also interferes with maintaining adequate nutrition, either through stimulation or suppression of appetite or through neglecting nutrition because of drug-seeking behaviour. Thus, nutrition interventions should be specific and relevant to the individual's circumstances and mental health. In addition, recommended daily allowances are important in the promotion of physical and mental health, and nurses should consider them when planning care.

Some psychiatric symptoms involve changes in perceptions of food, appetite, and eating habits. If a client believes that food is poisonous, he or she may eat sparingly or not at all. Interventions are then necessary to address the suspiciousness as well as to encourage adequate intake of recommended daily allowances. Allowing clients to examine foods, to participate in preparations, and to test the safety of the meal by eating slowly or after everyone else may be necessary.

Obesity can be a problem for individuals being treated for a mental disorder. Antipsychotics, antidepressants, and mood stabilizers are associated with weight gain, which is thought to be related to changes in metabolism and appetite caused by some of these medications. Many clients stop taking medications because of the weight gain. Excessive weight gain can be especially stressful to the individual's emotional well-being, as well as detrimental to physical health. However, nurses should encourage clients to avoid quick weight-loss programs because they are not effective. Furthermore, hypoglycemia can exacerbate a depressed mood and lead to suicidal thoughts. If weight gain is a problem, the best approach is to assist the client to monitor current intake and develop realistic strategies for changing eating patterns combined with a healthy lifestyle.

RELAXATION INTERVENTIONS

Relaxation promotes comfort, reduces anxiety, alleviates stress, eases pain, and prevents aggression. It can diminish the effects of hallucinations and delusions. The many different relaxation techniques used as mental health interventions range from simple deep breathing to biofeedback to hypnosis. Although some techniques such as biofeedback require additional training and, in some instances, certification, nurses can easily apply simple relaxation, distraction, and imagery techniques.

Simple relaxation techniques encourage and elicit relaxation to decrease undesirable signs and symptoms. **Distraction** is the purposeful focusing of attention away from undesirable sensations. See Table 13-1 for a description of the implementation of these techniques.

Table 13.1 Relaxation Techniques: Descriptions and Implementation	
Simple Relaxation Techniques	**Distraction**
• Create a quiet, nondisrupting environment with dim lights and a comfortable temperature.	• Distraction techniques include music, counting, television, reading, play, and exercise, among others. Help the client choose a technique that will work for him or her. Keep in mind what may or may not be appropriate for the client based on factors such as energy level, age, literacy level, and developmental level.
• Instruct the client to assume a relaxed position, wearing loose and comfortable clothing.	• Advise the client to practice the distraction technique before he or she will need to use it.
• Instruct the client to relax and to let the sensations happen.	• Have the client develop a specific plan for how and when he or she will use distraction. Distraction can be used alone or in conjunction with other techniques.
• Use a low tone of voice with a slow, rhythmic pace of words.	• Teach the techniques to family members or significant others.
• Instruct the client to take an initial slow, deep breath (abdominal breathing) while thinking about pleasant events.	• Evaluate and document the client's response to distraction.
• Use soothing music (without words) to enhance relaxation.	
• Reinforce the use of relaxation by praising efforts and helping the client to schedule time regularly for it.	
• Evaluate and document the client's response to relaxation.	

Adapted from McCloskey, J., & Bulechek, G. (2000). *Nursing interventions classification (NIC)* (3rd ed.). St. Louis, MO: Mosby.

Guided imagery is the purposeful use of imagination to achieve relaxation or to direct attention away from undesirable sensations. It is especially useful in stress management. With this technique, clients imagine themselves doing something pleasurable and relaxing, such as lying on the beach or watching snow fall. They are encouraged (with permissive directions from the nurse, such as "If you wish....") to slowly experience the scene and to express how they feel and think about it. Slow, deep breathing is also encouraged (McCloskey & Bulechek, 2000). Guided imagery can be considered an independent nursing intervention (Giedt, 1997), but as clients may experience unexpected, albeit therapeutic, reactions (e.g., crying) during guided imagery, students should not attempt this technique with clients unless supervised.

As a direct care provider, the nurse may teach the client relaxation exercises. As a case manager, nurses can include relaxation exercises in the plan of care. The unit leader can be responsible for ensuring that appropriately prepared staff members implement relaxation exercises. Relaxation techniques that involve physical touch (e.g., back rubs) must be used particularly carefully, if at all, for people with mental disorders. Touching and massaging are often not appropriate for clients who have a history of physical or sexual abuse. Such clients may find touching too stimulating or misinterpret it as being sexual or aggressive.

▇ HYDRATION INTERVENTIONS

Assessing fluid status and monitoring fluid intake and output are often important interventions. Overhydration or underhydration can be a symptom of a psychiatric disorder. For example, some clients with psychotic disorders experience chronic fluid imbalance. For these individuals, a treatment protocol that includes a target weight procedure can help prevent both overhydration and water intoxication and promote self-control (see Chapter 18). The nurse functions as the direct care provider (teaching client), unit leader (delegating weighing of the client to staff), or coordinator of the protocol.

Many psychiatric medications affect fluid and electrolyte balance (see Chapter 10). For example, when taking lithium carbonate, clients must have adequate fluid intake, with special attention paid to serum sodium levels. When sodium levels drop through perspiration, lithium is used in place of sodium, which in turn leads to lithium toxicity. Many psychiatric medications cause dry mouth, which in turn causes individuals to drink fluids excessively. Interventions that help clients understand the relationship of medications to fluid and electrolyte balance are important in their overall care.

▇ THERMOREGULATION INTERVENTIONS

Many psychiatric disorders can disturb the body's normal temperature regulation. Thus, clients cannot sense temperature increases or decreases and consequently cannot protect themselves from extremes of hot or cold. This problem is especially difficult for people who are homeless or live in substandard housing, such as some rooming houses. In addition, many psychiatric medications can also affect the ability to regulate body temperature.

Interventions include educating clients about the problem of thermoregulation, identifying potential extremes in temperatures, and developing strategies to protect the client from the adverse effects of temperature changes. For example, community nurses often engage in active outreach to at-risk clients during extreme weather alerts.

▇ PAIN MANAGEMENT

Emotional reactions are often manifested as pain. For instance, chronic, unexplained pain is one of the main symptoms of somatization disorder (see Chapter 22). Chronic pain is particularly problematic because often no cause for it is found.

PMH nurses are more likely to provide care to clients experiencing chronic pain than acute pain. However, a single intervention is seldom successful for relieving chronic pain. In some instances, pain is managed by medication; in other instances, nonpharmacologic techniques, such as simple relaxation techniques, distraction, or imagery, are used. Indeed, relaxation is one of the most widely used cognitive and behavioural approaches to pain. Psychoeducation, stress management techniques, and biofeedback are also used in pain management.

The key to managing pain is engaging the client in identifying how it is disrupting his or her personal, social, professional, and family life. Education focusing on the pain, the use of medications for treatment, and the development of cognitive skills are important pain management components. In some cases, redefining treatment success as improvement in functioning, rather than alleviation of pain, may be necessary. The interaction between stress and pain is important; that is, increased stress leads to increased pain. Clients can better manage their pain when stress is reduced.

▇ MEDICATION MANAGEMENT

The PMH nurse uses many medication management interventions to help clients maintain therapeutic regimens. Medication management involves more than the actual administration of medications. Nurses also assess medication effectiveness and side effects and consider drug–drug interactions. In addition, nurses assess any factors that may affect the client's adherence to a medication regimen, such as concerns regarding weight gain or reproductive ability, attitude toward taking medication, or cost issues. Education regarding medication must be made available to the client in appropriate ways, including information regarding the recognition and reporting of side effects. Suggesting strategies to assist the client in taking medication on time can be helpful. Treatment with psychopharmacologic agents can be lengthy because of the chronic nature of many disorders; many clients remain on medication regimens for years, never becoming medication free. Thus, medication education is an ongoing intervention that requires careful documentation. Medication follow-up may include home visits as well as telephone calls.

Interventions for the Psychological Domain

A major emphasis in PMH nursing is on the psychological domain: emotion, behaviour, and cognition. The nurse–client relationship serves as the basis for interventions directed toward the psychological domain. Because the therapeutic relationship is discussed extensively in Chapter 9, it is not covered in this chapter. This section covers counselling, conflict resolution, recovery orientation, reminiscence, behaviour therapy, cognitive interventions, psychoeducation, health teaching, and spiritual interventions. Chapter 8 presents the theoretic basis for many of these interventions.

Nurses in the direct care role will use all of the psychological interventions to respond to the health care problems of their clients. Nurses in case manager roles will also frequently use interventions from the psychological domain to promote recovery and to empower the client to make changes. Case management relationships are based on trust. The nurse manager oversees the use of the psychological interventions and evaluates the staff's ability to use the interventions and assess outcomes.

■ COUNSELLING INTERVENTIONS

Counselling interventions are specific, time-limited interactions between a nurse and a client, family, or group experiencing immediate or ongoing difficulties related to their health or well-being. Counselling is usually short-term and focuses on improving coping abilities, reinforcing healthy behaviours, fostering positive interactions, or preventing illnesses and disabilities.

Counselling strategies are discussed throughout the text. Psychotherapy is generally a long-term approach aimed at improving or helping clients regain previous health status and functional abilities. Mental health specialists, such as advanced practice nurses, use psychotherapy.

■ CONFLICT RESOLUTION

A conflict involves an individual's perceptions, emotions, and behaviours. In a conflict, a person believes that his or her own needs, interests, wants, or values are incompatible with someone else's (Boggs, 2003). The individual experiences fear, sadness, bitterness, anger, hopelessness, or some combination of these emotions in response to the perceived threat. Misunderstandings, poor communication, value or goal differences, personality issues, and stress can interplay to contribute to this conflict and impact its resolution (Boggs).

Conflict resolution is a specific type of intervention through which the nurse helps clients resolve disagreements or disputes with family, friends, or other clients. Conflicts can be positive if individuals see the problem as solvable and providing an opportunity for growth and interpersonal understanding. The nurse may be in the position of actually resolving a family conflict or teaching family members how to resolve their own conflicts positively. In addition, because nurses are frequently in positions of leadership, they often need conflict resolution skills to settle employee conflicts.

Conflict Resolution Process

Calmness and objectivity are important in resolving any client or family conflict. The desired outcome of conflict resolution is a "win-win" situation—that is, each party feels good about the outcome. Conflict resolution includes the following steps:

1. Identifying conflict issues.
2. Knowing your own response to the conflict.
3. Separating the problem from the people involved.
4. Staying focused on the issue and the underlying motivations behind the position the other person took.
5. Identifying available options.
6. Trying to identify established standards to guide the decision-making process (Boggs, 2003).

It is important to be aware of what is causing the conflict. This can be difficult to discern at times, and open, honest, and respectful communication is necessary to facilitate this awareness. It is helpful when all parties involved are able to reflect on their reactions to the conflict and what triggers their emotional responses. It is best and most constructive when all involved are able to focus on the issue at hand and not be critical of the people involved. The focus needs to be on the here and now of the problem, without dwelling on issues that have occurred in the past. Once all parties understand the underlying reasons for the dispute, attention can be given to developing options on how to appropriately address it. As much as possible, this development should be a collaborative process with all parties contributing fairly to the outcome (Boggs, 2003).

Cultural Brokering in Client–System Conflicts

Clients may be marginalized within the health care system due to potentially stigmatizing factors, such as poverty, sexual orientation, lack of formal education, race, or ethnicity. Differences in cultural values and languages between clients and health care organizations can contribute to clients' feelings of powerlessness. For example, new immigrants, people who are homeless, and people who need to make informed decisions under stressful conditions may be unable to navigate the health care system. The nurse can help to resolve such conflicts through **cultural brokering,** or the use of culturally appropriate strategies that aid in bridging or mediating between the client's culture and the health care system (McCloskey & Bulechek, 2000). The health care system can be understood as a culture in and of itself, with culture shock being a potential experience for clients and families new to it.

For the "nurse-as-broker" to be effective, he or she establishes and maintains a sense of connectedness or relationship with the client. In turn, the nurse also establishes and cultivates networks with other health care facilities and resources. Cultural sensitivity enables the nurse to be aware of and sensitive to the needs of clients from a variety of cultures. Cultural competence is necessary for the brokering process to be effective (see Chapter 3).

◼◗ RECOVERY ORIENTATION

Recovery-focused interventions are becoming more prevalent in PMH nursing practice. Nurses apply this orientation to their everyday interactions with their clients. For individuals struggling with addictions, self-help 12-step programs frequently refer to recovery as the abstinence from the addictive behaviour. For individuals with schizophrenia or bipolar disorder, a recovery orientation means helping the person regain functioning or "get on with life," despite having ongoing symptoms of the psychiatric illness. Recovery may refer to what the client does, how the nurse functions, or how the mental health system is organized. Research suggests that **recovery** involves an ongoing process of:

- Refining oneself and learning to accept one's vulnerabilities.

- Working to overcome the stigma and discrimination one may experience.
- Looking beyond what is lacking in one's life.
- Looking to regain hope, control, and responsibility in and for one's life.
- Exercising citizenship to become active members in one's community.
- Engaging in meaningful social activities.

People accomplish recovery and learn how to manage recurrent or ongoing health concerns with the love and support of significant others in their lives (Davidson, 2003).

One approach to recovery, the Tidal Model (Buchanan-Barker & Barker, 2006), emphasizes the importance of a collaborative relationship between the nurse and the client. The client's perspectives and individual experiences are accepted and valued. Recovery is contingent on the health professional having a genuine interest in the client and his or her experiences. The process is open, transparent, and based on the mutual establishment of goals that both parties work together to achieve. It is recognized that recovery requires time and commitment from both the nurse and the client, and that the process of change is enhanced through a genuine therapeutic relationship. (See Chapter 8 for more information on this model.)

◼◗ REMINISCENCE

Reminiscence, the thinking about or relating of past experiences, is used as a nursing intervention to enhance life review for older adults. Reminiscence encourages clients, either in individual or in group settings, to discuss their past and review their lives. Through reminiscence, individuals can identify past coping strategies that can support them in current stressful situations. Clients can also use reminiscence to maintain self-esteem, stimulate thinking, and support the natural healing process of life review. Activities that facilitate reminiscence include writing an account of past events, making a tape recording and playing it back, explaining pictures in old family albums, drawing a family tree, and writing to old friends. (See Chapter 29 for health promotion with the older adult.)

◼◗ BEHAVIOUR THERAPY

Behaviour therapy interventions focus on reinforcing or promoting desirable behaviours or altering undesirable ones. The basic premise is that because most behaviours are learned, new functional behaviours can also be learned. Behaviours—not internal psychic processes—are the targets of the interventions. The models of behavioural theorists serve as a basis for these interventions (see Chapter 8).

Behaviour Modification

Behaviour modification is a specific, systematized behaviour therapy technique that can be applied to individuals, groups, or systems. The aim of behaviour modification is to reinforce desired behaviours and extinguish undesired ones. Desired behaviour is rewarded to increase the likelihood that clients will repeat it and, over time, replace the problematic behaviour with it. Behaviour modification is used for various problematic behaviours, such as dysfunctional eating and addictions, and often is used in the care of children and adolescents.

Token Economy

Used in inpatient settings, a **token economy** applies behaviour modification techniques to multiple behaviours. In a token economy, clients are rewarded with tokens for selected desired behaviours. They can use these tokens to purchase meals, leave the unit, watch television, or wear street clothes, for example. In less restrictive environments, clients use tokens to purchase additional privileges, such as attending social events. Token economy systems have been especially effective in reinforcing positive behaviours in people who are developmentally disabled. The strategy has also been shown to work with aggressive inpatients (Bisconer, Green, Mallon-Czajka, & Johnson, 2006).

■ COGNITIVE INTERVENTIONS

Cognitive interventions are verbally structured interventions that reinforce and promote desirable, or alter undesirable, cognitive functioning. The belief underlying this approach is that thoughts guide emotional reactions, motivations, and behaviours. Cognitive interventions do not solve problems for clients but help clients develop new ways of viewing situations so that they can solve problems themselves. Nurses may use several models as the basis for cognitive interventions, but all models assume that by changing the cognitive appraisal of a situation (view of the world) and by examining the meaning of events, clients can reinterpret situations. In turn, emotional changes will follow the cognitive changes, and, ultimately, behaviours will change.

> **• CRNENOTE**
> Use the principles of teaching/learning in health promotion. This applies across all areas of nursing.

Because people develop their thinking patterns throughout their lifetime, many thoughts become so automatic that they are outside individuals' awareness. Thus, a person may be unaware of the automatic thoughts that influence his or her actions or other thoughts. **Automatic thinking** is often subject to errors or tangible distortions of reality that contradict objective appraisals. For example, a client with depression may be convinced that no one cares about him when, in fact, his family and friends are deeply concerned. **Illogical thinking,** another thinking error, occurs when a person draws a faulty conclusion. For example, a college student is so devastated by failing an examination that she perceives her college career to be over.

To engage in cognitive treatment, the client must be capable of introspection and reflection about thoughts and fantasies. Cognitive interventions are used in a wide range of clinical situations, from short-term crises to persistent mental disorders. Cognitive interventions also include thought stopping, contracting, and cognitive restructuring. These specific interventions are discussed in Chapter 15.

■ PSYCHOEDUCATION

Psychoeducation uses educational strategies to teach clients the skills they lack because of a psychiatric disorder. The goal of psychoeducation is a change in knowledge and behaviour. Nurses use psychoeducation to meet the educational needs of clients by adapting teaching strategies to their disorder-related deficits. As clients gain skills, functioning improves. Some clients may need to learn how to maintain their morning hygiene. Others may need to understand their illness and cope with hearing voices that others do not hear.

Specific psychoeducation techniques are based on adult learning principles, such as beginning at the point the learner is currently at and building on his or her current experiences. Thus, the nurse assesses the client's current skills and readiness to learn. From there, the nurse individualizes a teaching plan for each client. He or she can conduct such teaching in a one-to-one situation or in a group format.

Psychoeducation is a continuous process of assessing, setting goals, developing learning activities, and evaluating for changes in knowledge and behaviour. Nurses use it with individuals, groups, families, and communities. Psychoeducation serves as a basis for psychosocial rehabilitation, a service-delivery approach for those with severe and persistent mental illness (see Chapter 18).

> **• CRNENOTE**
> Nursing competencies include intervening in mental health crises and facilitating the client's reintegration with the family and community.

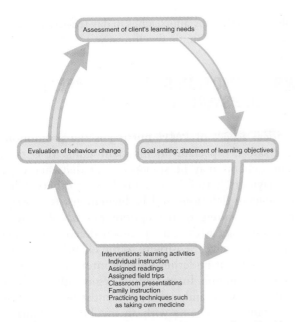

FIGURE 13.2 Teaching evaluation model. (Adapted from Rankin, S. H., Stallings, K. D., & London, F. [2005]. *Patient education.* Philadelphia, PA: Lippincott Williams & Wilkins.)

HEALTH TEACHING

Teaching-coaching is one of the standards of care for the PMH nurse (CFMHN, 2006; see Chapter 6). According to this standard, the PMH nurse "attempts to understand the life experience of the client and uses this understanding to support and promote learning related to health and personal development" (CFMHN, p. 13). Based on principles of teaching, health teaching involves collaborating with the client to determine learning needs and transmitting new information, "while considering the context of the client's life experiences. [The nurse] considers readiness, culture, literacy, language, preferred learning style, and resources available" (CFMHN, p. 13). According to the *Canadian Standards of Psychiatric-Mental Health Nursing,* "all interactions between the nurse and patient are potentially teaching/learning situations" (CFMHN, p. 13). Thus, in health teaching, the PMH nurse attends to potential healthcare problems in addition to mental disorders and emotional problems. For example, if a person has diabetes mellitus and is taking insulin, the nurse provides healthcare teaching related to diabetes and the interaction of this problem with the mental disorder (Fig. 13-2).

Interventions for the Social Domain

The social domain includes the individual's environment and its effect on his or her responses to mental disorders and distress. Interventions within the social domain are geared toward couples, families, friends, and large and small social groups, with special attention given to ethnicity and community interactions. In some instances, nurses design interventions that affect a client's environment, such as helping a family member decide to place a loved one in long-term care. In other instances, the nurse actually modifies the environment to promote positive behaviours through providing opportunities for clients to interact with others. For example, this can be accomplished through group or recreational activities for holidays or other special events which clients can attend. Group and family interventions are discussed in Chapters 16 and 17, respectively.

MILIEU THERAPY

Milieu therapy provides a stable and coherent social organization to facilitate an individual's treatment. (The terms *milieu therapy* and *therapeutic environment* are often used interchangeably.) In milieu therapy, the design of the physical surroundings, structure of client activities, and promotion of a stable social structure and cultural setting enhance the setting's therapeutic potential. A therapeutic milieu facilitates client interactions and promotes personal growth. Milieu therapy is the responsibility of the nurse in collaboration with the client and other health care providers. The key concepts of milieu therapy include safety and security, validation, open communication, and structured interaction.

Safety and Security

The milieu should be a healing place in which clients feel safe, secure, and cared for while dealing with their illness. The physical surroundings are important in this process and should be clean and comfortable, with special attention paid to promoting a noninstitutionalized environment. Pictures on walls, comfortable furniture, and soothing colours help clients relax. Most facilities encourage clients and nursing staff to wear street clothes, which helps decrease the formalized nature of hospital settings and promotes nurse–client relationships. Research suggests the absence of a therapeutic milieu can be experienced by clients and nurses in parallel ways (Shattell, Andes, & Thomas, 2008). For instance, nurses can feel caged in by an enclosed nursing station, while clients experience similar feelings by locked unit doors.

Therapeutic milieus emphasize client involvement in treatment decisions and operation of the unit. Too often, the stigma of mental illness can exist within institutional walls, and clients can be treated in a paternalistic manner. On most inpatient psychiatric units, clients participate in maintaining the quality of the physical surroundings, assuming responsibility for making their own beds, attending to their own belongings, and keeping an acceptable living area. Families are viewed as a part of the client's life; family involvement is encouraged. Thus, family members should feel welcomed and safe in the milieu, as well.

Validation

In a therapeutic environment, **validation** is another process that affirms a client's individuality. Clients should feel validated as persons of worth and deserving of respect. Staff–client interactions should constantly reaffirm the client's humanity and his or her human rights. The importance of the client's personal story, history, experience, and understanding of his or her illness must be recognized in all aspects of care.

Open Communication

In **open communication,** health and treatment information is shared with clients and families. Client self-disclosure is invited within the support of a nurse–client relationship, with attention paid to the parameters of confidentiality that exist within that therapeutic relationship. These parameters may change with the care situation. For instance, if the client is undergoing a forensic assessment, information disclosed may be shared with the justice system (e.g., law courts). The client needs to understand this (see Chapter 34). Further, the environment is shaped to facilitate optimal interaction and resocialization. Support, attention, praise, and reassurance given to clients improve self-esteem and increase confidence. Client education is also a part of this support, including guidance regarding effective coping skills. Nurses and other team members should strive to role model effective communication when interacting with one another as well as with clients and families. The dynamics of team interactions can affect the milieu in both positive and negative ways.

Structured Interaction

Structured interaction is a purposeful interaction that is intended to help clients cope with particular behaviours or to learn better ways of interaction. For instance, the treatment team may assign structured interactions to specific clients as part of their treatment. Specific attitudes or approaches are assumed with individual clients or in response to particular client behaviour if beneficial to the client. These approaches include indulgence, flexibility, passive or active friendliness, matter-of-fact attitude, casualness, watchfulness, or kind firmness. For example, if and when a client becomes overexcited by daily events, the team may provide a matter-of-fact attitude when responding; or if a client's illness includes delusions that lead him or her to engage in risky behaviour, the team may intervene with an attitude of kind firmness.

Milieu treatments are based on the individual needs of the clients and include relaxation groups, discussion groups, and medication groups. Spontaneous and planned activities are possible on a short-term unit as well as in a long-term setting. In the community, it is possible to apply milieu therapy approaches in day treatment centres, group homes, and single dwellings.

■■■ PROMOTION OF CLIENT SAFETY ON PSYCHIATRIC UNITS

A critical aspect of PMH nursing is the promotion of client safety, especially in inpatient units. It is critical because clients may be so severely ill that they engage in behaviours harmful to themselves or others. Clients experiencing delusions and hallucinations, for instance, can be responding to perceptions not based in reality. They can react with fear or in self-defence to dangers only they perceive. Sensitivity to the client's world as she or he is living it underlies nursing interventions used to keep the client safe. Interventions begin with observation and de-escalation and may evolve to the use of seclusion or restraints for clients with an involuntary status. See Chapter 6 for a discussion of ethical issues related to the use of behaviour control and restraint.

Observation

Like all hospitalized clients, individuals hospitalized on a psychiatric unit are observed by the nurses caring for them. **Observation** is the ongoing assessment of the client's status to identify and subvert any potential problem. The nature of mental disorders shapes the focus of the nurses' observations. In psychiatric settings, for instance, clients are ambulatory and thus more susceptible to environmental hazards. In addition, judgment and cognition impairment are symptoms of many psychiatric disorders. The reason for clients' admission may be, in fact, that they pose a danger to themselves or others. In PMH nursing, observation involves thoughtful, knowledgeable regard of the persons and consistent, responsible monitoring for any potential harm to themselves or others.

The intensity of the observation of the client depends on the assessed level of risk. Clients may be simply asked to "check in" at different times of the day, whereas other clients may be observed every 15 minutes by an assigned staff member. Some clients, such as those seen as at risk for suicide, may be constantly observed by a staff member assigned to only them. Mental health facilities have policies that specify levels of observation for clients at varying degrees of risk.

De-escalation

De-escalation is an interactive process of calming and redirecting a client who has an immediate potential for violence directed toward self or others. This intervention involves assessing the situation and preventing it from escalating to one in which injury occurs to the client or others. Once the nurse has assessed the situation, he or she responds matter-of-factly to it, using various interventions that can include a request for the client and/or others to leave the situation, distraction, and conflict resolution. Psychiatric staff members are usually trained in responding to situations of aggression as a team and, thus, are often able to de-escalate such situations effectively. See Chapter 36 for information on the management of aggression and violence. Nurses can use various interventions in this situation, including distraction, conflict resolution, and cognitive interventions.

Seclusion

Seclusion is the involuntary confinement of a person in a room from which the person is physically prevented from leaving (Department of Human Services, 2006). A client is placed in seclusion for purposes of safety or behavioural management. The seclusion room has no furniture except a mattress and a blanket. The walls may be padded. The room is environmentally safe, with no hanging devices, electrical outlets, or windows from which the client could jump. Once a client is placed in seclusion, he or she is observed at all times.

Seclusion can be an extremely negative client experience; consequently, its use is seriously questioned and many facilities have completely abandoned its practice. Clients have disputed the calming effects of seclusion and have perceived it as an instrument of power and control (Holmes, Kennedy, & Perron, 2004; Meehan, Bergen, & Fjeldsoe, 2004). Client outcomes may actually be worse if seclusion is used (Box 13-2). If units are adequately staffed and personnel are trained in dealing with assaultive clients, seclusion is rarely needed.

If seclusion is used, it must follow the same guidelines as the use of restraints (discussed next).

Restraints

In Canada, the laws for restricting the freedom of clients against their will are specific to each province. Restraint is the most restrictive safety intervention and is only used in the most extreme circumstances and as a measure of last resort. Provincial mental health acts govern the situations under which restraint may be used in their jurisdiction.

Chemical restraint is the use of medication to control clients or manage their behaviour. This is distinct from medication used to treat their psychiatric illness. In several provinces, it is possible for a client to be competent to refuse medical treatment but be required to stay in the hospital for psychiatric assessment.

A **physical restraint** is any human or mechanical method that restricts the freedom of movement or normal access to one's body, material, or equipment and cannot be easily removed (National Alliance on Mental Illness, 2008). Different types of physical restraints are available. Wrist restraints restrict arm movement. Four-point restraints are applied to the wrists and ankles in bed. When five-point restraints are used, all extremities are secured, and another restraint is placed across the chest (see Fig. 13-3).

In addition to the following provincial law, the nurse must also adhere to hospital policies regarding restraint. A physician's order is necessary for restraint, and nurses should document all of the previously tried de-escalation interventions before the application of restraint. Nurses should limit the use of restraints to times when an individual is judged to be a danger to self or others; they should

---

BOX 13.2

Research for Best Practice: The Mentally Ill and Social Exclusion: A Critical Examination of the Use of Seclusion From the Patient's Perspective

Holmes, D., Kennedy, S. L., & Perron, A. (2004). The mentally ill and social exclusion: A critical examination of the use of seclusion from the patient's perspective. Issues in Mental Health Nursing, 25, 559–578.

QUESTION: What are patients' perceptions and experiences of seclusion?

METHOD: Six patients with severe, persistent mental illness, who were hospitalized in a Canadian psychiatric unit, were asked during semistructured interviews to share, in their own words, their experience of seclusion. Phenomenology, a method that involves gaining a rich description of an experience, guided the research.

FINDINGS: The findings yielded three themes: the emotional impact of seclusion room experiences, the patients' perceptions of seclusion, and coping strategies used while in seclusion. Patients identified their emotional responses to being in

seclusion, ranging from fear and anger to sadness, shame, and feelings of abandonment. Patients identified the need to be in seclusion as a result of their being "bad." They felt alone and isolated from others. Patients described learning to cope with these experiences through a variety of means that included maladaptive coping strategies such as regression, anger, or rage. Others described being calmer in their reaction to seclusion and said that they used the time to re-establish relationships with the staff.

IMPLICATIONS FOR PRACTICE: This research identifies the need for nurses to critically examine the use of seclusion with patients and to recognize the way this intervention affects patients as individuals, as well as how it affects the therapeutic relationship. The research challenges nurses to reconceptualize the inpatient psychiatric milieu from one of control to one of care.

FIGURE 13.3 Bed with five-point restraints. (Courtesy of Alberta Hospitals, Photographer Pat Morrison.)

apply restraints only until the client has gained control over his or her behaviour. When a client is in physical restraints, the nurse should closely observe the client and protect him or her from self-injury.

Given the negative consequences to the client and the impact on the nurse–client relationship, it is essential that nurses treat the client with respect and dignity at all times during a psychiatric emergency that necessitates seclusion or restraint. Every incident should be followed up by a thorough debriefing to identify how the situation might have been avoided. Education on the ethical, clinical, and legal issues related to restraint practices is very important (Kontio et al., 2009).

■ HOME VISITS

Clients usually have been hospitalized or have received treatment for acute psychiatric symptoms before being referred to a home care service. The goal of **home visits**, the delivery of nursing care in the client's living environment, is to maximize the client's functional ability within the nurse–client relationship and with the family or partner, as appropriate. The PMH nurse who makes home visits needs to be able to work independently, is skilled in teaching clients and families, can administer and monitor medications, and uses community resources for the client's needs. Traditional home visits are regaining popularity, particularly when the client has concomitant psychiatric and physical illnesses.

Home visits can be especially useful when helping reluctant clients to enter therapy, conducting a comprehensive assessment, strengthening a support network, and maintaining clients in the community when their condition deteriorates. Home visits are also useful in helping individuals adhere to their medication regimen. The nurse, for instance, can gain a better understanding of the barriers to taking medication as prescribed and assists the client and family to address them. One major advantage of home visits is the opportunity to provide family members with information and education and to engage them in planning and interventions.

Home visits also offer the nurse an opportunity to develop cultural sensitivity to families from a variety of backgrounds. Home-based interventions require the nurse to gain an understanding, as much as possible, of the family structure and interactions, including the roles various members play, how the family functions in terms of responsibilities, and the family life cycle (see Chapter 17). A family's cultural background influences all of these factors, and culture is important to consider when planning interventions. The home visit also allows the nurse to identify clients who lack support from others in their daily lives.

The home visit process consists of three steps: the previsit phase, the home visit, and the postvisit phase. During previsit planning, the nurse sets goals for the home visit based on data received from other health care providers or the client. Any safety precautions that should be taken for the visit should be identified and acted upon. For instance, road conditions in winter time for a rural home visit or crime levels in an urban district to be visited may need to be considered. The nurse and the client agree on the time of the visit. While the nurse travels to the home, a general assessment can be made of the neighbourhood for access to services, socioeconomic factors, safety, and other factors relevant to the client's well-being within the community.

The actual visit can be divided into four parts. The first is the greeting phase, usually brief, in which the nurse begins to connect with the client and family members in their home setting. Greetings are important as they set the atmosphere for the visit and, on the part of the nurse, should be friendly but professional. In some cultures, the greeting phase may involve more formal interactions, such as taking food or tea with family members. The second phase establishes the focus of the visit. Sometimes, the purpose of the visit is medication administration, health teaching, or counselling. The client and family must be clear regarding the purpose. The implementation of the service is the next phase and should use most of the visit time. If the purpose of the visit is problem solving or decision making, the family's cultural values may determine the types of interaction and decision-making approaches. Closure is the last phase, the end of the home visit. It is a time to summarize and clarify important points. The nurse should also schedule any additional visits and reiterate client expectations between visits. Usually, the nurse is the only provider to see the client regularly. The nurse should acknowledge family members when leaving if they were not a part of the visit.

The postvisit phase includes documentation, reporting, and follow-up planning. This time is also when the nurse meets with the supervisor and presents data from the home visit at the team meeting.

■■■ COMMUNITY ACTION

Nurses have a unique opportunity to promote mental health awareness and support humane treatment for people with mental disorders. Activities range from being an advisor to support groups to participating in the political process through lobbying efforts and serving on community mental health boards. These unpaid activities are usually outside the realm of a particular job. However, an important role of professionals is to provide community service in addition to services through income-generating positions.

Interventions for the Spiritual Domain

Spiritual care cannot be readily separated from the bio/psycho/social components of care. It involves, rather, attention to all aspects of the client's life and life circumstances and takes direction from the client's reality (Sawatzky & Pesut, 2005). The integrative nature of spirituality, and therefore of spiritual care, can make it difficult to isolate and identify spiritual needs, document spiritual interventions, and stipulate outcomes. Although spirituality always has been a core aspect of nursing care, nurses can be hesitant to address this component of their practice. However, a Canadian study of nurses' experiences of spiritual nursing care found that there was a common dimension across all the nurses' descriptions:

"[S]piritual nursing care is about developing caring relationships through fostering connections to promote spiritual comfort and well-being" (Carr, 2008, p. 690). An attitude of respect and concern for the client's comfort, dignity, and well-being and recognition of the client as a person with a past, present, and future were seen as core to connection, even with individuals who appeared not to want the connection or who could not communicate. Four critical qualities for spiritual care emerged from the research data: *receptivity, humanity, competency,* and *positivity. Receptivity* involves being open to clients as a person and being genuinely present to them. It may mean simply "being with" (not just doing for) the client. *Humanity* is about being human, or put another way, being "real." It can be offering "the little things" that reveal thoughtful caring, such as knocking before entering the client's room, offering a favourite food to stimulate a client's poor appetite, or taking time to view family photos on display. *Competency* is enabling the client to know that she or he is in good hands. It reflects the integrative aspect of spiritual care that includes good bio/psycho/social care. *Positivity* describes the positive approach necessary to spiritual care. The nurse's attitude is one of hope and determination, of encouragement and good humour. Positivity is not about smiling all the time or insisting on only happy feelings being expressed. It is about fostering a positive spirit in others through one's own hopeful energy (Carr; see Box 13-3). These qualities of spiritual care underscore the importance of the nurse's own well-being and of the therapeutic environment (see Chapter 5).

■■■ BOX 13.3

Fostering Hope in Recovery

The fostering and maintenance of hope is an integral component to recovery from mental illness. Many of the symptoms of mental illness can contribute to feelings of hopelessness and despair. In addition, the chronic nature of many mental health concerns can contribute to strain and difficulty in maintaining a positive outlook for future recovery.

These feelings are experienced by individuals with mental illness as well as their families and loved ones. Families often provide considerable support over many years. Nurses must take the approach of family as client whenever possible and appropriate. This is necessary not only in the acute phase of the mental illness but also in maintaining recovery and intervening in relapses.

In a study that explored the experiences of families during recovery from mental illness, participants spoke of their hopes and fears in being a part of this ongoing process. Families reported on their cautious optimism that recovery would last and that the family members would return to how they were before the mental illness. There were concerns regarding the uncertainty of what the future held for the

individual with mental illness. As one parent noted, "I am not going to be here forever you know. So what is going to happen to her after I'm gone?" The challenges with providing such support often influenced family relationships both in positive and negative ways. Bonds were strengthened for some; while for others, they were strained.

Nurses need to have an understanding of these issues in providing comprehensive care for individuals with mental illness and their families. Nurses must also be aware of the importance of hope in recovery from mental illness. It is important to include the family in the timely provision of information, program referrals, and other interventions. In this approach, the nurse must use a strengths perspective in providing such interventions, and not focus solely on the deficits and negative impact that mental illness can have. While the nurse must allow for the family to grieve and cope with the diagnosis of mental illness, she or he must be mindful of the possibility that families can lose hope and fall into despair. Nurses too must be hopeful in order to foster hope in others.

From Tweedell, D., Forchuk, C., Jewell, J., & Steinnagel, L. (2004). Families' experiences during recovery or nonrecovery from psychosis. *Archives of Psychiatric Nursing, 18*(1), 17–25.

Times of illness and crisis can be opportunities for personal or spiritual growth for a person. The person may seek to connect or reconnect with others, with nature, with a power greater than himself or herself (that may be named in various ways, such as God, the Creator, or Allah, or not named out of respect), or with some aspect of the sacred (Baldacchino & Draper, 2001). Nurses can support clients in their spiritual growth by such means as listening to them as they describe their seeking; by responding to any requests for meeting with a religious leader/guide such as a minister, priest, rabbi, imam, lama, or elder; or by facilitating the use of religious ritual, such as a smudging ceremony for an Aboriginal client who requests it. Aspects of care for the spiritual domain relevant to particular disorders or age of human development may be found in the units on Care of Persons with Psychiatric Disorders, Children and Adolescents, and Older Adults.

SUMMARY OF KEY POINTS

◻ Nurses should work collaboratively with clients and families in determining interventions.

◻ Nurses develop interventions from assessment data and may organize them around nursing diagnoses. The client's needs, values, and preferred outcomes and the *Canadian Standards of Psychiatric-Mental Health Nursing* (CFMHN, 2006) guide the selection of interventions.

◻ A client's ability to manage self-care activities can fluctuate with symptom severity. The Orem self-care model can be used to conceptualize client needs (related to attitude, knowledge, and skill) and choose appropriate interventions.

◻ Interventions focusing on the biologic domain include activity and exercise; sleep, nutrition, relaxation, hydration, and thermoregulation interventions; pain management; and medication management. Nutritional interventions are used with most clients with psychiatric disorders. Medication management is a priority because of the long-term nature of the disorders and the importance of medication compliance.

◻ Interventions focusing on the psychological domain include counselling, behaviour therapy, cognitive interventions, psychoeducation, health teaching, and others. Implementation of these interventions requires a broad theoretic knowledge base.

◻ Interventions focusing on the social domain include group and family approaches, milieu therapy, safety interventions, home visits, and community action. On an inpatient psychiatric unit, the nurse uses milieu therapy to maximize the treatment effects of the client's environment.

◻ Interventions focusing on the spiritual domain involve a relationship and connection with the client that encompass the qualities of receptivity, humanity, competency, and positivity.

CRITICAL THINKING CHALLENGES

1 Tom, a 25-year-old man with schizophrenia, lives with his parents who want to retire to Vancouver Island. Tom goes to work each day but relies on his mother for meals, laundry, and reminders to take his medication. Tom believes that he can manage living on his own, but his mother is concerned. She asks the nurse for advice about leaving her son to manage on his own. Identify a nursing diagnosis and interventions that would meet some of Tom's potential responses to his changing lifestyle.

2 Joan, a 35-year-old married woman, is admitted to an acute psychiatric unit for stabilization of her mood disorder. She is extremely depressed but refuses to consider a recommended medication change. She asks the nurse what to do. Using a nursing intervention, explain how you would approach Joan's problem.

3 A nurse reports to work for the evening shift. The unit is chaotic. The television in the day room is loud; two clients are arguing about the program. Visitors are mingling in clients' rooms. The temperature of the unit is hot. One client is running up and down the hall yelling, "Help me, help me." Using a milieu therapy approach, what would you do to calm the unit?

WEB LINKS

www.arnnl.nf.ca/PDF/2008/role_of_the_psychiatric_mental_health_nurse_working_in_the_comm_policy_paper_apr_08.pdf The Association of Registered Nurses of Newfoundland and Labrador have developed a position statement concerning the role of the PMH nurse in community mental health settings.

www.camh.net This is the site of the Centre for Addiction and Mental Health.

www.ccmhi.ca This is the site of the Canadian Collaborative Mental Health Initiative where their charter can be accessed.

www.cfmhn.ca This is the site of the Canadian Federation of Mental Health Nurses (CFMHN), an associate member of the Canadian Nurses Association. The website contains conference information and standards related to psychiatric nursing practice in Canada.

www.cfmhn.ca/standards.html This site identifies the CFMHN Standards of Practice.

www.cmha.ca This is the site of the Canadian Mental Health Association, which contains information for health professionals and the general public about a broad range of mental health issues.

cna-aiic.ca/cna/documents/pdf/publications/CERT_Psych_e.pdf This document provides a list of the Canadian Nurses Association's Psychiatric/Mental Health Nursing Certification competencies.

cna-aiic.ca/CNA/documents/pdf/publications/ Code_of_Ethics_2008_e.pdf   The Canadian Nurses Association has released a new Code of Ethics to guide nursing.

www.crpnbc.ca/competency.html   This site outlines the competencies and standards of the College of Registered Psychiatric Nurses of British Columbia.

www.health.gov.nl.ca/health/mhcta   This is the site of the Government of Newfoundland and Labrador's Mental Health and Addictions Division, which includes the Mental Health Care and Treatment Act.

www.health.gov.sk.ca/mental-health-personal-rights   This is a site of the Saskatchewan Government outlining personal rights and mental health. It also includes a link to the province's Mental Health Services Act.

www.ispn-psych.org   This is the site of the International Society of Psychiatric-Mental Health Nurses, which is an international organization that promotes competent ethical psychiatric nursing practice.

www.mentalhealthcommission.ca   This is the site of the Mental Health Commission of Canada, which examines mental health care system issues in Canada.

www.mooddisorderscanada.ca   This is the site of the Mood Disorders Society of Canada, an organization that provides support for individuals with depression, bipolar disorder, and other associated mood disorders.

www.nedic.ca/index.shtml   This is the site of the National Eating Disorder Information Centre, which provides information on eating disorders such as bulimia and anorexia nervosa.

www.parl.gc.ca/39/1/parlbus/commbus/senate/ com-e/soci-e/rep-e/pdf/rep02may06high-e. pdf   This is a link to the report *Out of the Shadows at Last*, also known as the Kirby Report. This report is the result of extensive consultations with clients, families, health care providers, and the public concerning mental health in Canada.

www.phac-aspc.gc.ca/publicat/miic-mmac/pdf/men_ ill_e.pdf   This is a link to the *Report on Mental Illnesses in Canada*, which provides a comprehensive overview of the incidence and prevalence of mental illness in Canada.

www.rnao.org/bestpractices   This is the site of the Registered Nurses' Association of Ontario, which publishes best practice guidelines related to all aspects of nursing.

www.schizophrenia.ca   This is the site of the Schizophrenia Society of Canada, which acts as an advocacy group for individuals and families affected by schizophrenia.

REFERENCES

Baldacchino, D., & Draper, P. (2001). Spiritual coping strategies: A review of the nursing research literature. *Journal of Advanced Nursing, 34*(6), 833–841.

Bisconer, S. W., Green, M., Mallon-Czajka, J., & Johnson, J. S. (2006). Managing aggression in a psychiatric hospital using a behaviour plan: A case study. *Journal of Psychiatric and Mental Health Nursing, 13*(5), 515–521.

Boggs, K. (2003). Resolving conflict between nurse and client. In E. Arnold & K. Boggs (Eds.), *Interpersonal relationships: Professional communication skills for nurses* (4th ed., pp. 368–388). Philadelphia, PA: W. B. Saunders.

Buchanan-Barker, P., & Barker, P. J. (2006). The ten commitments: A value base for mental health recovery. *Journal of Psychosocial Nursing and Mental Health Services, 44*(9), 29–33.

Canadian Collaborative Mental Health Initiative. (2006). *Canadian collaborative mental health care charter*. Retrieved December 12, 2008, from http:// www.ccmhi.ca/en/products/charter.html

Canadian Federation of Mental Health Nurses. (2006). *Canadian standards of psychiatric- mental health nursing* (3rd ed.). Toronto, ON: Author.

Carr, T. (2008). Mapping the processes and qualities of spiritual nursing care. *Qualitative Health Research, 18*(5), 686–700.

Davidson, L. (2003). *Living outside mental illness: Qualitative studies of recovery in schizophrenia*. New York, NY: New York University Press.

Department of Human Services. (2006, October). *Seclusion*. Retrieved November 26, 2009, from http://www.health.vic.gov.au/mentalhealth/ cpg/seclusion.htm

Giedt, J. (1997). Guided imagery: A psychoneuroimmunological intervention in holistic nursing practice. *Journal of Holistic Nursing, 15*(2), 112–127.

Holmes, D., Kennedy, S. L., & Perron, A. (2004). The mentally ill and social exclusion: A critical examination of the use of seclusion from the patient's perspective. *Issues in Mental Health Nursing, 25*, 559–578.

Kontio, R., Välimäki, M., Putkonen, H., Cocoman, A., Turpeinen, S., Kuosmanen, L. & Joffe, G. (2009). Nurses' and physicians' educational needs in seclusion and restraint practices. *Perspectives in Psychiatric Care, 45*(3), 198–207.

Meehan, T., Bergen, H., & Fjeldsoe, K. (2004). Staff and patient perceptions of seclusion: Has anything changed? *Journal of Advanced Nursing, 47*(1), 33–38.

McCloskey, J., & Bulechek, G. (2000). *Nursing interventions classifications* (NIC), 3rd ed., St. Louis: Mosby.

National Alliance on Mental Illness. (2008). *Policy topics: What are restraints and seclusion?* Retrieved March 9, 2009, from http://www.nami.org/ Template.cfm?Section = Issue_Spotlights&template = /ContentManagement/ContentDisplay.cfm&ContentID = 7803

Orem, D. (1991). *Nursing concepts of practice* (4th ed.). St. Louis: MO: Year Book.

Rankin, S. H., Stallings, K. D., & London, F. (2005). *Patient education*. Philadelphia, PA: Lippincott Williams & Wilkins.

Sawatzky, R., & Pesut, B. (2005). Attributes of spiritual care in nursing practice. *Journal of Holistic Nursing, 23*(1), 19–33.

Shattell, M., Andes, M., & Thomas, S. (2008). How patients and nurses experience the acute care psychiatric environment. *Nursing Inquiry, 15*(3), 242–250.

Tweedell, D., Forchuk, C., Jewell, J., & Steinnagel, L. (2004). Families' experiences during recovery or nonrecovery from psychosis. *Archives of Psychiatric Nursing, 18*(1), 17–25.

CHAPTER
14

Psychopharmacology and Other Biologic Treatments

Kathleen Hegadoren

Adapted from the chapter "Psychopharmacology" by Susan McCabe

KEY CONCEPTS

- psychopharmacology
- receptors

LEARNING OBJECTIVES

After studying this chapter, you will be able to:

- Explain the key role of neurotransmitter chemicals and their receptor sites in the action of psychopharmacologic medications.
- Explain the role of receptors in the brain and other organ systems in the actions of psychotropic medications.
- Define the three properties that determine the strength and effectiveness of a medication.
- Describe hypothesized mechanisms of action for major classes of psychopharmacologic medication.
- Describe the major therapeutic effects as well as prevalent side effects of various classes of psychotropic medications.
- Suggest appropriate nursing methods to administer medications that facilitate efficacy.
- Implement interventions to minimize side effects of psychopharmacologic medications.
- Differentiate acute and chronic medication-induced movement disorders.
- Identify aspects of patient teaching that nurses must implement for successful maintenance of patients using psychotropic medications.
- Analyze the potential benefits and risks associated with other forms of somatic treatments, including electroconvulsive therapy, light therapy, and nutrition therapy.
- Evaluate potential causes of nonadherence and implement interventions to improve adherence with treatment regimens.

KEY TERMS

- absorption • adherence • adverse reactions • affinity • agonists • akathisia
- antagonists • bioavailability biotransformation • desensitization • distribution
- dystonia • efficacy • excretion • first-pass effect • half-life • intrinsic activity
- kindling • metabolism • pharmacogenomics • phototherapy • protein binding
- pseudoparkinsonism • selectivity • side effects • solubility • tardive dyskinesia
- target symptoms • therapeutic index • tolerance • toxicity • untoward effects

*T*hroughout history, treatment choices for mental disorders have been linked to the prevailing assumptions about the aetiology of these illnesses. In the early 1900s, Emil Kraeplin classified mental disorders based on clusters of observed symptoms, providing the basic tenets of the contemporary biologic approach to understanding and treating psychiatric disorders. However, this approach fell out of favour as psychoanalytic, psychodynamic, interpersonal, and other therapies flourished and mental disorders were increasingly assumed to have primarily a psychological aetiology. In the 1950s, when it was discovered that the phenothiazine medications, such as chlorpromazine (Thorazine), relieved many of the symptoms of psychosis, and that iproniazid, a medication for treating tuberculosis, elevated mood, there was renewed interest in neurophysiology and biologic treatments for treating mental disorders.

Recent scientific and technologic developments have renewed awareness of the biologic basis of mental disorders, leading to a proliferation of new medications that act at the cellular level, producing major behavioural and psychological change. These medications provide relief from debilitating symptoms in millions of individuals with psychiatric disorders. They have become the dominant form of treatment and are the cornerstones of all psychiatric treatment.

Most psychiatric and mental health (PMH) nurses work with individuals who are receiving psychopharmacologic agents as part of their treatment. As awareness of the prevalence of mental disorders increases, these medications are increasingly prescribed in primary care settings, and even nurses working in nonpsychiatric settings now need an in-depth knowledge of these medications to care for their patients in any setting (Hegadoren, 2004).

> **KEY CONCEPT Psychopharmacology** is a subspecialty of pharmacology that studies medications that affect the brain and behaviours and that are used to treat psychiatric and neurodegenerative disorders. It is important to remember, however, that many drugs used to treat other conditions, such as pain syndromes and heart disease, have powerful effects in the brain.

This chapter reviews the major classes of psychopharmacologic drugs used in treating mental disorders, including antipsychotics, mood stabilizers, antidepressants, antianxiety medications, and stimulants, and provides a basis for understanding the specific biologic treatments of psychiatric disorders that are described more fully in later chapters.

The target for psychiatric medications is predominantly the central nervous system (CNS) at the cellular and synaptic levels, although the autonomic nervous system often contributes to the pharmacologic profile of

psychiatric drugs. For this reason, this chapter focuses on understanding the impact of psychotropic medications on the basic unit of CNS functioning, the synapse, and on receptors embedded in neuronal cell membranes. This basic understanding allows the PMH nurse to accept the role and responsibilities of administering medications, proactively monitoring and treating side effects, and educating the patient and family, which are all crucial to successful psychopharmacologic therapy. In addition to psychopharmacologic therapy, other biologic treatments (sometimes referred to as *somatic treatments*) are used. These therapies include electroconvulsive therapy (ECT), light therapy, and nutritional therapy and are discussed later in this chapter.

■ PHARMACODYNAMICS

A comparatively small amount of medication can have a significant and large impact on cell function and resulting behaviour. When tiny molecules of medication are compared with the vast amount of cell surface in the human body, the fraction seems disproportionate. Yet the drugs used to treat mental disorders often have profound effects on behaviour. To understand how this occurs, one needs to understand both where and how drugs work.

Targets of Drug Action: Where Drugs Act

Drug molecules do not act on the entire cell surface, but rather at receptor sites. Many psychopharmacologic drugs, especially older classes, act at multiple receptors. Newer agents are more specific to one type of receptor, but none are exclusive to one type of receptor. Another key to understanding drug effects is the distribution of receptors within the body. Different types and subtypes of receptors can be concentrated in specific brain regions. Thus, there is a close relationship between the drug effects and the functions associated with a brain region.

> **KEY CONCEPT Receptors** are associated with the work of German chemist Paul Erhlich, who in 1900 suggested that a receptive substance exists within the cell membrane. The biologic action of a drug depends on how its structure interacts with a specific receptor. Thus, a basic understanding of how receptors work is key to understanding how most drugs work in the body.

Receptors are proteins that are embedded within the cell membrane and have binding sites for both naturally occurring chemicals (called *endogenous substances*) and administered drugs. Endogenous brain chemicals involved in neurotransmission, such as dopamine and serotonin, adhere to specific groups of receptors. Administered drugs may compete with neurotransmitters for these receptors by mimicking or blocking the action of the neurotransmitter. In this chapter, *receptor* refers only to those membrane proteins to which a neurotransmitter can specifically adhere to produce a change in the cell membrane, serving a physiologic regulatory function (such as those discussed in Chapter 10). These include ligand-gated ion channels or the G-protein–coupled receptors.

Receptors

Many drugs have been developed to act specifically at the receptor sites. Their chemical structure is similar to the neurotransmitter substance for that receptor. When attached, these drugs act as **agonists**—chemicals producing the same biologic action as the neurotransmitter itself—or as **antagonists**—chemicals blocking the biologic action of an agonist at a given receptor. Figure 14-1 illustrates the action of an agonist and an antagonist drug at a receptor site. A drug's ability to interact with a given receptor type may be judged by three properties: selectivity, affinity, and intrinsic activity.

Selectivity

The first property, called **selectivity,** is the ability of the drug to be specific for a particular receptor. If a drug is highly selective, it will interact only with its specific receptors in the areas of the body where these receptors occur and, therefore, not affect tissues and organs where its receptors do not occur. Using a "lock-and-key" analogy,

FIGURE 14.1 Agonist and antagonist drug actions at a receptor site. This schematic drawing represents drug–receptor interactions. At *top*, drug D has the correct shape to fit receptor R, forming a drug–receptor complex, which results in a conformational change in the receptor and the opening of a pore in the adjacent membrane. Drug D is an agonist. At *bottom*, drug A also has the correct shape to fit the receptor, forming a drug–receptor complex, but in this case, there is no conformational change and, therefore, no response. Drug A is, therefore, an antagonist.

only a specific, highly selective key will fit a given lock. The more selective or structurally specific a drug is, the more likely it will affect only the specific receptors for which it is meant. The more receptors for other neurochemicals are affected, the more unintended effects, or **side effects,** are produced. Selectivity is important to understand because it helps explain the concept of side effects caused by medications, a major cause of concern in medication treatment. The distribution of receptors in specific brain regions also plays a role in the side-effect profile. For example, dopamine antagonists can produce dystonic movements because high concentrations of dopamine receptors are found in the region of the brain that controls fine motor movement.

Affinity

The second property is that of **affinity,** which is the degree of attraction or strength of the bond between the drug and its receptor. Normally, these bonds are produced by relatively weak electrochemical attractions. Basic to the action of most drugs within the body is their ability to bind to a receptor, produce a response, and then easily move off the receptor. Although most drugs used in psychiatry have this on–off property in relation to their target receptors, some drugs, specifically the monoamine oxidase inhibitors (MAOIs) (discussed later in this chapter), have a different type of bond, called a *covalent bond.* This type of bond is stronger and irreversible at normal temperatures. The effects of the drugs that form covalent bonds are often called "irreversible" because new receptors must be produced, a process taking several weeks.

Intrinsic Activity

The final property of a drug's ability to interact with a given receptor is that of **intrinsic activity,** or the ability of the drug to produce a biologic response once it becomes attached to the receptor. Some drugs have selectivity and affinity but produce no biologic response; therefore, an important measure of a drug is whether it produces a change in the cell containing the receptor. Drugs that act as agonists have all three properties: selectivity, affinity, and intrinsic activity. However, antagonists have only selectivity and affinity because they produce no biologic response by attaching to that receptor. However, in complex biologic systems such as the brain, preventing an agonist from binding can yield multiple cellular and ultimately behavioural responses. An example of this is the antipsychotic class, all members of which are antagonists.

Some drugs act as *partial agonists.* When a stronger agonist with high intrinsic activity is combined with a weaker agonist (low intrinsic activity) that has high affinity for a given receptor, the net effect is that the weaker agonist will act as an antagonist to the stronger agonist. Because it has some intrinsic activity (although weak), it is referred to as a *partial agonist*. A drug may act as an agonist at one receptor and an antagonist at another. For some drugs, their activity is dose dependent: at low doses they act as agonists, but at higher doses they act more as antagonists. Medications that have both agonist and antagonist effects are called *mixed agonist–antagonists*.

Ion Channels

Some drugs act directly on ion channels imbedded in the nerve cell membrane. Examples include local anaesthetics that block the entry of sodium into the cell, preventing a nerve impulse, and nicotine, which acts as an agonist at nicotinic acetylcholine receptors. In psychiatry, the utility of calcium-channel blockers has been investigated for use with the symptoms of mania, a state of increased activity, euphoria, difficulty sleeping, racing thoughts, and rapid and forced speech (see Chapter 20). Operating on the hypothesis that mania is related to too much neurotransmitter released into the synapse, researchers suggested that modulating the influx of calcium (which stimulates the vesicles to release neurotransmitter) might decrease the symptoms of mania. Although this theory is overly simplistic, it is an example of how neurotransmission may be changed by different drug actions (Pacheco & Jope, 1996).

The benzodiazepine drugs, frequently used in psychiatry, decrease the symptoms of anxiety and are an example of drugs that affect the ion channels of the nerve cell membrane. The benzodiazepine molecule, in such drugs as diazepam (Valium), works by binding to a region of the gamma-aminobutyric acid (GABA)-receptor chloride channel complex. The binding site for these drugs is different from where GABA itself binds. When bound, these drugs increase the frequency and duration of chloride efflux mediated by GABA. The overall effect is helping GABA to decrease the ability of that cell to conduct a nerve impulse. Thus, they are referred to as being indirect agonists and are used as anticonvulsants, antianxiety, and hypnotic drugs.

Enzymes

Enzymes are complex proteins that catalyze specific biochemical reactions within cells and are the targets for some drugs used to treat mental disorders. For example, monoamine oxidase is the enzyme required to break down most bioamine neurotransmitters, such as norepinephrine, serotonin, and dopamine, and can be inhibited by medications from a group of antidepressants called MAOIs. The inhibitory effect is greater for norepinephrine and serotonin than it is for dopamine. This increase in available norepinephrine and serotonin is thought to initiate the cascade of cellular changes that ultimately relieve the symptoms of depression. Strong covalent bonds are formed between the medication and the enzyme, which inhibit the ability of the enzyme to inactivate the bioamine neurotransmitters after they have been used, resulting in increased amounts of these neurotransmitters ready for release in the nerve terminals. New enzyme molecules must be produced before any activity is restored. Although they have similar effects, some enzyme inhibitors (e.g., moclobemide) do not form covalent bonds, so are called reversible.

Carrier Proteins: Uptake Receptors

Neurotransmitters are small organic molecules that are released in response to a change in the polarity of the cell membrane (called an action potential), interact with receptors, and then are transported back into the neuronal cell by carrier proteins. In much the same way as receptors, these transporters (also referred to as *uptake receptors*) have recognition sites specific for the type of molecule to be transported. After a neurotransmitter, such as serotonin, has activated receptors in the synapse, its actions are terminated by these transporters that take serotonin back up into the presynaptic cell. Medications specific for this site may block or inhibit this transport and, therefore, increase the amount of the neurotransmitter in the synaptic space available for action on the receptors.

A primary action of most of the antidepressants is to increase the amount of neurotransmitters in the synapse by blocking their reuptake. Older antidepressants block the reuptake of more than one neurotransmitter. Some antidepressants, such as fluoxetine (Prozac) and sertraline (Zoloft), are more selective for serotonin, whereas reboxetine is more selective for norepinephrine. These medications are called selective serotonin reuptake inhibitors (SSRIs) and selective norepinephrine reuptake inhibitors, respectively. Newer antidepressants that are selective to both serotonin and norepinephrine are called SNRIs (e.g., venlafaxine [Effexor] and duloxetine [Cymbalta]). These more selective medications have reduced the number of side effects experienced by the patients. Figure 14-2 illustrates the reuptake blockade of serotonin by an SSRI.

FIGURE 14.2 Reuptake blockade of a transporter for serotonin by a SSRI.

Efficacy and Potency: How Drugs Act

Efficacy is another characteristic of medications to be considered when selecting a drug for the treatment of a particular set of symptoms. **Efficacy** is the ability of a drug to produce a desired response. It is important to remember that the degree of receptor occupancy contributes to efficacy, yet it is not the only variable. A drug may occupy a large number of receptors but not produce a response. In contrast, *potency* considers the amount of drug required to produce the desired biologic response. One drug may be able to achieve the same clinical effect as another drug but at a lower dose, making it more potent. Although the drug given at the lower dose is more potent, because both drugs achieve similar effects, they may be considered to have equal efficacy. However, side effects are often related to dose, so a potent drug that can produce a therapeutic response at a lower dose may be preferable.

Loss of Effect: Biologic Adaptation

In some instances, the effects of medications diminish with time, especially when they are given repeatedly, as in the treatment of chronic psychiatric disorders. This loss of effect can be a form of physiologic adaptation that may develop as the cell attempts to regain homeostatic control to counteract the effects of the drug. **Desensitization** is a rapid decrease in drug effects that may develop in a few minutes of exposure to a drug. This process is rare with most psychiatric medications but can occur with some medications used to treat serious side effects (e.g., physostigmine, sometimes used to relieve severe anticholinergic side effects). **Tolerance** is a gradual decrease in the action of a drug at a given dose or concentration in the blood. This decrease may take days or weeks to develop and results in the loss of therapeutic effect of a drug. This loss of effect is often called *treatment refractoriness*. There are many reasons for decreased drug effectiveness (Box 14-1). A rapid decrease can occur with some drugs because of immediate transformation of the receptor when the drug molecule binds to the receptor. Other drugs cause a decrease in the number of receptors. Some drugs may deplete cellular stores of neurotransmitters. Examples include D-amphetamine, which depletes dopamine stores, and the recreational drug "Ecstasy," which depletes serotonin stores. Drug tolerance is also caused by an increase in the *metabolism* (breakdown) of the medication, such as with barbiturates, which trigger an increase in the amount of hepatic enzymes responsible for their metabolism and results in a significant decrease in the blood level of the anticonvulsant carbamazepine (Tegretol) if used in combination with phenobarbital, for example. Cycling female hormones can also affect response to drugs. Progesterone and its metabolites bind to the same GABA receptor as do the benzodiazepines and can affect the efficacy and potency of benzodiazepines at certain stages of the menstrual cycle.

Other forms of physiologic adaptation result in a gradual tolerance that may be helpful in the case of unpleasant side effects, such as drowsiness or nausea. This information is important for the nurse to communicate to patients experiencing such side effects so that they can be reassured that the effects will subside. The PMH nurse must also know when tolerance will not occur and when a lack of tolerance to a significant side effect warrants discontinuation of the medication.

Target Symptoms and Side Effects

Psychiatric medications are indicated for specific symptoms, referred to as **target symptoms**. Target symptoms are those measurable specific symptoms expected to improve with medication use. The target symptoms for each class of medication are discussed more fully in later sections of this chapter. Because receptors for neurotransmitters such as serotonin are found in all regions of the brain and in the periphery, serotonin-related drugs produce widespread effects in many body systems. For example, these drugs interact with receptors in the gastrointestinal tract and in facial motor nerves, causing gastrointestinal upset and bruxism (clenching and grinding of teeth). These unwanted effects of medications are called **side effects** (or **untoward effects**). Some unwanted effects may have serious physiologic consequences, referred to as **adverse reactions**. Although technically different, these three terms are often used interchangeably in the literature.

Knowledge of a medication's affinity for receptors and subtypes of receptors may give some indication of the likelihood that specific target symptoms might improve and what side effects might be predicted. Table 14-1 provides a brief summary of possible physiologic effects from drug actions on specific neurotransmitters. For example, antagonists with high affinity for acetylcholine receptors of the muscarinic subtype will be more likely to cause such side effects as dry mouth, blurred vision, constipation, urinary hesitancy or retention, and nasal congestion. This

---

BOX 14.1

Mechanisms Causing Decrease in Medication Effects

- Change in receptor affinity
- Loss of receptors
- Depletion of neurotransmitter supply
- Increased metabolism of the drug
- Physiologic adaptation
- Interaction with female hormones

Table 14.1	Drug Affinity for Specific Neurotransmitters and Receptors and Subsequent Effects	
Neurotransmitter/ Receptor Action	**Physiologic Effects**	**Example of Drugs That Exhibit High Affinity**
Receptor Blockade		
Norepinephrine reuptake inhibition	Antidepressant action Potentiation of pressor effects of norepinephrine Interaction with guanethidine Side effects: tachycardia, tremors, insomnia, erectile and ejaculation dysfunction	desipramine reboxetine
Serotonin reuptake inhibition	Antidepressant action Antiobsessional effect Increase or decrease in anxiety, dose dependent Side effects: gastrointestinal distress, nausea, headache, nervousness, motor restlessness, and sexual side effects, including anorgasmia	fluoxetine paroxetine
Dopamine reuptake inhibition	Antidepressant action Antiparkinsonian effect Side effects: increase in psychomotor activity, aggravation of psychosis	buproprion
Reuptake Inhibition		
Histamine receptor blockade (H$_1$)	Side effects: sedation, drowsiness, hypotension, and weight gain	quetiapine imipramine clozapine olanzapine
Acetylcholine receptor blockade (muscarinic)	Side effects: anticholinergic (dry mouth, blurred vision, constipation, urinary hesitancy and retention, memory dysfunction), and sinus tachycardia	imipramine amitriptyline thioridazine clozapine
Norepinephrine receptor blockade (α_1 receptor)	Potentiation of antihypertensive effect of prazosin and terazosin Side effects: postural hypotension, dizziness, reflex tachycardia, sedation	amitriptyline clomipramine clozapine amitriptyline
Norepinephrine receptor blockade (α_2 receptor)	Increased sexual desire (yohimbine) Interactions with antihypertensive medications, blockade of the antihypertensive effects of clonidine Side effect: priapism	clomipramine clozapine trazodone yohimbine
Norepinephrine receptor blockade (β_1 receptor)	Antihypertensive action (propranolol) Side effects: orthostatic hypotension, sedation, depression, sexual dysfunction (including impotence and decreased ejaculation)	propranolol
Serotonin receptor blockade (5-HT$_{1a}$)	Antidepressant action Antianxiety effect Possible control of aggression	trazodone risperidone ziprasidone
Serotonin receptor blockade (5-HT$_2$)	Antipsychotic action Some antimigraine effect Decreased rhinitis Side effects: hypotension, ejaculatory problems, weight gain, metabolic disorders	risperidone clozapine olanzapine ziprasidone haloperidol
Dopamine receptor blockade (D$_2$)	Antipsychotic action Side effects: extrapyramidal symptoms, such as tremor, rigidity (especially acute dystonia and parkinsonism); endocrine changes, including elevated prolactin levels	ziprasidone

information should serve only as a guide in predicting side effects because of considerable interindividual variability in drug responses and not all underlying mechanisms have been elucidated. The PMH nurse should use this information to focus assessment on these areas. If the symptoms are mild, simple nursing interventions suggested in Table 14-2 should be implemented. If symptoms persist or are severe, the prescriber should be notified immediately.

Table 14.2	Managing Common Side Effects of Psychiatric Medications
Side Effect or Discomfort	**Intervention**
Blurred vision	Reassurance (generally subsides in 2–6 weeks)
Dry eyes	Warn ophthalmologist; no eye examination for new glasses for at least 3 weeks after a stable dose
	Artificial tears may be required; an increased use of wetting solutions for those wearing contact lenses
Dry mouth and lips	Frequent rinsing of mouth, good oral hygiene, sucking sugarless candies, lozenges, lip balm, lemon juice, and glycerin mouth swabs
Constipation	High-fiber diet, encourage bran, fresh fruits, and vegetables
	Metamucil (must consume at least 16 oz of fluid with dose)
	Increase hydration
	Exercise, increase fluids
	Mild laxative
Urinary hesitancy or retention	Monitor frequently for difficulty with urination, changes in starting or stopping stream
	Notify prescriber if difficulty develops
	A cholinergic agonist, such as bethanechol, may be required
Nasal congestion	Nose drops, moisturizer, *not* nasal spray
Sinus tachycardia	Assess for infections
	Monitor pulse for rate and irregularities
	Withhold medication and notify prescriber if resting rate exceeds 120 bpm
Decreased libido and ejaculatory inhibition	Reassurance (reversible)
	Consider change to another drug in same class or change class of drug
Postural hypotension	Frequent monitoring of lying-to-standing blood pressure during dosage adjustment period, immediate changes and accommodation, measure pulse in both positions
	Advise patient to get up slowly, sit for at least 1 minute before standing (dangling legs over side of bed), and stand for 1 minute before walking or until light-headedness subsides
	Increase hydration, avoid caffeine
	Elastic stockings if necessary
	Notify prescriber if symptoms persist or significant blood pressure changes are present; medication may have to be changed if patient does not have impulse control to get up slowly
Photosensitivity	Protective clothing
	Dark glasses
Dermatitis	Use of sun block, remember to cover *all* exposed areas
	Stop medication usage
	Consider medication change, may require a systemic antihistamine
	Initiate comfort measures to decrease itching
Impaired psychomotor functions	Advise patient to avoid dangerous tasks, such as driving
	Avoid alcohol, which increases this impairment
Drowsiness or sedation	Encourage activity during the day to increase accommodation
	Avoid tasks that require mental alertness, such as driving
	May need to adjust dosing schedule or, if possible, give single daily dose at bedtime
	May need a cholinergic medication if sedation is the problem
	Avoid driving or operating potentially dangerous equipment
	May need change to less-sedating medication
	Provide quiet and decreased stimulation when sedation is the desired effect
Weight gain	Exercise and diet teaching
	Caloric control and regular monitoring of blood glucose levels
Edema	Check fluid retention
	Reassurance
	May need a diuretic
Irregular menstruation	Reassurance (reversible)
Amenorrhea	May need to change class of drug
	Reassurance and counselling (does not indicate lack of ovulation)
	Instruct patient to continue birth control measures
Vaginal dryness	Instruct in use of lubricants

Drug Toxicity

All drugs have the capacity to be harmful as well as helpful. **Toxicity** generally refers to the point at which concentrations of the drug in the bloodstream are high enough to become harmful or poisonous to the body. However, what is considered harmful? Side effects can be harmful but not toxic, and individuals vary widely in their responses to medications. Some patients experience adverse reactions more readily than others. For example, women are more likely to experience side effects than men. **Therapeutic index,** a concept often used to discuss the toxicity of a drug, is a ratio of the maximum nontoxic dose to the minimum effective dose. A high therapeutic index means that there is a large range between the dose at which the drug begins to take effect and a dose that would be toxic to the body. Drugs with a low therapeutic index have a narrow range and are often carefully monitored through routine assessment of blood levels. This concept has some limitations. The concept of toxicity is only vaguely defined. The range can also be affected by drug tolerance. For example, individuals increasing their dosages of barbiturates as they became increasingly more tolerant to the effects and requiring larger doses to make them sleep have caused accidental deaths. The therapeutic index of a medication also may be greatly changed by the coadministration of other medications or drugs. For example, alcohol consumed with most CNS depressant drugs will have added depressant effects, greatly increasing the likelihood of toxicity or death.

Despite the limitations of the therapeutic index, it is a helpful guide for nurses, particularly when working with potentially suicidal individuals. PMH nurses must be aware of the potential for overdose and closely monitor the availability of drugs for these patients. In some cases, prescriptions may have to be dispensed every few days or each week until a suicidal crisis has passed to ensure that patients do not have a lethal dose available to them.

■ PHARMACOKINETICS: HOW DRUGS MOVE THROUGH THE BODY

The field of pharmacokinetics describes, often in mathematical models, how a drug moves throughout the body to get to its target receptors and then is eliminated. The processes of absorption, distribution, metabolism, and excretion are of central importance. Overall, the goal in pharmacokinetics is to describe and predict the time course of drug concentrations throughout the body and factors that may interfere with these processes. Together with the principles of pharmacodynamics, this information can be helpful to the psychiatric nurse in ways such as facilitating or inhibiting drug effects and predicting behavioural response.

Absorption and Routes of Administration

The first phase of drug disposition in the human body is **absorption,** defined as the movement of the drug from the site of administration into the plasma. It is important to consider the impact of routes by which a drug is administered on the process of absorption.

Not all potential routes of administration are available for medications used to treat psychiatric disorders. The primary routes available include oral (both tablet and liquid), sublingual, intramuscular (IM) (short- and long-acting agents), and intravenous (used for rapid treatment of adverse reactions and rarely for the treatment of the primary psychiatric disorder). The PMH nurse needs to know about the advantages and disadvantages of each route and the subsequent effects on absorption (Table 14-3).

Drugs taken orally are usually the most convenient for the patient; however, this route is also the most variable because absorption can be slowed or enhanced by a number of factors. Taking certain drugs orally with food or antacids may slow the rate of absorption or change the amount of the drug absorbed. For example, the β-receptor antagonist propranolol exhibits increased blood levels when taken with food. Antacids containing aluminium salts decrease the absorption of most antipsychotic drugs; thus, antacids must be given at least 1 hour before administration or 2 hours after.

Oral preparations absorbed from the gastrointestinal tract into the bloodstream first go to the liver through the portal vein. There, they may be metabolized in such a way that most of the drug is inactivated before it reaches the rest of the body. Some drugs are also subjected to metabolism in the gastrointestinal wall. These losses of orally administered drugs before entering the systemic circulation are termed the **first-pass effect.** The consequence of first-pass effect is that the fraction of the drug reaching systemic circulation is reduced, sometimes substantially. Drugs that commonly undergo first-pass effect include nortriptyline, meperidine, and propranolol. First-pass effect explains why the dose of propranolol given intravenously is so much less than the oral dose.

Other factors affecting absorption should also be considered when administering drugs with known first-pass effect. Liver disease and dysfunction can alter the first-pass effect and result in increased drug levels and thus an increased risk for side effects. Gastric motility also affects how the drug is absorbed. Increasing age, many disease states, and concurrent medications can reduce motility and slow absorption. Other factors, such as blood flow in the gastrointestinal system, drug formulation, and chemical factors, may also interfere with absorption. Nurses must be aware of a patient's physical condition and use of medications or other substances that can interfere with drug absorption.

In full strength, many liquid preparations, especially antipsychotics, irritate the mucosal lining of the mouth, oesophagus, and stomach and must be adequately diluted. Nurses must be careful when diluting liquid medications because some liquid concentrate preparations are incompatible with certain juices or other liquids. If a drug is mixed with

Table 14.3	Selected Forms and Routes of Psychiatric Medications		
Preparation and Route	Examples	Advantages	Disadvantages
Oral tablet	Basic preparation for most psychopharmacologic agents, including antidepressants, antipsychotics, mood stabilizers, anxiolytics, etc.	Convenience	Variable rate and extent of absorption, depending on the drug May be affected by the contents of the intestines May show first-pass metabolism effects May not be easily swallowed by some individuals
Oral liquid	Also known as concentrates Many antipsychotics, such as haloperidol, chlorpromazine, thioridazine, risperidone The antidepressant fluoxetine Antihistamines, such as diphenhydramine Mood stabilizers, such as lithium citrate	Ease of incremental dosing Easily swallowed In some cases, more quickly absorbed	More difficult to measure accurately Depending on drug: • Possible interactions with other liquids such as juice, forming precipitants • Possible irritation to mucosal lining of mouth if not properly diluted
Rapid-dissolving tablet	Atypical antipsychotics, such as olanzapine	Dissolves almost instantaneously in mouth Handy for people who have trouble swallowing or for patients who let medication linger in the cheek for later expectoration Can be taken when water or other liquid is unavailable	Patient needs to remember to have completely dry hands and to place tablet in mouth immediately Tablet should not linger in the hand
Sublingual	Lorazepam	Rapid action, no first-pass metabolism	Increased risk for tolerance and psychological dependance
Intramuscular	Some antipsychotics, such as haloperidol, chlorpromazine, and risperidone Anxiolytics, such as lorazepam Anticholinergics, such as diphenhydramine and benztropine mesylate No antidepressants No mood stabilizers	More rapid acting than oral preparations No first-pass metabolism	Injection-site pain and irritation Some medications may have erratic absorption if heavy muscle tissue at the site of injection is not in use High-potency antipsychotics in this form may be more prone to adverse reactions, such as NMS
IM depot (or long-acting)	Haloperidol decanoate, fluphenazine decanoate, risperidone	May be more convenient for some individuals who have difficulty following medication regimens	Significant pain at injection site
Intravenous	Anticholinergics, such as diphenhydramine, benztropine mesylate Anxiolytics, such as diazepam, lorazepam, and chlordiazepoxide The antipsychotic haloperidol (unlabelled use)	Rapid and complete availability to systemic circulation	Inflammation of tissue surrounding site Often inconvenient for patient and uncomfortable Continuous dosage requires use of a constant-rate IV infusion

an incompatible liquid, a white or grainy precipitant usually forms, indicating that some of the drug has bound to the liquid and inactivated. Thus, the patient actually receives a lower dose of the medication than intended. Precipitants can also form from combining two liquid medications in one diluent, such as juice. Sometimes, precipitants may be difficult to see, such as in orange juice, so nurses must be aware of the compatibilities of liquid preparations. If a precipitant forms in a medication cup, it will also form in the stomach, causing additional inactivation of the drugs. Therefore, some medications should be given at least an hour apart. With new technologies come novel administration routes and drug forms, one of which is the rapid-dissolving oral pill. Manufacturers have different procedures for developing rapid-dissolving drugs, and these are patented with unique names. Common forms include the DuraSolv and QuickTab technologies. Many drugs are currently available in rapid-dissolving form, including the atypical antipsychotic olanzapine (Zyprexa, Zydis), risperidone (Risperdal M-Tab), and mirtazapine (Remeron SolTab). Nurses need to be aware of the special administration and patient-teaching requirements of the rapid-dissolving drug forms.

To take an orally disintegrating tablet, the nurse or patient should use dry hands to peel back the foil packaging, immediately take out the tablet, and place it into the mouth. The tablet will quickly dissolve and can be swallowed with saliva. No water is needed to swallow disintegrating tablets. This is advantageous when a patient cannot swallow well or is unwilling to swallow pills, or when water is not readily available.

Bioavailability

Bioavailability describes the amount of the drug that actually reaches systemic circulation. The route by which a drug is administered significantly affects bioavailability. With some oral drugs, the amount of drug entering the bloodstream is decreased by first-pass metabolism and bioavailability is lower (Pandolfi et al., 2003). On the other hand, some rapid-dissolving oral medications have increased bioavailability.

Bioavailability is a concept often used to compare one drug with another, obviously implying that increased bioavailability makes one drug "better" than another. The US Food and Drug Administration (FDA) uses bioavailability as one measure for comparing the equivalency of the drugs when generic forms of a drug are developed. Although increased bioavailability of a drug may sound impressive, it is important to remember that this is not a characteristic solely of the drug preparation. It may be low if absorption is incomplete. Wide individual variations in the enzyme activity of the intestine or liver, gastric pH, and intestinal motility will all affect it. In practice, bioavailability is difficult to quantify.

PMH nurses must remember that many factors on any particular occasion may affect the absorption and bioavailability of the drug for an individual patient.

Distribution

Even after a drug enters the bloodstream, several factors affect how it is distributed in the body. **Distribution** of a drug reflects how easy it is for a drug to pass out of the systemic circulation and move into other types of tissues, such as brain, abdominal organs, skin, or bone, where target receptors are found. Factors that affect medication distribution to specific tissues in the body include the amount of blood flow or perfusion within the tissue; how lipophilic ("fat-loving") the drug is; plasma protein binding; and anatomic barriers, such as the blood–brain barrier, that the drug must cross. A drug may have rapid absorption and high bioavailability, but if it cannot cross the blood–brain barrier to reach the CNS, it is of little use in psychiatry. Table 14-4 provides a summary of how some significant factors affect distribution. Two of these factors, ionic characteristics and protein binding, warrant additional discussion with regard to how they relate to psychiatric medications.

Ionic Characteristics of Drugs

Drugs in the bloodstream can be charged molecules (in the form of positive or negative ions) or can be uncharged. There are many charged components within cell membranes. Thus, drugs that have an electrical charge cannot passively cross through a cell membrane; instead, they must be transported by carrier proteins. Uncharged drugs

Table 14.4	Factors Affecting Distribution of a Drug
Factor	**Effect on Drug Distribution**
Size of the organ	Larger organs require more drug to reach a concentration level equivalent to other organs and tissues.
Blood flow to the organ	The more blood flow to and within an organ (perfusion), the greater the drug concentration. The brain, for example, has high perfusion.
Ionic characteristics	Drugs with no electrical charge move easily across cell membranes and thus will be widely distributed.
Plasma protein binding	If a drug binds well to plasma proteins, particularly to albumin, it will stay in the body longer but have a slower distribution.
Anatomic barriers	Both the gastrointestinal tract and the brain are surrounded by layers of cells that control the passage or uptake of substances. Lipid-soluble substances are usually readily absorbed and pass the blood–brain barrier.

(also called lipophilic or "fat-loving" drugs) can move easily across cell membranes. Most psychiatric drugs are very lipophilic and can move into major organ systems, as well as cross the blood–brain barrier. However, this characteristic means that psychopharmacologic agents can also cross the placenta. It also means that these agents can be taken into fat stores. Drugs stored in fatty tissue are only slowly released back into the systemic circulation for eventual elimination. This is why a lipophilic drug can be detected long after discontinuation in older women and overweight individuals. This effect may also account for unexpected drug–drug interactions when substitute drugs regimes are initiated quickly.

Protein Binding

Many drugs bind to large carrier proteins in the bloodstream, referred to as **protein binding**. The degree to which a drug is bound to these plasma proteins affects the drug's ability to interact with receptors. Only unbound or "free" drugs can move across membranes to their target receptors. High protein binding can prolong the duration of action of the drug. Many of the psychiatric drugs are more than 90% protein bound. Chronic disease and normal aging can decrease the amounts of plasma protein, shifting the ratio of bound drug to free drug. For highly bound drugs like the classic antipsychotics, a decrease of only 10% of bound drug (e.g., from 90% to 80%) would translate into a doubling of free drug and significantly increase the risk for side effects.

Metabolism

The duration of drug action depends to a large degree on the body's ability to change or alter a drug chemically. **Metabolism,** also called **biotransformation,** is the process by which the drug is altered, often broken down into smaller substances known as *metabolites*. Through the processes of metabolism, lipid-soluble drugs become more water soluble so that they may be excreted more readily.

Most metabolism occurs in the liver, but it can also occur in the kidneys, lungs, and intestines. The outcome of this process is usually an inactive metabolite. However, metabolism can also change a drug to an active metabolite with either similar or very different actions as the parent compound. For instance, the antidepressant imipramine is metabolized to a pharmacologically active substance, desipramine, which also has antidepressant effects. This becomes important when measuring the therapeutic blood level of imipramine. It is more clinically relevant and accurate to obtain both imipramine and desipramine levels, even though the patient may be taking only the drug imipramine. Prozac (fluoxetine), an SSRI antidepressant, is metabolized in the liver and forms an active metabolite, norfluoxetine, which has a very long half-life. Metabolism may also change an inactive drug (called a prodrug) to an active one or an active drug to a toxic metabolite. Codeine is an example of a prodrug that must be metabolized before having analgesic properties. N-hydroxyacetaminophen is formed with an acetaminophen overdose and is further oxidized to a toxic chemical that can destroy liver cells.

The cytochrome P-450 superfamily of metabolic enzymes (or CYP450s) is responsible for most drug metabolism. The classification of the CYP450 superfamily uses a combination of numbers and letters to denote families, subfamilies, and individual enzymes. Specific genes encode each enzyme, but polymorphisms are common. Most psychiatric drugs are metabolized by members of the 1A, 2D, and 3A subfamilies of CYP450 enzymes. The 3A family is the most abundant, constituting more than 60% of the liver enzyme weight. The metabolizing activity of some of the CYP450 enzymes can be altered by drugs and environmental chemicals. Some drugs like phenobarbital induce CYP450 activity. This increases enzymatic action and thus decreases drug levels of any drug taken concomitantly with phenobarbital. Subthreshold drug levels may affect efficacy. Other common substances, such as tobacco smoke, alcohol, and coal tar in charcoal-broiled foods can induce the CYP450 enzyme system. Alternately, drugs can inhibit CYP450 activity and thus increase drug levels, potentially into toxic ranges. A CYP enzyme that is responsible for a wide variety of therapeutic agents and is often inhibited is CYP2D6. Acute alcohol ingestion and the anti-ulcer medication cimetidine (Tagamet), available over the counter, can inhibit CYP2D6. Some of the SSRIs are also potent inhibitors of CYP2D6. Grapefruit juice is an inhibitor of CYP3A enzymes. Not all SSRIs are equal in their potency to inhibit CYP2D6. Paroxetine (Paxil) is the most potent, producing more than 90% inhibition of this enzyme subfamily, whereas sertraline exhibits mild effects, with only 20% to 50% inhibition (Dalfen & Stewart, 2001). The newer SSRI citalopram has minimal inhibiting properties.

The metabolism of many of the older drugs has not been thoroughly investigated. Indeed, information about the specific CYP450 enzyme responsible for metabolism is available for only about 20% of commonly prescribed medications. In addition, a drug can be metabolized by more than one CYP450. A minor route of metabolism can become the major route under conditions of liver disease or dysfunction or if the individual has a genetic mutation of that enzyme, rendering it with only low intrinsic activity.

CYP450 enzymes contribute to the enormous differences in the reaction of individuals to medications. More than 100,000 people die in American hospitals each year of adverse reactions to medications that are safe and beneficial to others (Lazarou, Pomeranz, & Corey, 1998). Another 2.2 million experience serious side effects, whereas others experience no response to the same medications. Differences and changes in CYP450 enzymatic activity among people alter how individuals experience response to medications. These differences in the enzymes often are caused by genetic variations (Dahl, 2002). DNA variants in the CYP450 system and the enzymes encoded by these genes have been investigated for several CYP enzymes in relation to specific ethnic and racial groups. For example, about 3% of Caucasians and more than 20% of Japanese are poor metabolizers of CYP2C19. About 2% of Chinese, but up to 10% of Caucasians, are poor metabolizers of CYP2D6 (Baker, Urichuk, & Coutts, 1998).

The emerging science of **pharmacogenomics** blends pharmacology with genetic knowledge and is concerned with understanding and determining an individual's specific CYP450 makeup, then individualizing medications to match the person's CYP450 profile. Increasingly, psychiatric medications are prescribed after testing to determine the patient's CYP450 genotype to guide treatment with the most effective drugs for the patient, and to drastically reduce potential drug–drug interactions. For example, dextromethorphan is used to assess intrinsic activity of CYP2D6 and classify the individual into low, normal, or extensive metabolizers. Within the next decade, it is expected that scientists will begin to connect DNA variants with individual responses to medical treatments, identify particular subgroups of patients, and develop drugs customized for those populations.

Nurses should remain alert to the possibilities of drug–drug interactions when patients are receiving more than one medication. Pharmacology texts and dedicated websites are helpful reference sources. In addition, if an individual receiving a medication experiences an unusual reaction or suddenly loses effect from a medication that had previously been working, the nurse should carefully assess other substances that the person has recently consumed, including prescription medications, nonprescription remedies, dietary supplements or changes, and substances of abuse (including alcohol and tobacco). The widespread use of herbal products has introduced another potential source of drug–drug interaction. A good example of this is St. John's wort, a botanical product used extensively for mild depression. Drug–drug interactions have been reported for St. John's wort and alprazolam, amitriptyline, and cyclosporine (Izzo, 2004).

Excretion

Excretion refers to the elimination of drugs from the body either unchanged or as metabolites. *Clearance* refers to the total volume of blood, serum, or plasma from which a drug is completely removed from the bloodstream per unit of time. The driving force that determines the time required to eliminate a drug is the concentration of drug and the clearance rate. The elimination **half-life** ($t_{1/2}$) refers to the time required for plasma concentrations of the drug to be reduced by 50%. For example, 50% of a drug is cleared in one $t_{1/2}$. In the next $t_{1/2}$, 50% of the remaining concentration would be eliminated (leaving 25% of the original concentration), then after the third $t_{1/2}$, there would be 12.5% remaining. Thus, it usually takes four to seven half-lives for a drug to be completely eliminated from the body. Notable exceptions to this decrease by percent concentration include alcohol and acetylsalicylic acid, in which the specific enzymes responsible for metabolism limit the speed at which elimination can occur. For this reason, elimination is at a set rate irrespective of concentration, which is why in the case of alcohol, it can be calculated how many drinks it takes per hour to reach a blood alcohol level of 0.8 (a common legal level indicative of impairment) and the time required to eliminate all alcohol from the system. In the case of acetylsalicylic acid overdose, increasing the renal clearance through changes in pH or increasing fluid volume will not affect the time required for elimination because it is determined by enzyme activity, not blood flow.

As indicated previously, the goal of most metabolic processes is to decrease the lipophilic nature of drugs by increasing their ionic characteristics. Drugs that are in a more ionic form in the bloodstream can be easily removed by the kidney and excreted through urine. However, many psychiatric medications are large molecules and thus can also be removed through bile and eliminated in feces. Lithium, a mood stabilizer, is a notable exception. It is a very small cation and is dependent on renal excretion. Any impairment in renal function or renal disease, or even temporary dehydration (e.g., from flu symptoms or even strenuous exercise) may lead to severe toxic symptoms. Biliary elimination can lead to "enteroportal recirculation," a process by which active drug or metabolites that were excreted in bile into the small intestine are reabsorbed into the portal circulation, go through the liver again, and end up back into the systemic circulation. A well-known example of this is oral contraceptives. Oral antibiotics change the intestinal environment, can decrease recirculation, and thus affect the contraceptive efficacy. This same process of reabsorption may also contribute to the plasma concentration of psychiatric drugs over time.

Dosing refers to the administration of medication over time so that therapeutic levels may be achieved or maintained without reaching toxic levels. In general, it is necessary to give a drug at intervals no greater than the half-life of the medication to avoid excessive fluctuation of concentration in the plasma between doses. With repeated dosing, a certain amount of the drug is accumulated in the body. This accumulation slows as dosing continues and plateaus when absorption equals excretion. This is called *steady-state plasma concentration* or simply *steady state*. The rate of accumulation is determined by the half-life of the drug. Drugs generally reach steady state in four to five times the elimination half-life. However, because elimination or excretion rates may vary significantly, fluctuations may still occur, and dose schedules may need to be individualized.

The nurse should remember that although these principles can support best practice, they are not substitutes for ongoing individual assessment of indicators of treatment response or unwanted effects and recording individual perceptions about drug effects.

Individual Variations in Drug Effects

Many factors affect drug absorption, distribution, metabolism, and excretion. These factors may vary among individuals, depending on their age, genetics, and ethnicity. Nurses must be aware of and consider these individual variations in the effects of medications.

Age

Pharmacokinetics is influenced by life cycle stages. For example, gastric absorption changes with age. Gastric pH in a newborn is 6 to 8 and decreases to 1 to 3 over the first 24 hours (the pH remains elevated in a premature infant). This significantly affects drug absorption. Changes in drug absorption are also seen in older adults because of increased gastric pH, decreased gastric emptying, slowed gastric motility, and reduced splanchnic circulation. Normally, these changes do not significantly impair the oral absorption of a medication, but addition of common conditions, such as diarrhoea, may significantly alter and reduce absorption. The use of multiple drug therapies (termed *polypharmacy*) in older adults can also significantly alter pharmacokinetic properties of each individual drug (Hogan, Ebly, & Fung, 1995; Spina & Scordo, 2002; Turkoski, 1999).

Renal function is also altered in both very young and older adult patients. Infants who are exposed in utero to medications that are excreted through the kidneys may experience toxic reactions to these medications because renal function in the newborn is only about 20% of that of an adult. In less than a week, renal function develops to adult levels, but in premature infants, the process may take longer. Renal function also declines with age. Creatinine clearance in a young adult is normally 100 to 120 mL per minute, but after the age of 40, this rate declines by about 10% per decade. Medical illnesses, such as diabetes and hypertension, may further the loss of renal function. When creatinine clearance falls below 30 mL per minute, the excretion of drugs by the kidneys is significantly impaired, and potentially toxic levels may accumulate.

Metabolism changes across the life span, especially in infancy and childhood. At birth, many of the liver enzymes are not fully functional, whereas in early childhood, there is evidence of increased activity compared with adulthood. For example, CYP1A2 activity is reduced in the first 4 months, but increased between ages 1 and 2 years; CYP2D6 activity is reduced until ages 3 to 5 years, and CYP3A4 is reduced in the 1st month of life, but increased between ages 1 and 4 (Kearns, 2000; Kearns & Winter, 2004; Leeder & Kearns, 1997). Thus, paediatric pharmacotherapeutics cannot be simply based on relative dosing by weight. With age, blood flow to the liver and the mass of liver tissue both decrease. The activities of hepatic enzymes also slow with age. As a result, the ability of the liver to metabolize medications may show as much as a fourfold decrease between the ages of 20 and 70. Again, the use of multiple drugs in older adults adds to metabolic burden, potentially increasing drug levels of each individual drug.

Most psychiatric medications are bound to proteins. Albumin is one of the primary circulating proteins to which drugs bind. The production of albumin by the liver is lower in neonates and generally declines with age. In addition, a number of medical conditions change the ability of medications to bind to albumin. Malnutrition, cancer, and liver disease decrease the production of albumin, which translates to more free drug available to interact with target receptors and an increased risk for adverse or toxic effects.

Less information is known about age-related changes in pharmacodynamics. There is evidence of pharmacodynamic differences in cyclosporine effects in infants (Marshall & Kearns, 1999). Higher digoxin doses are required in infants because of lower affinity in target myocardial receptors (Soldin & Soldin, 2002). Changes in the parasympathetic nervous system produce a greater sensitivity in older adult patients to the anticholinergic side effects of specific psychiatric drugs.

Ethnicity and Genetic Makeup

Although only a small amount of information is available at this time, it is clear that genetics plays a significant role in the metabolism of medications. Studies of identical and nonidentical twins show that much of the individual variability in elimination half-life of a given drug is genetically determined (Vesell, 1977). Individuals of Asian descent have decreased activities of enzymes involved in the metabolism of ethanol compared with Caucasians and thus produce higher concentrations of acetaldehyde, resulting in such adverse symptoms as flushing, palpitations, and headache. Asian research subjects have been found to be more susceptible to the effects of drugs such as mephenytoin than are Caucasian individuals, whereas individuals of African descent were less sensitive (Klotz, 2007). Several case reports indicate that Asians require one half to one third the dose of antipsychotic medications required by Caucasians and that they may be more sensitive to side effects because of higher blood levels (Zhou, 2003). Lower doses of antidepressant medications are also often required for individuals of Asian descent. Although many of these variations appear to be related to the cytochrome P-450 genetic differences discussed earlier, more research is needed to understand fully the underlying mechanisms and to identify groups that may require different approaches to medication treatment.

PHASES OF DRUG TREATMENT

The PMH nurse is involved in all the phases of medication treatment. Considerations in terms of assessment, treatment issues such as **adherence** (keeping with the therapeutic regimen), prevalence and severity of side effects, and expected time lines for symptom relief vary across the phases of treatment, but all involve potential nursing actions. These phases include initiation, stabilization, maintenance, and discontinuation of the medication. PMH nurses must be concerned with treatment phases as a guide for what may be expected as they administer medications and monitor individuals receiving medications across each of these phases. The following subsections discuss some of the knowledge required and the assessments and interventions to be performed by the PMH nurse within each phase.

Initiation Phase

Before beginning to take medications, patients must undergo several assessments.

- A psychiatric evaluation, including past history and previous medication treatment response, will clarify diagnosis and determine target symptoms for medication use.
- An open discussion regarding adherence issues, such as attitudes toward drug treatments, patient-specific goals for the drug therapy, any lifestyle issues that affect the structuring of a drug regimen (e.g., shift work, type of occupation and current job responsibilities, reproductive issues), and any health insurance issues related to prescription benefits, will help to identify barriers to the patient's willingness and ability to comply with the medication regimen.
- Physical examination and indicated laboratory tests, often including baseline determinations such as a complete blood count (CBC), liver and kidney function tests, electrolyte levels, urinalysis, and possibly thyroid function tests and electrocardiogram (ECG), will help

determine whether a physical condition may be causing the symptoms and establish that it is safe to initiate use of a particular medication.
- Any other current medications, including over-the-counter medications, herbal remedies and mixtures from health food stores or naturopathic or homeopathic visitations, and alcohol, tobacco, and other recreational drug use should be identified to prevent harmful drug interactions.

Nurses should perform their own premedication evaluations, including physical assessments that focus on pre-existing symptoms, such as gastrointestinal distress, or restrictions in range of motion that may later be confused with side effects. Side effects are difficult to assess if baseline status has not been evaluated. An assessment of cognitive functioning will assist the nurse in assessing whether memory aids or other supports are necessary to assist the individual in accurately completing the medication regimen. Information from the psychosocial and lifestyle assessment should be reviewed in consultation with the prescriber and other members of the multidisciplinary team to develop a plan that is acceptable to the patient and will improve functioning, minimize side effects, and improve quality of life.

In all situations, recommendations and treatment alternatives should be developed and reviewed with input from the individual seeking treatment. Doing so will allow the patient to ask questions and receive complete information about target effects and the most common adverse effects, thus allowing for fully informed consent to the selected approach. Patients are often overwhelmed during the initial phases of treatment and may have symptoms that make it difficult for them to participate fully in treatment planning. Information is often forgotten or may need to be repeated and provided in written form for ongoing reference. Nurses must keep their detailed drug knowledge current to be able to answer questions and provide ongoing education.

When use of the medication is initiated, PMH nurses should treat the first dose as if it were a "test" dose. They should observe the patient closely for sensitivity to the medication, such as changes in blood pressure, pulse, or temperature; changes in mental status; allergic reactions; dizziness; ataxia; or gastric distress. Other common side effects that may occur with even one dose of medication should also be closely monitored. A protocol for reporting side effects and determining which ones should trigger immediate contact should be in place.

Stabilization Phase

During stabilization, the medication dosage is often adjusted to achieve the maximum amount of improvement with a minimum number of side effects. This process is sometimes referred to as *titration*. PMH nurses must continue to assess target symptoms, looking for change or improvement and side effects. If medications are being increased rapidly, such as in a hospital setting, nurses must closely monitor temperature, blood pressure, pulse, mental status, common side effects, and unusual adverse reactions.

On an outpatient basis, nurses must provide both verbal and written materials to individuals who are receiving the medication as to the expected outcome and potential side effects. This educational support should include factors that may influence the effectiveness of the medication, such as whether to take the medication with food, common interventions that may minimize side effects if they develop, and what side effects require immediate attention. Again, a plan is needed to clearly identify what to do if adverse reactions develop. The plan should include emergency telephone numbers or available emergency treatment and should be reviewed frequently.

Therapeutic drug monitoring is important in this phase of treatment for drugs with narrow therapeutic windows, such as lithium, valproate, and carbamazepine. Nurses must be aware of when and how these levels are to be determined and assist patients in learning these procedures. Plasma levels of other psychiatric medications can be evaluated, for example, to rule them out as a potential source of treatment nonresponse related to increased metabolism. Unfortunately, the first medication chosen often does not adequately improve the patient's target symptoms. In treatment of depression, for example, studies have shown that up to 60% of individuals fail to respond to any given antidepressant (Thase, 2002). This can be very discouraging, particularly in a population in which powerlessness and hopelessness are inherent in the disorder. This possibility must be discussed before initiating antidepressant drug therapy. Most of the time, a substitute drug from the same class or a drug from a new class will be given. Medications may also be changed when adverse reactions or seriously uncomfortable side effects occur or these effects substantially interfere with the individual's quality of life. Nurses should be familiar with the pharmacokinetics of both drugs to be able to monitor side effects and possible drug–drug interactions during this transition period.

At times, an individual may show only partial improvement from a medication, and the prescriber may try an augmentation strategy. *Augmentation* refers to the addition of another medication to enhance or potentiate the effects of the first medication. For example, a prescriber may add a mood stabilizer, such as lithium, to an antidepressant to improve the overall efficacy of the antidepressant. These strategies are often used with so-called treatment-resistant situations. *Treatment resistance* has various definitions, but most often it means that after several medication trials, the individual has gained, at best,

only partial improvement. Treatment-resistant symptoms often require multiple medications. Multiple medications may affect different physiologic processes and, in combination, provide overall synergistic or additive pharmacologic effects. Nurses must be familiar with the potential effects, side effects, drug interactions, and rationale for this type of complex treatment regimen.

Maintenance Phase

Once the individual's target symptoms have improved, medications may be continued to prevent relapse or reoccurrence. *Relapse* usually refers to reemerging symptoms in response to premature discontinuation of treatment, whereas *reoccurrence* refers to an entirely new episode that occurs over time after full remission was achieved. Higher risk for relapse in depression is associated with individuals who are older, have chronic episodes, have severe symptoms or psychotic symptoms, or have three or more previous or more frequent episodes (Viguera, Baldessarini, & Friedberg, 1998). Other reasons for reemerging symptoms, despite continued use of medication, include the loss of efficacy, metabolic induction, comorbid medical illness, psychosocial stressors, and concurrent use of prescription or nonprescription medications. Whatever the reason, patients must be educated about their target symptoms and have a plan of action if the symptoms return. The PMH nurse has a central role in assisting individuals to monitor their own symptoms, manage psychosocial stressors, and avoid other factors that may cause the exacerbation of symptoms that were previously under control.

Some side effects or adverse reactions emerge only after the individual has been receiving the medication for an extended period. Specific examples are discussed in later sections of this chapter.

Discontinuation Phase

Many psychiatric medications require a tapered discontinuation. Tapering involves slowly reducing dosage while monitoring closely for reemergence of key symptoms, such as a drop in mood, increased anxiety, sleep disturbance, thought disorder, or decreased level of self-care. Some psychiatric disorders, such as mild depression or adjustment disorder, may respond to several months of treatment and not reoccur. Other disorders, such as bipolar disorder, chronic major depressive disorder, and schizophrenia, usually require continued medication treatment for extended periods of time. A withdrawal syndrome, affecting up to 25% of individuals after abrupt cessation of the SSRIs, has been described and includes such symptoms as dizziness, restlessness, increased anxiety and mood lability, GI upset, and fatigue (Ditto, 2003). The restoration of the drug therapy relieves the symptoms within 24 hours. Untreated, the symptoms can last

1 to 3 weeks. Withdrawal effects have also been described for abrupt discontinuation of benzodiazepines.

Nurses must be aware of the potential for these symptoms, monitor them closely, and implement measures to minimize their effects. They should support individuals throughout this process, whether they can successfully stop taking the medication or must continue the treatment. Even if patients can successfully discontinue use of the medication without a return of symptoms, nurses may help implement preventive measures to avoid the reocurrence of the psychiatric disorder. In the roles of advocate, patient educator, and provider of interpersonal support, PMH nurses often have a central role in helping patients incorporate preventive mental health strategies into their daily routine.

ANTIPSYCHOTIC MEDICATIONS

It is hard to image how psychiatric illnesses were treated before the development of psychopharmacologic medications. Antipsychotic medications were among the very first drugs ever used to treat psychiatric disorders. First synthesized by Paul Charpentier in 1950, chlorpromazine became the interest of Henri Lorit, a French surgeon, who was attempting to develop medications that controlled preoperative anxiety. Administered in intravenous doses of 50 to 100 mg, chlorpromazine produced drowsiness and indifference to surgical procedures. At Lorit's suggestion, a number of psychiatrists began to administer chlorpromazine to agitated psychotic patients. In 1952, Jean Delay and Pierre Deniker, two French psychiatrists, published the first report of chlorpromazine's calming effects with psychiatric patients (Granger, 1999). They soon discovered it was especially effective in relieving hallucinations and delusions associated with schizophrenia. As more psychiatrists began to prescribe the medication, the use of restraints and seclusion in psychiatric hospitals dropped sharply, ushering in a revolution in psychiatric treatment.

Since that time, numerous antipsychotic medications have been developed. Older, typical antipsychotic medications, available since 1954, are equally effective, inexpensive drugs that vary in the degree to which they cause certain groups of side effects. Table 14-5 provides a list of selected antipsychotics grouped by the nature of their chemical structure and indicating the likelihood of certain side effects. These medications treat the symptoms of psychosis, such as hallucinations, delusions, bizarre behaviour, disorganized thinking, and agitation.

Typical and Atypical Antipsychotics

Initially, the term *major tranquilizer* was applied to this group of medications. Later, major tranquilizers were known as *neuroleptics*, which more accurately describes the action of drugs such as chlorpromazine and haloperidol.

Neuroleptic means "to clasp the neuron." The term reflects the common and often significant neurologic side effects produced by these types of drugs. The development of newer antipsychotic drugs that have less significant neurologic side effects has led to these older agents being used as secondary, not first-line, drugs. The term *typical antipsychotic* now identifies the older antipsychotic drugs with greater risk for neurologic side effects, and *atypical antipsychotic* identifies the newer generation of antipsychotic drugs with fewer adverse neurologic effects.

Indications and Mechanisms of Action

Antipsychotic medications generally are indicated for treating acute psychosis or severe agitation. Possible target symptoms for antipsychotics include hallucinations, delusions, paranoia, agitation, assaultive behaviour, bizarre ideation, disorientation, social withdrawal, catatonia, blunted affect, thought blocking, insomnia, and anorexia when these symptoms are the result of a psychotic process. (These symptoms are described more fully in later chapters.)

In general, the older, typical antipsychotics, such as haloperidol (Haldol), chlorpromazine, and thioridazine (Mellaril), are equally effective in relieving hallucinations, delusions, and bizarre ideation, termed "positive" symptoms of schizophrenia. The "negative" symptoms—blunted affect, social withdrawal, lack of interest in usual activities, lack of motivation, poverty of speech, thought blocking, and inattention—do not respond as well to the typical antipsychotics and in some cases may even be worsened by such agents. Newer atypical antipsychotics, such as clozapine, risperidone (Risperdal), olanzapine (Zyprexa), quetiapine (Seroquel), and ziprasidone (Geodon), are more effective at improving negative symptoms. Although antipsychotic medications are the primary treatment for schizophrenia and related illnesses, such as schizoaffective disorder, schizophreniform disorder, and brief psychotic disorder, they are increasingly being used to treat other psychiatric and medical illnesses. Psychotic symptoms that occur during a major depressive episode, anxiety, or bipolar affective disorder can be treated with antipsychotics, primarily on a short-term basis. These medications reduce agitation, aggressiveness, and inappropriate behaviour in pervasive developmental disorders, such as autism or severe mental retardation. Within the typical antipsychotics, haloperidol and pimozide are approved for treating Tourette's syndrome, reducing the frequency and severity of vocal tics. Some of the typical antipsychotics, particularly chlorpromazine, are used as antiemetics or for postoperative intractable hiccoughs.

Off-label uses of the drug have also been effective. Chlorpromazine and haloperidol are both effective in

Table 14.5	Side-Effect Comparison of Selected Antipsychotic Medications			
Drug Category Drug Name	Sedation	Extrapyramidal	Anticholinergic	Orthostatic Hypotension
Standard (Typical) Antipsychotics				
PHENOTHIAZINES				
ALIPHATICS				
chlorpromazine (Thorazine)	+4	+2	+3	+4
PIPERIDINES				
thioridazine (Mellaril)	+3	+1	+4	+4
mesoridazine (Serentil)	+3	+1	+4	+3
PIPERAZINES				
fluphenazine (Prolixin)	+1	+4	+1	+1
perphenazine (Trilafon)	+2	+3	+2	+2
trifluoperazine (Stelazine)	+1	+3	+1	+1
THIOXANTHENES				
thiothixene (Navane)	+1	+4	+1	+1
DIBENZOXAZEPINES				
Loxapine (Loxitane)	+2	+3	+2	+3
BUTYROPHENONES				
haloperidol (Haldol)	+1	+4	+1	+1
DIHYDROINDOLONES				
molindone (Moban)	+2	+3	+2	+1
Atypical Antipsychotics				
DIBENZODIAZEPINES				
clozapine (Clozaril)	+4	+/0	+4	+4
BENZISOXAZOLE				
risperidone (Risperdal)	+1	+/0	+/0	+2
THIENOBENZODIAZEPINE				
olanzapine (Zyprexa)	+4	+/0	+2	+1
DIBENZOTHIAZEPINE				
quetiapine fumarate (Seroquel)	+4	+/0	+/0	+3
MONOHYDROCHLORIDE				
ziprasidone HCl (Geodon)	+1	+/0	+1	+2
DIHYDROCARBOSTYRILS				
aripiprazole (Abilify)	+1	+/0	+/0	+1

treating drug-related psychosis, such as that caused by phencyclidine. Atypical antipsychotics have also been used to treat agitation and aggression seen in those acutely ill in intensive care units (often termed ICU psychosis) and with neurodegernative disorders like Alzheimer's disease (Kirbach, Simpson, Nietert, & Mintzer, 2008; Philip, Mello, Carpenter, Tyrka, & Price, 2008; Riker & Fraser, 2005). Some evidence exists for their efficacy at very small doses in treating psychiatric sequelae of trauma, especially in the case of significant dissociation and mood reactivity arising from childhood interpersonal abuse (Grootens & Verkes, 2005). Antipsychotic medications may also be useful in treating migraine headaches, Huntington's chorea, and some other neurologic disorders.

The typical antipsychotic drugs generally are effective in decreasing the so-called positive target symptoms because they are potent postsynaptic dopamine antagonists. Chapter 18 discusses the link between dopamine and disorders, such as schizophrenia, and provides additional details about how lowering dopamine levels helps reduce target symptoms. The atypical antipsychotic medications differ from the typical antipsychotics in that they block serotonin receptors as well as dopamine receptors. The differences between the mechanism of action of the typical and atypical antipsychotics helps to explain their differences in efficacy in relation to both positive and negative symptoms and side-effect profiles.

Pharmacokinetics

Antipsychotic medications administered orally have a variable rate of absorption complicated by the presence of food, antacids, smoking, and even the coadministration of anticholinergics, which slow gastric motility. Clinical effects begin to appear in about 30 to 60 minutes. Absorption after IM administration is less variable because this method avoids the first-pass effects. Therefore, IM administration produces greater bioavailability, but increases risk for side effects. It is

Table 14.6	Chemical Interactions With Antipsychotic Medications
Agent	**Effect**
Alcohol	Phenothiazines potentiate CNS depressant effects Extrapyramidal reactions may occur
Barbiturates	Speed action of liver microsomal enzymes so that antipsychotic is metabolized more quickly, reducing phenothiazine and haloperidol plasma levels; barbiturate levels may also be reduced by phenothiazines; potentiate CNS depressant effect
Tricyclic antidepressants	Can lead to severe anticholinergic side effects; some antipsychotics (especially phenothiazines or haloperidol) can raise the plasma level of the antidepressant, probably by inhibiting metabolism of the antidepressant
Hydrochlorothiazide and hydralazine	Can produce severe hypotension
Guanethidine	Antihypertensive effect is blocked by phenothiazines, haloperidol, and possibly thiothixene
Aluminum salts (antacids)	Impair gastrointestinal absorption of the phenothiazines, possibly reducing therapeutic effect Administer antacid at least 1 hour before or 2 hours after the phenothiazine
Tobacco	Heavy consumption requires larger doses of antipsychotic because of hepatic microsomal enzyme induction
Charcoal (and charbroiled food)	Decreases absorption of phenothiazines
Anticholinergics	May reduce the therapeutic actions of the phenothiazines, increase anticholinergic side effects, lower serum haloperidol levels, worsen symptoms of schizophrenia, increase symptoms of tardive dyskinesia
Meperidine	May result in excessive sedation and hypotension when coadministered with phenothiazines
Fluoxetine	Case report of serious extrapyramidal symptoms when used in combination with haloperidol
Lithium	May induce disorientation, unconsciousness, extrapyramidal symptoms, or possibly the risk for NMS when combined with phenothiazines or haloperidol
Carbamazepine	Decreases haloperidol serum levels, decreasing its therapeutic effects
Phenytoin	Increase or decrease in phenytoin serum levels; thioridazine and haloperidol serum levels may be decreased
Methyldopa	May potentiate the antipsychotic effects of haloperidol or may produce psychosis Serious elevations in blood pressure may occur with methyldopa and trifluoperazine
General anesthesia (barbiturates)	Antipsychotic may potentiate effect of anesthetic; may increase the neuromuscular excitation or hypotension

important to remember that IM medications are absorbed more slowly when patients are immobile, such as when restrained for long periods of time, because erratic absorption may occur when muscles are not in use. For example, the patient's arm may be more mobile than the buttocks. The deltoid has better blood perfusion, and thus medications are more readily absorbed. The nurse must also remember that plastic syringes may absorb some medications. This is true of the antipsychotics, and injectable medications should never be allowed to remain in the syringe longer than 15 minutes.

The metabolism of these drugs occurs almost entirely in the liver, where hepatic microsomal enzymes convert these highly lipid-soluble substances into water-soluble metabolites that can be excreted through the kidneys. Therefore, these medications are subjected to the effects of other drugs that induce or inhibit the cytochrome P-450 system described earlier. Table 14-6 summarizes many of the possible medication interactions with antipsychotics, including those resulting from changes in hepatic enzymes. Careful observance of concurrent medication use, including prescribed, over the counter, and substances of abuse, is required to avoid drug–drug interactions.

Excretion of these substances tends to be slow because the drugs can easily accumulate in fat stores. Most antipsychotics have a half-life of 24 hours or longer, but many also have active metabolites with longer half-lives. These two effects make it difficult to predict elimination time, and metabolites of some of these agents may be found in the urine months later. If a patient experiences side effects from a medication severe enough to discontinue the use of the drug and begin use of a new one, the adverse effects of the first drug may not necessarily immediately subside. The patient may continue to experience and sometimes need treatment for the adverse effects for several days. Similarly, patients who have discontinued use of antipsychotic drugs may still derive therapeutic benefit for several days to weeks after drug discontinuation.

Table 14.7	Antipsychotic Medications			
Generic (Trade) Drug Name	Usual Dosage Range (mg/day)	Half-Life (hours)	Therapeutic Blood Level	Approximate Equivalent Dosage (mg)
Standard (Typical) Antipsychotics				
PHENOTHIAZINES				
ALIPHATICS				
chlorpromazine (Thorazine)	50–1200	2–30	30–100 mg/mL	100
PIPERIDINES				
thioridazine (Mellaril)	50–600	10–20	1–1.5 ng/mL	100
mesoridazine (Serentil)	50–400	24–48	Not available	50
PIPERAZINES				
fluphenazine (Prolixin)	2–20	4.5–15.3	0.2–0.3 ng/mL	2
perphenazine (Trilafon)	12–64	Unknown	0.8–12.0 ng/mL	10
trifluoperazine (Stelazine)	5–40	47–100	1–2.3 ng/mL	5
THIOXANTHENES				
thiothixene (Navane)	5–60	34	2–20 ng/mL	4
DIBENZOXAZEPINES				
loxapine (Loxitane)	20–250	19	Not available	15
BUTYROPHENONES				
haloperidol (Haldol)	2–60	21–24	5–15 ng/mL	2
DIHYDROINDOLONES				
molindone (Moban)	50–400	1.5	Not available	10
Atypical Antipsychotics				
DIBENZODIAZEPINES				
clozapine (Clozaril)	300–900	4–12	141–204 ng/mL	50
BENZISOXAZOLE				
risperidone (Risperdal)	2–8	20	Not available	1
THIENOBENZODIAZEPINE				
olanzapine (Zyprexa)	5–10	21–54	Not available	Not available
DIBENZOTHIAZEPINE				
quetiapine fumarate (Seroquel)	150–750	7	Not available	Not available
MONOHYDROCHLORIDE				
ziprasidone HCl (Geodon)	40–160	7	Not available	Not available
DIHYDROCARBOSTYRILS				
aripiprazole (Abilify)	10–30	75–94	Not available	Not available

Typical antipsychotics are best administered in divided doses to minimize side effects, but the long elimination time does allow the medication to be given in once-daily dosing. This schedule increases adherence and reduces the impact of the peak occurrence of some side effects, such as sedation during the day.

High lipid **solubility**, accumulation in the body, and other factors have also made it difficult to correlate blood levels with therapeutic effects. Dose–response curves have not been established, and the dose required for an individual to experience treatment effects varies widely. Plasma levels of these medications are only partially helpful. Although these can be measured for a number of antipsychotics, their correlation with therapeutic response has been inconsistent. Haloperidol and clozapine correlate well and may be helpful in determining whether an adequate blood level has been reached and maintained during a trial of medication. Table 14-7 shows the therapeutic ranges available for some of the antipsychotic medications. Plasma levels may also be helpful in identifying absorption problems or metabolic differences (high or low metabolizer), determining adherence, and identifying adverse reactions from drug–drug interactions.

The potency of the antipsychotics also varies widely and is of specific concern when considering typical antipsychotic drugs. As Table 14-7 indicates, 100 mg chlorpromazine is roughly equivalent to 2 mg haloperidol and 5 mg trifluoperazine. Although drugs that are more potent are not inherently better than less potent drugs, differentiating low-potency versus high-potency antipsychotics may be somewhat helpful in predicting side effects. Roughly speaking, high-potency medications, such as haloperidol and fluphenazine, produce a greater frequency of extrapyramidal symptoms, and low-potency antipsychotics, such as chlorpromazine and thioridazine, produce more sedation and hypotension.

Ultimately, selection of medication from the group of typical antipsychotics depends predominately on predicted side effects, prior history of treatment response, whether or not a depot preparation will be needed during maintenance, concurrent medications, and other medical conditions.

Drug Formulations: Long-Acting Preparations

Currently in Canada, two typical antipsychotic drugs, haloperidol and fluphenazine, are available in long-acting, depot forms. These two antipsychotics may be administered by injection once every 2 to 4 weeks. After administration, the drug is slowly released from the injection site; therefore, these forms of the drugs are referred to as *depot preparations.* Long-acting injectable medications maintain a fairly constant blood level between injections. Because they bypass problems with gastrointestinal absorption and first-pass metabolism, this method may enhance therapeutic outcomes for the patient. Lower rates of relapse have been reported for patients receiving long-acting injectable medication compared with those taking oral medications (Bond, Pratoomsri, & Yatham, 2007). Depot preparations are used when individuals have difficulty remembering to take their oral medications and are able to keep appointments reliably or attend a program regularly where the injection may be administered. Fluphenazine decanoate and haloperidol decanoate are equally effective in treating the symptoms of psychosis. Long-acting forms of fluphenazine are available as fluphenazine decanoate and fluphenazine enanthate. The latter has a markedly increased risk for extrapyramidal side effects and is rarely used. Nurses should be aware that the injection site may become sore and inflamed if certain precautions are not taken. The liquids are viscous, and a large-gauge needle (at least 21-gauge) should be used to withdraw the drug from the ampoule. However, there is emerging evidence that glass particles can be drawn up with the liquid, especially if using an 18-gauge needle, and thus a filtered needle is preferred for the long-term use of depot medications (Preston & Hegadoren, 2004). See Box 14-2 for relevant research. Because the medication is meant to remain in the injection site, the needle should be dry, and a deep IM injection should be given by the Z-track method. (Note: Do not massage the injection site. Rotate sites and document in the patient's record.) A change to depot preparation from oral antipsychotic is done on a gradual basis after the patient is fully informed and consents and has taken several oral doses to ensure that no significant immediate adverse reactions are likely to occur.

Recently, an atypical antipsychotic, risperidone, has become available in a long-acting formulation. It differs from the conventional depot form in that it is aqueous based and thereby better tolerated. Long-acting risperidone is unique in that microspheres (encapsulated polymers containing the medication) gradually break down, releasing the active form of the medication. This medication is administered intramuscularly every 2 weeks.

BOX 14.2

Research for Best Practice: Glass Contamination in Parenterally Administered Medication

From Preston, S. T., & Hegadoren, K. (2004). Glass contamination in parenterally administered medication. Journal of Advanced Nursing, 48(3), 266–270.

THE QUESTION: Does the use of larger bore unfiltered needles increase the risk of aspirating more glass and other particles?

METHOD: A computer microscope was used to compare the number and size of glass particles aspirated into a syringe between two needle sizes [18 gauge (G) (130 μm lumen diameter) and 21G (90 μm lumen diameter)] without filters and 19G (110 μm lumen diameter) filtered needles. $N = 18$ in each group.

FINDINGS: At least one glass particle was found in 22% of the 1-mL ampoules, and 56% and 39% of the 2-mL ampoules, using 18G and 21G needles, respectively, had glass contaminants. Many of the 2-mL ampoules produced multiple glass particles on opening. Use of 19G filtered needles resulted in no glass particles. There was a significant difference in mean particle size between the 18G and 21G groups of 2-mL ampoules.

IMPLICATIONS FOR PRACTICE: The IM administration of glass particles is clinically problematic. Current nursing practice standards do not adequately address this issue in terms of aspiration or filtration techniques that can minimize risk to patients. The findings support the use of filtered needles in administering IM medications to patients who receive ongoing scheduled IM injections.

Initiation of this medication regimen requires that an oral antipsychotic be given during the first 3 weeks to reach a therapeutic blood level.

Side Effects, Adverse Reactions, and Toxicity

Various side effects and interactions can occur with antipsychotics (see Tables 14-6 and 14-7), with the typical antipsychotics producing more significant side effects than the atypical antipsychotics. The side effects vary largely based on their degree of attraction to different neurotransmitter receptors and their subtypes.

Cardiovascular Side Effects

Cardiovascular side effects, such as orthostatic hypotension, depend on the degree of blockade of α-adrenergic receptors. Low-potency typical antipsychotics, such as chlorpromazine and thioridazine, and the atypical antipsychotic clozapine have a high degree of affinity for α-adrenergic receptors and, therefore, produce considerable orthostatic hypotension. Other cardiovascular side effects from typical antipsychotics have been rare, but occasionally they cause ECG changes that have a benign or undetermined clinical effect. Thioridazine (Mellaril) and ziprasidone (Geodon) have both been associated with prolonged QT intervals and should be used cautiously in patients who have increased QT intervals or are taking other medications that may prolong the QT interval (Taylor, 2003).

Anticholinergic Side Effects

Anticholinergic side effects resulting from the blockade of acetylcholine are another common concern with the typical and some of the atypical antipsychotic drugs. Dry mouth, slowed gastric motility, constipation, urinary hesitancy or retention, vaginal dryness, blurred vision, dry eyes, nasal congestion, and confusion or decreased memory are examples of these side effects. Interventions for decreasing the impact of these side effects are outlined in Table 14-2. This group of side effects occurs with many of the medications used for psychiatric treatment. Sometimes a cholinergic medication, such as bethanechol, may reduce the peripheral effects but not the CNS effects. Using more than one medication with anticholinergic effects often increases the symptoms. Older adult patients are often most susceptible to a potential toxicity that results from high blockade of acetylcholine. This toxicity is called an *anticholinergic* crisis and is described, along with its treatment, in Chapter 18. The likelihood of anticholinergic side effects, along with sedation and extrapyramidal side effects, from antipsychotics is explored in Table 14-5.

Weight Gain

Other clinically important effects also occur with the antipsychotic medications. Weight gain from increased appetite is common with the low-potency antipsychotics but occurs in highest proportion with clozapine and olanzapine. Weight gain has been associated with antipsychotic drugs since chlorpromazine was developed and is of increasing concern with the increased use of atypical drugs such as clozapine and olanzapine. The weight gain related to antipsychotic medications is linked to an increased risk for diabetes, heart disease, and hyperlipidemia. Those at higher risk for developing metabolic or cardiovascular disorders are those individuals who show more rapid weight gain in the first weeks of drug treatment. A Quebec study ($N = 19,582$) showed that the risk for initiation of a pharmacologic treatment for diabetes or dyslipidemia is significantly higher with olanzapine than risperidone (Moisan, Gregoire, Gaudet, & Cooper, 2005). Awareness of these risks emphasizes the need for early preventive intervention with diet and exercise, as well as careful consideration in the choice of the specific atypical agent for at-risk populations (Henderson, 2008). The chronic health problems of diabetes and cardiovascular illness occur much more often in individuals with

mental illness than in the general population, making it essential for nurses to assist patients in dealing effectively with issues of weight gain. Guides and food diaries have been developed to help those who are maintained on long-term atypical antipsychotic drugs.

Endocrine and Sexual Side Effects

Endocrine and sexual side effects result primarily from the blockade of dopamine in the tuberoinfundibular pathways of the hypothalamus. As a result, blood levels of prolactin may increase with almost all the typical antipsychotics but less commonly with the atypical antipsychotics. Increased prolactin causes breast enlargement and rare but potential galactorrhoea (milk production and flow), decreased sexual drive, amenorrhea, menstrual irregularities, and increased risk for growth in preexisting breast cancers. Bromocriptine, a dopamine agonist, may be helpful, but more likely these symptoms necessitate a change in medication. The prescriber should be notified immediately. Endocrine side effects can occur in males as well. Retrograde ejaculation (backward flow of semen) is rare, but it may be painful and can occur with all of the antipsychotics. A more common side effect is erectile dysfunction, including difficulty achieving and maintaining an erection. Anorgasmia, or the inability to achieve orgasm, may develop in women.

Blood Disorders

Blood dyscrasias are rare but have received renewed attention since the introduction of clozapine. Agranulocytosis is an acute reaction that causes the individual's white blood cell count to drop to very low levels, and concurrent neutropenia, a drop in neutrophils in the blood, develops. In the case of the antipsychotics, the medication suppresses the bone marrow precursors to blood factors. The exact mechanism by which the drugs produce this effect is unknown. The most notable symptoms of this disorder include high fever, sore throat, and mouth sores. Although benign elevations in temperature have been reported in individuals taking clozapine, no fever should go uninvestigated. Untreated agranulocytosis can be life threatening. Although agranulocytosis can occur with any of the antipsychotics, the risk with clozapine is 10 to 20 times greater than with the other antipsychotics (Bilici, Tekelioglu, Efendioglu, Ovali, & Ulgen, 2003). Therefore, prescription of clozapine requires weekly blood samples for the first 6 months of treatment, and then every 2 weeks after that for as long as the drug is taken. Drawing of these samples must continue for 4 weeks after clozapine use has been discontinued. If sore throat or fever develops, medications should be withheld until a leukocyte count can be obtained. Hospitalization, including reverse isolation to prevent infections, is usually required. Agranulocytosis is more likely to develop during the first 18 weeks of treatment. Some research indicates that it is more common in women (Iqbal et al., 2003). The requirement for regular blood monitoring and added cost of laboratory services with clozapine has limited its use in community psychiatry with chronically mentally ill populations.

Miscellaneous

Photosensitivity reactions to antipsychotics, including severe sunburns or rash, most commonly develop with the use of low-potency typical medications. Sun block must be worn on all areas of exposed skin when taking these drugs. In addition, sun exposure may cause pigmentary deposits to develop, resulting in the discoloration of exposed areas, especially the neck and face. This discoloration may progress from a deep orange colour to a blue grey. Skin exposure should be limited and skin tone changes reported to the prescriber. Pigmentary deposits may also develop on the retina of the eye, especially with high doses of thioridazine, even for a few days. This condition is called *retinitis pigmentosa* and can lead to significant visual impairment. Therefore, thioridazine should never be administered in doses greater than 800 mg per day.

Antipsychotics may also lower a patient's seizure threshold. Patients with an undetected seizure disorder may experience seizures early in treatment. Those who have a preexisting condition should be monitored closely.

Neuroleptic malignant syndrome (NMS) and water intoxication are two serious complications that may result from antipsychotic medications. Characterized by rigidity and high fever, NMS is a rare condition that may occur abruptly with even one dose of medication. Temperature must always be monitored when administering antipsychotics, especially high-potency medications. Water intoxication may develop gradually with long-term use. This condition is characterized by the patient's consumption of large quantities of fluid (polydipsia) and the resulting effects of sodium depletion (hyponatremia). Both of these conditions are discussed more fully in Chapter 18.

Medication-Related Movement Disorders

Medication-related movement disorders are a group of side effects or adverse reactions that are commonly caused by typical antipsychotic medications but less commonly with atypical antipsychotic drugs. These disorders of abnormal motor movements can be divided into two groups: acute extrapyramidal syndromes (EPS), which are acute abnormal movements developing early in the course of treatment (sometimes after just one dose), and chronic syndromes, which develop from longer exposure to antipsychotic drugs. The atypical antipsychotic drugs are most likely to cause movement disorders.

Acute Extrapyramidal Syndromes

Acute EPS occurs in as many as 90% of all patients receiving typical antipsychotic medications (Chouinard & Chouinard, 2008). These syndromes include dystonia, parkinsonism, and akathisia (an involuntary movement disorder). They develop early in treatment, sometimes from as little as one dose. Although the abnormal movements are treatable, they are at times dramatic and frightening, causing physical and emotional impairments that often prompt patients to stop taking their medication. Some milder forms of EPS may occur with classes of medication other than antipsychotics, including the SSRIs. The acute EPS often are mistaken for aspects of anxiety, rather than medication side effects. Nurses play a vital role in the early recognition and treatment of these syndromes. Early recognition can save the patient considerable discomfort, fear, and impairment. All nurses must be aware of these symptoms, notifying the prescriber as soon as possible and implementing selected medication changes and other interventions. Several medications can control acute EPS (Table 14-8).

Dystonia, sometimes referred to as an *acute dystonic reaction*, is impaired muscle tone that generally is the first extrapyramidal symptom to occur, usually within a few days of initiating use of an antipsychotic. Dystonia is characterized by involuntary muscle spasms, especially of the head and neck muscles. Patients usually first complain of a thick tongue, tight jaw, or stiff neck. The syndrome can progress to a protruding tongue, oculogyric crisis (eyes rolled up in the head), torticollis (muscle stiffness in the neck, which draws the head to one side with chin pointing to the other), and laryngopharyngeal constriction. Abnormal postures of the upper limbs and torso may be held briefly or sustained. In severe cases, the spasms may progress to the intercostal muscles, producing more significant breathing difficulty for patients who already have respiratory impairment from asthma or emphysema.

Drug-induced parkinsonism is sometimes referred to as **pseudoparkinsonism** because its presentation is identical to Parkinson's disease without the same destruction of dopaminergic cells. These symptoms include the classic triad of rigidity, slowed movements (akinesia), and tremor. The rigid muscle stiffness is usually seen in the arms. Akinesia can be observed by the loss of spontaneous movements, such as the absence of the usual relaxed swing of the arms while walking. In addition, masklike facies or loss of facial expression and a decrease in the ability to initiate movements also are present. Usually, tremor is more pronounced at rest, but it can also be observed with intentional movements, such as eating. If the tremor becomes severe, it may interfere with the patient's ability to eat or maintain adequate fluid intake. Hypersalivation is possible as well. Pseudoparkinsonism symptoms may occur on one or both sides of the body

Table 14.8	Drug Therapies for Acute Medication-Related Movement Disorders		
Agents	**Typical Dosage Ranges**	**Routes Available**	**Common Side Effects**
Anticholinergics			
benztropine (Cogentin)	2–6 mg/day	PO, IM, IV	Dry mouth, blurred vision, slowed gastric motility causing constipation, urinary retention, increased intraocular pressure; overdose produces toxic psychosis
trihexyphenidyl (Artane)	4–15 mg/day	PO	Same as benztropine, plus gastrointestinal distress. Older adults are most prone to mental confusion and delirium
biperiden (Akineton)	2–8 mg/day	PO	Fewer peripheral anticholinergic effects. Euphoria and increased tremor may occur
Antihistamines			
diphenhydramine (Benadryl)	25–50 mg qid to 400 mg daily	PO, IM, IV	Sedation and confusion, especially in older adults
Dopamine Agonists			
amantadine (Symmetrel)	100–400 mg daily	PO	Indigestion, decreased concentration, dizziness, anxiety, ataxia, insomnia, lethargy, tremors, and slurred speech may occur on higher doses. Tolerance may develop on fixed dose
β-Blockers			
propranolol (Inderal)	10 mg tid to 120 mg daily	PO	Hypotension and bradycardia. Must monitor pulse and blood pressure. Do not stop abruptly as this may cause rebound tachycardia
Benzodiazepines			
lorazepam (Ativan)	1–2 mg IM / 0.5–2 mg PO	PO, IM	All may cause drowsiness, lethargy, and general sedation or paradoxical agitation. Confusion and disorientation in older adults
diazepam (Valium)	2–5 mg tid	PO, IV	Most side effects are rare and will disappear if dose is decreased
clonazepam (Klonopin)	1–4 mg/day	PO	Tolerance and withdrawal are potential problems

and develop abruptly or subtly, but usually within the first 30 days of treatment.

Akathisia is characterized by the inability to sit still. The person will pace, rock while sitting or standing, march in place, or cross and uncross the legs. All these repetitive motions have an intensity that is frequently beyond the explanation of the individual. In addition, akathisia may be present as a primarily subjective experience without obvious motor behaviour. This subjective experience includes feelings of anxiety, jitteriness, or the inability to relax, which the individual may or may not be able to communicate. It is extremely uncomfortable for a person experiencing akathisia to be forced to sit still or be confined. These symptoms are sometimes misdiagnosed as agitation or an increase in psychotic symptoms, but if the nurse administers an antipsychotic medication PRN (from the Latin *pro re nata*, which roughly translated means "as needed"), the symptoms will not abate and will often worsen. Differentiating akathisia from agitation

may be aided by knowing the person's symptoms before the introduction of medication. Psychotic agitation does not usually begin abruptly after antipsychotic medication use has been started, whereas akathisia may occur after administration. In addition, the nurse may ask the patient if the experience is felt primarily in the muscles (akathisia) or in the mind or emotions (agitation).

Akathisia is the most difficult acute medication-related movement disorder to relieve. It does not usually respond well to anticholinergic medications and is uncommon in patients receiving atypical antipsychotics. It is thought that the pathology of akathisia may involve more than just the extrapyramidal motor system. It may include serotonin changes that also affect the dopamine system (Kulkarni & Naidu, 2003). A number of medications have been used to reduce symptoms, including β-adrenergic blockers, anticholinergics, antihistamines, and low-dose antianxiety agents (Pierre, 2005). The usual approach to treatment is to change to an atypical antipsychotic if possible. If not, reducing the dose of typical antipsychotic medication can be tried. During this time, PMH nurses must closely assess for worsening of symptoms. β-Adrenergic blockers, such as propranolol (Inderal), given in doses of 30 to 120 mg per day, have been most successful (Miller & Fleischhacker, 2000). Nurses must monitor the patient's pulse and blood pressure because propranolol can cause hypotension and bradycardia. If the patient's pulse falls below 60 bpm, propranolol should be withheld and the prescriber notified. Normal signs of hypoglycaemia may be blocked by propranolol; therefore, patients with diabetes must monitor their blood or urine glucose levels carefully, especially because they are under physical stress from the disorder.

A number of nursing interventions may reduce the impact of these syndromes. Individuals with acute EPS need frequent reassurance that this is not a worsening of their psychiatric condition but instead is a treatable side effect of the medication. They also need validation that what they are experiencing is real and that the nurse is concerned and will be responsive to changes in these symptoms. Physical and psychological stress appears to increase the symptoms and further frighten the patient; therefore, decreasing stressful situations becomes important. These symptoms are often physically exhausting for the patient, and nurses should ensure that the patient receives adequate rest and hydration. Because tremors, muscle rigidity, and motor restlessness may interfere with the individual's ability to eat, the nurse may need to assist the patient with eating and drinking fluids to maintain nutrition and hydration.

Risk factors for acute EPS include previous episodes of EPS. Listen closely when patients say they are "allergic" or have had "bad reactions" to antipsychotic medications. Often, they are describing one of the medication-related movement disorders, particularly dystonia, rather than a rash or other allergic symptoms. About 90% of the individuals who have experienced EPS in the past will again have these symptoms if the use of an antipsychotic medication is restarted (Meyer, 2007; Nasrallah, 2002). High-potency medications, such as haloperidol and fluphenazine, are more likely to cause EPS. Age and gender appear to be risk factors for specific syndromes. Acute dystonia occurs most often in young men, adolescents, and children; akathisia is more common in middle-aged women. Older adult patients are at the greatest risk for experiencing pseudoparkinsonism (Sibon, Fenelon, Quinn, & Tison, 2004). Although the occurrence of EPS is decreasing as atypical medications are more commonly used, acute EPS remains a serious clinical concern.

Chronic Syndromes

Chronic syndromes develop from the long-term use of antipsychotics. They are serious and afflict about 20% of the patients who receive typical antipsychotics for an extended period (Pierre, 2005). These conditions are typically irreversible and cause significant impairment in self-image, social interactions, and occupational functioning. Early symptoms and mild forms may go unnoticed by the person experiencing them because they frequently remain beyond the individual's awareness. Therefore, PMH nurses in contact with individuals who are taking antipsychotic medications for months or years must be vigilant for symptoms of these typical chronic conditions.

First identified in 1957, **tardive dyskinesia** is the most well known of the chronic syndromes. It involves irregular, repetitive involuntary movements of the mouth, face, and tongue, including chewing, tongue protrusion, lip smacking, puckering of the lips, and rapid eye blinking. Abnormal finger movements are common as well. In some individuals, the trunk and extremities are also involved, and in rare cases, irregular breathing and swallowing lead to belching and grunting noises. These symptoms usually begin no earlier than after 6 months of treatment or when the medication is reduced or withdrawn. Once thought to be irreversible, considerable controversy now exists as to whether or not this is true.

Part of the difficulty in determining the irreversibility of tardive dyskinesia is that any movement disorder that persists after the discontinuation of antipsychotic medication has been described as tardive dyskinesia. Atypical forms are now receiving more attention because some researchers believe that they may have different underlying mechanisms of causation. Some of these forms of the disorder appear to remit spontaneously. Symptoms of what is now called *withdrawal tardive dyskinesia* appear when use of an antipsychotic medication is reduced or discontinued and remit spontaneously in 1 to 3 months. *Tardive dystonia* and *tardive akathisia* have also been described. Both appear in a manner similar to the acute syndromes but continue after the antipsychotic medication has been withdrawn. More research is needed to determine whether these syndromes are distinctly different in origin and outcome.

The risk for experiencing tardive dyskinesia increases with age. Although the prevalence of tardive dyskinesia averages 15% to 20%, the rate rises to 50% to 70% in older adults receiving antipsychotic medications (Tariot, Salzman, Yeung, Pultz, & Rak, 2000). Cumulative incidence of tardive dyskinesia appears to increase 5% per year of continued exposure to antipsychotic medications (Levy et al., 2002). Women are at higher risk than men. Individuals with affective disorders, particularly depression, are at higher risk than are those who have schizophrenia. Any individual receiving antipsychotic medication may experience tardive dyskinesia; therefore, nurses must be particularly alert to individuals at higher

BOX 14.3

Risk Factors for Tardive Dyskinesia

- Age older than 50 years
- Female
- Affective disorders, particularly depression
- Brain damage or dysfunction
- Increased duration of treatment
- Standard antipsychotic medication
- Possible—higher doses of antipsychotic medication

risk. Risk factors are summarized in Box 14-3. The causes of tardive dyskinesia remain unclear. Lack of a consistent theory of aetiology for the chronic medication-related movement disorder syndromes has led to inconsistent and disappointing treatment approaches. No one medication relieves the symptoms. Dopamine agonists, such as bromocriptine, and many other drugs have been tried. Even dietary precursors of acetylcholine, such as lethicin, and nutritional therapies, such as vitamin E supplements, may prove to be beneficial.

The best approach to treatment remains avoiding the development of the chronic syndromes. Preventive measures include use of atypical antipsychotics, using the lowest possible dose of typical medication, minimizing use of PRN medication, and closely monitoring individuals in high-risk groups for development of the symptoms of tardive dyskinesia. All members of the mental health treatment team who have contact with individuals taking antipsychotics for longer than 3 months must be alert to the risk factors and earliest possible signs of chronic medication-related movement disorders.

Monitoring tools, such as the Abnormal Involuntary Movement Scale (AIMS; Simpson & Angus, 1970), should be used routinely to standardize assessment and provide the earliest possible recognition of the symptoms. Standardized assessments should be performed at a minimum of 3- to 6-month intervals. The earlier the symptoms are recognized, the more likely they will resolve if the medication can be changed or its use discontinued. Newer, atypical antipsychotic medications have a much lower risk for causing tardive dyskinesia and are increasingly being considered first-line medications for treating schizophrenia. Other medications are under development to provide alternatives that limit the risk for tardive dyskinesia.

▪ CRNENOTE

Nurses need to be particularly vigilant concerning the side effects, adverse reactions, and toxicity that may occur with antipsychotic medications when patients are unable to distinguish such reactions from their psychotic symptoms.

▪ MOOD STABILIZERS (ANTIMANIA MEDICATIONS)

Mood stabilizers, or antimania medications, are psychopharmacologic agents used primarily for stabilizing mood swings, particularly those of mania in bipolar affective disorders. For a number of years, lithium was the only drug known to stabilize the symptoms of mania. Although it remains the gold standard of treatment for acute mania and maintenance of bipolar affective disorders, not all individuals experience response to lithium, and increasingly other drugs are being used as first-line agents. In the 1970s, carbamazepine (Tegretol) and later valproate, both anticonvulsants approved for treating epilepsy, were found to have mood-stabilizing effects. Other medications, such as calcium-channel blockers, have been used as adjunctive treatment for the symptoms of mania. At present, three drugs have Health Canada approval for the short-term treatment of acute mania. They include lithium, olanzapine (Zyprexa), and valproic acid (Depakote). Lithium is the only drug with approved Health Canada indication for the prevention and treatment of both manic and depressive episodes. Many other drugs, including other anticonvulsants, atypical antipsychotics, adrenergic blocking agents, and calcium-channel blockers, are frequently used to treat bipolar disorder (Yatham et al., 2006).

Lithium

Lithium, a naturally occurring element, was first discovered in the early 1800s. It has been in medical use in a variety of forms, including tonics and elixirs, since that time. As an element that acts as a salt substitute, the unregulated use of lithium produced a number of cases of toxicity and, as a result, lost favour in the 1940s. Rediscovered in 1949 by the Australian John Cade, lithium was found to reduce agitation in some patients experiencing psychosis, and in the 1950s, Schou (1978) published reports that lithium controlled and prevented the symptoms of mania. In 1970, the FDA approved lithium for use in treating manic episodes in bipolar affective disorder. Since then, it has become a mainstay in psychopharmacology. Lithium is effective in only about 40% of patients with bipolar disorder, and patients who do experience response often have limited clinical improvement. Although lithium is not a perfect drug, a great deal is known regarding its use—it is inexpensive, it has restored stability to the lives of thousands of people, and it remains the gold standard of bipolar pharmacologic treatment.

Indications and Mechanisms of Action

The target symptoms for lithium are the symptoms of mania, such as rapid speech, jumping from topic to topic (flight of ideas), irritability, grandiose thinking, impulsiveness, and agitation. Other psychiatric indications include using lithium for its mild antidepressant effects in treating depressive episodes of bipolar illness and in patients experiencing major depression that has only partially responded to antidepressants alone. Used in patients who have experienced only partial response, lithium has been used in augmentation as a potentiator (enhancing the effects) of antidepressant medications. It has also been shown to be helpful in reducing impulsivity and aggression in certain psychiatric patients.

Lithium has been effective in treating several nonpsychiatric disorders, such as cluster headaches. Because lithium stimulates leukocytosis, it often improves the neutrophil counts of patients who are undergoing chemotherapy or who have other conditions that cause neutropenia. In addition, lithium has been investigated as an antiviral agent because it appears to inhibit the replication of several DNA viruses, including herpes virus. Additional research is needed to fully understand the mechanisms of these effects.

Lithium is actively transported across cell membranes, altering sodium transport in both nerve and muscle cells. It replaces sodium in the sodium–potassium pump and is retained more readily than sodium inside the cell. Conditions that alter sodium content in the body, such as vomiting, diuresis, and diaphoresis, also alter lithium retention. The results of lithium influx into the nerve cell lead to increased storage of catecholamines within the cell, reduced dopamine neurotransmission, increased norepinephrine reuptake, increased GABA activity, and increased serotonin receptor sensitivity (Bschor et al., 2003; Solomon, Keitner, & Ryan, 2000). Lithium also alters the distribution of calcium and magnesium ions and inhibits second messenger systems within the neuron. The specific mechanisms by which lithium improves the symptoms of mania are complex, most likely involving the sum of all or part of these actions and more. Genetic research in bipolar disorder considers lithium response as an important criterion for subgrouping the bipolar population (Alda, 2004).

Pharmacokinetics

Lithium carbonate is available orally in capsule, tablet, and liquid forms. Slow-release preparations are also available. Lithium is readily absorbed in the gastric system and may be taken with food, which does not impair absorption. Peak blood levels are reached in 1 to 4 hours, and the medication is usually completely absorbed in 8 hours. Slow-release preparations are absorbed at a slower, more variable rate.

Lithium is not protein bound, and its distribution into the CNS across the blood–brain barrier is slow. The onset of action is usually 5 to 7 days and may take as long as 2 weeks. The elimination half-life is 8 to 12 hours, and

18 to 36 hours in individuals whose blood levels have reached steady state and whose symptoms are stable. Lithium is almost entirely excreted by the kidneys but is present in all body fluids. Conditions of renal impairment or decreased renal function in older adults decrease lithium clearance and may lead to toxicity. Several medications affect renal function and therefore change lithium clearance. See Chapter 20 for a list of these and other medication interactions with lithium. About 80% of lithium is reabsorbed in the proximal tubule of the kidney along with water and sodium. In conditions that cause sodium depletion, such as dehydration caused by fever, strenuous exercise, hot weather, increased perspiration, and vomiting, the kidney attempts to conserve sodium. Because lithium is a salt, the kidney retains lithium as well, leading to increased blood levels and potential toxicity. Significantly increasing sodium intake causes lithium levels to fall.

Lithium is usually administered in doses of 300 mg two to three times daily. During the acute phases of mania, blood levels of 0.8 to 1.4 mEq/L are usually attained and maintained until symptoms are under control. During maintenance, the dosage is reduced, and dosages are adjusted to maintain blood levels of 0.4 to 1 mEq/L. As a drug with a narrow therapeutic range or index, blood levels are monitored frequently during acute mania, while the dosage is increased every 3 to 5 days. These increases may be slower in older adults or patients who experience uncomfortable side effects. Blood levels should be monitored 12 hours after the last dose of medication. In the hospital setting, nurses should withhold the morning dose of lithium until the serum sample is drawn to avoid falsely elevated levels. Individuals who are at home should be instructed to have their blood drawn in the morning about 12 hours after their last dose and before they take their first dose of medication.

Lithium clears the body relatively quickly after the discontinuation of its use. Withdrawal symptoms are rare, but occasional anxiety and emotional lability have been reported. It is important to remember that almost half of the individuals who discontinue lithium treatment abruptly experience a relapse of symptoms within a few weeks (Goodwin & Ghaemi, 2000; Kennedy et al., 2003). Some research suggests that discontinuation of the use of lithium for individuals whose symptoms have been stable may lead to lithium losing its effectiveness when use of the medication is restarted (Kennedy et al., 2003). Patients should be warned of the risks in abruptly discontinuing their medication and should be advised to consider the options carefully in consultation with their prescriber.

Side Effects, Adverse Reactions, and Toxicity

At lower therapeutic blood levels, side effects from lithium are relatively mild. These reactions correspond with peaks in plasma concentrations of the medication after administration, and most subside during the first few weeks of therapy. Frequently, individuals taking lithium complain of excessive thirst and an unpleasant metallic-like taste. Sugarless throat lozenges may be useful in minimizing this side effect. Other common side effects include an increased frequency of urination, fine head tremor, drowsiness, and mild diarrhoea. Weight gain occurs in about 20% of the individuals taking lithium. Nausea may be minimized by taking the medication with food or by use of a slow-release preparation. However, slow-release forms of lithium increase diarrhoea. Muscle weakness, restlessness, headache, acne, rashes, and exacerbation of psoriasis have also been reported. See Chapter 20 for a summary of selected nursing interventions to minimize the impact of common side effects associated with lithium treatment. Patients most frequently discontinued their own medication use because of concerns with mental slowness, poor concentration, and memory problems.

As blood levels of lithium increase, the side effects of lithium become more numerous and severe. Early signs of lithium toxicity include severe diarrhoea, vomiting, drowsiness, muscular weakness, and lack of coordination. Lithium should be withheld and the prescriber consulted if these symptoms develop. Lithium toxicity can easily be resolved in 24 to 48 hours by discontinuing the medication, but haemodialysis may be required in severe situations. See Chapter 20 for a summary of the side effects and symptoms of toxicity associated with various blood levels of lithium.

Monitoring of creatinine concentration, thyroid hormones, and CBC every 6 months during maintenance therapy helps to assess the occurrence of other potential adverse reactions. Kidney damage is considered an uncommon but potentially serious risk for long-term lithium treatment. This damage is usually reversible after discontinuation of the lithium use. A gradual rise in serum creatinine and decline in creatinine clearance indicate the development of renal dysfunction. Individuals with preexisting kidney dysfunction are susceptible to lithium toxicity.

Lithium may alter thyroid function, usually after 6 to 18 months of treatment. About 30% of the individuals taking lithium exhibit elevations in thyroid-stimulating hormone, but most do not show the suppression of circulating thyroid hormone. Thyroid dysfunction from lithium treatment is more common in women, and some individuals require the addition of thyroxine to their care. During maintenance, thyroid-stimulating hormone levels may be monitored. Nurses should observe for dry skin, constipation, bradycardia, hair loss, cold intolerance, and other symptoms of hypothyroidism. Other endocrine system effects result from hypoparathyroidism, which increases parathyroid hormone levels and calcium. Clinically, this change is not significant, but elevated calcium levels may cause mood changes, anxiety, lethargy, and sleep disturbances. These symptoms may erroneously be attributed to depression if hypocalcaemia is not investigated.

Lithium use must be avoided during pregnancy because it has been associated with birth defects, especially when administered during the first trimester. If lithium is given during the third trimester, toxicity may develop in a newborn, producing signs of hypotonia, cyanosis, bradykinesia, cardiac changes, gastrointestinal bleeding, and shock. Diabetes insipidus may persist for months. Lithium is also present in breast milk, and women should not breast-feed while taking lithium. Women expecting to become pregnant should be advised to consult with their physician before discontinuing the use of birth control methods.

Anticonvulsants

Six anticonvulsants are commonly used to treat bipolar disorder: valproic acid, carbamazepine, gabapentin (Neurontin), topiramate (Topamax), lamotrigine (Lamictal), and oxcarbazepine (Trileptal). Although lithium alone has provided tremendous relief to thousands of individuals experiencing bipolar affective disorder, 20% to 40% of those affected by the disorder do not respond, most often those with rapid cycling episodes. The psychopharmacologic properties of some anticonvulsant medications have been reported since the 1960s, but it was not until the 1970s in Japan that carbamazepine was demonstrated to have mood-stabilizing effects in patients with bipolar affective disorders. Concern about blood dyscrasias delayed its release in the USA, and the increased risks for aplastic anaemia and agranulocytosis with carbamazepine use still require a close monitoring of CBCs during treatment. Valproate and its derivatives have had a similar course of development. With the exception of gabapentin (Neurontin), for which little evidence exists, the benefit of anticonvulsant use in bipolar disorder has been well established (Melvin et al., 2008).

Indications and Mechanisms of Action

Anticonvulsant medications in general are primarily indicated for treating seizure disorders. Target symptoms for the use of anticonvulsants with bipolar affective disorder include all the symptoms of mania discussed earlier. However, anticonvulsants are often used for individuals who have not experienced response to lithium or who are identified as having rapid cycling. Studies have shown some common traits in these individuals. Those who do not experience response to lithium most often are those who have a dysphoric or mixed mania. These individuals experience an increase in physical activity during manic episodes without any elevation in mood. They often are referred to as *mixed states* because they have elements of both depression and mania. These individuals exhibit symptoms of high anxiety, agitation, and irritability, which are then target symptoms for the use of anticonvulsants. Empirical data show carbamazepine and valproic acid to be effective in mood stabilization. The data are less clear for gabapentin, which for that reason is often an adjunctive, not primary, medication for treating patients with bipolar disorder (Grunze & Walden, 2002).

The term *rapid cycling* is applied when individuals experience four or more episodes of either depression or mania during a 12-month period. This occurs more often in women than in men. These patients make up a group of individuals who experience poor response to lithium treatment. Mood instability is also a target symptom of anticonvulsant medications. The theory of the mechanism of action of the anticonvulsants involves the concept of kindling as it applies to mood disorders.

Kindling refers to the emergence of spontaneous firing of nerve cells in response to repeated subthreshold electrical stimulation. Once brain regions, such as the amygdala, have been "kindled," it takes considerably less stimulation to initiate a seizure. In the case of mood disorders, it is hypothesized that "kindled" brain regions include the areas associated with emotional regulation. The stimulation of these regions by increasingly minor stressors or other environmental factors produces mood swings instead of a seizure.

Anticonvulsants have "antikindling" properties and decrease the sensitization of affected cells, making them less easy to stimulate. In general, the anticonvulsant mood stabilizers have many actions, but it is their effects on ion channels, reducing repetitive firing of action potentials in the nerves, that most directly decreases manic symptoms. In addition, drugs such as carbamazepine affect the release and reuptake of several neurotransmitters, including norepinephrine, GABA, dopamine, and glutamate. They also change several second messenger systems. No single mechanism has yet accounted for the anticonvulsants' ability to stabilize mood. Divalproex sodium also has been shown to have numerous neurotransmission effects. The most widely held theory of how it stabilizes mood swings relates to its effects on GABA. As the major inhibitory neurotransmitter in the CNS, increased levels of GABA and improved responsiveness of the neurons to GABA lead to the control of epileptic activity. Divalproex sodium increases levels of GABA in the CNS by activating its synthesis, inhibiting the catabolism (destructive metabolism) of GABA, increasing its release, and increasing receptor density (Loscher, 2002; Solomon et al., 2000). Although the exact mechanisms of action for the anticonvulsants remain unknown, these theories related to kindling and the enhanced functioning of GABA hold promise for the future of new developments in treatment.

Pharmacokinetics

Carbamazepine is an unusual drug and is absorbed in a somewhat variable manner. The liquid suspension is absorbed more quickly than the tablet form, but food does not appear to interfere with absorption. Peak plasma levels occur in 2 to 6 hours. Because high doses influence peak plasma levels and increase the risk for side effects, carbamazepine should be given in divided doses two or three times a day. The suspension, which has higher peak plasma levels and lower trough levels, must be given more frequently than the tablet form.

Valproic acid is more rapidly absorbed, but the enteric coating of divalproex sodium adds a delay of as long as 1 hour. Peak serum levels occur in about 1 to 4 hours. The liquid form (sodium valproate) is absorbed more rapidly and peaks in 15 minutes to 2 hours (Loscher, 2002). Food appears to slow absorption, but does not lower bioavailability of the drug. Valproate is a good example of the importance of considering *bioequivalence*, a term referring to the abilities of two formulations of the same drug to induce a therapeutic response of similar magnitude and duration (Zintzaras, 2005). For example, divalproex, an enteric-coated formulation, has a half-life of 12 to 16 hours; is not affected by food intake and achieves more consistent plasma levels than valproic acid, which has a shorter half-life (8 hours); should not be taken with food; and produces gastrointestinal irritation in about 40% of patients.

Carbamazepine and valproic acid are highly protein bound; therefore, patients who are older, medically ill, or malnourished may experience the effects of increased unbound levels of both drugs. When given with other drugs that are competing for the same protein-binding sites, higher levels of unbound drug may occur. In both cases, these individuals risk more side effects and fluctuations in medication plasma levels. Newer agents for the treatment of bipolar affective disorder, such as gabapentin, have little protein binding and therefore are not subject to some of these effects. Carbamazepine and valproic acid also cross easily into the CNS and move into the placenta as well. Both are associated with an increased risk for birth defects, including spina bifida, and carbamazepine accumulates in foetal tissue. Carbamazepine and valproic acid are metabolized by the cytochrome P-450 system of microsomal hepatic enzymes. However, one of the metabolites of carbamazepine is potentially toxic. When other concurrent medications inhibit the enzymes that break down this toxic metabolite, severe adverse reactions are often the result (e.g., decreased prothrombin times and hepatotoxicity; Kalapos, 2002). Medications that inhibit this breakdown include erythromycin, verapamil, and cimetidine (now available in nonprescription form).

Carbamazepine activates its own metabolism through induction of the P-450 microsomal hepatic enzymes.

Patients receiving carbamazepine may experience a precipitant drop in therapeutic blood levels and a relapse in symptoms, requiring a dosage increase for as long as 2 to 3 months after steady state has been achieved. Although valproic acid is also affected by other medications that stimulate the P-450 system, it does not enhance its own metabolism. Both carbamazepine and valproic acid are available in slow-release, extended-action forms, allowing for decreased daily dosing and improved adherence.

Nurses need to educate patients about potential drug interactions, especially with nonprescription medications. Nurses can also inform other health care practitioners who may be prescribing medication that these patients are taking carbamazepine. It is important to note that oral contraceptives may become ineffective, and female patients should be advised to use other methods of birth control.

Side Effects, Adverse Reactions, and Toxicity

The most common side effects of carbamazepine are dizziness, drowsiness, tremor, visual disturbance, nausea, and vomiting. These side effects may be minimized by initiating treatment in low doses. Patients should be advised that these symptoms will diminish, but care should be taken when changing positions or performing tasks that require visual alertness. Giving the drug with food may diminish nausea. Valproic acid also causes gastrointestinal disturbances, tremor, and lethargy. In addition, it can produce weight gain and alopecia (hair loss). These symptoms are transient and should diminish with the course of treatment. Dietary supplements of zinc and selenium may be helpful to patients experiencing hair loss. Constipation and urinary retention occur in some individuals. Nurses should monitor urinary output and assist patients to increase fluid consumption to decrease constipation.

Transient elevations in liver enzymes occur with both carbamazepine and valproic acid, but rarely do symptoms of hepatic injury occur. If the patient reports abnormal pain or shows signs of jaundice, the prescriber should be notified immediately. Several blood dyscrasias are associated with carbamazepine, including aplastic anaemia, agranulocytosis, and leucopenia. Patients should be advised to report fever, sore throat, rash, petechiae, or bruising immediately. In addition, advise patients of the importance of completing routine blood tests throughout treatment.

Both valproic acid and carbamazepine may be lethal if high doses are ingested. Toxic symptoms appear in 1 to 3 hours and include neuromuscular disturbances, dizziness, stupor, agitation, disorientation, nystagmus, urinary retention, nausea and vomiting, tachycardia, hypotension or hypertension, cardiovascular shock, coma, and respiratory depression. Carbamazepine appears to be more lethal at lower doses, but valproic acid is absorbed rapidly, and gastric lavage may be ineffective, depending on time from ingestion.

Of the newer anticonvulsant drugs, gabapentin (Neurontin) has relatively few side effects. Lamotrigine (Lamictal) in rare cases produces severe, life-threatening rashes that usually occur within 2 to 8 weeks of treatment. This risk is highest in children. The use of lamotrigine should be immediately discontinued if a rash is noted. Topamax (Topiramate) carries an increased risk for kidney stone formation. It can also cause a decrease in serum digoxin levels and may decrease effectiveness of oral birth control agents. In addition, ongoing ophthalmologic monitoring is required because of reports of acute myopia with secondary glaucoma. Trileptal (oxcarbazepine) has the potential for causing hyponatremia and may also decrease the effectiveness of oral birth control agents. Because of the potentially significant adverse reactions that the anticonvulsants can produce, careful patient teaching and monitoring are required.

▆▆ ANTIDEPRESSANT MEDICATIONS

Researchers in the 1950s who were investigating other drugs related to the phenothiazines for the treatment of psychosis discovered that imipramine, a related compound, relieved the symptoms of depression. Imipramine was the first of a number of medications that contained a three-ring structure in their chemical makeup and produced improvement in depression. These medications became known as tricyclic antidepressants (TCAs). Table 14-9 lists other related TCAs still in use today.

Concurrent with the discovery of TCAs, an antibiotic, iproniazid, used in treating tuberculosis, alleviated the symptoms of depression. Iproniazid increased the bioamine neurotransmitters by inhibiting monoamine oxidase, the enzyme that breaks down these neurotransmitters inside the nerve cell. Iproniazid is no longer used, but related, more effective drugs, phenelzine and tranylcypromine, make up a subgroup of antidepressants called the MAOIs.

TCAS, MAOIS, and More

Throughout the 1960s and 1970s, the TCAs and MAOIs were the primary medications for treating depression. Research continued to develop new agents with increased effectiveness, while decreasing the side effects and potential lethal effects. In the 1980s, several medications that were significantly different in chemical structure were introduced. Bupropion (Wellbutrin), introduced in 1987, had actions that were significantly different from those of

Table 14.9 Antidepressant Medications

Generic (Trade) Drug Name	Usual Dosage Range (mg/day)	Half-Life (hours)	Therapeutic Blood Level (ng/mL)
Tricyclic—Tertiary Amines			
amitriptyline (Elavil)	50–300	31–46	110–250
clomipramine (Anafranil)	25–250	19–37	80–100
doxepin (Sinequan)	25–300	8–24	100–200
imipramine (Tofranil)	30–300	11–25	200–350
Tricyclics—Secondary Amines			
amoxapine (Asendin)	50–600	8	200–500
desipramine (Norpramin)	25–300	12–24	125–300
nortriptyline (Aventyl)	30–100	18–44	50–150
protriptyline (Vivactil)	15–60	67–89	100–200
Selective Serotonin Reuptake Inhibitors			
fluoxetine (Prozac)	20–80	2–9 days	72–300
sertraline (Zoloft)	50–200	24	Not available
paroxetine (Paxil)	10–50	10–24	Not available
fluvoxamine (Luvox)	50–300	17–22	Not available
citalopram (Celexa)	20–50	35	Not available
escitalopram (Lexapro)	10–20	27–32	Not available
Other Antidepressant Medications			
PHENETHYLAMINE			
venlafaxine (Effexor)	75–375	5–11	100–500
TETRACYCLIC			
maprotiline (Ludiomil)	50–225	21–25	200–300
TRIAZOLOPYRIDINE			
trazodone (Desyrel)	150–600	4–9	650–1,600
PHENYLPIPERAZINE			
nefazodone (Serzone)	100–600	2–4	Not available
AMINOKETONE			
bupropion (Wellbutrin)	200–450	8–24	10–29
PIPERAZINOAZEPINES			
mirtazapine (Remeron)	15–45	20–40	Not available
Monoamine Oxidase Inhibitors			
moclobemide (Manerix)	300–600	6–10	Not available
phenelzine (Nardil)	15–90	24 (effect lasts 3–10 days)	Not available
tranylcypromine (Parnate)	10–60	24 (effect lasts 3–10 days)	Not available

previous antidepressants, but concern about the risk for seizures and other side effects limited initial excitement about its use. In 1988, the release of fluoxetine (Prozac) received much public attention and resulted in an increased awareness of depression and its treatment. Fluoxetine was the first of a class of drugs that acted "selectively" on one group of neurotransmitters, in this case serotonin. Other similarly selective medications, sertraline (Zoloft), paroxetine (Paxil), and fluvoxamine (Luvox), soon followed and together make up the SSRIs. The newest SSRIs include citalopram (Celexa) and escitalopram oxalate (Lexapro). Reboxetine is the only norepinephrine selective reuptake inhibitor available in Canada.

Citalopram is a racemate, which means it contains equal proportions of two isomers. Isomers are molecules with the same chemical formula but with a different spatial arrangement of the atoms, which may cause different effects in the human body or have different side-effect profiles. The two isomers of citalopram have been separated, and escitalopram, one of the isomers, is marketed as an antidepressant in its own right.

Since the initial introduction of the SSRIs, several new chemical compounds have been introduced that have unique structure or actions, making them difficult to categorize. These medications differ in which neurotransmitters they affect and in what side effects are common. This subgroup of antidepressants includes drugs such as mirtazapine (Remeron) and venlafaxine (Effexor). In the Canadian clinical guidelines for the treatment of depressive disorders developed by the CANMAT Depression Working Group (Kennedy, Lam, Cohen, Ravindran, & the CANMAT Depression Work Group, 2001), first-line treatment for a major depressive episode is either an SSRI or venlafaxine.

Indications and Mechanisms of Action

The TCAs have multiple effects on a variety of receptors in the CNS, including reuptake inhibition at serotonin and norepinephrine transporters; down-regulation of specific serotonin and noradrenergic receptors; and blockade of cholinergic, adrenergic, and histamine receptors. On the other hand, the MAOIs are more specific in their actions. They inhibit MAO, an enzyme that breaks down biogenic amines, such as serotonin, thereby increasing synaptic neurotransmission, resulting in clinical improvement.

The primary indication for antidepressant medications is depression, thus the name "antidepressant." Symptoms such as loss of interest in the person's usual activities (anhedonia), depressed mood, lethargy or decreased energy, insomnia, decreased concentration, loss of appetite, and suicidal ideation usually respond (see Chapter 20 for a more complete discussion of the symptoms of depression). Antidepressants are also used to treat other symptoms and disorders, and increasingly the name antidepressant might be somewhat misleading.

Antidepressants are prescribed to treat the whole range of anxiety disorders (see Chapter 21). Antidepressants are also used to treat eating disorders (see Chapter 23), depression in bipolar affective disorders, dysthymia, chronic pain disorders, and premenstrual syndrome. More sedating antidepressants are sometimes used in small doses to improve sleep disturbance. Trazodone, amitriptyline, mirtazapine, and other agents have been used alone or as adjunctive interventions for sleep disturbance. Antidepressants are also used for other sleep disorders, such as sleep apnoea. Symptoms of some psychiatric disorders of childhood (see Chapter 28), such as attention deficit hyperactivity disorder (ADHD), enuresis (bed wetting), and school phobia, often respond to antidepressant medication.

At times, the symptoms of depression present in an "atypical" manner, which is called *atypical depression*. Individuals with atypical depression have a mixture of anxiety and depression, hypersomnia, mood swings, worsening of the symptoms in the evening, and oversensitivity to such interpersonal feelings as rejection. These target symptoms of atypical depression often respond better to the MAOIs, such as phenelzine (Nardil), or to the mixed action antidepressants (those that have both direct neurotransmitter receptor action and reuptake properties), such as trazodone or nefazedone (Riederer, Lachenmayer, & Laux, 2004).

Pharmacokinetics

All of the antidepressant medications are well absorbed from the gastrointestinal system; however, some individual variations exist. For example, food slightly increases the amount of trazodone absorbed but decreases its maximum blood concentrations and lengthens the time to peak effects from 1 hour on an empty stomach to 2 hours with food. Food also increases the maximum concentrations of sertraline in the bloodstream and decreases the time to peak plasma levels, whereas fluoxetine and fluvoxamine are unaffected, although food may delay the absorption of fluoxetine. Food has little effect on the TCAs.

PMH nurses should review pharmacokinetic information as it applies to each individual medication. They must consider how this information will affect the patient's use of the medication given the target symptoms for which the drug is intended. For example, if trazodone is being used on a continuous dose schedule for its antidepressant effect, the effects of food probably matter very little. However, if trazodone is being used in a small dose at bedtime to assist a patient to sleep, an empty stomach becomes important because food would lengthen the time of onset of clinical effects, in this case, sleep.

The TCAs undergo considerable first-pass metabolism but reach peak plasma concentrations in 2 to 4 hours. The TCAs are highly bound to plasma proteins, which make the association between blood levels and therapeutic clinical effects difficult. However, some plasma ranges have been established. Table 14-9 includes the available ranges for therapeutic blood levels of the TCAs. In addition, times to steady-state plasma levels have wide variations, and the effective dose of medication must be individualized. Other antidepressants are also highly protein bound, which means that drugs that compete for these binding sites may cause fluctuations in blood levels of the antidepressants. Venlafaxine has the lowest protein binding; therefore, drug interactions of this type are not expected with this medication. Blood level changes caused by the presence of other drugs competing with binding sites are not expected.

The onset of action also varies considerably, depending on specific symptoms. For example, an improvement in sleep often occurs earlier than effects on overall mood or anhedonia. Complete relief of symptoms may take several weeks (Machado-Vieira, Salvadore, Luckenbaugh, Manji, & Zarate, 2008). Full enzyme inhibition with the MAOIs may take as long as 2 weeks, but the energizing effects may be seen within a few days. Overcoming issues such as social stigma, viewing depression as a personal failing, fear about taking a medication, and the decreased energy and motivation associated with depression have made deciding to seek treatment a major hurdle. Indeed, in both United States and Canadian community surveys, only about one third of individuals with depression had sought treatment for their symptoms (Patten & Beck, 2004; Rust et al., 2005). The variable onset of action may add to their sense of discouragement and powerlessnesss. PMH nurses and families are often involved in providing encouragement and other supportive interventions to assist the patient in "getting through" this period of time.

Although antidepressants are primarily excreted by the kidneys, their routes of metabolism vary. Most of the TCAs have active metabolites that act in much the same manner as the parent drug. Therefore, in determining the rate of elimination, one must consider the half-lives of these metabolites. Most of these antidepressants may be given in a once-daily single dose. If the medication causes sedation, this dose should be given at bedtime. The SSRIs frequently cause more activation of energy and are often given in the morning. Venlafaxine, nefazodone, and bupropion are examples of antidepressants whose shorter half-life periods and other factors require administration two or three times per day. Fluoxetine and its active metabolite have particularly long half-lives, remaining present for as long as 5 to 6 weeks. This may affect a number of decisions. For example, women who wish to have children and are taking fluoxetine ideally should discontinue use of the agent at least 6 weeks before attempting to conceive. They should be advised to consult their prescriber before making this decision. Fluoxetine would also not be a good choice for intermittent use for premenstrual dysphoric disorder. Table 14-9 provides information about the average elimination half-lives of most of the antidepressants.

Most of the antidepressants are metabolized by the P-450 enzyme system so that drugs that induce this system tend to decrease blood levels of the antidepressants, and inhibitors of this system increase antidepressant blood levels. This effect varies according to the subfamily that is induced. For example, fluvoxamine (Luvox) substantially inhibits CYP1A2. Thus, other drugs that are metabolized by the system experience slower metabolism. These include such medications as amitriptyline, clomipramine, imipramine, clozapine, propranolol, theophylline, and caffeine (Armstrong, Cozza, & Oesterheld, 2002). Paroxetine and fluoxetine are very potent inhibitors of CYP2D6, as well as mild inhibitors of CYP2C19 and CYP2C9.

Side Effects, Adverse Reactions, and Toxicity

Side effects of the antidepressant medications vary considerably. Because the TCAs act at several types of receptors, in addition to serotonin and norepinephrine receptors, these drugs have many unwanted effects. Conversely, the SSRIs are more selective for serotonin and have comparatively fewer and better tolerated side effects. Attention to a patient's ability to tolerate side effects is critical because uncomfortable side effects are the primary reason patients discontinue medication treatment. With the TCAs, sedation, orthostatic hypotension, and anticholinergic side effects are the most common sources of discomfort for patients receiving these medications. See Chapter 20 for a comparison of side effects of antidepressant medications.

Receptor affinities may be helpful in predicting which side effects are most likely to occur with a given medication. Table 14-1 provides a summary of major receptor targets for common antidepressants. Using this table in conjunction with Chapter 20, nurses may be able to predict which side effects will be most common with each medication. Interventions to assist in minimizing these side effects are listed in Table 14-2.

Tolerance develops gradually to the sedation and anticholinergic side effects caused by TCAs, but these may be minimized when the prescriber begins with a low dose and increases gradually. Other side effects of the TCAs include tremors, restlessness, insomnia, nausea and vomiting, confusion, pedal edema, headache, and seizures. Blood dyscrasias may also occur, and any fever, sore throat, malaise, or rash should be reported to the prescriber.

Sexual dysfunction is a relatively common side effect with most antidepressants. Erectile and ejaculation disturbances occur in men and anorgasmia in women. This side effect is often difficult to assess if the nurse has not obtained a sexual history before the initiation of use of the medication. Anorgasmia is particularly common with the SSRIs and often goes unreported, frequently because nurses and other health care providers do not ask. Bupropion and nefazodone (Serzone) appear to be least likely to cause sexual disturbance. In addition, when sexual dysfunction is related to the medication, several treatment options are available. These include a change in dose or type of antidepressant or, less frequently, using other medications to treat this side effect. Nurses must take responsibility for discussing the potential for sexual side effects before initiation of drug treatment and for continuing to reassess during follow-up visits. The TCAs have the potential for cardiotoxicity, which limits their use in older adults. Symptoms include prolongation of cardiac conduction that may worsen preexisting cardiac conduction problems. TCAs are contraindicated with second-degree atrioventricular block and should be used cautiously in patients who have other cardiac problems. Occasionally, they may precipitate heart failure, myocardial infarction, arrhythmias, and stroke. The newer antidepressants, such as the SSRIs and bupropion, are less cardiotoxic, and nefazodone currently exhibits no evidence of cardiotoxicity.

Antidepressants that block the dopamine (DB_{2B}) receptor, such as amoxapine, have produced symptoms of NMS. Mild forms of extrapyramidal symptoms and endocrine changes, including galactorrhea and amenorrhea, may develop. Amoxapine should be avoided in older adult patients because it may be associated with the development of tardive dyskinesia with this age group. Rare occurrences and only mild forms of extrapyramidal symptoms, such as tightness in the jaw and muscle spasms, may occur with any of the TCAs or SSRIs (Zullino, Delacrausaz, & Baumann, 2002).

The most common side effects of the SSRIs include headache, anxiety, insomnia, transient nausea, vomiting, and diarrhoea. Sedation may also occur, especially with fluvoxamine. Most often, these medications are given in the morning, but if daytime sedation occurs, they may be given in the evening. Higher doses, especially of fluoxetine, are more likely to produce sedation.

Venlafaxine (Effexor) has little effect on acetylcholine and histamine; thus, the risks for sedation and anticholinergic symptoms are low. However, higher doses are associated with sexual dysfunction, sedation, diastolic hypertension, increased perspiration, constipation, dry mouth, tremors, blurred vision, and asthenia or muscle weakness. Elevations in blood pressure have been described, and nurses should monitor blood pressure, especially in patients who have a preexisting history of hypertension. Nurses need to be very familiar with nefazodone (Serzone) and the clinical issues related to its side effects. Nefazodone is a phenylpiperazine antidepressant that is structurally related to trazodone. Its most common side effects include sedation, dizziness, orthostatic hypotension; less common is increased risk for seizures. Drug–drug interactions between nefazodone and triazolam and alprazolam have been reported, with increased plasma levels of these benzodiazepines, resulting in an enhancement of the psychomotor impairment caused by these agents. Bupropion (Wellbutrin) has a chemical structure unlike any of the other antidepressants. Some of its pharmacologic profile is due to effects on dopamine systems, in addition to effects on serotonin and norepinephrine.

Bupropion's activating effects may be experienced as agitation or anxiety by some patients. Others also experience insomnia and appetite suppression. Rarely, bupropion has produced psychosis, including hallucinations and delusions. Most likely, this is secondary to the stimulation of dopamine systems. Dopamine is also associated with reward and motivated behaviour, which accounts for the increasingly common use of bupropion, under the trade name of Zyban, as a smoking cessation agent. The slightly increased risk for experiencing seizures with bupropion use has received the most attention. It has been found that if the total daily dose of bupropion is no more than 450 mg and no individual dose is greater than 150 mg, the risk for seizures with bupropion is no greater than the risk with the other TCAs (Ferry & Johnston, 2003). Most important, bupropion has not been found to cause sexual dysfunction and often is used in individuals who are experiencing these side effects.

The MAOIs can produce anticholinergic side effects (dizziness, dry mouth, blurred vision, constipation, nausea, peripheral edema, urinary hesitancy), but at a much reduced rate compared with the TCAs. Orthostatic hypotension is common; thus, frequent assessment of lying and standing blood pressures is required, especially with older adults, who may be at risk for falls and subsequent bone fractures and require assistance in changing position.

Sexual dysfunction, including decreased libido, impotence, and anorgasmia, can occur with MAOIs.

The most serious side effect of the MAOIs is their interaction with food and certain medications. The food interaction occurs because MAOIs block the breakdown of tyramine, a trace amine with vasoconstrictor properties. Increased levels of tyramine can cause severe headaches and hypertension; stroke; and, in rare instances, death. Patients who are taking MAOIs are placed on a low-tyramine diet. This diet has been difficult for some individuals to follow, and concerns about the risk for severe hypertension have led many clinicians to rarely use the MAOIs (see Table 14-10).

MAOIs currently in use in Canada include phenelzine (Nardil) and tranylcypromine (Parnate). These are considered irreversible MAOIs because they form unbreakable covalent bonds with monoamine oxidase. It takes at least 2 weeks to produce replacement enzyme molecules after discontinuation of use of the medication. Moclobemide is an example of a reversible MAOI that is available in Europe and Canada. Although it acts in the same way as the irreversible MAOIs, moclobemide forms weaker bonds that are short lasting. Therefore, a less restrictive diet may be used with moclobemide. In addition to food restrictions, many prescription and nonprescription medications that stimulate the sympathetic nervous system (sympathomimetics) produce the same risk for hypertensive crisis as do foods containing tyramine. The nonprescription medication interactions involve primarily diet pills and cold remedies. Patients should be advised to check the labels of any nonprescription drugs carefully for a warning against use with antidepressants, especially tvhe MAOIs, and then consult their prescriber or pharmacist before consuming these medications. In addition, symptoms of other serious drug–drug interactions may develop, such as coma, hypertension, and fever, which may occur when patients receive meperidine (Demerol) while taking an MAOI. Patients should notify other health care providers, including dentists, that they are taking an MAOI before being prescribed or given any other medication.

Suicide is a major concern when working with individuals who are depressed. Systematic suicide risk assessment should be done routinely before initiating antidepressant therapy, in the first 2 to 4 weeks of treatment and for longer if indicated. Some of these medications are more lethal than others. For example, the TCAs pose a significant risk for overdose and are more lethal in children. Symptoms of overdose and treatment are discussed more fully in Chapter 20, but for now, it is important to remember that this potential exists. Sometimes, the prescriber will provide the patient with only small amounts of the medication, requiring more frequent visits, and will closely monitor use. In general, newer antidepressant medications, such as the SSRIs, are associated with less risk for toxicity and lethality in overdose. Box 14-4 highlights some of the newest antidepressants being tested in clinical trials.

Table 14.10	Example of a Tyramine-Restricted Diet	
Category of Food	Food to Avoid	Food Allowed
Cheese	All matured or aged cheeses All casseroles made with these cheeses, pizza, lasagna, etc. *Note:* All cheeses are considered matured or aged except those listed under the "Foods Allowed" column	Fresh cottage cheese, cream cheese, ricotta cheese, and processed cheese slices. All fresh milk products that have been stored properly (e.g., sour cream, yogurt, ice cream)
Meat, fish, and poultry	Fermented/dry sausage: pepperoni, salami, mortadella, summer sausage, etc. Improperly stored meat, fish, or poultry Improperly stored pickled herring	All fresh packaged or processed meat (e.g., chicken loaf, hot dogs), fish, or poultry Refrigerate immediately and eat as soon as possible
Fruits and vegetables	Fava or broad bean pods (not beans) Banana peel	Banana pulp All others except those listed in the "Food to Avoid" column
Alcoholic beverages	All tap beers	Alcohol: No more than two domestic bottled or canned beers or 4-fluid-oz glasses of red or white wine per day; this applies to nonalcoholic beer also; please note that red wine may produce a headache unrelated to a rise in blood pressure
Miscellaneous foods	Marmite concentrated yeast extract Sauerkraut Soy sauce and other soybean condiments	Other yeast extracts (e.g., brewer's yeast) Soy milk

Adapted from Gardener, D. M., Shulman, K. I., Walker, S. E., & Tailor, S. A. N. (1996). The making of a user-friendly MAOI diet. *Journal of Clinical Psychiatry, 57,* 99–104

BOX 14.4
Novel Antidepressant Drug Development

Research into the neurobiology of depression has implicated other neurotransmitter and neuroendocrine systems in the etiology of depression. This has led to the development of new antidepressants, many of which are currently in clinical trials.

For example, the hypothalamic-pituitary-adrenal (HPA) axis, a major stress hormone system, shows evidence of overactivity and blunted feedback control in depression. The principal activator of the HPA axis is a hormone called *corticotropin-releasing hormone* (CRH). This hormone is produced in the hypothalamus and stimulates the pituitary to release adrenocorticotrophic hormone (ACTH), which stimulates the release of cortisol from the adrenal gland. In depression, excessive CRH leads to increased levels of cortisol. Increased levels of cortisol are associated with some of the symptoms in depression, such as difficulty concentrating, sleep disturbance, and lowered energy. This led to the CRH theory of depression (Holsboer & Ising, 2008) and prompted the development of CRH antagonists and glucocorticoid receptor antagonists as potential antidepressants.

Glutamate is the major excitatory neurotransmitter and has been implicated in many psychiatric and neuropsychiatric disorders, including depression. Some evidence exists for increased glutamate in depression (Krystal et al., 2002). Thus, glutamate antagonists are also being tested for any antidepressant properties.

ANTIANXIETY AND SEDATIVE-HYPNOTIC MEDICATIONS

Sometimes called *anxiolytics*, antianxiety medications and sedative-hypnotic medications come from various pharmacologic classifications, including benzodiazepines, nonbenzodiazepines, and nonbarbiturate sedative-hypnotics, such as chloral hydrate. These drugs represent some of the most widely prescribed medications today for the short-term relief of anxiety or anxiety associated with depression.

Benzodiazepines

Commonly prescribed benzodiazepines include chlordiazepoxide (Librium), diazepam (Valium), lorazepam (Ativan), flurazepam (Dalmane), oxazepam (Serax), clonazapam (Rivotril), and triazolam (Halcion).

Indications and Mechanisms of Action

Benzodiazepines act as positive modulators at GABA ion channels, increasing the ease of GABA binding to its binding site. This enhancement of GABA binding increases both the duration and frequency of channel opening and decreases the firing rate of the nerve cell. This inhibition of nerve cell firing allows this class of drugs to act as anticonvulsants, antianxiety medications, or hypnotics, depending on dose and pharmacokinetic properties. Other neurotransmitter systems are also involved in the effects of benzodiazepines. Of the various benzodiazepines in use to relieve anxiety (and treat insomnia), oxazepam (Serax) and lorazepam (Ativan) are often preferred for patients with liver disease and for older adult patients because of their short half-lives.

Pharmacokinetics

The variable rate of absorption of the benzodiazepines determines the speed of onset. Table 14-11 provides relative indications of the speed of onset, from very fast to slow, for some of the commonly prescribed benzodiazepines.

Chlordiazepoxide (Librium) and diazepam (Valium) are slow, erratic, and sometimes incompletely absorbed when given IM, whereas lorazepam (Ativan) is rapidly and completely absorbed when given IM. Lorazepam is also well absorbed by the sublingual route.

All the benzodiazepines are highly lipid soluble and highly protein bound. They are distributed throughout the body and enter the CNS quickly. Other drugs that compete for protein-binding sites may produce drug–drug interactions. The degree to which each of these drugs is lipid soluble affects its duration of action. Most of these drugs have active metabolites, but the degree of activity of each metabolite affects the duration of action and elimination half-life. Most of these drugs vary markedly in the length of half-life. Oxazepam, which is itself an active metabolite of diazepam, and lorazepam have no active metabolites and thus have shorter half-lives. Sustained presence of these drugs after discontinuation may be observed in older adult or obese patients.

Side Effects, Adverse Reactions, and Toxicity

The most commonly reported side effects result from the sedative and CNS depression effects of these medications. Drowsiness, intellectual impairment, anterograde memory impairment, ataxia, and reduced motor coordination are common adverse effects. If used for sleep, many of these medications, especially long-acting benzodiazepines, produce significant "hangover" effects experienced on awakening. Flunitrazepam (Rohypnol), otherwise known as the "date rape" drug because of its ability to impair anterograde memory, is illegal in Canada. Older adults receiving repeated doses of medications, such as flurazepam (Dalmane), at bedtime may experience paradoxical confusion, agitation, and delirium, sometimes after the first dose. In addition, daytime fatigue, drowsiness, and cognitive impairments may continue while the person is awake. Current clinical guidelines for drug treatments in older adults suggest avoiding benzodiazepine use in this population (Cumbler, Guerrasio, Kim, & Glasheen, 2008). For most patients, the effects subside as tolerance develops; however, alcohol increases all these symptoms and potentiates the CNS depression. Individuals using these medications should be warned to be cautious when driving or performing other tasks that require mental alertness. If these tasks are part of the person's work requirements, another medication may be chosen. Administered intravenously, benzodiazepines often cause phlebitis and thrombosis at the intravenous sites, which should be monitored closely and changed if redness or swelling develops.

Because tolerance develops to most of the CNS depressant effects, individuals who wish to experience the feeling of "intoxication" from these medications may be tempted to increase their own dosage. Psychological

Table 14.11 Antianxiety and Sedative-Hypnotic Medications			
Generic (Trade) Drug Name	Usual Dosage Range (mg/day)	Half-Life (hours)	Speed of Onset After Single Dose
Benzodiazepines			
diazepam (Valium)	4–40	30–100	Very fast
chlordiazepoxide (Librium)	15–100	50–100	Intermediate
clorazepate (Tranxene)	15–60	30–200	Fast
prazepam (Centrax)	20–60	30–200	Very slow
flurazepam (Dalmane)	15–30	47–100	Fast
lorazepam (Ativan)	2–8	10–20	Slow-intermediate
oxazepam (Serax)	30–120	3–21	Slow-intermediate
temazepam (Restoril)	15–30	9.5–20	Moderately fast
triazolam (Halcion)	0.25–0.5	2–4	Fast
alprazolam (Xanax)	0.5–10	12–15	Intermediate
clonazepam (Livotril)	1.5–20	18–50	Intermediate
Nonbenzodiazepines			
buspirone (BuSpar)	15–30	3–11	Very slow
zolpidem (Ambien)	5–10	2.6	Fast

dependence is more likely to occur when using these medications for a longer period, as well as for the short-acting forms. Abrupt discontinuation of the use of benzodiazepines may result in a recurrence of the target symptoms, such as rebound insomnia or anxiety. Other withdrawal symptoms appear rapidly, including tremors, increased perspiration, palpitations, increased sensitivity to light, abdominal discomfort or pain, and elevations in systolic blood pressure. These symptoms may be more pronounced with the short-acting benzodiazepines, such as lorazepam. Gradual tapering is recommended for discontinuing the use of benzodiazepines after long-term treatment. When tapering short-acting medications, the prescriber may switch the patient to a long-acting benzodiazepine before discontinuing use of the short-acting drug.

Individual reactions to the benzodiazepines appear to be associated with sensitivity to their effects. Some patients feel apathy, fatigue, tearfulness, emotional lability, irritability, and nervousness. Benzodiazepines do little for depression symptoms, except for sleep disturbance, and may even exacerbate anhedonia and difficulties concentrating. As such, their use in depression, even with significant comorbid anxiety, should be closely monitored. Gastrointestinal disturbances, including nausea, vomiting, anorexia, dry mouth, and constipation, may develop. These medications may be taken with food to ease the gastrointestinal distress.

Older adults are particularly susceptible to incontinence, memory disturbances, dizziness, and increased risk for falls when using benzodiazepines. Pregnant patients should be aware that these medications cross the placenta and are associated with an increased risk for birth defects, such as cleft palate, mental retardation, and pyloric stenosis. Infants born addicted to benzodiazepines often exhibit flaccid muscle tone, lethargy, and difficulties sucking. All the benzodiazepines are excreted in breast milk, and breast-feeding women should avoid using these medications. Infants and children metabolize these medications more slowly; therefore, more drug accumulates in their bodies.

Toxicity can develop with liver dysfunction or disease. Symptoms include worsening of the CNS depression, ataxia, confusion, delirium, agitation, hypotension, diminished reflexes, and lethargy. Rarely do the benzodiazepines cause respiratory depression or death. In overdose, these medications have a high therapeutic index and rarely result in death unless combined with another CNS depressant drug, such as alcohol.

Nonbenzodiazepines: Buspirone and Zolpidem

One of the nonbenzodiazepines, buspirone (BuSpar), was first synthesized in 1968 by Michael Eison, who was searching for an improved antipsychotic medication. Later, it was found that buspirone was effective in controlling the symptoms of anxiety but had no effect on panic disorders and little effect on obsessive-compulsive disorder. Another nonbenzodiazepine, zolpidem (Ambien), is a medication for sleep that acts on the benzodiazepine–GABA receptor complex.

Indications and Mechanisms of Actions

These drugs are effective for treating anxiety disorders without the CNS depressant effects or the potential for abuse and withdrawal syndromes. Buspirone is indicated for treating generalized anxiety disorder; therefore, its target symptoms include anxiety and related symptoms, such as difficulty in concentrating, tension, insomnia, restlessness, irritability, and fatigue. Because buspirone does not add to depression symptoms, it has been tried for treating anxiety that coexists with depression. In some instances, it is thought to potentiate the antidepressant actions of other medications.

Buspirone has no effect on the benzodiazepine–GABA complex but instead appears to control anxiety by blocking the serotonin subtype of receptor, 5-HT_{1a}, at both presynaptic reuptake and postsynaptic receptor sites. It has no sedative, muscle relaxant, or anticonvulsant effects. It also lacks potential for abuse.

Zolpidem (Ambien), which is indicated for short-term insomnia treatment, appears to increase slow-wave (deep) sleep and to modulate GABA receptors in a similar fashion to benzodiazepines, but with less risk for tolerance or withdrawal issues.

Pharmacokinetics

Buspirone is rapidly absorbed but undergoes extensive first-pass metabolism. Food slows absorption but appears to reduce first-pass effects, increasing the bioavailability of the medication. Buspirone is given on a continual dosing schedule of three times a day because of its short half-life of 2 to 3 hours. Clinical action depends on reaching steady-state concentrations; taking this medication with food may facilitate this process.

Buspirone is highly protein bound but does not displace most other medications. However, it does displace digoxin and may increase digoxin levels to the point of toxicity. It is metabolized in the liver and excreted predominantly by the kidneys but also through the gastrointestinal tract. Patients with liver or kidney impairment should be given this medication with caution.

Buspirone cannot be used on a PRN basis; rather, it takes 2 to 4 weeks of continual use for symptom relief to occur. It is more effective in reducing anxiety in patients who have never taken a benzodiazepine.

Buspirone does not block the withdrawal of other benzodiazepines. Therefore, a switch to buspirone must be initiated gradually to avoid withdrawal symptoms. Nurses should closely monitor patients who are undergoing this change of medication for emergence of withdrawal symptoms from the benzodiazepines and report such symptoms to the prescriber.

Zolpidem is metabolized by the liver; it crosses the placenta, and enters breast milk. It has a short half-life of 3 hours, which makes it an ideal hypnotic and is excreted in the urine.

Side Effects, Adverse Reactions, and Toxicity

Common side effects from higher-dose buspirone include dizziness, drowsiness, nausea, excitement, and headache. Most other side effects occur at an incidence of less than 1%. There have been no reports of death from an overdose of buspirone alone. Older adults, pregnant women, and children have not been adequately studied. For now, buspirone can be assumed to cross the placenta and is present in breast milk; therefore, its use should be avoided in pregnant women, and women who are taking this medication should not breast-feed.

Rebound effects, such as insomnia and anxiety, from zolpidem are minimal. There are minimal effects on respiratory function and little potential for abuse. Although very rare, there have been cases of sleepwalking, sleep-driving, and other complex behaviors while asleep attributed to zolpidem use (Dolder & Nelson, 2008).

■■■■ STIMULANTS

Amphetamines were first synthesized in the late 1800s but were not used for psychiatric disorders until the 1930s. Initially, amphetamines were prescribed for a variety of symptoms and disorders, but their high abuse potential soon became obvious.

Methylphenidate, Pemoline, and Modafinil

Among the medications known as stimulants are methylphenidate (Ritalin), used for attention deficit disorders; pemoline (Cylert), a CNS stimulant also used for hyperactivity and attention deficit disorders; and modafinil (Provigil), used for narcolepsy, a sleep disorder.

Indications and Mechanisms of Action

Medical use of these drugs is now restricted to a few disorders, including narcolepsy, ADHD—particularly in children—and obesity unresponsive to other treatments. However, stimulants are increasingly being used as an adjunctive treatment in depression and other mood disorders to address the anhedonia and low energy common to these conditions.

Dextroamphetamine (or D-amphetamine, indicating the D-isomer; Dexadrine) indirectly stimulates the sympathetic nervous system, producing alertness, wakefulness, vasoconstriction, suppressed appetite, and hypothermia. Tolerance develops to some of these effects, such as suppression of appetite, but the CNS stimulation continues. Although the exact mechanism of action is not completely understood, stimulants cause a release of catecholamines, particularly norepinephrine and dopamine, into the synapse from the presynaptic nerve cell. They also block the reuptake of these catecholamines. Methylphenidate is structurally similar to the amphetamines but produces a milder CNS stimulation. Pemoline is structurally dissimilar from the amphetamines but produces the same pharmacologic actions. Pemoline predominantly affects the dopamine system and therefore has less effect on the sympathetic nervous system.

Although the stimulant effects of these medications may seem logically indicated for narcolepsy, a disorder in which the individual frequently and abruptly falls asleep, the indications for childhood ADHD seem less obvious. The aetiology and neurobiology of ADHD remain unclear, but psychostimulants produce a paradoxic calming of the increased motor activity characteristic of ADHD. Studies show that medication decreases disruptive activity during school hours, reduces noise and verbal activity, improves attention span and short-term memory, improves ability to follow directions, and decreases distractibility and impulsivity. Although these improvements have been well documented in the literature, the diagnosis of ADHD and subsequent use of psychostimulants with children remains a matter of controversy (see Chapter 28).

Off-Label Use

Psychostimulants have also been used for other psychiatric disorders, and nurses must be aware that these medications are outside of Health Canada–approved indications for the medications. Used alone, stimulants are not indicated for treating depression. However, research has found that these medications may be beneficial as adjunctive medications, especially in those with severe psychomotor retardation (Candy, Jones, Williams, Tookman, King, 2008). All appetite depressants are stimulants, but most are not related to the amphetamines and have a low potential for abuse. However, psychostimulants have been used for treating obesity when other treatments have failed. In addition, these medications have relieved lethargy, boosted mood, and reduced cognitive deficits associated with chronic medically debilitating conditions, such as chronic fatigue syndrome, acquired immunodeficiency syndrome, and some types of cancer, but more research is needed. Increasingly, psychostimulants are being used to improve the residual symptoms of attention deficit disorder in adults, such as inattention, impulsivity, decreased concentration, anxiety, and irritability. This use remains a matter of controversy, and psychostimulants should be used very cautiously in individuals who have a history of substance abuse.

Modafinil (Alertec) is a new wake-promoting agent used for treating excessive daytime sleepiness (EDS) associated with narcolepsy and other health states. Patients with EDS cannot stay awake in the daytime, even after getting enough night-time sleep. They fall asleep when they want to stay awake. Although modafinil is approved by Health Canada only for treating narcolepsy, it is being used for people with EDS and general fatigue found in many diverse disorders, including fibromyalgia and major depression. Its use by long distance truckers and shift workers has created controversy, and more research is needed.

Pharmacokinetics

Psychostimulants are rapidly absorbed from the gastrointestinal tract and reach peak plasma levels in 1 to 3 hours. Considerable individual variations occur between the drugs in terms of bioavailability, plasma levels, and half-life. Table 14-12 compares the primary psychostimulants used in psychiatry. Some of these differences are age dependent because children metabolize these medications more rapidly, producing shorter elimination half-lives. Methylphenidate (Ritalin) is available in a sustained-release form and should not be chewed or crushed.

The psychostimulants appear to be unaffected by food in the stomach and should be given after meals to reduce the appetite-suppressant effects when indicated. However, changes in urine pH may affect the rates of excretion.

Excessive sodium bicarbonate alkalizes the urine and reduces amphetamine secretion. An increased vitamin C or citric acid intake may acidify the urine and increase its excretion. Starvation from appetite suppression may have a similar effect. All these drugs are highly lipid soluble, crossing easily into the CNS and the placenta. Psychostimulants undergo metabolic changes in the liver, where they may affect, or be affected by, other drugs. They are primarily excreted through the kidneys; therefore, renal dysfunction may interfere with excretion.

The precise action of modafinil (Alertec) in promoting wakefulness is unknown. It does appear to have wake-promoting actions similar to sympathomimetic agents such as amphetamine and methylphenidate, although the pharmacologic profile is not identical. It is absorbed rapidly and reaches peak plasma concentration in 2 to 4 hours. The absorption of modafinil may be delayed by 1 to 2 hours if taken with food. Modafinil is eliminated through liver metabolism, with subsequent excretion of metabolites through renal excretion. Modafinil may interact with drugs that inhibit, induce, or are metabolized by CYP2C19 isoenzymes, including phenytoin, diazepam, and propranolol. Concurrent use of modafinil and other drugs metabolized by CYP2C19 may lead to increased circulating blood levels of the other drugs.

Psychostimulants are usually begun at a low dose and increased weekly, depending on improvement of symptoms and occurrence of side effects. Initially, children with ADHD are given a morning dose so that their school performance may be compared from morning to afternoon. Rebound symptoms of excitability and talkativeness may occur when use of the medication is withdrawn or after

Table 14.12 Psychostimulant Medications		
Generic (Trade) Name and Half-Life	**Usual Dosage Drug Range (mg/day)**	**Side Effects**
Dextroamphetamine (Dexedrine); 6–7 hours	5–40	Overstimulation Restlessness Dry mouth Palpitations Cardiomyopathy (with prolonged use or high dosage) Possible growth retardation (greatest risk); risk reduced with drug holidays
Methylphenidate (Ritalin); 2–4 hours	10–60	Nervousness Insomnia Anorexia Tachycardia Impaired cognition (with high doses) Moderate risk for growth suppression
Pemoline (Cylert); 12 hours (mean)	37.5–112.5	Insomnia Anorexia with weight loss Elevated liver function tests (ALT, AST, LDH) Jaundice Least risk for growth suppression

ALT, alanine aminotransferase; AST, aspartate aminotransferase; LDH, lactic dehydrogenase.

dose reduction. These symptoms also begin about 5 hours after the last dose of medication, which may affect the dosing regimen for some individuals. The return of symptoms in the afternoon for children with ADHD may require that a second dose be given at school. Prescribers should work with parents to implement other interventions after school and on weekends when the psychostimulants are not used. Severity of symptoms may require that the medications be continued during these times, but this dosing schedule should be determined after careful evaluation on an individual basis. Use of these medications should not be stopped abruptly, especially with higher doses, because the rebound effects may last for several days.

Side Effects, Adverse Reactions, and Toxicity

Side effects associated with psychostimulants typically arise within 2 to 3 weeks after beginning the medication. From most to least common, these side effects include appetite suppression, insomnia, irritability, weight loss, nausea, headache, palpitations, blurred vision, dry mouth, constipation, and dizziness. Because of the effects on the sympathetic nervous system, some individuals experience blood pressure changes (both hypertension and hypotension), tachycardia, tremors, and irregular heart rates. Blood pressure and pulse should be monitored initially and after each dosage change. Pemoline is associated with elevated liver enzymes and produces hepatotoxicity in 1% to 3% of children taking the medication; therefore, liver function tests should be obtained at least every 6 months. Liver function returns to normal when use of the medication is discontinued.

Rarely, psychostimulants suppress growth and development in children. These effects are a matter of controversy, and research has produced conflicting results. Although the suppression of height seems unlikely to some researchers, others have indicated that psychostimulants may have an effect on cartilage. More reports of suppressed growth have occurred with D-amphetamine (Dexedrine) and methylphenidate (Ritalin) than pemoline (Schertz, Adesman, Alfeiri, & Bienkowski, 1996). Height and weight should be monitored several times annually for children taking these medications and compared with prior history of growth. Weight should be monitored especially closely during the initial phases of treatment. These effects also may be minimized by drug "holidays," such as during school vacations.

Rarely, individuals may experience mild dysphoria, social withdrawal, or mild to moderate depression. These symptoms are more common at higher doses and may require discontinuing the medication. Abnormal movements and motor tics may also increase in individuals who have a history of Tourette's syndrome. Psychostimulants should be avoided by patients with Tourette's symptoms or a positive family history of the disorder. In addition,

dextroamphetamine has been associated with an increased risk for congenital abnormalities. Because there is no compelling reason for a pregnant woman to continue to take these medications, patients should be informed and should advise their prescriber immediately if they plan to become pregnant or if pregnancy is a possibility.

Death is rare from overdose or toxicity of the psychostimulants, but a 10-day supply may be lethal, especially in children. Symptoms of overdose include agitation, chest pain, hallucinations, paranoia, confusion, and dysphoria. Seizures may develop, along with fever, tremor, hypertension or hypotension, aggression, headache, palpitations, rashes, difficulty breathing, leg pain, and abdominal pain. Maximum dosage for children is 40 mg per day, with potential death resulting from a 400-mg dose. Parents should be warned regarding the potential lethality of these medications and take preventive measures by keeping the medication in a safe place.

Side effects associated with modafinil include nausea, nervousness, headache, dizziness, and trouble sleeping. If the effects continue or are bothersome, patients should consult the prescriber. Modafinil is generally well tolerated, with few clinically significant side effects. It is potentially habit forming and must be used with great caution in individuals with a history of substance abuse or dependence.

NEW MEDICATIONS

Each country has its own approval process for new medications. In Canada, this process is controlled by Health Canada. Through various phases of drug testing, a new drug must be determined to have therapeutic benefit based on known physiologic processes, animal testing, and laboratory models of human disease and its potential toxicity predicted at doses likely to produce clinical improvement in humans (see Box 14-5 for more information). Then, the pharmaceutical company can begin research with human volunteers after filing an *investigational new drug* (IND) application. Many new psychiatric medications, particularly the atypical antipsychotics and novel antidepressants, are in various phases of clinical testing and are expected to be released in the coming years. Keeping the phases of new drug development in mind will assist the PMH nurse in understanding what to expect from drugs newly released to the market.

OTHER BIOLOGIC TREATMENTS

Biological treatment is the term applied to treatments that work at a somatic, physical level but are nonpharmacologic in nature. There is a long history of using somatic therapies to treat neuropsychiatric illnesses. Throughout

Phases of New Drug Testing

- *Phase I*: Testing defines the range of dosages tolerated in healthy individuals.
- *Phase II*: Effects of the drug are studied in a limited number of individuals with the target disorder.
- *Phase III*: Extensive clinical trials are conducted at multiple sites throughout the country with larger numbers of patients. Efforts focus on corroborating the efficacy identified in phase II. Phase III concludes with a new drug application (NDA) being submitted to Health Canada.
- *Phase IV*: Postmarketing surveillance continues to detect new or rare adverse reactions and potentially new indications. During this period, adverse reactions from the new medication are required to be reported to Health Canada.

IMPLICATIONS FOR MENTAL HEALTH NURSES
Throughout the phases, side effects and adverse reactions are monitored closely. The studies are tightly controlled, and strict regulations are enforced at each step.

Clinical trials for new drugs usually involve patient populations that have no other health problems but the one under study. This is important to test the drug's effectiveness, but in clinical practice, many patients have other health problems, and postmarketing surveillance helps identify unforeseen benefits or adverse effects in most heterogeneous patient populations.

A newly approved drug is approved only for the indications for which it has been tested. However, there is often a widening of application for other health problems over time (called *off-label* uses).

In Canada, the pharmaceutical companies must follow strict guidelines in terms of product advertising and interaction with health professionals. For example, the companies are not permitted to advertise directly to the public, and there are stringent guidelines regarding any potential sales incentives offered to health professionals. This is to address potential ethical issues around influencing prescriber preferences.

history, numerous treatments have been developed and used to change the biologic basis of what was thought, at the time, to cause psychiatric disorders. Insulin coma, atropine coma, hemodialysis, hyperbaric oxygen therapy, continuous sleep therapy, and ether and carbon dioxide inhalation therapies are examples of some of the treatments that seemed to relieve some symptoms, but results could not be replicated, or potential adverse effects proved too great a risk. Although the primary biologic interventions remain pharmacologic, some somatic treatments continue to show efficacy, whereas others have gained acceptance, remain under investigation, or show promise for the future. Common somatic treatments include the following: ECT; phototherapy; nutritional therapy; and most recently, transcranial magnetic stimulation and vagus nerve stimulation (VNS).

Electroconvulsive Therapy

For hundreds of years, seizures have been known to produce improvement in some psychiatric symptoms. Camphor-induced seizures were used in the 16th century to reduce psychosis and mania. With time, other substances, such as inhalants, were tried, but most were difficult to control or produced adverse reactions, sometimes even fatalities. ECT was formally introduced in Italy in 1938. It is one of the oldest medical treatments available and remains safely in use today. Every year, over one million people in the world receive ECT as treatment (Payne & Prudic, 2009b). It is one of the most effective treatments for severe depression but has been used for other disorders, including mania and schizophrenia, when other treatments have failed. Although individuals with a severe form of depression, where delusions and/or paranoia are present, seem the best candidates for ECT, research has yet to determine accurate predictors of a person's response to ECT (Kellner, 2008). With ECT, a brief electrical current is passed through the brain to produce generalized seizures lasting 25 to 150 seconds. The patient does not feel the stimulus or recall the procedure. A short-acting anaesthetic and a muscle relaxant are given before induction of the current. A brief pulse stimulus, administered unilaterally on the nondominant side of the head, is associated with less confusion after ECT. However, some individuals require bilateral treatment for the effective resolution of depressive symptoms. Induction of a seizure is necessary to produce positive treatment outcomes. Because individual seizure thresholds vary and increase with age, the electrical impulse and treatment method also may vary. In general, the lowest possible electrical stimulus necessary to produce seizure activity is used. Blood pressure and the ECG are monitored during the procedure. This procedure is repeated two or three times a week, usually for a total of 6 to 12 treatments. Because there is no particular difference in treatment efficacy and a twice-weekly regimen produces less accumulative memory loss, this treatment course is often chosen. After symptoms have improved, antidepressant medications are used to prevent relapse. Some patients who cannot take or do not experience response to antidepressant treatment may go on maintenance ECT treatments. Usually, once-weekly treatments are gradually decreased in frequency to once monthly. The number and frequency of treatments vary depending on the individual's response.

Although ECT produces rapid improvement in depressive symptoms, its exact mechanism of antidepressant action remains unclear. It is known to down-regulate β-adrenergic receptors in much the same way as antidepressant medications. However, unlike antidepressant therapy, ECT produces an up-regulation in serotonin, especially 5-HT_2. ECT also has several other actions on neurochemistry, including increased influx of calcium and effects on second messenger systems.

Brief episodes of hypotension or hypertension, bradycardia or tachycardia, and minor arrhythmias are among the adverse effects that may occur during and immediately after the procedure but usually resolve quickly. Common aftereffects from ECT include headache, nausea, and muscle pain. Memory loss or disturbance is the most troublesome effect of ECT. Such cognitive side effects include *transient postictal* ("after seizure") *disorientation* that clears in minutes to hours and *anterograde amnesia* (amnesia for events occurring during and soon after a course of ECT) that varies in severity and for which use of a diary is helpful (Payne & Prudic, 2009a). Other possible cognitive effects are *short-term retrograde amnesia* (gaps in memory about things occurring a few weeks or months before the ECT) that usually clears within weeks, and *retrograde memory loss* (persistent, severe memory deficits) which occurs rarely (Payne & Prudic, 2009a). Many patients experience no amnesia at all. Memory loss occurring as part of the symptoms of untreated depression presents a confounding factor in determining the exact nature of the memory deficits from ECT. It is important to remember that patient surveys are positive, with most individuals reporting that they were helped by ECT and would have it again (Hirose, 2002).

ECT is contraindicated in patients with an increased intracranial pressure. Risk also increases in patients with recent myocardial infarction, recent cerebrovascular accident, retinal detachment, or pheochromocytoma (a tumor on the adrenal cortex) and in patients at high risk for complications from anaesthesia.

· CRNENOTE

Patients may be temporarily confused following ECT. Nurses need to monitor any confusion and reorient patients to the immediate environment as necessary.

Although ECT is a safe and effective treatment, its use carries substantial social stigma, and nurses need to provide education and support, including allowing patients and their families to share their concerns and beliefs. Although the actual procedure is usually completed by a physician and anaesthetist, nurses are involved in many aspects of care. These various roles are listed in Boxes 14-6 and 14-7.

Light Therapy (Phototherapy)

Human circadian rhythms are set by time clues (zeitgebers) inside and outside the body. One of the most powerful regulators of these body patterns is the cycle of daylight and darkness.

Research findings indicate that some individuals with depressive symptoms that worsen at specific times of the year (have a seasonal pattern) may experience disturbance in these normal body patterns or of circadian rhythms

---

BOX 14.6

Interventions for the Patient Receiving ECT

- Discuss treatment alternatives, procedures, risks, and benefits with patient and family. Make sure that informed consent for ECT has been given in writing.
- Provide initial and ongoing patient and family education.
- Assist and monitor the patient who must take nothing by mouth (NPO) after midnight the evening before the procedure.
- Make sure that the patient wears loose, comfortable, nonrestrictive clothing to the procedure.
- If the procedure is performed on an outpatient basis, ensure that the patient has someone to accompany him or her home and stay with him or her after the procedure.
- Ensure that pretreatment laboratory tests are complete, including CBC, serum electrolytes, urinalysis, ECG, chest radiograph, and physical examination.
- Teach the patient to create memory aids, such as lists and notepads, before the ECT.
- Explain that no foreign or loose objects can be in the patient's mouth during the procedure. Dentures will be removed, and a bite block may be inserted.
- When the patient is fully conscious and vital signs are stable, assist him or her to get up slowly, sitting for some time before standing.
- Monitor confusion closely; the patient may need reorientation to the bathroom and other areas.
- For outpatients, advise family members to observe how the patient manages at home, provide assistance as needed, and report any problems.
- Assist the patient to keep or schedule follow-up appointments.

(Steinhausen, Gundelfinge, & WinklerMetzke, 2008). For example, some individuals are more depressed during the winter months, when there is less light, and they improve spontaneously in the spring. (Refer to Chapter 20 for a complete description of depression and mood disorders.) These individuals usually have symptoms that are somewhat different from classic depression, including fatigue, increased need to sleep, increased appetite and weight gain, irritability, and carbohydrate craving. Administering artificial light to these patients during winter months has reduced these depressive symptoms.

Light therapy, sometimes called **phototherapy**, involves exposing the patient to an artificial light source to relieve seasonal depression. Artificial light is believed to trigger a shift in the patient's circadian rhythm to an earlier time. Research remains ongoing. The light source must be very bright, full-spectrum light, usually 2,500 lux, which is about 200 times brighter than normal indoor lighting. Harmful ultraviolet light is filtered out. Exposure to this light source has produced improvement and relief of depressive symptoms for significant numbers of seasonally depressed individuals. It produces no change for individuals who are not seasonally depressed.

BOX 14.7

Research for Best Practice: PMH Nurses and ECT

Gass, J. (2008). *Electroconvulsive therapy and the work of mental health nurses: A grounded theory study.* International Journal of Nursing Studies, 45, 191–202.

THE QUESTION: How do PMH nurses work with patients having ECT?

METHOD: With Grounded Theory as the method used, PMH nurses (20) and students (4) in mental health settings in the Scottish Health Board participated in unstructured interviews about their work and role with patients having ECT. Nonparticipant observation was also part of data collection.

FINDINGS: Two types of roles were identified: relational roles (information-giver, persuader, supporter, and sustaining the relationship) and treatment roles (support to medical staff and "forcing" involuntary patients to have ECT). A core category was "being there," conceived along a continuum of "engaged, present, and detached." Two dilemmas of nurses emerged: difficulty assuming a treatment role when an ECT nurse was present and role dissonance when "forcing" a patient to undergo ECT.

IMPLICATIONS FOR PRACTICE: Nurses who are at the "engaged" level of "being there" may slip to the level of "being present" when in a situation of forcing a patient to have ECT. While this may enable the nurse to fulfill her treatment role, it can create a personal dilemma. The "detached" nurse avoids this dilemma, but is not providing patient-centred care, a core element of PMH nursing. Being detached in one's relationship with a person undergoing ECT may be a sign of burnout and is a cause for concern.

Studies have shown that morning phototherapy produces a better response than either evening or morning and evening timing of the phototherapy session (Prasko, 2008). Light banks with full-spectrum light may be put together by the individual or obtained from various companies now producing these light sources. Light visors, visors containing small, full-spectrum light bulbs that shine on the eyelids, have also been developed. The patient is instructed to sit in front of the lights at a distance of about 3 feet, engaging in a variety of other activities, but glancing directly into the light every few minutes. This should be done immediately on arising and is most effective before 8 AM. The duration of administration may begin with as little as 30 minutes and increase to 2 to 5 hours. One to two hours is usually sufficient, and the antidepressant response begins in 1 to 4 days, with the full effect usually complete after 2 weeks. Full antidepressant effect is usually maintained with daily sessions of 30 minutes.

Side effects of phototherapy are rare, but eye strain, headache, and insomnia are possible. An ophthalmologist should be consulted if the patient has a preexisting eye disorder. In rare instances, phototherapy has been reported to produce mania. Irritability is a more common complaint. Follow-up visits with the prescriber or therapist are needed to help manage side effects and assess positive results. Phototherapy should be implemented only by a provider knowledgeable in its use.

Nutritional Therapies

The neurotransmitters necessary for normal healthy functioning are produced from amino acids taken in with the foods we eat. Many nutritional deficiencies may produce symptoms of psychiatric disorders. Fatigue, apathy, and depression are caused by deficiencies in iron, folic acid, pantothenic acid, magnesium, vitamin C, or biotin. Logically, treating these deficiencies with nutritional supplements should improve the psychiatric symptoms. The question becomes, Can nutritional supplements actually treat psychiatric disorders?

In 1967, Linus Pauling espoused the theory that ascorbic acid deficiency produced many psychiatric disorders. He implemented a treatment for schizophrenia that included large doses of ascorbic acid and other vitamins. This treatment was referred to as *megavitamin therapy* or *orthomolecular therapy*. Many psychiatrists showed interest in Pauling's proposal, but his research and claims could never be substantiated, and most researchers and clinicians became highly sceptical of this hypothesis. Nonetheless, a small group remains committed to orthomolecular approaches.

Older theories and related diets are based on the belief that food controls behaviour. High sugar intake was once thought to produce hyperactivity in children, and Benjamin Feingold developed a diet to eliminate food additives that he believed increased hyperactivity. More recently, advances in technology have led research to new investigations regarding dietary precursors for the bioamines. For example, tryptophan, the dietary precursor of serotonin, has been most extensively investigated as it relates to low serotonin levels and increased aggression. Individuals who have low tryptophan levels are prone to have lower levels of serotonin in the brain, resulting in depressed mood and aggressive behaviour (Young & Leyton, 2002). Some individuals with mild depression do respond to large amounts of tryptophan, and tryptophan has been used as an adjunct to antidepressant drugs. Many individuals are turning to dietary herbal preparations to address psychiatric symptoms. More than 17% of the adult population has used herbal preparations to address their mood or emotions. From St. John's wort for depression, to ginkgo for cognitive impairment, to kava for anxiety, herbal preparations are increasingly being used (McCabe, 2002). Nurses need to include an assessment of these agents into their overall patient assessment to understand the needs of the patient.

Medications may also influence the development of nutritional deficiencies that may worsen psychiatric symptoms. For example, drugs with strong anticholinergic activity often produce impaired or enhanced gastric motility, which may lead to the generalized malabsorption of vitamins and minerals. In addition, many nutritional supplements have toxicities of their own when given in excess. For example, daily ingestion of more than 100 mg pyridoxine (vitamin B_6) can produce neurotoxic symptoms, photosensitivity, and ataxia. More research is needed to identify the underlying mechanisms and relationships of dietary supplements and dietary precursors of the bioamines to mood and behaviour and psychopharmacologic medications. For now, it is important for the PMH nurse to recognize that diet can have a significant impact on behaviour in sensitive individuals and that supplements can be a potential source of drug–drug interaction.

New Somatic Therapies

Repetitive transcranial magnetic stimulation (rTMS) and VNS are two emerging somatic treatments for psychiatric disorders. Both are ways to directly affect brain activity by stimulating nerve cell firing rates. Transcranial magnetic stimulation was introduced in 1985 as a noninvasive, painless method to stimulate the cerebral cortex. Undergirding this procedure is the hypothesis that a time-varying magnetic field will induce an electrical field, which, in brain tissue, activates the inhibitory and excitatory neurons (Kanno, Matsumoto, Togashi, Yoshioka, & Mano, 2003), thereby modulating neuroplasticity in the brain. The low-frequency electrical stimulation from rTMS triggers lasting anticonvulsant effects in rats, and the therapeutic benefits of rTMS in humans are thought to be related to action similar to that produced by anticonvulsant medication. rTMS has been used for both clinical and research purposes. rTMS stimulation of the brain's prefrontal cortex may help some depressed patients in much the same way as ECT but without its side effects (Martin et al., 2003). Thus, it has been proposed as an alternative to ECT in managing symptoms of depression. rTMS treatment is administered daily for at least a week, much like ECT, except that subjects remain awake. Although proven effective for depression, rTMS does have some side effects, including mild headaches.

VNS is the newest of the currently available somatic treatments (Martin et al., 2003). For years, scientists have been interested in identifying how autonomic functions modulate activity in the limbic system and higher cortex. The vagus nerve has traditionally been considered a parasympathetic efferent nerve that was responsible only for regulating autonomic functions, such as heart rate and gastric tone. However, the vagus nerve (cranial X) also carries sensory information to the brain from the head, neck, thorax, and abdomen, and research has identified that the vagus nerve has extensive projections of its sensory afferent connections to many brain areas (Armitage, Husain, Hoffmann, & Rush, 2003). Although the basic mechanism of action of VNS is unknown, incoming sensory, or afferent, connections of the left vagus nerve directly project into many of the very same brain regions implicated in neuropsychiatric disorders. These connections help us to understand how VNS is helpful in treating psychiatric disorders. VNS changes levels of several neurotransmitters implicated in the development of major depression, including serotonin, norepinephrine, GABA, and glutamate (Forbes, Macdonald, Eljamel, & Roberts, 2003).

■◖ PSYCHOSOCIAL ISSUES IN BIOLOGIC TREATMENTS

Many factors influence successful medication and other biologic therapies. Of particular importance are issues related to adherence. Adherence refers to following the therapeutic regimen, self-administering medications as prescribed, keeping appointments, and following other treatment suggestions. Adherence exists on a continuum and can be conceived of as full, partial, or nil. Partial adherence, whereby a patient either attempts to take medications but misses doses or takes more than prescribed, is by far the most common. Recent estimates indicate that on the average, 50% or more of the individuals with schizophrenia taking antipsychotic medications stop taking the medications or do not take them as prescribed (Weiden, 2007). It should be remembered that problems with adherence are an issue with many chronic health states, including diabetes and arthritis, not just psychiatric disorders. Box 14-8 lists some of the common reasons for nonadherence.

The most often cited reasons for nonadherence are related to side effects of the medication. Improved functioning may be observed by health care professionals but not felt by the patient. Side effects may interfere with

---

BOX 14.8

Common Reasons for Nonadherence with Medication Regimens

- Uncomfortable side effects and those that interfere with quality of life, such as work performance or intimate relationships
- Lack of awareness of or denial of illness
- Stigma
- Feeling better
- Confusion about dosage or timing
- Difficulties in access to treatment and cost of newer drug therapies
- Substance abuse

work performance or other important aspects of the individual's life. For example, a construction worker cannot afford to be drowsy and sedated while operating a crane at a construction site, or a woman in an intimate relationship may find anorgasmia intolerable. Nurses need to be sensitive to the patient's ability to tolerate side effects and to the impact that side effects have on the patient's life. Medication choice, dosing schedules, and prompt treatment of side effects may be crucial factors in helping patients to continue their treatment, even if the symptoms for which they initially sought help have improved.

Cognitive deficits associated with some psychiatric disorders may make it difficult for the individual to self-monitor, develop insight, make choices, remember to fill prescriptions, or keep appointments. Family members may have beliefs and attitudes that influence the individual not to take the medication. They may misunderstand or deny the illness; for example, "My wife's better, so she doesn't need that medicine anymore." Family members may be distressed when observable side effects occur. Akinesia, which has been linked to suicidal thoughts as a way to relieve the subjective discomfort, may be the most distressing side effect for family members of individuals who have schizophrenia (Meltzer, 2000; Niedermeyer, 2008). Patients may also be reluctant to disclose financial constraints, especially in relation to the cost of newer agents, and may try to stretch out the prescription or just not fill their prescription. Adherence concerns must not be dismissed as the patient's or family's problem. PMH nurses should actively address this issue. A positive therapeutic relationship between the nurse and the patient and family must provide a strong sense of trust that side effects and other difficulties in treatment will be addressed and minimized. When individuals report distressing side effects, the nurse should immediately respond with assessment and interventions to reduce these effects. It is important to assess adherence often, asking questions in a nonthreatening, nonjudgmental manner. It also may be helpful to seek information from others who are involved with the patient.

Adherence can be improved by psychoeducation. This approach is most helpful if it addresses the individual's specific symptoms and concerns. For example, if the patient is having difficulty with understanding the purpose of the medication, it may be helpful to link taking it to a reduction of specific unwanted symptoms or improved functioning, such as continuing to work. Family members should also be included in these discussions.

Other factors that interfere with adherence should also be assessed and plans developed to minimize their effect. For example, an individual who is being considered for clozapine therapy may have missed a number of appointments in the past. On assessment, the nurse may discover that it takes the individual 2 hours on three different busses each way to reach the clinic. The nurse can then assist with arranging for a home health nurse to visit the patient's apartment, draw blood samples for analysis, and assess side effects, thus decreasing the number of trips the patient must make to the clinic.

SUMMARY OF KEY POINTS

☐ Psychopharmacology is the study of medications used to treat psychiatric disorders, including the drug categories of antipsychotics, mood stabilizers, antidepressants, antianxiety medications, and psychostimulants.

☐ Pharmacodynamics refers to the actions of drugs on living tissue and the human body, with the focus primarily on drug actions at receptor sites and transporters and on ion channel sites and enzyme activity.

☐ The importance of receptors is recognized in current psychopharmacology. Biologic action of many drugs depends on how their structure interacts with a specific receptor, functioning either as an agonist, reproducing the same biologic action as a neurotransmitter, or as an antagonist, blocking the response.

☐ A drug's ability to interact with a given receptor type may be judged on three qualities: selectivity—the ability to interact with specific types of receptors; affinity—the attraction the drug has for the binding site; and intrinsic activity—the ability to produce a certain biologic response.

☐ Many characteristics of specific drugs affect how well they act and how they affect patients. PMH nurses must be familiar with characteristics, adverse reactions, and toxicity of certain drugs to administer psychotropic medications safely, educate patients regarding their safe use, and encourage therapeutic adherence.

☐ Pharmacokinetics refers to how drugs move within the human body to get to their target tissues and how drugs are removed from the body. Bioavailability describes the amount of the drug that actually reaches the systemic circulation. The wide variations in pharmacokinetic properties across individuals are related to physiologic differences caused by age, genetic makeup, other disease processes, and chemical interactions.

☐ Antipsychotic medications are drugs used in treating psychotic disorders, such as schizophrenia. They act primarily by blocking dopamine or serotonin postsynaptically. In addition, they have a number of actions on other neurotransmitters. Older typical antipsychotic drugs work on positive symptoms and are inexpensive, but they produce many side effects. Newer atypical antipsychotic drugs work on positive and negative symptoms; are much more expensive, but have far fewer anticholinergic side effects; and are better tolerated by patients, but increase risk for metabolic disorders.

▫ Medication-related movement disorders are a particularly serious group of side effects that principally occur with the typical antipsychotic medications and that may be acute syndromes, such as dystonia, pseudoparkinsonism, and akathisia, or chronic syndromes, such as tardive dyskinesia.

▫ The mood stabilizers, or antimania medications, are drugs used to control wide variations in mood related to mania, but these agents may also be used to treat other disorders. Lithium and the anticonvulsants are chemically unrelated and act in different ways to stabilize mood.

▫ Antidepressant medications are drugs used primarily for treating symptoms of depression, but are also used extensively for anxiety disorders and eating disorders. They act by blocking the reuptake of one or more of the bioamines, especially serotonin and norepinephrine. These medications vary considerably in their structure and action. Newer antidepressants, such as the SSRIs, have fewer side effects and are less lethal in overdose than the older TCAs.

▫ Antianxiety medications also include several subgroups of medications, but benzodiazepines and nonbenzodiazepines are those principally used in psychiatry. Benzodiazepines act by enhancing the actions of GABA, whereas the nonbenzodiazepine buspirone acts on serotonin. Benzodiazepines can be used on a PRN basis, whereas buspirone must be taken regularly.

▫ Psychostimulants enhance neurotransmitter activity, acting at a number of different receptor sites. These medications are most often used for treating symptoms related to ADHD and narcolepsy.

▫ ECT uses the application of an electrical pulsation to induce seizures in the brain. These seizures produce a number of effects on neurotransmission that result in the fairly rapid relief of depressive symptoms.

▫ rTMS and VNS are two emerging somatic treatments for psychiatric disorders. They are both means to directly affect brain function through the stimulation of the nerves that are direct extensions of the brain.

▫ Phototherapy involves the application of full-spectrum light in the morning hours, which appears to reset circadian rhythm delays related to seasonal affective disorder and other forms of depression. Nutritional therapies are in various stages of investigation.

▫ Adherence refers to the ability of an individual to self-administer medications as prescribed and to follow other instructions related to medication treatment. It can be either full, partial, or nil. Nonadherence is related to factors such as medication side effects, cost, stigma, and family influences. Nurses play a key role in educating patients and helping them to improve adherence.

CRITICAL THINKING CHALLENGES

1 Discuss why it is essential that nurses have knowledge of the following concepts: neurotransmitter, receptor, agonist, and antagonist.

2 Discuss how the concepts of affinity with selectivity and intrinsic activity have meaning for nurses.

3 Discuss the usefulness of the concept of bioavailability for nurses. What does it mean to nurses, and how would nursing actions change if it were considered?

4 Delineate the ethical issues of nursing management activities associated with each phase of drug treatment: initiation, stabilization, maintenance, and discontinuation.

5 Discuss how you would go about identifying the target symptoms for a specific patient for the following medications: antipsychotic, antidepressant, and antianxiety drugs.

6 Discuss the ways in which you might explain to a patient the differences between typical and atypical antipsychotic medications.

7 Explain the health problems associated with anticholinergic side effects of the antipsychotic medications.

8 Compare the type of movements that characterize tardive dyskinesia with those that characterize akathisia and dystonia, and explore which one is easier for a patient to experience.

9 Explain how your nursing care would be different for a male patient taking lithium carbonate than for a female patient.

10 Discuss contrasting views why the antidepressant class of medications has become so commonly prescribed.

11 Discuss the efficacy of anticonvulsive therapy and its mechanism of action.

12 Compare different approaches that you might use with a patient with schizophrenia who has decided to stop taking his or her typical antipsychotic medication because of intolerance to side effects.

REFERENCES

Alda, M. (2004). The phenotype spectra of bipolar disorder. *European Neuropsycopharmacology, 14*(Suppl. 1), S94–S99.

Armitage, R., Husain, M., Hoffmann, R., & Rush, A. J. (2003). The effects of vagus nerve stimulation on sleep EEG in depression: A preliminary report. *Journal of Psychosomatic Research, 54*(5), 475–482.

Armstrong, S. C., Cozza, K. L., & Oesterheld, J. R. (2002). Med-psych drug-drug interactions update. *Psychosomatics, 43*(1), 77–81.

Baker, G. B., Urichuk, L. J., & Coutts, R. T. (1998). Drug metabolism and metabolic drug-drug interactions in psychiatry. *Child and Adolescent Pharmacology News Suppl, 1*, 1–8.

Bilici, M., Tekelioglu, Y., Efendioglu, S., Ovali, E., & Ulgen, M. (2003). The influence of olanzapine on immune cells in patients with schizophrenia. *Progress in Neuropsychopharmacology and Biological Psychiatry, 27*(3), 483–485.

Bond, D. J., Pratoomsri, W., & Yatham, L. N. (2007) Depot antipsychotic medications in bipolar disorder: A review of the literature. *Acta Psychiatrica Scandinavia Suppl, 434*, 3–16.

Bschor, T., Baethge, C., Adli, M., Lewitzka, U., Eichmann, U., & Bauer, M. (2003). Hypothalamic-pituitary-thyroid system activity during lithium augmentation therapy in patients with unipolar major depression. *Journal of Psychiatry Neuroscience*, 28(3), 210–216.

Candy, M., Jones, L., Williams, R., Tookman, A., & King, M. (2008). Psychostimulants for depression. *Cochrane Database for Systematic Reviews*, 16(2), CD006722.

Chouinard, G., & Chouinard, V. A. (2008). Atypical antipsychotics: CATIE study, drug-induced movements disorder and resulting iatrogenic psychiatric-like symptoms, supersentivitiy rebound psychosis and withdrawal syndromes. *Psychotherapies and Psychosomatics*, 77(2), 69–77.

Cumbler, E., Guerrasio, J., Kim. J., & Glasheen, J. (2008). Use of medications for insomnia in the hospitalized geriatric population. *Journal of the American Geriatric Society*, 56(3), 579–581.

Dahl, M. L. (2002). Cytochrome p450 phenotyping/genotyping in patients receiving antipsychotics: Useful aid to prescribing. *Clinical Pharmacokinetics*, 41(7), 453–470.

Dalfen, A. K., & Stewart, D. E. (2001). Who develops severe or fatal adverse drug reactions to selective serotonin reuptake inhibitors? *Canadian Journal of Psychiatry*, 46(3), 258–263.

Ditto, K. E. (2003). SSRI discontinuation syndrome: Awareness as an approach to prevention. *Postgraduate Medicine*, 114, 79–84.

Dolder, C. R., & Nelson, M. H. (2008). Hypnosedative-induced complex behaviors: Incidence, mechanisms and management. *CNS Drugs*, 22(12), 1021–1036.

Ferry, L., & Johnston, J. A. (2003). Efficacy and safety of bupropion SR for smoking cessation: Data from clinical trials and five years of postmarketing experience. *International Journal of Clinical Practice*, 57(3), 224–230.

Forbes, R. B., Macdonald, S., Eljamel, S., & Roberts, R. C. (2003). Cost-utility analysis of vagus nerve stimulators for adults with medically refractory epilepsy. *Seizure*, 12(5), 249–256.

Gardener, D. M., Shulman, K. I., Walker, S. E., & Tailor, S. A. N. (1996). The making of a user-friendly MAOI diet. *Journal of Clinical Psychiatry*, 57, 99–104.

Gass, J. (2008). Electroconvulsive therapy and the work of mental health nurses: A grounded theory study. *International Journal of Nursing Studies*, 45, 191–202.

Goodwin, F. K., & Ghaemi, S. N. (2000). The impact of mood stabilizers on suicide in bipolar disorder: A comparative analysis. *CNS Spectrums*, 5(2), 12–19.

Granger, B. (1999). The discovery of haloperidol. *Encephale*, 25(1), 59–66.

Grootens, K. P., & Verkes, R. J. (2005). Emerging evidence for the use of atypical antipsychotics in borderline personality disorder. *Pharmacopsychiatry*, 38(1), 20–23.

Grunze, H., & Walden, J. (2002). Relevance of new and newly rediscovered anticonvulsants for atypical forms of bipolar disorder. *Journal of Affective Disorders*, 72(Suppl. 1), S15–S21.

Hegadoren, K. M. (2004). Assessment and treatment of depression: A review in high risk populations. *Journal of Wound, Ostomy and Continence Nursing*, 31, 100–112.

Henderson, D. C. (2008). Managing weight gain and metabolic issues in patients treated with atypical antipsychotics. *Journal of Clinical Psychiatry*, 69(2), e04.

Hirose, S. (2002). ECT for depression with amnesia. *Journal of ECT*, 18(1), 60.

Hogan, D., Ebly, E., & Fung, T. (1995). Regional variations in use of potentially inappropriate medications by Canadian seniors participating in the Canadian Study of Health and Aging. *Canadian Journal of Clinical Pharmacology*, 2(4), 167–174.

Holsboer, F., & Ising, M. (2008). Central CRH system in depression and anxiety: Evidence from clinical studies with CRH(1) receptor antagonists. *European Journal of Pharmacology*, 583(2), 350–357.

Iqbal, M. M., Rahman, A., Husain, Z., Mahmud, S. Z., Ryan, W. G. & Feldman, J. M. (2003). Clozapine: A clinical review of adverse effects and management. *Annals of Clinical Psychiatry*, 15(1), 33–46.

Izzo, A. A. (2004). Drug interactions with St. John's Wort (Hypericum perforatum): A review of the clinical evidence. *International Journal of Pharmacology and Therapeutics*, 42(3), 139–148.

Kalapos, M. P. (2002). Carbamazepine-provoked hapatotoxicity and possible aetiological role of glutathione in the events. *Adverse Drug Reactions and Toxicology Reviews*, 21(3), 123–141.

Kanno, M., Matsumoto, M., Togashi, H., Yoshioka, M., & Mano, Y. (2003). Effects of repetitive transcranial magnetic stimulation on behavioural and neurochemical changes in rats during an elevated plus-maze test. *Journal of the Neurological Sciences*, 211(1–2), 5–14.

Kearns, G. L. (2000). Impact of developmental pharmacology on pediatric study design: Overcoming the challenges. *Journal of Allergy and Clinical Immunology*, 106(3), 128–138.

Kearns, G. L., & Winter, H. S. (2004). Proton pump inhibitors in pediatrics: Relevant pharmacokinetics and pharmacodynamics. *Journal of Pediatric Gastroenterology and Nutrition*, 37(Suppl. 1), S52–S59.

Kellner, C. H. (2008). ECT response prediction: From good to great. *Psychiatric Times*, 25(6), 21.

Kennedy, S. H., Lam, R. W., Cohen, N. L., Ravindran, A. V., & the CANMAT Depression Work Group. (2001). Clinical guidelines for the treatment of depressive disorders. IV. Medications and other biological treatments. *Canadian Journal of Psychiatry*, 46(S1), 38S–58S.

Kennedy, S. H., Segal, Z. V., Cohen, N. L., Levitan, R. D., Gemar, M., & Bagby, R. M. (2003). Lithium carbonate versus cognitive therapy as sequential combination treatment strategies in partial responders to antidepressant medication: An exploratory trial. *Journal of Clinical Psychiatry*, 64(4), 439–444.

Kirbach, S., Simpson, K., Nietert, P. J., & Mintzer, J. (2008). A markov model of the cost effectiveness of olanzapine treatment for agitation and psychosis in Alzheimer's disease. *Clinical Drug Investigation*, 28(5), 291–303.

Krystal, J. H., Sancora, G., Blumberg, H., Anand, A., Charney, D. S., Marek, G., et al. (2002). Glutamate and GABA systems as targets for novel antidepressant and mood-stabilizing treatments. *Molecular Psychiatry*, 7(Suppl. 1), S71–S80.

Klotz, U. (2007). The role of pharmacogenetics in the metabolism of antiepileptic drugs: Pharmacokinetic and therapeutic implications. *Clinical Pharmacokinetics*, 46(4), 271–279.

Kulkarni, S. K., & Naidu, P. S. (2003). Pathophysiology and drug therapy of tardive dyskinesia: Current concepts and future perspectives. *Drugs Today (Barc)*, 39(1), 19–49.

Lazarou, J., Pomeranz, B. H., & Corey, P. N. (1998). Incidence of adverse drug reactions in hospitalized patients: a meta-analysis of prospective studies. *Journal of the American Medical Association*, 279(15), 1200–1205.

Leeder, J. S., & Kearns, G. L. (1997). Pharmacogenetics in pediatrics. *Pediatric Clinics of North America*, 44(1), 55–77.

Levy, G., Schupf, N., Tang, M. X., Cote, L. J., Louis, E. D., Mejia, H., et al. (2002). Combined effect of age and severity on the risk of dementia in Parkinson's disease. *Annals of Neurology*, 51(6), 722–729.

Loscher, W. (2002). Basic pharmacology of valproate: A review after 35 years of clinical use for the treatment of epilepsy. *CNS Drugs*, 16(10), 669–694.

Machado-Vieira, R., Salvadore, G., Luckenbaugh, D. A., Manji, H. K., & Zarate, C. A. (2008). Rapid onset of antidepressant action: A new paradigm in the research and treatment of major depressive disorder. *Journal of Clinical Psychiatry*, 22, e1–e13.

Marshall, J. D., & Kearns, G. L. (1999). Developmental pharmacodynamics of cyclosporine. *Clinical Pharmacology and Therapeutics*, 66, 66–75.

Martin, J. L., Barbanoj, M. J., Schlaepfer, T. E., Thompson, E., Perez, V., & Kulisevsky, J. (2003). Repetitive transcranial magnetic stimulation for the treatment of depression: Systematic review and meta-analysis. *British Journal of Psychiatry*, 182, 480–491.

McCabe, S. (2002). Complementary herbal and alternative drugs in clinical practice. *Perspectives in Psychiatric Care*, 38(3), 98–107.

Meltzer, H. Y. (2000). Introduction. Side effects of antipsychotic medications: Physician's choice of medication and patient compliance. *Journal of Clinical Psychiatry*, 61(Suppl. 8), 3–4.

Melvin, C. L., Carey, T. S., Goodman, F., Oldham, J. M., & Ranney, L. M. (2008). Effectiveness of antiepileptic drugs for the treatment of bipolar disorder: Findings from a systematic review. *Journal of Psychiatric Practice*, 14(Suppl. 1), 9–14.

Meyer, J. M. (2007). Antipsychotic safety and efficacy concerns. *Journal of Clinical Psychiatry*, 68(Suppl. 14), 20–26.

Miller, C. H., & Fleischhacker, W. W. (2000). Managing antipsychotic-induced acute and chronic akathisia. *Drug Safety*, 22, 73–81.

Moisan, J., Gregoire, J., Gaudet, M., & Cooper, D. (2005). Exploring the risk of diabetes mellitus and dyslipidemia among ambulatory users of atypical antipsychotics: A population-based comparison of risperidone and olanzapine. *Pharmacoepidemiology and Drug Safety*, 14, 427–436.

Nasrallah, H. A. (2002). Pharmacoeconomic implications of adverse effects during antipsychotic drug therapy. *American Journal of Health-System Pharmacy*, 59(22 Suppl. 8), S16–S21.

Niedermeyer, E. (2008). Akinesia and the frontal lobe. *Clinical EEG and Neuroscience, 39*(1), 39–42.

Pacheco, M. A., & Jope, R. S. (1996). Phosphoinositide signaling in human brain. *Progress in Neurobiology, 50*(2–3), 255–273.

Pandolfi, A., Grilli, A., Cilli, C., Patruno, A., Giaccari, A., DiSilvestre, S., et al. (2003). Phenotype modulation in cultures of vascular and smooth muscle cells from diabetic rats: Association with increased nitric oxide synthase expression and superoxide anion generation. *Journal of Cellular Physiology, 196*(2), 378–385.

Patten, S. B., & Beck, C. A. (2004). Major depression and mental health care utilization in Canada. *Canadian Journal of Psychiatry, 49*(5), 303–309.

Payne, N., & Prudic, J. (2009a). Electroconvulsive therapy Part 1. A perspective on the evolution and current practice of ECT. *Journal of Psychiatric Practice, 15*(5), 346–368.

Payne, N., & Prudic, J. (2009b). Electroconvulsive therapy Part II. A biopsychosocial perspective. *Journal of Psychiatric Practice, 15*(5), 369–390.

Philip, N. S., Mello, K., Carpenter, L. L., Tyrka, A. R., & Price, L. H. (2008). Patterns of quetiapine use in psychiatric inpatients: An examination of off-label use. *Annals of Clinical Psychiatry, 20*(1), 15–20.

Pierre, J. M. (2005). Extrapyrimidal symptoms with atypical antipsychotics: Incidence, prevention and management. *Drug Safety, 28*(3), 191–208.

Prasko, J. (2008). Bright light therapy. *Neurology and Endocrinology Letters, 23*:29(Suppl. 1) [Epub ahead of print].

Preston, S. T., & Hegadoren, K. (2004). Glass contamination in parenterally administered medication. *Journal of Advanced Nursing, 48*(3), 266–270.

Riederer, P., Lachenmayer, L., & Laux, G. (2004). Clinical applications of MAO-inhibitors. *Current Medicinal Chemistry, 11*, 2033–2043.

Riker, R. R., & Fraser, G. L. (2005). Adverse events associated with sedatives, analgesics, and other drugs that provide patient comfort in the intensive care unit. *Pharmacotherapy, 25*(5 Pt 2), 8S–18S.

Rust, G., Daniels, E., Sacher, D., Bacon, J., Storhters, H., & Bornemann, T. (2005). Ability of community health centers to obtain health services for uninsured patients. *Journal of the American Medical Association, 293*(5), 554–556.

Schertz, M., Adesman, A. R., Alfieri, N. E. & Bienkowski, R. S. (1996). Predictors of weight loss in children with attention deficit hyperactivity disorder treated with stimulant medication. *Pediatrics, 98*(4), 763–769.

Schou, M. (1978). Lithium treatment. *Western Journal of Medicine, 128*(6), 535–536.

Sibon, I., Fenelon, G., Quinn, N. P., & Tison, F. (2004). Vascular parkinsonism. *Journal of Neurology, 252*(12), 513–524.

Simpson, G. M., & Angus, J. W. S. (1970). A rating scale for extrapyramidal side effects. *Acta Psychiatrica Scandinavica, 212* (Suppl.), 11–19.

Soldin, O. P., & Soldin, S. J. (2002). Review: Therapeutic drug monitoring in pediatrics. *Therapeutic Drug Monitoring, 24*, 1–8.

Solomon, D. A., Keitner, G. I., Ryan, C. E., Miller, I. W., Shea, M. T., Kazim, A., et al. (2000). Lithium plus valproate as maintenance polypharmacy for patients with bipolar I disorder: A review. *CNS Spectrums, 5*(2), 19–28.

Spina, E., & Scordo, M. G. (2002). Clinically significant drug interactions with antidepressants in the elderly. *Drugs Aging, 19*(4), 299–320.

Steinhausen, H. C., Gundelfinger, R., & WinklerMetz, C. (2008). Prevalence of self-reported affective and the validity of the seasonal pattern assessment questionnaire in young adults. *Journal of Affective Disorders, Oct 21* [Epub ahead of print].

Tariot, P. N., Salzman, C., Yeung, P. P., Pultz, J., & Rak, I. W. (2000). Long-term use of quetiapine in elderly patients with psychotic disorders. *Clinical Therapeutics, 22*(9), 1068–1084.

Taylor, D. (2003). Ziprasidone in the management of schizophrenia: The QT interval issue in context. *CNS Drugs, 17*(6), 423–430.

Thase, M. (2002). Studying new antidepressants: If there were a light at the end of the tunnel, could we see it? *Journal of Clinical Psychiatry, 63*(Suppl. 2), 24–28.

Turkoski, B. (1999). Meeting the challenge of medications reactions in the elderly. *Orthropaedic Nursing, 7*, 85–95.

Vesell, E. S. (1977). Genetic and environmental factors affecting drug disposition in man. *Clinical Pharmacology and Therapeutics, 22*, 659–665.

Viguera, A. C., Baldessarini, R. J., & Friedberg, J. (1988). Discontinuing antidepressant treatment in major depression. *Harvard Reviews in Psychiatry, 5*, 293–306.

Weiden, P. J. (2007). Understanding and addressing adherence issues in schizophrenia: From theory to practice. *Journal of Clinical Psychiatry, 68*(Suppl. 14), 14–19.

Yatham, L. N., Kennedy, S. H., O'Donovan, C., Parikh, S. V., MacQueen, G., McIntyre, R. S., et al. (2006). Canadian Network for Mood and Anxiety Treatments (CANMAT) guidelines for the management of patients with bipolar disorder: Update 2007. *Bipolar Disorders, 8*(6), 721–739.

Young, S. N., & Leyton, M. (2002). The role of serotonin in human mood and social interaction: Insight from altered tryptophan levels. *Pharmacology, Biochemistry and Behavior, 71*, 857–865.

Zhou, H. (2003). Pharmacokinetic strategies in deciphering atypical drug absorption profiles. *Journal of Clinical Pharmacology, 43*(3), 211–227.

Zintzaras, E. (2005). Statistical aspects of bioequivalence testing between two medicinal products. *European Journal of Drug Metabolism and Pharmacokinetics, 30*(1–2), 41–46.

Zullino, D., Delacrausaz, P., & Baumann, P. (2002). The place of SSRIs in the treatment of schizophrenia. *Encephale, 28*(5 Pt 1), 433–438.

Cognitive-Behavioural Therapy

Wendy Austin

Adapted from the chapter "Cognitive-Behavioural Therapy" by Tracey Tulley and Ruth Gallop

After studying this chapter, you will be able to:

- Describe the cognitive model.
- Discuss the levels of cognition, including core beliefs, intermediate beliefs, automatic thoughts, and their interrelationship.
- Identify and describe the ten principles of cognitive-behavioural therapy.
- Discuss cognitive treatment techniques.
- Discuss behavioural treatment techniques.

KEY CONCEPTS

- cognitive-behavioural therapy
- cognitive restructuring

KEY TERMS

• automatic thoughts • cognitive schema • core beliefs • intermediate beliefs

One of the more exciting and significant achievements in modern psychotherapy is the advancement of cognitive-behavioural therapy (CBT). CBT is a form of psychotherapy that emphasizes the centrality of thought or cognition in the development of core beliefs about self and the world. The aim of CBT is to identify, analyze, and ultimately change the habitually inflexible and negative cognitions about oneself, others, and the world at large that contribute to distressing emotional states and problematic behaviours (Ingram, Miranda, & Segal, 1998). Through modifying thinking, emotion and behaviour also change. CBT is the most widely researched form of psychotherapy and, given the robust findings from numerous controlled clinical trials, is recognized by many as the treatment of choice for many mental disorders, including posttraumatic stress disorder, bulimia nervosa, panic disorder, and depression. It is being studied for its efficacy in treating social anxiety disorder (Hofmann, 2007), work-related stress (Ruwaard, Lange, Bouwman, Broeksteeg, & Schrieken, 2007), late-life anxiety disorders (Hendriks, Oude Voshaar, Keijsers, Hoogduin, & van Balkom, 2008), insomnia (Erman, 2008), and social phobia (Ashbaugh, Anthony,

Liss, Summerfeldt, McCabe, Swinson, 2007). Current challenges include investigating the effects of CBT on brain activation (Straube, Glauer, Dilger, Mentzel, & Miltner, 2006), its delivery via the Internet (Tillfors et al., 2008), and its potential for use in primary prevention programs (Kuyken, Dalgleish, & Holden, 2007).

> **KEY CONCEPT** **Cognitive-behavioural therapy** is a psychotherapy focused on identifying, analyzing, and ultimately changing the habitually inflexible and negative cognitions about oneself, others, and the world that contribute to distress and problematic behaviours.

Although the assumptions underlying CBT can be traced back to ancient times and the Stoic philosopher, Epictetus, Aaron Beck, a psychiatrist, and Albert Ellis, a psychologist, are acknowledged with the founding of CBT as we know it today. From the mid-1950s to the early 1960s, when experimental and clinical psychology and psychiatry were ruled by behaviourism and psychoanalytic theory, Ellis and Beck, independently of each other, became increasingly dissatisfied with both the ability of

BOX 15.1

Research for Best Practice: Treating University Students with Social Phobia and Public Speaking Fears

Tillfors, M., Carlbring, P., Furmark, T., Lewen haupt, S., Spark, M., Eriksson, A., et al. (2008). Treating university students with social phobia and public speaking fears: Internet delivered self-help with or without live group exposure sessions. Depression and Anxiety, 25, 708–717.

THE QUESTION: Is Internet-based self-help CBT (with minimal therapist contact via e-mail) more effective if combined with live group exposure sessions?

METHODS: Thirty-eight university students meeting the *DSM-IV-TR* criteria for social phobia were randomized into two treatment groups: Internet-delivered CBT with five group exposure sessions or Internet program alone. Social anxiety, general anxiety, depression levels, and quality of life were measured pretreatment and posttreatment and at a 1-year follow-up.

FINDINGS: Both treatment groups showed significant improvement from pretest to posttest and from pretest to 1-year follow-up on all measures. The addition of group exposure sessions did not improve the outcome significantly.

IMPLICATIONS: Internet-based self-help programs alone with augmentation by live group sessions can be efficient in the treatment of university students with social phobia.

psychoanalysis to explain the struggles of their patients and its lack of scientific rigor. In treating their patients, they noted certain biases toward irrational and inflexible thought patterns that negatively influenced mood and behaviour. They proposed that if these rigid and negative thought patterns could be changed, mood would improve and behaviour would become more functional. Although this theory is now widely accepted, at that time, a cognitively focused psychotherapy was viewed as radical. Beck and Ellis remain international leaders in clinical practice, teaching and training, and empirical study of CBT. Although CBT is a mental health treatment, it is based on a cognitive model that is applicable to the experience of all humans in all situations. Beck and Ellis envisioned that future generations would be educated in the foundations of CBT so as to provide important life skills for coping with distress and problem solving (see Box 15-1).

THE COGNITIVE MODEL

The cognitive model forms the foundation of CBT, the essence of which is that humans respond primarily to cognitive representations of the environment, and that cognition mediates affect and behaviour (Ingram et al.,

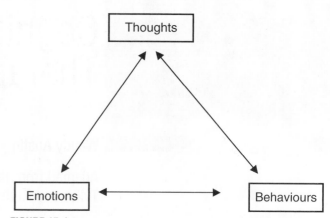

FIGURE 15.1 Interconnection between thoughts, emotions, and behaviours.

1998). In simpler terms, the way we *think* about situations influences our *emotions* and our *behaviour*. Our emotions, behaviours, and thoughts all interact in complex and interconnected ways; however, the cognitive model places particular importance on thoughts as the "director" of our experiences (Fig. 15-1).

Cognitive theory suggests that one's perception of situations and events is particularly salient in guiding emotional and behavioural responses (Beck, 1995). Events in and of themselves do not cause us to feel and act in particular ways; rather, it is how we *understand* or think about what happens to us that affects how we feel about it and what we do about it. For example, think about what would go through your mind if you entered a party where the only other guest you knew had not yet arrived. Would you think, "This is a great opportunity to introduce myself to others. Maybe I'll meet some interesting people," or would you think, "Everyone is staring at me because I'm alone. If my friend does not show up in the next 15 minutes, I'm leaving"? The party itself is a relatively neutral event, but how you interpret the event will affect how you feel at the party and what you do or how you act. If your thought process tends toward the former, your emotions of excitement and enjoyment will propel you to stay and mingle with the other partygoers (your behaviour). If your thought process is more consistent with the latter, your anxiety and uncertainty will compel you to flee (your behaviour).

The different ways that individuals evaluate and respond to a particular situation or event are as varied as the individuals themselves. The particular reasons why individuals are so varied in their perceptions of situations, and thereby their emotional and behavioural responses, are in part accounted for by their core beliefs. See Box 15-2 for an example of students responding differently to the same situation. In summary, the cognitive model posits that when an emotion is felt, a thought is behind it and when behaviour is enacted, a thought is behind it.

BOX 15.2

Effect of Cognition on Feelings and Behaviour

In this example, four student nurses in the same clinical group respond to the same situation in four different ways, owing to different patterns of thinking, feeling, and acting.

THE SITUATION: A nursing instructor informs the clinical group that by the end of their shift today, each student is expected to seek out an opportunity to insert their first intravenous line. All students received the appropriate classroom teaching and lab practice with this skill.

SUSAN thinks, "I have been waiting so long to perform advanced clinical skills. I can hardly wait to give it a try." She feels excited and responds behaviourally by informing all staff in morning report of her learning opportunity. She requests that any new intravenous starts be directed to her.

DAVID thinks, "I understand the theory behind intravenous insertion, but I did not have much success in the lab. I know I need to fulfill this requirement, but I am not sure how I am going to do it without hurting someone and embarrassing myself." He feels anxious and uncertain and responds behaviourally by reluctantly informing his buddy

nurse, midway through the shift, that he is required to meet this expectation.

JENNIFER thinks, "There is absolutely no way I am ready for this. I do not have the confidence or skill set to perform this task." She feels terrified and responds behaviourally by speaking to the clinical instructor privately informing her that she is feeling nauseous and must return home for the day.

PAULINE thinks, "Once again I'm being told what to do without any regard for my own learning needs. No one can force me to comply." She feels outraged and angry and responds behaviourally by refusing to complete the skill as required.

All the students were presented with the identical situation, and all received similar training to perform the required skill. The way in which each student *thought about* the situation, however, was very different and consequently led to emotions as varied as excitement and terror and behaviours as varied as approach and avoidance. It is not the situation itself that influenced how each of the students responded, but rather each individual's unique interpretation of the situation.

■ LEVELS OF COGNITION

At this point, it has been established that cognition is given primary importance in CBT. Now, the three levels of cognition that are considered in CBT are explored, beginning with the deepest level and moving toward the most superficial.

Core Beliefs

Cognitive theory posits the existence of core knowledge structures that hold, organize, and interpret all information about one's view of self, others, and the world (Hollon & Kriss, 1984; Needleman, 1999; Sperry, 1999). These structures, referred to as **core beliefs** or **cognitive schema**, comprise basic beliefs so fundamental that they are often not articulated in explicit words but rather are accepted as absolute truths (Beck, 1995). Core beliefs assist in evaluating and assigning meaning to events and influencing the subsequent range of affective and behavioural responses (Beck & Emery, 1985). The deeply rooted nature of core beliefs and their difficulty in being accessed, or explicitly identified, mean that they are difficult to change. Examples of core beliefs are I am inadequate; I am unlovable; Others are not trustworthy; and The world is an unsafe place.

Core beliefs hold both general and specific information about the self, others, and the world and influence the manner in which one negotiates one's way through life. If, for example, an individual holds the belief that she is a person worthy of love, she will likely engage in mutually

respectful and fulfilling relationships. Conversely, if the world is believed to be a hostile place in which people are not to be trusted, she may have an approach of hypervigilance and suspiciousness and may experience relationships as potentially dangerous. As one moves through life gathering and considering information, beliefs are processed in a way that is consistent with the view of self, others, and the world and become solidified (Hollon & Kriss, 1984). As such, core beliefs are self-confirming and self-perpetuating in nature which contribute to their rigidity and global application (Beck, 1995).

Intermediate Beliefs

Existing at a more accessible level than core beliefs are cognitive products, which are often separated into two categories: **intermediate beliefs** and **automatic thoughts** (Beck, 1995; Hollon & Kriss, 1984). Intermediate beliefs consist of attitudes, rules or expectations, and assumptions that influence one's perceptions, affect, and behaviours. They often take the form of "if... then," "should," or "must" statements that are rigid and unrealistic. Assumptions, rules, and expectations may have arisen from the direct teaching or observation of important others early in life. One's cultural background also plays a role in one's understanding and tolerance of what is acceptable. Examples of intermediate beliefs include

• If I'm not liked by everyone, it means I've failed.
• Assume the worst will happen because it usually does.
• If I show my vulnerability, I make myself open to attack.

- I must be the best in everything that I endeavour.
- Relationships make you open to rejection.

Automatic Thoughts

At an even more superficial level than intermediate, beliefs are automatic thoughts. Automatic thoughts are the "knee-jerk" in-the-moment words and images generated in a particular situation (Beck, 1995). They may not be logical and are often difficult to "shut off." Automatic thoughts are the most superficial and accessible of the levels of cognition and thus are generally the first to be targeted in treatment. Although automatic thoughts are accessible, we are not always immediately conscious of their presence. Instead, we may be more aware of the accompanying emotion rather than the preceding spontaneous thought. In fact, the presence of a strong emotion is often a signal that an important thought is present. For example, when a car cuts you off on the freeway, you might be more likely to respond with anger than to be aware of the thought behind the emotion of anger ("Who do you think you are? You put the safety of my family at risk."). Part of the early therapeutic work of CBT is to bring automatic thoughts into our awareness.

Relationship Between Levels of Cognition

The relationship between automatic thoughts, intermediate beliefs, and core beliefs is demonstrated in the following two examples. There is a situation in which an individual is standing in a line and someone steps into the position in front of her. In the moment, the individual tells herself, "This person must not have realized I was already in line. I will tell him that I was first in line so that he can take his place behind me." These automatic thoughts occur spontaneously and reside at the most superficial level of cognition. The deeper intermediate beliefs, rules, and expectations that support these automatic thoughts may be "People do not intend to be malicious but can cause inconvenience," "It is necessary to follow social norms," and "The ability to assert oneself is important." Underlying these automatic thoughts and intermediate rules and expectations is a core belief, the deepest level of cognition, of "I am a valuable person who is worthy of respect." This example of the relationship between the three levels of cognition is illustrated in Figure 15-2. Another individual may process this same situation very differently. The same three levels of cognition still exist, although the content of each level is different. She may tell herself, "This person saw me standing here, and he intentionally stepped in front of me. He must think I am someone that can be easily exploited." The intermediate beliefs and rules that gave rise to these automatic thoughts are "I am not capable of speaking up for myself," "I expect that people will treat me with a lack of respect," and "I can't speak up for myself; therefore, I'll never get anywhere in life." In this example, the automatic thoughts and expectations are driven by core beliefs rooted in a sense of unworthiness, such as "I'm not deserving of respect."

Situation: I am standing in line and someone steps into the position in front of me.

Automatic thoughts: This person must not have realized I was already in line.

I will tell him that I was first in line so that he can take his place behind me.

Intermediate beliefs, rules, expectations: People do not intend to be malicious, but can cause inconvenience.

It is necessary to follow social norms.

The ability to assert myself is important.

Core belief: I am a valuable person worthy of respect.

FIGURE 15.2 The relationship between levels of cognition.

Early experiences, past events, messages from others, and direct observations contribute to the formation of core beliefs and subsequent intermediate beliefs and automatic thoughts. In the individual whose early experiences were primarily nurturing, reliable, and positive, core beliefs are generally an accurate, realistic, and functional reflection of reality. However, the individual who experienced inconsistency, emotional unavailability, and cruelty may develop hypercritical beliefs about the self, others, and the world that are rigid, overgeneralized, and an inaccurate reflection of the current reality. These core beliefs contribute to emotions and behaviours that are intensely negative and harmful.

CRNENOTE

Understanding the way thinking affects emotions and behaviours can be helpful in working with clients who are having difficulty adhering to treatment regimens.

PRINCIPLES OF COGNITIVE-BEHAVIOURAL THERAPY

CBT is grounded in a set of specific principles. The particular treatment strategies employed in CBT are specific to the disorder being treated; however, the basic principles remain common across all disorders. The 10 principles that appear in Box 15-3 and discussed below are based on the work of Beck (1995), Beck and Emery (1985), and Fennell (1989).

BOX 15.3

Ten Principles of CBT

1. CBT is based on a cognitive-behavioural formulation of the client.
2. CBT requires a strong therapeutic alliance.
3. CBT is time limited and brief.
4. CBT is goal oriented, problem focused, and change oriented.
5. CBT is structured and directive.
6. CBT is educative.
7. CBT requires therapeutic collaboration.
8. CBT employs inductive reasoning.
9. CBT uses Socratic questioning.
10. CBT uses self-reflective exercises to apply and hone skills learned from therapy in day-to-day situations.

From Beck, J. (1995). *Cognitive therapy: Basics and beyond.* New York, NY: Guilford Press; Beck, A. T., & Emery, G. (1985). *Anxiety disorders and phobias: A cognitive perspective.* New York, NY: Basic Books; Fennell, M. J. V. (1989). Depression. In K. Hawton, P. M. Salkovskis, J. Kirk, & D. M. Clark (Eds.), *Cognitive behaviour therapy for psychiatric problems* (pp. 169–234). Oxford, UK: Oxford University Press.

Cognitive-Behavioural Formulation

A cognitive-behavioural formulation begins during the initial assessment of the client and is reviewed and revised over the course of therapy. It outlines the typical thoughts and problematic behaviours that contribute to the current distress. The client who presents with social anxiety may have the thoughts, "Showing my nervousness is a sign of weakness" and "I appear incompetent when I make presentations." Problematic behaviours that flow from these negative thoughts may include avoidance of any situation in which he might be the centre of attention (e.g., speaking up in meetings), overpreparing (e.g., memorizing a brief statement to be made during a meeting), and use of alcohol (e.g., reliance on several glasses of beer before attending a party where socializing is an expectation). The next component of the formulation involves collecting information on the factors that precipitated the onset of the current problem. The precipitating factor for the socially anxious client may be starting a new job where there is an expectation to chair meetings, conduct staff training, and give presentations to outside agencies. A cognitive-behavioural formulation also outlines the developmental issues that contributed to and continue to reinforce the current problem. For example, harsh criticism by parents for being less than perfect, being ridiculed and mocked by students while speaking in front of the class, and receiving below-average grades on oral presentations may all be predisposing factors for the socially anxious client. Over his life, he may have systematically ignored his multiple successes and amplified his perceived social failures, which served to strengthen his beliefs about weakness and inadequacy.

The cognitive-behavioural formulation is shared with the client as part of the collaborative relationship (see Box 15-3, principle 7). It is presented as a working framework that can be added to and changed by both the therapist and the client as new information becomes available. In addition to providing both a framework for guiding treatment and a means to enhancing therapeutic collaboration, it also demonstrates to the client how part of one's experience can be broken down in order to gain a better understanding of the whole, and that one's seemingly overwhelming problems are composed of smaller and more manageable parts.

Strong Therapeutic Alliance

Much of the emphasis of CBT is on therapy technique and strategies; however, therapeutic change would not be achievable without a strong therapeutic relationship consisting of trust, mutual respect, safety, empathy, warmth, and acceptance. Most clients enter therapy afraid, uncertain, and perhaps unsure if it will be helpful. Many have struggled for years on their own, perhaps too ashamed to seek help. Further, the personal histories of some clients render them highly mistrustful of those in positions of perceived power. It is the primary task of the therapist to create an environment in which clients feel free to disclose their anxieties and take risks, in which they feel attended to, listened to, and understood. The therapeutic relationship is discussed further in Chapter 8.

Time Limited and Brief

Some forms of psychotherapy, in particular the insight-oriented psychotherapies, are open-ended with respect to the length of treatment (see Chapter 7). Given the nature and goals of psychodynamic therapy, treatment may not be completed for a number of years. In contrast, CBT is a short-term form of treatment. For example, a maximum of 25 sessions of CBT are recommended for depression (Fennell, 1989; Kaplan, Sadock, & Greeb, 1994), whereas 5 to 20 sessions are recommended for anxiety disorders (Clark, 1998). The treatment guidelines for panic disorder recommend 12 sessions of CBT (American Psychiatric Association, 1998). The standard number of sessions for social phobia when it is delivered in group CBT, as determined by Heimberg's extensive study in the field, is 12 (Heimberg & Becker, 2002). Individuals who present with simple phobias generally require even fewer sessions, as few as one or two sessions in certain cases. When determining the number of sessions required, the therapist considers the severity and duration of the presenting problem, client motivation, and the client's ability to form and maintain a therapeutic relationship.

The *Suitability for Short-term Cognitive Therapy Rating Scale (SRS)*, developed at the Clarke Institute of Psychiatry[1] in Toronto by Safran, Segal, Shaw, and Vallis (1990), uses 10 criteria to determine suitability: accessibility of automatic thoughts (i.e., capacity to report on their own thinking), awareness and differentiation of emotion, acceptance of personal responsibility for a change, compatibility with cognitive rationale (i.e., sees values in examining links between thoughts, emotions, and behaviours), alliance potential (in-session evidence and out-of-session evidence), chronicity (duration of problems), security operations (intensity of efforts to block exploration of anxiety-producing content), focality (ability to remain focused), and general optimism/pessimism regarding therapy. The SRS has been shown to have the predictive value of potential to succeed in CBT (Myhr, Talbot, Annable, & Pinard, 2007).

Goal Oriented, Problem Focused, and Change Oriented

Clients enter CBT with a clear idea of that with which they are struggling. The therapist and client collaboratively set realistic and measurable goals to be attained within the treatment period. Using cognitive and behavioural strategies (to be discussed), the client works toward analyzing the current accuracy and logic of negative thinking patterns. Distortions in thinking are tested and are replaced with more accurate and flexible ways of evaluating self, others, and the world. Potential barriers to goal attainment are considered, and methods to overcome these obstacles are planned.

Structured and Directive

Although the content of each therapy session changes from week to week, sessions follow a similar structure throughout the course of treatment. The structure of CBT provides clarity, reassurance, and a sense of control to the client as well as maintains focus and maximizes the ability to use the session effectively. An additional benefit of the structured nature of CBT is that it supports the client to be his or her own therapist upon therapy termination.

The therapist begins the session with a mood check, asks for a brief summary of the client's week, collaboratively decides which problem areas will be discussed in the session (often referred to as agenda setting), requests feedback about the previous session, reviews and discusses the self-reflective exercise (see Box 15-3, principle 10), addresses the agenda items, provides new self-reflective exercises, and elicits feedback about the session. Throughout the session, the therapist offers summaries of key areas. As the therapy progresses, the client takes on the responsibility of providing these summaries and managing the structure in general.

Educative

The initial sessions of CBT are more therapist-directed than later sessions and include education about the client's presenting problem and the cognitive model of his or her particular disorder in addition to socializing the client to CBT. For example, the first four sessions of a group CBT intervention for self-injuring women who have a history of sexual abuse included therapist-led content on the cognitive model of childhood sexual abuse and self-injury; the cognitive, affective, and behavioural patterns that emerge from early experiences of abuse; and the functions and purposes of self-injury (Tully, 2005). Further on in CBT, therapists teach clients how to engage in cognitive restructuring, the process whereby habitually negative thought patterns are identified, evaluated, and modified. Providing clients information on the nature and course of their disorder not only helps them to understand their current struggles but also empowers clients to engage in a collaborative approach to their care. An additional benefit of the educative nature of CBT is that it assists in preparing clients for the process of self-therapy; that is, it helps ensure that clients adopt the skills necessary to continue to change and prevent relapse after the specific therapy has ended.

Therapeutic Collaboration

Cognitive-behavioural therapists practice from the stance that therapy is a collaborative effort. The client and therapist each bring essential and different ingredients to the relationship, and both are vital in achieving therapeutic change. The client assumes the role of equal partner in agenda setting, problem solving, and generating self-reflective exercises (see Box 15-3, principle 10). Because the content and the process of CBT are demystified and made transparent, it is possible for clients to truly take on a collaborative role. The therapist remains an active participant in the treatment; neither a neutral nor authoritative stance would be appropriate in CBT.

Inductive Reasoning

Clients entering therapy often view their thoughts and feelings as facts and unshakeable truths; for example, "I know I am a stupid person. When I'm depressed, it means I'm weak." Clients of CBT are encouraged to view their thoughts and feelings as hypotheses; they are not rigid facts but are plausible explanations that will be put to test and revised as needed. The goal is to assist clients in attending to all the available facts and information in their hypothesis testing, not merely the "old ruts" of thinking in which they generally find themselves stuck. Clients are encouraged to "think like a scientist and search for objective facts" or "play detective to find all the evidence" when examining the validity and accuracy of their thoughts.

Socratic Questioning

Cognitive-behavioural therapists adopt a questioning stance, referred to as Socratic questioning, as a method to reveal information about negative thought patterns and to aid in developing balanced thoughts. When a question is posed by the therapist, possible answers are generated. The client is encouraged to view these answers as hypotheses capable of being examined and tested in the therapy. The intention of Socratic questioning is not for the client to feel interrogated; rather, it is for the client to come to his or her own broader perspective about the validity, accuracy, and functionality of his or her thought process.

Self-Reflective Exercises

One of the most effective ways of helping clients reflect on and practice newly developed skills and monitor progress is through the use of self-reflective exercises, sometimes referred to as homework exercises. Extensive empirical study indicates that homework compliance is a significant predictor of positive treatment outcome (Kazantzis, Deane, & Ronan, 2000). Self-reflective exercises are provided at the end of each session with the expectation that the client will work on them throughout the week and be prepared to discuss them at the beginning of the following session. Providing the client with materials that facilitate recollection of the assignment promotes homework completion. It is essential that therapists review the assigned exercise with the client at the following session because this reinforces the therapist's commitment and investment in the process. Clients will be less likely to complete the exercises if they have little accountability and if they do not observe the therapist valuing the assignments. Review of the exercises also provides the therapist with clinically useful information. If clients state that they do not feel like completing the exercise, are too busy, or do not see the point, this provides the therapist with clinically relevant material that should be explored further in the therapy. For example, a client may avoid attempting the exercises because he does not feel as though it will be done "right" or "good enough" or that he will appear "stupid, just like I always do," which would lead to humiliation. The therapist would then take the opportunity to explore these thoughts, as they may represent negative patterns of thinking that are generalized to situations beyond the completion of the exercises and warrant analyzing and modification. If the client indicates an inability to complete the exercises because time is lacking, further exploration may reveal that either the exercises as assigned were in fact too detailed and labour intensive or that the client has difficulty committing the personal time necessary to effect therapeutic change. It is also equally important for the therapist to know whether the client is experiencing new insights and a sense of accomplishment through completing the exercises because this assists in gauging where next to direct the therapy.

TREATMENT STRATEGIES

CBT uses both cognitive and behavioural techniques to effect change. The strategies outlined here represent those basics to CBT. Additional strategies are used but, because of their advanced application, are beyond the scope of this text. Training in CBT is generally obtained at the graduate level and, although treatment strategies are described here, advanced training through course work, clinical practicum, and clinical supervision is essential before delivery of the treatment.

Cognitive Techniques

Cognitive techniques revolve primarily around cognitive restructuring, which is a process that follows a particular path of identifying, analyzing, and modifying the three levels of cognition, beginning with automatic thoughts and working through to core beliefs.

> **KEY CONCEPT** **Cognitive restructuring** is a process in which cognitions (automatic thoughts, intermediate and core beliefs) are identified, analyzed, and modified to effect positive change in mood and behaviour.

Identifying Automatic Thoughts

Awareness of one's thinking is the first step toward change. Early in treatment, clients are often unaware of their running internal negative dialogues about themselves, others, and the world. As previously discussed, the accompanying emotion may be much more apparent to clients than the underlying negative and inflexible thought process. When introducing clients to the skill of identifying automatic thoughts, a useful place to begin is to have them attend to shifts in or intensification of their emotions. When a strong emotion is felt or a new emotion is experienced, a question is asked, "What was going through your mind just then?" (Beck, 1995). This question often helps clients to attend to their thinking that drives their emotional experience. Another technique to elicit automatic thoughts is to ask the client to recount a very recent problematic situation. The client is encouraged to play back the situation in his or her mind using all the senses. As the client visualizes the details of what happened, he or she is asked, "What does this situation say about you?" "What does it mean for how others will view you?" "What is the most distressing aspect of this situation?" "If the worst case scenario came from this situation, what do you think would happen?" (Greenberger & Padesky, 1995). Once automatic thoughts are identified, the next step of evaluating their accuracy and usefulness is undertaken.

Evaluating Automatic Thoughts

The goal of evaluating automatic thoughts is to examine thoughts in detail to determine their accuracy. Clients consider both the evidence that supports and the evidence that does not support their automatic thoughts. It is important that clients focus on objective facts rather than interpretations, assumptions, or opinions when generating evidence that supports their automatic thoughts, although this may be difficult initially (Greenberger & Padesky, 1995). The task of finding evidence that does not support automatic thoughts can be aided by key questions such as, "What experiences have I had that show this thought is not always completely true?" "If someone I cared deeply about had this thought, what would I tell

them?" "If someone who cared deeply about me knew I was thinking this, what would they say to me?" "What evidence is there that this thought is not 100% true?" (Greenberger & Padesky). When evaluating automatic thoughts, often clients conclude that the evidence for the automatic thought is weaker than the evidence against and therefore that the thought is no longer as accurate and valid as it was once believed to be.

The following case example illustrates the process of evaluating automatic thoughts. A situation occurred in which a client, Elizabeth, was reprimanded by her employer for not completing her monthly report, an essential part of her job. After exploring the emotions she experienced in this situation (fear and shame), she identified several negative automatic thoughts, including, "My boss hates me," "I might lose my job," "He thinks I'm incompetent," "I'm not a responsible or trustworthy employee," and "I'm nothing but a screwup." The therapist helped Elizabeth determine which automatic thought was most distressing to her ("I'm nothing but a screwup"), and it was this thought that became the one to be evaluated. Elizabeth was asked to find evidence to support the thought, "I'm nothing but a screwup." Given that she was instructed to consider only objective information, and not her opinion, the following evidence was generated: "I failed two courses in one semester during my first year of university because I partied more than I studied," "I am sometimes late paying my credit card bill," and "I once had a boyfriend who told me I wouldn't get anywhere in life." Elizabeth's next task was to find evidence that does not support her thought, "I'm nothing but a screwup." In reviewing the key questions with her therapist, she was able to find the following nonsupporting evidence: "I generally receive above average yearly performance appraisals from my boss," "In addition to working this job, I volunteer in my son's classroom two times a month where I have been called invaluable," and "My best friend tells me that I'm a very organized mother."

Another aspect of the process of evaluating one's automatic thoughts involves identifying cognitive distortions. Cognitive distortions, also referred to as thinking errors or problematic thinking styles, are the characteristic and habitual ways in which people make errors in thinking about themselves or others (Burns, 1989). Thinking errors are problematic because they keep people locked into patterns of negative thinking and behaviour. Burns initially identified 10 types of thinking errors, a list that has been adapted and added to by others over time (Box 15-4). People have a tendency to engage in patterns of thinking errors that are similar across a variety of situations. All people engage in distorted thinking; it is not a phenomenon limited to people with mental disorders. In CBT, the therapist works with the client to first identify which thinking errors are being used. Clients are commonly given a handout listing all the cognitive errors with

BOX 15.4

Ten Thinking Errors

1. **All-or-nothing thinking:** The tendency to see things in black-and-white categories, with no shades of grey. Things are seen in extremes, either very good or very bad. "If I don't get a perfect evaluation, I'm a failure."
2. **Overgeneralization:** The assumption that one error/problem means a lifetime of the same error/problem. "If I lose this job, I will never succeed in making a living."
3. **Mental filter:** Filtering out the good things that happen and retaining only the negative. "When I received that award, I could see that Jane didn't think I deserved it."
4. **Magnification/minimization:** Overexaggeration of fears, imperfections, or errors. "There is absolutely no way I could have passed that exam. I've totally blown the course."
5. **Jumping to conclusions:** Concluding things that are not justified based on available evidence. "I saw Peter yawn during my presentation. Everyone was bored." It includes **mind reading:** "My coworker didn't say hello to me today because she's starting to dislike me" and

fortune telling: "He didn't call me tonight. That's it. He'll never call again."
6. **Labeling:** Putting a negative label on yourself or others, a way to believe that no one can change. "My roommate is a slob. I have to keep everything tidy."
7. **Personalization and blame:** Making yourself feel responsible for things out of your control. "It is my fault our team lost the game. If only I hadn't dropped the ball in the first half."
8. **Should/must statements:** Thinking in terms of "should" and "must." "I must make no mistakes during the skill laboratory, no matter what."
9. **Discounting the positives:** Refusing to credit the positive aspects of situations. "John said that I looked great today. He must think that I look terrible most days."
10. **Emotional reasoning:** Believing something must be true because one "feels" it so strongly, ignoring any evidence to the contrary. "I know I've had people in my life who say I'm a good person, but it's hard to believe because I feel like I'm so bad."

From Burns, D. D. (1989). *The feeling good handbook: Using the new mood therapy in everyday life.* New York, NY: Morrow.

relevant examples of each. This handout guides clients through the process of identifying and labeling thinking errors. The next step is to examine the usefulness and validity of this style of thinking so that clients can respond to their thoughts in a more realistic and balanced manner, thus achieving a more accurate view of themselves and others. Through the process of correcting thinking errors, clients see that the negative automatic thoughts and beliefs they held about themselves, others, and the world at large are no longer valid. It is important to catch oneself when making the errors and inject a clearer way of looking at the situation. When we give ourselves more options for how to think, we give ourselves more options for how to feel and how to respond.

Returning to the previous case of Elizabeth, she identified that she routinely engages in distorted thinking by jumping to conclusions ("I might lose my job." "He thinks I'm incompetent.") and overgeneralization ("I'm not a responsible or trustworthy employee. I'm nothing but a screwup"). Elizabeth worked with her therapist to increase her awareness of how frequently she engages in this style of thinking. Further, her therapist helped Elizabeth to realize the inaccuracy and destructiveness of this style of thinking.

Modifying Automatic Thoughts

Identifying and evaluating automatic thoughts are two important aspects of CBT; however, given the focus on change in CBT, modification of automatic thoughts is an essential component of the treatment. The client makes

use of everything he has learned and acquired in identifying and evaluating automatic thoughts to move toward modification. Modifying thoughts involves weighing both the evidence for and the evidence against an automatic thought in an effort to generate a new and more balanced way of thinking. It must be emphasized that this new way of thinking does not simply involve replacing negative thoughts with positive ones. Unquestioning acceptance of a positive stance can be as destructive as negative thinking because it does not take into account all available evidence (Greenberger & Padesky, 1995). The new way of thinking considers all aspects of one's experience so that one can arrive at a more broadened way of viewing oneself, others, or the world. In Elizabeth's case, she examined all her available evidence and recognized an alternative way of understanding her situation: "I have exceedingly high expectations of myself and find it very hard to give myself a break when I've done something I perceive as less than acceptable. I have screwed up in the past, but it's been relatively infrequently, and I do learn from my mistakes." It can also be useful for clients to make a summary statement of all the evidence that supports and does not support their automatic thought to help develop balanced thinking. For example, Elizabeth summarized her evidence by saying, "I've done things that are not responsible and have received negative messages from others of the same kind, but I also am currently successful in juggling many demanding roles and receive praise for my efforts." With this expanded view, clients generally report that they experience a positive shift in mood.

One very useful and commonly used tool to achieve the goals of identifying, evaluating, and modifying automatic thoughts is the Thought Record (Greenberger & Padesky, 1995). The Thought Record is a structured worksheet that records all the pertinent information about problematic and distressing situations and helps clients to make sense of why they feel and react in particular ways. Thought Records take all aspects of one's experience and organize them into information presented in seven columns: the situation, moods, automatic thoughts, evidence that supports the thoughts, evidence that does not support the thoughts, formation of balanced or alternative thoughts, and rerating of moods. At various points throughout the Thought Record, thoughts and emotions are rated and rerated on their degree of strength and believability (0% to 100%). Once the Thought Record is completed, the goal is for clients to experience a balanced or alternative thought that is rated as more believable than their original negative automatic thought accompanied by a decrease in the intensity of their originally identified emotions. Thought Records are often completed during therapy sessions as well as between sessions when problematic or distressing situations arise.

Students undergoing cognitive-behavioural training are generally required to routinely complete their own Thought Records to gain an increased awareness of their own thinking patterns and resulting emotions and behaviours and to encourage self-reflection and self-monitoring. Thought Records are often shared with supervisors and discussed in supervision sessions. Completing Thought Records is also very important for helping students in training become intimately acquainted with the process of completing the record. Although deceptively simple, Thought Records require much practice to achieve mastery.

Identifying and Modifying Intermediate Beliefs

Many of the same techniques used for identifying and modifying automatic thoughts are also used with intermediate beliefs or assumptions. There are some additional techniques that are employed, given that assumptions exist at a deeper level than automatic thoughts. Identifying assumptions can be aided by attending to the patterns of negative thoughts that emerge over the course of therapy. These themes suggest an underlying assumption or perhaps even a core belief. It can also be useful to help clients identify the rules that they live by and expect of others. A commonly used method to uncover assumptions behind an automatic thought is the downward arrow technique (Burns, 1980), in which the therapist questions the meaning of the client's thought until an assumption, or a core belief, about self, others, or the world is revealed.

BOX 15.5

A Dialogue Using the Downward Arrow Technique

Client: I didn't do the self-reflective exercise this week because it was too hard.

Therapist: What does that say about you that you found it too hard?

Client: It says that I didn't pay enough attention in the session last week.

Therapist: And if that were true, that you didn't pay enough attention last week, what would that say about you?

Client: It would say that I'm lazy.

Therapist: If it was true that you were lazy, what would that say about you?

Client: It would say that I'm useless.

See Box 15-5 for an example. This technique can also be used to reveal assumptions about others (What does *x* mean about other people?) or the world in general (What does *x* say about how the world works?). Once the assumption is revealed, the process of restructuring the assumption is initiated wherein the evidence for and against the assumption and alternative responses are considered. Behavioural experiments (to be discussed) are also an effective means to modify assumptions because they allow clients to use real-life situations to test the accuracy of beliefs.

Identifying and Modifying Core Beliefs

All the techniques discussed thus far, especially the downward arrow technique, are useful for identifying core beliefs. Additional strategies may be required because of the deeply rooted nature of core beliefs. Discussing the early life experiences of the client can often facilitate the identification of core beliefs. Through this process, the client and the therapist examine the influence of early experiences in developing and maintaining core beliefs. Often, core beliefs are better understood when the context in which they developed is considered. However, this is an advanced technique beyond the scope of this chapter. The exploration must be approached with care and conducted in a manner that is containing for the client; in-depth exploration wherein clients relive painful early experiences is not appropriate in CBT.

Beck (1995) encourages the use of Core Belief Worksheets to identify core beliefs, to strengthen the believability of new core beliefs, and to weaken the influence of old core beliefs. The client first identifies his old core belief and rates it out of 100 (e.g., "I'm undesirable," 70%), followed by his new core belief ("Once people get to know me, they can see that I'm a likeable person," 40%). Similar to the process of evaluating automatic thoughts, the client gathers evidence that contradicts his old belief and supports his new belief ("Last week someone in my running group gave me her number so we can arrange to go for a run together." "I have one friend who has stayed by my side despite all the things I've been through"). The final step is to gather evidence that supports the old belief with the addition of a cognitive reframe ("When my last girlfriend broke up with me, she said she could never love a person like me, but I was struggling with depression during our relationship; therefore, I couldn't bring much to the relationship," "People don't readily seek out my friendship, but I'm now realizing that I have given off signals to people to stay away. This was my way of protecting myself from the rejection I believed was inevitable"). A broader perspective is achieved through this process, one that takes into account both past and current experiences.

Behavioural Techniques

Increasingly, practitioners of CBT recognize the importance of behavioural experiments if core beliefs are to be modified. The validity and accuracy of old core beliefs are tested in real-life situations, thus strengthening new ones.

Behavioural strategies are primarily utilized in CBT as a way to test and challenge both old maladaptive thinking patterns and newly acquired rational thoughts. They may also be used to modify symptoms when conducted in a manner that supports a change in cognition (Wells, 1997). Behavioural techniques must be considered and implemented within the larger scope of CBT. They are not employed in isolation, nor are they implemented without being linked back to the cognitive model of the particular disorder being treated.

Behavioural Strategies to Test Beliefs

Behavioural experiments to test and challenge core beliefs have always been considered an essential treatment strategy in CBT; however, recent evidence suggests that they are more important for promoting and solidifying change than Thought Records (Bennett-Levy, 2003; Bennett-Levy et al., 2004). Behavioural experiments offer clients the opportunity to put their newly modified cognitions to test in real-life situations, thereby increasing the believability of alternative thoughts (Bennett-Levy, 2003). Without this behavioural component, the process of challenging the accuracy and validity of old thoughts and generating new thoughts may be little more than an intellectual exercise and may not lead to meaningful cognitive, emotional, or behavioural change. Behavioural experiments can be challenging for clients

because the prospect of putting new thoughts into action and testing old destructive ways of thinking can be anxiety producing.

Behavioural experiments can be presented to clients as an opportunity to "test-drive" their new thoughts to see what will really happen as a result. A typical behavioural experiment consists of the therapist and the client collaboratively constructing an experiment to test a new belief. For example, the new belief, "I'm a likeable person" could be tested by constructing an experiment in which the client plans to call an acquaintance from his running group and invite her to go for a run. The client makes a prediction about what might happen in the course of the experiment ("She'll agree to go with me, but she'll find me a bit uninteresting"). Potential obstacles are considered ("I will become very nervous and talk very little; therefore, she'll think I'm boring"), as well as action that can be taken to manage the obstacles ("Remind myself that being nervous is okay when you are getting to know people for the first time. Remind myself that even if I don't talk much, I can't jump to the conclusion that she will think I'm boring"). The actual result of the experiment is reported ("We ran together for one hour and talked about our interests. I found out that we have many things in common, including that we both like classic films and we're both shy people. She told me that *Citizen Kane* is playing in 2 weeks and suggested that we see it together"). The client then rates how much the result of the experiment supports his new belief (90%) and finally reflects on what was learned in the process of the experiment ("If I take more risks and show people who I really am, they can see that I'm a nice person and worth getting to know better"). Behavioural experiments are a powerful means of altering beliefs because they compel clients to take action on a thought. When clients are able to directly see the outcome of testing their beliefs, they are more likely to actually modify their beliefs.

Behavioural Strategies to Modify Symptoms

Numerous types of behavioural strategies for symptom reduction are available, including exposure techniques, relaxation training, and activity monitoring. Exposure therapies, including in vivo exposure, interoceptive exposure, graded exposure, and imaginal flooding, are utilized in panic disorder, panic disorder with agoraphobia, post-traumatic stress disorder, social phobia, and obsessive-compulsive disorder. The common thread among all types of exposure is that they put the client in contact with feared or avoided thoughts, emotions, behaviours, or situations (Needleman, 1999). Through this process, three possible outcomes may occur: the client's anticipated catastrophic outcome may be disconfirmed, the client may become desensitized to the feared response,

BOX 15.6

Research for Best Practice: Cognitive-Behavioural Therapy for Asthma and Coexisting Panic Disorder

Ross, C. J. M., Davis, T. M. A., & MacDonald, G. F. (2005). Cognitive-behavioural treatment combined with asthma education for adults with asthma and coexisting panic disorder. Clinical Nursing Research, 14, 131–157.

THE QUESTION: Does group-administered CBT, combined with asthma education for adults with coexisting asthma and panic disorder, lead to statistically significant changes in panic and asthma outcome measures?

METHODS: Forty-eight participants diagnosed with both panic disorder and asthma were randomly assigned to a treatment group or a wait-list control group. The CBT treatment occurred in 12 sessions over 8 weeks and was focused on four areas: anxiety and panic education; CBT techniques to identify, analyze, and modify cognitions related to anxiety and panic; breathing retraining; and interoceptive exposure. The asthma education focused on six components: airway inflammation and bronchospasm, medication, inhaler techniques, self-monitoring symptoms and peak flow,

asthma triggers and strategies for control, and action plans. Outcomes were measured by standardized panic disorder measures, a panic diary, asthma-related symptoms diaries, and an asthma quality-of-life measure.

FINDINGS: Statistically significant posttreatment improvements were demonstrated by CBT participants as compared with the control group, on measures of panic frequency (88% were panic free at posttreatment), general anxiety, and anxiety sensitivity as well as on measures of asthma-related quality of life and morning peak expiratory flow.

IMPLICATIONS: CBT combined with asthma education has potential as treatment for individuals with panic disorder with comorbid asthma. Nurses can assist patients in differentiating between panic episodes, asthma episodes, and combined panic–asthma episodes as well as preventing and/or controlling these episodes. The treatment is cost-effective and can be delivered by nurses with the appropriate level of training.

and the client's ability to cope with the feared situation may be improved (Needleman). Exposure-based techniques are very specific to the disorder being treated, and the protocols are extensive and comprehensive. Several treatment manuals for specific disorders are available and clearly outline the rationale and steps for conducting exposure therapy. The following authors may be referred to for further reading on exposure techniques: Antony and Swinson (2000), Taylor (2000), Foa and Rothbaum (1998), Swinson, Antony, Rachman, and Richter (1998).

Relaxation strategies, such as breathing retraining and progressive muscle relaxation, may be employed with clients who have generalized anxiety disorder, panic disorder, and posttraumatic stress disorder. Breathing retraining is the practice of learning how to breath at an appropriate pace and depth so that this skill can be called on when faced with feared stimuli. Clients are also educated about how the physiologic effects of hyperventilation or breath holding, such as increased blood pressure and disturbance of the oxygen–carbon dioxide balance, may worsen anxiety symptoms (Needleman, 1999). Progressive muscle relaxation, or Jacobsonian relaxation (Jacobson, 1938), involves the practice of deliberately tensing and relaxing 12 groups of muscles, beginning with the feet and moving upward to the face. The technique teaches clients how to relax muscles and induce a sense of physical and mental calmness. Other relaxation techniques may be employed, although they are not discussed here, such as mindfulness-based meditation and guided imagery.

Depressed individuals often benefit from activity scheduling, wherein daily activities and accompanying moods are recorded in a diary format (Beck, 1995). Many depressed clients become immobilized and believe that they must wait to feel better before engaging in activities. Activity monitoring encourages depressed individuals to instead engage in activity as a way to improve mood. Activity scheduling is useful for scheduling both pleasurable and avoided tasks and monitoring moods (Beck). It is also beneficial for challenging beliefs ("There isn't anything that I enjoy doing," "I'm not good at doing anything") (Beck, Rush, Shaw, & Emery, 1979). See Box 15-6 for an example of CBT research.

■ CONCLUSION

The simple idea that emotion and behaviour are influenced by cognition has generated decades of empirical study, which indicates that CBT is a highly effective and cost-efficient treatment for individuals struggling with certain mental disorders. The active and collaborative nature of CBT, combined with its orientation toward change, makes it an easy fit with nursing, as is evidenced by the interest and broad appeal of CBT among nurses. Psychiatric and mental health nurses are strong advocates of self-reflection and awareness of how one's own experiences influence the therapeutic relationship. With appropriate training, nurses will find CBT to be useful to their therapeutic repertoire. CBT offers an empirically and theoretically sound means to improve the mental health of their clients.

SUMMARY OF KEY POINTS

◻ The cognitive model is based on the idea that the way we think about situations influences our emotion and behaviour.

◻ Cognitive-behavioural therapy (CBT) is based on changing negative thought patterns as a means to improve mood and behaviour.

◻ CBT is the most widely researched form of psychotherapy used to treat many mental disorders, including posttraumatic stress disorder, bulimia nervosa, panic disorder, and depression.

◻ There are 10 principles of cognitive-behavioural therapy: cognitive-behavioural formulation; strong therapeutic alliance; time limited and brief; goal oriented, problem focused, and change oriented; structured and directive; educative; therapeutic collaboration; inductive reasoning; Socratic questioning; and self-reflective exercises.

◻ Cognitive techniques involve cognitive restructuring, a process that follows the steps of identifying, analyzing, and modifying automatic thoughts through to core beliefs.

◻ Behavioural techniques are used within the cognitive model and are seen as opportunities to test new beliefs.

CRITICAL THINKING CHALLENGES

1 How would you explain the cognitive model to a fellow student with no previous knowledge of CBT? What aspects of the model do you think are most important to emphasize?

2 Think about an incident that you experienced in the past week that caused you mild upset. Using the cognitive model, how would you differentiate between various aspects of your experience?

3 Describe the differences and interplays between core beliefs and automatic thoughts. Are there automatic thoughts that you routinely experience?

4 How do thinking errors contribute to emotional distress?

5 Why are behavioural experiments an essential aspect of CBT?

6 How are the principles of CBT different from and similar to other forms of psychotherapy you have studied?

WEB LINKS

www.camh.net/ The Centre for Addiction and Mental Health website contains information about CBT programs and the like.

www.cognitivetherapynyc.com This is the website of the American Institute for Cognitive Therapy, a group of clinical psychologists and psychotherapists that provide CBT which was founded in 1985.

www.cognitivetherapy.com/basics.html This website is supervised by John Winston Bush, PhD of the New York Institute for Cognitive and Behavioural Therapies and contains basic information about cognitive therapy.

MOVIES, NOVELS, AND BIOGRAPHIES

The Matrix: 1999. This science fiction story stars Keanu Reeves as Thomas Anderson, a computer hacker who learns that human life on Earth is not what it seems. Humans like Thomas think that they are living at the end of the 20th century. The truth is that it is actually two centuries later, and the world has been taken over by forms of cyber intelligence. These machines exist by "farming" the energy of captured humans, placating them by manipulating their minds into believing they are leading ordinary lives. A few humans, led by Morpheus, know the truth, and they lead Thomas to reality and to a new identity as Neo, The One.

VIEWING POINTS: Consider the way in which this movie illustrates the power of the mind to create and shape our reality and thus our actions. How difficult is it for Thomas to change his ideas about his life? Relate the premise of this movie to the assumptions underlying cognitive-behavioural theory.

REFERENCES

American Psychiatric Association. (1998). *Practice guidelines for the treatment of panic disorder.* Arlington, VA: American Psychiatric Publishing.

Antony, M. M., & Swinson, R. P. (2000). *Phobic disorders and panic in adults: A guide to assessment and treatment.* Washington, DC: American Psychological Association.

Ashbaugh, A., Anthony, M., Liss, A., Summerfeldt, L., McCabe, R., & Swinson, R. (2007). Changes in perfectionism following cognitive-behavioral treatment for social phobias. *Depression & Anxiety, 24,* 169–177.

Beck, J. (1995). *Cognitive therapy: Basics and beyond.* New York, NY: Guilford Press.

Beck, A. T., & Emery, G. (1985). *Anxiety disorders and phobias: A cognitive perspective.* New York, NY: Basic Books.

Beck, A. T., Rush, A. J., Shaw, B. F., & Emery, G. (1979). *Cognitive therapy of depression.* New York, NY: Guilford Press.

Bennett-Levy, J. (2003). Mechanisms of change in cognitive therapy: The case of automatic thought records and behavioural experiments. *Behavioural and Cognitive Psychotherapy, 31,* 261–277.

Bennett-Levy, J., Westbrook D., Fennell, M, Cooper, M., Rouf, K., & Hackmann, A. (2004). Behavioural experiments: Historical and conceptual underpinnings. In J. Bennett-Levy, G. Butler, M. Fennell, A. Hackmann, M. Mueller, & D. Westbrook (Eds.), *Oxford guide to behavioural experiments in cognitive therapy* (pp. 1–20). Oxford, UK: Oxford University Press.

Burns, D. D. (1980). *Feeling good: The new mood therapy.* New York, NY: Morrow.

Burns, D. D. (1989). *The feeling good handbook: Using the new mood therapy in everyday life.* New York, NY: Morrow.

Clark, D. M. (1998). Anxiety states: Panic and generalized anxiety. In K. Hawton, P. M. Salkovskis, J. Kirk, & D. M. Clark (Eds.), *Cognitive behaviour therapy for psychiatric problems* (pp. 52–96). Oxford, UK: Oxford University Press.

Erman, M. (2008). Cognitive behavior therapy for insomnia: Can I incorporate it into my practice? *Primary Psychiatry, 15*(3), 35–37.

Fennell, M. J. V. (1989). Depression. In K. Hawton, P. M. Salkovskis, J. Kirk, & D. M. Clark (Eds.), *Cognitive behaviour therapy for psychiatric problems* (pp. 169–234). Oxford, UK: Oxford University Press.

Foa, E. B., & Rothbaum, B. O. (1998). *Treating the trauma of rape: Cognitive behavioral therapy for PTSD.* New York, NY: Guilford Press.

Greenberger, D., & Padesky, C. A. (1995). *Mind over mood.* New York, NY: Guilford Press.

Heimberg, R. G., & Becker, R. E. (2002). *Cognitive-behavioral group therapy for social phobia.* New York, NY: Guilford Press.

Hendriks, G., Oude Voshaar, R., Keijsers, G., Hoogduin, C., & van Balkom, A. (2008). Cognitive-behavioural therapy for late-life anxiety disorders: A systemic review and meta-analysis. *Acta Psychiatrica Scandinavica, 117,* 403–411.

Hofmann, S. (2007). Cognitive factors that maintain social anxiety disorder: A comprehensive model and its treatment implications. *Cognitive Behaviour Therapy, 36*(4), 193–209.

Hollon, S., & Kriss, M. (1984). Cognitive factors in clinical research and practice. *Clinical Psychology Review, 4,* 35–76.

Ingram, R. E., Miranda, J., & Segal, Z. V. (1998). *Cognitive vulnerability to depression.* New York, NY: Guilford Press.

Jacobson, E. (1938). *Progressive relaxation.* Chicago, IL: University of Chicago Press.

Kaplan, H. I., Sadock, B. J., & Grebb, J. A. (1994). *Kaplan and Sadock's synopsis of psychiatry: Behavioral sciences, clinical psychiatry.* Baltimore, MD: Williams & Wilkins.

Kazantzis, N., Deane, F. P., & Ronan, K. R. (2000). Homework assignments in cognitive and behavioral therapy: A meta-analysis. *Clinical Psychology: Science & Practice, 7,* 189–202.

Kuyken, W., Dalgleish, T., & Holden, E. (2007). Advances in cognitive-behavioural therapy for uni-polar depression. *The Canadian Journal of Psychiatry, 52*(1), 5–13.

Myhr, G., Talbot, J., Annable, L., & Pinard, G. (2007). Suitability for short-term cognitive-behavioral therapy. *Journal of Cognitive Psychotherapy: An International Quarterly, 21*(4), 334–345.

Needleman, L. D. (1999). *Cognitive case conceptualization.* Mahwah, NJ: Lawrence Erlbaum.

Ruwaard, J., Lange, A., Bouwman, M., Broeksteeg, J., & Schrieken, B. (2007). E-mailed standardized cognitive behavioural treatment of work-related stress: A randomized controlled trial. *Cognitive Behaviour Therapy, 36*(3), 179–192.

Safran, J., Segal, Z., Shaw, B., & Vallis, T. (1990). Patient selection for short-term cognitive therapy. In J. D. Afran & Z. Segal (Eds.), *Interpersonal process in cognitive therapy* (pp. 236–247). New York, NY: Basic Books.

Sperry, L. (1999). Cognitive *behavior therapy of DSM-IV personality disorders.* Philadelphia, PA: Brunner/Mazel.

Straube, T., Glauer, M., Dilger, S., Mentzel, H-J., & Miltner, W. (2006). Effects of cognitive-behavioral therapy on brain activation in specific phobia. *NeuroImage, 29,* 125–135.

Swinson, R. P., Antony, M. M., Rachman, S., & Richter, M. A. (Eds.). (1998). *Obsessive compulsive disorder: Theory, research, and treatment.* New York, NY: Guilford Press.

Taylor, S. (2000). *Understanding and treating panic disorder: Cognitive and behavioral approaches.* New York, NY: Wiley.

Tillfors, M., Carlbring, P., Furmark, T., Lewenhaupt, S., Spak, M., Eriksson, A., et al. (2008). Treating university students with social phobia and public speaking fears: Internet delivered self-help with or without live group exposure sessions. *Depression and Anxiety, 25,* 708–717.

Tully, T. L. (2005). The development and pilot testing of a cognitive-behavioural group psychotherapy intervention for women with a history of childhood sexual abuse who engage in self-injury (Doctoral dissertation, University of Toronto, 2003). *Dissertation Abstracts International 66/06,* 3064.

Wells, A. (1997). *Cognitive therapy of anxiety disorders.* Chichester, UK: John Wiley & Sons.

CHAPTER 16

Interventions With Groups

Carol Ewashen

Adapted from the chapter "Interventions with Groups" by Mary Ann Boyd

LEARNING OBJECTIVES

After studying this chapter, you will be able to:

- Discuss group concepts that are useful in understanding and leading groups.
- Compare the different roles and responsibilities of group members.
- Identify the important aspects of leading a group, such as member selection, leadership skills, seating arrangements, and ways of dealing with challenging group members.
- Differentiate types of groups: psychoeducational, cognitive-behavioural therapy, supportive therapy, psychotherapy, and self-help.
- Compare different nursing intervention groups.

KEY CONCEPTS

- group
- group process

KEY TERMS

• closed group • formal group roles • group • group cohesion • group dynamics • group leadership • groupthink • informal group roles • interactive groups • leadership styles • maintenance functions • open group • self-help groups • structured groups • task functions • therapeutic factors

*P*articipation in therapeutic groups has powerful treatment effects. Group treatment is effective and efficient for patients to further understand themselves in relation to others through interaction, gain new knowledge and social skills, conquer unwanted thoughts and feelings, and change behaviour. For effective interventions, the nurse must possess leadership skills that can shape, enhance, and monitor group interactions. The decisions regarding which interventions fit best are complex and dependent upon the purpose of the group. Competent group skill development for the psychiatric and mental health (PMH) nurse requires the ability to critically select and modify techniques to best accommodate the particular practice conditions. This applies across diverse situations from providing patient education or conducting support groups to direct care provision, case management, and unit leadership. Understanding group skills and dynamics is also increasingly relevant to contemporary health care service delivery with emphasis on effective interprofessional practice collaboration and

teamwork. A challenge in group intervention is the shift from a primarily individual focus to a consideration of interpersonal and whole-group interactions. This chapter presents relevant group concepts for PMH nurses. **Group leadership** is explored with special emphasis on the groups relevant to PMH nursing practice.

GROUP: DEFINITIONS AND CONCEPTS

There are many different definitions of a group. Psychoanalytic tradition draws from the work of Sigmund Freud and considers group interaction as a recapitulation of the family of origin, interpreting unconscious conflicts, and reexamining them. Contemporary psychodynamic theories consider groups a combination of group dynamics and interpersonal and intrapsychic transactions (Rutan & Stone, 2001). Yalom (1983, 1998) and Yalom and Leszcz (2005) suggest that a group is a social microcosm of interpersonal dynamics and advocates a here-and-now, self-reflective approach. The cognitive-behavioural approach considers a group a social arena for corrective change in maladaptive thinking and behaviour patterns; whereas, according to systems theory, a group consists of parts or components that exist to perform some activity or purpose. As group members interact, subsystems form challenging leaders to understand boundary realignments and the effects of subcomponents on the system and to improve interpersonal communication. A global, but rather simple, definition of a group is two or more people who are in an interdependent relationship with one another. The simplicity of the definition is misleading because interactions within groups, or **group dynamics**, are anything but simple. Group dynamics influence the group's development and process. In fact, it takes an astute observer to determine the real dynamics of a group and the effects. No matter the type of group, its theoretic orientation, or its purpose, group dynamics influence the effectiveness of a group intervention.

In this text, a **group** is defined as "a social system with structure, norms, and usual ways of doing things" (Dimock & Devine, 1994, p. 54). Groups can be further defined according to the number of people or the relationship of members. A *dyad* is a group of two people, such as a married couple, siblings, or parent and child. A *triad* is a group of three people. A family is a special type of group and is discussed in Chapter 17.

 KEY CONCEPT A **group** is "a social system with structure, norms, and usual ways of doing things." (Dimock & Devine, 1994, p. 54).

Open Versus Closed Groups

A group can be viewed as either an open or a closed system. In an **open group**, new members are welcomed and provided time to learn group norms and expectations. For example, a newly admitted patient may join an anger management group that is part of an ongoing program in an inpatient unit. With new members, it is important to help them engage with the group by inviting member-to-member interaction. The advantage of an open group is that participants can join at any time. In addition, these groups can function on an ongoing basis and thus can be available to more people.

In a **closed group**, members begin the group at one time, and no new members are admitted. If a member of a closed group leaves, no replacement joins. Advantages of a closed group are that the participants get to know one another at the same time, the group is more cohesive, and members move through the group process concurrently. However, implementing closed-group interventions is often difficult, especially in tertiary settings, because patients are not always available at the same time.

Group Size

Group size is an important consideration in forming group programs. Many mental health professionals favour small groups, but large groups can also be effective. Whether to form a large or small group depends on the purpose, abilities, and availability of the participants and the skills of the leader. Small groups (usually no more than 8 to 10 members) become more cohesive, are less likely to form subgroups, and can provide a richer interpersonal experience than large groups. Small groups may function with one group leader, although many small groups are led by two people. An ideal small group is about seven to eight people in addition to the leader or leaders (Yalom & Leszcz, 2005).

CRNENOTE

The size of a group will depend on the overall patient goals and abilities. Patients with challenging behaviours should be carefully screened and assigned to smaller groups.

Small groups often are used for patients who are trying to deal with complex emotional issues, such as depression, anxiety, sexual abuse, eating disorders, or trauma. They are also ideal for individuals who require more individualized intervention. These groups work best if they are closed to new members or if new members are gradually introduced. One disadvantage of small groups relates to the loss of members. If places are unfilled, the group's dynamics change, which may interfere with the therapeutic process.

A large group (more than 10 members) can also be therapeutic as well as cost-effective in clinical settings. Some research suggests that large treatment groups are effective for specific problems, such as smoking, or settings, such as the workplace (Moher, Hey, & Lancaster, 2005). A large group can be ongoing and open-ended. In large group intervention, a challenge for the nurse leader is to include all members in discussion, preventing a sense of alienation with the potential for member dropout.

Leading a group, whether large or small, is complex because of the number of potential interactions, relationships, and conflicts that can form. The leader needs both presentation and group leadership skills. Posthuma (2001) suggests that it is insufficient to be purely a leader—a leader must practice in a therapeutic or facilitative manner. Practitioners who take on *leadership* of groups require education and training for competent, accountable group practices. In large groups, the leader is often both a presenter of educative information and a facilitator of experiential learning among participants. In-depth reflection on participants' feelings and thoughts may not be the focus of group work. Depending on the theoretic orientation and the purpose of the group, leadership style and interventions must change to be effective in meeting the goals of small or large groups.

Group Development

In the same way that the development of the therapeutic relationship is a process (see Chapter 9), so is the development of a group. Many researchers view group development as a sequence of phases, particularly in small groups (Table 16-1). Although models of group development differ, most follow a pattern of a beginning, middle, and ending stage (Alvarez, 2002). These stages should be thought of not as a straight line with one preceding another, but as a dynamic process that is constantly revisiting and reexamining group interactions and behaviours as well as progressing forward.

KEY CONCEPT Group process is the "what is happening" in the group, how members are interacting and relating as individuals and as a whole group, including nonverbal communications.

Beginning Stage

When a group begins, group members get to know one another and the group leader. The length of the beginning stage depends on, among other variables, the purpose of the group, the number of members, and the skill of the leader. It may last for only a few sessions or several. "Honeymoon" behaviour characterizes this stage in the beginning, but "conflict" dominates at the end. During the initial sessions, members usually display polite, congenial behaviour typical of those in new social situations. They are "good patients" and often intellectualize their problems; that is, these patients deal with emotional conflict or stress by excessively using abstract thinking or generalizations to minimize disturbing feelings. Members are usually anxious and sometimes display

behaviour that does not truly represent their feelings. In the first few sessions, members test whether they can trust one another. Sometime after the initial sessions, group members usually experience a period of conflict, either among themselves or with the leader. This conflict is a normal part of group development, and many believe that negotiating conflict satisfactorily is necessary to move into a productive working phase. Sometimes, one or more group members become the scapegoat. Such situations challenge the leader to guide the group during this period by avoiding taking sides and treating all members respectfully.

Middle (Working) Stage

The middle, or working, stage of groups involves a real sharing of ideas and the development of closeness. A group-as-a-whole culture may emerge that is distinct from the individual personalities of its members. The group develops its own rules and rituals and has its own behavioural norms—for example, groups develop regular patterns of seating and interaction. During this stage, the group realizes its purpose. If the purpose is education, the participants engage in learning new content or skills. If the aim of the group is to share feelings and experiences, these activities consume group meetings. During this stage, the group starts on time, and the leader often needs to remind members when it is time to stop.

Ending (Termination) Stage

Ending or termination can be difficult for a group, especially a successful therapeutic one. During the final stages, members begin to separate and may grieve for the loss of the group's closeness and begin to reestablish themselves as individuals. Individuals terminate from groups as they do from any relationship (see Chapter 9). One person may

Table 16.1 Comparison of Models of Group Development		
Tuckman (1965)	**Garland, Jones, and Kolodny (1973)**	**Corey and Corey (2006)**
Forming: Get to know one another and form a group	*Theme in all stages*: Closeness *Preaffiliation*: Approach and avoidance; ambivalence around involvement	*Pregroup Forming*: Preparing for and deciding if this is the right group
Storming: Tension and conflict occur; subgroups form and clash with each other	*Power and Control*: Testing out and vying for status, authority, autonomy, influence and connection	*Initial Stage*: Orienting; forming relations; establishing group structure and climate of trust
Norming: Develop norms for how to work with each other	*Intimacy*: More intense personal involvement and recognition of others; emergent growth	*Transition*: Emerging differences and potential for conflict
Performing: Reach consensus and develop cooperative relationships	*Differentiation*: Accept uniqueness of each with interdependence; cohesion	*Working*: Involved, interactive, and committed to engaging in productive group work
Adjourning: End of relationships and orientation to the future; sadness and appreciation	*Separation*: Moving apart; review and evaluation	*Final Stage*: Consolidation of learning; sadness and anxiety with leaving

not show up at the last session, another person may bring up issues that the group has already addressed, and others may demonstrate anger or hostility. Most members of successful groups are sad as the group terminates. During the last meetings, members may make arrangements for meeting after the group ends. These plans rarely materialize or continue. Leaders should recognize these plans as part of the farewell process—saying good-bye to the group.

Roles of Group Members

There are two **formal group roles**, the leader and the members. In small groups, however, members often assume **informal group roles** or positions in the group with rights and duties that are directed toward one or more group members. Informal roles can be categorized as task, maintenance, or individual roles. One way to think of group roles is as the different hats members try on and learn from while involved in a group (Benne & Sheats, 1948; Myers & Anderson, 2008). These roles can either help or hinder the group's process.

Task functions involve the business of the group or "keeping things focused." Individuals who provide this function keep the group focused on a main purpose. For any group to be successful, it must have members who assume some of these task roles, such as *information seeker* (asks for clarification), *coordinator* (spells out relationships between ideas), and *recorder* (keeper of the minutes). **Maintenance functions** help the group stay together by ensuring it starts on time, assisting individuals to compromise, and determining membership. These individuals are interested in maintaining group cohesiveness and may have difficulty with group conflict and differentiation. The *harmonizer* (keeps the peace), *compromiser* (gives and takes), and *standard setter* (sets expectations) are examples of maintenance roles. In a successful group, members take on and learn from both group task and maintenance functions (Table 16-2). Leader and member responsibilities and functions shift depending upon the group stage and task.

Individual roles are those member roles that enhance or detract from group functioning. These roles may detract from the group purpose and cohesion; for example, someone who monopolizes the group conversation inhibits group interaction and work on task. When individual roles dominate, the risk is that neither the group task nor group maintenance is accomplished.

In selecting members and analyzing group progress, the leader must pay attention to the dynamic among task and maintenance functions. If too many group members assume task functions and too few assume maintenance functions, the group may have difficulty developing cohesion. If too many members assume maintenance functions, the group may never finish its work. It is important for the leader to track the group functions including how much actually gets done.

Group Communication

One of the responsibilities of *group leadership* is to facilitate both verbal and nonverbal communication to meet the treatment goals of the individual members and the entire group. Because of the number of people involved, developing trusting relationships within groups is more complicated than is developing a single relationship with a patient. The communication techniques used in establishing and maintaining individual relationships are similar for groups, but the leader also attends to the communication patterns among the members.

Verbal Communication

Group interaction can be viewed as a communication network that becomes patterned and predictable. In a group, verbal comments are linked in a chain formation.

Communication Network

Asking a colleague to observe and record the content and interaction is a useful technique in determining the interaction pattern within a group; the leader may also use an audio or video recorder. In some groups, one person may always change the subject when another raises a sensitive topic. One person may always speak after another. People who sit next to each other tend to communicate among themselves. By analyzing the content and patterns, the leader can determine the existence of communication pathways—who is most liked in the group, who occupies a position of power, what subgroups have formed, and who is isolated from the group. Burtis and Turman's (2006) network analysis for group discussion provides a way to diagram connections amongst members and to identify stars, isolates, and overchosen and underchosen group members. Usually, those who are well liked or display leadership abilities tend to be chosen for interactions more often than do those who are less well liked (Fig. 16-1). In one study of communication networks, members who exhibited more dominant behaviours or who the group perceived as being dominant emerged as more central to the group's communication networks and both sent and received more messages. The study also found that the task at hand affects the communication network. Groups that worked on low-complexity tasks had more centralized communication than when they worked on high-complexity tasks (Brown & Miller, 2000).

Group Themes

Group themes are the collective socio-emotional and conceptual underpinnings of a group and express the

Table 16.2   Leader and Member Responsibilities and Functions

Group Stage	Leader	Member
Pregroup: Formation of a group *Informed decision making*: How does this group fit with this member this purpose?	*Design and plan the group*: Purpose, structure, process, evaluation methods. Solicit group membership. Conduct pregroup screening interviews. Determine the group composition. Provide orientation to members.	To determine: Is the group right for me? Do I have enough knowledge to understand the group purpose and process? What do I want from the group experience? How do my expectations fit with the group expectations?
Initial Stage Orientation, exploration, and setting the structure of the group Creating a safe place Sharing information Engaging each other and as a whole group around purpose	Orient group members. Establish ground rules, norms, and expectations. Encourage all members to be involved and express expectations, reactions, and concerns. Clarify understandings. Be open with members' concerns and questions. Provide guidance yet encourage member interaction and initiative.	To work through: Will I be accepted? What will the leader think of me? What is expected of me? Establish trust. Form relations with others. Express thoughts, feelings, expectations, and reservations. Become involved. Set goals for self and self-in-relation to others. Be respectful of others. Learn well and share understandings.
Transition Increased anxiety and emergence of differences with potential for conflict Reluctance to voice concerns or frustrations	Teach members the value of recognizing conflict, naming the issue, and negotiating a win-win situation. Practice directness and tactfulness in naming issues in the here and now. Encourage members to share reactions while maintaining a safe environment. Intervene with sensitivity and prevent scapegoating of a particular member. Encourage participatory interaction. Reinforce learning of self in relation to others negotiating difference/conflict in group.	Recognize own defences and resistances. Recognize and express reactions to the group. Learn to constructively confront issues. Work through conflicts and differences rather than withdraw or form subgroups.
Working High trust High group cohesion High productivity Interactive with willingness to take risks Supportive hopeful climate	Exemplify caring confrontation, disclosure of issues, support to others. Encourage member risk taking. Interpret meanings of behaviours and interpersonal patterns in group. Explore group themes. Encourage translating insight into action in daily living.	Practice openness with issues. Offer feedback to others. Practice new skills and behaviours in daily life. Initiate constructive challenge and support to others. Initiate active involvement with others.
Final Stage Saying good-byes Reflection on learning, relations, changes made, and challenges ahead	Encourage saying of good-byes to each other. Provide opportunity for members to provide feedback to each other. Reinforce changes made. Ensure members have the resources to enable further progress. Reemphasize the importance of confidentiality.	Acknowledge thoughts and feelings with leaving the group. Say good-bye to each member and to the leader. Review gains made and complete unfinished business. Evaluate the impact of the group. Plan for the future.

Adapted from Corey, M., & Corey, G. (2006). *Groups: Process and practice* (7th ed.). Toronto, ON: Thomson Brooks/Cole.

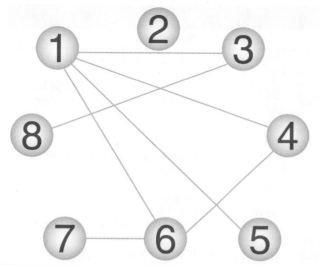

FIGURE 16.1 Network analysis of group discussion. In this analysis, response pattern was recorded during member interaction. Group members interacted with number 1 the most. Therefore, number 1 is the overchosen person. Numbers 5 and 7 are underchosen. Number 2 is never chosen and is determined to be the isolate.

members' underlying concerns or feelings, regardless of the group's purpose. Themes that emerge in groups help members to understand group dynamics. Different groups have different themes. For example, three themes emerged for a support group for grieving children, including vulnerability, the importance of maintaining memories, and the contribution of the group to the process of grieving (Graham & Sontag, 2001). Although some predictable themes occur in groups, the obvious or assumed themes at the beginning may actually wind up differing as the process continues. In one hospice support group, the members seemed to be focusing on the memories of their loved ones. However, upon closer examination of the thematic content of group interactions, the discussion was revolving around financial planning for the future.

Nonverbal Communication

Nonverbal communication is important to understanding group behaviour. All members, not just the group leader, observe the eye contact, posture, and body gestures of the participants. What is expressed is the result of individual and group, as well as internal and external, processes. For example, if one member is explaining a painful experience and another member looks away and tries to engage still another, the self-disclosing member may feel devalued and rejected because he or she interprets the disruptive behaviour as disinterest. However, if the leader interprets the disruptive behaviour as anxiety over the topic, he or she may try to engage the other member in discussing the source of the anxiety.

The leaders should remain attune to the nonverbal behaviour of group members during each session and the effect on group climate and process. Often, one or two people can set the overall mood of the group. Someone who comes to a session very sad or angry can set a tone of sadness or anger for the whole group. An astute group leader recognizes the effects of an individual's mood on the total group. If the purpose of the group is to deal with emotions, the group leader may invite the member to discuss emotional issues at the beginning of the session. The leader thus acknowledges the mood of the one person experiencing it and encourages discussion regarding the effect on other group members. If the group's purpose is inconsistent with self-disclosure of personal problems, the nurse should acknowledge the individual member's distress yet set limits while maintaining the group focus. In this instance, the nurse would limit repeated episodes of self-disclosure from that member or others and redirect discussion to the group task.

Group Norms and Standards

Groups develop norms or rules and standards that establish acceptable group behaviours. Some norms are formalized, such as beginning group on time, but others are never really formalized. These standards encourage conformity of behaviour among group members. The group discourages deviations from these established norms. A group member has four options in relation to norms: conform, change the norm, be deviant, or leave the group (Posthuma, 2001). Open discussion that encourages healthy interacting while addressing unhelpful or problematic behaviours is one of the most successful ways of renegotiating group norms. *Leadership* is critical in establishing group norms consistent with the group goals to effect desired changes.

Group Cohesion

One of the goals of most group leaders is to foster **group cohesion**, a sense of "we-ness" as a group, with high levels of participation and involvement among members. Group cohesion is analogous to the therapeutic alliance in one-to-one relationships (MacKenzie, 1997). One of the first tasks of a good leader is to develop group cohesion through engaging all members in the group process. This involves close monitoring of the group climate or atmosphere to develop a sense of belonging and commitment to the group goals. A particularly effective intervention for enhancing group cohesion is encouraging member-to-member interaction. In supportive and educational groups, leaders can promote social interaction with minimal supervision through organizing refreshment periods and team-building exercises. Cohesiveness is especially important in health education groups that focus on health maintenance behaviours such as exercise and weight control. These groups typically have high dropout rates, but members are more likely to attend when a group is cohesive (Annesi, 1999).

Dimock and Devine (1994) state that cohesion is like the glue that holds the group together and that if cohesion decreases, the group may begin to fall apart. Cohesion is a powerful force that motivates members and correlates with outcomes. In cohesive groups, members are committed to the existence of the group. In large heterogeneous groups, cohesiveness tends to be decreased, with subsequent decreased performance among group members in completing tasks. When members are strongly committed to completing a task and the leader encourages equal participation, cohesiveness promotes job satisfaction and higher performance (Steinhardt, Dolbier, Gottlieb, & McCalister, 2003). However, cohesiveness can be a double-edged sword. In very cohesive groups, members are more likely to transgress personal boundaries. Too much cohesiveness can exert powerful social pressure to conform to group standards with low tolerance for difference, while too little cohesiveness can result in mistrust, lack of engagement, and eventual disbanding of the group.

Groupthink and Decision Making

Groups that are strong and healthy encourage creativity, risk taking, and change while remaining respectful of all members. Healthy groups encourage conformity to group norms and standards while remaining respectful of each member's unique contributions. In a healthy group, conformity to group norms does not mean uniformity of member behaviour because a cohesive group is both productive and constructive (Dimock & Devine, 1994). However, if feelings of unity become too intense and members are overly invested in maintaining the status quo, a phenomenon of groupthink can occur (Kurtz, 1992). **Groupthink** is the tendency of many groups to avoid conflict, maintain cohesion, and adopt a closed-minded thinking that is often consistent with the ideas of the impartial group leader (Janis, 1982; Myers & Anderson, 2008). In groupthink, striving for unanimity overrides realistic, fair and just appraisal of alternative courses of action. Members may not give honest feedback to each other for fear of censure. Many catastrophes, such as the *Challenger* explosion, the Bay of Pigs invasion, and the Enron scandal, have been attributed to groupthink, but the empiric evidence of groupthink's negative implications in organizations is small. Studies have shown that a closed *leadership* style and an external threat, particularly time pressure, appear to promote symptoms of groupthink and defective decision making (Neck & Moorhead, 1995). The relationship between cohesiveness and groupthink is still inconclusive. In one study, groupthink was positively associated with group activities and team performance and negatively associated with concurrence (pressure for everyone to agree) and defective decision making (Choi & Kim, 1999).

Nurse leaders are responsible for mobilizing **therapeutic factors** to support healthy group development and prevent a stagnating groupthink. Which factors to mobilize and when depend on the type, purpose, and developmental stage of the group. Supportive factors often emerge spontaneously and include universality, altruism, hope, and acceptance (MacKenzie, 1997). Other **therapeutic factors** proposed by Yalom and Leszcz (2005) are imparting information, corrective recapitulation of the primary family group, development of socializing techniques, imitative behaviours, catharsis, existential factors, cohesiveness, and interpersonal learning (Box 16-1).

GROUP LEADERSHIP

In the beginning stage of a group, the group leader establishes the presence of each member; constructs a working environment; builds a working relationship with the group and among participants; and clarifies outcomes, processes, and skills related to the group's purpose (Alf & Wilson, 2001). While attempting to understand the group process, the leader must also consider when and how to participate. Depending on the purpose of the group and the stage of development, the leader position shifts, for example, from a primarily supportive role to educative with provision of information to interpretive of group dynamics. The leader reflects on, evaluates, and responds to promote effective group work. Leader intervention skills include attention to process while considering timing of interventions, when to clarify and when to interpret, when to intervene at the individual level, and when to intervene at the whole-group level. The use of various techniques enhances the leader's ability to lead the group effectively and to help the group meet its goals (Table 16-3).

One of the most important *leadership* skills is listening. A leader who practices active listening provides group members with someone who is responsive to what they say. A group leader who listens also models listening behaviour for others, helping them improve their skills. Listening enables the leader to process events and track interactions. The leader should be able to listen to the group members and formulate responses based on an understanding of the discussion. Members may need to learn to listen to one another, track discussions without changing the subject, and not speak while others are talking.

BOX 16.1

Research for Best Practice: Using the CORE-R Battery to Improve Group Practices

From Burlingame, G., Strauss, B., Joyce, A. S., MacNair-Semands, R., MacKenzie, R., Ogrodniczuk, J., et al. (2005). The American Group Psychotherapy Association's CORE Battery – Revised (CORE-R). *Draft report submitted at the 62nd Annual meeting of the AGPA, New York City, March 7–12, 2005.*

THE PROJECT: Collaborative project (Humboldt Foundation and the American Group Psychotherapy Association Research Special Interest Group) with the aim to revise and update the AGPA CORE battery (Clinical Outcomes Results Standardized measures), to develop clinically useful measures sensitive to patient change, to graph patient change, and to provide immediate feedback on patient status.

QUESTIONS: Does this group treatment work for this diagnostic category? What group treatment components are most important? Is this treatment working for this patient?

METHOD: Extensive review and metasynthesis of group literature from an empirical and a clinical perspective. The original CORE battery as well as AGPA Roy MacKenzie and Gary Burlingame course on group process and outcome instruments were reviewed. The CORE-R battery, an international tool to measure group processes and outcomes, was developed.

FINDINGS: Meta-analysis indicates that empirically supported treatment techniques explain only 10% of patient improvement. The claim of superior outcomes on one treatment over another has little empirical support. Recommend evidence-based models coupled with patient-focused treatment that consider patient response and therapist variability. Specific areas addressed by the CORE-R battery include selection of patients for group; pregroup preparation; and an extensive, empirically validated selection of group process and outcome measures.

IMPLICATIONS FOR PRACTICE: Clinical uses of the CORE-R *process measures* include gauging the quality of the group therapeutic environment, frequent process assessments to clarify the nature of group development over time, clarifying process dimensions that may be absent or negatively affect individual participants or the group as a whole, and increasing awareness of group dynamics. Clinical use of CORE-R *outcome measures*: It supplements clinical judgment, expands patient communication through written and verbal involvement, and provides ongoing feedback to the group leader regarding how much change as well as clinically significant changes.

The leader tracks the verbal and nonverbal interactions throughout the group. Depending on the group's purpose, the leader may keep this information to himself or herself to understand the group process or may share the observations with the group. For example, if the purpose of the group is psychoeducational, the leader may use the information to facilitate the best learning environment. If the purpose of the group is to improve the self-awareness and interaction skills of members, the leader may point out the observations. The leader needs to be clear about the purpose of the group and tailor *leadership* strategies accordingly.

Understanding different group **leadership styles** can be useful in deciding which style fits which group situation. Often leaders have a dominant style that fits more comfortably with who they are; however, developing a repertoire of different styles offers a wider range of interventions. Regardless of style, a leader remains fair and respectful, avoiding favouritism and encouraging participation and involvement of all members with each other. Other important skills include providing everyone with an opportunity to contribute and respecting everyone's ideas. A leader must also consider the degree of neutrality warranted in each situation. In supportive and educative groups, leaders tend to be more expressive and interactive. A good rule of thumb in relation to leader self-disclosure is to consider whether the disclosure furthers the purposes of the group. A leader is responsible for understanding the intent and impact of leader self-disclosure on both individual members and the group as a whole.

Some generally accepted guidelines in leading groups include setting start and stop times, arranging for the introduction of new members, and listening while other people talk. Leaders should explain these rules at the first group meeting and reemphasize them at different points. A group should always begin at its scheduled time; otherwise, members who tend to be late will not change their behaviour, and those who are on time will resent waiting for the others. A group should also end on time. Members should understand from the beginning that either new people can attend without the group knowing about it or that the group will discuss the introduction of new members before their attendance. Whatever the group decides, the leader must also follow the rules.

Choosing Leadership Styles

A group is led within the context of the group leader's theoretic background and the group's purpose. For example, a leader with training in cognitive-behavioural therapy may focus on treating depression by asking members to think differently about situations, which in turn leads to feeling better. A leader with a psychodynamic orientation may focus on the feelings of depression by examining situations that generate the same feelings. Whatever the leader's theoretic background, leadership

Table 16.3	Techniques in Leading Groups	
Technique	**Purpose**	**Example**
Support: giving feedback that provides a climate of emotional support	Helps a person or group continue with ongoing activities Informs group about what the leader thinks is important Creates a climate for expressing unpopular ideas Helps the more quiet and fearful members speak up	"We really appreciate your sharing that experience with us. It sounds like it was quite painful."
Confrontation: challenging a participant (needs to be done in a supportive environment)	Helps individuals learn something about themselves Helps reduce some forms of disruptive behaviour Helps members deal more openly and directly with one another	"Tom, this is the third time that you have changed the subject when we have talked about spouse abuse. Is something going on?"
Advice and suggestions: sharing expertise and knowledge that the members do not have	Provides information that members can use once they have examined and evaluated it Helps focus group's task and goals	"The medication that you are taking may be causing you to be sleepy."
Summarizing: statements at the end of the session that highlight the session's discussion, any problem resolution, and unresolved problems	Provides continuity from one session to the next Brings to focus still-unresolved issues Organizes past in ways that clarify Brings to focus themes and patterns of interaction	"This session we discussed Sharon's medication problems, and she will be following up with her physicians."
Clarification: restatement of an interaction	Checks on the meanings of the interaction and communication Avoids faulty communication Facilitates focus on substantive issues rather than allowing members to be side tracked into misunderstandings	"What I heard you say was that you are feeling very sad right now. Is that correct?"
Probing and questioning: a technique for the experienced group leader that asks for more information	Helps members expand on what they were saying (when they are ready to) Gets at more extensive and wider range of information Invites members to explore their ideas in greater detail	"Could you tell us more about your relationship with your parents?"
Repeating, paraphrasing, highlighting: a simple act of repeating what was just said	Facilitates communication among group members Corrects inaccurate communication or emphasizes accurate communication	*Member*: "I forgot about my wife's birthday." *Leader*: "You forgot your wife's birthday."
Reflecting feelings: identifying feelings that are being expressed	Orients members to the feelings that may lie behind what is being said or done Helps members deal with issues they might otherwise avoid or miss	"You sound upset."
Reflecting behaviour: identifying behaviours that are occurring	Gives members an opportunity to see how their behaviour appears to others and to evaluate its consequences Helps members to understand others' perceptions and responses to them	"I notice that when the topic of sex is brought up, you look down and shift in your chair."

Adapted from Sampson, E., & Marthas, M. (1990). *Group process for the health professions* (p. 222–224). Albany, NY: Delmar.

behaviour can be viewed as a continuum from direct to indirect. In *direct leadership behaviour*, the leader is an authoritarian and controls the interaction by giving directions and information and allowing little discussion. The leader literally tells the members what to do. On the other end of the continuum is *indirect leadership*, a form of laissez-faire, where the leader primarily reflects the group members' discussion and offers little guidance or information to the group. Effective *group leadership* is flexible and considers the group task. The challenge of providing leadership is to give sufficient direction that the group can meet its goals and develop its own group process but enough freedom that members can make mistakes and recover from their thinking errors in a supportive, caring learning environment.

Selecting the Members

Individuals can self-refer or be referred to groups by treatment teams or clinicians. The leader is responsible for assessing the individual's suitability to the group. In instances when a new group is forming, the leader pre-plans, sets criteria for group membership, and invites members so that the group can be well functioning and successful. The leader should consider the following criteria when selecting members:

- Does the purpose of the group match the treatment goals of the potential member?
- Does the potential member have the social skills to function comfortably in the group?
- Can the potential member make a commitment to attending group meetings?

Arranging Seating

Spatial seating arrangements contribute to group comfort and interactive group communication. Over time, group members tend to sit in the same places. Where a person sits may offer different insights into group interaction. For example, those who consistently sit close to the group leader may desire power more so than those who sit far away, or those sitting closer to the leader may feel safer. Arranging a group in a circle with chairs comfortably close to one another without a table focuses group work on relations with each other and on communication. In therapeutic interactive groups, no one should sit outside the group, as this often indicates exclusion and/or resistance. If a table is necessary, a round table is preferable to a rectangular one which spatially identifies two distinct positions of power for those who sit at the ends.

Ideally, the session is held in a quiet, pleasant room with no distractions, adequate space, and the assurance of privacy and confidentiality. Holding a session in too large or too small a room may inhibit engaged communication and a sense of comfort.

Dealing With Challenging Group Behaviours

Behaviours problematic to the group task can occur in all groups. They can be challenging to the most experienced group leaders and frustrating to new leaders. In dealing with any problematic behaviour or situation, the leader must remember to support the integrity of the individual members and the group as a whole. It is important for the group leader to remember that challenging or deviant members may serve a function for the group and are not necessarily a negative influence (American Group Psychotherapy Association, 2007). This could include releasing uncomfortable tension, speaking the unspeakable, or deflecting anger.

Monopolizer

Some people tend to monopolize a group by constantly talking or interrupting others. This behaviour is common in the beginning stages of group formation and usually represents anxiety that the member displaying such behaviour is experiencing. Within a few sessions, this person usually relaxes and no longer attempts to monopolize the group. However, for some people, monopolizing discussions is part of their interpersonal style and will continue. Other group members usually find the behaviour mildly irritating in the beginning and extremely annoying as time passes. Members may drop out of the group to avoid that person. The leader needs to decide if, how, and when to intervene. The best case scenario is when savvy group members remind the monopolizer to let others speak. The leader can then support the group in reinforcing rules that allow everyone the opportunity to participate. However, the group often waits for the leader to act. There are a couple of ways to manage the situation. The leader can interrupt the monopolizer by acknowledging the member's contribution but redirecting the discussion to others, or the leader can become more directive and limit the discussion time per member.

"Yes, But…"

Some people have a patterned response to any suggestions from others. Initially, they agree with suggestions others offer them, but then they add "yes, but…" and give several reasons why the suggestions will not work for them. Leaders and members can easily identify this patterned response. In such situations, it is best to avoid problem solving for the member and encourage the person to develop his or her own solutions. The leader can role model problem-solving behaviour for the other members and encourage them to let the member develop a solution that would work specifically for him or her.

Disliked Member

In some groups, members clearly dislike one particular member. This situation can be challenging for the leader because it can result in considerable tension and conflict. This person could become the group scapegoat. Depending on the group structure and purpose, one solution may be to move the person to a better-matched group. Whether the person stays or leaves, the group leader must stay neutral and avoid displaying negative verbal and non-verbal behaviours that indicate that he or she too dislikes the group member or that he or she is displeased with the other members for their behaviour. Often, the group leader can manage the situation by showing respect for the disliked member and acknowledging his or her contribution. In some instances, getting supervision from a more experienced group leader is useful. Defusing the situation may be possible by using conflict resolution strategies and discussing the underlying issues.

Group Conflict

Most groups experience periods of conflict. It is the avoidance of conflict that is problematic for a group. It is important that conflicts be acknowledged and then the leader must decide how best to address the issues. Member-to-member conflict can be negotiated by using the conflict resolution process discussed in Chapter 13. Leader-to-member conflict is more complicated and often difficult for members to express because the leader has the hierarchical position of greater power. In this instance, the leader can use conflict resolution strategies, including encouraging members to directly express concerns, while remaining sensitive to the power differential. Group cohesion often increases as conflictual issues are effectively addressed.

▬▬ TYPES OF GROUPS

Different types of groups are identified by the group goals and interactive processes or dynamics. The group leader assumes responsibility for ensuring group processes are in keeping with the group goals. Not every type of group is a therapy group.

Structured Groups

Structured groups have an explicit structure predetermined by the group leader. These groups are often short-term, oriented to education, and focus on a specific theme such as smoking prevention, substance abuse prevention, stress management, self-esteem for children, and parenting skills. Group goals focus primarily on education, psychosocial skill development, and task completion.

Psychoeducational Groups

Psychoeducational groups are directed to specific concepts and teaching-learning aims. The process is primarily didactic with opportunity for questions, discussions, and activities related to the topic. The group leader primarily imparts information, promotes discussions, and facilitates experiential learning through structured activities. Psychoeducational groups include task groups that focus on completion of specific activities (e.g., planning a week's menu) and teaching groups that are used to enhance knowledge, improve skills, or solve problems. Other examples include medication groups, anger management groups, and stress management groups. Psychoeducational groups are formally planned, and members are purposefully selected. Members are asked to join specific groups because of the focus of the group. These groups are time limited and last for only a few sessions (Box 16-2).

BOX 16.2

Research for Best Practice: Psychoeducational Codependency Support Groups for Older Adults

From McInnis-Perry, G. J., & Good, J. M. (2006). A psychoeducational codependency support group for older adults who reside in the community: Friends supporting friends. Journal of Gerontological Nursing, 32, 32–42.

QUESTION: What are the benefits of a psychoeducational support group for older adults with codependency issues?

METHOD: To promote well-being and reduce adverse effects of codependency among older adults, a pilot psychoeducational codependency support group curriculum was developed by the authors. A convenience sample of 22 older adults (age 65 years and older) who resided in an eastern Canadian community participated in six 90-minute psychoeducational group sessions held over a 2-month period. Most were females (68%). All participants had a loved one with an addiction (82% an adult child; 18% a spouse). A pretest and posttest were administered. Irvin Yalom's (1998) Therapeutic Factors were used to evaluate the group process.

FINDINGS: Results indicated that older adults do benefit from a psychoeducational support group format. Twenty-one participants demonstrated positive change post group intervention. A majority improved on knowledge and learning of addictions, effective communication, and establishing healthy boundaries. Increased self-esteem, reduced personal isolation, and a reduction in codependency issues were seen. Some participants continued to struggle with finding ways to nurture self. Strengths of the group process included identification and support regarding the suffering of each in having an addicted family member, gain in information, the sharing of emotions, and the instillation of hope.

IMPLICATIONS FOR PRACTICE: Using a time-limited psychoeducational group model to promote self-care for older adults who live in a codependent relationship can be effective. Providing a supportive group environment in which life experiences and coping strategies are shared allows older adults to work through sensitive and painful issues while supporting each other. Considerations for future research include using a larger sample size, a more diverse group of seniors, and standardized pretest and posttest instruments.

Cognitive-Behavioural Groups

The leader in cognitive groups identifies specific distorted thought patterns as the focus of change, whereas in behavioural groups, the leader targets specific behaviours to be modified. Cognitive and behavioural interventions may be combined to offer cognitive-behavioural group interventions. Cognitive interventions aim to modify distortions in attitudes and beliefs about self, the situation, and the future. Behavioural interventions modify behavioural excess, such as overly aggressive or sexual behaviour; behavioural deficits, such as social isolation or extreme passivity; and behaviours interfering with living, such as phobias and panic attacks (see Chapter 15). Cognitive-behavioural groups are often very structured with homework expectations for members.

Interactive Groups

Interactive groups include counselling and therapy groups. They may be focused and short-term or long-term experiential. Although some structure is predetermined by the group leader, group work primarily emphasizes dynamic, interactive group processes to allow for personal and interpersonal growth through experiential teaching and learning. The group becomes a microcosm of society. Group goals focus on addressing personal and interpersonal problems in living as well as modifying and changing more long-standing maladaptive patterns of behaviour.

Supportive Therapy Groups

Supportive therapy groups are usually less intense than psychotherapy groups and focus on helping individuals cope with their illnesses and problems as well as build interpersonal connections. Implementing supportive therapy groups is one of the basic functions of the PMH nurse. In conducting this type of group, the nurse focuses on helping members cope with situations that are common for other group members. Counselling strategies are used. For example, a group of patients with bipolar illness, whose illness is stable, may discuss at a monthly meeting how to tell other people about the illness or how to cope with a family member who seems insensitive to the illness. Family caregivers of people with mental illnesses benefit from the support of the group as well as additional information about providing care for an ill family member.

Psychotherapy Groups

Groups that rely primarily on interpretive interventions are known as group psychotherapies. Psychotherapy groups differ depending on the theoretic perspective, including psychodynamic, interpersonal, and existential. These groups focus primarily on increasing cognitive and emotional insight as well as improving interpersonal relations to help members face their life situations. In group psychotherapy, "therapeutic change is an enormously complex process" (Yalom, 1998, p. 7). At times, these groups can be extremely intense. Psychotherapy groups provide an opportunity for members to examine and resolve psychological and interpersonal issues within a safe environment. Mental health specialists who have a minimum of a master's degree and are trained in group psychotherapy lead such groups. When providing nursing care, communication with the group therapist is important for continuity and collaboration of care.

Self-Help Groups

Self-help groups are led by lay people, often a mental health consumer who has experienced a specific problem or life crisis. These groups are generally structured, with supportive interaction among members. These groups do not explore psychodynamic issues in depth. Professionals usually do not attend these groups or serve as consultants. Alcoholics Anonymous, Overeaters Anonymous, and One Day at a Time (a grief group) are examples of self-help groups.

■ COMMON NURSING INTERVENTION GROUPS

Common intervention groups led by nurses include medication, symptom management, anger management, self-care, and reminiscence groups. In addition, nurses lead many other groups, including stress management, relaxation groups, and women's groups. The key, as a nurse, to being a good group leader is to critically select and modify group interventions to best accommodate the primary focus of therapeutic change in relation to the unique conditions of the clinical setting and the group membership (Garrick & Ewashen, 2001).

Medication Groups

Nurse-led medication groups are common in psychiatric nursing. Not all medication groups are alike, so the nurse must be clear regarding the purpose of each specific medication group (Box 16-3). A medication group can be used primarily to transmit information about medications, such as action, dosage, and side effects, or it can focus on issues related to medications, such as compliance, management of side effects, and lifestyle adjustments. Many nurses incorporate both perspectives.

Assessing a member's medication knowledge is important before he or she joins the group to determine what the individual would like to learn. People with mental

---

BOX 16.3

Medication Group Protocol

PURPOSE: Develop strategies that reinforce a self-medication routine.

DESCRIPTION: The medication group is an open, ongoing group that meets once a week to discuss topics germane to self-administration of medication. Members will not be asked to disclose the names of their medications.

MEMBER SELECTION: The group is open to any person taking medication for a mental illness or emotional problem who would like more information about the medication, side effects, and staying on a regimen. Referrals from mental health providers are encouraged. Each person will meet with the group leader before attending the group to determine if the group will meet the individual's learning needs.

STRUCTURE: Format is a small group, with no more than eight members and one PMH nurse group leader

facilitating a discussion about the issues. Topics are rotated.

TIME AND LOCATION: 2–3 PM, every Wednesday at the Mental Health Center

COST: No charge for attending

TOPICS:
- How Do I Know if My Medications are Working?
- Side Effect Management: Is it Worth it?
- Hints for Taking Medications Without Missing Doses!
- Health Problems that Medication Affects
- (Other topics will be developed to meet the needs of group members.)

EVALUATION: Short pretest and posttest for instructor's use only.

---

illness may have difficulty remembering new information, so assessment of cognitive abilities is important. Assessing attention span, memory, and problem-solving skills gives valuable information that nurses can use in designing the group. The nurse should determine the members' reading and writing skills to select effective patient education materials.

An ideal group is one in which all members use the same medication. In reality, this situation is rare. Usually, the group members use various medications. The nurse should know which medications each member is taking, but to avoid violating patient confidentiality, the nurse needs to be careful not to divulge that information to other patients. If group members choose, they can share the names of their medications with one another. A small-group format works best, and the more interaction, the better. Using a lecture method of teaching is less effective than involving the members in the learning process. The nurse should expose the members to various audio and visual educational materials, including workbooks, videotapes, and handouts. The nurse should ask members to write down information to help them remember and learn through various modes. Evaluation of the learning outcomes begins with the first class. Nurses can develop and give pretests and posttests, which in combination can measure learning outcomes.

Symptom Management Groups

Nurses often lead groups that focus on helping patients deal with a severe and persistent mental illness. Handling hallucinations, being socially appropriate, and staying motivated to complete activities of daily living are a few common topics. In symptom management groups,

members also learn when a symptom indicates that relapse is imminent and what to do about it. Within the context of a symptom management group, patients can learn how to avoid relapse.

Anger Management Groups

Anger management is another common topic for a nurse-led group, often in the inpatient setting. The purposes of an anger management group are to discuss the concept of anger, identify antecedents to aggressive behaviour, and develop new strategies to deal with anger other than verbal and physical aggression (see Chapter 36). The treatment team refers individuals with a history of being verbally and physically abusive, usually to family members, to these groups to help them better understand their emotions and behavioural responses. Impulsiveness and emotional lability are problems for many of the group members. Anger management usually includes a discussion of associated stressful situations, events that trigger anger, feelings about the situation, and unmet personal needs.

Self-Care Groups

Another common nurse-led psychiatric group is a self-care group. People with psychiatric illnesses often have self-care deficits and benefit from the structure that a group provides. These groups are challenging because members usually know how to perform these daily tasks (e.g., bathing, grooming, performing personal hygiene), but their illnesses cause them to lose the motivation to complete them. The leader not only reinforces the basic self-care skills but also, more importantly, helps identify strategies that can motivate the patients and provide structure to their daily lives.

Reminiscence Groups

Reminiscence therapy has been shown to be a valuable intervention for older adults. In this type of group, members are encouraged to remember events from past years. Such a group is easily implemented. Usually, a simple question about an important family event will spark memories. Reminiscence groups are usually associated with people who have dementia and are having difficulty with recent memory. Recalling distant memories is comforting to older people and improves well-being. Reminiscence groups can also be used in caring for people with depression (Jones & Beck-Little, 2002) and in conjunction with cognitive therapy for affective symptoms in older adults (Puentes, 2004).

SUMMARY OF KEY POINTS

☐ The definition of group can vary according to theoretic orientation. A general definition of group is "a social system with structure, norms, and usual ways of doing things" (Dimock & Devine, 1994, p. 54). Group dynamics are the interactions within a group that constitute group development and process.

☐ Groups can be *open*, with every session available to new membership, or *closed*, with membership determined at the first session. Leading a group, whether small or large, is complex because dynamics change depending on different sizes of groups and clinical conditions.

☐ The group development process occurs in stages: beginning, middle (working), and ending (termination). These stages are not fixed but dynamic. Each stage challenges the leader to intervene in different ways. Success at the beginning stage prepares the group to take responsibility for addressing its purpose during the middle (working) stage.

☐ Although there are only two formal group roles, leader and member, there are many informal group roles. These roles are usually categorized according to purpose—task functions, maintenance functions, and individual roles. Members who assume task functions encourage the group members to stay focused on the group's task. Those who assume maintenance functions concern themselves more with the group working together than the actual task itself. Individual roles can either enhance or detract from the work of the group.

☐ Verbal communication includes the communication network and group themes. Nonverbal communication is more complex and involves eye contact, body posture, and mood of the group.

☐ Nurse leaders are responsible for mobilizing therapeutic factors to support healthy group development and prevent a stagnating groupthink. Which factors to mobilize and when depend on the type, purpose, and developmental stage of the group.

☐ Seating arrangements affect group interaction. The fewer physical barriers there are, such as tables, the better the potential for interactive communication. Everyone should be engaged as a member of the group and be invited to join in. Interactive groups should take place in a comfortable space with members facing one another in a circle arrangement.

☐ Leadership skills involve listening, tracking verbal and nonverbal behaviours, remaining fair and respectful, avoiding favouritism, and encouraging participation and involvement of all members with each other.

☐ The leader should address challenges to the leadership, group process, or other members to determine whether to intervene and how. In some instances, the leader redirects a monopolizing member; at other times, the leader supports the group to deal with the behaviour. Periods of group conflict occur in most groups during the transition from the beginning to the middle (working) phase.

☐ There are many different types of groups. PMH nurses lead psychoeducational and supportive therapy groups. Mental health specialists who are trained to provide intensive therapy lead psychotherapy groups and cognitive-behavioural groups. Consumers lead self-help groups, and professionals assist only as requested.

☐ Medication, symptom management, anger management, self-care, and reminiscence groups are common nurse-led groups.

CRITICAL THINKING CHALLENGES

1 Group members are very polite to one another and are superficially discussing topics. You would assess the group as being in which phase? Explain your answer.

2 After three sessions of a supportive therapy group, two members begin to share their frustration with having a mental illness. The group is moving into which phase of group development? Explain your answer.

3 Define the roles of the task and maintenance functions in groups. Observe your clinical group and identify classmates who are assuming task functions and maintenance functions.

4 Observe a patient group for at least five sessions. Discuss the seating pattern that emerges. Identify the communication network and the group themes. Then identify the group's norms and standards.

5 Discuss the conditions that lead to groupthink. When is groupthink positive? When is groupthink negative? Explain.

6 List at least six characteristics that are important for effective group leadership. Justify your answers.

7 During the first meeting, one member seems very anxious and tends to monopolize the conversation. Discuss how you would assess the situation and whether you would intervene.

8 At the end of the fourth meeting, one group member angrily accuses another of asking too many questions. The other members look on quietly. How would you assess the situation? Would you intervene? Explain.

WEB LINKS

www.agpa.org This is the site of the American Group Psychotherapy Association (AGPA), an interdisciplinary association for enhancing practice, theory, and research in group therapy. Extensive resources are available for members and nonmembers.

www.camh.net This is the site for the Centre for Addiction and Mental Health, which offers valuable practical, group, and research-based resources for health professionals in the field of addictions and mental health, including resources related to concurrent disorders, trauma, policy research, and health promotion.

www.cgpa.ca This is the site of the Canadian Group Psychotherapy Association (CGPA), a national organization dedicated to the promotion of group therapy practice and the enhancement of clinical knowledge and skills through training, continuing education, and research. CGPA is multidisciplinary, resulting in a rich and diverse membership. The association is responsible for setting national training standards and for accrediting regional training programs. CGPA has three levels of membership, reflecting a broad range of expertise and experience, from internationally acclaimed members to students of the mental health professions.

www.mentalhelp.net/selfhelp This is the site of the American Self-Help Group Clearinghouse, which serves as an online self-help resource containing information on many different self-help groups.

www.princeton.edu/main/tools/search/?q=group+dynamics+and+leadership This Outdoor Action Guide to Group Dynamics and Leadership, which appears on the Princeton website, illustrates a contemporary form of group that emphasizes team building, leadership, and outdoor activism.

www.projectmainstream.net This valuable website offers a national interdisciplinary electronic communications resource to improve health professionals' education on substance abuse. Numerous links to group interventions are available.

MOVIES, NOVELS, AND BIOGRAPHIES

Juno: 2007. A thought-provoking film in which a teenage girl becomes pregnant and struggles to decide whether or not to keep the baby. Group dynamics are apparent on several levels: her family (stepmom and dad), her peers at school, the adoptive parents, and her boyfriend and his family. This offers an excellent study of different family constellations, differing value conflicts, and discriminations as well as resilience in the face of adversity.

VIEWING POINTS: What are the dominant themes for each group and how do these change over time? Which relations offer the most learning for Juno and in what ways? Where is conflict most evident and how is it negotiated? Which individual, interpersonal, and group practices best supported resilience?

12 Angry Men: 1998. In this excellent film, a young man stands accused of fatally stabbing his father. A jury of his "peers" is deciding his fate. At first, the case appears to be "open and shut." This film depicts an intense struggle to reach a verdict and is an excellent study of group process and group dynamics.

VIEWING POINTS: Identify the leaders in the group. How does leadership change throughout the film? Do you find any evidence of groupthink? How does the group handle conflict?

REFERENCES

Alf, L., & Wilson, K. (2001). Facilitating group beginnings. 1. A practice model. *Groupwork*, *13*(1), 6–30.

Alvarez, A. (2002). Pratfalls, pittfalls, shortfalls and windfalls: Reflection on forming and being formed by groups. *Social Work With Groups*, *25*(1), 93–105.

American Group Psychotherapy Association. (2007). *Practice guidelines for group psychotherapy*. New York, NY: Sage.

Annesi, J. (1999). Effects of minimal group promotion on cohesion and exercise adherence. *Small Group Research*, *30*(5), 542–557.

Benne, K., & Sheats, P. (1948). Functional roles of group members. *Journal of Social Issues*, *4*(2), 41–49.

Brown, T., & Miller, C. (2000). Communication networks in task-performing groups: Effects of task complexity, time, pressure, and interpersonal dominance. *Small Group Research*, *31*(2), 131–157.

Burlingame, G., Strauss, B., Joyce, A. S., MacNair-Semands, R., MacKenzie, R., Ogrodniczuk, J., et al. (2005). *American Group Psychotherapy Association's CORE Battery—Revised (CORE-R)*. New York, NY: American Group Psychotherapy Association.

Burtis, J., & Turman, P. (2006). *Group communication pitfalls: Overcoming barriers to an effective group experience*. Thousand Oaks, CA: Sage.

Choi, J., & Kim, M. (1999). The organizational application of groupthink and its limitations in organizations. *Journal of Applied Psychology*, *84*(2), 297–306.

Corey, M., & Corey, G. (2006). *Groups: Process and practice* (7th ed.). Toronto, ON: Thomson Brooks/Cole.

Dimock, H. G., & Devine, I. (1994). *Making workgroups effective* (3rd ed.). North York, ON: Captus Press.

Garland, J., Jones, H., & Kolodny, R. (1973). A model of stages of development in social work groups. In S. Bernstein (Ed.), *Explorations in group work: Essays in theory and practice* (pp. 17–71). Boston, MA: Milford House.

Garrick, D., & Ewashen, C. (2001). An integrated model for adolescent inpatient group therapy. *Journal of Psychiatric and Mental Health Nursing, 8*, 165–171.

Graham, M., & Sontag, M. (2001). Art as an evaluative tool: A pilot study. *Art Therapy, 18*(1), 37–43.

Janis, I. (1982). *Groupthink* (2nd ed.). Boston, MA: Houghton-Mifflin.

Jones, E. D., & Beck-Little, R. (2002). The use of reminiscence therapy for the treatment of depression in rural-dwelling older adults. *Issues in Mental Health Nursing, 23*, 279–280.

Kurtz, L. F. (1992). Group environment in self-help groups for families. *Small Group Research, 23*, 199–215.

MacKenzie, R. K. (1997). *Time-managed group psychotherapy: Effective clinical applications*. Washington, DC: American Psychiatric Press.

McInnis-Perry, G. J., & Good, J. M. (2006). A psychoeducational codependency support group for older adults who reside in the community: Friends supporting friends. *Journal of Gerontological Nursing, 32*, 32–42.

Moher, M., Hey, K., & Lancaster, T. (2005). Workplace interventions for smoking cessation. *Cochrane Database of Systematic Reviews*.

Myers, S., & Anderson, C. (2008). *The fundamentals of small group communication*. Thousand Oaks, CA: Sage.

Neck, C. P., & Moorhead, G. (1995). Groupthink remodeled: The importance of leadership, time pressure, and methodical decision-making procedures. *Human Relations, 48*(5), 537–557.

Posthuma, B. (2001). *Small groups in counseling and therapy: Process and leadership* (4th ed.). Boston, MA: Pearson Education Canada.

Puentes, W. J. (2004). Cognitive therapy integrated with life review techniques: An eclectic treatment approach for affective symptoms in older adults. *Journal of Clinical Nursing, 13*, 84–89.

Rutan, J. S., & Stone, W. N. (2001). *Psychodynamic group psychotherapy* (3rd ed.). New York, NY: Guilford Press.

Sampson, E., & Marthas, M. (1990). *Group process for the health professions*. Albany, NY: Delmar.

Steinhardt, M. A., Dolbier, C. L., Gottlieb, N. H., & McCalister, K. T. (2003). The relationship between hardiness, supervisor support, group cohesion, and job stress as predictors of job satisfaction. *American Journal of Health Promotion, 17*(6), 382–389.

Tuckman, B. W. (1965). Development sequence in small groups. *Psychological Bulletin, 63*, 384–399.

Yalom, I. D. (1998). *The Yalom reader: Selections from the work of a master therapist and storyteller*. New York, NY: Basic Books.

Yalom, I. D. (1983). *Inpatient group psychotherapy*. New York, NY: Basic Books.

Yalom, I. D., & Leszcz, M. (2005). *The theory and practice of group psychotherapy* (5th ed.). New York, NY: Basic Books.

CHAPTER 17

Family Assessment and Interventions

Peggy Simpson

Adapted from the chapter "Family Assessment and Interventions" by Mary Ann Boyd and Lori Houger Limacher

LEARNING OBJECTIVES

After studying this chapter, you will be able to:

- Discuss the influence of mental illness on family functioning and how family functioning influences mental health.
- Develop a genogram that depicts family history, relationships, and physical and mental health patterns across three generations.
- Develop a plan for a comprehensive family assessment.
- Apply family nursing diagnoses to families who need nursing care.
- Discuss nursing interventions that are useful in caring for families.

KEY CONCEPTS

- comprehensive family assessment
- family

KEY TERMS

• extended family • family development • family life cycle • family structure • genogram • multigenerational transmission process • nuclear family • sibling position • subsystems • transition times

The Canadian census data (Statistics Canada, 2007) indicate that the portrait of Canadian families is changing. Although marriage and the traditional family structure remain important, there is more diversity in the way families are configured. More adult children are living at home with their parents, and more youngsters are living with their grandparents. Common-law couples and same sex couples are increasing in number. There are more couples living without children at home than with them, reflecting both the aging population and the lower fertility rates among younger couples. More Canadian adults are single rather than married (Statistics Canada, 2007). These characteristics are important when we begin to conceptualize **family** in the current Canadian context.

In the past, definitions of family have primarily focused on the structure and function of families. Traditional definitions of family suggest that families are unique in that, unlike other organizations, they generally incorporate new members by birth, adoption, or marriage, and members leave only by divorce or death. Nuclear families were defined as two or more people living together and related by blood, marriage, or adoption. An **extended family** consisted of several nuclear families whose members may or may not live together but function as one group. A more inclusive definition that focuses on belonging, affection, and durability of the relationships in the context of a person's life is conceptualized by Wright and Leahey (2005) as "the family is who they say they are." More recently, family relational practice has been defined as a complex process where economics, emotion, context, and experiences are interwoven and multilayered (Doane & Varcoe, 2005). The last two conceptualizations seem to be an appropriate "fit" for the changing portrait of Canadian families.

KEY CONCEPT **Family** is a group of people defined as "who they say they are" and involved relationally in a complex process where economics, emotion, context, and experiences are interwoven and multilayered (Doane & Varcoe, 2005; Wright & Leahey, 2005).

The psychiatric and mental health (PMH) nurse interacts with families in various ways. Because of the interpersonal and chronic nature of many mental illnesses, PMH nurses may have frequent and long-term contact with families. Involvement may range from meeting family members only once or twice to treating the whole family as a patient. Unlike a therapeutic group (see Chapter 16), the family system has a history and continues to function when the nurse is not there. The family relationships are influenced by past, present, and anticipated future relationships within at least a three-generation family system. This chapter explains how PMH nurses can integrate important family concepts into the nursing process when working together with families experiencing mental health problems.

Family Mental Health

In healthy families, members live in harmony with themselves and within society. These families support and nurture their members throughout their lives. However, mental illness can affect a family's overall health and daily functioning.

All families have strengths, resources, and capabilities. When families experience the crisis of overwhelming stress or acute or prolonged mental illness, they may not have the coping skills to manage the situation. It is inappropriate to term the family *dysfunctional*. It is more important for the PMH nurse to explore the contextual issues around the family situation and illness management, including the family perception of the problem, their strengths, resources, and capabilities, as well as their challenges and difficulties.

▬▬◗ EFFECTS OF MENTAL ILLNESS ON FAMILY FUNCTIONING

Any illness, including mental illness, influences the way families function. Families of people with a mental illness can provide a circle of care that both protects the individual with mental illness and supports his/her independence. Unfortunately, inadequate system supports may interrupt the circle of care and create a disruptive cycle of caregiving as family members witness the effects of system inadequacies that promote anger, frustration, and fear. They may be able to work "behind the scenes" and try to create a better, more hopeful world for their ill member (Ward-Griffin, Shofield, Vos, & Coatsworth-Puspoky, 2005). Families need strategies and solutions to help them in their efforts to care for a member with mental illness. The World Health Report (2001) identified six categories of needs of families of persons with mental disorders. These included skills for care of the ill member, enhancing family cohesion, assisting them to

network with other families experiencing mental illness, crisis support, financial support, and respite care.

Skills for care: Families require information about the illness, treatment modalities, symptom recognition, symptom management, monitoring, and rehabilitation strategies.

Family cohesion: The outcome for patients living with their families is better than for those living in institutions. Moderating the family's emotional response to the illness symptoms can reduce relapse in many mental illnesses. Supporting the family's problem-solving and coping strategies can strengthen family functioning.

Networking with other families: Families attain mutual support through networks. Many networks develop an advocating capacity, the goals of which include educating the general public, increasing support by policy makers, and fighting stigma and discrimination.

Crisis support: Families need to know the resources to contact in the event of a relapse or when increased symptoms warrant immediate intervention. They also need support in the event of a family member's suicide attempt or completion.

Financial support: Common mental disorders are twice as frequent among the poor as among the rich. Poverty is associated with unemployment, low education level, deprivation, and homelessness. Families may be able to advocate for affordable housing and supportive housing options.

Respite care: People with mental illness often have difficulty maintaining nonfamilial support networks and may rely exclusively on their families. Family caregiving roles, if not supported, can negatively influence the health of other members of the family. Opportunities for respite from caregiving can help sustain family efforts. Planning for future caregiving is a significant issue for many families: they are concerned about who will assume caregiving roles upon their death. Nevertheless, few families actually plan for this difficult eventuality (Smith, Hatfield, & Miller, 2000), potentially leaving the person with mental illness vulnerable to a difficult, even traumatic, time of transition.

It is important that nurses know how to help families discuss these issues and help them to explore alternatives in a context of trust and respect.

▬▬◗ INFLUENCE OF CULTURAL BELIEFS AND VALUES ON FAMILY FUNCTIONING

Families develop the roles and relationships among their members and the outside world in unique ways. Canada is a rich and diverse society (see Chapter 3). It is important that nurses engage in culturally safe and appropriate practice with families. Understanding cultural difference can be facilitated by following the lead of the family. Respectful interest in the family's problems and individual members' points of view is the best way to build trust. If asked, families will let nurses know what has meaning, significance, and importance for them (Doane & Varcoe, 2005; Turner, Weiling, & Allen, 2004). Inquiring how the mental illness is influencing all members of the family will help the nurse understand the reciprocity between the illness and family functioning. In this way, PMH nurses can gain understanding of the complex dynamics of familial context as it is shaped by culture and can learn about the way a particular family thinks about and organizes themselves around their member's mental illness, including how they interpret the illness, manage the symptoms, and access and utilize mental health care resources.

Comprehensive Family Assessment

A comprehensive family assessment involves the collection of all relevant data related to family health, psychological and spiritual well-being, and social functioning necessary to identify problems for which the nurse can enhance family strengths and generate nursing interventions. The assessment usually consists of a face-to-face interview with family members (although telephone- or videoconferencing may be an alternative) and may be conducted over several sessions. A comprehensive family assessment is appropriate when an individual is admitted to the hospital for psychiatric or mental health treatment. If the individual's admission status is voluntary and he or she is deemed competent to make treatment decisions, permission to contact the family is in order (Box 17-1).

BOX 17.1

Family Mental Health Assessment

FAMILY NAME: _____

FAMILY MEMBERS PRESENT AT INTERVIEW: _____
_____
_____
_____

NURSE INTERVIEWER: _____

1. Referral route and presenting problem (include psychiatric diagnosis and current treatment): _____
_____

2. Family composition (complete and attach a family genogram)
3. Family life cycle stage (include stage and any pertinent transitional issues): _____
_____

4. Pertinent history of the problem:
   a. Explore why the family is presenting for assistance at this point in time.
   b. Explore the effects of the mental health concern on all family members.
   c. Developmental history (including family of origin, health or medical events)
   d. Communication patterns (for solving day-to-day issues or problems)
   e. Previous solutions
   f. Ethnicity/culture
   g. Social supports (informal and formal programs)
   h. Financial and legal status
5. Strengths and problems (identify the family strengths, resources and capabilities): _____
_____

6. Summary (include a hypothesis about the presenting problem, any pertinent history, patterns of communicating, subsystems, or boundary issues): _____
_____

7. Goals/plans (list interventions and family responses): _____
_____

8. Nursing diagnosis: _____
_____
_____

Adapted from Wright, L. M., & Leahey, M. (2005). *Nurses and families: A guide to family assessment and intervention.* Philadelphia, PA: F. A. Davis.

KEY CONCEPT A **comprehensive family assess-ment** is the collection of all relevant data related to family health, psychological well-being, and social functioning to identify problems for which the nurse can generate nursing interventions and enhance family strengths.

RELATIONSHIP BUILDING

In preparing for a family assessment, the nurse must take steps to promote a positive nurse–family relationship by enabling an atmosphere of trust, respect, comfort, and cooperation. Many families do not know what to expect from the nurse. Each family is unique and its needs, its understanding of the situation, its expectations for care, and its previous experiences with the health care system are just some factors that should be explored at the beginning of a therapeutic relationship. More than the initial meeting may be necessary to build the relationship and complete the assessment.

The nurse must show understanding, competence, and caring. Listening to family members, acknowledging their expertise and knowledge, and addressing their immediate needs build confidence and trust with them. For example, a family that needs shelter or food is not ready to discuss a member's medication regimen until these basic needs are met.

GENOGRAMS

Families possess various structural configurations (e.g., single-parent, multigenerational, same-gender relationships). The **genogram** is a structural assessment tool that may be used by the nurse to collect information about the family members, their relationships, and health and illness patterns over time. The genogram may be used as a tool for engagement as well as a tool for family assessment, planning, and intervention. The tool is simple to use requiring only a pencil and paper or alternatively some computer programs have this feature.

Genograms are schematic diagrams of families, listing family members and their relationships to one another. A genogram includes the age, dates of marriage and death, and geographic location of each member. Squares represent men and circles represent women; ages are listed inside the figures. Horizontal lines represent marriages (including common-law marriage) with the date written on the line; vertical lines connect parents and children. Genograms can be particularly useful in understanding family history, composition, relationships, and illnesses (Fig. 17-1).

Genograms vary from simple to complex. The needs of the patient and family guide the level of assessment

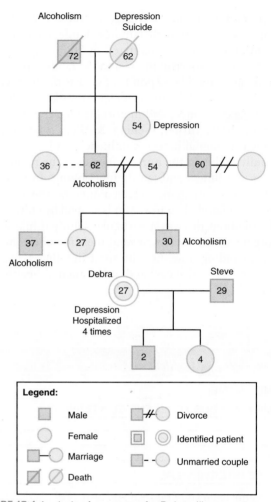

FIGURE 17.1 Analysis of genogram for Debra. Illness patterns are depression (maternal aunt, grandmother [suicide]) and alcoholism (brother, father, grandfather). Relationship patterns show that parents are divorced and neither sibling is married.

detail. In a small family with few concerns, the genogram can be simple. In a larger family with multiple concerns, the genogram can reflect these complexities. Nurses can explore important events such as marriages, divorces, deaths, and geographic movements in relation to the presenting concern. They can include cultural or religious affiliations, education and economic levels, and the nature of the work of each family member. PMH nurses should always include mental health issues and other significant health problems in the genogram. Questions should be designed to address the family's particular area of concern rather than a general exploration. The nurse can begin the interview by informing family members they will be having a conversation so the nurse can gain a better understanding of their situation, their concerns, and their family or support network. The genogram as a tool should be explained and the offer made to provide family members with a copy should they desire one.

Analyzing and Using Genograms

For a genogram to be useful in assessment, the nurse needs to analyze the data for family composition, relationship strengths and problems (particularly related to the mental health concern), and patterns of mental health in the family. Nurses can begin with family composition. Who is considered to be family? How large is the family? Where do family members live? In what way do the family members show support? A large family whose members live in the same city may have more support than a family in which distance separates members. Of course, this is not always the case. The nurse should also study the genogram for relationship and illness patterns. Who in the family are closer and further apart? How might marriage and divorce influence the relationships? What illness patterns might be observed across relationships or generations? For example, depression, gambling, or alcohol addiction might be evident in past generations and may be risk factors for present and future generations. Exploring the significance and meaning of these health issues with the family is important. This can lead to conversations with the family about family strengths and solution strategies that they have tried. It can further their understanding of health promotion and illness prevention related to family health risks.

■■ FAMILY BIOLOGIC DOMAIN

In the family biologic domain, the family assessment includes a discussion of family members' physical and mental health status and how the status affects family functioning. A family with multiple health problems, both physical and mental, will be trying to manage the symptoms and treatments as well as obtain the many financial and health care resources it needs.

Physical Health Status

The family health status involves the physical illnesses and disabilities of the current family, but information on that of past generations is also relevant. The nurse can record family health status information on the genogram. The current health status is an indication of the members' physical status and the stress currently being placed on the family and its resources. It is important for the nurse to explore how the health problems are affecting family functioning. For example, if a member requires frequent visits to a provider or hospitalizations, the whole family may feel the effects of focusing more time and financial resources on that member.

Mental Health Status

Exploring a family's history and experience with a mental disorder must be approached with respect and sensitivity.

In most cultures, mental health problems are associated with stigma and shame (WHO, 2001). How and with whom families share information about their ill member vary greatly.

Directly and matter-of-factly, the nurse should ask the family to identify any members who have had or have a mental illness. The nurse should record the information on the genogram as well as in narrative form. If family members do not know whether anyone in the family has or had a mental illness, the nurse should ask if anyone was treated for "nerves" or had a "nervous breakdown." Overall, a comprehensive family history of mental illness across multiple generations helps the nurse understand the significance of mental illness in the current generation. If one family member has a serious mental illness, the whole family can be affected. Exploring how this is unique to each family is important to planning care.

■■ FAMILY PSYCHOLOGICAL DOMAIN

Assessment of the family's psychological domain focuses on the family's development and life cycle, communication patterns, stress and coping abilities, and problem-solving skills. One aim of the assessment is to understand how family members communicate with each other as they negotiate developmental and life transitions, including illness. It is important for the nurse to explore coping styles and problem-solving abilities of family members relevant to the management of both crisis and long-term issues associated with their relative's mental illness.

> **• CRNENOTE**
>
> Identifying stressful events and coping mechanisms should be a priority in a family assessment.

Family Development

Family development is a broad term that refers to all the processes connected with the growth of a family, including changes associated with its economic situation, geographic location, migration, acculturation, and serious illness. In optimal family development, family members are relatively differentiated (capable of autonomous functioning) from one another, anxiety is low, and the parents have good emotional relationships with their own families of origin.

Family Life Cycles

There is a distinction between family life cycles and family development (Carter & McGoldrick, 1999). Family development refers to the unique path constructed by a family that is shaped by predictable and unpredictable events, such as illness, environmental disasters, and societal trends, such as an economic downturn. Family life cycle refers to a "typical" path most families go through related to the arrival and departure of family members through birth and death, couple unions and separations, and the raising and launching of children. It is important for PMH nurses to model inclusivity and respect for diversity of family forms in their practice with families. As well as the traditional **nuclear family** of father, mother, and children, a family may comprise lesbian and gay couples, single parents and their children, or children raising children without a parent. The parents may be unmarried, separated, or divorced; the children, biologic, adopted, or fostered. The family may be extended, including several generations in the same home. The nurse's focus regarding family development is not on categorizing the family but rather on understanding the relational processes that occur as the family evolves and responds to its member's mental illness.

The **family life cycle** is a process of expansion, contraction, and realignment of relationship systems to support the entry, exit, and development of family members in a functional way (Carter & McGoldrick, 1999) (Table 17-1). A family's life cycle is conceptualized in terms of stages throughout the years. To move from one stage to the next, the family system undergoes changes. Structural and potential structural changes within stages can usually be handled by rearranging the family system (first-order changes), whereas transition from one stage to the next requires changes in the system itself (second-order changes). In first-order changes, the family system is rearranged, such as when the youngest child enters schooling and the stay-at-home parent returns to work.

Table 17.1　Stages of the Family Life Cycle		
Family Life Cycle Stage	**Emotional Transition**	**Required Family Changes**
1. Leaving home: single young adults	Accepting emotional and financial responsibility for self	Differentiation of self in relation to family of origin Development of intimate peer relationships Establishment of self regarding work and financial independence
2. The joining of families through marriage: the new couple	Commitment to new system	Formation of marital system Realignment of relationships with extended families and friends to include spouse
3. Families with young children	Accepting new members into the system	Adjusting marital system to make space for children Joining in child-rearing, financial, and household tasks Realignment of relationships with extended family to include parenting and grandparenting roles
4. Families with adolescents	Increasing flexibility of family boundaries to include children's independence and grandparents frailties	Shifting of parent–child relationships to permit the adolescent to move in and out of system Refocus on midlife marital and career issues Beginning shift toward joint caring for older generation
5. Launching children and moving on	Accepting multitude of exits from and entries into the family system	Renegotiation of marital system as a dyad Development of adult–adult relationships between grown children and their parents Realignment of relationships to include in-laws and grandchildren Dealing with disabilities and death of parents (grandparents)
6. Families in later life	Accepting the shifting of generational roles	Maintaining own and couple functioning interests in face of physiologic decline, exploring new familial and social role options Support for a more central role of middle generation Making room in the system for the wisdom and experience of the elderly, supporting the older generation without overfunctioning for them Dealing with loss of spouse, siblings, and other peers and preparation for own death

From Carter B., & McGoldrick, M. (1999). Overview: The expanded family life cycle. In B. Carter & M. McGoldrick (Eds.). *The expanded family life cycle* (p. 2). New York, NY: Allyn & Bacon.

Table 17.2	The Divorcing Family	
Family Life Cycle Stage	**Prerequisite Attitude**	**Developmental Issues**
Divorce		
1. Decision to divorce	Acceptance of inability to resolve marital tensions sufficiently to continue relationship	Acceptance of one's own part in the failure of the marriage
2. Planning the breakup of the system	Supporting viable arrangements for all parts of the system	Working cooperatively on problems of custody, visitation, and finances
		Dealing with extended family about the divorce
3. Separation	Willingness to continue cooperative co-parental relationship and joint financial support of children	Mourning loss of intact family
		Restructuring marital and parent–child relationships and finances, adapting to living apart
	Work on resolution of attachment to spouse	Realignment of relationships with extended family, staying connected with spouse's extended family
4. The divorce	More work on emotional divorce: overcoming hurt, anger, guilt, etc.	Mourning loss of intact family: giving up fantasies of reunion
		Retrieval of hopes, dreams, and expectations from the marriage
		Staying connected with extended families
Postdivorce Family		
1. Single parent (custodial household or primary residence)	Willingness to maintain financial responsibilities, continue parental contact with ex-spouse, and support contact of children with ex-spouse and his or her family	Making flexible visitation arrangements with ex-spouse and family
		Rebuilding own financial resources
		Rebuilding own social network
2. Single parent (noncustodial)	Willingness to maintain parental contact with ex-spouse and support custodial parent's relationship with children	Finding ways to continue effective parenting relationship with children
		Maintaining financial responsibilities to ex-spouse and children
		Rebuilding own social network

From Carter, B., & McGoldrick, M. (1999). The divorce cycle: A major variation in the American family life cycle. In B. Carter & M. McGoldrick (Eds.), *The expanded family life cycle* (p. 375). New York, NY: Allyn & Bacon.

The system is rearranged, but the structure remains the same. In second-order changes, the family structure does change, such as when a member moves away from the family home to live independently. Families may be transitioning through more than one stage depending on the family configuration. As suggested, the nurse may use this model to explore potential areas of stress related to the family transitions. Multiple transitions can trigger or exacerbate symptoms of mental illness.

Variations of the family life cycle are presented for the divorced family (Table 17-2) and the remarried family (Table 17-3).

Transition times are any times of addition, subtraction, or change in status of family members. During transitions, family stresses are more likely to cause symptoms or difficulties. Significant family events, such as the death of a member or the introduction of a new member, also affect the family's ability to function. During these times, families may need help from the mental health system.

Culture, Ethnicity, and Race

The terms *culture*, *ethnicity*, and *race* are often used interchangeably in discussions about diversity in psychiatric settings. This mingling of terms can create confusion, given that these words can mean very different things (Doane & Varcoe, 2005). Culture generally refers to the beliefs, values, and norms that guide and shape the way a family lives, whereas ethnicity is associated with more distinctive traits, such as national heritage, social class, race, and religion. Race is generally considered a biologic dimension.

Given Canada's multicultural climate, it is important for nurses in psychiatric settings to consciously attend to diversity. One method for increasing sensitivity to culture has been by trying to identify distinctive characteristics or responses to life cycle transitions or disruptions such as mental illness within specific ethnic communities. Becoming conscious of the characteristics of particular ethnic groups is an important step toward developing an appreciation for diversity, as long as these norms are remembered to be gross generalizations. Labelling and categorizing ethnic groups' behaviours according to general rules can help raise our awareness of difference, but it can equally obscure the uniqueness of each family that we encounter. For the nurse, appreciating and validating ethnic differences, while at the same time acknowledging similarities, can feel like a delicate balancing act (McGoldrick, 2003).

Table 17.3	Remarried Family Formulations	
Family Life Cycle Stage	**Prerequisite Attitude**	**Developmental Issues**
1. Entering a new relationship	Recovery from loss of first marriage (adequate "emotional divorce")	Recommitment to marriage and to forming a family with readiness to deal with the complexity and ambiguity
2. Conceptualizing and planning new marriage and family	Accepting one's own fears and those of new spouse and children about remarriage and forming a stepfamily. Accepting need for time and patience for adjustment to complexity and ambiguity of multiple new roles Boundaries: space, time, membership, and authority Affective issues: guilt, loyalty conflicts, desire for mutuality, and irresolvable past hurts	Work on openness in the new relationships to avoid pseudomutuality Plan for maintenance of cooperative financial and co-parental relationships with ex-spouses Plan to help children deal with fears, loyalty conflicts, and membership in two systems Realignment of relationships with extended family to include new spouse and children Plan for maintenance of connections for children with extended family of ex-spouses
3. Remarriage and reconstitution of family	Final resolution of attachment to previous spouse and ideal of "intact" family Acceptance of a different model of family with permeable boundaries	Restructuring family boundaries to allow for inclusion of new spouse-stepparent Realignment of relationships and financial arrangement throughout subsystems to permit interweaving of several systems Making room for relationships of all children with biologic (noncustodial) parents, grandparents, and other extended families Sharing memories and histories to enhance stepfamily integration

From Carter, B., & McGoldrick, M. (1999). The divorce cycle: A major variation in the American family life cycle. In B. Carter & M. McGoldrick (Eds.), *The expanded family life cycle* (p. 377). New York, NY: Allyn & Bacon.

For example, if a nurse anticipates that an Indo-Canadian, Italian-Canadian, or Aboriginal-Canadian's extended family (aunts, uncles, and cousins) will be more involved in mental health treatment decisions and hospital visitation (Doane & Varcoe, 2005) or assumes that Chinese-Canadian families will be less likely to seek mental health treatment because they will not recognize or attend to mental illness in the same way (Casado & Leung, 2001), a generalization based on ethnicity is likely occurring. In the clinical example provided in Box 17-2, a particular generalization is at play in the description of Judy's rich familial connections and her location in a particular geographic region of Canada. This is another example of a cultural assumption.

Developing sensitivity to one's own beliefs about what constitutes normalcy and functionality in a family is a challenging and important endeavour. It is only in this process of self-reflection that the nurse will develop an awareness of the cultural norms and values that are guiding and creating the template against which the nurse is judging and assessing even the family life cycle (Doane & Varcoe, 2005). It is the dominant, white, middle-class, cultural rules that generally become the gold standard, the norm against which all other ethnic groups are measured and assessed. This can be problematic if the nurse is not aware of the power, and hence oppression, that might accompany these norms. Developing and maintaining sensitivity to ethnicity, culture, and power are important in helping the nurse to recognize issues of diversity (see Chapter 3).

Families in Poverty

The family life cycle of those living in poverty may vary from those with adequate financial means. People living in poverty struggle to make ends meet, and members may face difficulties in meeting their own or other members' basic developmental needs. They may be homeless or living in unsafe conditions. To be poor does not mean that a family is dysfunctional. But poverty is an important factor that can force even the healthiest families to crumble. In a study of families living in poverty, Hines (1999) observed four distinguishing characteristics: condensed life cycle, female-headed households of the extended-family type, chronic stress and untimely losses, and reliance on institutional supports.

When the life cycle is condensed, family members leave their home, mate, have children, and become grandparents at much earlier ages than their working-class and middle-class counterparts. Consequently, many individuals in such families assume new roles and responsibilities before they are developmentally capable. The condensed life

BOX 17.2

John and Judy Jones

John and Judy Jones were married 3 years ago, after their graduation from a small University in Eastern Canada. Judy's career choice required that she live on the East Coast, where she should be near her large family. John willingly moved with her and quickly found a satisfying position. After about 6 months of marriage, John became extremely irritable and depressed. He kept saying that his life was not his own. Judy was very concerned but could not understand his feelings of being overwhelmed. His

job was going well, and they had a very busy social life, mostly revolving around her family, whom John loved. They decided to seek counselling and completed the following genogram:

After looking at the genogram, both John and Judy began to realize that part of John's discomfort had to do with the number of family members who were involved in their lives. Judy and John began to redefine their social life, allowing more time with friends and each other.

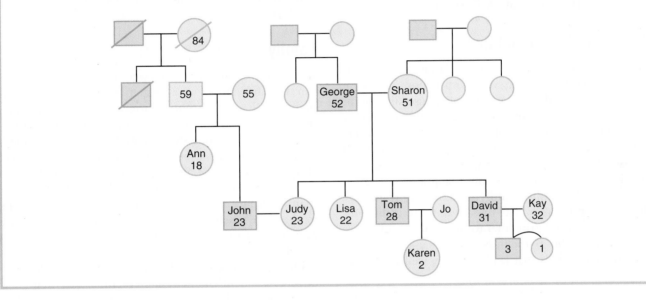

cycle creates adolescents whose educational opportunities are compromised (no time to complete school given the family demands), limiting their employment skills. Therefore, the cycle of poverty is reinforced.

The second characteristic that Hines observed is female-headed households of the extended-family type, in which a woman, her children, and her daughter's children often live together without clear delineation of their respective roles. This scenario can create economic and emotional burdens for the older woman who is the principal breadwinner and difficulty for the younger women in assuming parental responsibilities. Despite possible poor health, elderly family members continue to work to support their children and grandchildren into later life (Hines, 1999).

The third characteristic is chronic stress and untimely losses. Families living in poverty are subject to disruption via abrupt loss of members, loss of unemployment compensation, illness, death, imprisonment, or alcohol or drug addiction. Men may die relatively young compared with their middle-class counterparts. Ordinary problems, such as transportation or a sick child, can become major crises because of a lack of resources.

Reliance on institutional supports is the final distinguishing characteristic. Poor families are often forced to seek public assistance, which ultimately can result in additional stress in having to deal with a governmental agency.

Communication Patterns

Family communication patterns develop over a lifetime. Some family members communicate more openly and freely than others. In addition, family subgroups may have unique communication patterns with one another. Just as in any assessment interview, the nurse should observe the verbal and nonverbal communication of the family members. Who sits next to each other? Who talks to whom? Who answers most questions? Who volunteers information? Who changes the subject? Which subjects seem acceptable to discuss? Which topics are not discussed? How are partners intimate with each other? How are the family secrets or sensitive topics revealed? Does the nonverbal communication match the verbal communication? PMH nurses can use this information to help identify family problems, strengths, and communication issues.

Nurses should also assess the family for its daily communication patterns. Identifying which family members confide in one another is a place to start examining ongoing communication. Other areas include how often children talk with parents, which child talks to the parents most, and who is most likely to discipline the children. Another question considers how family members express positive and negative feelings. In determining how open or closed the family is, the nurse explores the type of information the family shares with nonfamily members. For example, one family may tell others about a member's mental illness, whereas another family may not discuss any illnesses with those outside the family.

Stress and Coping Abilities

One of the most important assessment tasks is to determine how family members deal with major and minor stressful events and their available coping skills. Some families seem able to cope with overwhelming stresses, such as the death of a member, major illness, or severe conflict, whereas other families seem to fall apart over relatively minor events. It is important for the nurse to listen to which situations a family appraises as stressful and help the family identify usual coping responses. The nurse can then evaluate these responses. If the family's responses are detrimental to health (e.g., substance abuse, physical abuse), the nurse may discuss the need to develop coping skills that lead to family well-being (see Chapter 35).

· CRNENOTE

Consider the following two questions.
How might a family transitioning through various life cycle stages experience the emotional process and second-order changes when one family member is experiencing an acute mental illness episode?
How might a family be affected when several life cycle stages are interrupted at the same time? For example, the death of a parent, job loss, and separation from a partner?

Problem-Solving Skills

Nurses assess family problem-solving skills by focusing on the more recent problems the family has experienced and determining the process that members used to solve them. For example, a child is sick at school and needs to go home. Does the mother, father, grandparent, or babysitter receive the call from the school? Who then cares for the child? Underlying the ability to solve problems is the decision-making process. Who makes and implements decisions? How does the family handle conflict? All these data provide information regarding the family's problem-solving abilities. Once these abilities are identified, the nurse can build on these strengths in helping families deal with additional problems.

■ FAMILY SOCIAL DOMAIN

An assessment of the family's social domain provides important data about the operation of the family as a system and its interaction within its environment. Areas of concern include the system itself, power dynamics, social and financial status, and formal and informal support networks.

Family Systems

Just as any group can be viewed as a system, a family can be understood as a system with interdependent members. Family system theories view the family as an open system whose members interact with their environment as well as among themselves. One family member's change in thoughts or behaviour can cause a ripple effect and change everyone else's. For example, a mother who decides to reinforce her child's positive efforts rather than focusing on negative actions may notice a change in the child's behaviour which may in turn result in a reduction of the stress she feels when interacting with the child.

One common scenario in the mental health field is the effect of a patient's improvement on the family. With new medications and treatment, patients are more likely to be able to live independently, which subsequently changes the responsibilities and activities of family caregivers. Although family members may be relieved that their caregiving burden is lifted, they will be also adjusting to changes in the demands on their time and energies. This transition may not be easy because it is often less stressful to maintain familiar activities than to venture into uncharted territory. Families may seem as though they want to keep an ill member dependent but, in reality, they are struggling with the change in their family system.

Mental health nursing has been influenced by several system models used in helping families. Three important examples are Wright-Leahey Calgary model (Wright, Watson, & Bell, 1996; Wright & Leahey, 2005), Bowen's family systems (1978), and Minuchin's structural family therapy (1981, 1996). These models have shaped the perspectives and language of family nursing.

The Calgary Family Assessment and Intervention Model

The Calgary Family Assessment Model (CFAM) and the Calgary Family Intervention Model (CFIM) are relational practice nursing models based on postmodernism, systems, cybernetics, communication and change theories, and the biology of cognition (Wright & Leahey, 2005). These two models are multidimensional frameworks that conceptualize the family into structural, developmental, and functional categories. Each assessment category contains several subcategories. Structure is further categorized into internal (family, gender, sexual orientation, etc.), external (extended family and larger systems), and contextual (ethnicity, race, social class, religion, spirituality, environment). Family developmental assessment is organized according to stages, tasks, and attachments. Functional assessment areas include instrumental (activities of daily living) and expressive (communication, problem-solving, roles, beliefs, influence, power, and alliances).

When the nurse uses CFAM/CFIM, relational practice develops and evolves during four stages: engagement, assessment, intervention, and termination. There is reciprocity in the relationship where the nurse and the family each bring specialized expertise in managing health problems, as well as strengths and resources, to the nurse–family relationship.

The *engagement* stage is the initial stage in which the family is greeted and made comfortable. In the *assessment* stage, problems are identified, and relationships between family and health providers develop. During this stage, the nurse opens space for the family to tell its story. The nurse asks key questions and listens to the patient and family members' expectations, hopes, questions, and ideas. The *intervention* stage is the core of the clinical work and involves providing a context in which the family can make changes (see the Family Interventions section in this chapter). The nurse considers the family knowledge and expertise in planning care. The nurse communicates regularly with the family to discuss information, ideas, and recommendations for treatment and involves the family to its satisfaction in making decisions about the treatment plan. The *termination* phase refers to the process of ending the therapeutic relationship (Wright & Leahey, 2005).

Bowen's Family Systems Model

Murray Bowen (1978) developed several system concepts used by professionals working with families. Four of these concepts, **sibling position, multigenerational transmission process, triangles,** and **family projection process,** are described here.

Multigenerational transmission process: Bowen believed that one generation transfers its emotional processes to the next generation. Certain basic patterns, including conflicts, between parents and children are replicas of those of past generations, and generations to follow will repeat them as well. For example, a spouse may stay emotionally distant from his partner, just as his father was with his mother.

Sibling position: Children can develop attitudes and behaviours based on their **sibling position** in their families. For example, a first-born child may readily accept responsibility, have more confidence, and be more outgoing than the second-born child, who has grown up in the older child's shadow. Conversely, the second-born child may be more inclined to identify with the oppressed and be more open to other experiences than the first-born child. Knowledge of these general responses to sibling position can be helpful in understanding the family's processes and patterns.

Triangles: According to Bowen, the triangle is a three-person system and the smallest stable unit in human relations. Cycles of closeness and distance characterize a two-person relationship. When anxiety is high during periods of distance, one party "triangulates" a third person or thing into the relationship. For example, two partners may have a stable relationship when anxiety is low. When anxiety and tension rise, one partner may be so uncomfortable that he or she confides in a friend instead of the other partner. In these cases, triangulating reduces the tension but freezes the conflict in place. In families, triangulating occurs when a husband and wife diffuse tension by focusing on the children. To maintain the status quo and avoid the conflict, one of the parents develops an overly intense relationship with one of the children.

Family projection process: Through this process, the triangulated member becomes the centre of the family conflicts; that is, the family projects its conflicts onto the child or other triangulated person. This projection appears as anxious, enmeshed concern. The triangulated member may be the person identified by the family as having the problem that caused the family to seek help. For example, a husband and wife are having financial worries and disagreeing about expenses. Their teenage son is having difficulty with interpersonal relationships in school. Instead of the parents resolving their differences over money, one or both parents become intensely focused on their son's difficulty.

The Bowen model offers one way for the nurse to understand the family system of relationships. For instance, are family interactions similar to those of the previous generation? Is the father of the family interacting with his children the way his father interacted with him? Does he recognize this? Do his children know what life was like for their father as a child? How do the personalities of older siblings compare with those of younger siblings? What would be the next problem this family needs to address once the presenting problem is successfully resolved? Is this "next" problem what is actually driving family conflicts? and so on.

Minuchin's Family Structure Model

Salvador Minuchin emphasizes the importance of family structure. In his model, the family consists of three essential components: structure, subsystems, and boundaries (Minuchin, Lee, & Simon, 1996).

Family structure is the organized pattern in which family members interact. As two adult partners come together to form a family, they develop the quantity of their interactions or how much time they spend interacting. For example, a newly married couple may establish their evening interaction pattern by talking to each other during dinner but not while watching television. The quality of the interactions also becomes patterned. Some topics are appropriate for conversation during their evening walk (e.g., reciting daily events), whereas controversial or emotionally provocative topics are relegated to other times and places.

Family rules are important influences on interaction patterns. For example, "family problems stay in the family" is a common rule. Both the number of people in the family and its development also influence the interaction pattern. For instance, the interaction between a single mother and her children changes when she remarries and introduces a stepfather. Over time, families repeat interactions, which develop into enduring patterns. For example, if a mother tells her son to straighten his room and the son refuses until his father yells at him, the family has initiated an interactional pattern. If this pattern continues, the child may come to see the father as the disciplinarian and the mother as incompetent.

Subsystems develop when family members join together for various activities or functions. Minuchin views each member as belonging to several different subgroups. Obvious groups are parents and children. Sometimes, there are "boy" and "girl" systems. Such systems become obvious in an assessment when family members talk about "the boys going fishing with dad" and "the girls going shopping with mother." A mother may also be a wife, sister, and daughter. Sometimes, these roles can conflict. It may be acceptable for a woman to be very firm as a disciplinarian in her role as a mother, while in her sister, wife, or daughter role, similar behaviour would provoke anger and resentment.

Boundaries are invisible barriers with varying permeabilities that surround each subsystem. They regulate the amount of contact a person has with others and protect the autonomy of the family and its subsystems. For instance, when family members do not take telephone calls at dinner, they are protecting themselves from outside intrusion. When parents do not allow children to interrupt them, they are establishing a boundary between themselves and their children. According to Minuchin, the spouse subsystem must have a clear boundary that separates it from parents, children, and the outside world.

Boundaries vary from rigid to diffuse. Rigid boundaries permit independence, growth, and mastery within the subsystem (e.g., parents are not overly involved with their children's activities), but too rigid boundaries can foster disengagement among family members (e.g., parents do not know their children's friends.) Diffuse boundaries promote enmeshed subsystems; that is, they promote interdependence that prevents age-appropriate independence to develop. For instance, children with "overinvolved" parents may struggle to learn to make their own decisions. Enmeshment issues can occur when parents want their children to see them as friends and peers. For Minuchin, the well-functioning family has clear, flexible boundaries with a strong parental subsystem. It is not the absence of problems that makes a family well functioning; it is the existence of functional family structure to handle them.

Some Recent Perspectives on Understanding Families

Recently, PMH nurses have been looking to the ideas of postmodernism and social constructivism to enrich their understanding of families. These ideas support exploring how families make meaning in their lives and how they construct their reality in relation to their social environment. For instance, the constructivist influence invites PMH nurses to understand that what they are seeing is a product of their own assumptions about people, families, and problems and their interactions with families. It is recognized that people are highly influenced by their current relationships and environments in constructing their realities. Thus, persons with mental illness and their families should be encouraged to express their perspectives (their own "truth") on their situation to the nurse. Nurses need to be respectful of family stories and viewpoints, within the parameters of values about human safety and rights, including self-determination and protection from interpersonal violence.

As well, PMH nurses are using a critical lens derived from feminist, poststructural, and postcolonial theories that support considerations of power, oppression, culture, economic conditions of life, social change, and emancipation. This critical perspective draws the nurses' attention to the sociopolitical, economic, and language contexts within which families are situated and constituted. The focus can then be on exposing underlying sociopolitical structures that are advantaging some people/families and disadvantaging others. Exploring social conditions and revising structures in ways that inequities are addressed become the goals.

Social and Financial Status

Social status is often linked directly to financial status. The nurse should identify the occupations of the family members. Who works outside the home and inside the home? Who is primarily responsible for the family's financial support? Families of low social status are more likely to have limited financial resources, which can place additional stresses on the family. Nurses can use information regarding the family's financial status to determine whether to refer the family to social services.

Cultural expectations and beliefs about acceptable behaviours may cause additional stress. For example, in one qualitative study of 12 black West Indian depressed women who immigrated to Canada or were first-born Canadians, the women rarely sought professional help because of the strong culturally defined stigma against mental disorders. Instead, they managed depression by "being strong," which meant that they tried not to dwell on their feelings, focused on diversions, tried to regain composure, or used other approaches. The researchers concluded that "being strong" may be a factor in inducing depression or slowing or preventing recovery for some women (Schreiber, Noerager Stern, & Wilson, 2000).

Formal and Informal Support Networks

According to balance theory (see Chapter 8), both formal and informal networks are important in providing support to individuals and families. These networks are the link among the individual, family, and the community. Assessing the extent of formal support (e.g., hospitals, agencies) and informal support (e.g., extended family, friends, neighbours) gives a clearer picture of the availability of support. In assessing formal support, the nurse should ask about the family's involvement with government institutions and self-help groups such as alcoholics anonymous. Assessing the informal network is particularly important in cultural groups with extended family networks or close friends because these individuals can be major sources of support to patients. If the nurse does not ask about the informal network, these important people may be missed. Nurses can inquire whether family members volunteer at schools, local hospitals, or nursing homes. They can also ask whether the family attends religious services or activities.

◼◼◼◼ FAMILY SPIRITUAL DOMAIN

Family members' spiritual and religious beliefs can influence how the family copes and manages mental health concerns. For many families, their religious affiliations will play a key role in their everyday lives. These affiliations can influence the family's understanding of health and illness and of healing and treatment. Religious and spiritual practices can foster family and community support and may be a major resource to families. It is increasingly recognized that, in all faith groups, the help and

guidance of clergy are frequently sought by families who have a mentally ill member (Aaron, 2008). Yet, research suggests that a majority of clergy (Christian clergy were studied) feel inadequate regarding their knowledge of mental illness (Farrell & Goebert, 2008). Unfortunately, clergy are not usually viewed in a collaborative way by mental health professionals (Leavey, Lowenthal, & King, 2007). Collaboration, however, could be of significant use to both groups, especially to individuals and families requiring assistance. Clergy can provide community-based support and assist health professionals, such as nurses, to understand patients' beliefs, important to informing treatment planning and to improving response to crisis. Nurses and their colleagues can, in turn, assist clergy to understand mental disorders and mental health problems and their treatment. Open communication can facilitate, for instance, appropriate use of complementary healing practices that can be a part of a group's religious beliefs. It may promote better trust in psychiatric treatment and care.

In addressing the spiritual domain of family nursing, it is important for the PMH nurse to recognize that family members may differ widely in their religious beliefs and in their approach to spirituality. Such variation among members' perspectives, if it exists, should inform the family assessment. It may be a source of enrichment or of distress or both for the family.

Family Nursing Diagnoses

From the assessment data, nurses can choose several possible nursing diagnoses. Interrupted Family Processes; Ineffective Therapeutic Regimen Management; or Compromised, Disabling, or Ineffective Family Coping are all possibilities. Nurses choose Interrupted Family Processes if a usually supportive family is experiencing stressful events that challenge its previously effective functioning. They choose Ineffective Family Therapeutic Regimen Management if the family is experiencing difficulty integrating into daily living a program for the treatment of illness and the sequela of illness that meets specific health goals. They select Ineffective Family Coping when the primary supportive person is providing insufficient, ineffective, or compromised support, comfort, or assistance to the patient in managing or mastering adaptive tasks related to the individual's health challenge (Carpenito, 2003).

Family Interventions

Family interventions focus on supporting the bio/psycho/social/spiritual integrity and functioning of the family as defined by its members. Although family therapy is reserved for mental health specialists, the generalist PMH nurse can implement several bio/psycho/social/spiritual interventions, such as counselling, promotion of self-care activities, supportive therapy, education and health teaching, and the use of genograms. Marshall and Harper-Jaques (2008) worked together with a family experiencing depression using psychoeducation, circular pattern diagrams, and therapeutic letters to illustrate just some ways PMH nurses can promote healing in families experiencing mental illness.

In implementing any family intervention, flexibility is essential, particularly when working with culturally diverse groups. To implement successful, culturally competent family interventions, nurses need to be open to modifying the structure and format of the sessions. Longer sessions are often useful, especially when a translator or an interpreter is used. Nurses also need to respect and work with the changing composition of family and nonfamily participants (e.g., extended family members, intimate partners, friends and neighbours, community helpers) in sessions. Because of the stigma that some cultural groups associate with seeking help, nurses may need to hold intervention sessions in community settings (e.g., churches, schools) or at the family's home. Finally, termination may need to be gradual or delayed (Celano & Kaslow, 2000).

COUNSELLING

Nurses often use counselling when working with families because it is a short-term problem-solving approach that addresses current issues. If the assessment reveals complex, long-standing relationship problems, the nurse needs to refer the family to a family therapist. If the family is struggling with psychiatric problems of one or more family members or the family system is in a life cycle transition, the nurse should use short-term counselling. The counselling sessions should focus on specific issues, problems, and strengths using sound group process theory. Usually, a problem-solving approach works well once an issue has been identified (see Chapter 15).

PROMOTING SELF-CARE ACTIVITIES

Families often need support in changing behaviours that promote self-care activities. For example, families may inadvertently reinforce a family member's dependency out of fear of the patient being taken advantage of in work or social situations. A nurse can help the family explore how to meet the patient's need for work and social activity and at the same time help alleviate family fears.

Caregiver distress or role strain can occur in families responsible for the care of members with long-term illness. Family interventions can help families deal with the burden of caring for members with psychiatric disorders. An analysis of 16 studies indicated that family interventions can affect relatives' burden, psychological distress, and the relationship between patient and relative and family functioning. These interventions varied from education sessions to intensive family treatment. In most interventions, information on mental illness was presented, as well as discussion. Interventions with more than 12 sessions had more profound effects than did shorter interventions (Cuijpers, 1999). Identifying community resources, groups, and volunteers that can help care for the caregiver will assist in alleviating distress (Cuellar & Butts, 1999).

SUPPORTING FAMILY FUNCTIONING AND COHESIVENESS

Supporting family functioning involves various nursing approaches. In meeting with the family, the nurse should identify and acknowledge its values. In developing a trusting relationship with the family, the nurse should confirm that all members have a sense of self and self-worth. One way this can be accomplished is for the nurse to actively notice and distinguish the family's strengths, resources, and capabilities in the form of a verbal *commendation* (Houger Limacher & Wright, 2003; Wright et al., 1996). For a family that has been challenged, often for many years, with a serious mental health issue, experiencing a direct, specific comment about its positive actions and solutions can be a powerful intervention. It can be as simple as a nurse stating to a family, "I am impressed with your strength, your detailed knowledge about the medication regime, and the way that you have stuck together to support one another by visiting the hospital and attending this family meeting." Supporting family subsystems, such as encouraging the children to play while meeting with the spouses, reinforces family boundaries. Based on assessment of the family system's operation and communication patterns, the nurse can reinforce open, honest communication.

See Box 17-3 for a summary of a research study on the therapeutic relationship.

PROVIDING EDUCATION AND HEALTH TEACHING

One of the most important family interventions is education and health teaching, particularly in families with mental illness. Families have a central role in the treatment

BOX 17.3

Research for Best Practice: Mental Illness and the Dominant Cultural Discourse: Oral History Accounts of Family Members

From Boschma, G. (2007). Accommodation and resistance to the dominant cultural discourse on psychiatric mental health: Oral history accounts of family members. Nursing Inquiry, 14(4), 266–278.

QUESTION: How is the relational network of families tested, affected, and shaped by a larger cultural set of meanings, explanations, and beliefs about mental illness, vulnerability, and dependency?

METHOD: Oral history: History of mental health care is enriched by the analysis of family member's stories.

FINDINGS: Analysis of family stories revealed the social construction of mental illness and how the family served as a mediating context in which the meaning of mental illness was negotiated.

IMPLICATIONS FOR PRACTICE: Stories by families revealed their ambivalence about the dominant biomedical explanation of mental illness. How our culture frames mental illness may be liberating for some family members but have limited meaning for others. Reaching agreement in families about whether to frame the family member's behaviour as a mental illness was an important matter for open or secret family debate. Exploring meaning and beliefs surrounding the diagnosis with the family can help nurses understand how the family situates themselves with each other, their ill member, and the mental health service team.

of mental illnesses. Members need to learn about mental disorders, medications, actions, side effects, and overall treatment approaches and outcomes. For example, families are often reluctant to have members take psychiatric medications because they believe the medications will "drug" the patient or become addictive. The family's beliefs about mental illnesses and treatment will affect how patients manage their illness.

USING GENOGRAMS

Genograms not only are useful in assessment but also can be used as intervention strategies. Nurses can use genograms to help family members understand current feelings and emotions as well as the family's evolution over several generations. Genograms allow the family to examine relationships from a factual, objective perspective. Often, family members gain new insights and can begin to understand their problems within the context of their family system. For example, families may begin to view depression in an adolescent daughter with new seriousness when they see it as part of a pattern of several generations of women who have struggled with depression. A husband, raised as an only child in a small town,

may better understand his feelings of being overwhelmed after comparing his family structure with that of his wife, who comes from a large family of several generations living together in an urban centre (Box 17-2).

USING FAMILY THERAPY

Family therapy is useful for families who are having difficulty maintaining family integrity. Various theoretical perspectives are used in family therapy; more recently, therapies influenced by postmodernism, hermeneutics, and social constructionism have developed and focus on collaborative, conversational approaches and narrative and solution focused therapies. Family therapy can be short-term or long-term and is conducted by mental health specialists, including advanced practice PMH nurses.

SUMMARY OF KEY POINTS

☐ Family is a group of people defined as "who they say they are" and involved relationally in a complex process where economics, emotion, context, and experiences are interwoven and multilayered. Families come in various compositions, including nuclear, extended, multigenerational, single-parent, same-gender, and blended families. Cultural values and beliefs define family composition and roles.

☐ Nurses complete a comprehensive family assessment when they care for families for extended periods or if a patient has complex mental health problems.

☐ In building relationships with families, nurses must establish credibility and competence with the family. Unless the nurse listens and addresses the family's immediate needs first, the family will have difficulty engaging in the challenges of caring for someone with a mental disorder.

☐ The genogram is an assessment and intervention tool that is useful in understanding health, relationships, and social functioning across several generations.

☐ In assessing the family biologic domain, the nurse determines physical and mental health status and its effects on family functioning.

☐ Family members are often reluctant to discuss the mental disorders of family members because of the stigma associated with mental illness. In many instances, family members do not know whether mental illnesses were present in other generations.

☐ The family psychological assessment focuses on family development, the family life cycle, communication patterns, stress and coping abilities, and problem-solving skills. One assessment aim is to begin to understand family interpersonal relationships.

◻ The family life cycle is a process of expansion, contraction, and realignment of the relationship systems to support the entry, exit, and development of family members in a functional way. The nurse should determine whether a family fits any of the life cycle models. Families living in poverty may have a condensed life cycle.

◻ In assessing the family social domain, the nurse compiles data about the system itself, social and financial status, and formal and informal support networks.

◻ Clergy of all faiths may be a significant support to families with a mentally ill member. Collaboration between clergy, nurses, and other health professionals can result in improved treatment planning and response to family crises.

◻ Family interventions focus on supporting the family's bio/psycho/social/spiritual integrity and functioning as defined by its members. Family PMH nursing interventions include counselling, promotion of self-care activities, noticing strengths and resources, purposefully commending the family, supportive therapy, education and health teaching, and the use of genograms. Mental health specialists, including advanced practice nurses, conduct family therapy.

◻ Education of the family is one of the most useful interventions. Teaching the family about mental disorders, life cycles, family systems, and family interactions can help the family develop a new understanding of family functioning and the effects of mental disorders on the family.

CRITICAL THINKING CHALLENGES

1 Differentiate between a nuclear family, extended family, and "family is who they say they are." What would these three configurations have in common?

2 Interview a family with a member who has a mental illness and identify who provides support to the individual and family during acute episodes of illness.

3 Interview someone from a different ethnic background regarding family beliefs about mental illness. Compare them to your own.

4 Develop a genogram for your family. Analyze the genogram in terms of its pattern of health problems, relationship issues, and other contextual issues including social and economic functioning.

5 A female patient, divorced with two small children, reports that she is reluctant to tell anyone about her bipolar disorder. However, she worries about who will look after her children, ages 5 and 7, if she experiences another psychotic episode. Using ideas about family development and life cycle transitions, develop a plan for structuring the counselling session.

6 A family is finding it difficult to provide transportation to a support group for an adult member with mental illness. The family is committed to his treatment but is also experiencing severe financial stress because of another family illness. Using a problem-solving approach, outline a plan for helping the family explore solutions to the transportation problem.

7 Discuss with a local religious leader or clergy his or her experiences related to mentally ill members of the community and their families. What is this leader's perspective of existing relationships with mental health professionals and preferred relationships?

WEB LINKS

www.aamft.org The American Association for Marriage and Family Therapy website offers help in finding a therapist and information on families and health. Canadian members of AAMFT may post their information on this site. It also provides resources for practitioners.

www.fameforfamilies.com/ The Family Association for Mental Health Everywhere (FAME) "is an organization for family support when mental illness of any form is an issue." FAME is "run for and by families to reduce the stress of coping with mental illness by strengthening and supporting family members in their role as caregivers." It is based in Toronto.

www.vifamily.ca The Vanier Institute of the Family was established in 1965 to promote the well-being of Canadian families. This national charitable organization offers support for students, educators, policy makers, and families. This site offers a newsroom and a virtual library.

www.schizophrenia.on.ca This is a web page for the Schizophrenia Society of Ontario. It has a page specific to the needs of families and consumers including coping, educational resources, and networking to strengthen families together.

www.parl.gc.ca/38/1/parlbus/commbus/senate/com-e/soci-e/rep-e/report1/repintnov04vol1table-e.htm This is a report on mental health, mental illness, and addictions in the Canadian context. Chapter 2 focuses on family. The report is from the Standing Senate Committee on Social Affairs, Science and Technology, Report 1, November 2004.

www12.statcan.ca/census-recensement/2006/as-sa/97-553/index-eng.cfm This is the 2006 Canada census data revealing the changing portrait of contemporary Canadian families.

MOVIES, NOVELS, AND BIOGRAPHIES

Proof: 2005. Based on a Pulitzer Prize winning play by D. Auburn, this movie captures family tensions that can occur when a family member has a severe mental illness. Anthony Hopkins plays the role of a mathematical genius, Robert, who became ill with a psychotic illness at the height of his career, over 20 years ago. His daughter, Catherine (Gwyneth Paltrow), lives with him, having given up her own studies to do so. The movie captures the days surrounding Robert's funeral. Catherine's sister, Claire, has returned home to take charge of settling her father's affairs, and Hal (Jake Gyllenhaal), a former graduate student of Robert, is sorting through his old professor's notes. When Jake comes across a notebook with a brilliant mathematical proof and Catherine claims it is hers, her own mental stability is questioned.

VIEWING POINTS: What is revealed in the relational dynamics between the two sisters? How has their father's illness influenced these dynamics? Do you think worry regarding inheritance of mental illness is common for family members with a parent or sibling with a mental disorder? In what ways may the stigma of mental illness affect family members?

Flower and Garnet: 2002. This very engaging story of a family living in British Columbia reveals the confusion of a young boy, Garnet, as he tries to understand his family and his world. Garnet's mother died giving birth to him, and Flower, Garnet's sister, has taken over the mothering role. His father's grief at the death of his wife remains unresolved. This award-winning film is both funny and moving in its portrayal of family dynamics.

VIEWING POINTS: What are the issues facing this family? What kind of support from the health care system would be helpful? What kind of efforts at support might not be suitable for this family?

New Waterford Girl: 1999. Mooney Pottie, 15 years of age, lives in the coal-mining town of New Waterford on Cape Breton with her parents and four siblings. She feels confined within the bounds of her small-town life and yearns to leave. Her new friend, Lou, has moved with her mother from the Bronx to Cape Breton in an effort to get away from her boxer father. Though she sees the town and Mooney's warm family through different eyes, Lou helps Moonie with her plan to escape to the big city.

VIEWING POINTS: Consider the differences between Moonie's and Lou's families. How does the location and context of one's home and family influence family relationships? This story is set in the 1970s. Do you think things are different now in New Waterford?

REFERENCES

Aaron, M. (2008). Spirituality, the heart of caring. *A Life in the Day, 12*(4), 23–26.

Boschma, G. (2007). Accommodation and resistance to the dominant cultural discourse on psychiatric mental health: Oral history accounts of family members. *Nursing Inquiry, 14*(4), 266–278.

Bowen, M. (1978). *Family therapy in clinical practice*. Northvale, NJ: Jason Aronson.

Carpenito, L. (2003). *Nursing diagnosis: Application to clinical practice* (10th ed.). Philadelphia, PA: Lippincott Williams & Wilkins.

Carter, B., & McGoldrick, M. (1999). *The expanded family life cycle*. New York, NY: Allyn & Bacon.

Casado, B., & Leung, P. (2001). Migratory grief and depression among elderly Chinese American immigrants. *Journal of Gerontological Social Work, 36*(1/2), 5–26.

Celano, M., & Kaslow, N. (2000). Culturally competent family interventions: Review and case illustrations. *American Journal of Family Therapy, 28*, 217–228.

Cuellar, N., & Butts, J. (1999). Caregiver distress: What nurses in rural settings can do to help. *Nursing Forum, 34*(3), 24–30.

Cuijpers, P. (1999). The effects of family interventions of relatives' burden: A meta-analysis. *Journal of Mental Health, 8*(3), 275–285.

Doane, G., & Varcoe, C. (2005). *Family nursing as relational inquiry: Developing health-promoting practice*. Philadelphia, PA: Lippincott Williams & Wilkins.

Farrell, J., & Goebert, D. (2008). Collaboration between psychiatrists and clergy in recognizing and treating serious mental illness. *Psychiatric Services, 59*, 437–440.

Hines, P. M. (1999). The family life cycle of African American families living in poverty. In B. Carter & M. McGoldrick (Eds.), *The expanded family life cycle* (pp. 327–345). New York, NY: Allyn & Bacon.

Houger Limacher, L., & Wright, L. M. (2003). Commendations: Listening to the silent side of a family intervention. *Journal of Family Nursing, 9*(2), 130–150.

Leavey, G., Lowenthal, K., & King, M. (2007). Challenges to sanctuary. *Social Sciences and Medicine, 65*(3), 548–559.

Marshall, A., & Harper-Jaques, S. (2008). Depression and family relationships. *Journal of Family Nursing, 14*(1), 56–73.

McGoldrick, M. (2003). Culture: A challenge to concepts of morality. In F. Walsh (Ed.), *Normal family process: Growing diversity and complexity* (3rd ed., pp. 235–39). New York, NY: Guilford Press.

Minuchin, S., & Fishman, H. C. (1981). *Family therapy techniques*. Cambridge, MA: Harvard University Press.

Minuchin, S., Lee, W., & Simon, G. (1996). *Mastering family therapy: Journey of growth and transformation*. New York, NY: John Wiley & Sons.

Schreiber, R., Noerager Stern, P., & Wilson, C. (2000). Being strong: How Black West-Indian Canadian women manage depression and its stigma. *Journal of Nursing Scholarship, 32*(1), 39–45.

Smith, G. C., Hatfield, A. B., & Miller, D. C. (2000). Planning by older mothers for the future care of offspring with serious mental illness. *Psychiatric Services, 51*(9), 1162–1166.

Statistics Canada. (2007). *2006 Census: Family Portrait: Continuity and change in Canadian families and households in 2006: Findings*. Retrieved 3 November, 2009 from http://www12.statcan.ca/census-recensement/2006/as-sa/97-553/index-eng.cfm

Turner, W. L., Wieling, E., & Allen, W. D. (2004). Becoming culturally effective family-based research programs: Implications for family therapists. *Journal of Mental and Family Therapy, 30*(3), 257–270.

Ward-Griffin, C., Schofield, R., Vos, S., & Coatsworth-Puspoky, R. (2005). Canadian families caring for members with mental illness: A vicious cycle. *Journal of Family Nursing, 11*(2), 140–161.

Wright, L. M., & Leahey, M. (2005). *Nurses and families: A guide to family assessment and intervention*. Philadelphia, PA: F. A. Davis.

Wright, L. M., Watson, W. L., & Bell, J. M. (1996). *Beliefs: The heart of healing in families and illness*. New York, NY: Guilford Press.

World Health Organization. (2001). *The world health report 2001 - Mental health: New understanding, new hope*. Geneva, Switzerland: Author.

UNIT *IV*

Care of Persons With Psychiatric Disorders

CHAPTER 18

Schizophrenia

Jane Hamilton Wilson

Adapted from the chapter "Schizophrenia" by Hélène Provencher, Andrea C. Bostrom, and Mary Ann Boyd

LEARNING OBJECTIVES

After studying this chapter, you will be able to:

- Distinguish key symptoms of schizophrenia.
- Analyze the prevailing biologic, psychological, and social theories that are the basis for understanding schizophrenia.
- Analyze human response to schizophrenia with emphasis on hallucinations, delusions, and social isolation.
- Formulate nursing diagnoses based on a bio/psycho/social/spiritual assessment of people with schizophrenia.
- Formulate nursing interventions that address specific diagnoses based on a continuum of care.
- Analyze special concerns within the nurse–patient relationship common to treating those with schizophrenia.
- Identify the expected outcomes and their evaluation.

KEY CONCEPTS

- disorganized symptoms
- negative symptoms
- neurocognitive impairment
- positive symptoms

KEY TERMS

- affective flattening or blunting • affective lability • aggression • agitation
- agranulocytosis • akathisia • alogia • ambivalence • anhedonia • apathy
- avolition • catatonic excitement • confused speech and thinking • delusions
- echolalia • echopraxia • expressed emotion • extrapyramidal side effects
- first episode psychosis • flight of ideas • hallucinations • hypervigilance
- hypofrontality • illusions • neuroleptic malignant syndrome • oculogyric crisis
- paranoia • paranoid schizophrenia • polyuria • prodromal • recovery
- regressed behaviour • retrocollis • stereotypy • tangentiality • tardive dyskinesia
- torticollis • waxy flexibility • word salad

Schizophrenia has fascinated and confounded healers, scientists, and philosophers for centuries. It is one of the most severe complex mental illnesses and is present in all cultures, races, and socioeconomic groups. Its symptoms have historically been attributed to possession by demons, considered punishment by gods for evils done, or accepted as evidence of the inhumanity of its sufferers. These explanations have resulted in enduring stigma for people with diagnoses of this disorder. Today, such stigma persists despite numerous national efforts to educate the Canadian public. All nurses need to understand this disorder and advocate to correct stereotyping and misperceptions. The new Mental Health Commission of Canada (MHCC) has identified combating the stigma of mental illness and preventing discrimination as important priorities in improving the mental health of Canadians (MHCC, 2007). Educating the public and the media about mental illness is a priority.

Clinical Course

In the late 1800s, Emil Kraepelin first described the course of the disorder he called *dementia praecox*. In the early 1900s, Eugen Bleuler renamed the disorder *schizophrenia*, meaning *split minds*, and began to determine that there was not just one type of schizophrenia, but rather a group of schizophrenias. More recently, Kurt Schneider differentiated behaviours associated with schizophrenia as "first rank" symptoms (e.g., psychotic delusions, hallucinations) and "second rank" symptoms (all other experiences and behaviours associated with the disorder). These pioneering physicians had a great influence on the current diagnostic conceptualizations of schizophrenia that emphasize the heterogeneity of the disorder in terms of symptoms, course of illness, and positive and negative symptoms.

▨▨ OVERVIEW OF SCHIZOPHRENIA

The clinical picture of schizophrenia is highly variable and complex. Individual symptoms differ from one another, and the experience for a single individual may be different from episode to episode. For some individuals, the illness onset is slow and insidious; for others, it is sudden, seemingly coming from out of the blue. Similarly, the course of schizophrenia is also unique and unpredictable. About 25% to 30% of people with schizophrenia experience a complete remission after one or several psychotic episodes (Harrison et al., 2001). However, early intervention, including pharmacologic and phase-specific psychosocial interventions, is promising for increasing the rate of recovery in people with first-onset schizophrenia (Addington, Saeed, & Addington, 2005b; Malla, Norman, McLean, Scholten, & Townsend, 2003). It is important to note that **recovery** does not mean cure (see Box 18-1). Although schizophrenia is treatable, it remains a serious and potentially disabling illness. As is the case with most chronic illnesses, the emphasis must be upon maximizing wellness as much as possible, while minimizing the disability. Thornton (2000) suggests that there is not one predictable outcome for an individual with schizophrenia. There may be a variety of outcomes depending on how the illness impacts the person, his or her family, and the kind and type of treatment received. Nurses in both inpatient and community settings have an opportunity to help patients live well with schizophrenia.

Acute Illness Period

Initially, the illness behaviours may be both confusing and frightening to the patient and the family. At first, the changes (often called **prodromal** symptoms) may be subtle and, as they often begin in late adolescence, can even be confused with the anxiety and moodiness of teenage

---

BOX 18.1

Recovery From Schizophrenia

The pioneering work of individuals who have described their own "journey of recovery" from serious mental illness has significantly contributed to a better understanding of recovery from schizophrenia. Patricia Deegan (1992), a psychologist and a psychiatric consumer/advocate, in describing her own experience explains: "[R]ecovery is marked by an ever deepening acceptance of our limitations… we find our limitations are the ground from which spring our own unique possibilities. It is a way of life, an attitude of approaching the day's challenges" (p. 7). Recovery, however, does not mean cure. Rather, recovery is a highly individual process or journey that can involve the experience of growth in response to challenges and the development of a new identity that includes, but moves beyond, illness. Recovery, according to Deegan, refers to "the lived experiences of people as they accept and overcome the challenge of their disability. They experience themselves as recovering a new sense of self and of purpose within and beyond the limits of disability. Recovery is about growth. Recovery can and does happen without professional intervention. Recovery is not just specific to psychosis. Recovery is about taking back control. Recovery is about hanging in there through the long and often slow process of healing. Recovery is a process, not an end point or destination. Everyone's recovery journey is different and deeply personal. Hope is central to recovery" (p. 8).

Source: Deegan, P. (1992). The independent living movement and people with psychiatric disabilities: Taking back control over our own lives. *Psychosocial Rehabilitation Journal, 15*, 5–9.

---

years. However, at some point, the changes in thought and behaviour become so disruptive or bizarre that they can no longer be overlooked. These changes herald the beginning of psychosis. Typically, family and friends become aware that something is not right. Changes might include episodes of staying up all night for several nights, incoherent conversations, and irritability or aggressive acts against self or others. For example, one patient's parents reported their son walking around the apartment for several days holding his arms and hands as if they were a machine gun, pointing them at his parents and siblings, and saying "rat-a-tat-tat, you're dead." Another father described his son's first delusional–hallucination episode as so convincing that it was frightening. His son began visiting cemeteries and making "mind contact" with the deceased. He saw his deceased grandmother walking around in the home and was certain that there were pipe bombs in objects in his home. Another patient believed that he had been visited by space aliens who wanted to unite their world with Earth and assured him that he would become the leader of his country. These experiences are collectively referred to as indicators of **first episode psychosis,** or the initial episode of psychosis, which most often occurs in adolescence or early adult life (see Box 18-2). This early stage of illness, defined as the first 3 to 5 years following the onset

BOX 18.2

First Episode Psychosis

First episode psychosis simply refers to the first time someone experiences psychotic symptoms or a psychotic episode. A psychotic episode occurs in three phases. The length of each phase varies from person to person.

Phase 1. *Prodrome*: The early signs may be vague and hardly noticeable. There may be changes in the way some people describe their feelings, thoughts, and perceptions, which may become more difficult over time.

Phase 2. *Acute*: Clear psychotic symptoms are experienced, such as hallucinations, delusions, or confused thinking.

Phase 3. *Recovery*: Psychosis is treatable: Most people recover. The pattern of recovery varies from person to person. Despite common misperceptions, recovery from a first episode of psychosis is more probable than not. With help, many never have another psychotic episode.

Adapted from the Early Psychosis Prevention and Intervention Centre (http://www.eppic.org.au).

of symptoms, is considered a critical period for intervention (Birchwood, Todd, & Jackson, 1998). Excellent early intervention has been found to lead to more favourable recovery outcomes, leading to many early intervention programs being developed in Canada and around the world. In general, the threefold aim of these programs has been to reduce the duration of untreated psychosis (DUP), to intervene appropriately at this early stage of illness, and to prevent subsequent relapse and minimize the disability (Malla, Norman, & Joober, 2005). These efforts have led to new hope for individuals who develop schizophrenia.

As the DUP increases, patients are less and less able to care for basic needs, such as eating, sleeping, and bathing. Substance use is common. Functioning at school or work deteriorates. Dependence on family and friends increases, and those individuals recognize the need for treatment. In the acute phase, individuals with schizophrenia are at high risk for suicide and may require hospitalization to protect themselves or others.

Initial treatment for schizophrenia focuses upon thorough assessment and the alleviation of symptoms through the initiation of medications, decreasing the risk for suicide through safety measures, normalizing sleep, and reducing substance use. Functional deficits may persist during this period, and the patient and family must begin to learn to cope with these. Emotional blunting diminishes the ability and desire to engage in hobbies, vocational activities, and relationships. Limited participation in social activities spirals into numerous skill deficits, such as difficulty engaging others interpersonally. Cognitive deficits lead to problems recognizing patterns in situations and transferring learning and behaviours from one circumstance to another similar one.

Stabilization Period

After the initial diagnosis of psychosis and the initiation of treatment, stabilization of schizophrenia symptoms becomes the focus. Symptoms become less acute but may still be present. Treatment is intense during this period as medication regimens are established and patients adapt to various medication side effects. Patients and their families begin to adjust to the idea of a family member having a long-term mental illness. Ideally, the use of substances is eliminated. Socialization with others begins to increase, and rehabilitation begins.

Maintenance and Recovery Period

After the patient's condition is stabilized, the patient focuses upon recovery efforts to regain the previous level of functioning and quality of life. Medication treatment of schizophrenia has generally contributed to an improvement in the symptom remission of people with this disorder; however, no medication has cured it. Faithful medication management tends to make the impairments in functioning less severe when they occur and to diminish the extremes an individual might experience. As with any chronic illness, stresses of life and major crises can contribute to exacerbations of symptoms.

Clearly, family support and involvement are extremely important at this time. Once the initial diagnosis is made, patients and families can be educated to watch for early signs of potential relapse and know how to cope with it. This is one of the important themes throughout the nursing process for people with schizophrenia. One of the key goals in the treatment of schizophrenia is to avoid subsequent relapses after the remission of the first episode. This is a tall order indeed. The long-term prognosis with regard to relapse is most certainly influenced by a patient's willingness to remain on maintenance antipsychotic treatment and by appropriate supportive resources being in place.

Relapses

Relapses can occur at any time during treatment and recovery. Relapse is not inevitable; however, it occurs with sufficient regularity to be a major concern in the treatment of schizophrenia. Relapses can occur and are very detrimental to the successful management of this disorder. With each subsequent relapse, rehabilitation is prolonged and there is a longer period of time required to recover. Combining medications and psychosocial treatment greatly diminishes the severity and frequency of recurrent relapses (van Meijel, van der Gaag, Kahn, & Grypdonck, 2003).

One of the major reasons for relapse is nonadherence to the medication regimen. Even with newer medications, nonadherence leading to relapse continues to be a problem (Leucht et al., 2003). Stopping the use of medications almost certainly leads to a relapse and may actually be a stressor that causes a severe and rapid relapse (Baldessarini, 2002). Lower relapse rates are, for the most part, among groups who were following an effective continuing treatment regimen.

Several factors contribute to relapse reduction and to optimal prognostic outcomes and recovery (see Table 18-1). Patients, their families, and members of the treatment team need to be familiar with ways to enhance recovery. It is also important to provide a realistically hopeful attitude for the future.

Many other factors can trigger a relapse: the degree of impairment in cognition and coping that leaves patients vulnerable to stressors; the accessibility of community

Table 18.1	Fostering Recovery From Schizophrenia	
Factors That Encourage Recovery		**Factors That Hinder Recovery**
• Early detection • Short DUP • Optimal treatment including medication, education, individual counselling, and family education and support • Supportive social network • Stable and safe living environment • Access to meaningful activity • Companionship • Attention to physical health • Quick resolution of psychotic symptoms • Hope for the future		• Late detection • Long DUP • Fragmented, inadequate, or inaccessible care • Little support from the social environment • Excess stress, tension, and conflict in the personal environment • Idleness, boredom • Isolation, loneliness • Neglect of physical health and abuse of street drugs or other substances • Persistent, unremitting psychotic symptoms • Hopelessness and despair

Adapted from Mental Health Recovery: What helps and what hinders? *A National Research Project for the Development of Recovery Facilitating System Performance Indicators.* Retrieved November 18, 2009, from http://dare-to-dream.us/recovery/MentalHealthRecovery.pdf

Table 18.2	Key Diagnostic Characteristics of Schizophrenia	DSM IV
Diagnostic Criteria and Target Symptoms		**Associated Findings**
Diagnostic Criteria • Two or more of the following characteristic symptoms present for a significant portion of time during a 1-month period: delusions, hallucinations, disorganized speech, grossly disorganized or catatonic behaviour, and negative symptoms • One or more major areas of social or occupational functioning (such as work, interpersonal relations, and self-care) markedly below the previously achieved level • Continuous signs persisting for at least 6 months • Absence or insignificant duration of major depressive, manic, or mixed episodes occurring concurrently with active symptoms • Not a direct physiologic effect of a substance or medical condition • Prominent delusions or hallucinations present when a prior history of autistic disorder or another pervasive developmental disorder exists *Target Symptoms and Associated Findings* • Inappropriate affect • Loss of interest or pleasure • Dysphoric mood (anger, anxiety, or depression) • Disturbed sleep patterns		• Lack of interest in eating or refusal of food • Difficulty concentrating • Some cognitive dysfunction, such as confusion, disorientation, and memory impairment • Lack of insight • Depersonalization, derealization, and somatic concerns • Motor abnormalities *Associated Physical Examination Findings* • Physically awkward • Poor coordination or mirroring • Motor abnormalities • Cigarette-related pathologies, such as emphysema and other pulmonary and cardiac problems *Associated Laboratory Findings* • Enlarged ventricular system and prominent sulci in the brain cortex • Decreased temporal and hippocampal size • Increased size of basal ganglia • Decreased cerebral size • Slowed reaction times • Abnormalities in eye tracking

resources, such as public transportation, housing, entry-level and low-stress employment, and social services; income supports that buffer the day-to-day stressors of living; the degree of stigmatization that the community holds for mental illness, which attacks the self-concept of patients; and the responsiveness of family members, friends, and supportive others (e.g., peers and professionals) when patients need help.

DIAGNOSTIC CRITERIA

The current definition outlined in the American Psychiatric Association's (APA's) *Diagnostic and Statistical Manual of Mental Disorders*, 4th ed., Text revision (*DSM-IV-TR*; APA, 2000) states that schizophrenia is a mixture of positive and negative symptoms that present for a significant portion of a 1-month period but with continuous signs of disturbance persisting for at least 6 months.

Positive symptoms can be thought of as symptoms that exist but should not and negative symptoms as ones that should be there but are not.

> **KEY CONCEPT** **Positive symptoms** reflect an excess or distortion of normal functions, including delusions and hallucinations.

> **KEY CONCEPT** **Negative symptoms** reflect a lessening or loss of normal functions, such as restriction or flattening in the range and intensity of emotion (**affective flattening** or **blunting**), reduced fluency and productivity of thought and speech (**alogia**), withdrawal and inability to initiate and persist in goal-directed activity (**avolition**), and inability to experience pleasure (**anhedonia**).

The *DSM-IV-TR* criteria for diagnosing schizophrenia include necessary symptomatology, duration of symptoms, evaluation of functional impairment, and elimination of alternate hypotheses that might account for the symptoms (APA, 2000). Several schizophrenia subtypes are currently recognized: paranoid, disorganized, catatonic, undifferentiated, and residual. There is a growing belief that this subtyping is not useful for predicting the course and response to treatment. The diagnostic criteria and current subtypes are listed in Table 18-2 and Box 18-3, respectively.

Positive Symptoms of Schizophrenia

Delusions are erroneous fixed beliefs that usually involve a misinterpretation of experience. For example, the patient believes someone is reading his or her thoughts

---

BOX 18.3
Key Diagnostic Characteristics of Schizophrenia Subtypes

PARANOID TYPE: *DSM-IV-TR* 295.30
- Preoccupation with delusions or auditory hallucinations
- Absence of markedly disorganized speech, disorganized or catatonic behaviour, or flat or inappropriate affect

DISORGANIZED TYPE: *DSM-IV-TR* 295.10
- Disorganized speech, disorganized behaviour, and flat or inappropriate affect

CATATONIC TYPE: *DSM-IV-TR* 295.20
At least two of the following characteristics present:
- Motor immobility or stupor
- Excessive purposeless motor activity
- Extreme negativism
- Posturing, stereotyped movements, prominent mannerisms, or prominent grimacing
- Echolalia or echopraxia

UNDIFFERENTIATED TYPE: *DSM-IV-TR* 295.90
- Only characteristic symptoms present, but does not meet criteria for other subtypes

RESIDUAL TYPE: *DSM-IV-TR* 295.60
- Absence of prominent delusions, hallucinations, disorganized speech, and grossly disorganized or catatonic behaviour
- Negative symptoms persist, or two or more positive symptoms are present in attenuated form, such as odd beliefs or unusual perceptual experiences

---

or plotting against him or her. Various types of delusions include the following:

- *Grandiose*: the belief that one has exceptional powers, wealth, skill, influence, or destiny
- *Nihilistic*: the belief that one is dead or a calamity is impending
- *Persecutory*: the belief that one is being watched, ridiculed, harmed, or plotted against
- *Somatic*: beliefs about abnormalities in bodily functions or structures

Hallucinations are perceptual experiences that occur without actual external sensory stimuli. They can involve any of the five senses, but they are usually *visual* or *auditory*. Auditory hallucinations are more common than visual ones. For example, the patient hears voices carrying on a discussion about his or her own thoughts or behaviours.

Negative Symptoms of Schizophrenia

Negative symptoms are not as dramatic as positive symptoms, but they can interfere greatly with the patient's ability to function day to day. Because expressing emotion is difficult for them, people with schizophrenia laugh, cry, and get angry less often. Their affect is flat, and they show little or no emotion when personal loss occurs. They also suffer from **ambivalence**, which is the concurrent experience of equally strong opposing feelings so that it is impossible to make a decision. The avolition may be so profound that simple activities of daily living, such as dressing or combing hair, may not get done. Anhedonia prevents the person with schizophrenia from enjoying activities. People with schizophrenia have limited speech and difficulty saying anything new or carrying on a conversation. These negative symptoms cause the person with schizophrenia to withdraw and suffer feelings of severe isolation.

Neurocognitive Impairment

Neurocognitive impairment exists in schizophrenia and may be independent of positive and negative symptoms. Neurocognition includes short- and long-term memory; vigilance or sustained attention; verbal fluency or the ability to generate new words; and executive functioning, which includes volition, planning, purposive action, and self-monitoring behaviour. Working memory is a concept that includes short-term memory and the ability to store and process information.

KEY CONCEPT **Neurocognitive impairment** in memory, vigilance, and executive functioning is related to poor functional outcome in schizophrenia (Addington & Addington, 2006).

This impairment is independent of the positive symptoms. That is, cognitive dysfunction can exist even if the positive symptoms are in remission. Not all areas of cognitive functioning are impaired. Long-term memory and intellectual functioning are not necessarily affected. However, for many people with this disorder, symptoms may have interfered with completing educational opportunities. Neurocognitive dysfunction often is manifested in disorganized symptoms.

KEY CONCEPT **Disorganized symptoms** of schizophrenia are those things that make it difficult for the person to understand and respond to the ordinary sights and sounds of daily living. These include **confused speech and thinking** and **disorganized behaviour**.

Disorganized Thinking

Examples of disturbed speech and thinking patterns can be found in Chapter 11, specifically in Boxes 11-6 and 11-7.

Disorganized perceptions often create an oversensitivity to colors, shapes, and background activities. **Illusions** occur when the person misperceives or exaggerates stimuli that actually exist in the external environment. This is in contrast to hallucinations, which are perceptions in the absence of environmental stimuli. Ancillary symptoms that may accompany schizophrenia include anxiety, depression, and hostility.

Disorganized Behaviour

Disorganized behaviour (which may manifest as a very slow, rhythmic, or ritualistic movement), coupled with disorganized speech, makes it difficult for someone with schizophrenia to partake in daily activities. Examples of disorganized behaviour include the following:

- **Aggression**—behaviours or attitudes that reflect rage, hostility, and the potential for physical or verbal destructiveness (usually comes about if the person believes that someone is going to do him or her harm)
- **Agitation**—inability to sit still or attend to others, accompanied by heightened emotions and tension
- **Catatonic excitement**—a hyperactivity characterized by purposeless activities and abnormal movements such as grimacing and posturing
- **Echopraxia**—involuntary imitation of another person's movements and gestures
- **Regressed behaviour**—behaving in a manner of a less mature life stage; childlike and immature
- **Stereotypy**—repetitive, purposeless movements that are idiosyncratic to the individual and to some degree outside of the individual's control
- **Hypervigilance**—sustained attention to external stimuli as if expecting something important or frightening to happen
- **Waxy flexibility**—posture held in odd or unusual fixed position for extended periods of time

■ SCHIZOPHRENIA IN SPECIAL POPULATIONS

Children

The diagnosis of schizophrenia is rare in children prior to adolescence. When it does occur in children aged 5 or 6 years, the symptoms are essentially the same as in adults. In this age group, hallucinations tend to be visual and delusions less developed. Because disorganized speech and behaviour may be explained better by other disorders that are more common in childhood, those disorders should be considered before applying the diagnosis of schizophrenia to a child (APA, 2000).

However, new studies suggest that the likelihood of children later experiencing schizophrenia can be predicted. Developmental abnormalities in childhood, including delays in the attainment of speech and motor development, problems in social adjustment, and poorer academic and cognitive performance, have been found to be present in individuals who experience schizophrenia in adulthood. Specific factors that appear to predict schizophrenia in adulthood include problems in motor and neurologic development, deficits in attention and verbal short-term memory, poor social competence, positive formal thought disorder–like symptoms, and severe instability of early rearing environment (Niemi, Suvisaari, Tuulio-Henriksson, & Lonnqvist, 2003).

Older Adults

People with schizophrenia do grow old. For older persons who have had schizophrenia since young adulthood, this may be a time in which they experience some improvement in symptoms or relapse fluctuations. For instance, admission to general hospitals for older individuals (age 65 years or older) with schizophrenia is more likely to be for an associated condition (Health Canada, 2002). Their lifestyle probably is dependent on the effectiveness of earlier treatment, the support systems that are in place (including relationships with family members and professionals), and the interaction between environmental stressors and the patient's functional impairments.

In late-onset schizophrenia, the diagnostic criteria are met after the age of 45 years. Women are affected more than men. The presentation of late-onset schizophrenia is most likely to include positive symptoms, particularly paranoid or persecutory delusions. Cognitive deterioration and affective blunting occur less frequently. Social functioning is more intact. Many individuals with diagnoses of late-onset schizophrenia have disturbances in sensory functions, primarily hearing and vision losses (APA, 2000). The cost of caring for older persons with schizophrenia remains high because many are no longer cared for in an institution, and community-based treatment has developed more slowly for this age group than for younger adults.

Epidemiology

Schizophrenia occurs in all cultures and countries. The incidence and prevalence rates are similar across studies, with variations explained by the definition of schizophrenia and the sampling method used. Schizophrenia occurs in about 1.3% of the population, or more than 400,000 people in Canada (Goldner, Hsu, Waraich, & Somers, 2002). Its economic costs are enormous. Direct costs include treatment expenses, and indirect costs include lost wages, premature death, and incarceration. In addition, employment among people with schizophrenia is one of the lowest of any group with disabilities (Crowther, Marshall, Bond, & Huxley, 2004). The costs of schizophrenia in terms of individual and family suffering probably are inestimable.

People with schizophrenia tend to cluster in the lowest social classes in industrialized countries and urban communities. For some, the symptoms of the illness are so pervasive that it is difficult for these individuals to maintain any type of gainful employment. Homelessness is a problem for those with severe and persistent symptoms of mental illness (e.g., people with schizophrenia or bipolar illness). Somewhere between 30% and 40% of the homeless are estimated to be suffering from mental illness and, of those, 20% to 25% are living with concurrent disorders, that is, with addiction and other health problems (The Standing Senate Committee on Social Affairs, Science and Technology, 2006).

RISK FACTORS

Risk factors for schizophrenia include stresses in the perinatal period (e.g., starvation, poor nutrition, infections), obstetrical complications, and genetic and family susceptibilities. There also has been evidence that parental age may also be a risk factor (Byrne, Agerbo, Ewald, Eaton, & Mortensen, 2003). Birth cohort studies suggest that the incidence of schizophrenia may be higher among individuals born in urban settings than those born in rural ones and may be somewhat lower in later-born birth cohorts (Harrison et al., 2003). Infants affected by these maternal stressors may have conditions that create their own risk, such as low birth weight, short gestation, and early developmental difficulties. In childhood, stressors may include central nervous system infections.

AGE OF ONSET

Most people who suffer from schizophrenia have the disorder diagnosed in late adolescence and early adulthood. When schizophrenia begins prior to age 25, symptoms seem to develop more gradually, and negative symptoms predominate throughout the course of the disease. People with early-onset schizophrenia experience a greater number of neuropsychological problems. Disruptions occur in milestone events of early adulthood, such as achieving in education, work, and long-term relationships (Csernansky, 2003).

GENDER DIFFERENCES

Men are typically diagnosed with schizophrenia earlier than women. The median age of onset for men is in the middle 20s, whereas the median age of onset for women is in the late 20s (APA, 2000). These gender differences have received attention because of hypotheses about sex-linked genetic etiologies. For instance, estrogen may play a protective role against the development of schizophrenia that disappears as estrogen levels drop during menopause (Hafner, 2003). This would account for the higher median age of onset and a more favourable treatment outcome in women.

ETHNIC AND CULTURAL DIFFERENCES

Increasingly, efforts are being made to consider culture and ethnic origin when diagnosing the disorder and treating individuals with symptoms of schizophrenia (APA, 2000; U.S. Department of Health and Human Services [HHS], 2001). Although symptoms of schizophrenia appear to be clearly defined, it is possible to find cultures in which what appears to be a hallucination may be considered a vision or a religious experience. In addition, behaviours such as averting eyes during a conversation or minimizing emotional expression may be culturally bound yet easily misinterpreted by clinicians of a different cultural or ethnic background.

Individuals of various racial groups may have varying diagnosis rates of schizophrenia. These findings may represent a correct diagnosis or may reflect a misdiagnosis of the disorder based on a cultural bias of the clinician. Prevalence studies indicate a lower incidence of schizophrenia in Asian versus non-Asian countries. It is not known if this difference is due to methodologic, genetic, environmental, or sociologic variables, such as stigma and underreporting (Goldner et al., 2002).

FAMILIAL DIFFERENCES

First-degree biologic relatives (children, siblings, parents) of an individual with schizophrenia have a 10 times greater risk for schizophrenia than the general population (APA, 2000). Other relatives may have an increased risk for disorders within the "schizophrenia spectrum" (a group of disorders with some similarities of behaviour, such as schizoaffective disorder and schizotypal personality disorder; APA). It is still not clear whether genetic vulnerability is present in all cases of schizophrenia. It is possible that genetic vulnerabilities are in terms of psychosis in general and that the expression of these vulnerabilities can take various forms (Walker, Kestler, Bollini, & Hochman, 2004).

COMORBIDITY

Several somatic and psychological disorders coexist with schizophrenia. It is estimated that nearly 50% of patients with schizophrenia have a comorbid medical condition, but many of these illnesses are misdiagnosed or undiagnosed (Goldman, 1999). Recently, more attention has been paid to the causes of mortality among people with schizophrenia. Several physical disorders have been identified, including vision and dental problems, hypertension, diabetes, and sexually transmitted diseases (Muir-Cochrane, 2006).

Substance Abuse and Depression

Among the behavioural comorbidities, substance abuse is common (see Chapter 24). Cannabis use, in particular, has been associated with an increased risk of psychosis onset (Arseneault, Cannon, Wilton, & Murray, 2004). Depression may also be observed in patients with schizophrenia. This is an important symptom for several reasons. First, depression may be the evidence that the diagnosis of a mood disorder is more appropriate (see Chapter 20). Second, depression is not unusual in all stages of schizophrenia and deserves attention. Third, the suicide rate (10%) among individuals with schizophrenia is higher than that of the general population. Risk factors for suicide are male gender, chronic illness with frequent relapses, frequent short hospitalizations, a negative attitude toward treatment, impulsive behaviour, parasuicide (nonfatal self-harm or gesture), psychosis, and depression (De Hert, McKenzie, & Peuskens, 2001). More recently, periods of untreated psychosis exceeding 1 year and treatment with older typical antipsychotic drugs also have been associated with a higher risk for suicide attempts (Altamura, Bassetti, Bignotti, Pioli, & Mundo, 2003).

Diabetes Mellitus

There is a renewed interest in the relationship of diabetes mellitus and schizophrenia. Years ago, an association was established between glucose regulation and psychiatric disorders (Franzen, 1970; Schimmelbusch, Mueller, & Sheps, 1971). In fact, insulin shock therapy was used in treating severe disorders. Also of growing concern is the possibility that people with schizophrenia may be more prone to type II diabetes than is the general public. Some suggest that this may be attributable to inherent characteristics (Ryan, Collins, & Thakore, 2003). Evidence that supports this view includes a higher rate of type II diabetes in first-degree relatives of people with schizophrenia and higher rates of impaired glucose tolerance and insulin resistance among people with schizophrenia. However, obesity, which is associated with type II diabetes, is a growing problem in North America, in general, and is complicated in schizophrenia treatment by the tendency of individuals to gain weight once their disease is managed with medications. Weight gain in some individuals may be attributed to a return to a healthier living situation in which regular meals are available and symptoms that interfere with obtaining food regularly (e.g., delusions) are decreased. For other individuals, weight gain may result from the antipsychotic drug (either typical or atypical) selected for the treatment. Not surprisingly, weight gain is often cited as a reason for nonadherence to antipsychotic medications.

Disordered Water Balance

Patients with schizophrenia, particularly of early onset, may experience disordered water balance. Often, this takes the form of water intoxication characterized by abnormally high water intake, followed by a rapid drop in serum sodium levels. The alteration in sodium level leads to diverse neurologic signs, ranging from ataxia to coma and possibly death. The prevalence rates of disordered water balance remain unclear.

The cause of water intoxication is unknown. Disordered water balance generally precedes water intoxication. Patients characteristically begin compulsively drinking excessive amounts of water. Behaviourally, these patients seem to be "driven to drink" (polydipsia) and may consume between 4 and 10 L of fluid a day. They carry soda cans and water bottles with them, hoard cups or other water containers, and drink frequently from fountains and showers and sometimes from toilets. They make frequent trips to the bathroom because of the excessive need to urinate (**polyuria**). Water intoxication, a complication that is life threatening, occurs when unusually large volumes of ingested water overwhelm the kidneys' capacity to excrete water. As a result, serum sodium levels rapidly fall below the normal range of 135 to 145 mEq/L to a level of 120 mEq/L or less (acute hyponatremia). This rapid decrease in sodium produces muscle twitching and irritability and puts the patient at risk for increased irritability, seizures, or coma (Boyd & Lapierre, 1996).

Etiology

Since the 1970s, hypothetical causes of schizophrenia have changed dramatically (Gur & Gur, 2005; Murray & Bramon, 2005; Walker et al., 2004). Purely psychological theories have been replaced by a neurobiologic model that says that patients with schizophrenia have a biologic predisposition or vulnerability that is exacerbated by environmental stressors. Individuals with schizophrenia are thought to have a genetically or biologically determined sensitivity that leaves them vulnerable to an overwhelming onslaught of stimuli from without and within

BOX 18.4
Deficits That Cause Vulnerability in Schizophrenia

COGNITIVE DEFICITS
- Deficits in processing complex information
- Deficits in maintaining a steady focus of attention
- Inability to distinguish between relevant and irrelevant stimuli
- Difficulty forming consistent abstractions
- Impaired memory

PSYCHOPHYSIOLOGIC DEFICITS
- Deficits in sensory inhibition
- Poor control of autonomic responsiveness

SOCIAL SKILLS DEFICITS
- Impairments in processing interpersonal stimuli, such as eye contact or assertiveness
- Deficits in conversational capacity
- Deficits in initiating activities
- Deficits in experiencing pleasure

COPING SKILLS DEFICITS
- Overassessment of threat
- Underassessment of personal resources
- Overuse of denial

Adapted from McGlashan, T. H. (1994). Psychosocial treatments of schizophrenia: The potential relationships. In N. C. Andreasen (Ed.), *Schizophrenia: From mind to molecule* (pp. 189–215). Washington, DC: American Psychiatric Press.

(HHS, 2001). These inherent vulnerabilities include cognitive, psychophysiologic, social competence, and coping deficits that alter the individual's ability, both cognitively and emotionally, to manage life events and interpersonal situations (Box 18-4 and Fig. 18-1). This section describes the various observations and current theories about the cause of schizophrenia. However, the exact cause of schizophrenia remains elusive.

■ BIOLOGIC THEORIES

Theories and research about the biologic vulnerability for schizophrenia focus on incorporating multiple observations into a coherent explanation. These observations include the course of the illness already described, possible brain structure changes identified by postmortem and neuroimaging techniques, familial patterns, and pharmacologic effects on behaviour and neurotransmitter functions in the brain. One of the more recent theories about the cause of schizophrenic vulnerability focuses on neurodevelopment of the brain from the prenatal period through adolescence. Research efforts are making progress in depicting the neurobiologic substrate of schizophrenia (Keshavan, Tandon, Boutros, & Nasrallah, 2008).

Spiritual

1. Spiritual confusion as auditory hallucinations seem from a higher power
2. And delusions may be religious in content

Biologic

1. Genetic predisposition
2. Dopaminergic dysfunction
3. Hypofrontality
4. Cognitive deficits
5. Immune dysfunction
6. Neuroanatomic changes

Social

1. Decreased financial status
2. Family and caregiver stress
3. Homelessness
4. Stigma and community isolation

Psychological

1. Difficulties in relating
2. Affective blunting (decreased emotional expression)
3. Difficulties with decision making
4. Self-concept changes
5. Decreased stress response and coping
6. Loss of family relationships

FIGURE 18.1 Bio/psycho/social/spiritual etiologies for patients with schizophrenia.

Neuroanatomic Findings

Postmortem and neuroimaging brain studies of patients with schizophrenia show four consistent changes in brain anatomy:

- Decreased blood flow to the left globus pallidus early in the disease
- Absence of normal blood flow increase in frontal lobes during tests of frontal lobe functioning, such as working memory tasks
- Thinner cortex of the medial temporal lobe and a smaller anterior portion of the hippocampus
- Decreases in gray matter and enlarged lateral and third ventricles and widened sulci (Chance, Esiri, & Crow, 2003)

These findings are being used as a basis for exploring the influence of genetic loading, obstetric complications, and differences in familial and nonfamilial patients with schizophrenia (Falkai et al., 2003; McDonald et al., 2002).

Familial Patterns

Evidence supports a familial or genetic base for schizophrenia. First-degree relatives (including siblings and children) are 10 times more likely to experience schizophrenia than are individuals in the general population (APA, 2000; HHS, 1999). Concordance for schizophrenia is higher among monozygotic (identical) twins than among dizygotic (fraternal) twins, although the rate is not perfectly concordant.

Genetic researchers have sought to identify specific genes responsible for schizophrenia, but replicated results are emerging very slowly (Tsuang, Stone, & Faraone, 2001). The infrequency of reproducible results is likely attributable to the heterogeneity of the disorder, which may not be consistent with a single gene theory. A model that includes several genes is more likely to explain the development of schizophrenia (HHS, 1999). Two possible locations are on the long arm of chromosome 22 and on chromosome 6 (Kandel, Schwartz, & Jessell, 2000).

Neurodevelopment

Current theory and research attempt to explain how genes or events early in life (especially perinatal events such as infections or obstetric irregularities) would cause schizophrenia yet manifest symptoms only after years—in adolescence or young adulthood. The neurodevelopmental theory explains and reconciles the inconsistent neuroanatomic brain changes that have been found and links them to early development. Neurodevelopmental models of etiology remain dominant and are fueling advances in epidemiology, imaging, and genetics. It is likely that future whole genome association studies will further tease out the gene–gene and gene–environment interactions (Rapoport, Addington, & Frangou, 2005).

Brain development from prenatal periods through adolescence requires several coordinated molecular activities, including cell proliferation, cell migration, axonal outgrowth, pruning of neuronal connections, programmed cell death, and myelination. All these activities require coordinated development, usually through the activation and inactivation of proteins by genes. Any of these processes could be disrupted by (1) inherited genes that place the individual at risk for schizophrenia, (2) a wild-type allele of this gene that is activated in adolescence or early adulthood, or (3) genetic sensitizing that leaves the individual susceptible to environmental causes or lesioning during some adverse perinatal event. In addition, several maturational events normally occur during puberty that may affect brain development: (1) changes in dopaminergic, serotonergic, adrenergic, glutamatergic, gamma-aminobutyric acid (GABA)-ergic, and cholinergic neurotransmitter systems and substrates; (2) a complex combination of synaptic pruning along with substantial brain growth in some areas of the cortex; and (3) changes in the steroid-hormonal environment (Chou, Halldin, & Farde, 2003).

Neurotransmitters, Pathways, and Receptors

Theories about the cause and pathophysiology of schizophrenia have been generated from decades of pharmacologic research and management of the disorder. For years, the leading hypothesis about the neurobiology of schizophrenia has been based on observations of drug actions. The *dopamine hypothesis* of schizophrenia arose from observations that antipsychotic drugs (Table 18-3), which so successfully ameliorate or reduce the positive symptoms of schizophrenia, act primarily by blocking postsynaptic dopamine receptors in the brain. In addition, other drugs that enhance dopamine function, such as amphetamines or cocaine, cause behavioural symptoms similar to those of **paranoid schizophrenia** in humans and bizarre stereotyped behaviour in monkeys. Antipsychotic drugs stop these drug-induced behaviours. Based on these observations, researchers concluded that schizophrenia was a syndrome of hyperdopaminergic action in the brain.

Table 18.3	Selected Antipsychotic Drugs	
Generic Name	**Trade Name**	**Dosage Range for Adults (mg/day)**
Selected Conventional Antipsychotic Drugs Used to Treat Psychosis in the United States		
First Generation		
Chlorpromazine	Thorazine	30–800
Fluphenazine	Prolixin; Permitil	0.5–20
Haloperidol	Haldol	1–15
Loxapine	Loxitane	20–250
Mesoridazine	Serentil	100–300
Molindone	Moban	15–225
Perphenazine	Trilafon	4–32
Pimozide	Orap*	1–10
Prochlorperazine	Compazine†	15–25
Thiothixene	Navane	5–25
Trifluoperazine	Stelazine	5–25
Triflupromazine	Vesprin	60–150
Second Generation		
Clozapine	Clozaril	200–600
Risperidone	Risperdal	4–16
Olanzapine	Zyprexa	10–20
Quetiapine	Seroquel	300–400
Ziprasidone	Geodon	40–160

*Approved in the United States for Tourette's syndrome.

†Adapted from Stahl, S. (2000). *Essential psychopharmacology: Neuroscientific basis and practical application* (2nd ed.). Cambridge, UK: Cambridge University Press.

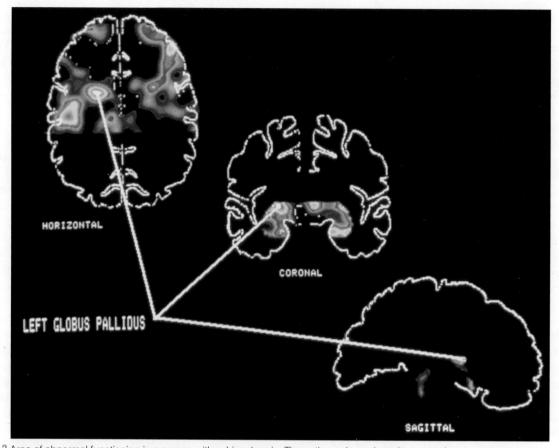

FIGURE 18.2 Area of abnormal functioning in a person with schizophrenia. These three views show the excessive neuronal activity in the left globus pallidus (portion of the basal ganglia next to the putamen). (Courtesy of John W. Haller, PhD, Departments of Psychiatry and Radiology, Washington University, St. Louis, MO.)

This old, straightforward hypothesis of dopamine hyperactivity is clearly complicated by recent findings. Positron emission tomography (PET) scan findings suggest that in schizophrenia, there is a general reduction in brain metabolism, with a relative hypermetabolism in the left side of the brain and in the left temporal lobe. Abnormalities exist in specific areas of the brain, such as in the left globus pallidus (Sedvall, 1994). These findings support further exploration of differential brain hemisphere function in schizophrenia (Fig. 18-2).

Other PET studies show **hypofrontality**, or a reduced cerebral blood flow and glucose metabolism in the prefrontal cortex of people with schizophrenia, and hyperactivity in the limbic area (Buchsbaum, 1990; Figs. 18-3 and 18-4). In addition, several types of dopamine receptors (labeled D_1, D_2, D_3, D_4, and D_5) and dopamine are found in four pathways (mesolimbic, mesocortical, nigrostriatal, and tuberoinfundibular) that innervate different parts of the brain (Kandel et al., 2000; see Chapter 10). Based on the current understanding of schizophrenia, the following discussion relates the neurobiologic changes to the clinical symptoms.

Positive Symptoms: Hyperactivity of Mesolimbic Tract

Positive symptoms of schizophrenia (hallucinations and delusions) are thought to be caused by dopamine *hyperactivity* in the mesolimbic tract, which regulates memory and emotion. It is hypothesized that this hyperactivity could result from an overactive modulation of neurotransmission from the nucleus accumbens (Kandel et al., 2000). Another explanation for dopaminergic hyperactivity in the mesolimbic tract is hypoactivity of the mesocortical tract, which normally inhibits dopamine activity in the mesolimbic tract by some type of feedback mechanism. In schizophrenia, the primary defect may be in the mesocortical tract, where dopaminergic function is diminished, thereby decreasing the inhibitory effects on the mesolimbic tract. This disinhibition may be responsible for the overactivity of dopamine in the mesolimbic tract, resulting in the positive symptom cluster (Kandel et al.,).

Support for this interconnection between the mesocortical and the mesolimbic tracts has been found in laboratory animals. Destruction of the mesocortical tract of animals resulted in increased activity in the mesolimbic tract, especially in the nucleus accumbens. A compensatory

FIGURE 18.3 Metabolic activity in a control subject (*left*), a subject with obsessive-compulsive disorder (*centre*), and a subject with schizophrenia (*right*). (Courtesy of Monte S. Buchsbaum, MD, The Mount Sinai Medical Center and School of Medicine, New York, NY.)

FIGURE 18.4 PET scan with ^{18}F-deoxyglucose shows metabolic activity in a horizontal section of the brain in a control subject (*left*) and in an unmedicated patient with schizophrenia (*right*). Red and yellow indicate areas of high metabolic activity in the cortex; green and blue indicate lower activity in the white-matter areas of the brain. The frontal lobe is magnified to show reduced frontal activity in the prefrontal cortex of the patient with schizophrenia. (Courtesy of Monte S. Buchsbaum, MD, The Mount Sinai Medical Center and School of Medicine, New York, NY.)

increase in mesolimbic neurons is a suggested mechanism by which this overactivity occurs.

Negative Symptoms and Cognitive Impairment: Hypoactivity of the Mesocortical Tract

Negative symptoms and cognitive impairment are thought to be related to hypoactivity of the mesocortical dopaminergic tract, which by its association with the prefrontal and neocortex contributes to motivation, planning, sequencing of behaviours in time, attention, and social behaviour (Jibson & Tandon, 2000; Kandel et al., 2000). Negative symptoms, such as poor motivation and planning and flat affect, are remarkably similar to the symptoms of patients who underwent lobotomy procedures in the late 1940s and early 1950s to disconnect the frontal cortex from the rest of the brain. Monkeys who have had dopamine in the prefrontal cortex depleted have difficulty with cognitive tasks. Finally, PET scans of energy metabolism suggest a reduced metabolism in frontal and prefrontal areas (Davidson & Heinrichs, 2003).

Role of Other Dopamine Pathways

The tuberoinfundibular dopaminergic tract is active in prolactin regulation and may be the source of neuroendocrine changes observed in schizophrenia. The nigrostriatal dopaminergic tract modulates motor activity and is believed to be the site of the **extrapyramidal side effects** of antipsychotic drugs, such as pseudoparkinsonism and **tardive dyskinesia** (abnormal involuntary movements). This may also be the site of some motor symptoms of schizophrenia, such as stereotypic behaviour.

Role of Other Receptors

Other receptors are also involved in dopamine neurotransmission, especially serotonergic receptors. It is becoming clear that schizophrenia does not result from the dysregulation of a single neurotransmitter or biogenic amine (e.g., norepinephrine, dopamine, serotonin). Investigators are also hypothesizing a role for glutamate and GABA (Ghose et al., 2003) because of the complex interconnections of neuronal transmission and the complexity and heterogeneity of schizophrenia symptoms. The N-methyl-D-aspartate (NMDA) class of glutamate receptor is being studied because of the actions of phencyclidine (PCP) at these sites and the similarity of the psychotic behaviours that are produced when someone takes PCP (see Figs. 18-2 to 18-4).

Neural Connectivity

Manifestations of poor mental coordination include difficulty in a variety of functions, such as measuring time or space; making inferences about relationships; and coordinating the processing, priority setting, retrieval, and expression of information. It is being hypothesized that there may be a basic developmental disorder of the neural connectivity involving multiple molecular mechanisms (Benes, 2000; Penn, 2001; Sallet et al., 2003).

■ PSYCHOLOGICAL THEORIES

Several psychological frameworks have been used to explain the etiology of schizophrenia. Before biologic and neurochemical discoveries, these psychological theories presented the primary cause of schizophrenia as dysfunctional parenting in early childhood development. Families often were blamed (e.g., the "schizophrenogenic mother" was suggested as a cause) and alienated by mental health professionals. These theories are no longer held valid, and neurochemical–biologic theories have replaced them.

■ SOCIAL THEORIES

There are no social theories believed to explain schizophrenia, but some theories focus on patterns of family interaction that seem to affect the eventual outcome and social adjustment of individuals with schizophrenia. The theory of **expressed emotion** (EE) correlates certain family communication patterns with an increase in symptoms and relapse in patients with schizophrenia. Families are classified as high-EE families when they make negative comments about family members; when there are aspects of speech that connote criticism, hostility, and negativity about the patient; and when they are emotionally "overly involved" with the patient, such as being overprotective or self-sacrificing. Low-EE families make fewer negative comments and show less overinvolvement with the patient. Families that rate high in the areas of criticism, hostility, and battles for control are hypothesized to be associated with increases in the patient's positive symptoms and relapse.

Research related to emotional expressiveness is contradictory and divisive. Although families categorized as low in EE have been shown to accept the patient as having a legitimate illness and have an understanding that interpersonal problems can exacerbate the illness (Weisman, Gomes, & Lopez, 2003), families high in EE have not been associated with either a greater family history of schizophrenia or the chronicity of the illness (Subotnik, Goldstein, Nuechterlein, Woo, & Mintz, 2002; Wuerker, Long, Haas, & Bellack, 2002).

Although this research might contribute to the understanding of how negative family interaction affects the patient, there are drawbacks to categorizing families in this dualistic manner. Professionals may tend to blame

BGW, born in 1973, spent most of his teenage years using drugs and alcohol, behaviour that started when he was 11. He and his small group of friends spent their teenage years outside of school running around on bicycles. He failed 8th grade, repeated it, and made it to 10th grade. He was removed permanently from school at the age of 16. His dress included a dirty denim jacket or Army fatigues, torn tee shirts with rock band logos, and tight-fitting jeans. At age 16, he was hospitalized for a psychotic episode initiated by LSD; it was the scariest moment of his life. His mind had been getting fuzzier every day; he had dabbled with black magic and Satanism. Later, he admitted that for years, he had been trapped in a fantasy land, only partially explained by his drug use.

Years of treatment followed, and even with abstinence from drugs, his mental status fluctuated. Once antipsychotic agents were prescribed, he began to feel like himself. He was motivated to complete his high school diploma and entered college. He kept his mental illness a secret. While in graduate school, his thoughts, feelings, and behaviours began to change. His thinking became delusional, his moods unpredictable, and his behaviours illogical. Finally, he was hospitalized once again, and his condition was stabilized with medications. Currently, he is reapplying to graduate school and this time vowing to keep people close to him aware of his mental status.

Adapted from Oxford University Press and the Maryland Psychiatric Research Center. (2002). Graduate student in peril: A first person account of schizophrenia. *Schizophrenia Bulletin, 28*(4), 745–755.

families for causing relapse or limit the patient's contact with the family, thus further alienating families who are so vital to the care and support of the patient.

There are numerous social barriers that prevent people with mental illness from getting the care they need. One of the major ones is the social stigma that surrounds mental illnesses (see Chapter 3). Box 18-5 describes the impact of living with a stigmatized illness. Another barrier is difficulty accessing recovery-oriented mental health services that provide comprehensive interventions, resources, and continuity of care. A Canadian study found that individuals experiencing symptoms of psychosis for the first time tried an average of 2.3 times to obtain help. The average length of time the psychosis remained untreated was almost 2 years (Addington, van Mastrigt, Jutchinson, & Addington, 2002; The Standing Senate Committee on Social Affairs, Science and Technology, 2006). Admittedly, mental health service delivery systems are often fragmented, with the quality and types of services varying between communities. Canada's remote rural regions present particular challenges to the provision of timely, comprehensive mental health care.

Interdisciplinary Treatment

The most effective treatment approach for individuals with schizophrenia involves a variety of disciplines, including nursing, psychiatry, psychology, social work, occupational and recreational therapies, pastoral counseling, and peer support workers. Pharmacologic management is the responsibility of the physicians and nurses; various psychosocial interventions can be implemented by all the members of the mental health team. Various professionals and paraprofessionals are necessary because of the complex nature of schizophrenia symptoms and the continuum of interventions required to enhance best outcomes. Inpatient teams are often the starting point, but the spectrum of interventions must include outpatient teams and community-based, recovery-oriented programs. Specialized assertive community teams are particularly helpful in fostering recovery from schizophrenia (see Chapter 4 for continuum of care).

A considerable amount of overlap exists among these professionals and the therapeutic interventions and services they perform. Individual, group, and family counseling may be performed by nurses, psychiatrists, psychologists, certified social workers, and pastoral counselors. Nurses, along with occupational and recreational therapists, can help patients with schizophrenia cope with the disruptions in their day-to-day functioning caused by cognitive and social deficits associated with negative symptoms. Teams of professionals working in partnership with self-help and peer-support programs can shape a favourable recovery environment for stabilizing and enhancing the lives of people who have schizophrenia. However, barriers to this type of treatment abound and include inadequate funding; limitations on physician fee reimbursements; staff shortages (in particular, skilled nurses); large caseloads; insufficient inpatient opportunities; and insufficient community supports, facilities, and social services. Despite these barriers, nurses can contribute significantly to interdisciplinary care given the nursing's emphasis on patients' responses to their illness, their functional adaptation, holistic needs, including physical and psychosocial requirements, and their orientation to family support.

Priority Care Issues

Several special concerns exist when working with people with schizophrenia. About 20% to 50% of people with the diagnosis of schizophrenia attempt suicide, and 10% commit suicide either as a result of psychosis in acute stages or in response to depression in the chronic phase (Canadian Psychiatric Association, 2005; De Hert et al., 2001). Suicide assessment always should be done with a person who is experiencing a first psychotic episode. In an inpatient unit, patient safety concerns extend to potential aggressive actions toward staff and other patients during episodes of psychoses. A priority of care during times of acute illness is treatment with antipsychotic medications.

During the chronic phase of schizophrenia, patients need help in accepting their illness and developing hopeful expectations for their future. They also need help to avoid social isolation through improved social and vocational skills and living arrangements that ensure contact with others (De Hert et al., 2001). Interventions that focus on these goals may address the hopelessness that leads to suicide.

Family Response to Disorder

Few families have had experience with mental illness to help them deal with the manifestations of schizophrenia. The first episode of psychosis is often accompanied by mixed emotions of disbelief, shock, fear, and care and concern for the family member. Hope that this is an isolated or transient episode may also be present. Families initially may seek reasons for the psychotic episode, attributing it to taking illicit drugs or to extraordinary stress or fatigue. Others, particularly parents, may even blame themselves. They often do not know how to comfort their disturbed family member and may find themselves fearful of his or her behaviours. If the patient is hostile and aggressive toward family members, the family may respond with anger and hostility along with fear, confusion, and anxiety. During these episodes, some families may have to seek help from police or a crisis response team to control the situation. Coming to terms with the mental illness of a loved one is often described as an experience of catastrophic proportions (Addington, McCleary, & Addington, 2005a).

The initial period of illness for a patient and family that receive a diagnosis of schizophrenia is extraordinarily difficult. Families may deny the severity and chronicity of the illness, engage in the activities of their previous lifestyle, and only partially engage in treatment within the mental health system. Often, during the initial phase of treatment, families are the primary caregivers for an ill relative. This necessitates that families have opportunities for explanation, education about the illness, and access to timely support. As families acknowledge the meaning of the diagnosis and the potential long-term rehabilitation required, they might feel overwhelmed, angry, and depressed.

◗ NURSING MANAGEMENT: HUMAN RESPONSE TO DISORDER

The nursing management of the patient with schizophrenia usually lasts many years. Different phases of the illness require various nursing interventions at varying intensity. During exacerbation of symptoms, many patients are hospitalized for stabilization. During periods of relative stability, the nurse helps the patient maintain a therapeutic regimen, develop positive mental health strategies, devise strategies to prepare for and cope with the stress, and reclaim his or her life as much as possible.

Because of the complexity of this major psychiatric disorder, the nursing management for each domain is discussed separately. In reality, the nursing process steps overlap in all domains. For example, medication management is a direct biologic intervention; however, the effects of medications also are seen in psychological functioning. In the clinical area, effective nursing management requires an integration of the assessment data from all domains into meaningful interventions. Nursing interventions should cover all domains, including biologic, psychological, social (including family functioning), and spiritual. See Nursing Care Plan 18-1 and Interdisciplinary Treatment Plan 18-1.

Many nursing diagnoses apply to a person with schizophrenia. This is particularly true given that schizophrenia affects so many aspects of an individual's functioning and that symptoms can be observed in cognitive, emotional, family, social, and physical functioning. The applicable diagnoses can be categorized into the phases in which they are most likely to appear. However, it is important to note that even though they have been sorted into these categories, they may still represent recovery challenges in other phases. It is also important to note that the periods between exacerbations of symptoms are actually very important phases for pursuing recovery goals.

Biologic Domain

Biologic Assessment

The following sections highlight the important assessment areas for people with schizophrenia.

Current and Past Health Status and Physical Examination

It is important to conduct a thorough history and physical examination to rule out medical illness or substance abuse that could cause the psychiatric symptoms. It is also important to screen for comorbid medical illnesses that need to be treated, such as diabetes mellitus, hypertension, and cardiac disease, or a family history of such disorders. People with schizophrenia have a higher mortality rate from physical illness and often have smoking-related illnesses, such as emphysema, and other pulmonary and cardiac problems. The nurse should determine whether the patient smokes or chews tobacco, which not only affects the patient's health but also can affect the clearance of medications.

Physical Functioning

The negative symptoms of schizophrenia are often manifested in terms of impairment in physical functioning.

Nursing Care Plan 18.1

Patient With First Episode Psychosis: Probable Schizophrenia

JT is a 19-year-old man who was brought to the hospital following his return from college, where he had locked himself in his room for 3 days. He was talking to nonexistent people in a strange language. His room was covered with small pieces of taped paper with single words on them. His parents immediately made arrangements for him to be assessed and, if necessary, subsequently hospitalized.

Setting: Psychiatric Intensive Care Unit

Baseline Assessment: JT is a 6′1″, 145-lb young man whose appearance is disheveled. He has not slept for 4 days and appears frightened. He is hypervigilant, pacing, and mumbling to himself. He is vague about past drug use, but his parents do not believe that he has used drugs. He appears to be hallucinating, conversing as if someone is in the room. He is confused and unable to write, speak, or think coherently. He is disoriented to time and place. Lab values are within normal limits except Hgb, 10.2, and Hct, 32. He has not eaten for several days.

Associated Psychiatric Diagnosis	Medications
Axis I: Schizophrenia, paranoid Axis II: None Axis III: None Axis IV: Educational problems (failing) 　　　Social problems (withdrawn from peers) GAF = Current 25 Potential?	Risperidone (Risperdal), 2 mg bid, then titrate to 3 mg if needed Lorazepam (Ativan), 2 mg PO or IM for agitation PRN

Nursing Diagnosis 1: Disturbed Thought Processes

Defining Characteristics	Related Factors
Inaccurate interpretation of stimuli (people thinking his thoughts) Cognitive impairment—attention, memory, and executive function impairment Suspiciousness Hallucinations	Uncompensated alterations in brain activity

Outcomes

Initial	Long Term
Decrease or eliminate hallucinations Accurate interpretation of the environment (stop thinking that people are thinking his thoughts) Improvement in cognitive functioning (improved attention, memory, and executive functioning)	Use coping strategies to deal with hallucinations or delusions if they reappear Communicate clearly with others Maintain cognitive functioning

Interventions

Interventions	Rationale	Ongoing Assessment
Initiate a nurse–patient relationship by using an accepting, nonjudgmental approach. Be patient.	A therapeutic relationship will provide patient support as he begins to deal with the realization that he has experienced a first episode psychosis and that diagnosis, although uncertain at this stage, could be the onset of schizophrenia. Be patient and offer information in small, gradual ways. Information processing is likely to be slow at this time.	Determine the extent to which JT is willing to trust and engage in a relationship.

Continued

Nursing Care Plan 18.1 *(Continued)*

Interventions

Interventions	Rationale	Ongoing Assessment
Administer risperidone as prescribed. Observe for effects, side effects, and adverse effects. Begin teaching about the medication and its importance, once symptoms subside.	Risperidone is a D2 and 5-HT2A antagonist and is indicated for the management of psychotic disorders.	Make sure JT swallows the pills. Monitor for relief of positive symptoms and assess side effects, especially extrapyramidal. Monitor BP for orthostatic hypotension and body temperature increase (NMS).
During hallucinations and delusional thinking, assess significance (is it frightening, voices telling him to hurt himself or others?). Reassure JT that you will keep him safe. (Do not try to convince JT that his hallucinations are not real.) Redirect to the here-and-now.	It is important to understand the context of the hallucinations and delusions to be able to provide the appropriate interventions. By avoiding arguments about the content, the nurse will enhance communication.	Assess the meaning of the hallucination or delusion to the patient. Determine whether he is a danger to himself or others. Determine whether the patient can be redirected.
Assess the ability for self-care activities.	Disturbed thinking may interfere with JT's ability to carry out ADLs.	Continue to assess: determine whether the patient can manage self-care.

Evaluation

Outcomes	Revised Outcomes	Interventions
Hallucinations and delusions began to decrease within 3 days. He is oriented to time, place, and person. Attention and memory are improving.	Participate in unit activities according to ITP. Agree to continue to take antipsychotic medications as prescribed.	Encourage attendance at treatment activities. Teach JT about medications. Teach JT about first episode psychosis initially and schizophrenia when diagnosis is confirmed.

Nursing Diagnosis 2: Risk for Violence

Defining Characteristics

Assaultive toward others, self, and environment
Presence of pathophysiologic risk factors: delusional thinking

Related Factors

Frightened, secondary to auditory hallucinations and delusional thinking
Poor impulse control
Dysfunctional communication patterns

Outcomes

Initial	Long Term
Avoid hurting self or assaulting other patients or staff. Decrease agitation and aggression.	Control behaviour with assistance from staff and parents.

Interventions

Interventions	Rationale	Ongoing Assessment
Acknowledge the patient's fears, hallucinations, and delusions. Be genuine and empathetic.	Hallucinations and delusions change an individual's perception of environmental stimuli. A patient who is frightened will respond because of his need to stay safe.	Determine whether the patient is able to hear you. Assess his response to your comments and his ability to concentrate on what is being said.
Offer the patient choices of maintaining safety: keeping distance from others, medication for relaxation, etc.	By having choices, he will begin to develop a sense of control over his behaviour.	Observe the patient's nonverbal communication for evidence of increased agitation.
Administer lorazepam, 2 mg, for agitation. Oral route is preferable over injection.	Exact mechanisms of action are not understood, but this medication is believed to potentiate the inhibitory neurotransmitter GABA, relieving anxiety and producing sedation.	Observe for a decrease in agitated behaviour.

Continued

Nursing Care Plan 18.1 (Continued)

Evaluation

Outcomes	Revised Outcomes	Interventions
JT gradually decreased agitated behaviour. Lorazepam was given regularly for the first 2 days.	Demonstrate control of behaviour by resisting hallucinations and delusions.	Teach JT about the effects of hallucinations and delusions. Problem-solve ways of controlling hallucinations if they occur. Emphasize the importance of taking medications.

INTERDISCIPLINARY TREATMENT PLAN 18.1

Patient With First Episode Psychosis: Probable Schizophrenia

Admission Date	Date of This Plan	Type of Plan: Check Appropriate Box					
05/03/10		☐ Initial	☐ Master	☐ 30	☐ 60	☐ 90	☐ Other

Treatment Team Present:
A. Barton, MD; J. Jones, RN; C. Anderson, RPN; B. Thomas, PhD; T. Toon, SW; J. Barker, LP; F. Huffern, OT, H. Kitchen, Peer Support Worker (PeerSW)

DIAGNOSIS (DSM-IV-TR):

AXIS I: Schizophreniform disorder, possible schizophrenia
AXIS II: None
AXIS III: None
AXIS IV: Educational problems (failing)
       Social problems (withdrawn from peers)
AXIS V: Current GAF: 25
       Highest-Level GAF This Past Year: 90

ASSETS (MEDICAL, PSYCHOLOGICAL, SOCIAL, EDUCATIONAL, VOCATIONAL, RECREATIONAL):

1. First episode of psychosis. No evidence of drug use.
2. Premorbid functional level appears to be normal.
3. Maintained good grades in high school.
4. Has supportive family members.

Prob. No.	Date	Problem/Need	Code	Code	Date
1	3/5/10	Is hallucinating and had delusional thoughts. Unable to communicate with parents or staff.		T	
2	3/5/10	Is aggressive and is striking out at staff and unfamiliar people.		T	
3	3/5/10	Dropped out of college because of thoughts and behaviours.		X	
4	3/5/10	Family members are very upset about their son's psychiatric symptoms.		T	

CODE   T = Problem must be addressed in treatment.
          N = Problem noted and will be monitored.
          X = Problem noted, but deferred/inactive/no action necessary.
          O = Problem to be addressed in aftercare/continuing care.
          I = Problem incorporated into another problem.
          R = Resolved.

Continued

INTERDISCIPLINARY TREATMENT PLAN 18.1 (*Continued*)

INDIVIDUAL TREATMENT PLAN PROBLEM SHEET

#1 Problem/Need	Date Identified	Problem Resolved Discontinuation Date
Is hallucinating and has delusional thoughts. Unable to communicate with parents or staff.	3/5/10	

Objective(s)/Short-Term Goals	Target Date	Achievement Date
1. Reduce report and observations of hallucinations and delusions.	3/15/10	

Treatment Interventions	Frequency	Person Responsible
1. Antipsychotic therapy for hallucinations and delusions. Administer and monitor for adherence, effect, and side effects.	As prescribed	MD/RN
2. Monitor the frequency of hallucinations and delusions.	Close observation for 24–48 hours, then according to RN judgment	RN/RPN, LPN
3. Attend Symptom Management group as symptoms subside.	Daily	PhD, RN, RPN

#2 Problem/Need	Date Identified	Problem Resolved/Discontinuation Date
Is aggressive and is striking out at staff and unfamiliar people.	3/5/10	

Objective(s)/Short-Term Goals	Target Date	Achievement Date
1. De-escalate aggressive behaviour.	3/15/10	

Treatment interventions	Frequency	Person Responsible
1. Keep the patient in a quiet, nonstimulating environment. Assign a private room.	Ongoing	RN/RPN/LPN
2. Administer antianxiety medication as needed.	PRN	MD/RN/RPN
3. Use de-escalation techniques when approaching the patient.	Ongoing	Everyone
4. Assign to anger management group, the if needed when psychotic symptoms decrease.	In 1 week	RN/RPN/LPN

#4 Problem/Need	Date Identified	Problem Resolved/Discontinuation Date
Family members are very upset about their son's psychiatric symptoms.	3/5/10	

Objective(s)/Short-Term Goals	Target Date	Achievement Date
Increase the family's comfort levels with mental illness.	3/15/10	

Treatment Interventions	Frequency	Person Responsible
1. Meet with the family members each time they visit. Provide counseling and education to the family.	Ongoing	RPN/RN/MD
2. Encourage the family to attend family support group.	Weekly	RN/PeerSW
3. Provide community resources for the treatment of mental illness.	When visiting	RN/RPN/Peer SW

Responsible QMHP		**Client or Guardian**		**Staff Physician**	
Signature	Date	Signature	Date	Signature	Date

Self-care often deteriorates, and sleep may be nonexistent during acute phases. Information regarding physical functioning may best be collected from family members.

Nutritional Assessment

A nutritional history should be completed to determine baseline eating habits and preferences. Medications can alter normal nutrition, and the patient may need to limit calories or fat consumption.

Fluid Imbalance Assessment

The nurse should remain alert for signs of polydipsia and polyuria to identify disordered water balance. Patients suspected of having disordered water balance should be assessed for signs and symptoms of hyponatremia, water intoxication, excessive urination, incontinence, or periodically elevated blood pressure. Signs and symptoms of hypervolemia that may be evident include puffiness of the face or eyes, abdominal distention, and hypothermia. These patients should be weighed daily, and their urine specific gravity and serum sodium levels should be monitored (Boyd & Lapierre, 1996).

Pharmacologic Assessment

Baseline information about the initial psychological and physical functioning should be obtained before the initiation of medication (or as early as possible). Side effects of medications should be assessed. Patients are often physically awkward and have poor coordination, motor abnormalities, and abnormal eye tracking. Before medication begins, standardized assessment of abnormal motor movements should be conducted using one of several assessment tools designed for that purpose, such as the Abnormal Involuntary Movement Scale (AIMS; Guy, 1976; see Appendix D), the Dyskinesia Identification System: Condensed User Scale (DISCUS; Sprague & Kalachnik, 1991; Table 18-4), or the Simpson-Angus Rating Scale (Simpson & Angus, 1970; see Appendix C), which is designed for Parkinson-like symptoms.

Nursing Diagnoses for Biologic Domain

Typical nursing diagnoses focusing on the biologic domain for the person during all phases of schizophrenia include self-care deficit and disturbed sleep pattern. During a relapse, ineffective therapeutic regimen management, imbalanced nutrition, excess fluid volume, and sexual dysfunction are possible diagnoses. Constipation may occur if the patient takes anticholinergic medications.

Interventions for Biologic Domain

Nursing interventions during the initial acute phase of schizophrenia include prompt, safe, and informed administration of antipsychotic medications. During any stage, attention to self-care needs and the patient's ability to maintain hygiene and adequate nutrition are important.

Promotion of Self-Care Activities

For many individuals with schizophrenia, the plan of care will include specific interventions to enhance self-care, nutrition, and overall health knowledge. Negative symptoms commonly leave patients unable to initiate these seemingly simple activities. Developing a daily schedule of routine activities (e.g., showering and shaving) can help the patient structure the day. Most patients actually know how to perform self-care activities (e.g., hygiene, grooming) but are not motivated (avolition) to carry them out consistently. Interventions include developing a schedule with the patient for various hygiene activities and emphasizing the importance of maintaining appropriate self-care activities. Given the problems related to attention and memory in people with schizophrenia, education about these areas requires careful planning.

Activity, Exercise, and Nutritional Interventions

Encouraging activity and exercise is necessary, not only to maintain a healthy lifestyle but also to counteract the side effects of psychiatric medications that cause weight gain. Because the diagnosis of schizophrenia is usually made in late adolescence or early adulthood, it is possible to establish solid exercise patterns early.

During episodes of acute psychosis, patients are unable to focus on eating. Often when patients begin antipsychotic medications, normal satiety and hunger responses change, and overeating or weight gain can become a problem. Promoting healthy nutrition is a key intervention. Maintaining healthy nutrition and monitoring calorie intake also become important because of the effect many medications have on eating habits. Patients report that appetite increases and cravings for food develop when some medications are initiated.

Weight gain is one of the reasons some patients become resistant to taking medication. It also may be a contributing factor to the development of type II diabetes

Table 18.4	**The Dyskinesia Identification System**

	NAME	**I.D.**

(HEALTH CARE FACILITY)
Dyskinesia Identification System:
Condensed User Scale (DISCUS)

CURRENT PSYCHOTROPICS/ANTI-
CHOLINERGIC AND TOTAL MG/DAY

_____ ____ mg
_____ ____ mg
_____ ____ mg
_____ ____ mg

See Instructions on the Other Side

EXAM TYPE (check one)
☐ 1. Baseline
☐ 2. Annual
☐ 3. Semi annual
☐ 4. D/C—1 month
☐ 5. D/C—2 months
☐ 6. D/C—3 months
☐ 7. Admission
☐ 8. Other

COOPERATION (check one)
☐ 1. None
☐ 2. Partial
☐ 3. Full

SCORING
0—**Not present** (movements not observed or some movements observed but not considered abnormal)
1—**Minimal** (abnormal movements are difficult to detect or movements are easy to detect but occur only once or twice in a short nonrepetitive manner)
2—**Mild** (abnormal movements occur infrequently and are easy to detect)
3—**Moderate** (abnormal movements occur frequently and are easy to detect)
4—**Severe** (abnormal movements occur almost continuously **and** are easy to detect)
NA—**Not assessed** (an assessment for an item is not able to be made)

ASSESSMENT
DISCUS Item and Score (circle one score for each item)

FACE	1. Tics..	0 1 2 3 4 NA
	2. Grimaces...	0 1 2 3 4 NA
EYES	3. Blinking..	0 1 2 3 4 NA
ORAL	4. Chewing/Lip Smacking.......................	0 1 2 3 4 NA
	5. Puckering/Sucking/ Thrusting Lower Lip.............................	0 1 2 3 4 NA
LINGUAL	6. Tongue Thrusting/ Tongue in Cheek.................................	0 1 2 3 4 NA
	7. Tonic Tongue.......................................	0 1 2 3 4 NA
	8. Tongue Tremor....................................	0 1 2 3 4 NA
	9. Athetoid/Myokymic/ Lateral Tongue.....................................	0 1 2 3 4 NA
HEAD/ NECK/ TRUNK	10. Retrocollis/Torticollis..........................	0 1 2 3 4 NA
	11. Shoulder/Hip Torsion..........................	0 1 2 3 4 NA
UPPER LIMB	12. Athetoid/Myokymic Finger–Wrist–Arm..................................	0 1 2 3 4 NA
	13. Pill Rolling...	0 1 2 3 4 NA
LOWER LIMB	14. Ankle Flexion/ Foot Tapping..	0 1 2 3 4 NA
	15. Toe Movement.....................................	0 1 2 3 4 NA

EVALUATION

1. Greater than 90 d neuroleptic exposure? : YES   NO
2. Scoring/intensity level met? : YES   NO
3. Other diagnostic conditions? : YES   NO
 (if yes, specify)
_____
_____

4. Last exam date: _____
 Last total score: _____
 Last conclusion: _____

Preparer signature and title for items 1–4 (if different from the physician):

5. Conclusion (circle one):

A. No TD (if scoring prerequisite met, list other diagnostic conditions or explain in comments)	D. Withdrawal TD
	E. Persistent TD
	F. Remitted TD
B. Probable TD	G. Other (specify in comments)
C. Masked TD	

6. Comments:
_____
_____
_____
_____
_____
_____
_____

COMMENTS/OTHER
_____
_____
_____
_____
_____

TOTAL SCORE
(items 1–15 only)

EXAM DATE

RATER SIGNATURE AND TITLE	**NEXT EXAM DATE**	**CLINICIAN SIGNATURE**	**DATE**

From Sprague, R. L., & Kalachnik, J. E. (1991). Reliability, validity, and a total score cutoff for the Dyskinesia Identification Scale System: Condensed User Scale (DISCUS) with mentally ill and mentally retarded populations. *Psychopharmacology Bulletin, 27*, 51–58.

mellitus. As such, this places patients at greater risk for several health complications and early death. Monitoring for diabetes and managing weight are important activities for all care providers (Stahl, 2002). Patients should be screened for risk factors of diabetes, such as family history, obesity as indicated by a body mass index (BMI) exceeding or equal to 27, and age older than 45 years. Patients' weight should be measured at regular intervals and their BMI calculated. Blood pressure readings should be taken regularly. Laboratory findings for triglycerides, HDL cholesterol, and glucose level should be monitored and reviewed regularly as well. All providers should be alert to the development of diabetic ketoacidosis, particularly in patients known to have diabetes who begin taking new antipsychotic agents. A program to address weight gain should be initiated at the earliest sign of weight gain (probably between 5 and 10 pounds over desired body weight). Reduced caloric intake may be accomplished by increasing the patient's access to affordable, healthful, and easy-to-prepare foods. Behavioural management of weight gain includes keeping a food diary, diet teaching, and exercise and weight management support groups.

Thermoregulation Interventions

Patients with schizophrenia may have disturbed body temperature regulation. In winter, they may seem to be oblivious to cold weather. In the heat of summer, they may dress for winter. Observing patients' responses to temperatures helps identify problems in this area. In patients who are taking psychiatric medications, body temperature needs to be monitored, and the patient needs to be protected from extremes in temperature. Sun safety is also important, and regular use of a sun screen product to avoid skin damage from sunburn should be recommended.

Promotion of Normal Fluid Balance and Prevention of Water Intoxication

Nursing interventions for disordered water balance include teaching and assisting the patient to develop self-monitoring skills. Fluid intake and weight gain should be monitored to control fluid intake and reduce the likelihood of developing water intoxication.

Pharmacologic Interventions

Early in the 20th century, somatic treatment of schizophrenia included hydrotherapy (baths), wet-pack sheets, insulin shock therapy, electroconvulsive therapy, psychosurgery, and occupational and physical therapies. But in the early 1950s, treatment of schizophrenia drastically changed with the accidental discovery that a drug, chlorpromazine, used to induce anesthesia also calmed patients with schizophrenia. Optimism persists as older medications continue to be used effectively while offering clues into the workings of the brain and

as new discoveries about the brain lead to more precise medications for treating schizophrenia.

Antipsychotic drugs have the general effect of blocking dopamine transmission in the brain by blocking D$_2$ receptors to some degree (see Chapter 14). Some also block other dopamine receptors and receptors of other neurotransmitters to varying degrees. For the most part, the antidopamine effects are not specific to the mesolimbic and mesocortical tracts associated with schizophrenia, but instead travel to all the dopamine receptor sites throughout the brain. This results in desirable antipsychotic effects but also creates some unpleasant and undesirable side effects. The effects of these drugs on other neurotransmitter systems account for additional side effects.

The newer antipsychotic drugs risperidone (Risperdal; Box 18-6), olanzapine (Zyprexa), quetiapine (Seroquel), and ziprasidone (Geodon) appear to be more efficacious and safer than conventional antipsychotics. They are available in a variety of formulations. Risperidone is also available in a long-acting injectable form (Consta). They are effective in treating negative and positive symptoms. These newer drugs also affect several other neurotransmitter systems, including serotonin. This is believed to contribute to their antipsychotic effectiveness (see Chapter 10).

Monitoring and Administering Medications

Antipsychotic medications are the treatment of choice for patients with psychosis. The use of conventional or typical antipsychotics (e.g., haloperidol, Thorazine) decreased dramatically with the introduction of the second generation of antipsychotics. Generally, it takes about 1 to 2 weeks for antipsychotic drugs to effect a change in symptoms. During the stabilization period, the type of drug selected should be given an adequate trial, generally 6 to 12 weeks, before considering a change in the drug prescription. If treatment effects are not seen, another antipsychotic agent may be tried. Clozapine (Clozaril) use may be initiated when no other atypical antipsychotic is effective (see Box 18-7 for more information about Clozaril).

Adherence to a prescribed medication regimen is the best approach to preventing relapse. Unfortunately, patient compliance with medication with atypical antipsychotic agents is not much different from that with conventional antipsychotic agents (Dolder, Lacro, Dunn, & Jeste, 2002). The use of long-acting injectables is expected to improve compliance outcomes. In these days of spending restraints and funding shortfalls, inpatient facilities are discharging patients before a judgment can be made about the efficacy of a given drug treatment. Nurses and other mental health professionals are charged to ensure the continuation of these stabilization protocols and to ensure that outpatient caregivers assume

BOX 18.6

Drug Profile: Risperidone (Risperdal; Consta, Long-Acting Injectable)

DRUG CLASS: Atypical antipsychotic.

RECEPTOR AFFINITY: Antagonist with high affinity for D_2 and 5-HT_2, also histamine (H_1) and α_1- and α_2-adrenergic receptors, weak affinity for D_1 and other serotonin receptor subtypes; no affinity for acetylcholine or β-adrenergic receptors.

INDICATIONS: Psychotic disorders such as schizophrenia, schizoaffective illness, bipolar affective disorder, and major depression with psychotic features.

ROUTES AND DOSAGE: 1-, 2-, 3-, and 4-mg tablets and liquid concentrate (1 mg/mL). 25, 50, and 75 mg long-acting IM.

Adult Dosage: Initial dose typically 1 mg bid. Maximal effect at 6 mg/day. Safety not established above 16 mg/day. Use lowest possible dose to alleviate symptoms.

Geriatric: Initial dose, 0.5 mg/day, increase slowly as tolerated.

Children: Safety and efficacy with this age group have not been established.

INJECTION: Initiate 25 or 50 mg with oral supplementation for 2–3 weeks. Then injections only, every 2–3 weeks. Given IM in gluteal area.

HALF-LIFE (PEAK EFFECT): mean, 20 hours (1 hour, peak active metabolite = 3–17 hours).

SELECT ADVERSE REACTIONS: Insomnia, agitation, anxiety, extrapyramidal symptoms, headache, rhinitis, somnolence, dizziness, headache, constipation, nausea, dyspepsia, vomiting, abdominal pain, hypersalivation, tachycardia, orthostatic hypotension, fever, chest pain, coughing, photosensitivity, and weight gain.

WARNING: Rare development of NMS. Observe frequently for early signs of tardive dyskinesia. Use caution with individuals who have cardiovascular disease; risperidone can cause ECG changes. Avoid its use during pregnancy or while breast-feeding. Hepatic or renal impairments increase plasma concentration.

SPECIFIC PATIENT/FAMILY EDUCATION

- Notify the prescriber if tremor, motor restlessness, abnormal movements, chest pain, or other unusual symptoms develop.
- Avoid alcohol and other CNS depressant drugs.
- Notify the prescriber if pregnancy is possible or planning to become pregnant. Do not breast-feed while taking this medication.
- Notify the prescriber before taking any other prescription or OTC medication.
- It may impair judgment, thinking, or motor skills; avoid driving or other hazardous tasks.
- During titration, the individual may experience orthostatic hypotension and should change positions slowly.
- Do not abruptly discontinue.

BOX 18.7

Drug Profile: Clozapine (Clozaril)

DRUG CLASS: Atypical antipsychotic

RECEPTOR AFFINITY: D_1 and D_2 blockade, antagonist for 5-HT_2, histamine (H_1), α-adrenergic, and acetylcholine. These additional antagonist effects may contribute to some of its therapeutic effects. It produces fewer extrapyramidal effects than standard antipsychotics with lower risk for tardive dyskinesia.

INDICATIONS: Severely ill individuals who have schizophrenia and have not responded to standard antipsychotic treatment. Unlabeled use for other psychotic disorders, such as schizoaffective disorder and bipolar affective disorder.

ROUTES AND DOSAGE: Available only in tablet form, 25- and 100-mg doses.

Adult Dosage: Initial dose of 25 mg PO bid or qid may gradually increase in 25–50 mg/day increments, if tolerated, to a dose of 300–450 mg/day by the end of the 2nd week. Additional increases should occur no more than once or twice weekly. Do not exceed 900 mg/day. For maintenance, reduce the dosage to the lowest effective level.

Children: Safety and efficacy with children younger than 16 years have not been established.

HALF-LIFE (PEAK EFFECT): 12 hours (1–6 hours).

SELECT ADVERSE REACTIONS: Drowsiness, dizziness, headache, hypersalivation, tachycardia, hypo/hypertension, constipation, dry mouth, heartburn, nausea/vomiting, blurred vision, diaphoresis, fever, weight gain, hematologic changes, seizures, tremor, and akathisia.

WARNING: Agranulocytosis, defined as a granulocyte count of <500 mm^3, occurs at about a cumulative 1-year incidence of 1.3%, most often within 4–10 weeks of exposure, but it may occur at any time. Required registration with the clozapine. *Patient Management System,* a WBC count before initiation, and weekly WBC counts while taking the drug and for 4 weeks after its discontinuation. Rare development of NMS. No confirmed cases of tardive dyskinesia, but it remains a possibility. Increased seizure risk at higher doses. Use caution with individuals who have cardiovascular disease; clozapine can cause ECG changes. Cases of sudden, unexplained death have been reported. Avoid its use during pregnancy or while breast-feeding.

SPECIFIC PATIENT/FAMILY EDUCATION

- Need informed consent regarding the risk for agranulocytosis. Weekly blood draws are required. Notify the prescriber immediately if lethargy, weakness, sore throat, malaise, or other flu-like symptoms develop.
- Notify the prescriber if pregnancy is possible or planning to become pregnant. Do not breast-feed while taking this medication.
- Notify the prescriber before taking any other prescription or OTC medication. Avoid alcohol or other CNS depressant drugs.
- It may cause drowsiness and seizures; avoid driving or other hazardous tasks.
- During titration, the individual may experience orthostatic hypotension and should change positions slowly.
- Do not abruptly discontinue.

Table 18.5	Nursing Interventions for Anticholinergic Side Effects
Effect	**Intervention**
Dry mouth	Sips of water; hard candies and chewing gum (preferably sugar free)
Blurred vision	Avoid dangerous tasks; teach the patient that this side effect will diminish in a few weeks
Decreased lacrimation	Artificial tears if necessary
Mydriasis	May aggravate glaucoma; teach the patient to report eye pain
Photophobia	Sunglasses
Constipation	High-fiber diet; increased fluid intake; laxatives as prescribed
Urinary hesitancy	Privacy; run water in sink; warm water over perineum
Urinary retention	Regular voiding (at least every 2–3 hours) and whenever urge is present; catheterize for residual; record intake and output; evaluate benign prostatic hypertrophy
Tachycardia	Evaluate for preexisting cardiovascular disease; sudden death has occurred with thioridazine (Mellaril)

the responsibility for maintaining this stabilization phase of treatment and continue to monitor and manage the patient's symptoms. Outpatient systems should avoid the immediate manipulation of dosages and drugs during the stabilization phase unless a medical emergency ensues.

Given the nature of a chronic illness like schizophrenia, patients generally face a lifetime of taking antipsychotic medications. Rarely is discontinuation of medications prescribed; however, many patients stop taking medications on their own. Some situations that require the cessation of medication use are **neuroleptic malignant syndrome** (NMS) (see Emergency! Box later in this chapter) and **agranulocytosis** (dangerously low level of circulating neutrophils). Discontinuation is an option when tardive dyskinesia develops. Discontinuation of medications, other than in circumstances of a medical emergency, should be achieved by gradually lowering the dose over time. This diminishes the likelihood of withdrawal symptoms, which include withdrawal dyskinesias and withdrawal psychosis.

Monitoring Extrapyramidal Side Effects

Parkinsonism that is caused by antipsychotic drugs is identical in appearance to Parkinson's disease and tends to occur in older patients. The symptoms are believed to be caused by the blockade of D_2 receptors in the basal ganglia, which throws off the normal balance between acetylcholine and dopamine in this area of the brain and effectively increases acetylcholine. The symptoms are managed by reestablishing the balance between acetylcholine and dopamine by reducing the dosage of the antipsychotic (increasing dopamine activity) or adding an anticholinergic drug (decreasing acetylcholine activity), such as benztropine (Cogentin) or trihexyphenidyl (Artane). Discontinuation of the use of anticholinergic drugs should never be abrupt, which can cause a cholinergic rebound and result in withdrawal symptoms, such as vomiting, excessive sweating, and altered dreams and nightmares. Thus, the anticholinergic drug dosage should be reduced gradually (tapered) over several days. If a patient experiences

akathisia (physical restlessness), an anticholinergic medication may not be particularly helpful. Table 18-5 lists the anticholinergic side effects of antiparkinson drugs and several antipsychotic medications and interventions to manage them.

Dystonic reactions are also believed to result from the imbalance of dopamine and acetylcholine, with the latter being dominant. Young men seem to be more vulnerable to this particular extrapyramidal side effect. This side effect, which develops rapidly and dramatically, can be very frightening for patients as their muscles tense and their body contorts. The experience often starts with stiffness experienced in the muscles and can rapidly escalate to **oculogyric crisis**, in which the muscles that control eye movements tense and pull the eyeball so that the patient is looking toward the ceiling. This may be followed rapidly by **torticollis**, in which the neck muscles pull the head to the side, or **retrocollis**, in which the head is pulled back, or orolaryngeal-pharyngeal hypertonus, in which the patient has extreme difficulty swallowing. The patient may also experience contorted extremities. These symptoms occur early in antipsychotic drug treatment, when the patient may still be experiencing psychotic symptoms. This compounds the patient's fear and anxiety and requires a quick response. The immediate treatment is to administer benztropine (Cogentin), 1 to 2 mg, or diphenhydramine (Benadryl), 25 to 50 mg, intramuscularly or intravenously. This is followed by daily administration of anticholinergic drugs and, possibly, by a decrease in antipsychotic medication (see Box 18-8 for more information about benztropine).

Akathisia appears to be caused by the same biologic mechanism as other extrapyramidal side effects. Patients are restless and report that they feel driven to keep moving. They are very uncomfortable. Frequently, this response is misinterpreted as anxiety or increased psychotic symptoms, and the patient may be inappropriately given increased dosages of the antipsychotic drug, which only perpetuates the side effect. If possible, the dose of the antipsychotic drug should be reduced. A beta-adrenergic blocker such as propranolol (Inderal),

BOX 18.8

Drug Profile: Benztropine mesylate (Cogentin)

DRUG CLASS: Antiparkinson agent

RECEPTOR AFFINITY: Blocks cholinergic (acetylcholine) activity, which is believed to restore the acetylcholine/dopamine balance in the basal ganglia.

INDICATIONS: Used in psychiatry to reduce extrapyramidal symptoms (acute medication-related movement disorders), including pseudoparkinsonism, dystonia, and akathisia (not tardive syndromes), due to neuroleptic drugs such as haloperidol. Most effective with acute dystonia.

ROUTES AND DOSAGE: Available in tablet form, 0.5-, 1-, and 2-mg doses, also injectable 1 mg/mL.

Adult Dosage: For acute dystonia, 1–2 mg IM or IV usually provides rapid relief. No significant difference in the onset of action after IM or IV injection. Treatment of emergent symptoms may be relieved in 1 or 2 days, with 1–2 mg orally two to three times per day. Maximum daily dose is 6 mg/day. After 1–2 weeks, withdraw the drug to see if continued treatment is needed. Medication-related movement disorders that develop slowly may not respond to this treatment.

Geriatric: Older adults and very thin patients cannot tolerate large doses.

Children: Do not use in children younger than 3 years. Use with caution in older children.

HALF-LIFE: 12–24 hours, very little pharmacokinetic information is available.

SELECT ADVERSE REACTIONS: Dry mouth, blurred vision, tachycardia, nausea, constipation, flushing or elevated temperature, decreased sweating, muscular weakness or cramping, urinary retention, urinary hesitancy, dizziness, headache, disorientation, confusion, memory loss, hallucinations, psychoses, and agitation in toxic reactions, which are more pronounced in elderly people and occur at smaller doses.

WARNING: Avoid its use during pregnancy or while breastfeeding. Give with caution in hot weather due to a possible heatstroke. Contraindicated with angle-closure glaucoma, pyloric or duodenal obstruction, stenosing peptic ulcers, prostatic hypertrophy or bladder neck obstructions, myasthenia gravis, megacolon, or megaesophagus. It may aggravate the symptoms of tardive dyskinesia or other chronic forms of medication-related movement disorder. Concomitant use of other anticholinergic drugs may increase the side effects and risk for toxicity. Coadministration of haloperidol or phenothiazines may reduce serum levels of these drugs.

SPECIFIC PATIENT/FAMILY EDUCATION
- Take with meals to reduce dry mouth and gastric irritation.
- Dry mouth may be alleviated by sucking sugarless candies, adequate fluid intake, or good oral hygiene; increase the intake of fiber and fluids in diet to avoid constipation; stool softeners may be required. Notify the prescriber if urinary hesitancy or constipation persists.
- Notify the prescriber if rapid or pounding heartbeat, confusion, eye pain, rash, or other adverse symptoms develop.
- It may cause drowsiness, dizziness, or blurred vision; use caution while driving or performing other hazardous tasks requiring alertness. Avoid alcohol and other CNS depressants.
- Do not abruptly stop this medication because a flu-like syndrome may develop.
- Use caution in hot weather. Ensure adequate hydration. It may increase the susceptibility to heatstroke.

---

20 to 120 mg, may be required. Failure to manage this side effect is a leading cause of patients ceasing to take antipsychotic medications.

Tardive dyskinesia (impaired voluntary movement, resulting in fragmented or incomplete movements), tardive dystonia, and tardive akathisia are less likely to appear in individuals taking atypical, rather than conventional, antipsychotics. Table 18-6 describes these and associated motor abnormalities. Tardive dyskinesia is late-appearing abnormal involuntary movements (dyskinesia). It can be viewed as the opposite of parkinsonism both in observable movements and in etiology. Whereas muscle rigidity and absence of movement characterize parkinsonism, constant movement characterizes tardive dyskinesia. Typical movements involve the mouth, tongue, and jaw and include lip smacking, sucking, puckering, tongue protrusion, the bon-bon sign (where the tongue rolls around in the mouth and protrudes into the cheek as if the patient were sucking on a piece of hard candy), athetoid (worm-like) movements in the tongue, and chewing.

Other facial movements, such as grimacing and eye blinking, also may be present.

Movements in the trunk and limbs are frequently observable. These include rocking from the hips, athetoid movements of the fingers and toes, jerking movements of the fingers and toes, guitar strumming movements of the fingers, and foot tapping. The long-term health problems for people with tardive dyskinesia are choking associated with loss of control of muscles used for swallowing and compromised respiratory function leading to infections and, possibly, respiratory alkalosis.

Because the movements resemble the dyskinetic movements of some patients who have idiopathic Parkinson's disease and who have received long-term treatment with L-dopa (a direct-acting dopamine agonist that crosses the blood–brain barrier), the suggested hypothesis for tardive dyskinesia includes the supersensitivity of the dopamine receptor in the basal ganglia.

There is no consistently effective treatment; however, antipsychotic drugs mask the movements of tardive

Table 18.6	Extrapyramidal Side Effects of Antipsychotic Drugs	
Side Effect	**Period of Onset**	**Symptoms**
Acute Motor Abnormalities		
Parkinsonism or pseudoparkinsonism	5–30 days	Resting tremor, rigidity, bradykinesia/akinesia, mask-like face, shuffling gait, and decreased arm swing
Acute dystonia	1–5 days	Intermittent or fixed abnormal postures of the eyes, face, tongue, neck, trunk, and extremities
Akathisia	1–30 days	Obvious motor restlessness evidenced by pacing, rocking, and shifting from foot to foot; subjective sense of not being able to sit or be still; these symptoms may occur together or separately
Late-Appearing Motor Abnormalities		
Tardive dyskinesia	Months to years	Abnormal dyskinetic movements of the face, mouth, and jaw; choreothetoid movements of the legs, arms, and trunk
Tardive dystonia	Months to years	Persistent sustained abnormal postures in the face, eyes, tongue, neck, trunk, and limbs
Tardive akathisia	Months to years	Persisting, unabating sense of subjective and objective restlessness

Adapted from Casey, D. E. (1994). Schizophrenia: Psychopharmacology. In J. W. Jefferson & J. H. Greist (Eds.), *The psychiatric clinics of North America: Annual of drug therapy* (Vol. 1, pp. 81–100). Philadelphia, PA: WB Saunders.

dyskinesia and have periodically been suggested as a treatment. This is counterintuitive because these are the drugs that cause the disorder. Newer antipsychotic drugs, such as clozapine, may be less likely to cause the disorder. The best management remains prevention through prescription of the lowest possible dose of antipsychotic drug over time that minimizes the symptoms of schizophrenia, prescription of these drugs for psychotic symptoms only, and early case finding by regular systematic screening of everyone receiving these drugs (see Table 18-6).

Orthostatic hypotension is another side effect of antipsychotic drugs. The primary antiadrenergic effect is decreased blood pressure, which may be general or orthostatic. Patients may be protected from falls by teaching them to rise slowly and by monitoring blood pressure before doses of the drug. The nurse should monitor and document lying, sitting, and standing blood pressures when any antipsychotic drug therapy begins.

Hyperprolactinemia can occur and is associated with the use of haloperidol and risperidone. When dopamine is blocked in the tuberoinfundibular tract, it can no longer repress prolactin, the neurohormone that regulates lactation and mammary function. The prolactin level increases and, in some individuals, side effects appear. Gynecomastia (enlarged breasts) can occur among both sexes and is understandably distressing to individuals who may be experiencing delusional or hallucinatory body image disturbances. Galactorrhea (lactation) also may occur. Menstrual irregularities and sexual dysfunction are also possible. If these symptoms appear, the medication should be reduced or changed to another antipsychotic agent. Evidence for long-term consequences of hyperprolactinemia is lacking.

Weight gain is related to antipsychotic agents, especially olanzapine and clozapine, which have major antihistaminic properties. Patients may gain as much as 20 or 30 pounds within 1 year. Increased appetite and weight gain are often distressing to patients. Diet teaching and monitoring may have some effect on this side effect. Another solution is to increase the accessibility of healthful, easy-to-prepare food. Although nausea and vomiting can occur with the use of these drugs, most often, these drugs mask nausea.

Sedation is another possible side effect of antipsychotic medication. Patients should be monitored for the sedating effects of antipsychotic agents that are antihistaminic. In elderly patients, sedation can be associated with falls.

New-onset diabetes should be looked for in patients taking antipsychotic drugs. Recently, an association was made between new-onset diabetes mellitus and the administration of atypical antipsychotic agents, especially olanzapine and clozapine. Patients should be assessed and monitored for clinical symptoms of diabetes. Fasting blood glucose tests are commonly ordered for these individuals.

Cardiac arrhythmias may also occur. Prolongation of the QT interval is associated with torsade de pointes (polymorphic ventricular tachycardia) or ventricular fibrillation. The potential for drug-induced prolonged QT interval is associated with many drugs. The newly approved antipsychotic agent ziprasidone (Geodon) may be more likely than other drugs to prolong the QT interval and change the heart rhythm. For these patients, baseline electrocardiograms may be ordered. Nurses should observe these patients for cardiac arrhythmias.

Agranulocytosis is a reduction in the number of circulating granulocytes and decreased production of granulocytes in the bone marrow that limits one's ability to fight infection. Agranulocytosis can develop with the use of all antipsychotic drugs, but it is most likely to develop with clozapine use. Although laboratory values below 500 cells/mm^3 are indicative of agranulocytosis, often granulocyte counts drop to below 200 cells/mm^3 with this syndrome.

Patients taking clozapine must have regular blood tests. White blood cell and granulocyte counts should be measured before the treatment is initiated and at least weekly or twice weekly after the treatment begins. Initial white blood cell counts should be above 3,500 cells/mm^3 before treatment initiation; in patients with counts of 3,500 to 5,000 cells/mm^3, cell counts should be monitored three times a week if clozapine is prescribed. Any time the white blood cell count drops below 3,500 cells/mm^3 or granulocytes drop below 1,500 cells/mm^3, the use of clozapine should be stopped, and the patient should be monitored for infections.

A faithfully implemented program of blood monitoring, however, should not replace careful observation of the patient. It is not unusual for blood cell counts to drop precipitously in a period of 2 to 3 days. This may not be discovered when the patient is on a strict weekly blood monitoring schedule. Any reported symptoms that are reminiscent of a bacterial infection (e.g., fever, pharyngitis, weakness) should be a cause for concern, and immediate evaluation of blood count status should be undertaken. Because patients are frequently discharged before the critical period of risk for agranulocytosis, patient education about these symptoms is also essential so that they will report these symptoms and obtain blood monitoring if necessary. In general, granulocytes return to normal within 2 to 4 weeks after discontinuing use of the medication.

Drug–Drug Interactions

Several potential drug–drug interactions are possible when administering antipsychotic medications. One of the cytochrome P450 enzymes responsible for the metabolism of olanzapine and clozapine is 1A2. If either olanzapine or clozapine is given with another medication that inhibits this enzyme, such as fluvoxamine (Luvox), the antipsychotic blood level would increase and possibly become toxic. On the other hand, cigarette smoking can also induce 1A2 and lower concentration of drugs metabolized by this enzyme, such as olanzapine and clozapine. Smokers may require a higher dose of these medications than do nonsmokers (Stahl, 2000).

Several atypical antipsychotic agents, including clozapine, quetiapine, and ziprasidone, are metabolized by the 3A4 enzyme. Weak inhibitors of this enzyme include the antidepressants fluvoxamine, nefazodone, and norfluoxetine (an active metabolite of fluoxetine). Potent inhibitors of 3A4 enzyme include ketoconazole (antifungal drug), protease inhibitors, and erythromycin. If these drugs are given with clozapine, quetiapine, or ziprasidone, the antipsychotic level will rise. In addition, the mood stabilizer carbamazepine (Tegretol) is a 3A4 inducer. When this drug is given with clozapine, quetiapine, or ziprasidone, the antipsychotic dose should be increased to compensate for the 3A4 induction. If the use of carbamazepine is discontinued, the dosage of the antipsychotic agent needs to be adjusted (Stahl, 2000).

Risperidone, clozapine, and olanzapine are substrates for the enzyme 2D6. Theoretically, antidepressants (fluoxetine and paroxetine) that inhibit this enzyme could increase these antipsychotics' levels. However, this is not usually clinically significant (Stahl, 2000).

Teaching Points

Nonadherence to the medication regimen is an important factor in relapse; the family must be made aware of the importance of the patient consistently taking medications. Medication education should cover the association between medications and the amelioration of symptoms (in general as well as individualized for the patient), side effects and their management, and interpersonal skills that help the patient and family report medication effects.

Emergency! Neuroleptic Malignant Syndrome

In NMS, severe muscle rigidity develops with elevated temperature and a rapidly accelerating cascade of symptoms (occurring during the next 48 to 72 hours), which can include two or more of the following: hypertension, tachycardia, tachypnea, prominent diaphoresis, incontinence, mutism, leukocytosis, changes in the level of consciousness ranging from confusion to coma, and laboratory evidence of muscle injury (e.g., elevated creatinine phosphokinase). NMS occurs in about 1% of those who receive antipsychotic drugs, especially the conventional antipsychotics such as haloperidol (and other drugs that block dopamine, such as metoclopramide; Montoya, Ocampo, & Torres-Ruiz, 2003). As many as one third of these patients may die as a result of the syndrome. NMS is probably underreported and may account for unexplained emergency room deaths of patients taking these drugs who do not have diagnoses because their symptoms do not seem serious. The presenting symptom is a temperature greater than 37.5 °C (usually between 38.3 °C and 39.4 °C) with no apparent cause.

BOX 18.9

Diagnostic Criteria for NMS*

1. Treatment with neuroleptics within 7 days of onset (2–4 weeks for depot neuroleptic medications)
2. Hyperthermia
3. Muscle rigidity
4. Five of the following:
   - Change in mental status
   - Tachycardia
   - Hypertension or hypotension
   - Tachypnea or hypoxia
   - Diaphoresis or sialorrhea
   - Tremor
   - Incontinence
   - Creatinine phosphokinase elevation or myoglobinuria
   - Leukocytosis
   - Metabolic acidosis
5. Exclusion of other drug-induced, systemic, or neuropsychiatric illnesses

* All five items are required concurrently.

From Caroff, S., & Mann, S. (1993). Neuroleptic malignant syndrome. *Medical Clinics of North America, 77,* 185–202, with permission.

The most important aspects of nursing care for patients with NMS relate to recognizing symptoms early, stopping the administration of any neuroleptic medications, and initiating supportive nursing care. In any patient with fever, fluctuating vital signs, abrupt changes in levels of consciousness, or any of the symptoms presented in Box 18-9, NMS should be suspected. The nurse should be especially alert for early signs and symptoms of NMS in high-risk patients, such as those who are agitated, physically exhausted, or dehydrated or those who have an existing medical or neurologic illness. Patients receiving parenteral or higher doses of oral neuroleptic drugs or lithium concurrently must also be carefully assessed. The nurse should carefully monitor fluid intake and fluid and electrolyte status.

CRNENOTE

Recognition of side effects, including movement disorders, tardive dyskinesia, and weight gain, should lead to interventions. NMS is a medication emergency.

To prevent NMS from developing in a patient with signs or symptoms of the disorder, the nurse should immediately discontinue the administration of any neuroleptic drugs and notify the physician. In addition, the nurse should hold any anticholinergic drugs that the patient may be taking. A common error made by nurses who fail to analyze the patient's total clinical picture (including vital signs, mental status changes, and laboratory values) is to continue the use of neuroleptic drugs. Figure 18-5 shows how to decide whether to withhold an antipsychotic medication. Medical treatment includes administering several medications. Dopamine agonist drugs, such as bromocriptine (modest success), and muscle relaxants, such as dantrolene or benzodiazepine, have been used. Antiparkinsonism drugs are not particularly useful. Some patients experience improvement with electroconvulsive therapy.

The vital signs of the patient with symptoms of NMS must be monitored frequently. In addition, it is important to check the results of the patient's laboratory tests for increased creatine phosphokinase, elevated white blood cell count, elevated liver enzymes, or myoglobinuria. The nurse must be prepared to initiate supportive measures or anticipate emergency transfer of the patient to a medical-surgical or an intensive care unit.

Treating high temperature (which frequently exceeds 39 °C) is an important priority for these patients. High body temperature may be reduced with a cooling blanket and acetaminophen. Because many of these patients experience diaphoresis, temperature elevation, or dysphagia, it is important to monitor fluid hydration. Another important aspect of care for patients with NMS is safety. Joints and extremities that are rigid or spastic must be protected from injury. The treatment of these patients depends on the facility and availability of medical support services. In general, patients in psychiatric inpatient units that are separated from general hospitals are transferred to medical-surgical settings for treatment.

Emergency! Anticholinergic Crisis

There is also a potential for abuse of anticholinergic drugs. Some patients may find the anticholinergic effects of these drugs on mood, memory, and perception pleasurable. Although at toxic dosages patients may experience disorientation and hallucinations, lesser doses may cause patients to experience greater sociability and euphoria. Anticholinergic crisis is a potentially life-threatening medical emergency caused by an overdose of or a sensitivity to drugs with anticholinergic properties. This syndrome (also called anticholinergic delirium) may result from an accidental or intentional overdose of antimuscarinic drugs, including atropine, scopolamine, or belladonna alkaloids, which are present in numerous prescription drugs and over-the-counter (OTC) medicines. The syndrome may also occur in psychiatric patients who are receiving therapeutic doses of anticholinergic drugs, especially when such agents are combined with other psychotropic drugs that produce

Drug category

Is patient on antipsychotic drug? — No → Not NMS

Yes

Risk factors

Does patient have any risk factors for NMS? Dehydration? History of NMS? Recent dosage increase? Psychomotor agitation?

Yes

Possible early signs and symptoms

Does patient have any early signs or symptoms of NMS? Low-grade fever? Tachycardia? Elevated BP? Catatonia? Diaphoresis?

Yes

Classic signs and symptoms

Does patient have any classic symptoms of NMS? Hyperthermia? "Lead pipe" rigidity? Mental status changes? Other autonomic CNS changes? — Hold drug →

Notify physician

FIGURE 18.5 Action tree for "holding" a neuroleptic drug because of suspected NMS.

anticholinergic side effects. Numerous drugs commonly prescribed in psychiatric settings produce anticholinergic side effects, including tricyclic antidepressants and some antipsychotics. As a result of either drug overdose or drug sensitivity, these anticholinergic substances may produce an acute delirium or a psychotic reaction resembling schizophrenia. More severe anticholinergic effects may occur in older patients, even at therapeutic levels (stahl, 2000).

The signs and symptoms of anticholinergic crisis are dramatic and physically uncomfortable (Box 18-10). This disorder is characterized by elevated temperature; parched mouth; burning thirst; hot, dry skin; decreased salivation; decreased bronchial and nasal secretions; widely dilated eyes (bright light is painful); decreased ability to accommodate visually; increased heart rate; constipation; difficulty urinating; and hypertension or hypotension. The face, neck, and upper arms may become flushed because of a reflex blood vessel dilation. In addition to peripheral symptoms, patients with anticholinergic psychosis may experience neuropsychiatric symptoms of anxiety, agitation, delirium, hyperactivity, confusion, hallucinations (especially visual), speech difficulties, psychotic symptoms, or seizures. The acute

BOX 18.10

Emergency: Signs and Symptoms of Anticholinergic Crisis

Neuropsychiatric signs: confusion; recent memory loss; agitation; dysarthria; incoherent speech; pressured speech; delusions; ataxia; periods of hyperactivity alternating with somnolence, paranoia, anxiety, or coma

Hallucinations: accompanied by "picking," plucking, or grasping motions; delusions; or disorientation

Physical signs: unreactive dilated pupils; blurred vision; hot, dry, flushed skin; facial flushing; dry mucous membranes; difficulty swallowing; fever; tachycardia; hypertension; decreased bowel sounds; urinary retention; nausea; vomiting; seizures; or coma

psychotic reaction that is produced resembles schizophrenia. The classic description of anticholinergic crisis is summarized in the following mnemonic: "Hot as a hare, blind as a bat, mad as a hatter, dry as a bone."

In general, episodes of anticholinergic crisis are self-limiting, usually subsiding in 3 days. However, if untreated, the associated fever and delirium may progress to coma or cardiac and respiratory depression.

Although rare, death is generally due to hyperpyrexia and brain-stem depression. Once the use of the offending drug is discontinued, improvement usually occurs within 24 to 36 hours.

A specific and effective antidote, physostigmine, an inhibitor of anticholinesterase, is frequently used for treating and diagnosing anticholinergic crisis. Administration of this drug rapidly reduces both the behavioural and the physiologic symptoms. However, the usual adult dose of physostigmine is 1 to 2 mg intravenously, given slowly during a period of 5 minutes because rapid injection of physostigmine may cause seizures, profound bradycardia, or heart block. Physostigmine is relatively short acting, so it may need to be given several times during the course of treatment. This drug provides relief from symptoms for a period of 2 to 3 hours. In addition to receiving physostigmine, patients who intentionally overdose on large amounts of anticholinergic drugs are treated by gastric lavage, administration of charcoal, and catharsis. The dose may be repeated after 20 or 30 minutes.

It is important for the nurse to be alert for signs and symptoms of anticholinergic crisis, especially in elderly people and children, who are much more sensitive to the anticholinergic effects of drugs, and in patients who are receiving multiple medications with anticholinergic effects. If signs and symptoms of the syndrome occur, the nurse should discontinue the use of the offending drug and notify the physician immediately.

Other Somatic Interventions

Electroconvulsive therapy is suggested as a possible alternative when the patient's schizophrenia is not being successfully treated by medication alone. Some research reports using electroconvulsive therapy as an augmentation to antipsychotic therapy (Ota et al., 2003; Tang & Ungvari, 2003). For the most part, this is not indicated unless the patient is catatonic or has a depression that is not treatable by other means.

Psychological Domain

Although schizophrenia is a brain disorder, the psychological manifestations are the most difficult to assess and treat. Many of these psychological manifestations improve with the use of medications, but they are not necessarily eliminated.

Psychological Assessment

Several assessment scales have been developed and received considerable reliability and validity testing to help evaluate positive and negative symptom clusters

BOX 18.11
Rating Scales For Use With Schizophrenia

Scale for the Assessment of Negative Symptoms (SANS)
Available from Nancy C. Andreasen, MD, PhD, Department of Psychiatry, College of Medicine, The University of Iowa, Iowa City, IA 52242. Copyright 1984 (see Box 18-13).

Scale for the Assessment of Positive Symptoms (SAPS)
Available from Nancy C. Andreasen (see above). (see Box 18-12).

Abnormal Involuntary Movement Scale (AIMS)
Guy, W. (1976), *ECDEU: Assessment manual for psychopharmacology* (DHEW Publication No. 76–338). Washington, DC: Department of Health Education and Welfare, Psychopharmacology Branch.

Brief Psychiatric Rating Scale (BPRS)
Overall, J. E., & Gorham, D. R. (1988). The Brief Psychiatric Rating Scale (BPRS): Recent developments in ascertainment and scaling. *Psychopharmacology Bulletin, 24,* 97–99.

Dyskinesia Identification System: Condensed User Scale (DISCUS)
Sprague, R. L., & Kalachnik, J. E. (1991). Reliability, validity, and a total score cutoff for the Dyskinesia Identification Scale System: Condensed User Scale (DISCUS) with mentally ill and mentally retarded populations. *Psychopharmacology Bulletin, 27*(1), 51–58 (see Table 18-4).

Simpson-Angus Rating Scale
Simpson, G. M., & Angus, J. W. S. L. (1970). A rating scale for extrapyramidal side effects. *Acta Psychiatrica Scandinavica, 212*(Suppl.), 11–19. Copyright 1970 Munksgaard International Publishers, Ltd.

in schizophrenia. Box 18-11 lists the standardized instruments used in assessing symptoms of patients with schizophrenia. These include the Scale for the Assessment of Positive Symptoms (SAPS; Box 18-12), the Scale for the Assessment of Negative Symptoms (SANS; Box 18-13), and the Positive and Negative Syndrome Scale (PANSS; Kay, Fiszbein, & Opler, 1987), which assesses both symptom clusters in the same instrument. Tools that list symptoms, such as the Brief Psychiatric Rating Scale (BPRS) (Overall & Gorham, 1988) (see Appendix B), SANS, or SAPS, can also be used to help patients self-monitor their symptoms.

Usually, information about prediagnosis experiences requires retrospective reporting by the patient or the family. This reporting is reliable for the frankly psychotic symptoms of delusions and hallucinations; however, negative symptoms are more difficult to date. In fact, negative symptoms vary from an imperceptive deviation from normal to a clear impairment. Negative symptoms probably occur earlier than positive symptoms and are less easily noted by the patient and significant others.

BOX 18.12

Scale for the Assessment of Positive Symptoms (SAPS)

0 = None 1 = Questionable 2 = Mild 3 = Moderate 4 = Marked 5 = Severe

HALLUCINATIONS

1. *Auditory Hallucinations*   0 1 2 3 4 5
The patient reports voices, noises, or other sources that no one else hears.
2. *Voices Commenting*   0 1 2 3 4 5
The patient reports a voice that makes a running commentary on his behaviour or thoughts.
3. *Voices Conversing*   0 1 2 3 4 5
The patient reports hearing two or more voices conversing.
4. *Somatic or Tactile Hallucinations*   0 1 2 3 4 5
The patient reports experiencing peculiar physical sensations in the body.
5. *Olfactory Hallucinations*   0 1 2 3 4 5
The patient reports experiencing unusual smells that no one else notices.
6. *Visual Hallucinations*   0 1 2 3 4 5
The patient sees shapes or people that are not actually present.
7. *Global Rating of Hallucinations*   0 1 2 3 4 5
This rating should be based on the duration and severity of the hallucinations and their effect on the patient's life.

DELUSIONS

8. *Persecutory Delusions*   0 1 2 3 4 5
The patient believes that he is being conspired against or persecuted in some way.
9. *Delusions of Jealousy*   0 1 2 3 4 5
The patient believes that his spouse is having an affair with someone.
10. *Delusions of Guilt or Sin*   0 1 2 3 4 5
The patient believes that he has committed some terrible sin or done something unforgivable.
11. *Grandiose Delusions*   0 1 2 3 4 5
The patient believes that he has special powers or abilities.
12. *Religious Delusions*   0 1 2 3 4 5
The patient is preoccupied with false beliefs of a religious nature.
13. *Somatic Delusions*   0 1 2 3 4 5
The patient believes that somehow his body is diseased, abnormal, or changed.
14. *Delusions of Reference*   0 1 2 3 4 5
The patient believes that insignificant remarks or events refer to him or have some special meaning.
15. *Delusions of Being Controlled*   0 1 2 3 4 5
The patient feels that his feelings or actions are controlled by some outside force.
16. *Delusions of Mind Reading*   0 1 2 3 4 5
The patient feels that people can read his mind or know his thoughts.
17. *Thought Broadcasting*   0 1 2 3 4 5
The patient believes that his thoughts are broadcast so that he or others can hear them.
18. *Thought Insertion*   0 1 2 3 4 5
The patient believes that thoughts that are not his own have been inserted into his mind.
19. *Thought Withdrawal*   0 1 2 3 4 5
The patient believes that thoughts have been taken away from his mind.
20. *Global Rating of Delusions*   0 1 2 3 4 5
This rating should be based on the duration and persistence of the delusions and their effects on the patient's life.

BIZARRE BEHAVIOUR

21. *Clothing and Appearance*   0 1 2 3 4 5
The patient dresses in an unusual manner or does other strange things to alter his appearance.
22. *Social and Sexual Behaviours*   0 1 2 3 4 5
The patient may do things considered inappropriate according to usual social norms (e.g., masturbating in public).
23. *Aggressive and Agitated Behaviour*   0 1 2 3 4 5
The patient may behave in an aggressive, agitated manner, often unpredictably.
24. *Repetitive or Stereotyped Behaviour*   0 1 2 3 4 5
The patient develops a set of repetitive actions or rituals that he must perform over and over.
25. *Global Rating of Bizarre Behaviour*   0 1 2 3 4 5
This rating should reflect the type of behaviour and the extent to which it deviates from social norms.

POSITIVE FORMAL THOUGHT DISORDER

26. *Derailment*   0 1 2 3 4 5
A pattern of speech in which ideas slip off track onto ideas obliquely related or unrelated.
27. *Tangentiality*   0 1 2 3 4 5
Replying to a question in an oblique or irrelevant manner.
28. *Incoherence*   0 1 2 3 4 5
A pattern of speech that is essentially incomprehensible at times.
29. *Illogicality*   0 1 2 3 4 5
A pattern of speech in which conclusions are reached that do not follow logically.
30. *Circumstantiality*   0 1 2 3 4 5
A pattern of speech that is very indirect and delayed in reaching its goal idea.
31. *Pressure of Speech*   0 1 2 3 4 5
The patient's distracted by nearby stimuli that interrupt his flow of speech.
32. *Distractible Speech*   0 1 2 3 4 5
The patient's speech is rapid and difficult to interrupt; the amount of speech produced is greater than that considered normal.
33. *Clanging*   0 1 2 3 4 5
A pattern of speech in which sounds, rather than meaningful relationships, govern word choice.
34. *Global Rating of Positive Formal Thought Disorder*   0 1 2 3 4 5
This rating should reflect the frequency of abnormality and the degree to which it affects the patient's ability to communicate.

INAPPROPRIATE AFFECT

35. *Inappropriate Affect*   0 1 2 3 4 5
The patient's affect is inappropriate or incongruous, not simply flat or blunted.

BOX 18.13

Scale for the Assessment of Negative Symptoms (SANS)

0 = None; 1 = Questionable; 2 = Mild; 3 = Moderate; 4 = Marked; 5 = Severe;

AFFECTIVE FLATTENING OR BLUNTING

1. *Unchanging Facial Expression*   0 1 2 3 4 5
   The patient's face appears wooden; it changes less than expected as the emotional content of discourse changes.
2. *Decreased Spontaneous Movements*   0 1 2 3 4 5
   The patient shows few or no spontaneous movements and does not shift position, move extremities, etc.
3. *Paucity of Expressive Gestures*   0 1 2 3 4 5
   The patient does not use hand gestures, body position, etc., as an aid to expressing ideas.
4. *Poor Eye Contact*   0 1 2 3 4 5
   The patient avoids eye contact or "stares through" interviewer even when speaking.
5. *Affective Nonresponsivity*   0 1 2 3 4 5
   The patient fails to smile or laugh when prompted.
6. *Lack of Vocal Inflections*   0 1 2 3 4 5
   The patient fails to show normal vocal emphasis patterns; is often monotonic.
7. *Global Rating of Affective Flattening*   0 1 2 3 4 5
   This rating should focus on the overall severity of symptoms, especially unresponsiveness, eye contact, facial expression, and vocal inflections.

ALOGIA

8. *Poverty of Speech*   0 1 2 3 4 5
   The patient's replies to questions are restricted in amount and tend to be brief, concrete, and unelaborated.
9. *Poverty of Content of Speech*   0 1 2 3 4 5
   The patient's replies are adequate in amount but tend to be vague, overconcrete, or overgeneralized, and they convey little information.
10. *Blocking*   0 1 2 3 4 5
    The patient indicates, either spontaneously or with prompting, that his train of thought was interrupted.
11. *Increased Latency of Response*   0 1 2 3 4 5
    The patient takes a long time to reply to questions; prompting indicates that the patient is aware of the question.
12. *Global Rating of Alogia*   0 1 2 3 4 5
    The core features of alogia are poverty of speech and poverty of content.
13. *Grooming and Hygiene*   0 1 2 3 4 5
    The patient's clothes may be sloppy or soiled, and the patient may have greasy hair, body odor, etc.

14. *Impersistence at Work or School*   0 1 2 3 4 5
    The patient has difficulty seeking or maintaining employment, completing school work, keeping house, etc. If an inpatient, he or she cannot persist at ward activities, such as OT, playing cards, etc.
15. *Physical Anergia*   0 1 2 3 4 5
    The patient tends to be physically inert. He or she may sit for hours and does not initiate spontaneous activity.
16. *Global Rating of Avolition–Apathy*   0 1 2 3 4 5
    Strong weight may be given to one or two prominent symptoms if particularly striking.

ANHEDONIA–ASOCIALITY

17. *Recreational Interests and Activities*   0 1 2 3 4 5
    The patient may have few or no interests. Both the quality and the quantity of interests should be taken into account.
18. *Sexual Activity*   0 1 2 3 4 5
    The patient may show a decrease in sexual interest and activity or in enjoyment when active.
19. *Ability to Feel Intimacy and Closeness*   0 1 2 3 4 5
    The patient may display an inability to form close or intimate relationships, especially with the opposite sex and family.
20. *Relationships With Friends and Peers*   0 1 2 3 4 5
    The patient may have few or no friends and may prefer to spend all of his or her time isolated.
21. *Global Rating of Anhedonia–Asociality*   0 1 2 3 4 5
    This rating should reflect the overall severity, taking into account the patient's age, family status, etc.

ATTENTION

22. *Social Inattentiveness*   0 1 2 3 4 5
    The patient appears uninvolved or unengaged. He or she may seem "spacey."
23. *Inattentiveness During Mental Status Testing*   0 1 2 3 4 5
    Tests of "serial 7s" (at least five subtractions) and spelling "world" backward: Score: 2 = 1 error; 3 = 2 errors; 4 = 3 errors.
24. *Global Rating of Attention*   0 1 2 3 4 5
    This rating should assess the patient's overall concentration, clinically and on tests.

From Nancy C. Andreasen, MD, PhD, Department of Psychiatry, College of Medicine, The University of Iowa, Iowa City, IA 52242. Copyright 1984 Nancy C. Andreasen. Reprinted with permission.

Responses to Mental Health Problems

Schizophrenia robs people of mental health and imposes social stigma. People with schizophrenia struggle to maintain control of their symptoms, which affect every aspect of their life. The person with schizophrenia displays a variety of interrelated symptoms and experiences deficits in several areas. More than half of patients report the following prodromal symptoms (in order of frequency): tension and nervousness, lack of interest in eating, difficulty concentrating, disturbed sleep, decreased enjoyment and loss of interest, rest-lessness, forgetfulness, depression, social withdrawal from friends, feeling laughed at, more religious thinking, feeling bad for no reason, feeling too excited, and hearing voices or seeing things.

Because schizophrenia is a disorder of thoughts, perceptions, and behaviour, it is sometimes not recognized as an illness by the person experiencing the symptoms. Many people with thought disorders do not believe that they have a mental illness. Their denial of mental illness and the need for treatment poses problems for the family and clinicians. Ideally, in lucid moments, patients recognize that their thoughts are really delusions, that their perceptions are hallucinations, and that their behaviour is disorganized. In reality, many patients do not believe that they have a mental illness but agree to treatment to please their family and clinicians.

Mental Status and Appearance

The patient with schizophrenia may look eccentric or disheveled or have poor hygiene and bizarre dress. The patient's posture may suggest lethargy or stupor.

Mood and Affect

Patients with schizophrenia often display altered mood states. In some cases, they may show heightened emotional activity; others may display severely limited emotional responses. Affect, the outward expression of mood, is categorized on a continuum: flat (emotional expression entirely absent), blunted (expression of emotions present but greatly diminished), and full range. Inappropriate affect is marked by incongruence between the emotional expression and the thoughts expressed. Other common emotional symptoms include the following:

- **Affective lability**—abrupt, dramatic, unprovoked changes in the type of emotions expressed
- **Ambivalence**—the presence and expression of two opposing feelings, leading to inaction
- **Apathy**—reactions to stimuli are decreased; diminished interest and desire

Speech

Speech patterns may reflect obsessions, delusions, pressured thinking, loose associations, or **flight of ideas** and neologisms. Speech is an indicator of thought content and other mental processes and is usually altered. An assessment of speech should note any difficulty articulating words (dysarthria) and difficulty swallowing (dysphagia) as indicators of medication side effects. In many instances, what an individual says is as important as how it is said. Both content and speech patterns should be noted.

Thought Processes and Delusions

Delusions can be distinguished from strongly held ideas by "the degree of conviction with which the belief is held despite clear contradictory evidence" (APA, 2000, p. 299). Culture must be considered when evaluating delusions. Delusional beliefs are those not sanctioned or held by a cultural or religious subgroup.

Bizarre delusions alone are sufficient to diagnose schizophrenia. It can often be difficult to distinguish between bizarre and nonbizarre delusions. Nonbizarre delusions generally have themes of jealousy and persecution and are derived from ordinary life experiences. For example, a woman believes that her husband, from whom she has recently separated, is trying to poison her, or a man believes that members of the Mafia are trying to kill him because, when he was in high school, he reported to the principal that several of his classmates were selling drugs at school (APA, 2000).

Bizarre delusions are those that are implausible, not understandable, and not derived from ordinary life experiences. Bizarre delusions often include delusions of control (that some outside force controls thoughts and actions), thought broadcasting (that others can read or hear one's thoughts), thought insertion (that someone has placed thoughts into one's mind), and thought withdrawal (that someone is removing thoughts from one's mind; APA, 2000). For example, a patient who has been with a hypnotist for 2 months reports that the hypnotist continued to read his mind and was "picking his brain away piece by piece." Another patient was convinced that a computer chip was placed in her vagina during a gynecologic examination and that this somehow directly influenced her physical movements and her thoughts.

Assessing and judging the content of the delusion and exploring other aspects of the delusional experience are helpful in understanding the significance of these false beliefs. The underlying feeling that accompanies the delusion should be identified. Other aspects to consider include the conviction with which the delusion is held; the extent other aspects of the individual's life are incorporated or affected by the delusion; the degree of internal consistency, organization, and logic evidenced in the delusion; and the amount of pressure (in terms of preoccupation and concern) individuals feel in their lives as a result of the delusion (see Box 18-14).

Hallucinations

Hallucinations are the most common example of disturbed sensory perception observed in patients with schizophrenia. Hallucinations can be experienced in all sensory modalities; however, auditory hallucinations are the most common in schizophrenia. Some specific hallucinations may be sufficient to diagnose schizophrenia, such as hearing voices conversing with each other or carrying on a discussion with someone who is not there. Because most individuals will not spontaneously share their hallucinatory experiences with an interviewer, the nurse may need to rely on indirect evidence in the patient's behaviour, such as (1) pauses during conversations in which the individual seems preoccupied or appears to be listening to someone other than the interviewer, (2) looking toward the perceived source of a voice, or (3) responding to the voices in some manner.

BOX 18.14

Therapeutic Dialogue: The Patient With Delusions

John joined the nurse in a game of pool. The following conversation occurred as they played.

INEFFECTIVE APPROACH

John: The RCMP put a transmitter in my molar, here (points to his right cheek).

Nurse: No one would put a transmitter in your tooth; come on, the RCMP isn't looking for you.

John: You get the striped ones. Yeah, they want to monitor me while I'm here. I know that they have the real Governor General here in the hospital. They are trying to get Stephen Harper to intervene with the Ontario Police. Mark from Ottawa told me that.

Nurse: The Governor General can't possibly be here; I saw her on television this morning.

John: Maybe—she does have lighter hair and has different coloured contacts to disguise her eyes, but they're just trying to keep people from knowing what they're doing.

Nurse: John, Michaelle Jean isn't in the hospital; if she were, I would know it because I work here.

John: (With anger) You don't know anything! You are probably from the RCMP also. I have nothing else to say to you.

EFFECTIVE APPROACH

John: The RCMP put a transmitter in my molar, here (points to his right cheek).

Nurse: Oh. Which balls are mine?

John: You get the striped ones. Yeah, they want to monitor me while I'm here. I know that they have the real Governor General here in the hospital. They are trying to get Stephen Harper to intervene with the Ontario Police. Mark from Ottawa told me that.

Nurse: Do you suppose that you saw someone who looks like the Governor General?

John: Maybe—she does have lighter hair and has different coloured contacts to disguise her eyes. But they're just trying to keep people from knowing what they're doing.

Nurse: You sound a little overwhelmed with all the information you have.

John: No, no. I can handle it. The RCMP can't do anything to me, I'll never talk. They are trying to confuse me so that I stay away from the Governor General. They all think they can keep me from my mission.

Nurse: Who is it that worries you, John?

John: Everyone in the government. The RCMP, CSIS, CRA—all those alphabets.

Nurse: It must be rather frightening to feel all these people are looking for you. You must be scared a lot of the time.

John: It's scary but I can handle it. I've handled it all my life.

Nurse: You've been in scary situations all your life?

John: Yeah. I don't know. Maybe not scary, just hard. I never seemed to be able to do as well as my parents wanted—or as I wanted.

CRITICAL THINKING CHALLENGE

- How did the nurse's argumentative responses cause the patient to react in the first scenario?
- What effective communication techniques did the nurse use in the second scenario?

Although patients may not spontaneously share their hallucinations, many validate observations of the examiner or admit to a history of hallucinations when asked (see Box 18-15).

Disorganized Communication

The other aspect of thought content and processes that may be altered in schizophrenia is the organization of expressed thoughts. Impaired verbal fluency (ability to produce spontaneous speech) is commonly present. Abrupt shifts in the focus of conversation are a typical symptom of disorganized thinking. The most severe shifts in focus may occur after only one or two words (**word salad**), after one or two phrases or sentences (flight of ideas or loose associations), or somewhat less severely as a shift that occurs when a new topic is repeatedly suggested and pursued from the current topic (**tangentiality**). In some individuals, speech may be a simple repetition of words or phrases spoken by others (**echolalia**).

Cognitive Impairments

Although cognitive impairments in schizophrenia vary widely from patient to patient, several primary problems have been identified:

- Attention may be increased and sustained on external stimuli over a period of time (hypervigilance).
- The ability to distinguish and focus on relevant stimuli may be diminished.
- Familiar cues may go unrecognized or be improperly encoded.
- Information processing may be diminished, leading to inappropriate or illogical conclusions from available observations and information (Cirillo & Seidman, 2003; Hartman, Steketee, Silva, Lanning, & Andersson, 2003).

Cognitive impairments are not easy to recognize. By relying only on clinical assessment, the nurse can miss the extent of the impairment. Using a standardized instrument such as the Mini-Mental Status Examination

BOX 18.15

Therapeutic Dialogue: The Patient With Hallucinations

The following conversation took place in a dayroom with several staff members in the room. The patient was potentially very violent. Although it is a good example of dealing with someone who is hallucinating, it is not a situation that should be taken lightly. Always make certain that you have a means to leave a situation (i.e., you are not in the corner of a room) and that you have sufficient staff members close by to ensure safety. Take careful note whether or not the patient has a potential weapon near at hand.

Jason approached the nurse and asked to play pool. The nurse debated about playing but chose to play because Jason appeared distracted and the game might give him something to focus on.

INEFFECTIVE APPROACH

Nurse: Shall I break?

Jason: (Had been looking off to his right, but turns and looks directly at the nurse.) Yeah, go ahead. (Looks at the table briefly and then turns to look out the door and down the hallway.)

Nurse: (Breaking the pool balls without putting any in a pocket.) It's your turn. You can hit any that you'd like.

Jason: (Turning back to the table.) Huh? (Shaking his head as he stared at the table.) What?

Nurse: You know, Jason, you really should pay attention.

Jason: (Hits a ball in and moves to the other side of the table. Stops in line with the next shot but doesn't bend down to take aim. Stands very still and then shakes his head slightly and quickly. Leans down to take aim and then stands up again.)

Nurse: Jason. (Looks at the nurse.) Jason! Are you going to play or not, I don't have all day.

Jason: Oh yeah. (Leans down, takes aim, and misses.)

Nurse: (Moves to where the next shot is. Position is near where Jason is standing. The nurse watches him carefully, moving closer to him.) Please move over, Jason.

Jason: No. (Doesn't move. In peripheral vision, the nurse sees Jason's lips move and he again looks to his right and shakes his head in a staccato motion, as if trying to shake something out of his head.)

EFFECTIVE APPROACH

Nurse: Shall I break?

Jason: (Had been looking off to his right, but turns and looks directly at the nurse.) Yeah, go ahead. (Looks at the table briefly and then turns to look out the door and down the hallway.)

Nurse: (Breaking the pool balls without putting any in a pocket.) Your turn; you can hit any that you'd like.

Jason: (Turning back to the table.) Huh? (Shakes his head as he stares at the table.) What?

Nurse: You can hit any ball you like. I didn't get any.

Jason: (Hits a ball in and moves to the other side of the table. Stops in line with the next shot but doesn't bend

down to take aim. Stands very still and then shakes his head slightly and quickly. Leans down to take aim and then stands up again.)

Nurse: Jason. (He looks at nurse.) Are you aiming at the 10 ball?

Jason: Oh yeah. (Leans down, takes aim, and misses.)

Nurse: (Moving to where her next shot is. The position is very close to where Jason is standing. The nurse watches him carefully while moving closer to him.) Here, let me take this shot.

Jason: Oh. (Moves back. In peripheral vision, the nurse sees Jason's lips move and again he looks to his right and shakes his head in a staccato motion, as if trying to shake something out of his head.)

Nurse: I missed again. (Moves away from the table and turns to Jason, who moves up to the table. He leans down and then stands up again. His lips move again as he turns his head to the right and then looks over his back toward the doorway.) Jason. Jason. (He looks at the nurse.) You have the striped ones.

Jason: (Nods and leans down to take a shot, which he makes. He then misses the next shot. He stands up and moves back from the table, again looking back toward the doorway. He shakes his head) "no."

Nurse: (Watches him closely and moves to the opposite side of the table, making the next shot. Lining up the next shot, Jason leans the pool cue against the table, looks past the nurse, and turns and walks away toward the door. Looks down the hallway, takes a few steps, stops for a minute or so, turns back into the room, and again looks past the nurse. Sits down and shakes his head again. Holds his head in his hands, with his hands covering his ears. The nurse picks up his pool cue and places both against the wall, out of the way. The nurse, recognizing that Jason is likely experiencing auditory hallucinations, remains where she can observe him, noting, as well, that another staff member is near at hand.)

CRITICAL THINKING CHALLENGE

- How did the nurse's impatience translate into Jason's behaviour in the first scenario?
- What effective communicating techniques did the nurse use in the second scenario?

(MMSE), the Cognitive Assessment Screening Instrument (CASI), or the 7-Minute Screen can provide a screening measurement of cognitive function (see Chapter 11). If impairment exists, neuropsychological testing by a qualified psychologist may be necessary.

Memory and Orientation

Impairments in orientation, memory, and abstract thinking may be observed. Orientation to time, place, and person may remain relatively intact unless the patient is particularly preoccupied with delusions and hallucinations. Although all aspects of memory may be affected in schizophrenia, registration or the recall within seconds of newly learned information may be particularly diminished. This affects the individual's short-term and long-term memories. The ability to engage in abstract thinking may be impaired.

Insight and Judgment

Individuals display insight when they display evidence of knowing their own thoughts, the reality of external objects, and their relationship to these. Judgment is the ability to decide or act on a situation. Insight and judgment are closely related to each other and depend on cognitive functions that are frequently impaired in people with schizophrenia.

Behavioural Responses

During periods of psychosis, unusual or bizarre behaviour often occurs. These behaviours can usually be understood within the context of the patient's disturbed thinking. The nurse needs to understand the significance of the behaviour to the individual. One patient moved the family furniture into the yard because he thought that evil spirits were hiding in the furniture. His bizarre behaviour was an attempt to protect his family. Another patient painted a sequence of numbers on his bedroom walls. He said that the numbers were the language of the angels. His bizarre thoughts were at the basis of his behaviour.

Because of the negative symptoms, specifically avolition, patients may not seem interested or organized to complete their normal daily activities. They may stay in bed most of the day or refuse to take a shower. Many times, they will agree to get up in the morning and go to work, but they never get around to it. Several specific behaviours are associated with schizophrenia, including stereotypy (idiosyncratic repetitive, purposeless movements), echopraxia (involuntary imitation of others' movements), and waxy flexibility (posture held in odd or unusual fixed position for extended periods). In some cases, certain behaviours need to be evaluated carefully to distinguish them from movements that are associated with medication side effects, such as grimacing, stereotypic behaviour, or agitation.

Self-Concept

In schizophrenia, self-concept is usually poor. Patients often are aware that they are hearing voices others do not hear. They recognize that they are different from others and are often scared of "going crazy." Many are aware of the loss of expectations for their future achievements. The pervasive stigma associated with having a mental illness contributes to the poor self-concept. Body image can be disturbed, especially during periods of hallucinations or delusions. One patient believed that her body was infected with germs and she could feel them eating away her insides.

Stress and Coping Patterns

Stressful events are often linked to psychiatric symptoms (see Chapter 8 for discussion of the diathesis-stress model). It is important to determine stresses from the patient's perspective because a stressful event for one may not be stressful for another (see Chapter 35). It is also important to determine typical coping patterns, especially negative coping strategies, such as the use of substances or aggressive behaviour.

Risk Assessment

Because of high suicide and attempted suicide rates among patients with schizophrenia, the nurse needs to assess the patient's risk for self-injury: Does the patient speak of suicide, have delusional thinking that could lead to dangerous behaviour, and have command hallucinations telling him or her to harm self or others? Does the patient have homicidal ideations? Does the patient have access to weapons? Does the patient lack social support and the skills to be meaningfully engaged with other people or a vocation? Substance-related disorders are also common among patients with schizophrenia, and nurses should assess for substance abuse.

Nursing Diagnoses for Psychological Domain

Many nursing diagnoses can be generated from data collected assessing the psychological domain. Disturbed thought processes can be used for delusions, confusion, and disorganized thinking. Disturbed sensory perception is appropriate for hallucinations or illusions. Other examples of diagnoses include disturbed body image, low self-esteem, disturbed personal identity, risk for violence, ineffective coping, and knowledge deficit.

Interventions for Psychological Domain

All the psychological interventions, such as counseling, conflict resolution, behaviour therapy, and cognitive interventions, are appropriate for patients with schizophrenia. The following discussion focuses on applying these interventions.

Special Issues in the Nurse–Patient Relationship

The development of the nurse–patient relationship with patients with schizophrenia centres on developing trust and accepting the person as a worthy human being. People with schizophrenia are often reluctant to engage in any relationship because of previous rejection and, in some instances, an underlying suspiciousness that is a part of the illness. If they are having hallucinations, their images of other people may be distorted and frightening. They struggle to trust their own thoughts and perceptions, and engaging in an interaction with another human being may prove too overwhelming.

The nurse should approach the patient in a calm and caring manner. Engaging the patient in a relationship may take time. Short, time-limited interactions are best for a patient who is experiencing psychosis. Being consistent in interactions and following through on promises will help establish trust within the relationship.

Establishing a therapeutic relationship is crucial, especially with patients who deny that they are ill. Patients are more likely to agree to treatment if these recommendations are made within the context of a safe, trusting relationship. Even if some patients deny having mental illness, they may take medication and attend treatment activities because they trust the nurse.

Management of Disturbed Thoughts and Sensory Perceptions

Although antipsychotic medications may relieve positive symptoms, they do not always eliminate hallucinations and delusions. The nurse must continue helping the patient develop creative strategies for dealing with these sensory and thought disturbances. Information about the content of the hallucinations and delusions is needed, not only to determine whether the medications are effective but also to assess safety and the meaning of these thoughts and perceptions to the patient. In caring for a patient who is experiencing hallucinations or delusions, nursing actions should be guided by three general patient outcomes:

- Decrease the frequency and intensity of hallucinations and delusions.
- Recognize that hallucinations and delusions are symptoms of a brain disorder.
- Develop strategies to manage the recurrence of hallucinations or delusions.

When interacting with a patient who is experiencing hallucinations or delusions, the nurse must remember that these experiences are real to the patient. The nurse should never tell a patient that these experiences are not real. Discounting the experiences blocks communication. It also is dishonest to tell the patient that you are having the same hallucinatory experience. It is best to validate the patient's experiences and identify the meaning of these thoughts and feelings to the patient. For example, a patient who believes that he or

she is under surveillance by the police probably feels frightened and suspicious of everyone. By acknowledging how frightening it must be to always feel like you are being watched, the nurse focuses on the feelings that are generated by the delusion, not the delusion itself. The nurse can then offer to help the patient feel safe within this environment. The patient, in turn, begins to feel that someone understands him or her.

Teaching Points

Teaching patients that hallucinations and delusions are part of the disorder becomes easier after the medication begins working. Once patients believe and acknowledge that they have a mental illness and that some of their thoughts are delusions and some of their perceptions are hallucinations, they can develop strategies to manage their symptoms.

Self-Monitoring and Relapse Prevention

Patients benefit greatly by learning techniques of self-regulation, symptom monitoring, and relapse prevention. By monitoring events, time, place, and stimuli surrounding the appearance of symptoms, the patient can begin to predict high-risk times for symptom recurrence. Cognitive behavioural therapy is often used in helping patients monitor and identify their emerging symptoms in order to prevent relapse (Gumley, O'Grady, McNay, Reilly, Power, Norrie, 2003).

Another important nursing intervention is to help the patient identify who and where to talk about delusional or hallucinatory material. Because self-disclosure of these symptoms immediately labels someone as having a mental illness, patients should be encouraged to evaluate the environment for negative consequences of disclosing these symptoms. It may be fine to talk about it at home but not at the grocery store.

Enhancement of Cognitive Functioning

After identifying deficits in cognitive functioning, the nurse and the patient can develop interventions that target specific deficits. The most effective interventions usually involve the whole treatment team. If the ability to focus or attend is an issue, patients can be encouraged to select activities that improve attention, such as computer games. For memory problems, patients can be encouraged to make lists and to write down important information.

Executive functioning problems are the most challenging for these patients. Patients who cannot manage daily problems may have planning and problem-solving impairments. For these patients, developing interventions that closely simulate real-world problems may help. Through coaching, the nurse can teach and support the development of problem-solving skills. For example, during hospitalizations, patients are given medications and reminded to take them on time. They are often instructed in a classroom setting but rarely have an opportunity to practice self-medication and figure out what to do if their prescription expires, the medications are lost, or they forget their medications. Yet, when discharged, patients are expected to take medication at the prescribed dose at the prescribed time. Interventions designed to have patients actively engage in problem-solving behaviour with real problems are needed.

Another approach to helping patients solve problems and learn new strategies for dealing with problems is solution-focused therapy, which focuses on the strengths and positive attributes that exist within each person. This is a therapy that involves years of training to master, but there are techniques that can be used. For example, patients can be asked to identify the most important problem from their perspective. This focuses the patient on an important issue for that patient.

Behavioural Interventions

Behavioural interventions can be very effective in helping patients improve motivation and organize routines and daily activities, such as maintaining a regular schedule and completing activities. Reinforcement of positive behaviours (e.g., getting up on time, completing hygiene, going to treatment activities) can easily be included in a treatment plan. In the hospital, patients gain ward privileges by following an agreed-on treatment plan.

Stress and Coping Skills

Developing skills to cope with personal, social, and environmental stresses is important to everyone, but particularly to those with a severe mental illness. Stresses can easily trigger symptoms that patients are trying to avoid. Establishing regular counseling sessions to support the development of positive coping skills is helpful for both the hospitalized patient and those in the community.

Patient Education

Cognitive deficits (difficulty in processing complex information, maintaining steady focus of attention, distinguishing between relevant and irrelevant stimuli, and forming abstractions) may challenge the nurse planning educational activities. Evidence indicates that people with schizophrenia may learn best in an errorless learning environment (O'Carroll, Russell, Lawrie, & Johnstone, 1999), that is, they are directly given correct information and then encouraged to write it down. Asking questions that encourage guessing is not as effective in helping them retain information. Trial-and-error learning is avoided. In one study, a group of people

with schizophrenia who were taught using an errorless learning approach improved work skill in two entry-level job tasks (index card filing and toilet-tank assembly) and performed better than the group that was instructed with conventional trial-and-error instructions (Kern, Green, Mintz, & Liberman, 2003; Kern, Liberman, Kopelowicz, Mintz, & Green, 2002).

Teaching and explaining should occur in an environment with minimal distractions. Terminology should be clear and unambiguous. Visual aids can supplement verbal information, but these materials should have simple information stated in simple language. The nurse takes care not to overcrowd the visual material or incorporate images that draw attention away from the important content. Teaching should occur in small segments with frequent reinforcement. Most important of all, teaching should occur when the patient is ready. Regular assessments of cognitive abilities with standardized instruments can help determine this readiness. These suggestions can be adapted for teaching during any phase of the illness.

Skill-training interventions should be designed to compensate for cognitive deficits. To help patients learn to process complex activities, such as catching a bus, preparing a meal, or shopping for food or clothing, nurses should break the activity into small parts or steps and list them for the patient's reference, for example,

- Make sure you have the correct bus fare in your pocket.
- Leave your apartment with keys in hand.
- Close the door.
- Walk to the corner.
- Turn right and walk three blocks to the bus stop.

Family Education

Because having a family member with schizophrenia is a life-changing event for the family and friends who provide care and support, educating patients and their families is crucial. It is a primary concern for the psychiatric and mental health nurse. Family support and education are crucial to help patients maintain their treatment. Education should include information about the disease course, treatment regimens, support systems, and life management skills (see Box 18-16). The most important factor to reinforce during patient and family education is the consistent taking of medication.

Social Domain

Social Assessment

Several difficulties with social functioning occur in schizophrenia. As the disorder progresses, individuals can become increasingly socially isolated. On a

Psychoeducation Checklist: Schizophrenia

When caring for the patient with schizophrenia, be sure to include the caregiver as appropriate and address the following topic areas in the teaching plan:

- Psychopharmacologic agents, including drug action, dosage, frequency, and possible adverse effects. Stress the importance of adherence to the prescribed regimen
- Management of hallucinations
- Coping strategies such as self-talk, getting busy
- Management of the environment
- Use of contracts that detail the expected behaviours, with goals and consequences
- Community resources

one-to-one basis, this occurs because the individual seems unable to connect with people in his or her environment. Several aspects of the symptoms already discussed can contribute to this, for example, emotional blunting and anhedonia (the inability to form emotional attachment and experience pleasure). Cognitive deficits that contribute to difficult social functioning include problems with face and affect recognition, deficiencies in recall of past interactions, problems with decision making and judgment in conflictual interactions, and poverty of speech and language. Poor functioning and the inability to complete activities of daily living are manifested in poor hygiene, malnutrition, and social isolation.

Functional Status

Functional status of patients with schizophrenia should be assessed initially and at regular periods. The usual assessment instrument is the Global Assessment of Functioning (GAF). If a patient's GAF score is less than 60, interventions should be designed to enhance social or occupational functioning.

Social Systems

In schizophrenia, support systems become very important in maintaining the patient in the community. The individual may become socially isolated if the treatment and management occur in long-term care facilities and group homes away from family and friends. One challenge in treating schizophrenia is to identify and maintain the patient's links with family and significant others. Assessment of the patient's formal support (e.g., family, providers) and informal support (e.g., neighbors, friends) should be conducted.

Quality of Life

People with schizophrenia often have a poor quality of life, especially older people, who may have spent many years in a long-term hospital. The nurse should assess the patient's quality of life and how it could be improved. Simple changes, such as arranging for a different roommate or improving access to social activities by meeting transportation needs, can greatly improve a patient's quality of life.

Family Assessment

The assessment of the family could take many forms, and the family assessment guide presented in Chapter 17 can be used. In some instances, the patient will be young and living with his or her parents. This is most often the case when a young person experiences the first episode psychosis. Often, the nurse's first contact with the patient and family is in the initial phases of the disorder. The family is dealing with the shock and disbelief of seeing a child with a mental illness that has lifelong consequences. Ideally in this instance, the assessment process may be extended over several sessions to provide the family with support and education about the disorder.

Because women with schizophrenia generally have better treatment outcomes than do men, many will marry and have children. These women experience the same life stresses as other women and may find themselves single parents, raising children in poverty-stricken conditions. Managing a psychiatric illness and trying to be an effective parent in a socially stigmatizing society are exceedingly challenging because of the lack of financial resources and social support. This family will need an extensive assessment of financial need and social support. The family life cycle model presented in Chapter 17 can also be used as a framework for the assessment.

Nursing Diagnoses for Social Domain

The nursing diagnoses generated from the assessment of the social domain are typically impaired social interaction, ineffective role performance, disabled family coping, and interrupted family processes. Outcomes will depend on the specific diagnostic area.

Interventions for Social Domain

Promoting Patient Safety

Although violence is not a consistent behaviour of people with schizophrenia, it is always a concern during the initial phase when hallucinations or delusions may put patients at risk for harming themselves or others. Nonviolent patients who are experiencing hallucinations and delusions can also be at risk for victimization by more aggressive patients. The patient who is hallucinating needs to be protected. This protection may include increased staff monitoring and, if necessary, a safer environment in a secluded area.

The nurse's best approach to avoiding violence or aggression is to demonstrate respect for the patient and the patient's personal space, assess and monitor for signs of fear and agitation, and use preventive interventions before the patient loses control. Medications should be administered as ordered. Because most antipsychotic and antidepressant medications take 1 to 2 weeks to begin moderating the patient's behaviour, the nurse must be vigilant during the acute illness.

Reducing environmental stimulation is particularly important for individuals who are experiencing hallucinations but can be helpful for all patients when signs of fear and agitation are observed. Allowing patients to use private rooms or seclusion for brief periods can be an important preventive method.

Other techniques of managing the environment (milieu management) have been found to be helpful in inpatient settings. One researcher who examined aggression and violence in psychiatric hospitals found violent behaviour to be associated with the following predictors: a history of violence, a coercive interaction style of using violence to obtain what is desired, and an environment in which violence is inadvertently rewarded,

for example, by gaining staff attention (Morrison, 1992, 1993; Morrison & Carney Love, 2003). Morrison proposed the following methods to help avoid acts of violence or aggression:

- Take a thorough history that includes information about the patient's past use of violence.
- Help the patient to talk directly and constructively with those with whom he or she is angry, rather than venting anger to staff about a third person.
- Set limits with consistent and justly applied consequences.
- Involve the patient in formulating a contract that outlines patient and staff behaviours, goals, and consequences.
- Schedule brief but regular time-outs to allow the patient some privacy without the attention of staff either before or after the time-out (these time-outs may be patient activated).

Staff members need to have planned sessions after all incidents of violence or physical management in which the event is analyzed. These sessions allow staff members to learn how to better manage these situations and evaluate patients' cues. With sensitive leadership, these sessions can help staff to learn more about the interaction of patient and staff characteristics that can contribute to these incidents. (See Box 18-17 for research that shows the way conflict and containment can be reduced on inpatient units.)

BOX 18.17

Research for Best Practice: Reducing Conflict and Containment on Acute Psychiatric Wards

Bowers, L., Brennan, G., Flood, C., Lipang, M., & Oladapo, P. (2006). Preliminary outcomes of a trial to reduce conflict and containment on acute psychiatric wards: City nurses. Journal of Psychiatric and Mental Health Nursing, 13, 22–27, 165–172.

QUESTION: This intervention study aimed to reduce conflict and containment on two acute psychiatric inpatient units through changes in nurses' beliefs, attitudes, and practices. This required that two nurses were employed to work with staff members on the two inpatient units for 1 year, assisting with the implementation of changes according to a previously developed model of conflict and containment. These changes focused upon (1) the positive appreciation of patients by staff members, (2) the ability of staff members to regulate their own natural reactions to patients, and (3) the creation of an effective structure (rules and regulations) of ward life. The model served to bring about enhanced ward expertise in a low conflict, low containment, and high-therapy nursing.

METHODS: Using a before-and-after study design, incorporating aspects of action research, the researchers determined if the working intervention model reduced the

incidents of conflict and containment on the units. It required establishing baseline (before intervention) measurement of conflict and containment as well as of both the nurses' attitudes and the ward atmosphere. These data were compared with measures of these dimensions obtained postintervention (after the implementation of the model).

FINDINGS: Outcome measures reflected significant reductions in verbal abuse (down 44%), physical violence (down 53%), self-harm (down 72%), and absconding (down 69%). Physical violence by patients was reduced by half. These results indicate that a low-conflict environment can be achieved through alterations in staff attitudes and working practices.

IMPLICATIONS FOR PRACTICE: High levels of containment are not required to reduce conflict in acute psychiatric settings. Nurses can use this model to enhance ward atmosphere and improve the number and quality of nurse–patient interactions. These clinical/ward activities have the potential to create positive benefits for both patients and nursing staff.

Convening Support Groups

People with mental illness benefit from support groups that focus on daily problems and the stress of dealing with a mental illness. These groups are useful throughout the continuum of care and help reduce the risk for suicide. In the hospital setting, the focus of the group can be simply sharing the experience of living with a mental illness. In the community, a regular support group can provide interaction with people with similar problems and issues and the opportunity to share stories of recovery. Friendships often develop from these groups.

Implementing Milieu Therapy

Individuals with schizophrenia can be hospitalized or live in group homes for a long period of time. Expecting people who have an illness that interferes with their ability to live with family members to live with complete strangers in peace and harmony is unrealistic. Arranging the treatment environment to maximize recovery is crucial to the rehabilitation of the patient.

Developing Psychiatric Rehabilitation Strategies

Rehabilitation strategies are used to support the individual's recovery and integration into the community (see Chapter 19). Community-based psychosocial rehabilitation programs usually offer long-term intensive case management services to adults with schizophrenia. Programs provide a continuum of services to meet the changing needs of people with psychiatric disabilities. Patients set rehabilitation goals, and services are then provided to help "clients" (most programs do not use the term "patients") reach their goals. Services range from daily home visits to providing transportation, occupational training, and group support. Social skills training shows much promise for patients with schizophrenia, both individually and in groups. This is a method for teaching patients specific behaviours needed for social interactions. The skills are taught by lecture, demonstration, role playing, and homework assignments (see Chapters 13 and 16). Nurses may be team members and involved in case management or provision of services. These and other psychological treatment approaches, combined with breakthroughs in biologic therapy, continue to help improve the functioning and quality of life for patients with schizophrenia.

Family Interventions

When schizophrenia first becomes apparent, the patient and family must negotiate the mental health system for the first time (in most cases), a challenge that almost equals that of confronting the family member's illness. In most provincial jurisdictions, the mental health system is huge and is usually ignored unless a family member becomes seriously mentally ill. The system includes inpatient and outpatient clinics supported by provincial health insurance and publicly funded community mental health clinics and hospitals.

Family members should be encouraged to participate in educational and support groups that help family members deal with the realities of living with a loved one with a mental illness. Family members should be given information about local community and provincial resources and organizations such as mental health associations and those that can help families negotiate the complex system. See Nursing Care Plan 18-2 for care of a patient with a more persistent form of schizophrenia.

Spiritual Domain

Many people living with schizophrenia find comfort in their spirituality, as well as the strength to deal with life events that interfere with their recovery journeys. Religious or spiritual beliefs can be a resource for both patients and their families. Such beliefs may help, for instance, to reappraise difficult events into a positive light (e.g., God gives us only difficulties that we are able to handle). A relationship with the sacred through ritual, prayer, worship, meditation, or other spiritual activities may offer solace, peace, and serenity. These activities may also help to structure the daily lives of individuals with schizophrenia, an important rehabilitation goal. The experience of living with a serious and chronic illness, however, can also cause a crisis of faith or lead one to question the purpose and meaning of one's life. This may be especially true if one's illness brings stigma and rejection by the members of one's community. The sense of connection and hope that supports spiritual growth may be diminished if one is labeled as "crazy" by others. Spiritual nursing care actively supports patients in their efforts to sustain and enhance their spirituality. This support can take many forms, from safeguarding the dignity of the patient to understanding the potential impact of hallucinations on spiritual needs, to ensuring spiritual activities can occur. In psychiatric and mental health settings, there may be reluctance on the part of staff to consider the spirituality of a patient who is experiencing the psychotic symptoms of delusions and hallucinations, especially if there are religious overtones to the "voices" and/or fixed beliefs. Knowledge of the patient and of the disease, along with a broad, rich understanding of spirituality, should, nevertheless, enable the nurse and other staff to address the spiritual domain of care.

Nursing Care Plan 18.2

Patient With Schizophrenia

MP is a 53-year-old woman who was brought to the crisis support clinic by her community nurse case manager. MP had made a number of telephone calls to her case manager and to the police in rapid succession in the previous 24 hours to report that her next door neighbour was spying on her. When the nurse case manager arrived, MP was very agitated and distrusting. The case manager also received a call from MP's landlord to report that MP has been making threatening hand gestures to neighbours from her apart- ment window. MP disclosed to her nurse case manager that her neighbours had tampered with her medications and that she had not been taking them for several days. MP was acutely paranoid and agreed to a hospitalization to keep herself safe. She had been attending the Community Club- house Program but had not been there for 2 weeks. She failed to attend her follow-up appointment at the mental health clinic to pick up her biweekly dosette of pills..

Setting: Crisis Support Team: Psychosocial Rehabilitation Unit

Baseline Assessment: MP is a 5'4", 155-lb woman whose appearance is disheveled. She has not slept for 2 days and appears frightened. She is hypervigilant, suspicious, irritable, and wringing her hands. She is vague about when she last took her treatment medications. She is oriented to time and place and person. Lab values are within normal limits. She has a history of at least 12 former admissions to the psychiatric ward for self-discontinuation of treatment medications.

Associated Psychiatric Diagnosis	Medications

Axis I: Schizophrenia, paranoid
Axis II: None
Axis III: None
Axis IV:
    Social problems: Landlord threatening to evict MP
        from her apartment.
    Estranged from her two adult sons.
    Support system limited to a few acquaintances at
        the clubhouse.
GAF = Current 30
	Olanzapine, 5 mg bid
	Lorazepam (Ativan), 2 mg PO or IM for agitation PRN

Nursing Diagnosis 1: Ineffective Health Maintenance

Defining Characteristics	Related Factors
MP does not remember when she last took her medications. Two weeks of pills are still in the dosette box. MP has not taken the pills for at least 2 weeks, possibly more. MP has not attended the Clubhouse program for 2 weeks. MP did not attend her appointment at the clinic to get a refill of pills in her dosette. MP has been calling the police and the case manager several times in the past 24 hours. MP has not been out shopping for food. MP is making threatening gestures to neighbours.	Paranoid delusions are contributing to her thought disturbance. Suspiciousness is contributing to her reluctance to leave her apartment. Inability to make thoughtful judgments. Ineffective individual coping.

Outcomes

Initial	Long Term
Restarts medications in the hospital. Agreement from MP to a referral to the ACT team. Increased ability to self-administer medications. Demonstrates willingness to take her medications independently while in hospital using a blister pack dosette.	MP will communicate her understanding of and demonstrate follow through with the mutually agreed on health maintenance plan. MP will show the ability to perform health maintenance activities needed to function in her apartment independently with ACT team assistance.

Continued

Nursing Care Plan 18.2 *(Continued)*

Interventions

Interventions	Rationale	Ongoing Assessment
Take initial steps to help MP feel safe in the hospital setting.	When a person feels safe, trust is more likely to develop.	Determine when MP's suspiciousness is diminishing. Assess when she is ready to discuss plans for discharge.
Listen carefully, making eye contact. Make efforts to clarify what MP is thinking and feeling.	Listening attentively will help MP to feel safe and cared for.	
Contact all community care providers and convene an interdisciplinary meeting to discuss possible changes to the current community care plan.	A meeting of all care providers will provide a forum to explore alternative support/treatment solutions to improve MP's health maintenance once discharged.	Assess MP's readiness for discharge and transition to the ACT team in addition to returning to the community clubhouse.
	ACT team will be able to increase visitation to MP's home at more frequent intervals. ACT team will provide a more intense level of support.	

Evaluation

Outcomes	Revised Outcomes	Interventions
MP's delusions begin to decrease.	MP meets with the ACT team and agrees to include this team in her follow-up health maintenance plan.	Problem-solve ways for MP to respond to ongoing worries and suspicions.
MP uses some distraction techniques to draw her away from focusing upon the neighbours.		Develop a written, mutually agreed on relapse prevention and crisis action plan and send to all community care partners.

Nursing Diagnosis 2: Disturbed Thought Processes

Defining Characteristics	Related Factors
Inaccurate interpretation of stimuli (neighbours tampering with her medications) Cognitive impairment—attention, memory, and executive function impairment Suspiciousness Hallucinations (hears voices telling her that her sons are in danger)	Uncompensated alterations in brain activity

Outcomes

Initial	Long Term
Decrease or eliminate hallucinations. Have accurate interpretation of the environment. Exhibits some reality-based thinking. Demonstrates improvement in cognitive functioning (improved attention, memory, and executive functioning). Interacts appropriately with others.	Use coping strategies to deal with hallucinations or delusions if they reappear. Communicate clearly with others. Maintain cognitive functioning.

Continued

Nursing Care Plan 18.2 (Continued)

Interventions

Interventions	Rationale	Ongoing Assessment
Initiate a nurse–patient relationship by using an accepting, nonjudgmental approach. Be patient.	A therapeutic relationship will provide patient support as she begins to deal with the realization that she is in hospital once again. Be patient and offer reassurance as required until MP feels safe. Do not argue with the false beliefs.	Determine the extent to which MP is willing to trust and engage in a relationship. Make every effort to help MP attend to real rather than internal stimuli, orient her to the real situation, and encourage MP to focus upon distracting concrete activities. Make determined efforts to steer thinking in alternate directions.
Administer Olanzapine as prescribed. Observe for effects, side effects, and adverse effects. Begin teaching about the potential switch to an injectable form of antipsychotic medication.	Olanzapine is a D2 and 5-HT$_{2A}$ antagonist and is indicated for the management of psychotic disorders.	Make sure MP swallows the pills. Monitor for relief of positive symptoms and assess side effects, especially extrapyramidal. Monitor BP for orthostatic hypotension and body temperature increase (NMS).
Assess the ability for self-care activities.	Disturbed thinking may interfere with MP's ability to carry out ADLs.	Continue to assess: determine whether the patient can manage self-care.

Evaluation

Outcomes	Revised Outcomes	Interventions
Delusions began to decrease within 6 days.	Participate in Community Clubhouse activities as soon as possible to bridge the transition from hospital back to the community.	Encourage attendance at the Clubhouse while in hospital to reconnect with the activity/recreational group which MP enjoys.

Nursing Diagnosis 3: Anxiety Related to Fears About Neighbours

Defining Characteristics	Related Factors
Constantly asking nurses for reassurance that her neighbours are not on the unit. Presence of pathophysiologic risk factors: delusional thinking.	Frightened, secondary to **paranoia** (feelings of being unsafe) and delusional thinking.

Outcomes

Initial	Long Term
MP is able to describe a reduction in anxiety. Decreased agitation, gesturing, and pacing.	MP will demonstrate decreased anxiety while at home. MP will refrain from gesturing at neighbours.

Interventions

Interventions	Rationale	Ongoing Assessment
Acknowledge MP's fear and paranoid delusions. Be genuine and empathetic.	Anxiety and delusions change an individual's perception of environmental stimuli. A patient who is frightened will respond because of her need to stay safe.	Assess her response to your comments and her ability to concentrate on what is being said.
Reassure MP verbally at frequent intervals. Make frequent brief supportive contacts. Acknowledge MP's distress.	It is helpful to validate the anxious feelings MP is experiencing.	Observe MP's nonverbal communication for evidence of increased anxiety and agitation.
Administer lorazepam, 2 mg, for agitation. Oral route is preferable over injection.	Exact mechanisms of action are not understood, but this medication is believed to potentiate the inhibitory neurotransmitter GABA, relieving anxiety and producing sedation.	Observe for a decrease in anxiety.

Continued

Nursing Care Plan 18.2 *(Continued)*

Evaluation

Outcomes	Revised Outcomes	Interventions
MP gradually decreased anxious behaviour. Lorazepam was given regularly for the first 4 days.	Demonstrate control of behaviour by resisting delusions.	Teach MP about the effects of delusions. Problem-solve ways of controlling hallucinations if they occur. Emphasize the importance of taking medications.

EVALUATION AND TREATMENT OUTCOMES

Outcome research related to schizophrenia has redefined previous ways of thinking about the course of the disorder. Schizophrenia was once considered to have a progressively long-term and downward course, but it is now known that schizophrenia can be successfully treated and managed. In one older, but significant study, the researchers interviewed patients 20 to 25 years after diagnosis and found that 50% to 66% experienced significant improvement or recovery (Harding, Zubin, & Strauss, 1987). This study is important because it occurred before the development of atypical antipsychotic agents. Today, we can be hopeful that even more people can experience improvement or recover from schizophrenia.

CONTINUUM OF CARE

Continuity of care has been identified as a major goal of community mental health systems for patients with schizophrenia because they are at risk for becoming "lost" to services if left alone after discharge. Careful attention to discharge planning encourages follow-up care in the community. In fact, many mental health systems require an outpatient appointment before discharge to better facilitate this transition. Treatment of schizophrenia occurs across a variety of settings. Not only inpatient hospitalization but also partial hospitalization, day treatment, and crisis stabilization and continuing community care can be used effectively.

Inpatient-Focused Care

Much of the previous discussion concerns care in the inpatient setting. Today, inpatient hospitalizations are brief and focus on patient stabilization. Many times, patients are involuntarily admitted for a short period. During the stabilization period, the status is changed to voluntary admission, whereby the patient agrees to treatment.

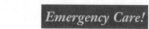 *Emergency Care!*

Emergency care ideally takes place in a hospital emergency room, but often the crisis occurs in the home. Patients are usually relapsing and do not recognize their bizarre or aggressive behaviours as symptoms. A specially trained crisis team is sent to assess the emergency and recommend further treatment. In the emergency room, patients are brought not only because of relapse but also because of medication side effects. Nurses should refer to the previous discussion for nursing management.

Community Care

Most of the care of patients with schizophrenia will be in the community through publicly supported mental health delivery systems. Community services include assertive community treatment; outpatient therapy; case management; and psychosocial rehabilitation, including clubhouse programs. For a very small number of patients with a community treatment order (CTO) in effect that delineates the conditions required to live in the community, services must be congruent with those conditions (see Chapter 3). For all patients in the community, health care should be integrated in a holistic manner with physical health care. Nurses should be especially vigilant that patients with mental illnesses receive proper primary and medical health care.

· CRNENOTE

Priorities in the patient with acute symptoms of schizophrenia include managing psychosis and keeping the patient safe and free from harming self or others. In the community, the priorities are preventing relapse, maintaining and improving psychosocial functioning, psychoeducation, and improving quality of life.

Mental Health Promotion

In some cases, it is not the disorder itself that threatens the mental health of the person with schizophrenia but

FIGURE 18.6 Bio/psycho/social/spiritual interventions for patients with schizophrenia.

the stresses of trying to receive care and services. Health care systems are complex and are often at the mercy of a system rule that is outdated. Development of assertiveness and conflict resolution skills can help the person in negotiating access to systems that will provide services. Developing a positive support system for stressful periods will help promote a positive outcome (Fig. 18-6).

SUMMARY OF KEY POINTS

◻ The patient with schizophrenia displays a complex myriad of symptoms typically categorized as positive symptoms (those that exist but should not), such as delusions or hallucinations and disorganized thinking and behaviour, and negative symptoms (characteristics that should be there but are lacking), such as alogia, avolition, anhedonia, and affective blunting.

◻ In the past, the diagnosis and treatment of schizophrenia focused on the more observable and dramatic positive symptoms (i.e., delusions and hallucinations), but recently scientists have shifted their focus to the disorganizing symptoms of cognition.

◻ The clinical presentation of schizophrenia occurs in three phases: phase 1, first episode psychosis, entails the initial diagnosis and first treatment; phase 2 includes periods of stabilization between episodes of overt signs and symptoms but during which the patient needs sustained treatment; and phase 3 includes periods of exacerbation or relapse that require hospitalization or more frequent contacts with mental health professionals and increased use of resources.

◻ Biologic theories of what causes schizophrenia include genetic, infectious-autoimmune, neuroanatomic, and dopamine hypotheses. The last is supported by the advanced technology of PET scan findings and the understanding of the mechanisms of antipsychotic medications.

◻ Biologic assessment of the patient with schizophrenia must include a thorough history and physical examination to rule out any medical illness or substance abuse problem that might be the cause of the patient's symptoms, assessment of risk for self-injury or injury to others, and documentation of baseline health information before medications are administered. Several standardized assessment tools are available to help assess characteristic abnormal motor movements.

▢ Several nursing interventions address the biologic domain—promotion of self-care activities; activity; exercise; and nutritional, thermoregulation, and fluid balance interventions. In general, the antipsychotic drugs used to treat schizophrenia block dopamine transmission in the brain but also cause some troublesome and sometimes serious side effects, primarily anticholinergic side effects and extrapyramidal side effects (motor abnormalities). Newer antipsychotic agents block serotonin as well as dopamine. The nurse should be familiar with these drugs, their possible side effects, and the interventions required to manage or control side effects.

▢ The extrapyramidal side effects of antipsychotic drugs can appear early in drug treatment and include acute parkinsonism or pseudoparkinsonism, acute dystonia, and akathisia, or they can appear late in treatment after months or years. The primary example of late-appearing extrapyramidal side effects is tardive dyskinesia, which is a severe syndrome of abnormal motor movements of the mouth, tongue, and jaw.

▢ Psychological assessment must include equal attention to manifestations of both positive and negative symptoms and a concentrated focus on the cognitive impairments that make it so difficult for patients to manage their disorder. Several standardized assessment tools assess for positive and negative symptoms. Development of the nurse–patient relationship becomes key in helping patients manage the disturbed thoughts and sensory perceptions. Interventions should be designed to enhance cognitive functioning. Patient and family education are critical interventions for the person with schizophrenia.

▢ Because schizophrenia is a lifetime disorder and patients require the continued support and care of mental health professionals and family or friends, one of the primary nursing interventions is ensuring that patients and families are properly educated regarding the course of the disorder, the importance of drug maintenance, and the need for consistent care and support. Research is demonstrating that interaction between patients and their families is key to the success of long-term treatments and outcomes.

CRITICAL THINKING CHALLENGES

1 Why are positive symptoms easier to track than negative symptoms?

2 Describe ways in which medical illness or substance abuse could cause a patient to show symptoms similar to schizophrenia.

3 Suggest reasons that a higher rate of schizophrenia is found in lower classes of people from urban, industrialized communities.

4 The physical environment is important to the patient with schizophrenia. Think of the typical hospital unit. What environmental factors could be stress

producing or misleading to the person with schizophrenia?

5 Compare therapeutic and nontherapeutic communication skills when dealing with a person with schizophrenia who is actively hallucinating.

6 Explore using a simulation exercise developed by Deegan (2006), *Hearing Voices that are Distressing*, with your student group. Research suggests that students find it a valuable experience that facilitates understanding and empathy (Hamilton Wilson et al., 2009).

WEB LINKS

www.cmha.ca   This is the site of the Canadian Mental Health Association, a charitable organization that promotes mental health and supports the resilience and recovery of those with mental illness.

www.eppic.org.au   This is the site of the Early Psychosis Prevention and Intervention Centre, Melbourne, Australia. It has excellent downloadable and printable fact sheets in multiple language formats for patient/family education.

www.mentalhealth.com   This is the site of Internet Mental Health, which provides extensive information on schizophrenia.

www.nami.org   This is the site of the National Alliance on Mental Illness, which is the largest grassroots organization for people with mental illness and their families in the United States.

www.narsad.org   This is the site of the U.S. National Alliance for Research on Schizophrenia and Depression, which is a national organization that raises and distributes money for research.

www.nimh.nih.gov   This is the site of the U.S. National Institute of Mental Health, which presents all aspects of the diagnosis and treatment of schizophrenia.

www.psychosissucks.ca   This is a British Columbia early psychosis intervention site with links to other excellent resources.

www.schizophrenia.ca   This is the site of the Schizophrenia Society of Canada, an organization committed to alleviating suffering caused by schizophrenia.

www.schizophrenia.com   This is a not-for-profit information, support, and education centre for families of individuals with schizophrenia.

MOVIES, NOVELS, AND BIOGRAPHIES

A Beautiful Mind: 2001. This academy award–winning movie starring Russell Crowe is based on the biography of the mathematician and Nobel Laureate John Nash by

Sylvia Nasar (1998). It presents the life and experiences of this man as he experienced schizophrenia. It shows how his life and work were altered and the effects on his relationships with family and colleagues. The movie depicts how this man came to terms with his illness.

VIEWING POINTS: How does the treatment John Nash received in the 1950s differ from treatment today? How would you classify his symptoms according to the *DSM-IV-TR*? What is typical and/or problematic about Mr. Nash's relationship with the medications prescribed for him?

Benny and Joon: 1993. Joon is a young woman with schizophrenia who lives with her overprotective brother. In an attempt to keep her safe, Joon's brother unsuccessfully hires one housekeeper after another. After winning a bet in a poker game, Joon's brother acquires Benny, played by Johnny Depp, who entertains and cares for Joon. A romance develops that results in Benny and Joon attempting to run away. Joon's symptoms reappear. After treatment, Joon struggles with becoming independent from both her brother and boyfriend.

VIEWING POINTS: How does Joon's brother's behaviour interfere with her normal growth and development? When Joon's symptoms appeared, how would you classify them according to the *DSM-IV-TR*? What advice would you like to give to Joon and her brother?

Strange Voices: 1987. This film, starring Nancy McKeon, depicts the impact of early psychosis upon the individual and the family. It shows how difficult it is to understand and accept the onset of illness and shows the early aspects of the journey of recovery.

VIEWING POINTS: What are the earliest signs that Nicole is becoming ill? What reactions/responses do you see in the family? What impact does Nicole's illness have on her sibling?

REFERENCES

Addington, J., & Addington, D. (2006). The impact of cognitive functioning on outcome. *Schizophrenia Research, 86*(S1), 27.

Addington, J., McCleary, A., & Addington, D. (2005a). Three year outcome of family work in an early psychosis program. *Schizophrenia Research, 79,* 107–116.

Addington, J., Saeed, H., & Addington, D. (2005b). The course of cognitive functioning on in first episode psychosis: Changes over time and impact on outcome. *Schizophrenia Research, 78,* 35–43.

Addington, J., van Mastrigt, S., Jutchinson, J., & Addington, D. (2002). Pathways to care: Help seeking behaviour in first episode psychosis. *Acta Psychiatrica Scandinavica, 106,* 358–364.

Altamura, A. C., Bassetti, R., Bignotti, S., Pioli, R., & Mundo, E. (2003). Clinical variables related to suicide attempts in schizophrenic patients: A retrospective study. *Schizophrenia Research, 60,* 47–55.

American Psychiatric Association. (2000). *Diagnostic and statistical manual of mental disorders* (4th ed., Text revision). Washington, DC: Author.

Arseneault, L., Cannon, M., Wilton, J., & Murray, R. (2004). Causal association between cannabis and psychosis: An examination of the evidence. *British Journal of Psychiatry, 184,* 100–117.

Baldessarini, R. J. (2002). *Clinical psychopharmacology: Overview and recent advances.* Symposium conducted at Cape Cod Symposia, Eastham, Massachusetts.

Benes, F. M. (2000). Emerging principles of altered neural circuitry in schizophrenia. *Brain Research Developmental Brain Research, 31*(2–3), 251–269.

Birchwood, M., Todd, P., & Jackson, C. (1998). Early intervention in psychosis: The critical period hypothesis. *British Journal of Psychiatry, 172,* 53–59.

Bowers, L., Brennan, G., Flood, C., Lipang, M., & Oladapo, P. (2006). Preliminary outcomes of a trial to reduce conflict and containment on acute psychiatric wards: City nurses. *Journal of Psychiatric and Mental Health Nursing, 13,* 22–27, 165–172.

Boyd, M., & Lapierre, E. (1996). Fluid imbalance and water intoxication: The elusive syndrome. In A. McBride, & J. Austin (Eds.), *Psychiatric mental health nursing: Integration of the biological into behavioural* (pp. 396–424). Philadelphia, PA: WB Saunders.

Buchsbaum, M. (1990). The frontal lobes, basal ganglia, and temporal lobes as a site for schizophrenia. *Schizophrenia Bulletin, 16,* 377–387.

Byrne, M., Agerbo, E., Ewald, H., Eaton, W. W., & Mortensen, P. B. (2003). Parental age and risk of schizophrenia: A case-control study. *Archives of General Psychiatry, 60*(7), 673–678.

Canadian Psychiatric Association. (2005). Clinical practice guidelines: Treatment of schizophrenia. *Canadian Journal of Psychiatry, 50*(S1), 1–48.

Caroff, S., & Mann, S. (1993). Neuroleptic malignant syndrome. *Medical Clinics of North America, 77,* 185–202.

Casey, D. E. (1994). Schizophrenia: Psychopharmacology. In J. W. Jefferson, & J. H. Greist (Eds.), *The psychiatric clinics of North America: Annual of drug therapy* (Vol. 1, pp. 81–100). Philadelphia, PA: WB Saunders.

Chance S. A., Esiri, M. M., Crow, T. J. (2003) Ventricular enlargement in schizophrenia: A primary change in the temporal lobe? *Schizophrenia Research, 62,* 123–131

Chou, Y. H., Halldin, C., & Farde, L. (2003). Occupancy of 5HT(1A) receptors in clozapine in the primate brain: A PET study. *Psychopharmacology, 166*(3), 234–240.

Cirillo, M. A., & Seidman, L. J. (2003). Verbal declarative memory dysfunction in schizophrenia: From clinical assessment to genetics and brain mechanisms. *Neuropsychology Review, 13*(2), 43–77.

Crowther, R., Marshall, M., Bond, G., & Huxley, P. (2004). *Cochrane Database of Systematic Reviews, 1,* 1–86.

Csernansky, J. G. (2003). Treatment of schizophrenia: Preventing the progression of disease. *Psychiatric Clinics of North America, 26*(2), 367–379.

Davidson, L. L., & Heinrichs, R. W. (2003). Quantification of frontal and temporal lobe brain-imaging findings in schizophrenia: A meta-analysis. *Psychiatry Research, 122*(2), 69–87.

De Hert, M., McKenzie, K., & Peuskens, J. (2001). Risk factors for suicide in young people suffering from schizophrenia: A long-term follow-up study. *Schizophrenia Research, 47*(2–3), 127–134.

Deegan, P. (1992). The independent living movement and people with psychiatric disabilities: Taking back control over our own lives. *Psychosocial Rehabilitation Journal, 15,* 5–9.

Deegan, P. (2006). *Hearing voices curriculum: Complete training and curriculum package.* Retrieved November 18, 2009, from http://www.power2u.org/mm5/merchant.mvc?

Dolder, C. R., Lacro, J. P., Dunn, L. B., & Jeste, D. V. (2002). Antipsychotic medication adherence: Is there a difference between typical and atypical agents? *American Journal of Psychiatry, 159*(1), 103–108.

Falkai, P., Schneider-Axmann, T., Honer, W. G., Vogeley, K., Schonell, H., Pfeiffer, U., et al. (2003). Influence on genetic loading, obstetric complications, and premorbid adjustment on brain morphology in schizophrenia: A MRI study. *European Archives of Psychiatry and Clinical Neuroscience, 253*(2), 92–99.

Franzen, G. (1970). Plasma free fatty acids before and after an intravenous insulin injection in acute schizophrenic men. *British Journal of Psychiatry, 116*(531), 173–177.

Ghose, S., Weickert, C. S., Colvin, S. M., Coyle, J. T., Herman, M. M., Hyde, T. M., et al. (2003). Glutamate carboxypeptidase II gene expression in the human frontal and temporal lobe in schizophrenia. *Neuropsychopharmacology, 29*(1), 117–125.

Goldman, L. S. (1999). Medical illness in patients with schizophrenia. *Journal of Clinical Psychiatry, 60*(Suppl. 21), 1015.

Goldner, E. M., Hsu, L., Waraich, P., & Somers, J. M. (2002). Prevalence and incidence studies of schizophrenia disorders: A systematic review of the literature. *Canadian Journal of Psychiatry, 47*(9), 833–843.

Gumley, A., O'Grady, M., McNay, L., Reilly, J., Power, K., & Norrie, J. (2003). Early intervention for relapse in schizophrenia: Results of a 12-month randomized controlled trial of cognitive behavioural therapy. *Psychological Medicine, 33*(3), 419–431.

Gur, R. E., & Gur, R. C. (2005). Neuroimaging in schizophrenia: Linking neuropsychiatric manifestations to neurobiology. In B. J. Sadock &

V. A. Sadock (Eds.), *Comprehensive textbook of psychiatry* (pp. 1396–1408). Philadelphia, PA: Lippincott Williams & Wilkins.

Guy, W. (1976). *ECDEU: Assessment manual for psychopharmacology* (DHEW Publication No. 76–338). Washington, DC: Department of Health Education and Welfare, Psychopharmacology Branch.

Hafner, H. (2003). Gender differences in schizophrenia. *Psychoneuroendocrinology, 23*(Suppl. 2), 17–54.

Hamilton Wilson, J., Azzopardi, W., Sager, S., Gould, B., Conroy, S., Deegan, P., & Archie, S. (2009). A narrative study of the experiences of student nurses who have participated in the Hearing Voices that are Distressing simulation. *International Journal of Nursing Education Scholarship, 6*(1), article 19.

Harding, C., Zubin, J., & Strauss, J. (1987). Chronicity in schizophrenia: Fact, partial fact or artifact? *Hospital and Community Psychiatry, 38*(5), 477–486.

Harrison, G., Fouskakis, D., Rasmussen, F., Tynelius, P., Sipos, A., & Gunnell, D. (2003). Association between psychotic disorder and urban place of birth is not mediated by obstetric complications or childhood socioeconomic position: A cohort study. *Psychological Medicine, 33*(4), 723–731.

Harrison, G., Hopper, K., Craig, T., Laska, E., Siegel, C., Wanderling, K., et al. (2001). Recovery from psychotic illness: A 15 and 25 year international follow-up study. *British Journal of Psychiatry, 178*, 506–517.

Hartman, M., Steketee, M. C., Silva, S., Lanning, K., & Andersson, C. (2003). Wisconsin Card Sorting Test performance in schizophrenia: The role of working memory. *Schizophrenia Research, 63*(3), 201–217.

Health Canada. (2002). *A report on mental illnesses in Canada: Chapter 3: Schizophrenia.* Retrieved August 31, 2005, from http://www.phac-aspc.gc.ca/publicat/miic-mmac/pdf/chap_3_e.pdf

Jibson, M. D., & Tandon, R. (2000). Treatment of schizophrenia. In D. L. Dunner, & J. E. Rosenbaum (Eds.), *The psychiatric clinics of North America annual of drug therapy* (Vol. 7, pp. 83–113). Philadelphia, PA: WB Saunders.

Kandel, E. R., Schwartz, J. H., & Jessell, T. M. (2000). *Principles of neural science* (4th ed.). New York, NY: McGraw-Hill.

Kay, S. R., Fiszbein, A., & Opler, L. A. (1987). The Positive and Negative Syndrome Scale (PANSS) for schizophrenia. *Schizophrenia Bulletin, 13*, 261–276.

Kern, R. S., Green, M. V., Mintz, J., & Liberman, R. P. (2003). Does 'errorless learning' compensate for neurocognitive impairments in the work rehabilitation of persons with schizophrenia? *Psychological Medicine, 33*(3), 433–442.

Kern, R. S., Liberman, R. P., Kopelowicz, A., Mintz, J., & Green, M. F. (2002). Applications of errorless learning for improving work performance in persons with schizophrenia. *American Journal Psychiatry, 159*(11), 1921–1926.

Keshavan, M., Tandon, R., Boutros, N., & Nasrallah, H. (2008). Schizophrenia, "just the facts": What we know in 2008. Part 3: Neurobiology. *Schizophrenia Research,* doi: 10.1016/jschres. 2008.07.020.

Leucht, S., Barnes, T. R., Kissling, W., Engel, R. R., Correll, C., & Kane, J. M. (2003). Relapse prevention in schizophrenia with new-generation antipsychotics: A systematic review and exploratory meta-analysis of randomized, controlled trials. *American Journal of Psychiatry, 160*(7), 1209–1222.

Malla, A., Norman, R., & Joober, R. (2005). First episode psychosis, early intervention and outcome: What have we learned? *Canadian Journal of Psychiatry, 50*(14), 881–891.

Malla, A., Norman, R., McLean, T., Scholten, D., & Townsend, L. (2003). A Canadian programme for early intervention in non-affective psychotic disorders. *Australian New Zealand Journal of Psychiatry, 37*, 407–413.

McDonald, C., Grech, A., Toulopoulou, T., Schulze, K., Chapple, B., Sham, P., et al. (2002). Brain volumes in familial and non-familial schizophrenia probands and their unaffected relatives. *American Journal of Medical Genetics, 114*(6), 616–625.

McGlashan, T. H. (1994). Psychosocial treatments of schizophrenia: The potential relationships. In N. C. Andreasen (Ed.), *Schizophrenia: From mind to molecule* (pp. 189–215). Washington, DC: American Psychiatric Press.

Mental Health Commission of Canada. (2007). A time for action: Tackling stigma and discrimination. Available at: http://www.mentalhealthcommission.ca/English/Pages/AntiStigmaCampaign.aspx

Mental Health Recovery: What helps and what hinders ? *A National Research Project for the Development of Recovery Facilitating System Performance Indicators.* NAMI SCC website, Retrieved from http://www.namiscc.org/Recovery/2002/MentalHealthRecovery.htm

Montoya, A., Ocampo, M., & Torres-Ruiz, A. (2003). Neuroleptic malignant syndrome in Mexico. *Canadian Journal of Clinical Pharmacology, 10*(3), 111–113.

Morrison, E. F. (1992). A coercive interactional style as an antecedent to aggression in psychiatric patients. *Research in Nursing and Health, 15*, 421–431.

Morrison, E. F. (1993). Toward a better understanding of violence in psychiatric settings: Debunking the myths. *Archives of Psychiatric Nursing, 7*, 328–335.

Morrison, E. F., & Carney Love, C. (2003). An evaluation of four programs for the management of aggression in psychiatric settings. *Archives in Psychiatric Nursing, 17*(4), 146–155.

Muir-Cochrane, E. (2006). Medical co-morbidity factors and barriers to care for people with schizophrenia. *Journal of Psychiatric & Mental Health Nursing, 13*(4), 447–452.

Murray, R. M., & Bramon, E. (2005). Developmental model of schizophrenia. In B. J. Sadock & V. A. Sadock (Eds.), *Comprehensive textbook of psychiatry* (pp. 1381–1396). Philadelphia, PA: Lippincott Williams & Wilkins.

Nasar, S. (1998). *A beautiful mind: The life of mathematical genius and Nobel Laureate John Nash.* New York, NY: Touchstone.

Niemi, L. T., Suvisaari, J. M., Tuulio-Henriksson, A., & Lonnqvist, J. K. (2003). Childhood developmental abnormalities in schizophrenia: Evidence from high-risk studies. *Schizophrenia Research, 60*(2–3), 239–258.

O'Carroll, R., Russell, H., Lawrie, S., & Johnstone, E. (1999). Errorless learning and the cognitive rehabilitation of memory-impaired schizophrenic patients. *Psychological Medicine, 29*, 105–112.

Ota, M., Mizukami, K., Katano, T., Sato, S., Takeda, T., & Asada, T. (2003). A case of delusional disorder, somatic type with remarkable improvement of clinical symptoms and single photon emission computed tomography findings following modified electroconvulsive therapy. *Progress in Neuro-Psychopharmacology & Biological Psychiatry, 27*(5), 881–884.

Overall, J. E., & Gorham, D. R. (1988). The Brief Psychiatric Rating Scale (BPRS): Recent developments in ascertainment and scaling. *Psychopharmacology Bulletin, 24*, 97–99.

Oxford University Press and the Maryland Psychiatric Research Center. (2002). Graduate student in peril: A first person account of schizophrenia. *Schizophrenia Bulletin, 28*(4), 745–755.

Penn, A. A. (2001). Early brain wiring: Activity-dependent processes. *Schizophrenia Bulletin, 27*(3), 336–347.

Rapoport, J., Addington, A., & Frangou, S. (2005). The neurodevelopmental model of schizophrenia: Update 2005. *Molecular Psychiatry, 10*, 434–449.

Ryan, M. C. M., Collins, P., & Thakore, J. H. (2003). Impaired fasting glucose tolerance in first-episode, drug-naive patients with schizophrenia. *American Journal of Psychiatry, 160*, 284–289.

Sallet, P. C., Elkis, H., Alves, T. M., Oliveira, J. R., Sassi, E., Campi de Castro, C., et al. (2003). Reduced cortical folding in schizophrenia: An MRI morphometric study. *American Journal of Psychiatry, 160*(9), 1606–1613.

Schimmelbusch, W. H., Mueller, P. S., & Sheps, J. (1971). The positive correlation between insulin resistance and duration of hospitalization in untreated schizophrenia. *British Journal of Psychiatry, 118*(545), 42–36.

Sedvall, G. (1994). Positron-emission tomography as a metabolic and neurochemical probe. In N. C. Andreasen (Ed.), *Schizophrenia: From mind to molecule* (pp. 147–155). Washington, DC: American Psychiatric Press.

Simpson, G. M., & Angus, J. W. S. L. (1970). A rating scale for extrapyramidal side effects. *Acta Psychiatrica Scandinavica, 212*(Suppl.), 11–19.

Sprague, R. L., & Kalachnik, J. E. (1991). Reliability, validity, and a total score cutoff for the Dyskinesia Identification Scale System: Condensed User Scale (DISCUS) with mentally ill and mentally retarded populations. *Psychopharmacology Bulletin, 27*, 51–58.

Stahl, S. (2000). *Essential psychopharmacology: Neuroscientific basis and practical application* (2nd ed.). Cambridge, UK: Cambridge University Press.

Stahl, S. M. (2002). The metabolic syndrome: Psychopharmacologists should weigh the evidence for weighing the patient. *Journal of Clinical Psychiatry, 63*, 1094–1095.

The Standing Senate Committee on Social Affairs, Science and Technology. (2006). Out of the shadows at last: Transforming mental health, mental illness and addiction services in Canada. Retrieved February 10, 2008, from http://www.parl.gc.ca/39/1/parlbus/commbus/senate/Com-e/SOCI-E/rep-e/rep02may06-e.htm

Subotnik, K. L., Goldstein, M. J., Nuechterlein, K. H., Woo, S. M., & Mintz, J. (2002). Are communication deviance and expressed emotion related to family history of psychiatric disorders in schizophrenia? *Schizophrenia Bulletin, 28*(4), 719–729.

Tang, W., & Ungvari, G. (2003). Efficacy of electroconvulsive therapy in treatment-resistant schizophrenia: a prospective, open trial. *Progress in Neuro-Psychopharmacology & Biological Psychiatry, 27,* 373–379.

Thornton, L. (2000). *Finding a hope in Schizophrenia Healing and Hope for everyone in the Family.* Washington, DC: APA Books.

Tsuang, M. T., Stone, W. S., & Faraone, S. V. (2001). Genes, environment and schizophrenia. *British Journal of Psychiatry, 178*(Suppl. 40), S18–S24.

United States Department of Health and Human Services. (2001). *Mental health: Culture, race, and ethnicity—A supplement to mental health: A report of the Surgeon General.* Rockville, MD: Author.

van Meijel, B., van der Gaag, M., Kahn, R. S., & Grypdonck, M. H. (2003). Relapse prevention in patients with schizophrenia: The application of an intervention protocol in nursing practice. *Archives of Psychiatric Nursing, 17*(4), 165–172.

Walker, E., Kestler, L., Bollini, A., & Hochman, K. M. (2004). Schizophrenia: Etiology and course. *Annual Review of Psychology, 55,* 401–430.

Weisman, A. G., Gomes, L. G., & Lopez, S. R. (2003). Shifting blame away from ill relatives: Latino families' reactions to schizophrenia. *Journal of Nervous and Mental Disease, 191*(9), 574–581.

Wuerker, A. K., Long, J. D., Haas, G. L., & Bellack, A. S. (2002). Interpersonal control, expressed emotion, and change in symptoms in families of persons with schizophrenia. *Schizophrenia Research, 58*(2–3), 281–292.

CHAPTER
19

Schizoaffective, Delusional, and Other Psychotic Disorders

Diana Clarke

Adapted from the chapter "Schizoaffective, Delusional, and Other Psychotic Disorders" by Nan Roberts and Roberta Stock

LEARNING OBJECTIVES

After studying this chapter, you will be able to:

- Define schizoaffective disorder and distinguish the major differences among schizophrenia, schizoaffective, and mood disorders.
- Discuss the important epidemiologic findings related to schizoaffective disorder.
- Explain the primary etiologic factors regarding schizoaffective disorder.
- Explain the primary elements involved in assessment, nursing diagnoses, nursing interventions, and evaluation of patients with schizoaffective disorder.
- Define delusional disorder and explain the importance of nonbizarre delusions in diagnosis and treatment.
- Explain the important epidemiologic findings regarding delusional disorder.
- Discuss the primary etiologic factors of delusional disorder.
- Explain the various subtypes of delusional disorder.
- Explain the nursing care of patients with delusional disorder.

KEY TERMS

• delusional disorder • delusions • erotomania • misidentification • nonbizarre delusions • persecutory delusions • psychosis • schizoaffective disorder • thymoleptic

*P*sychiatric and mental health (PMH) nurses care for patients who have psychiatric disorders involving underlying psychoses other than schizophrenia and mood disorders. This chapter introduces other psychotic disorders and describes the associated nursing care. Central to understanding the problems of these patients is the concept of **psychosis**, a term used to describe a state in which an individual experiences positive symptoms, also known as psychotic symptoms (hallucinations, delusions, or disorganized thoughts, speech, or behaviour) (see Chapter 18). Other psychotic disorders defined by the presence of psychosis include schizophreniform, schizoaffective, delusional, brief psychotic, and shared psychotic disorders. Other psychotic disorders may be induced by drugs or alcohol.

Schizoaffective disorder (SCA) is one of the more complex psychotic disorders but one of the more common diagnoses that the generalist nurse is likely to encounter.

The person with delusional disorder is more likely to be treated in a medical-surgical setting and is rarely seen by a psychiatrist. This disorder often remains undiagnosed; therefore, for nurses practicing in nonpsychiatric settings, recognizing and understanding it are crucial to providing meaningful care.

Schizoaffective Disorder

◼◼◖ CLINICAL COURSE

SCA is a complex and persistent psychiatric illness. This disorder was recognized in 1933 by Kasanin, who described varying degrees of symptoms of both schizophrenia (SCH) and mood disorders (MD), beginning in youth. All his patients were well-adjusted before the sudden onset of symptoms that erupted after the occurrence of a specific environmental stressor. Since Kasanin's time, debate and controversy about the status of this disorder have been extensive, resulting in many different definitions and classifications that remain under consideration (Maj, Pirozzi, Formicola, Bartoli, & Bucci, 2000). Box 19-1 reflects the history of this debate. The debate continues. A systematic review of clinical trial studies comparing SCA with SCH and MD suggests that SCA occupies an intermediate position between the latter disorders, but no clear cut distinctions between SCA and SCH or SCA and MD could be found (Cheniaux et al., 2008). A survey of psychiatrists' attitudes toward SCA found that while almost all had used the diagnosis in clinical practice and most considered the diagnosis to be clinically useful, there was little agreement about its nature, its relationship to other mental disorders, or its etiology (Rowe & Clark, 2008).

SCA is characterized by intervals of intense symptoms alternating with quiescent periods, during which psychosocial functioning is adequate. The episodic nature of this

disorder is characteristic. This disorder is at times marked by symptoms of schizophrenia; at other times, it appears to be a mood disorder. In other cases, both psychosis and pervasive mood changes occur concurrently.

Whether SCA is a schizophrenia spectrum disorder with mood symptoms or a mood disorder with psychotic symptoms is still open for debate although the current evidence leans toward the former (Evans et al., 1999). Furthermore, in an Ontario study of early signs of schizophrenia spectrum disorders (schizophrenia, SCA, and schizophreniform disorder), it was found that greater psychobiologic changes (in appetite, sleep, energy, and restlessness) during the prepsychotic phase were associated with a more emotionally reactive form of schizophrenia (Norman, Scholten, Malla, & Ballageer, 2005). Current clinical emphasis is on treatment of presenting symptoms and not necessarily on establishing a definitive diagnosis.

> **• CRNENOTE**
>
> Patients with schizoaffective disorder have many similar responses to their disorder as people with schizophrenia, with one exception. These patients have many more "mood" responses and are very susceptible to suicide.

Patients with SCA are more likely to exhibit persistent psychosis, with or without mood symptoms, than patients with a mood disorder. They feel that they are on a "chronic roller coaster ride" of symptoms that are often more difficult to cope with than the individual problem of either schizophrenia or mood disorder (Marneros, 2003). The diagnosis of this disorder is made only after these course-related characteristics are considered.

The long-term outcome of SCA is generally better than that of schizophrenia but worse than that of mood disorder (Moller et al., 2002). This group of patients resembles the mood disorder group in work function and the schizophrenia group in social function. In one study, compared with patients with a bipolar mood disorder, schizoaffective patients were less likely to recover and more likely to have persistent psychosis, with or without mood symptoms. Patients with SCA also have poorer executive function than do control subjects or patients with nonpsychotic bipolar disorder schizophrenia (Gooding & Tallent, 2002; Reichenberg et al., 2002).

◼◼◖ DIAGNOSTIC CRITERIA

Mental health providers find SCA difficult to conceptualize, diagnose, and treat because the clinical picture is often very complex and varies from episode to episode over time. Patients often have misdiagnoses of schizophrenia or conversely of depression with psychotic features or

---

BOX 19.1

History of the Diagnosis: Schizoaffective

1933:	Kasanin first coined the phrase *schizoaffective psychosis.*
1980:	*DSM-III* did not include diagnostic criteria for schizoaffective disorder.
1987:	Schizoaffective disorder was first recognized as a separate diagnosis in the *DSM-III-R*; the definition included the length of time in relation to symptoms.
1994:	Schizoaffective disorder was maintained as a separate disorder in the *DSM-IV.*
2000:	Schizoaffective disorder was maintained as a separate disorder in the *DSM-IV-TR.*

Table 19.1 Key Diagnostic Characteristics of Schizoaffective Disorder 295.70	
Diagnostic Criteria and Target Symptoms	**Associated Findings**
• Uninterrupted period of illness with concurrent major depressive episode, manic episode, or mixed episode • *Bipolar type*: manic or mixed episode or manic or mixed episode and major depressive episode • *Depressive type*: only major depressive episode • Characteristic symptoms of schizophrenia (two or more) during a 1-month period • Delusions • Hallucinations • Disorganized speech • Grossly disorganized or catatonic behaviour or negative symptoms • Delusions or hallucinations for at least 2 weeks without prominent mood symptoms • Symptoms of mood episode present for major portion of the active and residual periods of illness • Not a direct physiologic effect of a substance or medical condition	*Associated Behavioural Findings* • Poor occupational functioning • Restricted range of social contact • Difficulties with self-care • Increased risk for suicide

---

IN A LIFE

Louis Riel (1844–1885)
Metis Leader

Public Persona

Louis Riel, leader of the Metis in Manitoba and Saskatchewan, has been remembered as the man who negotiated for the establishment of Manitoba as a province and who led the fight for the protection of Metis and Aboriginal land and rights in Western Canada. Arrested for treason in 1884, he showed symptoms of grandiosity and paranoid delusions. He was declared "sane" by the superintendent of the Asylum for the Insane in Toronto, stood trial, and was hanged in 1885.

Personal Realities

Riel had numerous episodes of profound depression, apparent psychosis, and delusional thinking throughout his life. At times, he believed he had been substituted for the real Louis Riel who had died. At other times, he talked about his "mission" to form a new religion and replace the Pope. He was hospitalized and committed to insane asylums on numerous occasions. He has, retrospectively, variably been "diagnosed" in the literature with paranoid schizophrenia, schizoaffective disorder, and bipolar disorder.

From Perr, I. N. (1992). Religion, political leadership, charisma and mental illness: The strange story of Louis Riel. *Journal of Forensic Science*, *37*(2), 574–584; Waite, P. (1987). Between three oceans: Challenges of a continental destiny. In C. Brown (Ed.), *The illustrated history of Canada* (pp. 279–373). Toronto, ON: Lester & Orpen Dennys.

---

bipolar mood disorder. The difficulty in conceptualizing SCA is reflected in the controversy regarding the diagnostic criteria. For example, it has been argued that this disorder should be named either *schizophrenia with mood symptoms* or *mood disorder with schizophrenic symptoms*. More than 50 years after SCA was first described, the diagnosis was finally officially confirmed by the psychiatric community and included in the American Psychiatric Association's (APA, 1980) *Diagnostic and Statistical Manual of Mental Disorders*, 3rd ed., Revision (*DSM-III-R*).

To receive a diagnosis of SCA, a patient must have an uninterrupted period of illness when there is a major depressive, manic, or mixed episode along with two of the following symptoms of schizophrenia: delusions, hallucinations, disorganized speech, disorganized or catatonic behaviour, or negative symptoms (e.g., affective flattening, alogia, or avolition). In addition, although the person experiences problems with mood most of the time, the positive symptoms (delusions or hallucinations) must be present without the mood symptoms at some time during this period (for at least 2 weeks) (Table 19-1). Those with permanent delusions or auditory hallucinations report more basic symptoms (Fabisch et al., 2001). To clarify this disorder further, two related subtypes of SCA have been identified. In the bipolar type, the patient exhibits manic symptoms alone or a mix of manic and depressive symptoms. Patients with the depressive type display only symptoms of a major depressive episode (APA, 2000). The most common disorders from which SCA must be differentiated include mood disorders of manic, depressive, or mixed types and schizophrenia.

EPIDEMIOLOGY AND RISK FACTORS

The lifetime prevalence of SCA is estimated to be less than 1%, but there are no current studies (APA, 2000). This disorder occurs less commonly than does schizophrenia. The incidence of SCA is relatively constant across populations in varied geographic, climatic, industrial, and social environments. Environmental contributions are minimal.

Patients with schizoaffective disorder are at high risk for suicide. The risk for suicide in patients with psychosis is increased by the presence of depression. Risk for suicide is increased with the use of alcohol or substances, cigarette smoking, previous attempts at suicide, and previous hospitalizations (Potkin et al., 2003; Seguin et al., 2006).

Lack of regular social contact may be a factor that confers a long-term risk for suicidal behaviour, which may be reduced by treatments designed to enhance social networks and contact (Radomsky, Haas, Mann, & Sweeney, 1999) and help patients to protect themselves against environmental stressors (Huxley, Rendall, & Sederer, 2000). Cognition is more impaired with SCA than with nonpsychotic mood disorder (Evans et al., 1999).

Age of Onset

SCA can affect children and the elderly. In children, the disorder is rare and is often indistinguishable from schizophrenia. In the older adult, this disorder becomes complicated because of frequent comorbid medical conditions. The typical age of onset for this disorder is early adulthood, and the most common type presented is bipolar. Other studies have reported a relatively late onset of SCA of mainly the depressive type (APA, 2000). Earlier age of onset is associated with longer illness, more severe illness, and worse outcomes (APA).

Gender

This disorder is more likely to occur in women than in men, which may be accounted for by a greater incidence of the depressive type in women (APA, 2000). As with schizophrenia, the age of onset is later for women than for men (Sadock & Sadock, 2007).

Ethnicity and Culture

Although some reports have indicated a connection between SCA and social class, others support no specific association with race, geographic area, or class (Siris & Lavin, 1995).

Family

Some authorities support a familial association in SCA, but a clear familial pattern has not been established. Relatives of patients with diagnoses of SCA appear to be at increased risk for this disorder, schizophrenia, or both. There is some initial genome evidence that if there is a familial association, it is most likely related to the mother not the father (DeLisi et al., 2002).

Comorbidity

SCA may be associated with substance abuse. Men may be more likely to engage in antisocial behaviour. Twenty-five percent of patients with diagnoses of SCA experience postpsychotic depression and panic attacks (APA, 2000).

ETIOLOGY

Biologic Theories

Although the etiologies of schizophrenia and mood disorder have been investigated extensively, the etiology of SCA remains unresolved. Research to locate a biologic marker has been limited. Variables may be structural, as well as neurochemical.

Neuropathologic

Magnetic resonance imaging (MRI) and computed tomography (CT or CAT) scans have been used in the study of SCA for more than 10 years (Crow & Harrington, 1994; Lewine, Hudgins, Brown, Caudle, & Risch, 1995; Scott, Price, George, Brillman, & Rothfus, 1993). Midline brain abnormalities, especially in women, have been found. In SCA, changes in brain structure appear to be similar to those seen in bipolar disorder (Getz et al., 2002). Whether midline structural abnormality is directly causal, indirectly contributory, or an intriguing phenomenon in SCA is unclear. Research aimed at determining neuropsychological differences between SCH and SCA remains inconclusive, but it is argued that severity may be the difference between the disorders (Heinrichs, Ammari, Vaz, & Miles, 2008).

Genetic

The etiology is believed to be primarily genetic. Results from family, twin, and adoption studies vary but suggest that SCA may consist of phenotypic variations or expressions of a genetic interform between schizophrenia and affective psychoses (DeLisi et al., 2002).

Biochemical

Before 1999, the prevailing neurochemical hypothesis was overactivity of dopamine pathways. Whether this disturbance of dopaminergic transmission is primary remains unclear (Rietschel et al., 2000). In studies of deficit symptoms in SCA, altered patterns of glucose metabolism have been found that might cause neurobiologic and neurophysiologic impairments (Regenold, Thapar, Marano, Gavirneni, & Kondapavuluru, 2002).

Psychological and Social Theories

Psychological, psychodynamic, environmental, and interpersonal factors may have a precipitating role when they coincide with a biomedical diathesis that creates vulnerability to this disorder (see Chapter 8 for explanation of the diathesis-stress theory). No current psychodynamic behavioural, cognitive, or developmental theories of causation explain SCA. Family dynamics do not appear to affect the development of this disorder, except for the strong genetic predisposition, which is virtually unexplained.

▰ INTERDISCIPLINARY TREATMENT

Patients with SCA benefit from comprehensive treatment. Because this disorder is persistent, these individuals are constantly trying to manage complex symptoms. Ideally, most of the treatment occurs within the patient's natural environment, and hospitalizations are limited to times of symptom exacerbation, when symptoms are so severe or persistent that extended care in a protected environment is necessary.

Pharmacologic intervention is needed to stabilize the symptoms, and it presents specific challenges. Long-term atypical antipsychotic agents are as effective as the traditional combination of a standard antipsychotic agent and an antidepressant drug. Mood stabilizers, such as lithium or valproic acid, may also be used. A combination of antipsychotic and antidepressant agents is sometimes used (see Chapter 14).

After the patient's condition has stabilized (i.e., the patient exhibits a decrease in positive and negative symptoms), the treatment that led to remission of symptoms should be continued. Titrating antipsychotic agents to the lowest dose that provides suitable protection may enable optimal psychosocial functioning, while slowing recurrence of new episodes. Patients with SCA will likely need to remain on medication for the disorder. Electroconvulsive therapy (see Chapter 14) is considered when symptoms are refractory to other interventions or when the patient's life is at risk and a rapid response is required (Swoboda, Conca, Konig, Waanders, & Hansen, 2001).

The treatment plan is revised regularly, and symptoms are monitored to guide medication management. PMH nursing interventions in hospital and in community care are guided by the nursing diagnoses. Psychotherapy may help manage interpersonal relationships and mood changes. Social services are often needed to obtain disability benefits or services. Use of advanced practice clinicians helps to provide continuity of care (McCann & Baker, 2003).

▰ PRIORITY CARE ISSUES

Patients with SCA may be at least as susceptible to suicide (see Chapter 38) as those with mood disorder (Potkin et al., 2003). Living with a persistent psychotic disorder that has a mood component makes suicide a real risk. A recent review of completed suicides in New Brunswick has further suggested that comorbidity with substance abuse may amplify the risk (Sequin et al., 2006).

▰ NURSING MANAGEMENT: HUMAN RESPONSE TO SCHIZOAFFECTIVE DISORDER

Biologic Domain

Assessment

Assessment of patients with SCA is similar to assessment of those with schizophrenia and affective disorder. A careful history from the patient and family is crucial. The history should contain a description of the full range and duration of symptoms the patient has experienced and those observed by the family; this information is important for predicting outcomes. A patient who has had symptoms for a relatively long period of time has greater difficulty in overcoming effects of the psychosis, which may cause the function to deteriorate.

A thorough systems assessment is important to discover any physiologic problems the patient is experiencing, such as sleep pattern disturbances, difficulties with self-care, or poor nutritional habits.

Nursing Diagnoses for Biologic Domain

Common nursing diagnoses for the biologic domain are disturbed thought process, disturbed sensory perception, and disturbed sleep patterns. Because of the variety of problems in patients with SCA, almost any nursing diagnosis could be generated. The persistent nature of this disorder lends itself to numerous and varied problems that must all be addressed (see Nursing Care Plan 19-1).

Interventions for Biologic Domain

Patient Education

Interventions are based on the needs identified in the bio/psycho/social/spiritual assessment (Fig. 19-1). Helping the patient to establish a regular sleep pattern by using a routine can promote or reestablish normal rest patterns. Focusing with the patient on the principles of good nutrition and identifying any barriers to healthy eating can improve nutritional status. Working

Nursing Care Plan 19.1

Patient With Schizoaffective Disorder

Ms. B is a 28-year-old divorced woman with a 4-year-old daughter. They reside with Ms. B's parents. Ms. B is a hairdresser and tries to work, but she becomes stressed in the workplace, which results in her being fired. She has never applied for disability. Her parents are stressed because of the exacerbations of her illness and caring for her child.

Ms. B has had numerous hospitalizations for aggressive behaviour, noncompliance with medications, and receiving medications from various physicians, which results in inappropriate psychiatric management. She is medication seeking and is often prescribed benzodiazepines and diet pills by her primary care physician.

The patient has an ingrained delusional system that makes it hard to introduce reality orientation and feedback. She believes that her ex-husband has sexually abused their child. She has gone to numerous attorneys to try to prosecute her ex-husband to no avail because of the lack of evidence to prove any abuse.

For the last 2 years, Ms. B has believed that a bank guard is in love with her. She is adamant about him protecting her and her child. She states that he watches over them. They have no contact other than speaking to each other when she enters the bank. She has been seeing a man the past 9 months but states that she really does not care much for him and it is hard for her to move forward in the relationship because she loves the bank guard.

Medications have included antidepressants, neuroleptics (typical and atypical), mood stabilizers, benzodiazepines, sleep medications, and anticonvulsants. She often complains of being depressed and yet does not take the antidepressant medications when they are prescribed.

Setting: Intensive Care Psychiatric Unit in a General Hospital

Baseline Assessment: Ms. B is admitted to the hospital through the ER. She was hearing voices and was delusional. She has not been taking medications for several months. She is oriented in all spheres and well nourished but unkempt. She is verbalizing delusions about a man at the bank. She cannot sleep well and reportedly goes outdoors at night and yells at a bank guard. Reality feedback increases her agitation. She denies any problems.

Associated Psychiatric Diagnosis	Medications
Axis I: Schizoaffective disorder	None
Axis II: Deferred	
Axis III: None	
Axis IV: Social problem (maintaining relationships)	
Economic problem (no income)	
Occupational problem (unemployed)	
Axis V: Current, 28	
Potential, 60	

Nursing Diagnosis 1: Ineffective Individual Coping

Defining Characteristics	Related Factors
Inability to meet role expectations	Chronicity of the condition
Anxiety	Inadequate psychological resources secondary to delusions
Delusions	Inadequate coping skills
Inability to problem solve	Inadequate psychological resources to adapt to residential setting

Outcomes

Initial	Discharge
1. Identify coping patterns	5. Manage own behaviour
2. Identify stressors	6. Medication compliance
3. Identify personal strengths	7. Reduction of delusions
4. Accept support through the nursing relationship	

Continued

Nursing Care Plan 19.1 *(Continued)*

Interventions

Interventions	Rationale	Ongoing Assessment
Initiate a nurse–patient relationship to develop trust.	Through the use of the nurse–patient relationship, the patient will be able to maintain compliance with the treatment plan.	Determine whether the patient is able to relate to the nurse.
Facilitate the identification of stressors in the patient's environment.	To be able to cope with stressors, they need to be identified by the patient.	Assess whether the patient is able to identify and verbalize stressors.
Develop coping strategies to manage environmental stressors.	The patient needs to develop realistic strategies to handle environmental stressors.	Determine whether patient-identified strategies are realistic.
Help the patient to identify personal strengths.	By identifying personal strengths, the patient will increase confidence in using coping strategies.	Assess the patient's ability to incorporate coping strategies into her daily routine.
Assist the patient to understand the disorder and its management.	By understanding the disorder, the patient can develop ways to manage her disorder.	Assess the patient's level of understanding of the disease.
Facilitate emotional support for the family.	Supported family is better equipped to support the patient.	Assess the family's ability to seek emotional support from the staff.
Teach coping skills.	By developing positive coping skills, anxiety and agitation will decrease.	Assess the patient's ability to learn the skills to manage stressors.

Evaluation

Outcomes	Revised Outcomes	Interventions
Within the nursing relationship, Ms. B. was able to understand how coping skills can reduce stressors.	Support the patient's ability to recognize stressor and apply coping skills.	Discuss stressors and means of applying coping skills.
Increased insight into what behaviour is appropriate has helped the patient to decrease verbalization of delusions.	Provide ongoing support to maintain the present level of functioning.	Discuss behaviour and provide reality feedback.

Nursing Diagnosis 2: Disturbed Thought Processes

Defining Characteristics	Related Factors
Delusions	Ingrained delusions
Impulsivity	Decreased ability to process secondary to delusions
Medication noncompliance	

Outcomes

Initial	Discharge
1. Maintain reality orientation.	4. Identify situations that contribute to delusions.
2. Communicate clearly with others.	5. Identify how delusions affect life situations.
3. Express delusional material less frequently.	6. Use coping strategies to deal with delusions.
	7. Recognize changes in behaviour.

Interventions

Interventions	Rationale	Ongoing Assessment
Promote adherence to medication regimen.	Medication will reduce delusions.	Assess for side effects: heat intolerance, NMS, renal failure, constipation, dry mouth, increased appetite, salivation, nausea, vomiting, tardive dyskinesia, seizures, somnolence, agitation, insomnia, dizziness.

Continued

Nursing Care Plan 19.1 (Continued)

Interventions

Interventions	Rationale	Ongoing Assessment
Teach actions, effects, and side effects of medications.	The more knowledgeable patients are about medication, the more likely they will comply.	Assess ability to understand information.
Support reality testing through helping the patient to differentiate thoughts and feelings in relation to situations.	When comparing thoughts with the situations, patients can develop skills to refute delusions.	Assess for medication compliance.
Monitor verbalization of delusional material.	To determine whether medication is reducing delusional thoughts.	Assess verbalization of delusional material.
Identify stressors that promote delusions.	If the patient is able to identify stressors that promote delusions, she can manage the stressors to effectively decrease delusions.	Assess the patient's ability to recognize stressors when they occur. Encourage use of crisis planning or wellness planning tools.
Assist the patient in developing skills to deal with delusions (recognizing delusional themes can help the patient in distinguishing between reality-based and non–reality-based patterns).	Even though medication can reduce the occurrence of delusions, they may continue in some people with decreased intensity. Cognitive-behavioural skills are important in dealing with these altered thoughts.	Monitor the patient's ability to handle delusions.

Evaluation

Outcomes	Revised Outcomes	Interventions
Delusions will be less ingrained.	Continue to practice skills in reality orientation and communication.	Support verbalization of reality-based thoughts.
The patient verbalized action, effect, dosage, and side effects of medications.	Take prescribed medication regularly.	Give positive feedback for understanding of medication.
Medication compliance		Initiate pill counts to determine medication compliance.

Summary: Ms. B was discharged from the hospital. Verbalization of delusions had not decreased. She was less anxious. She is presently on Risperdal 2 mg AM and hs, Effexor XR 75 mg AM, Xanax 0.5 mg AM, and Seroquel 50 mg hs. Her mother is helping by filling a weekly medication box. At times, Ms B is questioning her delusions.

with the patient can help identify self-care deficits, especially those caused by lack of motivation. For deficits created by severe mood symptoms, establishing a routine and setting goals can be useful.

The collaborative development of a crisis plan or a "wellness" plan when the individual is well can help the patient identify triggers and prodromal symptoms of decompensation and allow them to preplan coping mechanisms and engaging of supports to mitigate the effects of illness (Copeland, 2005). Such plans have been well researched in the United Kingdom and have been shown to decrease the need for involuntary hospitalization (Papageorigiou, King, Jonhohamed, Davison, & Dawson, 2002; Sutherby et al., 1999). Preliminary evidence from a recent study in Manitoba suggests that giving patients a role in planning their community care through the use of a Wellness Planner which includes crisis planning and personal goal setting can increase their sense of empowerment and improve their quality of life (Marchinko, 2008).

Pharmacologic Interventions

An in-depth history of the patient's medication is important in evaluating response to past medications and predicting response to the present regimen. Investigate adherence to past treatment to determine the probability of successful intervention. Develop a plan to increase adherence based on any past problems or issues. For example, use medication boxes and calendars and get help from others in managing the medication. Some patients may need to receive their neuroleptics in a long-acting, injectable depot format. Recognizing medication side effects quickly and intervening promptly to alleviate them will help maintain adherence. Promoting understanding of the need for medications is essential.

FIGURE 19.1 Bio/psycho/social/spiritual interventions for patients with schizoaffective disorders.

Mood and psychotic symptoms are equally important and should be evaluated throughout treatment. Atypical antipsychotic agents are generally prescribed because of their efficacy and safe side effect profile. Clozapine, reported effective for SCA by several authorities, can reduce hospitalizations and risk for suicide (Potkin et al., 2003). A significant portion of patients whose symptoms have resisted other neuroleptic agents experience improvement with clozapine therapy (Volavka et al., 2002). Atypical antipsychotic agents may have **thymoleptic** (mood stabilizing), as well as antipsychotic, effects. Quetiapine has been found effective (Bech, 2001). Dosage is the same as that used for treating schizophrenia, but lower dosage ranges may also be effective.

• CRNENOTE

The medication regimen for patients with schizoaffective disorder will be complex and may include antipsychotics, mood stabilizers, antidepressants, and occasional antianxiety agents.

In many cases, symptoms of depression disappear when psychotic symptoms decrease. If depressive symptoms persist, adjunctive use of an antidepressant agent may be helpful. Successful use of anticonvulsant agents for this disorder has been documented in several clinical trials (Dietrich, Kropp, & Emrich, 2001). Mood stabilizers, which can decrease the frequency and intensity of episodes, may be an alternative adjunctive medication for mood states associated with the bipolar type.

Administering and Monitoring Medications

One of the greatest challenges in pharmacologic interventions is monitoring target symptoms and identifying changes in symptom pattern. Patients can switch from being relatively calm to being very emotional. Whether the patient is overreacting to an environmental event or mood symptoms have changed and the patient requires a medication change can be determined only through careful observation and documentation.

Adherence to medication regimens is critical to a successful outcome. Patients need an opportunity to discuss barriers to compliance.

Managing Side Effects

Monitoring medication side effects in patients with SCA is similar to that in patients with schizophrenia. Patients receiving antipsychotic medications need to be aware of extrapyramidal symptoms and the possibility of developing metabolic syndrome—a triad of diabetes, dyslipidemia, and hypertension with associated obesity (McIntyre, McCann, & Kennedy, 2001; Shirzadi & Ghaemi, 2006). Regular monitoring of abdominal obesity and fasting blood glucose has been shown to be a cost-effective screening test to detect patients at high risk for cardiovascular morbidity (Straker et al., 2005). Counselling regarding nutrition and healthy lifestyle choices (e.g., smoking cessation, physical exercise) is paramount with these patients.

Monitoring for Drug Interactions

Avoid using lithium with antipsychotic medications. A few patients taking haloperidol and lithium have experienced an encephalopathic syndrome, followed by irreversible brain damage. Lithium may interact similarly with other antipsychotic agents. It may also prolong the effects of neuromuscular blocking agents. Use of nonsteroidal anti-inflammatory drugs may increase plasma lithium levels. Diuretics and angiotensin-converting enzyme inhibitors should be prescribed cautiously with lithium, which is excreted through the kidney (see Chapter 10 for more information).

Teaching Points

- Instruct patients to take medications as prescribed.
- Determine whether the patient has sufficient resources to purchase and obtain medications.
- Have the patient write down the prescribed medication and time of administration.
- Explain the target symptom for each medication (e.g., psychosis and mood for atypical antipsychotic agents, mood for antidepressant and mood stabilizer drugs).
- Caution patients about orthostatic hypotension and instruct them to get up slowly from a lying or sitting position. Also advise them to maintain adequate fluid intake.
- Advise patients to contact their case coordinators or health care providers immediately if they experience dramatic changes in body temperature (neuroleptic malignant syndrome [NMS]), inability to control motor movement (dystonia), or dizziness.
- Advise patients to avoid over-the-counter medications unless a prescriber is consulted.
- Advise patients taking olanzapine and clozapine to monitor body weight and report rapid weight gains.
- Advise patients to report symptoms of diabetes mellitus (frequent urination, excessive thirst, etc.).

Psychological Domain

Assessment

The patient's level of insight into his or her illness may play a role in the course and treatment of SCA.

Patients with SCA tend to have better insight than those with schizophrenia (Pini, Cassano, Dell'Osso, & Amador, 2001). Stressors should be evaluated because they may trigger symptoms. Uncovering or exploratory techniques that may reveal, for example, past episodes of abuse should generally be avoided. Mental status and reality contact may be compromised. Assessment of anxiety level or reactions to stressful situations is important because the combination of these symptoms with psychosis increases the patient's risk for suicide.

Nursing Diagnoses for Psychological Domain

In SCA, individuals vacillate between mood dysregulation and disturbed thinking. Typical nursing diagnoses for this domain include hopelessness, powerlessness, ineffective coping, and low self-esteem.

Interventions for Psychological Domain

Using appropriate interpersonal modalities is important to help the patient, family, and social and vocational support networks cope with the onslaught of acute episodes and recuperative periods. Patients with SCA have fewer awareness deficits than do patients with schizophrenia. Structured, integrated, and problem-solving psychotherapeutic interventions should be used to develop or increase the patient's insight. Psychoeducational interventions can help to decrease symptoms, enhance recognition of early regression, and hone psychosocial skills (see Boxes 19-2 and 19-3.)

BOX 19.2

Psychoeducation Checklist: Schizoaffective Disorder

When caring for the patient with schizoaffective disorder, be sure to include the caregiver as appropriate and address the following topic areas in the teaching plan:

- Psychopharmacologic agents (antipsychotic or antidepressants), if used, including drug action, dosage, frequency, and possible adverse effects
- Methods to enhance adherence
- Sleep measures
- Consistent routines
- Goal setting
- Nutrition
- Support networks
- Problem solving
- Positive coping strategies
- Social and vocational skills training

BOX 19.3

Research for Best Practice: Helping Women Living with Schizophrenia or Schizoaffective Disorder

From Chernomas, W. M., Clarke, D. E., & Chisholm, F. A. (2000). Perspectives of women living with schizophrenia. Psychiatric Services, 51(12), 1517–1521.

THE QUESTION: What are women's perceptions of their experience with schizophrenia or schizoaffective disorder within the context of their life stages and corresponding health issues?

METHODS: Five focus groups totaling 28 women who self-identified as having schizophrenia or schizoaffective disorder and who were living in a community in Winnipeg, Manitoba, met to discuss their health-related needs, ranging from parenting and reproductive health to relationships and aging.

FINDINGS: This group of women led marginalized, deprived lives in the face of multiple losses, social stigma, limited interpersonal contacts, and poverty. Although reasonably well educated, the majority of the group was unemployed and living on social assistance. Relationships were fraught with challenges. Making new friends or reestablishing connections with old friends was socially difficult and could be emotionally threatening, but not making friends resulted in isolation and loneliness. Intimate relationships created

potential dangers of vulnerability and victimization. Women also struggled with their self-identity, whether to see themselves as women or as someone with a mental illness. Women felt, in many cases, that the health care system focused on their illness and that they had become invisible as women. They struggled with medications that controlled their symptoms but resulted in side effects. They frequently did not feel comfortable sharing their concerns about side effects such as weight gain and amenorrhea with their health care providers. Nevertheless, they conveyed a persistent sense of wanting life to improve and hoping that it could. A sense of hope and, in many cases, spirituality kept them going.

IMPLICATIONS FOR NURSING: The illness itself often takes precedence over other significant issues in women's lives, and practitioners may unwittingly contribute to diminished quality of life. Nurses can lessen the pain of a woman's dilemma by engaging her in discussions of options and providing support while she ponders which options are best for her; by monitoring her response to side effects of medications; by setting a climate that promotes discussion of sensitive subject matter; and by adopting an attitude of working with a woman in partnership.

Social Domain

Assessment

Social dysfunction is common in patients with diagnosis of SCA. Premorbid adjustment, such as marital status and adolescent social adjustment, may influence patients' level of functioning at the time of diagnosis and their prognoses. Assess for social skill deficits and problems with interpersonal conflicts, particularly in men. Assessment of an adult patient's childhood may give a clue to the patient's current level of social functioning. Assess the patient's use of fantasy and fighting as a means of coping. Patients who report the most severe peer rejection present with the angriest dispositions and display antisocial behaviours.

Nursing Diagnoses for Social Domain

Because of their mood and thought disturbances, these individuals will have significant problems in the social domain. Typical nursing diagnoses include compromised family coping, impaired home maintenance, and social isolation.

Interventions for Social Domain

Social skills training is useful for remediating social deficits and may result in positive social adjustment.

Positive results include improved interpersonal competence and decreased symptom severity. Help in identifying feelings and in developing realistic goals, along with supportive therapy, can integrate insight into the disease process. Crisis planning, engaged in collaboration between the patient and the mental health care provider, can help both the patient and the family recognize oncoming decompensation and take appropriate steps to improve coping. Education focusing on conflict-resolution skills, promoting compromise, negotiation, and expression of negative feelings, can help the patient achieve positive social adjustment. Social skills can be improved through role playing and assertiveness training. Supportive, nurturing, and nonconfrontational interventions help to minimize anxiety and improve understanding (see Box 19-4).

Helping the patient to develop coping skills is essential. Teach communication skills to decrease conflicts and environmental negativity. Memory is linked with development of social skills; psychotic symptoms may interfere with retention of these skills, resulting in slower learning. These patients require long-term, intense social training.

Families are at risk for ineffective coping. Family members face many of the same issues faced by families of patients with schizophrenia and are often puzzled by the patient's emotional overreaction to normal daily stresses. Frequent arguments may lead to verbal and physical abuse.

BOX 19.4

Therapeutic Dialogue: Ms. B's "Delusions"

INEFFECTIVE COMMUNICATION

Nurse: Hello, Ms. B, what has been happening?

Patient: The guy from the bank keeps me up all night.

Nurse: That's not possible.

Patient: He's there all the time to look after me.

Nurse: No, he's not. You just think that.

Patient: No, he really is. He is helping me.

Nurse: He does not even know who you are.

EFFECTIVE COMMUNICATION

Nurse: Hello, Ms. B. How have you been?

Patient: That guy from the bank is really bothering me.

Nurse: What is happening?

Patient: He keeps me up all night. I go out in the street to yell at him.

Nurse: Have you actually seen him at night?

Patient: No, but I know he is there.

Nurse: How can he be there when you cannot see him?

Patient: He can't.

Nurse: Does it seem that the thoughts about him come from your mind?

Patient: This might be.

Nurse: Your illness often causes thoughts that are not based in reality.

Patient: It seems real but yet so unreal. Those are sort of stupid thoughts.

CRITICAL THINKING CHALLENGE

- How could the nurse's approach in the first scenario have prevented development of a therapeutic relationship?
- How can the second scenario benefit the patient in developing insight into her delusions?
- Discuss the differences between the two approaches.

Spiritual Domain

As with persons living with schizophrenia, the spiritual domain of care is very significant for persons living with SCA (see Chapter 18). Finding meaningful ways to cope with such a serious illness, one that often brings social rejection and isolation, becomes a life challenge. Religious or spiritual beliefs may be a comfort, and a relationship with the sacred through ritual, prayer, or other activities may offer daily comfort. Spiritual nursing care can support patients particularly in times of despair. With SCA, more than with SCH, the person is likely to experience emotional turmoil that is seriously disruptive to a sense of serenity the person may have achieved. Spiritual support should be understood as an ongoing need. The nurse needs to strive, as well, to understand the potential impact of other symptoms, such as hallucinations and delusions, on spiritual needs and to assist persons with SCA to engage in spiritual activities that are satisfying to them.

■ EVALUATION AND TREATMENT OUTCOMES

Teaching skills to patients with SCA often takes longer than teaching other patients. When evaluating progress related to interventions, be patient if outcomes are not completely met. Psychoeducation results in increased knowledge of the illness and treatment, increased medication compliance, fewer relapses and hospitalizations, briefer inpatient stays, increased social function,

decreased family tension, and lighter family burdens (Andres, Pfammatter, Garst, Teschner, & Brenner, 2000). Maintain realistic outcomes and praise small successes to promote positive outcomes (Fig. 19-2).

■ CONTINUUM OF CARE

Inpatient Focus Care

Hospitalization may be required during acute psychotic episodes or when suicidal ideations are present. This structured environment protects the patient from self-harm (i.e., suicidal, assaultive, financial, legal, vocational, or social). During periods of acute psychosis, offering reassurance in a soft, nonthreatening voice and avoiding confrontational stances will help the patient begin to trust the staff and nursing care (see Chapter 9). Avoid seclusion and restraint and keep environmental stimulation to a minimum. Use the patient's coping capabilities to reinforce constructive aspects of functioning and enable a return to autonomy.

Emergency Care!

Emergency care is needed during symptom exacerbation. Psychosis, mood disturbance, and medication-related adverse effects account for most emergency situations. During an exacerbation of psychosis, patients may become agitated or aggressive. Assaultive behaviour can be managed by using therapeutic techniques (see Chapter 36) and pharmacologic management. If medications are

Spiritual

1. Increased hope
2. Comfort from sacred activities

Biologic

1. Improved sleep patterns
2. Increased participation in self-care activities
3. Improved nutrition
4. Increased compliance with medications
5. Decreased incidence of medication adverse effects

Social

1. Positive social adjustment
2. Improved conflict resolution
3. Improved communication skills
4. Increased use of community-related support systems
5. Improved home management

Psychological

1. Increased insight
2. Improved coping abilities
3. Decreased conflicts
4. Increased autonomy and self-esteem
5. Improved social and vocational skills
6. Increased awareness of personal strengths
7. Increased reality orientation
8. Decreased hallucinations and delusions

FIGURE 19.2 Bio/psycho/social/spiritual outcomes for patients with schizoaffective disorder.

used, benzodiazepines such as lorazepam are usually given. Patients are then evaluated for antipsychotic therapy. Possible medication-related adverse effects include NMS as a reaction to dopamine antagonists or serotonin intoxication, especially if the patient is taking an atypical antipsychotic agent and a selective serotonin reuptake inhibitor (see Chapter 18). Suicidality must always be assessed (see Chapter 38).

Family Intervention

Helping families support the patient at home or in a community placement is an integral part of nursing care. With the patient's permission, key family members can be included in home visits to learn about symptoms, medications, and side effects. By collaborating with family members, the nurse can strengthen the patient's willingness to follow treatment, monitor symptoms, and continue with rehabilitation and recovery.

Community Treatment

After the patient is released from the hospital, graduated levels of care (i.e., partial hospitalization, day treatment, group home) can help the patient to return to a more normal environment. Programs that foster building and practicing social and vocational skills are appropriate and should also incorporate the patient's natural skills, interests, and aspirations because they are as important as problems and deficits.

Because this illness is episodic, the person with SCA requires close and continued follow-up in the outpatient setting by psychiatrists, nurses, and therapists. These patients require ongoing medication management, supportive and cognitive therapy, and symptom management. If symptoms intensify, hospitalization may be required until they are brought under control.

Delusional Disorder

CLINICAL COURSE

Delusional disorder is a psychotic disorder characterized by nonbizarre, logical, stable, and well-systemized delusions that occur in the absence of other psychiatric disorders. **Delusions** are false, fixed beliefs unchanged by reasonable arguments. Although delusions are a symptom of many psychotic disorders, in delusional disorder, the delusions are **nonbizarre delusions**; that is, they are characterized by adherence to possible situations that could occur in real life and are plausible in the context of the person's ethnic and cultural background (APA, 2000).

Examples of real-life situations include being followed, poisoned, infected, loved at a distance, or deceived by a spouse or lover. A diagnosis of delusional disorder is based on the presence of one or more nonbizarre delusions for at least 1 month (APA, 2000). Delusions are the primary symptom of this disorder.

The course of delusional disorder is variable. Onset can be acute, or the disorder can occur gradually and become chronic. Patients with this disorder usually live with their delusions for years, rarely receiving psychiatric treatment. They are seldom brought to the attention of health care providers unless their delusion relates to their health (somatic delusion), or they act on the basis of their delusion and violate legal or social rules. Full remissions can be followed by relapses.

Apart from the direct impact of the delusion, psychosocial functioning is not markedly impaired. The person's clarity of thinking and behaviour and emotional responses are usually consistent with the delusional focus. In general, behaviour is not odd or bizarre. In fact, behaviour is remarkably normal, except when the patient focuses on the delusion. At that time, thinking, attitudes, and mood may change abruptly. Personality does not usually change, but the patient is gradually, progressively involved with the delusional concern (APA, 2000).

■◖ DIAGNOSTIC CRITERIA

Delusional disorder is characterized by the presence of nonbizarre delusions and includes several subtypes: erotomanic, grandiose, jealous, somatic, mixed, and unspecified (Table 19-2). These subtypes represent the prominent theme of the delusion. A patient who has met criteria A for schizophrenia does not receive a diagnosis of delusional disorder (see Chapter 18 for criteria A). Although hallucinations may be present, they are not prominent (APA, 2000).

If mood episodes occur with this disorder, the total duration of the mood episode is relatively brief compared with the total duration of the delusional period. The delusion is not caused by the direct physiologic effects of substances (i.e., cocaine, amphetamines, marijuana) or a general medical condition (i.e., Alzheimer's disease, systemic lupus erythematosus). Because delusional disorder is uncommon and possesses features that are characteristic of other illnesses, the differential diagnosis has a clear-cut logic. It is a diagnosis of exclusion requiring careful evaluation. Distinguishing this disorder from schizophrenia and mood disorders with psychotic features is difficult (APA, 2000).

The prevalence of delusion disorder is about 3 per 10,000 general population. It is a rare disease even in psychiatric samples (Meloy, 1999). Research data are limited because numbers of recorded case studies and participants are small, and the studies lack systematic description, assessment, and diagnosis.

Table 19.2 Key Diagnostic Characteristics of Delusional Disorder 297.1 DSM IV	
Diagnostic Criteria and Target Symptoms	**Associated Findings**

• Nonbizarre delusions of at least 1 month's duration
• No presence of characteristic symptoms of schizophrenia
• Functioning not markedly impaired; behaviour not odd or bizarre
• If concurrent with delusions, mood disorders relatively brief in comparison with delusional periods
• Not a direct physiologic effect of substance or medical condition
  Erotomanic type: delusions that another person of usually higher status is in love with the person
  Grandiose type: delusions of inflated worth, power, knowledge, identity, or special relationship to a deity or famous person
  Jealous type: delusions that the individual's sexual partner is unfaithful
  Persecutory type: delusions that the person or someone close to the person is being malevolently treated in some way
  Somatic type: delusion that person has some physical defect or general medical condition
  Mixed type: delusions characteristic of more than one of the above types; no one theme predominates
  Unspecified type: delusion cannot be clearly identified or described
	• Social, marital, or work problems
	• Ideas of reference
	• Irritable mood
	• Marked anger and violent behaviour (especially with jealous type)

Delusional disorder may be associated with dysfunction in the frontal-subcortical systems and with temporal dysfunction, particularly on the left side (Fujii, Ahmed, & Takeshita, 1999).

■ SUBTYPES

Erotomanic Delusions

The concept of **erotomania** dates to the 17th century. Erotomania rarely appears in the pure or primary form. Secondary erotomania, which occurs with other psychiatric conditions, is more common. Differential diagnosis is important for excluding other significant psychiatric disorders or histologic conditions.

The erotomanic subtype is characterized by the delusional belief that the patient is loved intensely by the "loved object," who is usually married, of a higher socioeconomic status, or otherwise unattainable. The patient believes that the loved object's position in life would be in jeopardy if his or her true feelings were known. In addition, the patient is convinced that he or she is in amorous communication with the loved object. The loved object is often a public figure (e.g., movie star, politician) but may also be a common stranger. The patient believes that the loved object was the first to make advances and fall in love. The patient may entertain some delusional beliefs about a sexual relationship with the loved object, yet the beliefs are unfounded. The delusion, which often idealizes romantic love and spiritual union, rather than sexual attraction (APA, 2000), becomes the central focus of the patient's existence.

The patient may have minimal or no contact with the loved object and often keeps the delusion secret, but efforts to contact the loved object through letters, telephone calls, gifts, visits, surveillance, and stalking are also common. The patient may in many cases transfer his or her delusion to another loved object. There is some evidence that celebrity worship is associated with cognitive deficits (McCutcheon, Ashe, Houran, & Maltby, 2003).

Patients with erotomanic delusional disorder are generally unattractive; are often lower-level employees; lead withdrawn, lonely lives; are single with poor interpersonal relationships; and have limited sexual contacts or are sexually repressed. Clinical patients are mostly women, who do not usually act out their delusions. Forensic patients are mostly men, who tend to be more aggressive and can become violent in pursuit of the loved object, although the loved object may not be the object of the aggression. Men in particular come into contact with the law in their pursuit of the loved object or in a misguided effort to rescue the loved object from some imagined danger. Orders of protection are generally ineffective, and criminal charges of stalking or harassment that lead to incarceration are ineffective as a long-term solution to the problem (Harmon, Rosner, & Owens, 1995; Munro, 1999). The result is repeated arrests and psychiatric examinations, followed by ineffective treatment. Patients are rarely motivated to seek psychiatric treatment. This disorder is difficult to control, contain, or treat. The patient seldom gives up the belief that he or she is loved by the loved object. Separation from the loved object is the only satisfactory means of intervention (APA, 2000). Cognitive rigidity arising from frontal-subcortical dysfunction may contribute to maintaining erotic delusions and result in inability to alter a belief system (Fujii et al., 1999).

Grandiose Delusions

Patients presenting with grandiose delusions are convinced they have a great, unrecognized talent or have made an important discovery. A less common presentation is the delusion of a special relationship with a prominent person (i.e., an adviser to the Prime Minister) or of actually being a prominent person (i.e., the Prime Minister). In the latter case, the person with the delusion may regard the actual prominent person as an impostor. Other grandiose delusions may be religious in nature, such as a delusional belief that he or she has a special message from a deity (APA, 2000; Munro, 1999).

Jealous Delusions

The central theme of the jealous subtype is the unfaithfulness or infidelity of a spouse or lover. The belief arises without cause and is based on incorrect inferences justified by "evidence" (i.e., rumpled clothing, spots on sheets) the patient has collected. The patient usually confronts the spouse or lover with a host of such evidence. An associated feature is paranoia. The patient may attempt to intervene in the imagined infidelity by secretly following the spouse or lover or by investigating the imagined lover (APA, 2000; Munro, 1999).

Delusions of jealousy are difficult to treat and may diminish only with separation, divorce, or the death of the spouse or lover. Except in the elderly, such patients generally are male. Jealousy is a powerful, potentially dangerous emotion. Aggression, even violent behaviour, may result. Litigious behaviour is common, and symptoms with forensic aspects are often seen. Care is essential in determining how to work with these patients.

Somatic Delusions

Somatic delusions, a mix of psychotic and somatic symptoms, have been described for more than 100 years. The central theme of somatic delusions involves bodily functions or sensations. These patients believe they have physical ailments. Delusions of this nature are fixed, inarguable, and intense, with the patient totally convinced of the physical nature of the somatic complaint. The delusion occurs in the absence of other medical or psychiatric conditions. Medication can cause tactile hallucinations that result directly from the physiologic effects of the medication; when the medication or drug is removed, the symptoms disappear. Somatic delusions are manifested in the following beliefs (APA, 2000):

- A foul odor is coming from the skin, mouth (delusions of halitosis), rectum, or vagina
- Insects have infested the skin (delusional parasitosis)
- Internal parasites have infested the digestive system
- A certain body part is misshapen or ugly (contrary to visible evidence)
- Parts of the body are not functioning (e.g., large intestine, bowels).

The delusion of infestation by insects cannot occur without sensory perceptions, which constitute tactile hallucinations. The patient vividly describes crawling, itching, burning, swarming, and jumping on the skin surface or below the skin. The patient maintains the conviction that he or she is infested with parasites in the absence of objective evidence to the contrary.

Patients with somatic delusions present a dilemma for health care systems because of their excessive use of health care resources. They seek repeated medical consultations with dermatologists, entomologists, infectious disease specialists, and general practitioners. They seek treatment from primary care physicians and refuse psychiatric referral. Even if they seek psychiatric help, these patients typically do not adhere to long-term psychiatric treatment. Patients often go through elaborate rituals to cleanse themselves or their surroundings of the perceived pests, collecting hair, scabs, and skin flakes as evidence of an infection. They insist on being given unnecessary medical tests and procedures and are consequently at risk for increased morbidity because of invasive evaluation. Anger and hostility are common among this group, and behavioural characteristics include shame, depression, and avoidance.

The somatic subtype is rare but may be under diagnosed. Both genders are affected equally, but when onset occurs in late middle age, female patients tend to predominate. Studies of somatic delusions have been marred by methodological uncertainties, and factors limiting investigation include rarity of the disease, lack of contact with psychiatrists, and noncompliance with the medication regimen. A variant of the somatic subtype is body dysmorphic disorder, which is classified under somatoform disorders in the *Diagnostic and Statistical Manual of Mental Disorders*, 4th ed., Text revision (*DSM-IV-TR*) (see Chapter 22).

Unspecified Delusions

In the mixed subtype, no one delusional theme predominates, and the patient presents with two or more types of delusions. In the unspecified subtype, the delusional beliefs cannot be clearly determined, or the predominant delusion is not described as a specific type. Patients are usually women who experience feelings of depersonalization and derealization and have negative-associated paranoid features. The delusions can be short-lived, recurrent, or persistent. This subtype also includes delusions of **misidentification** (i.e., illusions of doubles), wherein a familiar person is replaced by an impostor. For example, the patient may believe that close family members have assumed the persona of strangers or that people they know can change into other people at will. This type of delusion occurs rarely and is generally associated with schizophrenia, Alzheimer's disease, or other organic conditions (APA, 2000).

Persecutory delusions, the most common type seen, are not listed as a separate subtype in the *DSM-IV-TR*, but they are addressed as a subtype of delusional disorder in the text (APA, 2000). The central theme of persecutory delusions is the patient's belief that he or she is being conspired against, cheated, spied on, followed, poisoned, drugged, maliciously maligned, harassed, or obstructed in pursuit of long-term goals. The patient exaggerates small slights, which become the focus of the delusion.

The focus of persecutory delusions is often on some injustice that must be remedied by legal action (querulous paranoia). Patients often seek satisfaction by repeatedly appealing to courts and other government agencies (Harmon et al., 1995; Munro, 1999). These patients are often angry and resentful and may even behave violently toward the people the patient believes are persecuting him or her. The course may be chronic, although the patient's preoccupation with the delusional belief often waxes and wanes. The clarity, logic, and systematic elaboration of this delusional theme leave a remarkable stamp on this condition (APA, 2000).

■ EPIDEMIOLOGY AND RISK FACTORS

Delusional disorder is relatively uncommon in clinical settings (APA, 2000). The best estimate of its prevalence in the population is about 0.03%, but precise information is lacking (APA). Lifetime morbidity is between 0.05% and 0.1% because of the late age of onset.

Few risk factors are associated with delusional disorder. Patients can live with their delusions without psychiatric intervention because their behaviour is normal; although if delusions are somatic, patients risk unnecessary medical interventions. Acting on delusions carries a risk for intervention by law enforcement agencies or the legal system. Suicide attempts are neither more nor less common than in the general population (Grunebaum et al., 2001).

Age of Onset

Delusional disorder can begin in adolescence and occurs in middle to later adulthood. Onset occurs at a later age than among patients with schizophrenia. A prevalence of 2% to 4% has been reported in the elderly (APA, 2000).

Gender

Gender does not appear to affect the overall frequency of most delusional disorders (APA, 2000). Patients with erotomanic delusions are generally women; in forensic settings, most people with this disorder are men. Men also tend to experience more jealous delusions, except in the elderly population, in which women outnumber men.

Ethnicity and Culture

A person's ethnic, cultural, and religious background must be considered in evaluating the presence of delusional disorder. The content of delusions varies between cultures and subcultures (APA, 2000).

Family

An increased familial risk and familial genetic factors are unknown.

■■ COMORBIDITY

Mood disorders are frequently found in patients with delusional disorders, who typically have mild symptoms of depression such as irritable or dysphoric mood. Delusional disorder may also be associated with obsessive-compulsive disorder and paranoid, schizoid, or avoidant personality disorder (APA, 2000).

■■ ETIOLOGY

The cause of delusional disorder is unknown. The only major feature of this condition is the formation and persistence of the delusions. Few have investigated possible neurophysiologic and neuropsychological causes of delusional disorder, and theories of causation are contradictory. Delusion beliefs have been considered as dysfunctional extremes of cognitive and emotional mechanisms that have adaptive significance, although biased and lacking in flexibility. This argument places delusions on a continuum with "normalcy" and perhaps a function of high vigilance toward threat and a search for safety (Abdel-Hamid & Brüne, 2008). No social theories of causation are addressed in the literature.

Possible medical reasons for delusions, especially in cases of sudden onset, need to be carefully ruled out. Disorders of the basal ganglia, toxic-metabolic conditions, dementias, and substance-related disorders can produce delusions in some patients (Sadock & Sadock, 2007).

Biologic Theories

Neuropathologic

In patients with delusional disorder, MRI shows a degree of temporal lobe asymmetry. However, these differences are subtle, so delusional disorder may involve a neurodegenerative component (Ota et al., 2003). The tactile hallucinations of somatic delusions may arise from sensory alterations in the nervous system (Baker, Cook, & Winokur, 1995) or from sensory input that has been misinterpreted because of subtle cortical changes associated with aging.

Genetic and Biochemical

Delusional disorder is probably biologically distinct from other psychotic disorders, yet little or no attention has been paid to genetic factors. Delusions may involve faulty processing of essentially intact perceptions, whereby perceptions become linked with an interpretation that has deep emotional significance but no verifiable basis (Conway et al., 2002; McGuire et al., 2001). Alternately, a complex, malfunctioning dopaminergic system may lead to delusions (Morimoto et al., 2002). This explanation could lead to the argument that a particular delusion depends on the "circuit" that is malfunctioning. Denial of reality has been linked to right posterior cortical dysfunction. Some authors have proposed a combination of biologic and early life experiences as etiologic components (Bentall, Corcoran, Howard, Blackwood, & Kinderman, 2001).

■■ INTERDISCIPLINARY TREATMENT

Few, if any, interdisciplinary treatments are associated with delusional disorder because patients rarely receive attention from health care providers. Pharmacologic intervention is often based on symptoms. For example, patients with somatic delusions are treated for the specific complaints with which they present. Use of benzodiazepines may be common with this disorder because complaints are vague.

PRIORITY CARE ISSUES

By the time a patient with a diagnosis of delusional disorder is seen in a psychiatric setting, he or she has generally had the delusion for a long time. It is deeply ingrained and many times unshakable, even with psychopharmacologic intervention. These patients rarely comply with medication regimens.

Male patients who have the erotomanic subtype are likely to require special care because they are more likely than other patients to act on their delusions (e.g., by continued attempts to contact the loved object, or stalking). This group is generally seen in forensic settings.

NURSING MANAGEMENT: HUMAN RESPONSE TO DELUSIONAL DISORDER

Biologic Domain

Assessment

Body systems are assessed to evaluate any physical problems. In people with somatic delusional disorder, assessment may be difficult because of the number and variety of presenting symptoms. Complaints are explored to develop a complete symptom history and to determine whether symptoms have a physical basis or are delusional. Past history of each symptom should be determined because this information may affect outcome. The more recent the onset, the more favourable the prognosis.

> **CRNENOTE**
>
> By definition, delusions are fixed, false beliefs that cannot be changed by reasonable arguments. The nurse should assess the patient's delusion to evaluate its significance to the patient and the patient's safety and the safety of others. The nurse should not dwell on the delusion or try to change it.

Most patients who receive diagnoses of delusional disorder do not experience functional difficulties or impairments. Self-care patterns may be disrupted in patients with the somatic subtype by the elaborate processes used to treat perceived illness (e.g., bathing rituals, creams). Sleep may be disrupted because of the central and overpowering nature of the delusions.

A complete medication history, past and present, is also important to determine the patient's past response and what agents the individual perceives as effective. Examining the patient's records for tests and procedures may help to substantiate the individual's symptoms.

Nursing Diagnoses for the Biologic Domain

The nursing diagnoses for the biologic domain depend on the type of delusions that are manifested and the response to these symptoms. For example, for a woman with the somatic delusion that insects are crawling on her, disturbed sensory perception (Tactile) would be appropriate. For others who are fearful of poisoning, imbalanced nutrition, less than body requirements, may be a useful diagnosis. Refusal of all medication may support a nursing diagnosis of ineffective therapeutic regimen management.

Interventions for Biologic Domain

Interventions are based on the problems identified during assessment (Fig. 19-3). Each is addressed individually. The nurse helps the patient to establish routines that can resolve problems and promote healthy functioning. A mechanism for managing the patient's medication regimen is developed.

Somatic Interventions

Delusional disorder has a reputation of being chronic and resistant to treatment. Treating somatic disorder is difficult because of the patient's insistence that the problem is not psychiatrically related. Many patients with delusional disorder are seen only by nonpsychiatric specialists, who use expensive and ineffective treatments. Patients with this disorder may adhere poorly to psychiatric pharmacotherapy, which may be directly related to the lack of insight about their illness (Nose, Barbui, & Tansella, 2003). Realistic and modest goals are most sensible. Establishing a therapeutic relationship is a goal for which to strive.

Pharmacologic Interventions

The literature available about using psychiatric medications in delusional disorder is sparse, and the available reports conflict. Antipsychotic agents are useful in improving acute symptoms by decreasing agitation and the intensity of the delusion. They may also be effective in the long term, but little formal information exists to support this theory.

Administering and Monitoring Medications

Patients often do not adhere to medication regimens and require monitoring of target symptoms. Look for an opportunity to discuss medications and to identify issues the patient may have with them.

Managing Side Effects

Management of side effects is similar to that in other disorders that have a delusional component. The nurse assesses for NMS, extrapyramidal side effects, weight gain, and sedation.

FIGURE 19.3 Bio/psycho/social/spiritual interventions for patients with delusional disorder.

Monitoring for Drug Interactions

Interactions are similar to those seen with medications for other disorders. A detailed list of prior and current medications must be elicited from patients, especially those with somatic delusions, because they may be receiving medications from many different practitioners.

Teaching Points

Patients may need help and information in order to take the medication as prescribed. Determine whether the patient has sufficient resources to purchase and obtain medications, and explain target symptoms for each medication. Caution patients not to take over-the-counter medications without consulting their provider.

Psychological Domain

Assessment

Patients with delusional disorder show few, if any, psychological deficits, and those that do occur are generally related directly to the delusion. Use of the Minnesota Multiphasic Personality Inventory (MMPI), a clinical scale that identifies paranoid symptom deviation, may be useful in substantiating the diagnosis.

Mental status is not generally affected. Thinking, orientation, affect, attention, memory, perception, and personality are generally intact. Presenting reality-based evidence in an attempt to change the person's delusion can be helpful in determining whether the belief can be altered with sufficient evidence. If mental status is altered, this fact is generally brought to the health professional's attention by a third party, such as police, family member, neighbour, physician, or attorney. In these cases, the person has usually acted in some manner to draw attention to himself or herself. Talk with the person to grasp the nature of the delusional thinking: theme, impact on the person's life, complexity, systematization, and related features.

Nursing Diagnosis for Psychological Domain

Numerous nursing diagnoses could be generated based on the assessment of the psychological domain. Ineffective denial, impaired verbal communication, deficient knowledge, and risk for loneliness are some examples. Nursing diagnoses of disturbed self-concept, disturbed self-esteem, anxiety, fear, and powerlessness may also be generated.

BOX 19.5

*Psychoeducation Checklist: **Delusional Disorder***

When caring for the patient with delusional disorder, be sure to include the caregiver, as appropriate, and address the following topic areas in the teaching plan:

- Psychopharmacologic agents (antipsychotic or antidepressants), if used, including drug action, dosage, frequency, and possible adverse effects
- Identification of troubling experiences
- Consequences of delusions
- Realistic goal setting
- Positive coping strategies
- Safety measures
- Social training skills
- Family participation in therapy

Interventions for Psychological Domain

Patients with delusional disorder are treated most effectively in outpatient settings with supportive therapy that allays the person's anxiety. Initiating discussion of the troubling experiences and consequences of the delusion and suggesting a means for coping may be successful. Assisting the person toward a more satisfying general adjustment is desirable (see Box 19-5).

Insight-oriented therapy is not useful because there is no benefit in trying to prove the delusion is not true, arguing the person out of the delusion, or telling the individual that the delusion is imaginary. Cognitive therapy with supportive therapy that focuses on reasoning or reality testing to decrease delusional thinking, or modifying the delusion itself, may be helpful (see Chapter 15). Educational interventions can aid the patient in understanding how factors such as sensory impairment, social and physical isolation, and stress contribute to the intensity of this disorder.

In certain instances, hospitalization is needed in response to dangerous behaviour that could include aggressiveness, poor impulse control, excessive psychological tension, unremitting anger, and threats. Suicide can be a concern, but most patients are not at risk. If hospitalization is required, the person needs to be approached tactfully. Legal assistance may be necessary (Reid, 2005).

Social Domain

Assessment

A common characteristic of individuals with delusional disorder is normal behaviour and appearance unless their delusional ideas are being discussed or acted on. The cultural background of the person with delusional disorder has to be evaluated. Ethnic and cultural systems have different beliefs that are accepted within their individual context but not outside their group. Problems can occur in social, occupational, or interpersonal areas. In general, the person's social functioning and marital functioning are more likely to be impaired than his or her intellectual or occupational functioning. Most are employed, although generally they hold low-paying jobs. Supportive family members and friends can mean a more positive outcome for the person living with a delusional disorder.

Life difficulties are often related to the delusion. Thus, assessing the person's capacity to act in response to the delusion is important. What is the person's level of impulsiveness (i.e., related to behaviours of suicide, homicide, aggression, or violence)? Establishing as complete a picture of the person as possible, including the person's subjective private experiences and concrete psychopathologic symptoms, helps to reduce uncertainty in the assessment process.

Nursing Diagnoses for the Social Domain

Several nursing diagnoses can be generated from the assessment data for the social domain. Ineffective coping, interrupted family processes, and ineffective role performance are examples.

Interventions for Social Domain

People with diagnoses of delusional disorder often become socially isolated. The secretiveness of their delusions and the importance the delusions have in their lives are central to this phenomenon. Social skills training tailored to the patient's specific deficits can help to improve social adaptation. Family therapy can help the person reintegrate into the family; family education and patient education will enhance understanding of the patient and the disease process. However, group therapy is usually not beneficial because the patient lacks insight into the origin of the delusion. Families face many of the same issues as families of patients with other disorders involving delusions and are at risk for ineffective coping.

Spiritual Domain

Nurses may hesitate to address the spiritual domain of a person who is experiencing delusional thinking, especially if there are religious overtones to fixed beliefs. This hesitancy may lie in an awareness that another's religious beliefs may seem so different to one's own that they may seem "fixed" and "false." Trying to understand the way a person's religious or spiritual beliefs are being shaped by his or her delusional disorder may seem a daunting task. If the nurse's response, however, is to be as sensitive and receptive as possible to the person's values (as revealed in his or her general behaviour and expression of pleasure and fears as well as by preillness choices and goals), then spiritual care may begin. Attending to the person's ultimate need to find meaning in life is what is required. This is grounded in thoughtful caring and attention to "the little things" that matter to the person, as well as through a hopeful, encouraging attitude that may foster hope in the patient (Carr, 2008).

EVALUATION AND TREATMENT OUTCOMES

For patients with delusional disorders, the greater the lack of insight and the poorer the adherence to treatment regimens, the more difficult it is to teach the individual. The patient rarely, if ever, develops full insight, and the symptoms related to the original diagnosis are not likely to disappear completely. In evaluating progress, the nurse must remember that outcomes are often not met completely. The nurse should maintain realistic outcomes and praise small successes to promote positive outcomes (Fig. 19-4).

CONTINUUM OF CARE

Inpatient Focus Care

Hospitalization rarely occurs and is usually initiated by the legal or social violations. Insight-oriented interventions help the patient to understand his or her situation. Avoid confrontational situations; use the patient's coping abilities to reinforce constructive aspects of functioning to enable a return to autonomy.

Emergency Care!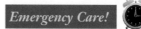

Emergency care is seldom required, unless the patient has had an incident with the law or legal system. The patient may be agitated or aggressive because the delusion, which is perceived as real, has been interrupted.

Family Intervention

Family therapy may be helpful. By helping the family to develop mechanisms to cope with the patient's delusions, nurses help the family to be more supportive and understanding of the patient.

FIGURE 19.4 Bio/psycho/social/spiritual outcomes for patients with delusional disorder.

Community Treatment

Patients with diagnosis of delusional disorder are treated most effectively in an outpatient setting. They should be encouraged to seek psychiatric treatment. Insight-oriented therapy to develop an understanding of the patient's delusion may be helpful. Medications are not often used with delusional disorder, but antipsychotic agents or benzodiazepines are helpful during exacerbations. Other treatments include supportive therapy, development of coping skills, cognitive therapy, and social skills training. Family therapy may be helpful.

Other Psychotic Disorders

Other disorders have psychoses as their defining features. The nursing care for patients with these disorders is not discussed specifically, but care used with other disorders can be applied to the disorders presented here (Table 19-3).

▄▄◗ SCHIZOPHRENIFORM DISORDER

The essential features of schizophreniform disorder are identical to those of criteria A for schizophrenia, with the exception of the duration of the illness, which can be less than 6 months (APA, 2000). However, symptoms must be present for at least 1 month to be classified as a schizophreniform disorder (Table 19-4). This diagnosis is also used as provisional if symptoms have lasted more than 1 month, but it is uncertain whether the person will recover before the end of the 6-month period. Some research has suggested that this illness may be an early manifestation of schizophrenia (Iancu, Dannon, Ziv, & Lepkifker, 2002).

Altered social or occupational functioning may occur but is not necessary. Most patients experience interruption in one or more areas of daily functioning (APA, 2000).

▄▄◗ BRIEF PSYCHOTIC DISORDER

In brief psychotic disorder, the length of the episode is at least 1 day but less than 1 month. The onset is sudden and includes at least one of the positive symptoms of criteria A for schizophrenia found in Chapter 18 (see also Table 19-4). Differentiating this illness from bipolar SCA is important (Marneros, Pillmann, Haring, Balzuweit, & Bloink, 2002).

The person generally experiences emotional turmoil or overwhelming confusion and rapid, intense shifts of affect (APA, 2000). Although episodes are brief, impairment can be severe, and supervision may be required to protect the person. Suicide is a risk, especially in younger patients. A predisposition to develop a brief psychotic disorder may include preexisting personality disorders (APA). The person's ethnic and cultural background should also be considered in relation to the social or religious context of the symptoms presented. This disorder is uncommon but usually appears in early adulthood (APA).

Table 19.3 Other Psychotic Disorders		DSM IV
Disorder	**Definition**
Schizophreniform disorder	This disorder is identical to schizophrenia except the total duration of the illness can be less than 6 months (must be at least 1 month) and there may not be impaired social or occupational functioning.
Schizoaffective disorder	This disorder is characterized by an uninterrupted period of illness during which at some time there is a major depressive, manic, or mixed episode along with two of the following symptoms of schizophrenia: delusions, hallucinations, disorganized speech, disorganized or catatonic behaviour, or negative symptoms (affective flattening, alogia, or avolition).
Delusional disorder	This disorder is characterized by the presence of nonbizarre delusion and includes several subtypes: erotomanic, grandiose, jealous, somatic, mixed, and unspecified.
Brief psychotic disorder	In this disorder, there is a sudden onset of at least one positive psychotic symptom that lasts at least 1 day but less than 1 month. Eventually, the individual has a full return to normal.
Shared psychotic disorders (*folie à deux*)	In this disorder, one person who is in a close relationship with another person who already has a psychotic disorder with prominent delusions also develops the delusion.
Other psychotic disorders due to substances such as drugs and alcohol	The prominent hallucinations or delusions are judged to be due to the physiologic effects of substances (drugs, alcohol).

Adapted from American Psychiatric Association. (2000). *Diagnostic and statistical manual of mental disorders* (4th ed., Text revision). Washington, DC: Author.

Table 19.4	Key Diagnostic Characteristics for Other Psychotic Disorders	DSM IV

Disorder	Diagnostic Characteristics and Target Symptoms
Schizophreniform disorder	Symptoms of schizophrenia present Delusions, hallucinations, disorganized speech, grossly disorganized or catatonic behaviour, and negative symptoms Not due to schizoaffective or mood disorders Not due to effects of substance or general medical condition Episode lasting at least 1 month but less than 6 months
Brief psychotic disorder	Presence of delusions, hallucinations, disorganized speech, and grossly disorganized or catatonic behaviour (at least one) Duration of at least 1 day but less than 1 month; returns to preillness level of functioning Not the direct physiologic effect of a substance or general medical condition; not better accounted for by other mental disorders
Shared psychotic disorder (folie à deux)	Delusion developing in a person who is in a close relationship with another person who already has an established delusion Delusion similar in content to that of the other person Not the direct physiologic effect of a substance or general medical condition; not better accounted for by other mental disorders
Psychotic disorder due to a general medical condition	Prominent hallucinations or delusions Evidence from history, physical examination, or laboratory studies that disturbance is a result of the physiologic consequences of a general medical disorder Not occurring exclusively during delirium
Substance-induced psychotic disorders	Prominent hallucinations or delusions Symptoms developed during or within 1 month of substance intoxication or withdrawal or medication use related to the disturbance Not better accounted for by other mental disorders Not occurring exclusively during delirium

SHARED PSYCHOTIC DISORDER

In shared psychotic disorder (*folie à deux*), a person develops a close relationship with another individual ("inducer" or "primary case") who has a psychotic disorder with prominent delusions (APA, 2000; Trabert, 1999) (see Table 19-4). With this disorder, the person believes and shares part or all of the inducer's delusional beliefs. The content of the delusions depends on the inducer, who is the dominant person in the relationship and imposes the delusions on the passive person (APA). This disorder is somewhat more common in women, and the age of onset is variable. Delusional beliefs are usually shared by people who have lived together for a long time in relative social isolation. However, family members rarely share the same delusional belief. When the relationship is interrupted, the passive person's delusional beliefs decrease or disappear (APA).

Treatment is sought infrequently (Trabert, 1999). When care is sought, the inducer usually brings the situation to clinical treatment (APA, 2000). When the passive person is removed from the setting, 93% have a favourable course even with no treatment (Trabert). If the inducer receives no intervention, the course is usually chronic.

PSYCHOTIC DISORDERS ATTRIBUTABLE TO SUBSTANCE

Patients with a psychotic disorder attributable to a substance present with prominent hallucinations or delusions that are the direct physiologic effects of a substance (e.g., drug abuse, toxin exposure; APA, 2000) (see Table 19-4). During intoxication, symptoms continue as long as the use of the substance continues. Withdrawal symptoms can occur for as long as 4 weeks. Differential diagnosis is recommended.

SUMMARY OF KEY POINTS

☐ Schizoaffective disorder has symptoms typical of both schizophrenia and mood disorders but is a separate disorder. Although these patients experience mood problems most of the time, the diagnosis of schizoaffective disorder depends on the presence of positive symptoms (i.e., delusions or hallucinations) without mood symptoms at some time during the uninterrupted period of illness.

☐ Although controversy and discussion continue about whether schizoaffective disorder is truly a separate disorder, the *DSM-IV-TR* identifies it as separate.

□ Patients with schizoaffective disorder have fewer awareness deficits and appear to have more insight than do patients with true schizophrenia, a fact that can be used in teaching patients to control symptoms, recognize early regression, and develop psychosocial skills.

□ Patients with schizoaffective disorder will likely never be medication free. Intermittent antipsychotic dosing is best for patients who can detect recurring symptoms and institute their own drug therapy.

□ Nursing care for patients with schizoaffective disorder is focused on minimizing psychiatric symptoms through promoting medication maintenance and on helping patients maintain optimal levels of functioning. Interventions centre on developing social and coping skills through supportive, nurturing, and nonconfrontational approaches. The nurse must be constantly attuned to the mood state of the patient and help the patient learn to solve problems, resolve conflict, and cope with social situations that trigger anxiety.

□ Delusional disorder is characterized by stable, well-systematized, and logical nonbizarre delusions that could occur in real life and are plausible in the context of the patient's ethnic and cultural background. These delusions may or may not interfere with an individual's ability to function socially. Patients typically deny any psychiatric basis for their problem and refuse to seek psychiatric care. Patients whose delusions relate to somatic complaints are often seen on medical-surgical units of hospitals. Diagnosis otherwise is often made only when patients act on the basis of their delusions and violate the law or social rules.

□ Delusional disorder is further classified as a particular subtype, depending on the nature and content of the patient's delusions, including erotomanic, grandiose, jealous, somatic, mixed, and unspecified.

□ Patients with delusional disorder usually do not experience functional difficulties or mental status impairments. Their thinking, orientation, affect, attention, memory, perception, and personality generally remain intact.

□ The therapeutic relationship is crucial to the successful treatment of the patient with delusional disorder. Nurses must be aware of the patient's fragile self-esteem and unusual sensitivities and anxieties and try to establish a trusting relationship through a flexible, nonjudgmental approach that promotes empathy, trust, and support.

CRITICAL THINKING CHALLENGES

1   Mr. J first received a diagnosis of schizophrenia but, after experiencing extreme mood disturbances, finally received a diagnosis of schizoaffective disorders. During a recent outpatient visit, he confides to a nurse that he just has stress and does not think that he really has any psychiatric problems. Identify assessment areas that should be pursued before the patient leaves his appointment. How would you confront the denial?

2   Ms. S believed that she had bipolar disorder. At a recent clinic visit, she was told that she most probably had schizoaffective disorder. The patient asked the nurse how a bipolar disorder could turn into schizoaffective disorder. Identify three appropriate responses to her question.

3   A patient with schizoaffective disorder is prescribed an antipsychotic agent (Risperdal) and a mood stabilizer (Depakene). The patient asks you why both medications are needed. Develop the best response for this question. Be thorough.

4   At an interdisciplinary treatment team meeting, the nurse recommends that a woman with schizoaffective disorder attends an anger management group. The rest of the team believes that only a mood stabilizer is needed. Develop the rationale for attendance at the anger management group in addition to medication supplementation.

5   A patient was prescribed olanzapine (Zyprexa) and an antidepressant citalopram (Celexa) for the treatment of schizoaffective disorder. Since her last monthly visit, she gained 15 pounds. She is considering discontinuing her medication regimen because of the weight gain. Develop a plan that addresses her weight gain and her intention to discontinue her medication regimen.

6   A has received a diagnosis of schizoaffective disorder, and B has received a diagnosis of delusional disorder. How would the symptoms differ? Would there be any similarities? If so, what would they be?

7   Identify and explain each of the subtypes of delusional disorder.

8   An elderly person in a nursing home has a delusion that her husband is having an affair with her sister. Discuss nonpharmacologic nursing interventions that should be implemented with this patient. How would you explain her delusion to her husband? Choose one of the subtypes of delusion and develop a plan for clinical management, focusing on psychiatric nursing care, for a patient experiencing this condition.

9   A patient convincingly informs you that she is having an affair with a famous actor. They both attended the same college at about the same time. How would you determine whether this patient's belief is a delusion or reality? Is it important that the nurse understands whether the relationship is real? Explain the rationale for your answer.

10   A patient informs a student nurse that he is a member of the Secret Service and that he is undercover.

He asks the nurse to keep the secret. The student considers several possible responses, including redirecting the patient to a different topic and confronting him with the reality of his hospitalization. Discuss the best response to this patient's comment.

WEB LINKS

www.cmha.ca   Website for the Canadian Mental Health Association, which is a nationwide, charitable organization that promotes the resilience and recovery of people experiencing mental illness.

www.schizophrenia.ca   Website for the Schizophrenia Society of Canada, which provides support and education for individuals living with schizophrenia and their families.

www.mooddisorderscanada.ca   Website for the Mood Disorders Society of Canada, which is a volunteer organization designed to improve the lives of people living with mood disorders.

www.surgeongeneral.gov   Website for Healthy People 2010 and Report of the USA's Surgeon General.

www.nami.org   National Alliance for the Mentally Ill website with advocacy information.

www.mentalhealth.com   Internet mental health website that provides the American and European description of schizoaffective disorder and its treatment.

www.geocities.com/CollegePark/Classroom/6237   Learn from a registered psychiatric nurse about schizoaffective and other disorders and about what psychiatric nurses do.

www.mhinfosource.com   Answers to questions about schizoaffective and other psychiatric disorders.

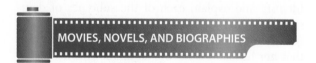

MOVIES, NOVELS, AND BIOGRAPHIES

Misery: 1990. This movie stars James Caan as Paul Sheldon and Kathy Bates as Annie Wilkes. Sheldon is the writer of a popular mystery series who finishes his last novel in a secluded cabin in Colorado. After being rescued in a blizzard by Annie Wilkes, he becomes her prisoner when she prevents him from leaving his cabin. Annie is in love with him but is demanding and possessive. She identifies with the heroine in his latest novel and is outraged at the conclusion of the novel.

SIGNIFICANCE: Annie demonstrates the thinking patterns associated with delusional disorder.

VIEWING POINTS: Identify the disturbed thinking that Annie demonstrates. Part of Annie's behaviour seems normal, and other behaviours are illogical. How are they linked?

REFERENCES

Abdel-Hamid, M., & Brüne, M. (2008). Neuropsychological aspects of delusional disorder. *Current Psychiatry Reports, 10,* 229–234.

American Psychiatric Association. (1980). *Diagnostic and statistical manual of mental disorders* (3rd ed.). Washington, DC: Author.

American Psychiatric Association. (2000). *Diagnostic and statistical manual of mental disorders* (4th ed., Text revision). Washington, DC: Author.

Andres, K., Pfammatter, M., Garst, F., Teschner, C., & Brenner, H. D. (2000). Effects of a coping-oriented group therapy for schizophrenia and schizoaffective patients: A pilot study. *Acta Psychiatrica Scandinavica, 101*(4), 318–322.

Baker, P. B., Cook, B. L., & Winokur, G. (1995). Delusional infestation: The interference of delusions and hallucinations. *Psychiatric Clinics of North America, 18*(2), 345–361.

Bech, P. (2001). The significance of delusions in depressive disorders. *Current Opinions in Psychiatry, 14*(1), 47–49.

Bentall, R. P., Corcoran, R., Howard, R., Blackwood, N., & Kinderman, P. (2001). Persecutory delusions: A review and theoretical integration. *Clinical Psychology Review, 21*(8), 1143–1192.

Carr, T. (2008). Mapping the processes and qualities of spiritual nursing care. *Qualitative Health Research, 18*(5), 686–700.

Cheniaux, E., Landeira-Fernandez, J., Telles, L., Lessa, J., Dias, A., Duncan, T., et al. (2008). Does schizoaffective disorder really exist? A systematic review of the studies that compared schizoaffective disorder with schizophrenia or mood disorders. *Journal of Affective Disorders, 106,* 209–217.

Chernomas, W., Clarke, D., & Chisholm, F. (2000). Perspectives of women living with schizophrenia. *Psychiatric Services, 51,* 1517–1521.

Conway, C. R., Bollini, A. M., Graham, B. G., Keefe, R. S., Schiffman, S. S., & McEvoy, J. P. (2002). Sensory acuity and reasoning in delusional disorder. *Comprehensive Psychiatry, 43*(3), 175–178.

Copeland, M. E. (2005). Mary Ellen Copeland: Mental health recovery and WRAP. Retrieved January 29, 2005, from http://www.mentalhelathrecovery.com/shop/index.php

Crow, T. J., & Harrington, C. A. (1994). Etiopathogenesis and treatment of psychosis. *Annual Review of Medicine, 45,* 219–234.

DeLisi, L. E., Shaw, S. H., Crow, T. J., Shields, G., Smith, A. B., Larach, V. W., et al. (2002). A genome-wide scan for linkage to chromosomal regions in 382 sibling pairs with schizophrenia or schizoaffective disorder. *American Journal of Psychiatry, 159*(5), 803–812.

Dietrich, D. E., Kropp, S., & Emrich, H. M. (2001). Oxcarbazepine in affective and schizoaffective disorders. *Pharmacopsychiatry, 34*(6), 242–250.

Evans, J. D., Heaton, R. K., Paulsen, J. S., McAdams, L. A., Heaton, S. C., & Jeste, D. V. (1999). Schizoaffective disorder: A form of schizophrenia or affective disorder? *Journal of Clinical Psychiatry, 60*(12), 874–882.

Fabisch, K., Fabisch, H., Langs, G., Macheiner, H., Fitz, W., & Honigl, D. (2001). Basic symptoms and their contribution to the differential typology of acute schizophrenic and schizoaffective disorders. *Psychopathology, 34*(1), 15–22.

Fujii, D. E., Ahmed, I., & Takeshita, J. (1999). Neuropsychologic implications in erotomania: Two case studies. *Neuropsychiatry, Neuropsychology and Behavioral Management, 12*(2), 110–116.

Getz, G. E., DelBello, M. P., Fleck, D. E., Zimmerman, M. E., Schwiers, M. L., & Strakowski, S. M. (2002). Neuroanatomic characterization of schizoaffective disorder using MRI: A pilot study. *Schizophrenia Research, 55*(1–2), 55–59.

Gooding, D. C., & Tallent, K. A. (2002). Spatial working memory performance in patients with schizoaffective psychosis versus schizophrenia: A tale of two disorders? *Schizophrenia Research, 15*(3), 209–218.

Grunebaum, M. F., Oquendo, M. A., Harkavy-Friedman, J. M., Ellis, S. P., Li, S., Haas, G. L., et al. (2001). Delusions and suicidality. *American Journal of Psychiatry, 158*(5), 742–747.

Harmon, R. B., Rosner, R., & Owens, H. (1995). Obsessional harassment and erotomania in a criminal court population. *Journal of Forensic Science, 41*(2), 188–196.

Heinrichs, R. W., Ammari, N., Vaz, S., & Miles, A. (2008). Are schizophrenia and schizoaffective disorder neuropsychologically distinguishable? *Schizophrenia Research, 99,* 149–154.

Huxley, N. A., Rendall, M., & Sederer, L. (2000). Psychosocial treatments in schizophrenia: A review of the past 20 years. *Journal of Nervous and Mental Disease, 188*(4), 187–201.

Iancu, I., Dannon, P. N., Ziv, R., & Lepkifker, E. (2002). A follow-up study of patients with *DSM-IV* schizophreniform disorder. *Canadian Journal of Psychiatry, 47*(1), 56–60.

Kasanin, J. (1933). The acute schizo-affective psychoses. *American Journal of Psychiatry, 13*, 97–126.

Lewine, R. R., Hudgins, P., Brown, F., Caudle, J., & Risch, S. C. (1995). Differences in qualitative brain morphology findings in schizophrenia, major depression, bipolar disorder, and normal volunteers. *Schizophrenia Research, 15*(3), 253–259.

Maj, M., Pirozzi, R., Formicola, A. M., Bartoli, L., & Bucci, P. (2000). Reliability and validity of the *DSM-IV* diagnostic category of schizoaffective disorder: Preliminary data. *Journal of Affective Disorders, 57*(1–3), 95–98.

Marchinko, S. (2008). The Wellness Planner: Testing an intervention designed to increase empowerment and improve quality of life in individuals with mental illness. Unpublished Master's thesis. University of Manitoba, Winnipeg, Manitoba.

Marneros, A. (2003). The schizoaffective phenomenon: The state of the art. *Acta Psychiatrica Scandinavica Supplementum, 418*, 29–33.

Marneros, A., Pillmann, F., Haring, A., Balzuweit, S., & Bloink, R. (2002). The relation of 'acute and transient psychotic disorder' (ICD-10 F23) to bipolar schizoaffective disorder. *Journal of Psychiatric Research, 36*(3), 165–171.

McCann, T. V., & Baker, H. (2003). Models of mental health nurse–general practitioner liaison: Promoting continuity of care. *Journal of Advanced Nursing, 41*(5), 471–479.

McGuire, L., Junginger, J., Adams, S. G. Jr., Burright, R., & Donovick, P. (2001). Delusions and delusional reasoning. *Journal of Abnormal Psychology, 110*(2), 259–266.

McCutcheon, L. E., Ashe, D. D., Houran, J., & Maltby, J. (2003). A cognitive profile of individuals who tend to worship celebrities. *Journal of Psychology, 137*(4), 309–322.

McIntyre, R. S., McCann, S. M., & Kennedy, S. H. (2001). Antipsychotic metabolic effects: Weight gain, diabetes, and lipid abnormalities. *Canadian Journal of Psychiatry, 46*, 273–281.

Meloy, J. R. (1999). Erotomania, triangulation and homicide. *Journal of Forensic Science, 44*(2), 421–424.

Moller, H. J., Bottlender, R., Gross, A., Hoff, P., Wittmann, J., Wegner, U., et al. (2002). The Kraepelinian dichotomy: Preliminary results of a 15-year follow-up study on functional psychoses: Focus on negative symptoms. *Schizophrenia Research, 56*(1–2), 878–894.

Morimoto, K., Miyatake, R., Nakamura, M., Watanabe, T., Hirao, T., & Suwaki, H. (2002). Delusional disorder: Molecular genetic evidence for dopamine psychosis. *Neuropsychopharmacology, 26*(6), 794–801.

Munro, A. (1999). *Delusional disorder.* Cambridge, MA: Cambridge University Press.

Norman, R., Scholten, D., Malla, A., & Ballageer, T. (2005). Early signs in schizophrenia spectrum disorders. *Journal of Nervous and Mental Disease, 193*, 17–23.

Nose, M., Barbui, C., & Tansella, M. (2003). How often do patients with psychosis fail to adhere to treatment programmes? A systematic review. *Psychological Medicine, 33*(7), 1149–1160.

Ota, M., Mizukami, K., Katano, T., Sato, S., Takeda, T., & Asada, T. (2003). A case of delusional disorder, somatic type with remarkable improvement of clinical symptoms and single photon emission computed tomography findings following modified electroconvulsive therapy. *Progress in Neuro-psychopharmacology & Biological Psychiatry, 27*(5), 881–884.

Papageorigiou, A., King, M., Jonhohamed, A., Davison, D., & Dawson, J. (2002). Advanced directives for patients compulsorily admitted to hospital with serious mental illness. *British Journal of Psychiatry, 181*, 513–519.

Perr, I. N. (1992). Religion, political leadership, charisma, and mental illness: The strange story of Louis Riel. *Journal of Forensic Sciences, 37*(2), 574–584.

Pini, S., Cassano, G. B., Dell'Osso, L., & Amador, X. F. (2001). Insight into illness in schizophrenia, schizoaffective disorder, and mood disorders with psychotic features. *American Journal of Psychiatry, 158*(1), 122–125.

Potkin, S. G., Alphs, L., Hsu, C., Krishnan, K., Anand, R., Young, F. K., et al. (2003). Predicting suicidal risk in schizophrenic and schizoaffective patients in a prospective two-year trial. *Biological Psychiatry, 54*(4), 444–452.

Radomsky, E. D., Haas, G. L., Mann, J. J., & Sweeney, J. A. (1999). Suicidal behavior in patients with schizophrenia and other psychotic disorders. *American Journal of Psychiatry, 156*(10), 1590–1595.

Regenold, W. T., Thapar, R. K., Marano, C., Gavirneni, S., & Kondapavuluru, P. V. (2002). Increased prevalence of type 2 diabetes mellitus among psychiatric inpatients with bipolar I affective and schizoaffective disorders independent of psychotropic drug use. *Journal of Affective Disorders, 70*(1), 19–26.

Reichenberg, A., Weiser, M., Rabinowitz, J., Caspi, A., Schmeidler, J., Mark, M., et al. (2002). A population-based cohort study of premorbid intellectual, language, and behavioral functioning in patients with schizophrenia, schizoaffective disorder and nonpsychotic bipolar disorder. *American Journal of Psychiatry, 159*(12), 2027–2035.

Reid, W. (2005). Delusional disorder and the law. *Journal of Psychiatric Pratice, 11*(2), 126–130.

Rietschel, M., Krauss, H., Muller, D. J., Schulze, T. G., Knapp, M., Marwinski, K., et al. (2000). Dopamine d3 receptor variant and tardive dyskinesia. *European Archives of Psychiatry and Clinical Neuroscience, 250*(1), 31–35.

Rowe, R., & Clark, T. (2008). A survey of psychiatrists' attitudes to schizoaffective disorder. *International Journal of Psychiatry in Clinical Practice, 12*(1), 25–30.

Sadock, B. J., & Sadock, V. A. (2007). *Kaplan and Sadock's synopsis of psychiatry* (10th ed.). Philadelphia, PA: Wolters Kluwer Health/Lippincott Williams & Wilkins.

Scott, T. F., Price, T. R., George, M. S., Brillman, J., & Rothfus, W. (1993). Midline cerebral malformations and schizophrenia. *Journal of Neuropsychiatry and Clinical Neurosciences, 5*(3), 287–293.

Seguin, J., Lesage, A., Chawky, N., Guy, A., Daigle, F., Girard, G., et al. (2006). Suicide cases in New Brunswick from April, 2002 to May 2003: The importance of better recognizing substance and mood disorder comorbidity. *Canadian Journal of Psychiatry, 51*, 581–586.

Shirzadi, A. A., & Ghaemi, S. N. (2006). Side effects of atypical antipsychotics: Extrapyramidal symptoms and the metabolic syndrome. *Harvard Review of Psychiatry, 14*, 152–164.

Siris, S. G., & Lavin, M. R. (1995). Other psychotic disorders. In H. Kaplan & B. Sadock (Eds.), *Comprehensive textbook of psychiatry* (6th ed.). Baltimore, MD: Williams & Wilkins.

Straker, D., Correll, L. U., Kramer-Ginsberg, E., Abdulhamid, N., Koshy, F., Rubens, E., et al. (2005). Cost-effective screening for metabolic syndrome in patients treated with second-generation antipsychotic medications. *American Journal of Psychiatry, 162*, 1217–1221.

Sutherby, K., Szmukler, G. I., Halpern, A., Alexander, M., Thornicroft, G., Johnson, C., et al. (1999). A study of 'crisis cards' in a community psychiatric service. *Acta Psychiatrica Scandinavica, 100*, 56–61.

Swoboda, E., Conca, A., Konig, P., Waanders, R., & Hansen, M. (2001). Maintenance electroconvulsive therapy in affective and schizoaffective disorder. *Neuropsychobiology, 43*(1), 23–28.

Trabert, W. (1999). Shared psychotic disorder in delusional parasitosis. *Psychopathology, 32*(1), 30–34.

Volavka, J., Czobor, P., Sheitman, B., Lindenmayer, J. P., Citrome, L., McEvoy, J. P., et al. (2002). Clozapine, olanzapine, risperidone, and haloperidol in the treatment of patients with chronic schizophrenia and schizoaffective disorder. *American Journal of Psychiatry, 159*(2), 255–262.

Waite, P. (1987). Between three oceans: Challenges of a continental destiny. In C. Brown (Ed.), *The illustrated history of Canada* (pp. 279–373). Toronto, ON: Lester Orpen Denys.

CHAPTER 20

Mood Disorders

Yvonne M. Hayne

Adapted from the chapter "Mood Disorders" by Sandra J. Wood and Katharine P. Bailey

The World Health Organization (WHO) predicts that mood disorders will be the number one public health problem in the 21st century. Data from the Canadian Community Health Survey (CCHS) on mental health and well-being report that as many Canadians suffer from major depression as from other leading chronic medical conditions such as heart disease, diabetes, or a thyroid condition. In a 12-month period, 4.9% of the Canadian population, or approximately 1.6 million people, are estimated to have experienced either a major depressive or manic episode (CCHS, 2003). Notable trends are to appreciable increases in these figures, such that escalating socioeconomic burdens to the nation can be anticipated. Latest figures pose costs for a 1-year period at $14.4 billion, nearly $500 for each Canadian citizen (Statistics Canada, 2004b). At national and personal levels, mood disorders are associated with high levels of impairment in occupational, social, and physical functioning. Mood disorders often go undetected and untreated. Studies suggest that more than two thirds of people with bipolar disorder are misdiagnosed (Hirschfeld, Lewis, & Vornik, 2003).

Canadian federal–provincial initiatives have developed a variety of collaborative approaches to mental health care, such as that demonstrated in the "Shared Mental Health Care" model, which aims at more effective diagnosis, assessment, and treatment of mental health patients in the context of the family physician's office (McElheran, Eaton, Rupcich, Basinger, & Johnston, 2004). Such collaborative endeavours are thought to increase efficiency in the utilization of health care resources by enhancing the prospect of astute identification of psychological and somatic complaints, making more apparent the correct diagnosis. Appropriate remedial care can then more readily be instituted to avert intensification of the illness. In mood disorders, the potential for suicide is significant. Accurate diagnosis is vital in establishing psychological and pharmaceutical treatment. Nurses practicing in any health care setting need to develop competence in assessing patients for the presence of a mood disorder and, should such a disorder be suspected, provide appropriate educational and clinical interventions or referral.

> **KEY CONCEPT** **Mood** is a pervasive and sustained emotion that colours one's perception of the world and how one functions in it. Normal variations in mood, such as sadness, euphoria, and anxiety, occur as responses to specific life experiences and are time limited, not associated with significant functional impairment.

> **KEY CONCEPT** **Mood disorders,** as defined in the *DSM-IV-TR* (APA, 2000b), are recurrent disturbances or alterations in mood that cause psychological distress and behavioural impairment.

The primary alteration is in mood rather than in thought or perception. Several terms describe observable expressions of mood (called **affect**; American Psychiatric Association [APA], 2000b), including the following:

- *Blunted*: significantly reduced intensity of emotional expression
- *Flat*: absent or nearly absent affective expression
- *Inappropriate*: discordant affective expression accompanying speech content or ideation
- *Labile*: varied, rapid, and abrupt shifts in affective expression
- *Restricted or constricted*: mildly reduced in range and intensity of emotional expression.

Primary mood disorders include both depressive (**unipolar**) and manic-depressive (**bipolar**) disorders. The *Diagnostic and Statistical Manual of Mental Disorders*, 4th ed., Text Revision (*DSM-IV-TR*; APA, 2000b) has

established specific criteria for the diagnostic classification of these disorders, including criteria for severity (a change from previous functioning), duration (at least 2 weeks), and clinically significant distress or impairment. Mood episodes are the "building blocks" for the mood disorder diagnoses. The *DSM-IV-TR* describes four categories of mood episodes: major depressive episode, manic episode, mixed episode, and hypomanic episode. This chapter focuses on the depressive disorders and bipolar disorder. The *DSM-IV-TR* categorizes mood disorders as follows:

- *Depressive disorders*: major depressive disorder, single or recurrent; dysthymic disorder; and depressive disorder not otherwise specified (NOS)
- *Bipolar disorders*: bipolar I disorder, bipolar II disorder, cyclothymic disorder, and bipolar disorder NOS
- *Mood disorder* caused by a general medical condition
- *Substance-induced mood disorder*
- *Mood disorder NOS*.

Two additional diagnoses within the category of mood disorders warrant mention. First, *postpartum onset specifier* is distinguished by the onset of an episode within 3 to 4 weeks postpartum (Gavin et al., 2005). Second, *seasonal pattern specifier* is particularly notable in Canada, where weather variations appear to dispose to the occurrence of symptoms (APA, 2000a).

The advantage of early diagnosis of a mood disorder (e.g., early intervention, community nursing support) can be constrained by the adverse effect of a psychiatric diagnosis as a negative social label. The prime intention of effective care can be sabotaged by the need to keep the diagnosis hidden, even from oneself (Barney, Griffiths, Jorm, & Christensen, 2006; Halter, 2004; see Box 20-9.)

Depressive Disorders

◼◼◼ CLINICAL COURSE

The primary *DSM-IV-TR* criterion for major depressive disorder is one or more major depressive episodes. In a major **depressive episode**, either a depressed mood or a loss of interest or pleasure in nearly all activities must be present for at least 2 weeks. Four of the following seven additional symptoms must also be present: disruption in sleep, appetite (or weight), concentration, energy; psychomotor agitation or retardation; excessive guilt or feelings of worthlessness; and suicidal ideation (see Table 20-1). Individuals often describe themselves as depressed, hopeless, discouraged, or "down in the dumps." If individuals complain of feeling sad and empty, a depressed mood can sometimes be inferred from their facial expression and demeanour (APA, 2000a; Health Canada, 2002). Depression may present with such behaviours as obsessive ruminating, phobias, and panic attacks.

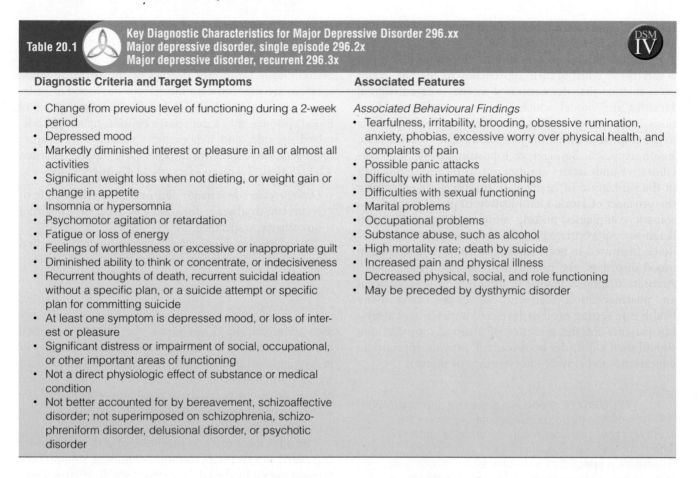

Table 20.1	Key Diagnostic Characteristics for Major Depressive Disorder 296.xx Major depressive disorder, single episode 296.2x Major depressive disorder, recurrent 296.3x	DSM IV

Diagnostic Criteria and Target Symptoms	Associated Features
• Change from previous level of functioning during a 2-week period • Depressed mood • Markedly diminished interest or pleasure in all or almost all activities • Significant weight loss when not dieting, or weight gain or change in appetite • Insomnia or hypersomnia • Psychomotor agitation or retardation • Fatigue or loss of energy • Feelings of worthlessness or excessive or inappropriate guilt • Diminished ability to think or concentrate, or indecisiveness • Recurrent thoughts of death, recurrent suicidal ideation without a specific plan, or a suicide attempt or specific plan for committing suicide • At least one symptom is depressed mood, or loss of interest or pleasure • Significant distress or impairment of social, occupational, or other important areas of functioning • Not a direct physiologic effect of substance or medical condition • Not better accounted for by bereavement, schizoaffective disorder; not superimposed on schizophrenia, schizophreniform disorder, delusional disorder, or psychotic disorder	*Associated Behavioural Findings* • Tearfulness, irritability, brooding, obsessive rumination, anxiety, phobias, excessive worry over physical health, and complaints of pain • Possible panic attacks • Difficulty with intimate relationships • Difficulties with sexual functioning • Marital problems • Occupational problems • Substance abuse, such as alcohol • High mortality rate; death by suicide • Increased pain and physical illness • Decreased physical, social, and role functioning • May be preceded by dysthymic disorder

Major depressive disorder is commonly a progressive illness. With time, episodes tend to occur more frequently, become more severe, and last longer. Complications in the form of alcohol abuse disorders and suicidality may be the most serious of occurrences associated with major depression (Goldstein & Levitt, 2006).

Dysthymic disorder is a milder but more chronic form of major depressive disorder. The *DSM-IV-TR* criteria for dysthymic disorder are depressed mood for most days for at least 2 years and two or more of the following symptoms: poor appetite or overeating, insomnia or oversleeping, low energy or fatigue, low self-esteem, poor concentration or difficulty making decisions, and feelings of hopelessness. The NOS category includes disorders with depressive features that do not meet strict criteria for major depressive disorder.

▬◖ DEPRESSIVE DISORDERS IN SPECIAL POPULATIONS

Children and Adolescents

Depressive disorders in children have manifestations similar to those seen in adults, with a few exceptions. In major depressive disorder, children are less likely to experience psychosis, but when they do, auditory hallucinations are more common than delusions. They are more likely to have anxiety symptoms, such as fear of separation, and somatic symptoms, such as stomach aches and headaches. Mood may be irritable, rather than sad, especially in adolescents. The risk for suicide is very real in children and adolescents, and peaks during the mid-adolescent years. In Canada, the suicide rate since the 1980s (12.2 per 100,000 people in 1999) has remained fairly constant for teens aged 15 to 19; for both sexes, it is recorded as the second-leading cause of teen death, surpassed only by motor vehicle crashes (Statistics Canada, 2004c).

Older Adults

Most older patients with symptoms of depression do not meet the full criteria for major depression. However, it is estimated that 8% to 20% of older adults in the community and as many as 37% in primary care settings experience depressive symptoms. Treatment is successful in 60% to 80%, but response to treatment is slower than in younger adults. Depression in older adults often is associated with chronic illnesses, such as heart disease, stroke, and cancer; symptoms may have a more somatic focus. Suicide is a very serious risk for older adults, especially men.

IN A LIFE

James Eugene Carrey (1962–)
Canadian-born Actor/Comedian

Public Persona

Jim Carrey grew up in Toronto, Canada. His fame as a comedian began on *The Carol Burnett Show* at the age of 10. His stage talents ripened through the comedy routines he performed for classmates throughout his school years. Carrey, a high school dropout, began his acting career in comedy clubs and with bit-part television and movie performances. Soon his unique on-screen characteristics were recognized and he became a box-office success. Jim Carrey is well known for his performances in such films as *The Mask, Eternal Sunshine of the Spotless Mind,* and *A Christmas Carol.* He was inducted into Canada's Walk of Fame in 2004.

Personal Reality

Carrey publicly discussed his struggle with depression on *60 Minutes* (November 2004), exposing a serious, complicated side of himself as a person who was continually questioning himself and the world. Carrey has been candid about periods of desperation in his life: the poverty, deprivation, and anger that marked some of his early childhood and adolescence; the struggles through two failed marriages; the highs and the lows bordering on despair; and the extended use of Prozac that helped him "out of a jam." Through it all, Jim, using the mask of *comedy* as a shield, maintains "life is beautiful" and that he is committed to giving full expression to the "realness" of his being.

Source: Leung, R. (Nov. 21, 2004). Carrey: Life is too beautiful. *60 Minutes,* CBS NEWS. Retrieved November 18, 2009, from http://www.cbsnews.com/stories/2004/11/18/60minutes/main656547.shtml

In Canada, the highest mortality rates due to suicide are found in people older than 80 years of age. Rates are the highest among men 85 years and older, at 31 suicides per 100,000 (Health Canada, 2002).

EPIDEMIOLOGY

The analysis of CCHS data reveals an estimated 3 million Canadians report experiencing major depression at some time in their lives. Approximately 1.2 million Canadians, aged 15 or older, had a diagnosable major depressive episode in 2002 (Statistics Canada, 2004a). In Canada, major depressive disorders are seen to affect twice as many women as men (Kovacs, 2001). The risk for the disorder increases 1.5 to 3.0 times if a first-degree relative has the disorder. Further, the highest rates of first-onset depression occur in the young-adult age group (12 to 24 years), with lower rates occurring in people 65 years of age and older (Remick, 2002).

In adolescence, major depressive disorder is twice as common in female as in male populations, while prepubertal boys and girls are noted to be equally affected. Major depressive disorders often co-occur with other psychiatric and substance-related disorders. Depression often is associated with a variety of medical conditions, particularly endocrine disorders, cardiovascular disease, neurologic disorders, autoimmune conditions, viral or other infectious diseases, certain cancers, and nutritional deficiencies, or as a direct physiologic effect of a substance (e.g., a drug of abuse, a medication, other somatic treatment for depression, or toxin exposure; APA, 2000a).

Ethnic and Cultural Differences

While prevalence rates in Canada are unrelated to race, culture can influence the experience and communication of the symptoms of depression. Canada is a country of vast regional differences and numerous "microidentities" populated by indigenous and nonindigenous peoples. Many groups of inhabitants, such as those of Ukrainian and Asian cultures, maintain "homeland" beliefs and ideologies that may influence how individuals experience and express emotional disturbances. Depressive symptoms evidenced among Canada's Aboriginal peoples may be quite distinct coming from respective cultures, such as the Inuit, Métis, Blackfoot, Algonquian, Iroquoian, and so on (King Blood, 2005). Culture may dictate an iron resolve to keep feelings in check or unexpressed. Native spirituality, inherent to many First Nations peoples, may add a complexity to detecting depression, with each group expressing and coping with feelings differently. In some cultures, somatic symptoms, rather than sadness or guilt, may predominate. Complaints of "nerves" and headaches (in Ukrainian cultures); weakness, tiredness, or "imbalance" (in Chinese and other Asian cultures); or problems of the "heart" (in Middle Eastern cultures) may be the way of expressing the depressive experience. Although culturally distinctive experiences must be distinguished from symptoms, it is imperative that a symptom not be dismissed merely because it may be viewed as the norm for a culture. The Canadian Nurses Association (CNA) recognizes that nurses must be equipped to care for an ever diverse population and value multiple ways of knowing, engaging, and expressing in order to make proper assessments and accurate diagnoses, and to provide culturally sensitive care (Edmunds & Kinnaird-Iler, 2005).

Risk Factors

Depression is so common that it is sometimes difficult to identify risk factors. The Adverse Childhood Experiences (ACE) study indicates devastating risk links between childhood emotional, physical, and sexual abuses and subsequent life experiences of depression (Felitti, 2007). Other generally acknowledged risk factors include the following:

- Prior episode of depression
- Family history of depressive disorder

- Lack of social support
- Stressful life event
- Current substance use
- Medical comorbidity
- Economic difficulties.

▬▬ ETIOLOGY

Genetics

Family, twin, and adoption studies suggest a hereditary component to the etiology of mood disorders, though strong genetic association to severe symptomatology is debated in the literature (Ebmeier, Donaghey, & Steele, 2006). Major depressive disorder, however, does demonstrate more commonly among first-degree biologic relatives of people with this disorder than among the general population, suggesting "gene–environment" interaction (Caspi et al., 2003). Additionally, positive correlates between "electrophysiologcal deficits" and "familial risk for depression" have been reported (Zhang, Hauser, Conty, Emrich, & Dietrich, 2007).

Neurobiologic Hypotheses

Neurobiologic theories of the etiology of depression emerged in the 1950s. These theories posit that major depression is caused by a deficiency or dysregulation in central nervous system (CNS) concentrations of the neurotransmitters norepinephrine, dopamine, and serotonin or in their receptor functions. These hypotheses arose in part from observations that some pharmacologic agents elevated mood, and subsequent studies identified their mechanisms of action. All antidepressants currently available have their therapeutic effects on these neurotransmitters or receptors. Current research focuses on the synthesis, storage, release, and uptake of these neurotransmitters, as well as on postsynaptic events (e.g., second-messenger systems; Donati & Rasenick, 2003).

Neuroendocrine and Neuropeptide Hypotheses

Major depressive disorder is associated with multiple endocrine alterations, specifically of the hypothalamic–pituitary–adrenal axis, the hypothalamic–pituitary–thyroid axis, the hypothalamic–growth hormone axis, and the hypothalamic–pituitary–gonadal axis. In addition, there is mounting evidence that components of neuroendocrine axes (e.g., neuromodulatory peptides such as corticotropin-releasing factor) may themselves contribute to depressive symptoms. Evidence also suggests that the secretion of these hypothalamic and growth hormones is controlled by many of the neurotransmitters implicated in the pathophysiology of depression (Hanley & Van de Kar, 2003).

Psychoneuroimmunology

Psychoneuroimmunology is a recent area of research into a diverse group of proteins known as *chemical messengers* between immune cells. These messengers, called cytokines, signal the brain and serve as mediators between immune and nerve cells. The work of Marques-Deak, Cizza, and Sternberg (2005) showed attendant effects between the brain, the immune system, and the neuroendocrine system. Dysregulation occurring between these can result in adverse effects and may manifest as symptoms of major depression and related disorders. The connection between brain–immune interactions and susceptibility to major depression is a complex and ongoing study.

Psychological Theories

Psychodynamic Factors

Most psychodynamic theorists acknowledge some debt to Freud's original conceptualization of the psychodynamics of depression, which ascribes etiology to an early lack of love, care, warmth, and protection, with resultant anger, guilt, and helplessness. Nolen-Hoeksem (2002) presents psychological variables related to avoidant coping styles as being relevant to the onset of depression. Distorted negative beliefs and thoughts about the self, the environment, and the future are all psychological variants that can induce and perpetuate depressive symptoms (see Chapter 15).

Behavioural Factors

Behaviourists hold that depression occurs primarily as the result of a severe reduction in rewarding activities or an increase in unpleasant events in one's life. The resultant depression then leads to further restriction of activity, thereby decreasing the likelihood of experiencing pleasurable activities, which, in turn, intensifies the mood disturbance (see Chapter 8).

Developmental Factors

Developmental theorists pose that depression results from the loss of a parent through death or separation or a lack of emotionally adequate parenting. These factors may delay or prohibit the realization of appropriate developmental milestones. Adolescence, in particular, is a time of transition that may dispose one to hopelessness about the future (Abela, Brozina, & Haigh, 2002).

Social Theories

Family Factors

Family theorists Wright and Leahey (2005) contend that "the family is who they say they are" (p. 60). Wright and

Leahey ascribe maladaptive "circular" patterns in family interactions as contributing to the onset of depression in family members. Disruption to family dynamics deriving from multiple causes can manifest as depression experienced by a single family member. Nurses should be vigilant in identifying whether the individual's depressive experience is symptomatic of family distress. In such cases, a "family unit" assessment and assistance may be warranted and, indeed, possibly the best predictor of a positive outcome for the individual (see Chapter 17).

Social Factors

Major depression may follow adverse or traumatic life events, especially those that involve the loss of an important human relationship or role in life. Social isolation, deprivation, and financial distress are risk factors (APA, 2002). In Canada (1999/2000), women between the ages of 35 and 45 years had the greatest number of hospitalizations for major depressive disorder (Health Canada, 2002).

■ INTERDISCIPLINARY TREATMENT OF DISORDER

Although depressive disorders are the most commonly occurring mental disorders, they are usually treated within the primary care setting, not the psychiatric setting. Individuals with depression enter mental health settings when their symptoms become so severe that hospitalization is needed, usually for suicide attempts, or if they self-refer because of incapacitation. Interdisciplinary treatment of these disorders, which are often lifelong, needs to include a wide array of health professionals in all areas. The specific goals of treatment are to

- Reduce/control symptoms and, if possible, eliminate signs and symptoms of the depressive syndrome
- Improve occupational and psychosocial function as much as possible
- Reduce the likelihood of relapse and recurrence.

■ PRIORITY CARE ISSUES

The overriding concern for people with mood disorders is safety. In depressive disorders, suicide risk should always be considered, and suicide assessments should be done frequently (see Chapter 38).

■ FAMILY RESPONSE TO DISORDER

Depression in one member affects the whole family. Spouses, children, parents, siblings, and friends experience frustration, guilt, and anger when the family member is immobilized and cannot function. It is often hard for others to understand the depth of the mood and how disabling it can be. Financial hardship can occur when the family member cannot go to work and spends days in bed. The lack of understanding and difficulty of living with a depressed person can lead to abuse. Research on families who have a member with a bipolar mood disorder reveals that families are profoundly affected by the social context of mental illness. They must manage crises, help the family member to control symptoms, and develop their own notion of "normal." Families use strategies such as being vigilant, setting limits, dealing with loss, and acknowledging the family member's strengths (Rea et al., 2003).

■ NURSING MANAGEMENT: HUMAN RESPONSE TO DEPRESSIVE DISORDER

The diagnosis of major depressive disorder is made when *DSM-IV-TR* criteria are met. An awareness of the risk factors for depression, a comprehensive biopsychosocialspiritual assessment, and a history of the patient's illness and any past treatment are key to formulating a treatment plan and to evaluating outcomes. Interviewing a family member or close friend about the patient's day-to-day functioning and specific symptoms may be helpful in determining the course of the illness, current symptoms, and level of functioning.

Biologic Domain

Assessment

Because some symptoms of depression are similar to those of some medical problems or side effects of medication therapies, biologic assessment must include a physical systems review and thorough history of medical problems, with special attention to CNS function, endocrine function, anemia, chronic pain, autoimmune illness, diabetes, or menopause. Additional medical history includes surgeries; medical hospitalizations; head injuries; episodes of loss of consciousness; and pregnancies, childbirths, miscarriages, and abortions. A complete list of prescribed and over-the-counter (OTC) medications should be compiled, including the reason for a medication's being prescribed or its use discontinued. A physical examination is recommended with baseline vital signs and baseline laboratory tests, including a comprehensive blood chemistry panel, complete blood counts, liver function tests, thyroid function tests, urinalysis, and electrocardiograms. Biologic assessment also includes evaluating the patient for the characteristic neurovegetative symptoms listed below.

- *Appetite and weight changes*: In major depression, changes from baseline include decrease or increase in appetite with or without significant weight loss or gain (i.e., a change of more than 5% of body weight in 1 month). Weight loss occurs when not dieting. Older adults with moderate to severe depression need to be assessed for dehydration as well as weight changes.
- *Sleep disturbance*: The most common sleep disturbance associated with major depression is insomnia. The *DSM-IV-TR* definitions of insomnia are divided into three categories: initial insomnia (difficulty falling asleep); middle insomnia (waking up during the night and having difficulty returning to sleep); or terminal insomnia (waking too early and being unable to return to sleep; APA, 2000b). Less frequently, the sleep disturbance is hypersomnia (prolonged sleep episodes at night or increased daytime sleep). The individual with either insomnia or hypersomnia complains of not feeling rested upon awakening.
- *Decreased energy, tiredness, and fatigue*: Fatigue associated with depression is a subjective experience of feeling tired regardless of how much sleep or physical activity a person has had. Even the smallest tasks require substantial effort.

In addition to a physical assessment including weight and appetite, sleep habits, and fatigue factors, an assessment of current medications should be completed. The frequency and dosage of prescribed and over-the-counter medications should be explored. In depression, the nurse must always assess the lethality of the medication being taken. For example, if a patient has sleep medications at home, the individual should be further queried about the number of pills in the bottle. Patients also need to be assessed for their use of alcohol, marijuana, and other mood-altering medications, as well as herbal substances because of the potential for drug–drug interactions. For example, patients taking antidepressants that affect serotonin regulation could also be taking St. John's wort (*Hypericum perforatum*) to fight depression. The combined drug and herb could interact to cause serotonin syndrome (altered mental status, autonomic dysfunction, and neuromuscular abnormalities).

Nursing Diagnoses for Biologic Domain

There are several nursing diagnoses that could be formulated based on assessment data, including Disturbed Sleep Pattern, Imbalanced Nutrition, Fatigue, Self-Care Deficit, and Nausea. Other diagnoses that should be considered are Disturbed Thought Processes and Sexual Dysfunction.

Interventions for Biologic Domain

Because weeks or months of disturbed sleep patterns and nutritional imbalance only make depression worse, counselling and education should aim to establish normal sleep patterns and healthy nutrition.

Teaching Physical Care

Encouraging patients to practice positive sleep hygiene and eat well-balanced meals regularly helps the patient move toward remission or recovery. Activity and exercise are also important for improving depressed mood state. Most people find that regular exercise is hard to maintain. People who are depressed may find it impossible. When teaching about exercise, it is important to start with the current level of patient activity and increase slowly. For example, if the patient is spending most of the time in bed, encouraging the patient to get dressed every day and walk for 5 or 10 minutes may be all that the patient can tolerate. Gradually, patients should be encouraged to have a regular exercise program and to maintain a healthy diet.

Pharmacologic Interventions

An antidepressant is selected based primarily on the particular patient's target symptoms and an individual agent's side-effect profile. Other factors that may influence choice include

- Prior medication response
- Drug interactions and contraindications
- Medication responses in family members
- Concurrent medical and psychiatric disorders
- Patient preference
- Age of patient
- Cost of medication.

Unlike many psychiatric disorders, depressive disorders may be time limited. As such, medication therapy should be reviewed periodically. The intensity of treatment and clinical management of psychiatric disorders is relative to the phase (acute, continuation, maintenance) of the presenting illness.

- *Acute phase.* The primary goal of therapy for the acute phase is symptom reduction or remission. The objective is to choose the right match of medication and dosage for the patient. Careful monitoring and follow up are essential during this phase to assess patient response to medications, adjust dosage if necessary, identify and address side effects, and provide patient support and education.
- *Continuation phase.* The goal of this treatment phase is to decrease the risk for relapse (a return of the current episode of depression). If a patient experiences a response to an adequate trial of medication, use of the medication generally is continued at the same dosage for at least 4 to 9 months after the patient returns to a clinically well state.
- *Maintenance phase.* For patients who are at high risk for recurrence (see Risk Factors section earlier in this chapter), the optimal duration of maintenance treatment is unknown but is measured in years, and full-dose therapy is required for effective prophylaxis (Schatzberg, Cole, & DeBattista, 2003).
- *Discontinuation of medication use.* The decision to discontinue active treatment should be based on the same factors considered in the decision to initiate maintenance treatment. These factors include the frequency and severity of past episodes, the persistence of dysthymic symptoms after recovery, the presence of comorbid disorders, and patient preference. Many patients continue taking medications for their lifetime.

• CRNENOTE

Patients may be reluctant to take prescribed antidepressant medications or may self-treat depression. Continuing medication and emphasizing the potential drug–drug interactions should be included in the teaching plan.

Administering Antidepressant Medication Therapy

Antidepressant medications have proved effective in all forms of major depression. To date, controlled trials have shown no single antidepressant drug to have greater efficacy in the treatment of major depressive disorder. Antidepressant medications can be grouped as follows:

- Cyclic antidepressants, which include the tricyclic antidepressants (TCAs) and maprotiline (a tetracyclic);
- Selective serotonin reuptake inhibitors (SSRIs), which currently include escitalopram oxalate (Lexapro), fluoxetine (Prozac), sertraline (Zoloft), fluvoxamine (Luvox), paroxetine (Paxil), and citalopram (Celexa; see Box 20-1 for more information);
- Monoamine oxidase inhibitors (MAOIs), which include phenelzine (Nardil) and tranylcypromine (Parnate);
- "Atypical" antidepressants, which include trazodone (Desyrel), bupropion (Wellbutrin), venlafaxine (Effexor), and mirtazapine (Remeron). Table 14-9 in Chapter 14 lists antidepressant medications, usual dosage range, half-life, and therapeutic blood levels.

The first-generation drugs, the TCAs and MAOIs, are being used less often than the second-generation drugs, the SSRIs and atypical antidepressants. Second-generation drugs selectively target the neurotransmitters and receptors thought to be associated with depression in order to minimize side effects. The side-effect profiles of the two generations of drugs are significantly different as well (Table 20-2). The efficacy of the MAOIs is well established. Evidence suggests their distinct advantage is treating a specific subtype of depression, so-called atypical depression (characterized by increased appetite, reverse diurnal mood variation, and hypersomnia), depression with panic symptoms, or social phobia (Schatzberg et al., 2003). Given the complexity of their use, MAOIs usually are reserved for patients whose depression fails to respond to other antidepressants or patients who cannot tolerate typical antidepressants.

Monitoring Medications

Patients should be carefully observed when taking antidepressant medications, not only for the anticipated side effects generally associated with them but also for their less common, sometimes even lethal possibilities. Although it is essential to know the valued benefits of antidepressants, it is equally important to be cognizant of the severe adverse effects these chemical agents can provoke. For example, some studies include evidence that both SSRIs and TCAs can induce the emergence of "medication activation syndrome" (extreme anxiety, hostility, agitation) and exacerbate suicidal ideation (Lam & Kennedy, 2004), the very things they are intended to avert. When observing patients taking antidepressants, nurses must be vigilant to the range of such possibilities, knowing also that, in the depths of depression, saving medication for a later suicide attempt is not uncommon (Box 20-2). During antidepressant treatment, there is ongoing monitoring of vital signs, plasma drug levels as appropriate, liver and thyroid function tests, complete blood counts, and blood chemistry. Responsibilities include ensuring that patients are receiving a therapeutic dosage, assessing adherence to the medication regimen, monitoring for side effects, and helping to prevent toxicity. Various pharmacologic

BOX 20.1

Drug Profile: Escitalopram Oxalate (Lexapro)

DRUG CLASS: Antidepressant

RECEPTOR AFFINITY: A highly selective serotonin reuptake inhibitor with low affinity for 5HT 1-7 or alpha and beta adrenergic, dopamine D1-5, histamine H1-3, muscarinic M1-5, and benzodiazepine receptors or for Na^+, K^+, Cl^-, and Ca^{++} ion channels that have been associated with various anticholinergic, sedative, and cardiovascular side effects.

INDICATIONS: Treatment of depression

ROUTES AND DOSAGES: Available as 5-, 10-, and 20-mg oral tablets.

Adults: Initially 10 mg once a day. May increase to 20 mg after a minimum of a week. Trials have not shown greater benefit at the 20-mg dose.

Geriatric: The 10-mg dose is recommended. Adjust dosage related to the drug's longer half-life and the slower liver metabolism of older adults.

Renal impairment: No dosage adjustment is necessary for mild to moderate renal impairment.

Children: Safety and efficacy not established in this population.

HALF LIFE (PEAK EFFECT): 27–32 hours (4–7 hours)

Source: RX List available at http://www.rxlist.com/cgi/generic/lexapro.htm

SELECTED ADVERSE REACTIONS: Most common adverse events include insomnia, diarrhea, nausea, increased sweating, dry mouth, somnolence, dizziness, and constipation. Most serious adverse events include ejaculation disorder in males; fetal abnormalities and decreased fetal weight in pregnant patients; serotonin syndrome if co-administered with MAOIs, St. John's wort, or SSRIs, including citalopram (Celexa), of which escitalopram (Lexapro) is the active isomer.

SPECIFIC PATIENT/FAMILY EDUCATION:
- Do not take in combination with citalopram (Celexa) or other SSRIs or MAOIs. A 2-week washout period between escitalopram and SSRIs or MAOIs is recommended to avoid serotonin syndrome.
- Notify prescriber if pregnancy is possible or being planned. Do not breast-feed while taking this medication.
- Use caution driving or operating machinery until certain escitalopram does not alter physical abilities or mental alertness.
- Notify prescriber of any OTC medications, herbal supplements, or home remedies being used in combination with escitalopram.
- Ingestion of alcohol in combination with escitalopram is not recommended, although escitalopram does not seem to potentiate mental and motor impairments associated with alcohol.

Table 20.2   Side Effects of Antidepressant Medications

Generic (Trade) Drug Name	Side Effects				
	Anticholinergic	Sedation	Orthostatic Hypotension	Gastrointestinal Distress	Weight Gain
Tricyclics: Tertiary Amines					
amitriptyline (Elavil)	+4	+4	+2	0	+4
clomipramine (Anafranil)	+3	+3	+2	+1	+4
doxepin (Sinequan)	+2	+3	+2	0	+3
imipramine (Tofranil)	+2	+2	+3	+1	+3
Tricyclics: Secondary Amines					
amoxapine (Asendin)	+3	+2	+1	0	+1
desipramine (Norpramin)	+1	+1	+1	0	+1
nortriptyline (Aventyl, Pamelor)	+2	+2	+1	0	+1
SSRIs					
fluoxetine (Prozac)	0/+1	0/+1	0/+1	+3	0
sertraline (Zoloft)	0	0/+1	0	+3	0
paroxetine (Paxil)	0	0/+1	0	+3	0
fluvoxamine (Luvox)	0/+1	0/+1	0/+1	+3	0
citalopram (Celexa)	0/+1	0/+1	0/+1	+3	0
escitalopram (Lexapro)	0/+1	0/+1	0/+1	+3	0
Atypical: Antidepressants					
venlafaxine (Effexor)	0	0	0	+3	0
trazodone (Desyrel)	0	+1	+3	+1	+1
bupropion (Wellbutrin)	+2	+2	+1	0	0/+1
mirtazapine (Remeron)	+3	+4	+3	+3	+2

0, absent or rare; 0/+1, lowest likelihood; +4, highest likelihood.

BOX 20.2

Guidelines: Monitoring and Administering Antidepressant Medications

Nurses should do the following in administering/monitoring antidepressant medications:

- Observe the patient for cheeking or saving medications for a later suicide attempt.
- Monitor vital signs: obtain baseline data (e.g., orthostatic vital signs and temperature) before the initiation of medications.
- Periodically monitor liver and thyroid function, blood chemistry, and complete blood count as appropriate, and compare with baseline values.
- Monitor patient symptoms for therapeutic response and report inadequate response to prescriber.

- Monitor patient for side effects and report to the prescriber serious side effects or those that are chronic and problematic for the patient. (Table 20-3 indicates pharmacologic and nonpharmacologic interventions for common side effects.)
- Monitor drug levels as appropriate. (Therapeutic drug levels for antidepressants are listed in Table 14-9 in Chapter 14.)
- Monitor dietary intake as appropriate, especially with regard to MAOI antidepressants.
- Inquire about patient's use of other medications, alcohol, street drugs, OTC medications, and/or herbal supplements that might alter the desired effects of prescribed antidepressants.

Table 20.3	Interventions to Relieve Side Effects of Antidepressants	
Side Effect	**Pharmacologic Intervention**	**Nonpharmacologic Intervention**
Dry mouth, caries, inflammation of the mouth	Bethanechol 10–30 mg tid Pilocarpine drops	Sugarless gum Sugarless lozenges 6–8 cups water per day Toothpaste for dry mouth
Nausea, vomiting	Cisapride 0.5 mg bid	Take medication with food Soda crackers, toast, tea
Weight gain	Change medication	Nutritionally balanced diet Daily exercise
Urinary hesitation Constipation	Bethanechol 10–30 mg tid Stool softener	6–8 cups water per day Bulk laxative Daily exercise 6–8 cups water per day Diet rich in fresh fruits and vegetables and grains
Diarrhea Orthostatic hypotension	OTC antidiarrheal	Maintain fluid intake Increase hydration Sit or stand up slowly
Drowsiness	Shift dosing time Lower medication dose Change medication	One caffeinated beverage at strategic time Do not drive when drowsy No alcohol or other recreational drugs Plan for rest time
Fatigue	Lower medication dose Change medication	Daily exercise
Blurred vision	Bethanechol 10–30 mg tid Pilocarpine eye drops	Temporary use of magnifying lenses until body adjusts to medication
Flushing, sweating	Terazosin 1 mg qd Lower medication dose Change medication	Frequent bathing Lightweight clothing
Tremor	β-Blockers Lower medication dose	Reassure patient that tremor may decrease with adjustments to medication. Notify caregiver if tremor interferes with daily functioning.

and nonpharmacologic interventions for the side effects of antidepressant medications are listed in Table 20-3. (Note: In Chapter 14, therapeutic blood levels for antidepressant medications can be found in Table 14-9 and MAOI diet restrictions in Table 14-10.)

Baseline vital signs should be obtained before the initiation of any medication (most particularly if administered to children, older adults, or those physiologically compromised). Thereafter, monitoring medication

effects should include objective observations, vital signs, the patient's subjective reports, and the administration of rating scales over the course of treatment. Special attention should be accorded in the case of those on medications known to have an impact on vital signs (e.g., TCAs, MAOIs, or venlafaxine).

Individualizing dosages is essential for achieving optimal efficacy. When the newer antidepressants are used, this is usually done by fine-tuning the dosage based on patient feedback. The TCAs, including imipramine (Tofranil), desipramine (Norpramin), amitriptyline (Elavil), and nortriptyline (Pamelor), have standardized valid plasma levels that can be useful in determining therapeutic dosages, although therapeutic plasma levels may vary from individual to individual. Blood samples should be drawn as close as possible to 12 hours from the last dose. The newer antidepressants do not have established standardized ranges, and optimal dosing is based on efficacy and tolerability.

Monitoring and Managing Side Effects

First-Generation Antidepressants: TCAs and MAOIs

The most common side effects associated with TCAs and MAOIs are the antihistaminic side effects (sedation and weight gain) and anticholinergic side effects (potentiating CNS drugs, blurred vision, dry mouth, constipation, urinary retention, sinus tachycardia, and decreased memory).

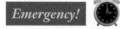

If possible, TCAs should not be prescribed for patients at risk for suicide. Lethal doses of TCAs are only three to five times the therapeutic dose, and more than 1 g of a TCA is often toxic and may be fatal. Death may result from cardiac arrhythmia, hypotension, or uncontrollable seizures.

Serum TCA levels should be evaluated when overdose is suspected. In acute overdose, almost all symptoms develop within 12 hours. Anticholinergic effects are prominent: dry mucous membranes, warm and dry skin, blurred vision, a decreased bowel motility, and urinary retention. CNS suppression (ranging from drowsiness to coma) or an agitated delirium may occur. Basic overdose treatment includes induction of emesis, gastric lavage, and cardiorespiratory supportive care. The most common side effects of MAOIs are headache, drowsiness, dry mouth, constipation, blurred vision, and orthostatic hypotension.

If co-administered with food or other substances containing tyramine (e.g., aged cheese, beer, red wine), MAOIs can trigger a hypertensive crisis that may be life threatening. Symptoms include sudden, severe pounding or explosive headache in the back of the head or temples, racing pulse, flushing, stiff neck, chest pain, nausea and vomiting, and profuse sweating.

MAOIs are more lethal in overdose than are the newer antidepressants and thus should be prescribed

with caution if the patient's suicide potential is elevated (see Chapter 14). An MAOI generally is given in divided doses to minimize side effects. Selected adverse effects of MAOIs include headache, drowsiness, dry mouth and throat, insomnia, nausea, agitation, dizziness, constipation, asthenia, blurred vision, weight loss, and postural hypotension. Although priapism was not reported during clinical trials, the MAOIs are structurally similar to trazodone, which has been associated with priapism (prolonged painful erection).

Second-Generation Antidepressants: SSRIS and Atypical Antidepressants

Serotonin syndrome is a potentially serious side effect caused by drug-induced excess of intrasynaptic serotonin (5-hydroxytryptamine [5-HT]). First reported in the 1950s, it was relatively rare until the introduction of the SSRIs. In most cases, serotonin syndrome occurs as a result of serotonin build-up when more than one drug acting on the serotonergic system (e.g., an SSRI and a TCA) is prescribed (Keogh & Doyle, 2008). Although serotonin syndrome can be life threatening, once differential diagnosis with neuroleptic malignant syndrome is made, supportive care measures generally serve in symptom recovery. Unlike neuroleptic malignant syndrome, which develops within 3 to 9 days after the introduction of neuroleptic medications (see Chapter 18), serotonin syndrome tends to develop within hours or days after initiating or increasing the dose of serotonergic medication or adding a drug with serotomimetic properties. The symptoms include altered mental status, autonomic dysfunction, and neuromuscular abnormalities. At least three of the following symptoms must be present for a diagnosis: mental status changes, agitation, myoclonus, hyperreflexia, fever, shivering, diaphoresis, ataxia, and diarrhea. In patients who also have peripheral vascular disease or atherosclerosis, severe vasospasm and hypertension may occur in the presence of elevated serotonin levels. In addition, in a patient who is a slow metabolizer of SSRIs, higher-than-normal levels of these antidepressants may circulate in the blood. In sum, vigilance is required to detect serotonergic symptoms that can result from varied and even uncommon causes, including medications such as meperidine prescribed for pain (Koczmara, Perri, Hyland, & Rousseaux, 2005).

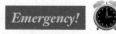

The most important emergency interventions are stopping use of the offending drug, notifying the physician, and providing necessary supportive care (e.g., intravenous fluids, antipyretics, cooling blanket).

Monitoring for Drug Interactions

Although SSRIs and newer atypical antidepressants produce fewer and generally milder side effects, which improve the patient's toleration and compliance, there are some side effects to note. Among the most common are

- Insomnia and activation
- Headaches
- Gastrointestinal symptoms
- Weight gain

Sexual side effects, primarily diminished interest and performance, are also reported with some SSRIs, particularly sertraline. The most potentially harmful, but preventable, side effect/interaction of SSRIs is serotonin syndrome (Box 20-3).

The atypical antidepressant nefazodone has been shown to raise hepatic enzyme levels in some patients, potentially leading to hepatic failure, and is no longer recommended for use in Canada. Trazodone administration has been associated with erectile dysfunction and priapism. Bupropion can cause seizures, particularly in patients at risk for seizures. Bupropion has also been associated with the development of psychosis because it is dopaminergic, and its use should be avoided in patients with schizophrenia. Venlafaxine can cause an increase in blood pressure, although this side effect appears to be dose related and can be controlled by lowering the dose (APA, 2002). For a listing of potential drug–drug interactions related to antidepressants, see Table 20-4.

BOX 20.3

Emergency: Serotonin Syndrome

CAUSE: Excessive intrasynaptic serotonin

HOW IT HAPPENS: Combining medications that increase CNS serotonin levels, such as SSRIs + MAOIs; SSRIs + St. John's wort; or SSRIs + diet pills, dextromethorphan; or alcohol, especially red wine; or SSRI + street drugs, such as LSD, MMDA, or Ecstasy.

SYMPTOMS: Mental status changes, agitation, ataxia, myoclonus, hyperreflexia, fever, shivering, diaphoresis, diarrhea.

TREATMENT: Assess all medication, supplements, foods, and recreational drugs ingested to determine the offending substances.

Discontinue any substances that may be causative factors. If symptoms are mild, treat supportively on outpatient basis with propranolol and lorazepam and follow up with prescriber.

If symptoms are moderate to severe, hospitalization may be needed with monitoring of vital signs and treatment with intravenous fluids, antipyretics, and cooling blankets.

FURTHER USE: Assess on a case-by-case basis and minimize risk factors for further medication therapy.

Teaching Points

If depression goes untreated or is inadequately treated, episodes can become more frequent, more severe, and of longer duration, and they can lead to suicide. Patient

Table 20.4	Drug–Drug Interactions: Antidepressants	
Antidepressant	**Other Drug**	**Effect of Interaction/Treatment**
Fluvoxamine	Theophylline	Increased theophylline level: seizures. Tx: Reduce theophylline levels when administering with fluvoxamine.
Fluoxetine, paroxetine	TCAs Benzodiazepines Phenothiazines	Increased plasma levels of TCA. Tx: Reduce TCA levels when giving with fluoxetine or paroxetine.
Fluoxetine, fluvoxamine, nefazadone, triazolam	Alprazolam Benzodiazepines	Increased plasma levels of alprazolam. Tx: Reduce dose of alprazolam when administered with benzodiazepines.
Fluvoxamine	Caffeine Nicotine	Lowered levels of fluvoxamine. Tx: Increase dose of fluvoxamine in smokers or patients whose coffee, tea, or caffeinated drink intake is high.
SSRIs	Warfarin	Increased prothrombin time, bleeding. Tx: Monitor closely, decrease the dose of warfarin if giving with SSRIs.
SSRIs	Lithium TCAs Barbiturates	Increased CNS effects of SSRIs. Tx: Adjust dosage of SSRI.
SSRIs	Phenytoin	Increased serum levels of phenytoin. Tx: Adjust dosage of phenytoin.

Data from McCuistion, L. E., & Gutierrez, K. J. (2002). *Real-world nursing survival guide: Pharmacology.* Philadelphia, PA: WB Saunders and Stahl, S. (2000). *Essential psychopharmacology: Neuroscientific basis and practical applications.* Cambridge, MA: Cambridge University Press.

education involves explaining this pattern and the importance of continuing medication use after the acute phase of treatment to decrease the risk of relapse.

The situation of patients discontinuing their prescribed medication prematurely is not uncommon. It may be natural for patients to assume that their experience of symptom relief, after short-term medication use, means their disorder has resolved. It is important for the nurse to recognize this erroneous assumption and to make clear to patients that "response" is not the same thing as "remission." Although immediate relief of symptoms may signify response, patients need to be carefully informed about the adverse possibility of depression recurring with the discontinuation of their medication. Medication should be continued for at least 6 months to 1 year after symptom relief (Markley, 2008). If the patient experiences a recurrence after tapering the first course of treatment, the regimen should be reinstituted for at least another year, and if the illness recurs, medication should be continued indefinitely (Schatzberg et al., 2003).

When on a regimen of antidepressants, patients should be cautioned about taking OTC medications such as those for hay fever and asthma or nasal decongestants. Herbal substances also pose problems. For example, the herb St. John's wort is particularly offensive in causing hypertension if taken in combination with agents containing monoamines. Consultation with a pharmacist is generally a wise course of action for patients considering impromptu combinations of medication.

Other Somatic Therapies

Electroconvulsive Therapy

Although its therapeutic mechanism of action is unknown, electroconvulsive therapy (ECT) is an effective treatment for severe depression. It is generally reserved for patients whose disorder is refractory or intolerant to initial drug treatments, or who are so severely ill that rapid treatment is required (e.g., patients with malnutrition, catatonia, or suicidality).

ECT is contraindicated for patients with an increased intracranial pressure. Other high-risk patients include those with recent myocardial infarction, recent cerebrovascular accident, retinal detachment, or pheochromocytoma (tumour on the adrenal cortex or other tumours), and those at risk for complications of anesthesia. Severely depressed older adults may have a more favourable response to ECT than to medication; however, the benefits of the treatment need to be considered carefully against its risks.

The CNA supports standards and best practices that uphold and effectively regulate professional nursing care for patients (CNA, 2005). For those undergoing ECT, the role of the nurse includes providing educational and emotional support for the patient and family; assessing baseline or pretreatment level of function; preparing the patient for the ECT process; and monitoring and evaluating the patient's response to the treatment, sharing it with the ECT team, and modifying treatment as needed. The actual procedure, possible therapeutic mechanisms of action, potential adverse effects, contraindications, and nursing interventions are described in detail in Chapter 14.

Light Therapy (Phototherpy)

Light therapy (described in Chapter 14) is acknowledged as an efficacious option for the treatment of seasonal affective disorder (SAD), through its effects on the circadian system. Indeed, support mounts for its value as "adjuvant" (i.e., modifies another agent with little or no direct effects by itself) to pharmacotherapy in treating nonseasonal depression as well (Even, Schroder, Friedman, & Rouillon, 2008).

Psychological Domain

Assessment

The mental status examination is an effective clinical tool to evaluate the psychological aspects of major depression because the focus is on disturbances of mood and affect, thought processes and content, cognition, memory, and attention. The comprehensive mental status examination is described in detail in Chapter 11.

Mood and Affect

The person with depression has a sustained period of feeling depressed, sad, or hopeless and may experience anhedonia (loss of interest or pleasure). The patient may report "not caring anymore" or not feeling any enjoyment in activities that were previously considered pleasurable. In some individuals, this may include a decrease in or loss of libido (sexual interest or desire) and sexual function. Depressed mood may be severe enough to provoke thoughts of suicide.

Numerous assessment scales are available for assessing depression. Easily administered self-report questionnaires can be valuable detection tools. These questionnaires cannot be the sole basis for making a diagnosis of major depressive episode, but they are sensitive to depressive symptoms. The Beck Depression Inventory (BDI) is one such commonly used self-report scale. The Hamilton Rating Scale for Depression (HAM-D; see Appendix F) is one of several clinician-completed rating scales used and, as such, may be somewhat more precise than self-report questionnaires in detecting depression.

Thought Content

Depressed individuals often have an unrealistic, negative evaluation of their worth or have guilty preoccupations or ruminations about minor past failings. Such individuals often misinterpret neutral or trivial day-to-day events as evidence of personal defects, and they have an exaggerated sense of responsibility for untoward events. As a result, they feel helpless, hopeless, worthless, and powerless. An exploration of the individual's perspective on self, the world, and the future should be included in the overall assessment, as should the possible occurrence of disorganized thought processes (e.g., tangential or circumstantial thinking) and perceptual disturbances (e.g., hallucinations, delusions).

Suicidal Behaviour

Patients with major depression are at an increased risk for suicide. Suicide risk should be assessed initially and throughout the course of treatment. Suicidal ideation includes thoughts that range from a belief that others would be better off if the person were dead or thoughts of death (passive suicidal ideation) to actual specific plans for committing suicide (active suicidal ideation). The frequency, intensity, and lethality of these thoughts can vary and can help to determine the seriousness of intent. The more specific the plan and the more accessible the means, the more serious is the intent. Risk factors that must be carefully considered are the availability and adequacy of social supports, past history of suicidal ideation or behaviour, presence of psychosis or substance abuse, and decreased ability to control suicidal impulses.

Cognition and Memory

Many individuals with depression report an impaired ability to think, concentrate, or make decisions. They may appear easily distracted or complain of memory difficulties. In older adults with major depression, memory difficulties may be the chief complaint and may be mistaken for early signs of a dementia (pseudodementia), thus complicating the diagnostic process (APA, 2000a; Fischer, 2002). When the depression is fully treated, the memory problem often improves or fully resolves.

Nursing Diagnoses for Psychological Domain

Nursing diagnoses focusing on the psychological domain of the patient with a depressive disorder are numerous. If patient data lead to the diagnosis of Risk for Suicide, the patient should be further assessed for plan, intent, and accessibility of means. Other nursing diagnoses include Hopelessness, Low Self-Esteem, Ineffective Individual Coping, Decisional Conflict, Spiritual Distress, and Dysfunctional Grieving.

Interventions for Psychological Domain

Although pharmacotherapy is usually the primary treatment method for major depression, patients also can benefit from psychosocial and psychoeducational treatments. The most effective therapies for patients with severe or recurrent major depressive disorder are combinations of psychotherapy (including interpersonal therapy, cognitive-behavioural therapy [CBT], behaviour therapy, or brief dynamic therapy) and pharmacotherapy. Adding a course of CBT may be an adjunct strategy for preventing relapse in patients who have had only a partial response to pharmacotherapy alone (APA, 2000a; see Chapter 15).

Clinical practice guidelines suggest that the combination of medication and psychotherapy may be particularly useful in more complex situations (e.g., depression in the context of concurrent, chronic general-medical or other psychiatric disorders, or in patients who fail to respond completely to either treatment alone). Recent studies suggest that short-term cognitive and interpersonal therapies may be as effective as pharmacotherapy in cases of milder depression. Psychotherapy in combination with medication may also be used to address collateral issues, such as medication adherence or secondary psychosocial problems (Casacalenda, Perry, & Looper, 2002).

CRNENOTE

A cognitive therapy approach is recommended for the acute phase of depression. This approach should be included in most nursing care plans for patients with depression.

Therapeutic Relationship

One of the most effective therapeutic tools for treating any psychiatric disorder is the therapeutic alliance, a helpful and trusting relationship between clinician and patient. The alliance is built from a number of activities, including the following:

- Establishment and maintenance of a supportive relationship
- Availability in times of crisis
- Vigilance regarding dangerousness to self and/or others
- Education about the illness and treatment goals
- Encouragement and feedback concerning progress
- Guidance regarding the patient's interactions with the personal and work environment
- Realistic goal setting and monitoring.

Interacting with depressed individuals is challenging because they tend to be withdrawn and have difficulty expressing feelings and engaging in interpersonal interactions. The therapeutic alliance partly depends

BOX 20.4

Therapeutic Dialogue: *Approaching the Depressed Patient*

George Sadder is a 70-year-old retired businessman who has been admitted to a day treatment program because of complaints of stomach pains, insomnia, and hopelessness. He has withdrawn from social activities he previously enjoyed, such as golfing and going out to eat with his wife and friends. This morning, rather than joining a group activity, he is sitting in a chair by himself.

INEFFECTIVE APPROACH

Nurse: "Hi, Mr. Sadder. My name is Sally. How are you feeling today?"

Mr. S: "Lousy, just lousy! I didn't sleep well last night, and my stomach is killing me!"

Nurse: "Oh, that's too bad! Have you had any breakfast?"

Mr. S: "No! Didn't I say that my stomach is killing me?"

Nurse: "Maybe eating breakfast would help your stomach pain."

Mr. S: "You don't know anything about my pain!" (gets up and walks away).

EFFECTIVE APPROACH

Nurse: "Hi. My name is Sally."

Mr. S: "Hello, Sally. My name is George Sadder."

Nurse: "I'd like to sit down with you, if that is OK."

Mr. S: "If you want, but I am not much of a talker."

Nurse: "That's OK. We can talk or not, whatever you wish."

Mr. S: (Patient winces)

Nurse: "You just winced. Are you in pain?"

Mr. S: "Yes, my stomach has been killing me lately."

Nurse: "What do you usually do to ease the pain?"

Mr. S: "I usually take an antacid with my meals but forgot this morning."

Nurse: "I'll see if I can get some for you now."

Mr. S: "Thanks. When my stomach settles down, maybe we can talk."

Nurse: "That would be fine. I'll check back with you in a few minutes."

CRITICAL THINKING CHALLENGE

- What ineffective techniques did the nurse use in the first scenario and how did they impair communication?
- What effective techniques did the nurse use in the second scenario and how did they facilitate communication?

---

on winning the patient's trust through a warm and empathic stance within the context of professional boundaries (see Chapter 9). Understanding the individual's personal experience of receiving a psychiatric diagnosis will enable the nurse to respond to the individual more effectively (see Box 20-4).

• CRNENOTE

Establishing the patient–nurse relationship with a person who is depressed requires an empathic, quiet approach. Too much enthusiasm can block communication.

Cognitive Therapy

Cognitive therapy has been successful in reducing depressive symptoms during the acute phase of major depression (APA, 2002; see Chapter 15). This therapy uses techniques such as thought stopping and positive self-talk to dispel irrational beliefs and distorted attitudes. The use of cognitive therapy in the acute phase of treatment, combined with medication, has grown in the past few years and now may be considered first-line treatment for mildly to moderately depressed outpatients. Varied modalities for implementing cognitive therapy have been made convenient through telephone and computer-assisted technology, with outcomes said to be similar to standard delivery modes (Corcoran & Walsh, 2009b).

Behaviour Therapy

Behaviour therapy has been effective in the acute treatment of patients with mild to moderately severe depression, especially when combined with pharmacotherapy. Therapeutic techniques include activity scheduling, self-control therapy, social skills training, and problem solving. The efficacy of behaviour therapy in the continuation and maintenance phase of depression has not been subjected to controlled studies (APA, 2002). Behaviour therapy techniques are described in Chapter 13.

Interpersonal Therapy

Interpersonal therapy seeks to recognize, explore, and resolve the interpersonal losses, role confusion and transitions, social isolation, and deficits in social skills that may precipitate depressive states (APA, 2002). It maintains that losses must be mourned and related affects appreciated, that role confusion and transitions must be recognized and resolved, and that social skills deficits must be overcome to acquire social supports. Some evidence in controlled studies suggests that interpersonal therapy is more effective in reducing depressive symptoms with certain populations, such as depressed patients with human immunodeficiency virus infection, and less successful with patients who have personality disorders (APA; see Chapter 25).

Family and Marital Therapy

Patients who experience high family stress are at risk for greater future severity of illness, higher use of health services, and higher health care expenses. Marital and family problems are common among patients with mood disorders; comprehensive treatment requires that these problems be assessed. They may be an outcome of major depression but may also increase susceptibility to depression and in some instances stop recovery. Research suggests that group intervention for couples may reduce depressive symptoms and increase partners' relational satisfaction through learned abilities in regulating mood and emotions (Kirby & Baucom, 2007). Assisting the adjustment of the nondepressed partner, and of all family members, may be invaluable in averting a relapse of depression for the recovering patient. Many family nursing interventions (discussed in detail in Chapter 17) may be used by the generalist psychiatric nurse in providing targeted family-centered care. These include

- Monitoring patient and family for indicators of stress
- Teaching stress management techniques
- Counselling family members on coping skills for their own use
- Providing necessary knowledge of options and support services
- Facilitating family routines and rituals
- Assisting family to resolve feelings of guilt
- Assisting family with conflict resolution
- Identifying family strengths and resources with family members
- Facilitating communication among family members.

Group Therapy

The role of group therapy in treating depression is based on clinical experience rather than on systematic, controlled studies. It may be particularly useful for depression associated with bereavement or chronic medical illness. Individuals may benefit from the example of others who have dealt successfully with similar losses or challenges. Survivors can gain self-esteem as successful role models for new group members. Medication support groups can provide information to the patient and to family members regarding prognosis and medication issues, thereby providing a psychoeducational forum.

Teaching Patients and Families

Patients with depression and their significant others often incorrectly believe that their illness is their own

fault and that they should be able to "pull themselves up by their boot straps" or "snap out of it." It is vital to educate patients and their families about the nature, prognosis, and treatment of depression to dispel these false beliefs and the unnecessary guilt that ensues.

Patients need to know the full range of suitable treatment options before consenting to participate in treatment. The nurse can provide opportunities for them to question, discuss, and explore their feelings about past, current, and planned use of medications and other treatments (CNA, 2005). Developing strategies to enhance adherence and to raise awareness of early signs of relapse can be important aids to making treatment more effective. See Box 20-5 for a checklist of important topics to discuss with patients who have a major depressive disorder.

Social Domain

Assessment

Social assessment focuses on patients' developmental history, family psychiatric history, patterns of relationship, education and work history, the quality of their support system, and the impact of physical or sexual abuse on their interpersonal functioning (see Chapter 11). Including a family member or close friend in the assessment process can be helpful. Changes in patterns of relating (especially social withdrawal) and changes in level of occupational functioning are commonly reported and may represent a significant deterioration from baseline behaviour. Increased use of "sick days" may occur. The family's level of support and understanding of the disorder also need to be assessed.

Nursing Diagnoses for Social Domain

Nursing diagnoses common for the social domain include Ineffective Family Coping, Ineffective Role Performance, Interrupted Family Processes, and Caregiver Role Strain (if the patient is also a caregiver).

Interventions for Social Domain

Individuals experiencing depression often withdraw from daily activities such as engaging in family routines, attending work, and participating in community events. During hospitalization, patients often withdraw to their rooms and refuse to participate in unit activities. Nurses are challenged to help the patient balance the need for privacy with the need to return to normal social functioning. Depressed patients should never be approached in an overly enthusiastic manner; this approach will irritate them and block communication. On the other hand, patients should be encouraged to set realistic goals to reconnect with family and community. Explaining to patients the importance of attending social activities, however much they may not feel like doing so, will promote the recovery process.

Milieu Therapy

While hospitalized, milieu therapy (see Chapter 13) helps depressed patients maintain socialization skills and continue to interact with others. When depressed, people are often unaware of their environment and withdraw into themselves. On a psychiatric unit, depressed patients should be encouraged to attend and participate in unit activities. These individuals have a decreased energy level and thus may be moving more slowly than others; however, their efforts should be acknowledged.

Safety

In many cases, patients are admitted to the psychiatric hospital because of a suicide attempt. Suicidality should continually be evaluated, and the patient should be protected from self-harm (see Chapter 11). During the depths of depression, patients may not have the energy to complete a suicide, but as they begin to feel better, and as their energy increases, they may be at a greater risk. If a previously depressed patient appears to have become energized overnight, he or she may have made the decision to commit suicide and thus may be relieved that the decision is finally made. The nurse may misinterpret the mood improvement as a positive move toward recovery; however, this patient may be very intent on suicide. These individuals should be carefully monitored to maintain their safety.

Other Interventions

Nurses are exceptionally well positioned to engage patients and their families in the active process of improving daily functioning, increasing knowledge and skill acquisition, and increasing independent living. Consumer-oriented support groups can help to enhance the self-esteem and the support network of participating patients and their families. Advice, encouragement, and the sense of group camaraderie may make an important contribution to recovery (CNA, 2005). Organizations providing support and information include the Canadian Mental Health Association (CMHA), the Canadian Alliance on Mental Illness and Mental Health (CAMIMH), the Mood Disorders Society of Canada, the Native Mental Health Association of Canada, and the Organization for Bipolar Affective Disorders (OBAD).

Interventions for Family Members

The family needs education and support during and after the treatment of a depressed family member. Nurses should be attentive to family distress and caregiver burden, and provide appropriate support and education. Because major depressive disorder is a recurring disorder, the family needs information about specific antecedents to a family member's depression and what steps to take. For example, one patient may routinely become depressed during the fall of each year, with one of the first symptoms being excessive sleepiness. For another patient, a major loss, such as a child going to college or the death of a pet, may precipitate a depressive episode. Families of older patients need to be aware of the possibility of depression and related symptoms, which may occur after the deaths of friends and relatives. Families of children who are depressed often misinterpret depression as behaviour problems.

Spiritual Domain
Assessment

Spirituality involves thoughts and feelings that contribute meaning and purpose to one's existence (Schmidt & Mauk, 2004). When a person experiences depression he or she may have despairing thoughts and express a lack of spiritual well-being. Spiritual assessment facilitates the implementation of holistic care (Massey, Gitchett, & Roberts, 2004). The intensely personal and intimate nature of this domain justifies a cautionary and tentative approach. Patients with mood disorders may feel especially guarded in discussing their spirituality, fearing clinicians may belittle or "pathologize" their experience. In attending to the spiritual domain, Massey et al. propose a mixture of subjective and objective methods, endorsing a three-phase itemized and progressive process, which entails basic spiritual screening, spiritual history taking, and if deemed advisable, an in-depth spiritual assessment.

Spiritual Screening

An initial screening is directed to determining basic needs related to a person's religious affiliation and/or his or her desire for additional spiritual attention. The topic can be broached by questions such as: Do you wish to identify a particular religion with which you are associated? Would you like to speak with a representative of that religion (e.g., minister, priest, chaplain, elder, imam, rabbi)? Queries posed tentatively and with sensitivity are more likely to have the desired effect of eliciting concerns, should they exist. This initial assessment gives an indication of whether spirituality is an organizing principle in the patient's life and whether further assessment is appropriate (Hodge, 2006).

Spiritual History Taking

Goals of spiritual history taking include identifying themes of the patient's spiritual concerns, recognizing the impact of those concerns on the patient's condition, establishing relevant care, and identifying appropriate referrals (Massey et al., 2004). One model of spiritual history taking is based on the HOPE acronym: "H–sources of **h**ope, meaning, comfort, strength, peace, love, and connection; O–**o**rganized religion; P–**p**ersonal spirituality and **p**ractice; E–**e**ffects on medical care and **e**nd of life issues" (Anandarajah & Hight, 2001).

Spiritual Assessment

The focus is directly on patients' understanding of spirituality and its importance in their lives. The intent is an in-depth exploration of their religious history and/or spiritual practice related to whether and how they might wish to have spiritual concerns included in their work of recovery (Fallot, 2007; Wong-McDonald, 2007). Within an interdisciplinary context, this multifaceted exploration may default to (or be done in consultation with) pastoral counsellors or clinicians deemed most proficient in addressing the spiritual dimension of a patient's experience.

Nursing Diagnoses for Spiritual Domain

Nursing diagnoses pertaining to the spiritual domain focus on distress of the spirit. Very often these are specified as situational. Within the realm of mood disorders, these are often expressed as disturbances in one's belief system related to the loss of hope, the meaning of life and suffering, and discouragement and despair.

Interventions for Spiritual Domain

Spiritual interventions can have positive outcomes for individuals suffering depression and other mood disorders. Where need presents, appropriate people can intervene with patients by way of guided conversations, personal life storytelling, and ritual experiences (Massey et al., 2004). Spiritual activities can be encouraged, including prayer, the reading of religious texts, meditation, attendance at devotional services or ceremonies, and so on. Such modalities of care may serve to relieve distress, make meaning of suffering, nurture hope, and promote spiritual resolution and wellness.

■ EVALUATION AND TREATMENT OUTCOMES

The major goals of treatment are to help the patient to be as independent as possible and to achieve stability, remission, and recovery from major depression. It is often a lifelong struggle for the individual. An ongoing evaluation of the patient's symptoms, functioning, and quality of life should be carefully documented in the patient's record in order to monitor treatment outcomes.

■ CONTINUUM OF CARE

Individuals with depressive disorders may initially present in inpatient and outpatient medical and primary care settings, emergency departments, and inpatient and outpatient mental health settings (see Chapter 4). Nurses should be able to recognize depression in these patients and make appropriate interventions or referrals. The continuum of care beyond these settings may include partial hospitalization or day treatment programs; individual, family, or group psychotherapy; home visits; and psychopharmacotherapy. Although most patients with major depression are treated in outpatient settings, brief hospitalization may be required if the patient is suicidal or psychotic.

Nurses working on inpatient units provide a wide range of direct services, including administering and monitoring medications and monitoring target symptoms; conducting psychoeducational groups; and, more generally, structuring and maintaining a therapeutic environment. Nurses providing home care can help individuals living with a mood disorder and their families to address the everyday challenges such an illness brings. Community nurses are well situated to detect undiagnosed depressive disorders and make appropriate referrals.

Nursing practice requires a coordinated, ongoing interaction among patients, families, and providers to deliver comprehensive services. This includes using the complementary skills of other disciplines for forming overall

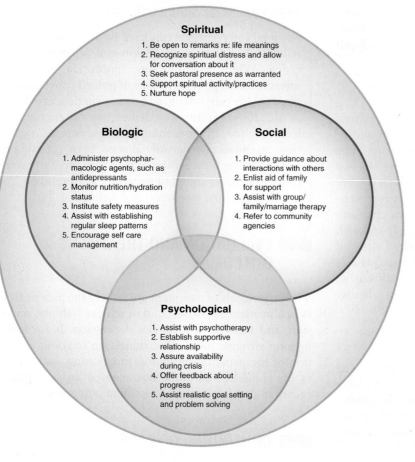

Spiritual

1. Be open to remarks re: life meanings
2. Recognize spiritual distress and allow for conversation about it
3. Seek pastoral presence as warranted
4. Support spiritual activity/practices
5. Nurture hope

Biologic

1. Administer psychopharmacologic agents, such as antidepressants
2. Monitor nutrition/hydration status
3. Institute safety measures
4. Assist with establishing regular sleep patterns
5. Encourage self care management

Social

1. Provide guidance about interactions with others
2. Enlist aid of family for support
3. Assist with group/ family/marriage therapy
4. Refer to community agencies

Psychological

1. Assist with psychotherapy
2. Establish supportive relationship
3. Assure availability during crisis
4. Offer feedback about progress
5. Assist realistic goal setting and problem solving

FIGURE 20.1 Holistic interventions for patients with major depressive disorder.

goals, plans, and decisions and for providing continuity of care as needed (CNA, 2005). Collaborative care of the patient is key to achieve the remission of symptoms and physical well-being, restoring baseline occupational and psychosocial functioning, and reduce the likelihood of relapse or recurrence (Fig. 20-1).

Bipolar Disorders (Manic-Depressive Disorders)

◼◼◼ DIAGNOSTIC CRITERIA

Bipolar disorders are distinguished from depressive disorders by the occurrence of manic or hypomanic (i.e., mildly manic) episodes in addition to depressive episodes. The *DSM-IV-TR* divides bipolar disorders into Bipolar I (characterized by one or more manic episodes generally with a major depressive occurrence); Bipolar II (periods of major depression accompanied by at least one incidence of hypomania); and **cyclothymic disorder** (periods of hypomanic episodes and depressive episodes that do not meet full criteria for a major depressive episode) (Table 20-5).

KEY CONCEPT **Mania** is primarily characterized by an abnormally and persistently elevated, expansive, or irritable mood for duration of at least 1 week (or less, if hospitalized; APA, 2000b).

A **manic episode** is characterized by **euphoria**, a state of elation experienced as a heightened sense of well-being. Osuji and Cullum (2005) elucidate that decreased inhibition, impulsivity, and distractibility negatively affect cognition in the areas of *attention* and *concentration* and alter the individual's ability to learn and effectively solve problems. During a manic episode, the individual may manifest an **expansive mood**, in which he or she shows an inappropriate lack of restraint in expressing feelings and frequently overvalues his or her own importance. Expansive qualities include an unceasing and indiscriminate enthusiasm for interpersonal, sexual, or occupational interactions. Manic episodes can also consist of irritable mood, in which the person is easily annoyed and provoked to anger, particularly when the person's wishes are challenged or thwarted. In addition, manic episodes can consist of alterations between euphoria and irritability (**lability of mood**). To meet full *DSM-IV-TR* criteria, three (or four if the mood is

| **Table 20.5** | **Key Diagnostic Characteristics of Bipolar I Disorder 296.xx**
296.0x—Bipolar I, single manic episode
296.40—Bipolar I, most recent episode hypomanic
296.4x—Bipolar I, most recent episode manic
296.5x—Bipolar I, most recent episode depressed
296.7—Bipolar I, most recent episode unspecified | DSM IV |

Diagnostic Criteria and Target Symptoms

- Presence of one or more manic episodes or mixed episodes, including one or more major depressive episodes

Manic episode
- Abnormally and persistently elevated, expansive, or irritable mood for at least 1 week
- Persistence of inflated self-esteem and grandiosity
- Decreased need for sleep
- More talkative than usual or pressure to keep talking
- Flight of ideas or racing thoughts
- Distractibility
- Increased goal-directed activity or psychomotor agitation
- Excessive involvement in pleasurable activities with high potential for painful results (e.g., unrestrained buying sprees, foolish business investments)
- Marked impairment in occupational functioning or in usual social activities or relationships; possible hospitalization to prevent harm; psychotic features

Major depressive episode (symptoms appear nearly every day)
- Depressed mood most of the day
- Markedly diminished interest or pleasure in all or most all activities for most of the day
- Significant weight loss when not dieting; weight gain or an increase or a decrease in appetite
- Insomnia or hypersomnia
- Psychomotor agitation or retardation
- Fatigue or loss of energy
- Feelings of worthlessness or excessive or inappropriate guilt
- Diminished ability to concentrate or indecisiveness
- Recurrent thoughts of death, suicidal ideation without a specific plan, suicide attempt or specific plan for committing suicide
- Not bereavement
- Clinically significant distress or impairment in social, occupational, or other important areas of functioning

Mixed episode
- Criteria for both manic and major depressive episodes nearly every day for at least 1 week
- Hospitalization to prevent harm; psychotic features

Hypomanic episode
- Distinct period of persistently elevated, expansive, or irritable mood through at least 4 days
- Clearly different from usual nondepressed mood
- Same symptoms as that for manic episode but does not cause impairment in social or occupational functioning or necessitate hospitalization
- Unequivocal change in function, uncharacteristic of person when asymptomatic
- Change observable by others

Associated Findings

Associated Behaviour Findings
Manic episode
- Resistive to efforts for treatment
- Disorganized or bizarre behaviour
- Change in dress or appearance
- Possible gambling and antisocial behaviour

Major depressive episode
- Tearfulness, irritability
- Obsessive rumination
- Anxiety
- Phobia
- Excessive worry over physical symptoms
- Complaints of pain
- Possible panic attacks
- Difficulty with intimate relationships
- Marital, occupational, or academic problems
- Substance abuse
- Increased use of medical services
- Attempted or complete suicide attempts

Mixed episode
- Similar to those for manic and depressive episodes

Hypomanic episodes
- Sudden onset with rapid escalation within 1–2 days
- Possibly precede or are followed by major depressive episode
- Increased cortisol secretion
- Absence of dexamethasone nonsuppression
- Possible abnormalities with norepinephrine, serotonin, acetylcholine, dopamine, or GABA neurotransmitter

Major depressive episode
- Sleep electroencephalogram abnormalities
- Possible abnormalities with norepinephrine, serotonin, acetylcholine, dopamine, or GABA neurotransmitter systems

Continued

Table 20.5	Key Diagnostic Characteristics of Bipolar I Disorder 296.xx *(Continued)* 296.0x—Bipolar I, single manic episode 296.40—Bipolar I, most recent episode hypomanic 296.4x—Bipolar I, most recent episode manic 296.5x—Bipolar I, most recent episode depressed 296.7—Bipolar I, most recent episode unspecified	DSM IV

Diagnostic Criteria and Target Symptoms	Associated Findings
• Not severe enough to cause marked impairment in social or occupational functioning or to require hospitalization; no psychotic features • Episode not better accounted for by other disorders such as schizoaffective disorder and not superimposed on schizophrenia, schizophreniform, delusional, or psychotic disorders • Not a direct physiologic effect of substance or other medical condition	

irritable) of seven additional symptoms must be present: inflated self-esteem or grandiosity, decreased need for sleep, being more talkative or having pressured speech, flight of ideas or racing thoughts, distractibility, increase in goal-directed activity or psychomotor agitation, and excessive involvement in pleasurable activities that have a high potential for painful consequences. The disturbance must be severe enough to cause marked impairment in social activities, occupational functioning, and interpersonal relationships, or require hospitalization to prevent self-harm.

During a manic episode, patients experience an increase in energy that can be described as hyperactivity, and they tend to require less sleep to feel rested. The individual often remains awake for long periods at night or wakes up several times a night, full of energy. Increased motor activity and agitation, which may be purposeful at first (e.g., cleaning the house), may deteriorate into inappropriate or disorganized actions. The individual may get involved unrealistically in several new endeavours, such as a spree of overspending, or in reckless sexual encounters, drug or alcohol use, or other high-risk activities such as driving too fast or taking up dangerous sports (see Box 20-6). The individual becomes overly talkative, feels pressured to continue talking, and at times is difficult to interrupt. Thoughts become disorganized and may skip rapidly among seemingly unrelated topics. This decreased logical connection between thoughts is termed *flight of ideas*. Patients with mania have inflated self-esteem, which may range from unusual self-confidence to grandiose delusions. Other psychiatric disorders can have symptoms that mimic a manic episode. Schizophrenia, schizoaffective disorder, anxiety disorders, some personality disorders (borderline personality disorder and histrionic personality disorder), substance abuse involving stimulants, and adolescent conduct disorders should be ruled out when making a diagnosis of mania.

BOX 20.6

Clinical Vignette: *The Patient with Mania*

Mr. Bell was a day-trader on the stock market. Initially he was quite successful and, as a result, upgraded his lifestyle with a more expensive car, a larger and more luxurious house, and a boat. When the stock market declined dramatically, Mr. Bell continued to trade, saying that if he could just find the "right" stock he could earn back all of the money he had lost. He spent his days and nights in front of his computer screen, taking little or no time to eat or sleep. He defaulted on his mortgage, car, and boat payments and was talking nonstop to his wife. She brought him to the hospital for evaluation

WHAT DO YOU THINK?
• What behavioural symptoms of mania does Mr. Bell exhibit?
• What cognitive symptoms of mania does Mr. Bell exhibit?

The *DSM-IV-TR* criteria for a **mixed episode** are met when the criteria for both a manic episode and a major depressive episode are met and are present for at least 1 week. Individuals who are having a mixed episode usually exhibit high anxiety, agitation, and irritability. The criteria for a **hypomanic episode** are the same as for a manic episode, except that the time criterion is at least 4 days, rather than 1 week, and no marked impairment in social or occupational functioning is present.

Secondary Mania

Mania can be caused by underlying medical disorders, precipitated by some medical treatments, or induced by certain substances of abuse (e.g., certain metabolic abnormalities, neurologic disorders, CNS tumours, and medications). Such precipitants might be particularly suspected in older persons who present with new onset manic symptoms (Hoblyn, 2004).

Rapid Cycling Specifier

Rapid cycling can occur in both bipolar I and bipolar II disorders. The concept of rapid cycling signifies four or more episodes of major depression, mania, mixed mania, or hypomania occurring in any combination or order within a 12-month period (APA, 2000b).

The *DSM-IV-TR* criteria for cyclothymic disorder are at least 2 years of numerous periods with hypomanic symptoms and numerous periods with depressive symptoms that do not meet full criteria for a major depressive episode.

 CLINICAL COURSE

Bipolar disorder is a chronic, cyclic disorder. An increased frequency of episodes or more continuous symptoms have been reported in patients who experienced onset at an earlier age and who have a significant family history of illness. Mixed mania and depression is noted in the categorizations of bipolar disorder. The description of this particular subtype, however, is less than clear, with associated symptoms described that tend (somewhat simultaneously) to both mania and depression. It would seem that mixed bipolar disorder refers to a nearly blended symptomatology, with indicators of disturbance agitating at the extreme ends of the mood spectrum. Extreme turmoil can correlate with mixed states, which have been associated with increased suicidal ideation, compared with states of pure mania (Maser et al., 2002). Bipolar disorders can lead to severe functional impairment as manifested by alienation from family, friends, and co-workers; indebtedness; job loss; divorce; and other problems of living (Rothbaum & Astin, 2000).

 EPIDEMIOLOGY

Distribution and Age of Onset

In Canada, the estimated 1-year prevalence for bipolar disorder (i.e., the estimated percentage of the population who have the disorder during any 1-year period) is between 0.2% and 0.6% among adults in the general population (Health Canada, 2002). The estimated mean age of onset is between 21 and 30 years.

Bipolar disorder in children has only recently been recognized. Although it is not well studied, depression usually appears first. Somewhat different than in adults, the hallmark of childhood bipolar disorder is intense rage. Children may display seemingly unprovoked rage episodes for as long as 2 to 3 hours. The symptoms of bipolar disorder reflect the developmental level of the child: Whereas children younger than 9 years exhibit more irritability and emotional lability, older children exhibit more classic symptoms, such as euphoria and grandiosity. The first contact with the mental health system often occurs when the behaviour becomes disruptive, possibly 5 to 10 years after its onset. These children often have other psychiatric disorders such as attention deficit hyperactivity disorder and conduct disorder (Kowatch & DelBello, 2005; see Chapter 28). There are no studies as yet to indicate whether or not children with bipolar disorder will have the disorder as adults.

Neurophysiologically, geriatric patients with mania demonstrate more abnormalities and cognitive disturbances (confusion and disorientation) than do younger patients. It generally was believed that the incidence of mania decreases with age because this population was thought to consist of only those individuals who had a diagnosis in younger years and managed to survive into old age. Recently, late-onset bipolar disorder was identified when researchers found evidence of an increased incidence of mania with age, especially in women older than 50 years and in men in the 8th and 9th decades. Late-onset bipolar disorder is more likely related to secondary mania (Hoblyn, 2004).

Gender, Ethnic, and Cultural Differences

Although no significant gender differences have been found in the lifetime prevalence of bipolar I disorder, the incidence of bipolar II disorder is reportedly 5% greater in females than males (Barnes & Mitchell, 2005). In addition, some data indicate female patients with bipolar disorder are at greater risk for depression whereas male patients are prone to manic episodes (Corcoran & Walsh, 2009a). No significant differences have been found based on race or ethnicity (APA, 2000a; CNA, 2005).

 COMORBIDITY

Medical comorbidity in patients with bipolar disorder is a significant issue as it complicates diagnosis and management of the illness and may have a negative impact on patient outcomes (Yatham et al., 2006). The two most common comorbid conditions are anxiety disorders (most prevalent: panic disorder and social phobia) and substance use (most commonly alcohol and marijuana). Individuals with a comorbid anxiety disorder are more likely to experience a more severe course. A history of substance use further complicates the course of illness and results in less chance for remission and poorer treatment compliance (Goldberg, Garno, Leon, Kocsis, & Portera, 1999).

 ETIOLOGY

Current theories of the etiology of mood disorders are associated with chronic abnormalities of neurotransmission, which are thought to result in compensatory but maladaptive changes in brain regulation. In addition, the use of controlled structural and functional imaging studies of patients with mood disorders have generated hypotheses that CNS dysfunction is associated with specific structural brain abnormalities and functional CNS alterations (Sheline, 2003).

Chronobiologic Theories

Sleep disturbance is an important aspect of depression and mania. Sleep patterns appear to be regulated by an internal biologic clock centred in the hypothalamus (see Chapter 10). Artificially induced sleep deprivation is known to precipitate mania in some patients with bipolar disorder (Grunze, Amann, Dittmann, & Walden, 2002). Because a number of neurotransmitter and hormone levels follow circadian patterns, sleep disruption may lead to biochemical abnormalities that affect mood. Seasonal changes in light exposure also trigger affective episodes in some patients, typically depression in winter and hypomania in the summer in the northern hemisphere (Cutler & Marcus, 1999).

Sensitization and Kindling Theory

Sensitization (increase in response to a drug with repetition of the same dosage) and the related phenomenon of kindling (subthreshold stimulation of a neuron generates an action potential; see Chapter 14) refer to animal models. Repeated chemical or electrical stimulation of certain regions of the brain produces stereotypical behavioural responses or seizures. The amount of the chemical or electricity required to evoke the response or seizure decreases with each experience. These phenomena have been used as models to explain why, over time, affective episodes, particularly those seen in patients with bipolar disorder, recur in shorter and shorter cycles and with less relation to environmental precipitants. It is hypothesized that repeated affective episodes might be accompanied by the progressive alteration of brain synapses that lower the threshold for future episodes and increase the likelihood of illness. The kindling theory also helps explain the value of using antiseizure medication, such as carbamazepine and valproic acid, for mood stabilization.

Genetic Factors

The genetic basis for the development of bipolar disorder is only beginning to be explored. Results from family, adoption, and twin studies indicate that bipolar disorder is highly heritable (McCuffin et al., 2003). Such results show a 1% incidence rate in the general population,

compared with a 7% incidence rate for first-degree relatives of a patient with bipolar disorder, and 60% for a monozygotic twin of a bipolar patient (Payne, Potash, & DePaulo, 2005). Modes of genetic transmission and the cumulative effects of multiple genes interacting with environmental influences have yet to be definitively identified.

Psychological and Social Theories

Most psychological and social theories of mood disorders focus on loss as the cause of depression in genetically vulnerable individuals. Mania is considered to be a biologically rooted condition, but when viewed from a psychological perspective, mania is usually regarded as a condition that arises from an attempt to overcompensate for depressed feelings, rather than a disorder in its own right. It is now generally accepted that environmental conditions contribute to the timing of an episode of illness, rather than cause the illness (Johnson, Andersson-Lundman, Aberg-Wistedt, & Mathe, 2000).

INTERDISCIPLINARY TREATMENT OF DISORDER

Patients with bipolar disorder have a complex set of issues and likely will be treated by an interdisciplinary team. Nurses, physicians, social workers, psychologists, and activity therapists all have valuable expertise for bipolar patients. For children with bipolar disorder, school teachers and counsellors are included in the team. For older adults, the primary care physician becomes part of the team. An important treatment goal is to minimize and prevent either manic or depressive episodes, which tend to accelerate over time. The fewer the episodes, the more likely the person can live a normal, productive life. Another important goal is to help the patient and family to learn about the disorder and manage it throughout a lifetime.

PRIORITY CARE ISSUES

During a manic episode, protection of the patient is a priority. It is during a manic episode that poor judgment and impulsivity result in risk-taking behaviours that can have dire consequences for the patient and family. For example, one patient withdrew all the family money from the bank and gambled it away. Risk for suicide is always a possibility. During a depressive episode, the patient may feel that life is not worth living. During a manic episode, the patient may believe that he or she has supernatural powers, such as the ability to fly. As patients recover from a manic episode, they may be so devastated by the consequences of the episode's impulsive behaviour and poor judgment that suicide seems like a reasonable option.

FAMILY RESPONSE TO DISORDER

Bipolar disorder can devastate families, who often feel that they are on an emotional merry-go-round, particularly if they have difficulty understanding the mood shifts. They can experience burden in relation to patient problem behaviour (e.g., impulsive behaviour during manic episodes, such as excessive debt, assault charges, and sexual infidelities) and in terms of the disruption of household routine (Perlick et al., 2007). Families, however, report developing coping strategies that allow them to address issues as they occur (Goossens, van Wijngaarden, Knoppert-van der Klein, & van Achterberg, 2008).

NURSING MANAGEMENT: HUMAN RESPONSE TO BIPOLAR DISORDER

The nursing care of patients with bipolar disorder is one of the most interesting yet greatest challenges in psychiatric nursing. In general, the behaviour of patients with bipolar disorder is normal between mood episodes. The ideal nursing care occurs during a period of time when the nurse can see the patient in the acute illness phase and in remission. The nursing care of bipolar depression should be approached in a manner similar to that used for major depressive disorder, as described previously.

Biologic Domain

Assessment

With regard to the biologic domain, the assessment emphasis is on evaluating symptoms of mania and, most particularly, changes in sleep patterns. The assessment should follow the guidelines in Chapter 11. In the manic phase of bipolar disorder, the patient may not sleep, resulting in irritability and physical exhaustion. Because eating habits usually change during a manic or depressive episode, the nurse should assess changes in diet and body weight. Because patients with mania may experience malnutrition and fluid imbalance, laboratory studies, such as monitoring of thyroid function, should be completed. Abnormal thyroid functioning can be responsible for the mood and behavioural disturbances. During a manic phase, patients often become hypersexual and engage in risky sexual practices. Changes in sexual practices should be explored.

Pharmacologic Assessment

When a patient is in a manic state, the previous use of antidepressants should be assessed because a manic episode may be triggered by antidepressant use. In such cases, the use of antidepressants should be discontinued. Many times, manic or depressive episodes occur after patients stop taking their mood stabilizer, at which time the reason for stopping the medication should be explored. Patients may stop taking their medications because of side effects or because they no longer believe they have a mental disorder. Special attention should also focus on the use of alcohol and other substances. Usually, a drug screen is ordered to determine current use of substances.

Nursing Diagnoses for Biologic Domain

Among nursing diagnoses in this domain are Disturbed Sleep Pattern, Sleep Deprivation, Imbalanced

Nutrition, Hypothermia, Deficient Fluid Volume, and Medication Non-Adherence. If patients are in the depressive phase of illness, the previously discussed diagnoses for depression should be considered.

Interventions for Biologic Domain

Physical Care

In a state of mania, the patient's physical needs are rest, adequate hydration and nutrition, and re-establishment of physical well-being. Self-care has usually deteriorated. For a patient who is unable to sit long enough to eat, snacks and high-energy foods should be provided that can be eaten while moving. Alcohol should be avoided. Sleep hygiene is a priority but may not be realistic until medications take effect. Limiting stimuli can be helpful in decreasing agitation and promoting sleep.

CRNENOTE
Protection of patients with mania is always a priority. Ongoing assessment should focus on irritability, fatigue, nutrition, and potential for harming self or others.

Teaching Points

Once the patient's mood stabilizes, the nurse should focus on monitoring changes in physical functioning in sleep or eating behaviour and teaching patients to identify antecedents to mood episodes. A regular sleep routine should be maintained if possible. High-risk times for manic episodes, such as changes in work schedule (day to night), should be avoided if possible. Patients should be taught to monitor the amount of their sleep each night and report decreases in sleep of more than 1 hour per night, as this may be a precursor to a manic episode.

Intervention With Mood Stabilizers

Pharmacotherapy is essential in bipolar disorder to achieve two goals: the rapid control of symptoms and the prevention of future episodes—or, at least, reduction in their severity and frequency. Pharmacotherapy

Table 20.6	Mood Stabilizing Medications	
Generic (Trade) Drug Name	Usual Dosage Range (Daily)	Half-Life (Hours)
lithium (Eskalith, Lithane)	600–1,800 mg	17–36
divalproex sodium (Depakote)	15–60 mg/kg	6–16
carbamazepine (Tegretol)	200–1,200 mg	25–65
olanzapine (Zyprexa)	5–20 mg	21–54
risperidone (Risperdol)	1–6 mg	20

BOX 20.7

Drug Profile: Lithium (Eskalith)

DRUG CLASS: Mood stabilizer

RECEPTOR AFFINITY: Alters sodium transport in nerve and muscle cells, increases norepinephrine uptake and serotonin receptor sensitivity, slightly increases intraneuronal stores of catecholamines, delays some second messenger systems. Mechanism of action is unknown.

INDICATIONS: Treatment and prevention of manic episodes in bipolar affective disorder. Used successfully in a number of unlabelled uses such as prophylaxis of cluster headaches, premenstrual tension, bulimia, etc.

ROUTES AND DOSAGE: 150-, 300-, and 600-mg capsules. Lithobid, 300-mg slow-release tablets; Eskalith CR, 450-mg controlled-release tablets. Lithium citrate, 300-mg/5 mL liquid form.

Adult: In acute mania, optimal response is usually 600 mg tid or 900 mg bid. Obtain serum levels twice weekly in acute phase. Maintenance: Use lowest possible dose to alleviate symptoms and maintain serum level of 0.6–1.2 mEq/L. In uncomplicated maintenance obtain serum levels every 2–3 months. Do not rely on serum levels alone. Monitor patient side effects.

Geriatric: An increased risk for toxic effects, use lower doses, monitor frequently.

Children: Safety and efficacy in children younger than 12 years has not been established.

HALF-LIFE (PEAK EFFECT): Mean, 24 hours (peak serum levels in 1–4 hours). Steady state reached in 5–7 days.

SELECT ADVERSE REACTIONS: Weight gain

WARNING: Avoid use during pregnancy or while breastfeeding. Hepatic or renal impairments increase plasma concentration.

SPECIFIC PATIENT/FAMILY EDUCATION:
- Avoid alcohol or other CNS depressant drugs.
- Notify prescriber if pregnancy is possible or planned. Do not breast-feed while taking this medication.
- Notify prescriber before taking any other prescription, OTC medication, or herbal supplements.
- May impair judgment, thinking, or motor skills; avoid driving or other hazardous tasks.
- Do not abruptly discontinue use.

continues through the various phases of bipolar disorder:

- *Acute phase.* The goal of treatment in the acute phase is symptom reduction and stabilization. Therefore, for the first few weeks of treatment, mood stabilizers may need to be combined with antipsychotics or benzodiazepines, particularly if the patient has psychotic symptoms, agitation, or insomnia. If the clinical situation is not an emergency, patients usually start on a low dose and gradually increase the dose until maximum therapeutic benefits are achieved. Once stabilization is achieved, the frequency of serum level monitoring should be every 1 to 2 weeks during the first 2 months and every 3 to 6 months during long-term maintenance. Medications most commonly used for mood stabilization in bipolar disorder are listed in Table 20-6 (also see Chapter 14).
- *Continuation phase.* The treatment goal in this phase is to prevent relapse of the current episode or cycling into the opposite pole. It lasts about 2 to 9 months after acute symptoms resolve. The usual pharmacologic procedure in this phase is to continue the mood stabilizer while closely monitoring the patient for signs or symptoms of relapse.
- *Maintenance phase.* The goal of treating this phase is to sustain remission and to prevent new episodes. The great weight of evidence favours long-term prophylaxis against recurrence after the effective treatment of acute episodes. It is recommended that long-term or lifetime prophylaxis with a mood stabilizer be instituted after two manic episodes or one severe manic episode, or if there is a family history of bipolar disorder.
- *Discontinuation of medication use.* Like the course of major depressive disorder, the course of bipolar disorder typically is recurrent and progressive. Therefore, the same issues and principles regarding the decision to continue or discontinue pharmacotherapy apply.

The mainstays of somatic therapy are the mood-stabilizing drugs. The three agents that show significant efficacy in controlled trials are lithium carbonate (Lithium), divalproex sodium (Depakote), and carbamazepine (Tegretol; Table 20-6). Lithium, divalproex sodium, and the atypical antipsychotic olanzapine (Zyprexa) are approved by Health Canada, under the authority of the Food and Drugs Act, for treating acute mania.

Lithium Carbonate

Lithium is the most widely used mood stabilizer (see Box 20-7). Combined response rates from five studies demonstrated that 70% of patients experienced at least partial improvement with lithium therapy. However, for most patients, lithium is not a fully adequate treatment for all phases of the illness, and particularly during the acute phase, supplemental use of antipsychotics and benzodiazepines is often beneficial. During acute depressive episodes, supplemental use of antidepressants is most often indicated (Keck et al., 2000). Because of its significant side-effect burden (Table 20-7), lithium is poorly tolerated in at least one third of treated patients and has the narrowest gap between therapeutic and toxic concentrations of any routinely prescribed psychotropic agent (Belmaker & Yaroslavsky, 2000). Predictors of poor response to lithium in acute mania include a history of poor response, rapid cycling, dysphoric symptoms, mixed symptoms of depression and mania, psychiatric comorbidity, and medical comorbidity (Alda & Grof, 2000).

Table 20.7	Lithium Blood Levels and Associated Side Effects
Plasma Level	**Side Effects or Symptoms of Toxicity**
<1.5 mEq/L Mild side effects	Metallic taste in mouth
	Fine hand tremor (resting)
	Nausea
	Polyuria
	Polydipsia
	Diarrhea or loose stools
	Muscular weakness or fatigue
	Weight gain
	Edema
	Memory impairments
1.5–2.5 mEq/L Moderate toxicity	Severe diarrhea
	Dry mouth
	Nausea and vomiting
	Mild to moderate ataxia
	Incoordination
	Dizziness, sluggishness, giddiness, vertigo
	Slurred speech
	Tinnitus
	Blurred vision
	Increasing tremor
	Muscle irritability or twitching
	Asymmetric deep tendon reflexes
	Increased muscle tone
>2.5 mEq/L Severe toxicity	Cardiac arrhythmias
	Blackouts
	Nystagmus
	Coarse tremor
	Fasciculations
	Visual or tactile hallucinations
	Oliguria, renal failure
	Peripheral vascular collapse
	Confusion
	Seizures
	Coma and death

Lithium is a salt, and the interaction between lithium levels and sodium levels in the body and the relationship between lithium levels and fluid volume in the body remain crucial issues in its safe, effective use. The higher the sodium levels are in the body, the lower the lithium level will be, and vice versa. Thus, changes in dietary sodium intake can affect lithium blood levels that, in turn, may affect therapeutic results or increase the incidence of side effects. The same applies to fluid volume. If body fluid decreases significantly because of a hot climate, strenuous exercise, vomiting, diarrhea, or drastic reduction in fluid intake, then lithium levels can rise sharply, causing an increase in side effects, progressing to lethal lithium toxicity. See Table 20-8 for lithium interactions with other drugs. See Chapter 14 for further discussion of lithium's possible mechanisms of action, pharmacokinetics, side effects, and toxicity.

Emergency!

If symptoms of moderate or severe toxicity (e.g., cardiac arrhythmias, blackouts, tremors, seizures) are noted, withhold additional doses of lithium, immediately obtain a blood sample to analyze the lithium level, and push fluids if the patient can take fluids. Contact the physician for further direction about relieving the symptoms. Mild side effects tend to subside or can be managed by nursing measures (see Table 20-9).

Divalproex Sodium

Divalproex sodium (Depakote), an anticonvulsant, has a broader spectrum of efficacy and has about equal benefit for patients with pure mania as for those with other forms of bipolar disorder (e.g., mixed mania, rapid cycling, comorbid substance abuse, secondary mania). Moreover, in one large placebo-controlled study, patients taking divalproex sodium experienced a longer period of stable mood than did patients taking lithium or placebo (Bowden et al., 2000). Whereas divalproex is usually initiated at 250 mg twice a day or lower, in the inpatient setting it can be initiated in an oral loading

Table 20.8	Lithium Interactions With Medications and Other Substances
Substance	**Effect of Interaction**
Angiotensin-converting enzyme inhibitors, such as: • Captopril • Lisinopril • Quinapril	Increases serum lithium; may cause toxicity and impaired kidney function
Acetazolamide	Increases the renal excretion of lithium, decreases lithium levels
Alcohol	May increase serum lithium level
Caffeine	Increases lithium excretion, increases lithium tremor
Carbamazepine	Increases neurotoxicity, despite normal serum levels and dosage
Fluoxetine	Increases serum lithium levels
Haloperidol	Increases neurotoxicity, despite normal serum levels and dosage
Loop diuretics, such as furosemide	Increases lithium serum levels, but may be safer than thiazide diuretics; potassium-sparing diuretics (amiloride, spirolactone) are safest
Methyldopa	Increases neurotoxicity without increasing serum lithium levels
Nonsteroidal anti-inflammatory drugs, such as: • Diclofenac • Ibuprofen • Indomethacin • Piroxicam	Decreases renal clearance of lithium Increases serum lithium levels by 30%–60% in 3–10 days Aspirin and sulindac do not appear to have the same effect
Osmotic diuretics, such as: • Urea • Mannitol • Isosorbide	Increases renal excretion of lithium and decreases lithium levels
Sodium chloride	High sodium intake decreases lithium levels; low sodium diets may increase lithium levels and lead to toxicity
Thiazide diuretics, such as: • Chlorothiazide • Hydrochlorothiazide	Promotes sodium and potassium excretion; increases lithium serum levels; may produce cardiotoxicity and neurotoxicity
TCAs	Increases tremor; potentiates pharmacologic effects of TCAs

Table 20.9	Interventions for Lithium Side Effects
Side Effect	**Intervention**
Edema of feet or hands	Monitor intake and output, check for possible decreased urinary output
	Monitor sodium intake
	Patient should elevate legs when sitting or lying
	Monitor weight
Fine hand tremor	Provide support and reassurance, if it does not interfere with daily activities
	Tremor worsens with anxiety and intentional movements; minimize stressors
	Notify prescriber if it interferes with patient's work and compliance will be an issue
	More frequent smaller doses of lithium may also help
Mild diarrhea	Take lithium with meals
	Provide for fluid replacement
	Notify prescriber if becomes severe; may need a change in medication preparation or may be early sign of toxicity
Muscle weakness, fatigue, or memory and concentration difficulties	Provide support and reassurance; this side effect will usually pass after a few weeks of treatment
	Short-term memory aids such as lists or reminder calls may be helpful
	Notify prescriber if becomes severe or interferes with the patient's desire to continue treatment
Metallic taste	Suggest sugarless candies or throat lozenges
	Encourage frequent oral hygiene
Nausea or abdominal discomfort	Consider dividing the medication into smaller doses, or give it at more frequent intervals
	Give medication with meals
Polydipsia	Reassure patient that this is a normal mechanism to cope with polyuria
Polyuria	Monitor intake and output
	Provide reassurance and explain nature of side effect
	Also explain that this causes no physical damage to kidneys
	Withhold medication
Toxicity	Notify prescriber
	Use symptomatic treatments

dose using 20 to 30 mg/kg body weight (see Box 20-8). This may speed the reduction of manic symptoms and diminish the need for antipsychotics early in the course of therapy (Hirschfeld, Baker, Wozniak, Tracy, & Sommerville, 2003).

Baseline liver function tests and a complete blood count with platelets should be obtained before starting therapy, and patients with known liver disease should not be given divalproex sodium. Optimal blood levels appear to be in the range of 50 to 150 ng/mL. Levels may be obtained weekly until the patient is stable, and then every 6 months. Divalproex sodium is associated with increased risk for birth defects. Cases of life-threatening pancreatitis have been reported in adults and children receiving valproate, either initially or after several years of use. Some cases were described as hemorrhagic, with a rapid progression from onset to death. If pancreatitis is diagnosed, valproate use should be discontinued.

Carbamazepine

Carbamazepine, an anticonvulsant, also has mood-stabilizing effects. Data from various studies suggest that it may be effective in patients who are unresponsive to lithium. The most common side effects of carbamazepine are dizziness, drowsiness, nausea, and vomiting, which may be avoided with slow incremental dosing. Carbamazepine has both benign and severe hematologic toxicities. Frequent clinically unimportant decreases in white blood cell counts occur. Estimates of the rate of severe blood dyscrasias vary from 1 in 10,000 patients treated to a more recent estimate of 1 in 125,000 (Schatzberg et al., 2003). Mild, nonprogressive elevations of liver function test results are relatively common. Carbamazepine is associated with increased risk for birth defects.

In patients older than 12 years, carbamazepine is begun at 200 mg once or twice a day. The dosage is increased by no more than 200 mg every 2 to 4 days, to 800 to 1,000 mg a day, or until therapeutic levels or effects are achieved. It is important to monitor for blood dyscrasias and liver damage. Liver function tests and complete blood counts with differential are minimal pretreatment laboratory tests and should be repeated about 1 month after initiating treatment, and at 3 months, 6 months, and yearly. Other yearly tests should include electrolytes, blood urea nitrogen, thyroid function tests, urinalysis, and eye examinations. Carbamazepine levels are measured monthly until the patient is on a stable dosage. Studies suggest that

BOX 20.8

Drug Profile: Divalproex Sodium (Depakote)

DRUG CLASS: Antimania agent

RECEPTOR AFFINITY: Thought to increase the level of inhibitory neurotransmitter, GABA, to brain neurons. Mechanism of action is unknown.

INDICATIONS: Treatment of bipolar disorders.

ROUTES AND DOSAGE: Available in 125-mg delayed-release capsules, and 125-, 250-, and 500-mg enteric-coated tablets.

Adult Dosage: Dosage depends on symptoms and clinical picture presented; initially the dosage is low and is gradually increased depending on the clinical presentation.

HALF-LIFE (PEAK EFFECT): 6–16 hours (1–4 hours)

SELECT ADVERSE REACTIONS: Sedation, tremor (may be dose related), nausea, vomiting, indigestion, abdominal cramps, anorexia with weight loss, slight elevations in liver enzymes, hepatic failure, thrombocytopenia, transient increases in hair loss.

WARNING: Use cautiously during pregnancy and lactation. Contraindicated in patients with hepatic disease or significant hepatic dysfunction. Administer cautiously with salicylates; may increase serum levels and result in toxicity.

SPECIFIC PATIENT/FAMILY EDUCATION:
- Take with food if gastrointestinal upset occurs.
- Swallow tablets or capsules whole to prevent local irritation of mouth and throat.
- Notify prescriber before taking any other prescription or OTC medications or herbal supplements.
- Avoid alcohol and sleep-inducing or OTC products.
- Avoid driving or performing activities that require alertness.
- Do not abruptly discontinue use.
- Keep appointments for follow up, including blood tests to monitor response.

Table 20.10	Selected Medication Interactions With Carbamazepine

Interaction	Drug Interacting With Carbamazepine
Increased carbamazepine levels	Erythromycin
	Cimetidine
	Propoxyphene
	Isoniazid
	Calcium-channel blockers (Verapamil)
	Fluoxetine
	Danazol
	Diltiazem
	Nicotinamide
Decreased carbamazepine levels	Phenobarbital
	Primidone
	Phenytoin
Drugs whose levels are decreased by carbamazepine	Oral contraceptives
	Warfarin, oral anticoagulants
	Doxycycline
	Theophylline
	Haloperidol
	Divalproex sodium
	TCAs
	Acetaminophen—increased metabolism, but also increased risk for hepatotoxicity

blood levels in the range of 8 to 12 ng/mL correspond to therapeutic efficacy. See Table 20-10 for carbamazepine's interactions with other drugs. See Chapter 14 for further discussion of carbamazepine's possible mechanisms of action, pharmacokinetics, side effects, and toxicity.

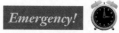 **Emergency!**

Both valproate and carbamazepine may be lethal if high doses are ingested. Toxic symptoms appear in 1 to 3 hours and include neuromuscular disturbances, dizziness, stupor, agitation, disorientation, nystagmus, urinary retention, nausea and vomiting, tachycardia, hypotension or hypertension, cardiovascular shock, coma, and respiratory depression.

Newer Anticonvulsants

In small clinical trials, case reports, and anecdotal evidence, newer anticonvulsants also show promise as mood stabilizers (Yatham et al., 2006). Lamotrigine (Lamictal) has efficacy in treating mania, both as a single agent and in combination with lithium or valproate (Bowden et al., 2003). Observations suggest that it may be particularly effective for rapid cycling and in the depressed phase of bipolar illness. Anecdotal evidence suggests that gabapentin (Neurontin) may be effective for acute mania, mood stabilization, and rapid cycling. Topiramate (Topamax) has been used mostly as add-on therapy in mixed patient samples with refractory mood disorders. A characteristic of topiramate is that it is more associated with weight loss than weight gain. Controlled trials are needed to evaluate further the efficacy of these and other anticonvulsants (Schatzberg et al., 2003).

Intervention With Antidepressants

Acute bipolar depression has received little scientific study in comparison with unipolar depression. Antidepressant drugs may cause either a switch to mania or a mixed state, and may induce rapid cycling.

Unfortunately, lithium or anticonvulsants are not as effective against depression as they are against mania. However, in a few patients, lithium or anticonvulsants can be used alone with good antidepressant effects. The most common treatment of bipolar depression is an antidepressant combined with a mood stabilizer to "protect" the patient against a manic switch. The antidepressant agents are the same as those used in unipolar illness, although they are sometimes given in lower dosages and for shorter periods of time as a precaution.

Intervention With Antipsychotics

Antipsychotics are prescribed for patients who experience psychosis as a part of bipolar disorder. If patients cannot tolerate mood stabilizers, antipsychotics may be given instead of antidepressants to stabilize the moods. Generally, the antipsychotic dosage is lower than what is prescribed for patients with schizophrenia.

Administering and Monitoring Medication

During acute mania, patients may not believe that they have a psychiatric disorder and refuse to take medication. Because their energy is still high, they can be very creative in avoiding medication. Once patients begin to take medications, symptom improvement should be evident. If a patient is very agitated, a benzodiazepine may be given for a short period.

Monitoring and Managing Side Effects

It is unlikely that patients will take only one medication; they may receive several. In some instances, one agent will be used to augment the effects of another, such as supplemental thyroid hormone to boost antidepressant response in depression. Possible side effects for each medication should be listed and cross-referenced. When a side effect appears, the nurse should document the side effect and notify the prescriber so that further evaluation can be made. In some instances, medications should be changed.

Monitoring for Drug Interactions

It is a well-established practice to combine mood stabilizers with antidepressants or antipsychotics. The previously discussed drug interactions should be considered when caring for a person with bipolar disorder. A big challenge is monitoring alcohol, drugs, OTC medications, and herbal supplements. A complete list of all medications should be maintained and evaluated for any potential interaction. (See Table 20-4 for specific drug interactions.)

Other Somatic Interventions: ECT

ECT may be a treatment alternative for patients with severe mania who exhibit unremitting, frenzied physical activity. Other indications for ECT include acute mania that is unresponsive to antimanic agents and high suicide risk. ECT is safe and effective in patients receiving antipsychotic medications. The use of valproate or carbamazepine will elevate the seizure threshold, requiring some adjustments in treatment.

Teaching Points

For patients who are taking lithium, it is important to explain that a change in salt intake can affect the therapeutic blood level. If there is a reduction in salt intake, the body will naturally retain lithium to maintain homeostasis. This increase in lithium retention can lead to toxicity. Once stabilized on a lithium dose, salt intake should remain constant. This is fairly easy to do, except during the summer, when excessive perspiration can occur. Patients should increase salt intake during periods of perspiration, increased exercise, and dehydration. As most mood stabilizers and antidepressants can cause weight gain, patients should be alerted to this and should be instructed to monitor any changes in eating, appetite, or weight. Weight reduction techniques may need to be instituted. As always, patients should be clearly instructed to check with the nurse or physician before taking any OTC medication or herbal supplements.

Psychological Domain

Assessment

The assessment of the psychological domain should follow the process explained in Chapter 11. Individuals with bipolar disorder can usually participate fully in this part of the assessment.

Mood

By definition, bipolar disorder is a disturbance of mood. If the patient is depressed, using an assessment tool for depression may help determine the severity of depression. If mania predominates, evaluating the quality of the mood (elated, grandiose, irritated, or agitated) becomes important. Usually, mania is determined by clinical observation.

Cognition

In a depressive episode, the individual may not be able to concentrate enough to complete cognitive tasks, such as those called for in the Mini-Mental State Exam (MMSE). During the acute phase of a manic or depressive episode, mental status may be abnormal, and in a manic phase, judgment is impaired by extremely rapid, disjointed, and distorted thinking. Moreover, feelings such as grandiosity can interfere with normal executive functioning.

Thought Disturbances

Psychosis commonly occurs in patients with bipolar disorder, especially during acute episodes of mania. Auditory hallucinations and delusional thinking are part of the clinical picture. In children and adolescents, psychosis may not be so easily detected.

Stress and Coping Factors

Stress and coping are critical assessment areas for a person with bipolar disorder. A stressful event often triggers a manic or depressive episode. In some instances, there may be no apparent stress precipitating the episode, but it is important to discuss the possibility of a specific trigger. Determining the patient's usual coping skills for stresses lays the groundwork for developing interventional strategies. Negative coping skills, such as substance use or aggression, should be identified because these skills need to be replaced with positive coping skills.

Risk Assessment

Patients with bipolar disorder are at high risk for injury to self (Dubovsky, 2005) and others, with 10% to 15% of patients completing suicide. Child abuse, spouse abuse, or other violent behaviours may occur during severe manic episodes; thus, patients should be assessed for suicidal or homicidal risk (APA, 2000a). The risk for relapse and poorer treatment outcomes are associated with obesity. Preventing and treating obesity in patients with bipolar disorder could decrease the morbidity and mortality related to physical illness, enhance psychological well-being, and possibly improve the course of the disorder (Fagiolini, Kupfer, Houck, Novick, & Frank, 2003).

Nursing Diagnoses for Psychological Domain

Nursing diagnoses associated with the psychological domain of bipolar disorder include Disturbed Sensory Perception, Disturbed Thought Processes, Defensive Coping, Risk for Suicide, Risk for Violence, and Ineffective Coping.

Interventions for Psychological Domain

Pharmacotherapy is the primary treatment for bipolar disorder, but it is often unsuccessful unless adjunctive psychosocial interventions are included in the treatment plan. An integration of psychotherapeutic techniques with pharmacotherapy is strongly recommended by clinicians *and* patients (Thase & Sachs, 2000). The most common psychotherapeutic approaches include psychoeducation, individual CBT, individual interpersonal therapy, and adjunctive therapies such as those for substance use (Rothbaum & Astin, 2000).

Several risk factors associated with bipolar disorders make patients more vulnerable to relapses and resistant to recovery. Among these are high rates of non-adherence to medication therapy, obesity, marital conflict, separation, divorce, unemployment, and underemployment. The goals of psychosocial interventions are to address risk factors and associated features that are difficult to address with pharmacotherapy alone. Particularly important are improving medication adherence, decreasing the number and length of hospitalizations and relapses, enhancing social and occupational functioning, improving quality of life, increasing the patient's and family's acceptance of the disorder, and reducing the suicide risk (Scott & Colom, 2005).

Psychoeducation

Psychoeducation is designed to provide information on bipolar disorder and successful treatment and recovery and usually focuses on medication adherence. Research suggests that individuals with bipolar disorder who adhere to their medication have fewer health problems and more life contentment (Darling, Olmstead, Lund, & Fairclough, 2008). The nurse can help by providing information about the illness and obstacles to recovery. Helping the patient to recognize warning signs and symptoms of relapse and to cope with residual symptoms and functional impairment are important interventions. Resistance to accepting the illness and to taking medication, the symbolic meaning of medication taking, and worries about the future can be discussed openly. In the interest of improved medication adherence, it is helpful to listen carefully to patients' concerns about the medication, its dosing schedules, any changes in dosage, and its side effects (see Box 20-8). Health teaching and weight management should be a component of any psychoeducation program. In addition to individual variations in body weight, many of the medications (divalproex sodium, lithium, antidepressants, olanzapine) are associated with weight gain. Monitoring weight and developing individual weight management plans can reduce the risk for relapse and increase the possibility of medication adherence. Overall, the plan to support adherence should be made to fit the attitude, knowledge, and skills of the individual patient.

Psychotherapy

Long-term psychotherapy may help prevent both mania and depression by reducing the stresses that trigger episodes and increasing the patient's acceptance of the need for medication. Patients should be encouraged to keep their appointments with the therapist, be honest and open, do the assigned homework, and give the therapist feedback on how the treatment is working (Kahn, Ross, Printz, & Sachs, 2000).

Social Domain

Assessment

One of the tragedies of bipolar disorder is its effect on social and occupational functioning. Cultural views of mental illness influence the patient's acceptance of the disorder. During illness episodes, patients often behave in ways that jeopardize their social relationships. Losing a job or going through a divorce are common events. When performing an assessment of social function, the nurse should identify changes resulting from a manic or depressive episode.

Nursing Diagnoses for Social Domain

Nursing diagnoses for adults can include Ineffective Role Performance, Interrupted Family Processes, Impaired Social Interaction, Impaired Parenting, and Compromised Family Coping. Diagnoses for children and adolescents can include Delayed Growth and Development and Caregiver Role Strain in family coping with a member with a bipolar disorder.

Interventions for Social Domain

Interventions focusing on the social domain are integral to nursing care for all ages. During mania, patients usually violate others' boundaries. Roommate selection for patients requiring hospital admittance needs to be carefully considered. If possible, a private room is ideal because patients with bipolar disorder tend to irritate others, who quickly tire of the intrusiveness. These patients may miss the cues indicating anger and aggression from others. The nurse should protect the patient with mania from self-harm, as well as harm from other patients.

Support groups are helpful for people with this disorder. Participating in groups allows the person to meet others with the disorder and learn management and preventive strategies. Support groups also are helpful in dealing with the stigma associated with mental illnesses.

Family Interventions

Marital and family interventions are often needed at different periods in the life of a person with bipolar disorder. For the family with a child with this disorder, additional parenting skills are needed to manage the behaviours. The goals of family interventions are to help the family understand and cope with the disorder.

Interventions may range from occasional counselling sessions to intensive family therapy.

Family psychoeducation strategies have been shown to be particularly useful in decreasing the risk for relapse and hospitalization. In a study of 53 patients with mania, half were assigned to a 9-month family-focused psychoeducational group and half to individually focused treatment. Those in family-focused treatment were less likely to be rehospitalized (Rea et al., 2003). For more information, see Box 20-9.

Spiritual Domain

The nursing approach to the spiritual domain in the care of the person with a bipolar disorder is the same as for the person with a major depressive disorder. See Research for Best Practice Box 20-10 for research describing the experience of receiving a psychiatric diagnosis.

◼ EVALUATION AND TREATMENT OUTCOMES

Desired treatment outcomes are stabilization of mood and enhanced quality of life. Primary tools for evaluating outcomes are nursing observation and patient self-report (see Nursing Care Plan 20-1).

◼ CONTINUUM OF CARE

Inpatient Management

Inpatient admission is the treatment setting of choice for patients who are severely psychotic or who are an immediate threat to themselves or others. In acute

BOX 20.10

Research for Best Practice

QUESTION: What is the lived experience of psychiatric diagnosis?

METHOD: Lived experience is an immediate, reflexive response to a happening in life. The experience (phenomenon) of interest in this study was the response to receiving a psychiatric diagnosis, as differentiated from experiencing the illness itself. This phenomenological study, therefore, involved gathering concrete, detailed accounts of participants' experience of diagnosis, including self drawings (before and after diagnosis) that provided an additional means of expressing this personal experience.

FINDINGS: Emphasized in the lived description of psychiatric diagnosis was the notion that the diagnosis places the individual in a context of reflective self-knowledge. Before and after drawings help exemplify participants' perceptions of a "legitimized/de-legitimized self." Below are excerpts, including drawings, of the experiences of two participants, Matt and Jeff.

Matt desperately wanted to avoid being "abnormal." A diagnosis spelled "insanity" and he shuddered at the prospect of it. Why not "bizarre experience" or something less caustic? The diagnosis threatened to reveal "a secret he held to himself about himself"; confronting him with, "I am flawed! Not, I have a flaw, but, I am flawed!" He sketches

"diagnosis" in "Before" and "After" self profiles. Pre-diagnosis self has a halo to arc dark (blue) hair (he interprets this as ominous). With diagnosis there is no evading the ill-fated knowledge and Matt accommodates the diagnosis, coloring his hair bright (green) to represent hope and "self-acceptance."

Jeff views embracing the diagnosis as central in to his mental illness experience in that it supplied him *"a battle-ground for living."* Prior to diagnosis he felt empty, forlorn, immobilized (*"a scarecrow, suspended in a field"*). *Diagnosis* resulted in *"knowledge made knowledgeable"* to him. With that he was able to reformulate (pictured as a snowman). Someone "cared" enough to assist this re-constituting (the therapeutic encounter). Therefore, he is not cold as a snowman (scarf); he wears a smile. Rediscovery of his personal significance (top hat) equips him to take up his future (hands outstretched).

IMPLICATIONS: Understanding what it is like to receive a psychiatric diagnosis is important knowledge for nurses who are caring for persons during this transformative time. With such knowledge, nurses may be better prepared to help patients sustain hope and self-acceptance. It is knowledge that may be transferred to understanding the potential life-changing ramifications of any medical diagnosis.

Diagnosis: Matt Before and After. (From *Hayne Y. [2001]. To be diagnosed – the experience of persons with chronic mental illness* [Unpublished Dissertation]. Edmonton, AB: University of Alberta.)

Diagnosis: Jeff Before and After. (From *Hayne Y. [2001]. To be diagnosed – the experience of persons with chronic mental illness* [Unpublished Dissertation]. Edmonton, AB: University of Alberta.)

Nursing Care Plan 20.1

The Patient with Bipolar Disorder

Steven was a young businessman in the oil sector. He was married with three young children living in a large metropolitan city. When his business began to fail, he lost millions of dollars within weeks. He describes feeling desperate and going into "overdrive" trying to save the company; trying to spare his employees from lay-off; trying to evade the inevitable bankruptcy. "I just wouldn't quit," he says. "Because I wouldn't quit my mind quit. And it just literally went into la-la-land. My mind just shut down. I kind of lost contact with everything." Steven unwittingly stepped in front of a car and was hit. "I jumped up and just carried on," he says. Bystanders, however, mobilized his transport to a hospital emergency department (ED). "The doctor looked at me for 8 seconds and said 'manic depressive!'"

Steven sees his condition as a gift: "I'm very likable ... and creative ... With mania you think faster and when you think faster you process more. So I just process more information quicker. ... "I have the energy that most people can only dream of ... I mean incredible energy ... I can do anything, anytime, anywhere ... And everything seems in its right space. And it can be you have no money, no house, no job, no family, no friends, no food, and you feel incredible. None of that matters! It's like the ultimate high!"

The first hospitalization established a medical regime for Steven and his health stabilized for a time. An initial manic episode very often involves treatment with lithium carbonate resulting in mood stabilization. Recurring mania with episodes of depression may benefit from treatment with TCAs and MAOIs, though this course of action was not necessary for Steven.

Steven found his psychiatric diagnosis was "a destructive (gift) of difference!" "I went from one day being gifted to the next day being mentally ill. That's a very large step." He depicts this in a before-diagnosis drawing, stating, "I had everything before: a wife, 3 children, a home! The sun shone in my world." This is contrasted in an after-diagnosis portrayal, where "the sun is gone." "I lost it all. There is just me! No job, no friends, no home, no family! My wife thought she married a gifted person. When she realized the mental illness, she took the kids and left." Within months of his discharge from the hospital, Steven became confused and disorganized. A restaurant owner reported him for causing a disturbance. When police arrived, he was incoherent and behaving erratically. He was transported to an ED.

From *Hayne Y. (2001). To be diagnosed – the experience of persons with chronic mental illness* (Unpublished Dissertation). Edmonton, AB: University of Alberta.

From *Hayne Y. (2001). To be diagnosed – the experience of persons with chronic mental illness* (Unpublished Dissertation). Edmonton, AB: University of Alberta.

Setting: Acute Care Psychiatric Unit in a General Hospital

Baseline Assessment: From the ED Steven is admitted to acute care inpatient services where he presents with symptoms of mixed bipolar mood disorder. His mood is brittle and he is easily irritated. His speech is pressured. He is unable to account for his behaviour and is exhibiting flight of ideas. Historical records indicate his prior admission and discharge on lithium, which he admits not taking. When asked why he stopped his medication he states, "I completely disagreed with it. I didn't think that my gift needed treatment."

Associated Psychiatric Diagnosis	Medications
Axis I: Bipolar I disorder, most recent episode mixed, severe	Lithium carbonate 300 mg tid × 2 years
Axis II: Deferred (none apparent)	L-Thyroxine 0.1 mg q am × 1 day
Axis III: Hypothyroidism	Clonazepam 0.5 mg bid for sleep and agitation
Axis IV: Social problems (Divorce finalized 18 months ago. Ex-wife has full custody of three children. Patient has supervised visitations.	Carbamazepine added on transfer to be titrated up to 400 mg tid
Axis V: GAF = Current 50 Potential 85	

Continued

Nursing Care Plan 20.1 (Continued)

Nursing Diagnosis 1: Risk for Self-Harm

Defining Characteristics	Related Factors
Potential for life-threatening injury Poor judgement and impulse control Lack of support system	Elation and expansive feelings Excitement vacillating with desolation Loss secondary to finances/job, divorce

Outcomes

Initial	Discharge
1. Will contract no self-harm. 2. Will comply with unit regulations. 3. Will participate in program activities. 4. Will achieve balance in activities of daily living (e.g., rest, hydration, nutrition).	5. Will discuss the complexity of his illness. 6. Will express antecedents of treatment related to mania and depression. 7. Will discuss need for adherence to meds. 8. Will identify antecedents and indicators of impending illness exacerbation.

Interventions

Interventions	Rationale	Ongoing Assessment
Initiate a nurse–patient relationship, demonstrate acceptance of patient as a worthwhile human being through the use of nonjudgmental statements and behaviour.	A sense of worthlessness often underlies despair. The positive therapeutic relationship can maintain the patient's dignity.	Assess the stages of the relationship and determine whether a therapeutic relationship is actually being formed. Identify indicators of trust.
Initiate suicide precautions per hospital policy. Apply vigilant observation routines.	Safety of the individual is a priority with people who have poor impulse control.	Determine risk of self harm.
Obtain a no self-harm contract.	A contract can help the patient maintain safety by encouraging the resistance of impulses.	Determine patient's ability to commit to a contract.

Evaluation

Outcomes	Revised Outcomes	Interventions
Has not harmed self, denies self-harm thoughts/intent. Made a no self-harm contract with nurse, agrees to keep it after discharge.	Absence of risk or self-harm intent will continue. Maintain a no self-harm contract with outpatient mental health provider.	Discontinue precautions incrementally; maintain ongoing assessment for safety. Support and reinforce this contract.

Nursing Diagnosis 2: Impaired Sense of Self and Self-Esteem

Defining Characteristics	Related Factors
Expressions of grandiosity vacillating with expressions of shame and guilt. Lack of success in business endeavours and relationships.	Labile mood (elation and despair noted). Feelings of abandonment secondary to separation from significant others. Feelings of failure secondary to bankruptcy and relationship problems. Unrealistic expectations of self.

Outcomes

Initial	Discharge
1. Realistic self appraisal. 2. Modify excessive and unrealistic self expectations.	3. Verbalize acceptance of personal limitations. 4. Report freedom from untoward symptoms. 5. Avoid behavioural risks.

Continued

Nursing Care Plan 20.1 (Continued)

Interventions

Interventions	Rationale	Ongoing Assessment
Enhance patient's sense of self by being attentive; validate interpretation of what is being said or experienced; help to make consistent, realistic verbalizations.	By showing respect and helping the patient frame happenings realistically, the nurse can support and help build the patient's sense of self.	Determine whether patient confirms realistic interpretation of situations and verbalizes with moderation in rate and volume.
Assist to reframe and redefine negative statements ("not a failure, but a setback").	Reframing an event positively can help the patient view the situation in an alternative way.	Assess whether the patient can actually view the world in a different way.
Problem solve with patient about how to approach finding satisfying employment.	Work is very important to adults. Bankruptcy can decrease self-esteem. Focusing on the possibility of a future job can provide hope.	Assess the patient's problem-solving ability. Note indicators of realistic plans.
Encourage positive physical habits (healthy eating patterns, exercise, adequate sleep).	A healthy lifestyle promotes well-being, increasing self-esteem.	Determine willingness to consider making lifestyle changes.
Teach patient to validate consensually with others.	Low self-esteem is generated by negative interpretations of the world. Through consensual validation, the patient can determine whether others view situations in the same way.	Assess patient's ability to participate in this process.
Teach constructive self appraisal. Helpful exercises might include self-affirmations, imagery, use of humour, meditation/prayer, relaxation.	There are many different approaches that can be practiced to increase self-esteem.	Assess patient's energy level and ability to focus on learning new skills.
Assist in establishing appropriate personal boundaries.	In an attempt to meet their own needs, people with a compromised sense of self often violate other people's boundaries and or allow others to take advantage of them. Helping patients establish their own boundaries will improve the likelihood of needs being met in an appropriate manner.	Assess patient's ability to understand the concept of boundary violation and its significance.
Provide an opportunity within the therapeutic relationship to express thoughts and feelings. Use open-ended statements and questions. Encourage expression of both positive and negative statements.	The individual with compromised self-esteem may have difficulty expressing thoughts and feelings. Varied outlets for expression may help improve how thoughts and feelings are expressed.	Monitor thoughts and feelings that are expressed in order to help the patient examine them.
Explore opportunities for positive socialization.	Individuals with insecurity issues may be in social situations that reinforce artificial self-evaluation. Helping the patient identify new positive situations will present other options.	Assess whether the new situations are potentially positive or are a re-creation of other negative (self-aggrandizing) situations.
Steven began to modify excessive and unrealistic expectations of self.	Strengthen ability to affirm realistic aspects and examine expectations related to work and relationships.	Refer to mental health clinic for cognitive behavioural psychotherapy.
Verbalized defeatist thinking related to finding worthwhile employment.	Identify important aspects of tentative employment so that he can begin looking for a job that has those characteristics.	Attend a support group that focuses on job interviewing skills.
As Steven's mood stabilized, he was able to sleep through the night, and he began eating again. He also expressed positive thoughts about his future.	Maintain a stable mood to promote a positive and realistic self-concept.	Monitor mood and identify antecedents to mood escalation and/or depression.

Continued

Nursing Care Plan 20.1 (Continued)

Nursing Diagnosis 3: Ineffective Individual Coping

Defining Characteristics	Related Factors
Verbalization in inability to cope or ask for help.	Altered mood (alternating mania and depression) caused by changes secondary to body chemistry (bipolar disorder)
Reported difficulty with life stressors	
Compromised ability to problem solve	Altered mood caused by changes secondary to intake of mood-altering substance (alcohol)
Alteration in social participation	
Disinhibited behaviour resulting in self-risk	Unsatisfactory support system
Distorted thought and self-control	Sensory overload secondary to excessive activity
Substance abuse	Unreliable psychological resources for consistency of employment.

Outcomes

Initial	Discharge
1. Accept support through the nurse–patient relationship.	6. Practice new coping skills.
2. Identify areas of ineffective coping.	7. Focus on realistic strengths.
3. Examine current efforts at coping.	
4. Identify realistic areas of strength.	
5. Learn new coping skills.	

Interventions

Interventions	Rationale	Ongoing Assessment
Identify current stresses in Steven's life, including the acceptance of bipolar disorder.	When areas of concern are verbalized by the patient, he will be able to focus on one issue at a time. If he identifies the mental disorder as a stressor, he will more likely be able to develop strategies to deal with it.	Determine whether Steven is able to identify problem areas realistically. Continue to assess for self-risk behaviours.
Identify Steven's strengths in dealing with past stressors.	By focusing on past successes, he can identify strengths and build on them in the future.	Assess if Steven can identify any previous successes in his life.
Assist Steven in discussing, selecting, and practicing positive coping skills (jogging, yoga, thought stopping).	New coping skills take a conscious effort to learn and will at first seem strange and unnatural. Practicing these skills will help build a repertoire of coping strategies.	Assess whether Steven follows through on learning new skills.
Educate patient on the use of alcohol and its relationship to bipolar disorder.	Alcohol is an ineffective coping strategy that can exacerbate the symptoms of bipolar disorder.	Assess for the patient's willingness to control drinking.
Assist patient in coping with bipolar disorder, beginning with education about it.	A mood disorder is a major stressor in a patient's life. To manage the stress, the patient needs a knowledge base.	Determine Steven's knowledge about bipolar disorder.
Administer lithium as ordered (give with food or milk). Reinforce the action, dosage, and side effects. Review laboratory results to determine whether lithium is within therapeutic limits. Assess for toxicity. Recommend a normal diet with normal salt intake; maintenance of adequate fluid intake.	Lithium carbonate is effective in the treatment of bipolar disorder, but it must be managed. Patient should have a thorough knowledge of the medication and side effects.	Assess for target action, side effects, and toxicity.
Administer carbamazepine as ordered, to be titrated up to 400 mg tid. Observe for presence of hypersensitivity to the drug. Teach about action, dosage, and side effects. Emphasize the possibility of drug interaction with alcohol, some antibiotics (and TCAs and MAOIs if these become a treatment option).	Carbamazepine can be effective in bipolar disorder; however, it can increase CNS toxicity when given with lithium carbonate.	Assess for target action, side effects, and toxicity.

Continued

Nursing Care Plan 20.1 (Continued)

Interventions

Interventions	Rationale	Ongoing Assessment
Administer thyroid supplement as ordered. Review laboratory results of thyroid functioning. Discuss the symptoms of hypothyroidism and how they are similar to depression. Emphasize the importance of taking lithium and L-thyroxine. Explain about the long-term effects of lithium on thyroid functioning.	Hypothyroidism can be a side effect of lithium carbonate and also mimics symptoms of depression.	Determine whether patient understands the relationship between thyroid dysfunction and lithium carbonate.

Evaluation

Outcomes	Revised Outcomes	Interventions
Clonazepam 0.5 mg bid for sleep and agitation.		
Steven is easily engaged in a therapeutic relationship. He examined the areas in his life where he coped ineffectively.	Establish a therapeutic relationship with a therapist at the mental health clinic.	Refer to mental health clinic.
He identified his strengths and how he coped with stressors, especially his illness, in the past.	Continue to view illness as a potential stressor that can disrupt life.	Seek advice immediately if there are any problems with medications.
He learned new problem-solving skills and reported that he learned a lot about his medication. He plans to adhere to medication regimen.	Continue to practice new coping skills as stressful situations arise.	Discuss with therapist the outcomes of using new coping skills.

mania, nursing interventions focus on patient safety, as such patients are prone to injury because of hyperactivity and are often unaware of injuries they sustain. Distraction may also be effective when a patient is talking or acting inappropriately. Removal to a quieter environment may be necessary if other interventions have not been successful, but the patient should be carefully monitored. Because patients are often impulsive, disinhibited, and interpersonally inappropriate during acute mania, the nurse should avoid direct confrontations or challenges.

Medication management (Fig. 20-2), including control of side effects and promotion of self-care, is a major nursing responsibility during inpatient hospitalization. Nurses should be familiar with drug–drug interactions (Table 20-4) and with interventions to help control side effects.

Intensive Outpatient Programs

Intensive outpatient programs for several weeks of acute-phase care during a manic or depressive episode are used when hospitalization is not necessary or in order to prevent or shorten hospitalization. These programs are usually called *partial hospitalization* or *day hospitalization*.

Close medication monitoring and milieu therapies that foster the restoration of a patient's previous adaptive abilities are the major nursing responsibilities in these settings.

Setting up frequent office visits and crisis telephone calls are additional nursing interventions that can help to shorten or prevent hospitalization during the acute phase of a manic episode. Psychoeducation that includes the patient and significant others are alternatives. Severely and persistently ill patients may need ongoing intensive treatment, but the frequency of visits can be decreased for patients whose conditions stabilize and who enter the continuation or the maintenance phase of treatment.

Spectrum of Care

In today's health care climate, with efforts to reduce hospitalization, most patients with bipolar disorder are treated as outpatients. Hospitalizations are usually brief, and treatment focuses on restabilization. Patients with mood disorders are likely to need long-term medication regimens and supportive psychotherapy to function in the community. Therefore, medication regimens and additional treatment planning need to be tailored to

Spiritual

1. Openness to remarks regarding life meanings
2. Recognize spiritual distress and allow for conversation about it
3. Seek pastoral presence as warranted
4. Support spiritual activity/practices
5. Nurture hope

Biologic

1. Administer psychopharmacologic agents, such as hthium
2. Obtain serum drug levels
3. Assist with measures to enhance sleep and rest
4. Institute safety precautions
5. Plan for medication adherence

Social

1. Integrate family therapeutic interventions
2. Promote use of appropriate social skills
3. Refer to community agencies for support
4. Institute protective environmental precautions

Psychological

1. Assist with psychotherapy treatment program
2. Monitor behaviour
3. Avoid confrontation
4. Psychoeducation

FIGURE 20.2 Holistic interventions for patients with bipolar I disorder.

individual needs. Patients need extended and continued follow up to monitor medication trials and side effects, reinforce self-care management, and provide continued psychosocial support (see Chapter 4).

Mental Health Promotion

Mental health promotion activities should be the focus during remissions. During this period, patients have an opportunity to learn new coping skills that promote positive mental health. Stress management and relaxation techniques can be practiced for use when needed. A plan for managing emerging symptoms can also be developed during this period.

SUMMARY OF KEY POINTS

▫ Mood disorders are characterized by persistent or recurring disturbances in mood that cause significant psychological distress and functional impairment. Moods can be broadly categorized as manic or dysphoric (typified by exaggerated feelings of elation or irritability) or depressive or dysthymic (typified by feelings of sadness, hopelessness, loss of interest, and fatigue).

▫ Primary mood disorders include both depressive disorders (unipolar depression) and manic-depressive disorders (bipolar disorders).

▫ Genetics undoubtedly play a role in the etiology of mood disorders. Risk factors include family history of mood disorders; prior mood episodes; lack of social support; stressful life events; substance abuse; and medical problems, particularly chronic or terminal illnesses.

▫ The recommended depression treatment guidelines include antidepressant medication, alone or with psychotherapeutic management or psychotherapy; ECT for severe depression; or light therapy (phototherapy) for patients with seasonal depressive symptoms.

▫ Nurses must be knowledgeable about antidepressant medications: their therapeutic effects and associated side effects, toxicity, dosage ranges, and contraindications. Nurses must also be familiar with ECT protocols and associated interventions. Patient education and the provision of emotional support during the course of treatment are also nursing responsibilities.

▫ Many symptoms of depression, such as weight and appetite changes, sleep disturbance, decreased energy, and fatigue, are similar to those of medical illnesses. Assessment includes a thorough medical history and physical examination to detect or rule out medical or psychiatric comorbidity.

□ Bio/psycho/social/spiritual assessment includes assessing mood; speech patterns; thought content and processes; suicidal or homicidal thoughts; cognition and memory; social factors such as patterns of relationship, quality of support systems, and changes in occupational functioning; and spiritual beliefs and practices. Several self-report scales are helpful in evaluating depressive symptoms.

□ Establishing and maintaining a therapeutic nurse–patient relationship is key to successful outcomes. Nursing interventions that foster the therapeutic relationship include being available in times of crisis, providing understanding and education to patients and their families regarding goals of treatment, providing encouragement and feedback concerning the patient's progress, providing guidance in the patient's interpersonal interactions (within the work environment, the community), and helping to set and monitor realistic goals.

□ Psychosocial interventions for mood disorders include self-care management, cognitive therapy, behaviour therapy, interpersonal therapy, patient and family education regarding the nature of the disorder and treatment goals, marital and family therapy, and group therapy that includes medication maintenance support groups and other consumer-oriented support groups.

□ Bipolar disorders are characterized by one or more manic episodes or mixed mania (co-occurrence of manic and depressive states) that cause marked impairment in social activities, occupational functioning, and interpersonal relationships and may require hospitalization to prevent self-harm.

□ Manic episodes are periods in which the individual experiences abnormally and persistently elevated, expansive, or irritable mood characterized by inflated self-esteem, decreased need to sleep, excessive energy or hyperactivity, racing thoughts, easy distractibility, and inability to stay focused. Other symptoms can include hypersexuality and impulsivity.

□ Similar to treatment of major depressive disorder, pharmacotherapy is the cornerstone of treatment of bipolar illness, but adjunctive psychosocial interventions are needed as well. Pharmacologic therapy includes treatment with mood stabilizers alone or in combination with antipsychotics or benzodiazepines if psychosis, agitation, or insomnia is present and antidepressants for unremitted depression. ECT is a valuable alternative for patients with severe mania that do not respond to other treatment.

□ Recent major advances in bipolar disorder treatment research validate the efficacy of integrated psychosocial and pharmacologic treatment involving family or couples therapies, psychoeducational programs, and individual cognitive-behavioural or interpersonal therapies.

CRITICAL THINKING CHALLENGES

1 A patient comes into a physician's office distraught and expressing concerns about her ability to cope with her current situation. Describe how you would assess this patient for suicide risk.

2 Describe how you would approach the patient described above if you determined that she was suicidal.

3 Discuss difficulties in the differential diagnosis of bipolar disorder in the manic phase and other medical and psychiatric disorders. List the information you would use to rule out the other diagnoses when dealing with a patient who appears to have mania.

4 Describe how you would approach a patient who is expressing concern that the diagnosis of bipolar disorder will negatively affect his or her social and work relationships.

5 Your depressed patient does not seem inclined to talk about his or her depression. Describe the measures you would take to initiate a therapeutic relationship.

6 Your patient with mania is experiencing physical hyperactivity that is interfering with his or her sleep and nutrition. Describe the actions you would take to meet the patient's needs for nutrition and rest.

7 Prepare a hypothetical discussion with a patient with potential bipolar disorder concerning the advantages and disadvantages of lithium versus divalproex sodium for treatment of bipolar disorder.

8 Prepare a hypothetical discussion with a depressed patient with potential unipolar disorder concerning the advantages and disadvantages of each of the major classifications of antidepressants.

WEB LINKS

www.bpkids.org   This is the site of the Child & Adolescent Bipolar Foundation (CABF), a parent-led, not-for-profit membership organization that maintains an extensive website of information and support for families and youth who have bipolar disorder. The organization has a large professional advisory board of experts in the field, including Kay Redfield Jamison, author of *An Unquiet Mind* (1995), a book about her own struggles with bipolar disorder. While much of the information is available to anyone visiting the website, for a donation families and professionals can obtain membership access to chat rooms and other resources.

www.canmat.org   The site of the Canadian Network for Mood and Anxiety Treatment with information for health professionals and the public, including guidelines for management and treatment.

www.camimh.ca   This is the site of the Canadian Alliance on Mental Illness and Mental Health (CAMIMH), which displays the services of member mental health organizations, including health care practitioners, consumers, and their families. The organization is committed to raising mental health awareness and making accessibility to care and support for the mentally ill and their families a priority for government and communities.

www.casp-acps.ca   This is the site of the Canadian Association for Suicide Prevention, which provides information regarding suicide and the resources related to its prevention, for example, the location of crisis centres, survivor support groups, and related library materials. Guidelines to minimize the suicide risk of loved ones are available here.

www.cmha.ca   This is the site of the Canadian Mental Health Association (CMHA), which uses a wellness model to approach such topics as mental fitness and how it is defined, acquired, and maintained across the life span.

www.cpa.ca   This is the site of the Canadian Psychological Association, which takes an advisory role to people wanting to know about issues and care alternatives. Areas of focus include mental health problems related to mood disorders and the psychological factors necessary to maintain wellness in the context of such mood-related disorders.

www.mooddisorderscanada.ca   This is the site of the Mood Disorders Society of Canada (MDSC), a volunteer organization with a commitment to optimizing the quality of life for people with mood disorders. The MDSC gives a voice to consumers by establishing a national research agenda and developing strategies of care.

www.nimh.nih.gov   This is the site of the National Institute of Mental Health (NIMH), which provides a forum for worldwide research into mental illness. In addition to offering a wealth of information on the latest research in the field, the site offers education information pamphlets on depression, bipolar disorder, and other mental illnesses that can be ordered or printed free of charge. These publications are in the public domain and can be reproduced without copyright infringement, as long as authorship is acknowledged.

www.nnmh.ca   This is the site of the National Network for Mental Health, which functions as an advocate and educational resource for Canadian mental health consumers and their families and friends. The organization's goal is to unite and empower individuals.

www.obad.ca   This is the site of the Organization for Bipolar Affective Disorders (OBAD). This organization offers peer support for anyone affected by mood disorders, aiming to assist them to be active in their recovery and gain a sense of resolution in their lives.

www.psychguides.com/bipolar   A copy of *Treatment of Bipolar Disorder: A Guide for Patients and Families* can be downloaded from this site.

MOVIES, NOVELS, AND BIOGRAPHIES

About Schmidt: 2002. Jack Nicholson plays Warren Schmidt, a 67-year-old man who retires from his job as an insurance company executive. He experiences work withdrawal and a lack of direction for his retirement. His is irritated by his wife and has no idea what to do to fill his days. He is moved by a television program to sponsor a child in Africa, with whom he begins a long, one-sided correspondence. When his wife dies unexpectedly, he is initially numb, then sad, and finally angry when he discovers that she had once had an affair with his best friend. He is estranged from his only daughter, whose wedding to a man he feels is beneath her, is imminent. The movie follows Warren as he searches for connection and meaning in his life. Warren Schmidt demonstrates a common phenomenon among older adults when they retire. He also shows the impact of grief superimposed on initial dysthymia or depression.

VIEWING POINTS: Look for the changes in Schmidt's manifestations of depression in different situations. Note how he experiences the various stages of grieving. What do you think about Schmidt's search for significance and meaning in his life?

Mad Love: 1995. Casey Roberts (Drew Barrymore), a pretty high-school student, experiences bipolar disorder; Matt Leyland (Chris O'Donnell) is a fellow student who falls in love with her. Matt, unaware of Casey's medical condition and struggling with his own family issues, becomes enraptured with Casey and perceives her as a free spirit. When Casey attempts suicide and is admitted to a psychiatric unit, Matt helps her escape. To evade their parents, they embark on a trip to Mexico, a journey filled with misadventure. Despite Casey's erratic behaviour, Matt doesn't develop insight into Casey's illness until her behaviour becomes so disorganized that he must face it and try to help her get treatment and become well.

VIEWING POINTS: The euphoria, irritability, risk taking, poor judgment, and labile mood that are hallmarks of bipolar disorder are well illustrated in this movie, as is the depression that underlies mania. We can see the impact of bipolar disorder on loved ones. Look for Casey's inability to control her behaviour. Note her heightened perception of the sensory stimulation occurring around her. What other psychiatric diagnoses might resemble bipolar disorder? Consider the symptoms of borderline personality disorder, narcissistic disorder, and attention deficit hyperactivity disorder.

Mr. Jones: 1993. This film is about a musician, Mr. Jones (Richard Gere), and his psychiatrist. In his manic state, Mr. Jones is a charismatic, charming individual who persuades a contractor to hire him, proceeds to the roof of the building, and prepares to fly off the roof. He withdraws large sums of money from the bank. He knows that he has bipolar disorder but refuses to take his medication because of the side effects. He has episodes of depression during which he becomes suicidal. Once hospitalized, he struggles with trying to find a life on medication.

Viewers can gain insight into the impact of mental illness on the promising career of a classical musician. This film illustrates the ways in which interpersonal relationships are affected by a psychiatric disorder. Unfortunately, the unethical romantic relationship between Mr. Jones and his psychiatrist detracts from the quality of the film's content.

VIEWING POINTS: Why does the diagnosis of paranoid schizophrenia not fit Mr. Jones' clinical picture in the admitting room? Identify the antecedents to the manic and depressive episodes. At what point is the physician–patient relationship first compromised? Are there early warning signs that should have alerted the psychiatrist that she was violating professional boundaries?

REFERENCES

Abela, J. R. Z., Brozina, K., & Haigh, E. P. (2002). An examination of the response styles theory of depression in third- and seventh-grade children: A short-term longitudinal study. *Journal of Abnormal Child Psychology, 30*(5), 515–527.

Alda, M., & Grof, P. (2000). Genetics and lithium response in bipolar disorders. In J. C. Soares & S. Gershon (Eds.), *Bipolar disorders: Basic mechanisms and therapeutic implications* (pp. 529–543). New York, NY: Marcel Dekker.

American Psychiatric Association. (2000a). *Desk reference to the diagnostic criteria from DSM-IV-TR.* Arlington, VA: Author.

American Psychiatric Association. (2000b). *Diagnostic and statistical manual of mental disorders* (4th ed., Text revision). Washington, DC: Author.

American Psychiatric Association. (2002). *Compendium of practice guidelines for the treatment of psychiatric disorders.* Washington, DC: Author.

Anandarajah, G., & Hight, E. (2001). Spirituality and medical practice: Using the HOPE questions as a practical tool for spiritual assessment, *American Family Physician, 63*(1), 81–89.

Barnes, C., & Mitchell, P. (2005). Considerations in the management of bipolar disorder in women. *Australian and New Zealand Journal of Psychiatry, 39*(8), 662–673.

Barney, L. J., Griffiths, K. M., Jorm, A. F., & Christensen, H. (2006). Stigma about depression and its impact on help-seeking intentions. *Australian & New Zealand Journal of Psychiatry, 40*(11), 51–54.

Belmaker, R. H., & Yaroslavsky, Y. (2000). Perspectives for new pharmacological interventions. In J. C. Soares & S. Gershon (Eds.), *Bipolar disorders: Basic mechanisms and therapeutic implications* (pp. 507–527). New York, NY: Marcel Dekker.

Bowden, C. L., Calabrese, J. R., McElroy S. L., Gyulai, L., Wassef, A., Petty, F., et al. (2000). A randomized placebo-controlled 12-month trial of divalproex and lithium in treatment of out patients with bipolar disorder. *Archives of General Psychiatry, 57,* 481–489.

Bowden, C. L., Calabrese, J. R., Sachs, G., Yatham, L. N., Asghar, S. A., Hompland, M., et al. (2003). A placebo-controlled 18-month trial of lamotrigine and lithium maintenance treatment in recently manic or hypomanic patients with bipolar 1 disorder. *Archives of General Psychiatry, 60*(4), 392–400.

Canadian Community Health Survey. (2003). *Mental health and well-being.* Retrieved August 24, 2005, from http://www.statcan.ca/Daily/English/030903/d030903a.htm

Canadian Nurses Association. (2005). *Standards and best practices.* Retrieved August 30, 2005, from http://www.cna-nurses.ca/CNA/practice/standards/default_e.aspx

Casacalenda, N., Perry, J. C., & Looper, K. (2002). Remission in major depressive disorder: A comparison of pharmacotherapy, psychotherapy, and control condition. *American Journal of Psychiatry, 159*(8), 1354–1360.

Caspi, A., Sudgen, K., Moffit, T.E., Taylor, A., Craig, I.W., Harrington, H., et al. (2003). Influence of life stress on depression: Moderation by a polymorphism in the 5-TT gene. *Science, 301*(5631), 386–389.

Corcoran, J., & Walsh, J. (2009a). Bipolar disorder. In J. Corcoran & J. Walsh (Eds.), *Mental health in social work* (pp. 216–241). Boston, MA: Pearson Education.

Corcoran, J., & Walsh, J. (2009b). Depressive disorders. In J. Corcoran & J. Walsh (Eds.), *Mental health in social work* (pp. 189–215). Boston, MA: Pearson Education.

Cutler, J. L., & Marcus, E. R. (1999). Mood disorders. In *Psychiatry.* Philadelphia, PA: W. B. Saunders.

Darling, C., Olmstead, S., Lund, V., & Fairclough, J. (2008). Bipolar disorder: Medication adherence and life contentment. *Archives of Psychiatric Nursing, 22*(3), 113–126.

Donati, R. J., & Rasenick, M. M. (2003). G protein signaling and the molecular basis of antidepressant action. *Life Science, 73*(1), 1–17.

Dubovsky, S. L. (2005). Treatment of bipolar depression. *Psychiatric Clinics of North America, 28*(2), 349–370.

Ebmeier, K. P., Donaghey, C., & Steele, J. D. (2006). Recent developments and current controversies in depression. *Lancet, 367,* 153–167.

Edmunds, K., & Kinnaird-Iler, E. (2005). In L. L. Stamler & L. Yiu (Eds.), *Community health nursing: A Canadian perspective* (pp. 247–264). Toronto, ON: Pearson Prentice Hall.

Even, C., Schroder, C. M., Friedman, S., & Rouillon, F. (2008). Efficacy of light therapy in nonseasonal depression: A systematic review. *Journal of Affective Disorders, 108,* 11–23.

Fagiolini, A., Kupfer, D. J., Houck, P. R., Novick, D. M., & Frank, E. (2003). Obesity as a correlate of outcome in patients with bipolar I disorder. *American Journal of Psychiatry, 160*(1), 112–117.

Fallot, R. (2007). Spirituality and religion in recovery: Some current issues. *Psychiatric Rehabilitation Journal, 30*(4), 261–270.

Felitti, V. (2007). The tragic imprint of childhood adversity. In *Alberta Mental Health Board (AMHB), Mending Minds: Information Supplement.* Proceedings of the Mental Health Research Showcase, Alberta, Canada.

Fischer, C. E. (2002). A clinician's guide to interpreting cognitive measures in clinical trials for Alzheimer's disease. *Canadian Journal of Psychiatry.* Retrieved August 31, 2005, from http://ww1.cpa-apc.org:8080/Publications/Archives/Bulletin/2002/june/geriatricPsych.asp

Gavin, N., Gaynes, B., Lohr, K., Meltzer-Brody, S., Gartlehner, G., & Swinson, T. (2005). Perinatal depression: A systematic review of prevalence and incidence. *Obstetrician Gynecology, 106,* 1071–1083.

Goldberg, J. F., Garno, J. L., Leon, A. C., Kocsis, J. H., & Portera, L. (1999). A history of substance abuse complicates remission from acute mania in bipolar disorder. *Journal of Clinical Psychiatry, 60,* 733–740.

Goldstein, B. I., & Levitt, A. (2006). Is current alcohol consumption associated with increased lifetime prevalence of major depression and suicidality? Results from a pilot community survey. *Comprehensive Psychiatry, 47*(5), 330–333.

Goossens, P., van Wijngaarden, B., Knoppert-van der Klein, E., & van Achterberg. (2008). Family caregiving in bipolar disorder: Caregiver consequences, caregiver coping styles, and caregiver distress. *International Journal of Social Psychiatry, 54*(4), 303–316.

Grunze, H., Amann, B., Dittmann, S., & Walden, J. (2002). Clinical relevance and possibilities of bipolar rapid cycling. *Neuropsychobiology, 45*(Suppl. 1), 20–26.

Halter, M. J. (2004). The stigma of seeking care and depression. *Archives of Psychiatric Nursing, 18*(5), 178–184.

Hanley, N. R., & Van de Kar, L. D. (2003). Serotonin and the neuroendocrine regulation of the hypothalamic-pituitary-adrenal axis in health and disease. *Vitamins and Hormones: Advances in Research and Applications, 66,* 189–225.

Health Canada. (2002). *A Report on mental illness in Canada.* Ottawa, ON: Author.

Hirschfeld, R. M., Baker, J. D., Wozniak, P., Tracy, K., & Sommerville, K. W. (2003). The safety and early efficacy of oral-loaded divalproex versus standard-titration divalproex, lithium, olanzapine, and placebo in the treatment of acute mania associated with bipolar disorder. *Journal of Clinical Psychiatry, 64*(7), 841–846.

Hirschfeld, R. M., Lewis, L., & Vornik, L. A. (2003). Perceptions and impact of bipolar disorder: How far have we really come? Results of the national depressive and manic-depressive association 2000 survey of individuals with bipolar disorders. *Journal of Clinical Psychiatry, 64*(2), 161–174.

Hoblyn, J. (2004). Bipolar disorder in later life: Older adults presenting with new onset manic symptoms usually have underlying medical or neurologic disorder. *Geriatrics, 59*(6), 41–44.

Hodge, D. R. (2006). A template for spiritual assessment: A review of the JCAHO requirements and guidelines for implementation. *Social Work, 51*(4), 317–326.

Johnson, L., Andersson-Lundman, G., Aberg-Wistedt, A., & Mathe, A. A. (2000). Age of onset in affective disorder: Its correlation with hereditary and psychosocial factors. *Journal of Affective Disorders, 59*(2), 139–148.

Kahn, D. A., Ross, R., Printz, D. J., & Sachs, G. S. (2000). Treatment of bipolar disorder: A guide for patients and families. In G. S. Sachs, D. J. Printz, D. A. Kahn, D. Carpenter, & J. P. Docherty (Eds.), *The expert consensus guideline series: Medication treatment of bipolar disorder 2000* (pp. 1–8). Retrieved November 18, 2009, from http://www.psychguides.com/Bipolar_2000.pdf

Keck, P. E., Mendlwicz, J., Calabrese, J. R., Fawcett, J., Suppes, T., Vestergaard, P. A., et al. (2000). A review of randomized controlled clinical trials in acute mania. *Journal of Affective Disorders, 59*(Suppl.1), 31–37.

Keogh, B., & Doyle, L. (2008). Psychopharmacological adverse effects. *Mental Health Practice, 11*(6), 28–30.

King Blood, R. J. (2005). Aboriginal Canadians. In L. L. Stamler & L. Yiu (Eds.), *Community health nursing: A Canadian perspective* (pp. 239–246). Toronto, ON: Pearson Prentice Hall.

Kirby, J. S., & Baucom, D. H. (2007). Treating emotion dysregulation in a couples context: A pilot study of a couples skills group intervention. *Journal of Marital and Family Therapy, 33*(3), 375.

Koczmara, C., Perri, D., Hyland, S., & Rousseaux, L. (2005). Meperidine (Demerol) safety issues. *Dynamics, 16*(1), 8–12.

Kovacs, M. (2001). Gender and the course of major depressive disorder through adolescence in clinically referred youngsters. *Journal of the American Academy of Child and Adolescent Psychiatry, 40*, 1079–1085.

Kowatch, R. A., & DelBello, M. P. (2005). Pharmacotherapy of children and adolescents with bipolar disorder. *Psychiatric Clinics of North America, 28*(2), 385–397.

Lam, R. W., & Kennedy, S. H. (2004). Prescribing antidepressants for depression in 2005: Recent concerns and recommendations. *Canadian Journal of Psychiatry, 49*(12), 1–6.

Leung, R. (Nov. 21, 2004). Carrey: Life is too beautiful. *60 Minutes*, CBS NEWS. Retrieved November 18, 2009, from http://www.cbsnews.com/stories/2004/11/18/60minutes/main656547.shtml

Markley, V. N. (2008). Mood disorders. In P. G. O'Brien, W. Z. Kennedy, & K. A. Ballard (Eds.), *Psychiatric mental health nursing: An introduction to theory and practice* (pp. 316–334). Mississauga, ON: Jones and Bartlett Publishers.

Marques-Deak, A., Cizza, G., & Sternberg, E. (2005). Brain-immune interactions and disease susceptibility. *Molecular Psychiatry, 10*(3), 239–250.

Maser, J. D., Akiskal, H. S., Schettler, P., Scheftner, W., Mueller, T., Endicott, J., et al. (2002). Can temperament identify affectively ill patients who engage in lethal or near-lethal suicidal behaviour? A 14-year prospective study. *Suicide and Life-Threatening Behavior, 32*(1), 10–32.

Massey, K., Gitchett, G., & Roberts, P. A. (2004). Assessment and diagnosis in spiritual care. In N. L. Mauk & K. L. Schmidt (Eds.), *Spiritual care in nursing practice* (pp. 209–242). Philadelphia, PA: Lippincott Williams & Wilkins.

McCuffin, P., Rijsdijk, F., Andrew, J., Sham, P., Katz, R., & Cardno, A. (2003). The heritability of bipolar affective disorder and the genetic relationship to unipolar depression. *Archives of General Psychiatry, 60*(5), 497–502.

McCuistion, L. E., & Gutierrez, K. J. (2002). *Real-world nursing survival guide: Pharmacology*. Philadelphia, PA: WB Saunders.

McElheran, W., Eaton, P., Rupcich, C., Basinger, M., & Johnston, D. (2004). Shared mental health care: The Calgary model. *Families, Systems, & Health, 22*(4), 424–438.

Nolen-Hoeksem, S. (2002). Gender differences in depression. In I. H. Gotlib & C. Hammen (Eds.), *Handbook of depression* (pp. 492–509). New York, NY: Guilford Press.

Official Robert Munsch website, retrieved November 19, 2009, from http://www.robertmunsch.com/

Osuji, I. J., & Cullum, C. M. (2005). Cognition in bipolar disorder. *Psychiatric Clinics of North America, 28*(2), 427–441.

Payne, J. L., Potash, J. B., & DePaulo, J. R. (2005). Recent findings on the genetic basis of bipolar disorder. *Psychiatric Clinics of North America, 28*(2), 481–498.

Perlick, D., Rosenheck, R., Miklowitz, D., Chessick, C., Wolff, N., Kaczynski, R., et al. (2007). Prevalence and correlates of burden among caregivers of patients with bipolar disorder enrolled in the Systematic Treatment Enhancement Program for Bipolar Disorder. *Bipolar Disorders, 9*, 262–273.

Rea, M. M., Tompson, M. C., Miklowitz, D. J., Goldstein, M. J., Hwang, S., & Mintz, J. (2003). Family-focused treatment versus individual treatment for bipolar disorder: Results of a randomized clinical trial. *Journal of Consulting Clinical Psychology, 71*(3), 482–492.

Remick, R. A. (2002). Diagnosis and management of depression in primary care: A clinical update and review. *Canadian Medical Association Journal, 167*(11), 1253–1260.

Rothbaum, B. O., & Astin, M. C. (2000). Integration of pharmacotherapy and psychotherapy for bipolar disorder. *Journal of Clinical Psychiatry, 61*(Suppl. 9), 68–75.

Schatzberg, A. F., Cole, J. O., & DeBattista, C. (2003). *Manual of clinical psychopharmacology* (4th ed.). Washington, DC: American Psychiatric Publishing.

Schmidt, K. L., & Mauk, N. L. (2004). Spirituality as a life journey. In N. L. Mauk & K. L. Schmidt (Eds.), *Spiritual care in nursing practice* (pp. 1–19). Philadelphia, PA: Lippincott Williams & Wilkins.

Scott, J., & Colom, F. (2005). Psychosocial treatments for bipolar disorders. *Psychiatric Clinics of North America, 28*(2), 371–384.

Sheline, Y. I. (2003). Neuroimaging studies of mood disorder effects on the brain. *Biological Psychiatry, 54*(3), 338–352.

Stahl, S. (2000). *Essential psychopharmacology: Neuroscientific basis and practical applications*. Cambridge, MA: Cambridge University Press.

Statistics Canada. (2004a). *Bipolar disorder, social support and work. Supplement to Health Reports*. Ottawa, ON: Author. Retrieved November 19, 2009, from http://www.statcan.ca/english/freepub/82–003-SIE/2004000/pdf/82–003-SIE20040007443.pdf

Statistics Canada. (2004b). *How healthy are Canadians? Focus on mental health*. Ottawa, ON: Author. Retrieved November 19, 2009, from http://www.statcan.ca/english/freepub/82–003-SIE/2004000/pdf/82–003-SIE2004000.pdf

Statistics Canada. (2004c). The people: Major causes of death. Ottawa, ON: Author. Retrieved November 19, 2009, from http://www43.statcan.ca/02/02b/02b_003_e.htm#t01

Thase, M. E., & Sachs, G. S. (2000). Bipolar depression: Pharmacotherapy and related therapeutic strategies. *Biological Psychiatry, 48*, 558–572.

Wong, J. (1999, May 26). Lunch with Robert Munsch. *The Globe and Mail*.

Wong-McDonald, A. (2007). Spirituality and psychosocial rehabilitation: Empowering persons with serious psychiatric disabilities at an inner-city community program. *Psychiatric Rehabilitation Journal, 30*(4), 295–300.

Wright, L. M., & Leahey, M. (2005). *Nurses and families: A guide to family assessment and intervention* (4th ed.). Philadelphia, PA: FA Davis.

Yatham, L., Kennedy, S., O'Donovan, C., Parikh, S., MacQueen, G., McIntyre, R., Sharma, V., & Beaulieu, S. (2006). Canadian Network for Mood and Anxiety Treatments (CANMAT) guidelines for the management of patients with bipolar disorder: update 2007. *Bipolar Disorders, 8*, 721–739.

Zhang, Y., Hauser, U., Conty, C., Emrich, H. M., & Dietrich, D. E. (2007). Familial risk for depression and P3b component as a possible neurocognitive vulnerability marker. *Neuropsychobiology, 55*, 14–20.

CHAPTER 21

Anxiety Disorders

Kathleen Hegadoren

Adapted from the chapter "Anxiety Disorders" by
Robert B. Noud and Kathy Lee

KEY CONCEPTS

- anxiety
- compulsions
- obsessions
- panic

LEARNING OBJECTIVES

After studying this chapter, you will be able to:

- Differentiate normal anxiety responses to stressors and fear from responses suggestive of an anxiety disorder.
- Describe anxiety disorders as a heterogeneous collection of disorders with anxiety as the core component.
- Discuss the similarities and differences in the epidemiology, etiology, symptomatology, and treatment of anxiety disorders.
- Discuss the relevant theories and neurobiologic correlates of the anxiety disorders.
- Discuss the bio/psycho/social/spiritual treatment approaches used for patients with anxiety disorders.
- Identify the key components of nursing care for patients with anxiety disorders.
- Develop a nursing care plan through the continuum of care for patients with panic disorder.
- Identify bio/psycho/social/spiritual indicators for four levels of anxiety and nursing interventions appropriate for each level.

KEY TERMS

•allostasis•anxiolytic•depersonalization•distraction•exposure therapy•existential anxiety•flooding•generalized anxiety disorder•interoceptive conditioning•obsessive-compulsive disorder•panic disorder•panic control treatment•phobia•positive self-talk•posttraumatic stress disorder•systematic desensitization

*A*nxiety is an uncomfortable feeling of apprehension or dread that occurs in response to internal or external stimuli and can result in physical, emotional, cognitive, and behavioural symptoms.

All symptoms of anxiety disorders can be found in healthy individuals given particular circumstances. It is the severity of the symptoms and the degree to which they impact on social, occupational, and interpersonal functioning that move anxiety symptoms from normal responses to an anxiety disorder. The anxiety disorders discussed in this chapter include generalized anxiety disorder, obsessive-compulsive disorder, posttraumatic stress disorder, acute stress disorder, social phobia, panic disorder, and specific phobias. Dissociation as a response to overwhelming anxiety is discussed as it pertains to panic disorder, acute stress disorder, and posttraumatic stress disorder. However, dissociative disorders will not be discussed (see Chapters 25 and 37 for further discussion on dissociative disorders).

KEY CONCEPT **Anxiety** is the apprehension or dread in response to internal or external stimuli that can be experienced in physical, emotional, cognitive, and/or behavioural ways.

The anxiety disorders as described in the *Diagnostic and Statistical Manual of Mental Disorders*, 4th ed., Text Revision (*DSM-IV-TR*; American Psychiatric Association [APA], 2000), are a heterogeneous collection of disorders, but all have anxiety symptoms as a dominant component of the clinical presentation. Many of these anxiety disorders are managed through outpatient clinics and private psychological treatment regimes. Hospitalization is usually limited to those with comorbid depressive disorder or acute deterioration of functioning. Anxiety disorders are often difficult to treat, and symptoms often persist over many years. Thus, these disorders are frequently chronic in their longitudinal course, with acute episodes occurring in response to stressors or other health problems.

NORMAL VERSUS ABNORMAL ANXIETY RESPONSE

Anxiety is an unavoidable human condition that takes many forms and serves different purposes. One's response to anxiety can be positive and motivate one to act, or it can produce paralyzing fear, causing inaction. Normal anxiety is described as being of realistic intensity and duration for the situation and is followed by relief behaviours intended to reduce or prevent more anxiety (Peplau, 1989). Normal anxiety response is appropriate to the situation, can be dealt with without repression, and can be used to help the patient identify what underlying problem has caused the anxiety. McEwen (2005) conceptualizes normal responses as **allostasis**, the adaptive processes that maintain homeostasis through the production of various brain and peripheral stress-related chemicals. These mediators of our stress responses promote adaptation to perceived threat or stress. However, they also contribute to allostatic overload, the cumulative wear and tear on biologic systems that can increase the risk for stress-related disorders and physical health problems like cardiovascular and metabolic disorders.

During a perceived threat, rising anxiety levels cause physical and emotional changes in all individuals. A normal emotional response to anxiety consists of three parts: physiologic arousal, cognitive processes, and coping strategies. Physiologic arousal, or the fight-or-flight response, is the signal that an individual is facing a threat. Cognitive processes decipher the situation and decide whether the perceived threat should be approached or avoided. Coping strategies are employed to resolve the threat. Table 21-1

summarizes many physical, affective, cognitive, and behavioural symptoms associated with anxiety.

OVERVIEW OF ANXIETY DISORDERS

Anxiety disorders are the most common mental health problem in Canada, according to Statistics Canada's (2003) Community Health Survey of Mental Health and Wellbeing, with approximately 4.7% of Canadians having such a disorder. Survey results confirm that women experience anxiety disorders more often than men: 5.8% versus 3.6%, respectively. Anxiety disorders affect individuals of all ages. Edmonton Alberta studies have found prevalence rates of anxiety disorder in adults (18 years and older) to be 6.5% (Bland, Newman, & Orn, 1988) and in elderly (65 years and older) to be 3.1% (Newman, Bland, & Orn, 1998). The lifetime prevalence rate of social anxiety disorder is reported to be about 10% (Sareen & Stein, 2000). Of depressed elderly patients, 35% will have at least one anxiety disorder diagnosis (Lenze et al., 2000). Anxiety disorders are the psychiatric disorders most frequently treated in children, with the percentage of children affected comparable to that of asthma (Castellanos & Hunter, 2000). In the Statistics Canada survey (2003), quoted above, 6.5% of persons aged 15 to 24 reported having an anxiety disorder during the past year; and 12% reported having an anxiety disorder over their lifetime. Some evidence suggests a relationship between childhood separation anxiety disorder and atopic disorders (asthma, hives, hay fever, and eczema) and adult-onset panic disorder (Slattery et al., 2002). Indeed, symptoms of obsessive-compulsive disorder (OCD) and social anxiety disorder often begin in adolescence (Regier, Rae, Narrow, Kaelber, & Schatzberg, 1998). Young patients with anxiety disorders often experience separation anxiety disorder, but this is often dismissed as fear of strangers and other signs of anxiety are considered developmentally appropriate. Children and adolescents with anxiety disorders have higher rates of suicidal behaviour, early parenthood, drug and alcohol dependence, and educational underachievement later in life (Woodward, 2001). Early life traumas, a history of physical or sexual abuse, socioeconomic or personal disadvantages, and behavioural inhibition by adults have been associated with an increased risk for anxiety disorders in children (Castellanos & Hunter, 2000; Friedman et al., 2002; Marshall et al., 2000; Woodward, 2001). Some anxiety disorders show evidence of genetic vulnerability, especially panic disorder, obsessive-compulsive disorder, and phobias (Hettema, Neale, & Kendler, 2001). Links have been shown between serotonin transporter and specific brain enzyme polymorphisms and anxiety-related personality in women (Enoch, Xu, Ferro, Harris, & Goldman, 2003; Melke et al., 2001).

Table 21.1	Symptoms of Anxiety		
		Physical	
Cardiovascular	**Neuromuscular**		**Gastrointestinal**
Sympathetic	Increased reflexes		Loss of appetite
Palpitations	Startle reaction		Revulsion toward food
Heart racing	Eyelid twitching		Abdominal discomfort
Increased blood pressure	Insomnia		Diarrhea and vomiting
	Unsteadiness		**Eyes**
Respiratory			Dilated pupils
Rapid breathing	**Skin**		
Difficulty getting air	Face flushed or pale		**Urinary Tract**
Shortness of breath	Sweating		Pressure to urinate
Pressure of chest	Feeling hot or cold		
Shallow breathing			
Lump in throat			
Choking sensations			
Gasping			
Affective	*Cognitive*		*Behavioural*
Edgy	**Sensory-Perceptual**		Inhibited
Impatient	Feeling dazed		Tonic immobility
Uneasy	Objects seem blurred/distant		Flight
Nervous	Environment seems different/unreal,		Avoidance
Wound up	feelings of depersonalization		Impaired coordination
Anxious	Self-consciousness		Restlessness
Fearful	Hypervigilance		Postural collapse
Apprehensive			Hyperventilation
Scared	**Thinking Difficulties**		Jumpy
Frightened	Cannot recall important things		Jittery
Alarmed	Confused		
Terrified	Difficulty focusing attention		
	Difficulty concentrating		
	Fear of losing control or not being able		
	to cope		
	Fear of physical injury or death		
	Fear of going crazy		
	Fear of negative evaluation		
	Frightening visual images		
	Repetitive fearful ideation		

Adapted from Beck, A. T., Emery, C., & Greenberg, R. L. (1985). *Anxiety disorders and phobias: A cognitive perspective* (pp. 23–27). New York, NY: Basic Books.

Generalized Anxiety Disorder

Transient anxiety is an integral part of the human condition and serves as a powerful behavioural motivator. Despite significant changes to this diagnostic category from earlier versions of the DSM, **generalized anxiety disorder** (GAD) remains a controversial diagnosis, with little empirical basis as to what is the boundary between GAD and normal worries. In contrast to everyday worries, GAD must be excessive, persistent, and pervasive, but there are no standards as to what constitutes reasonable versus excessive worrying. Thus, the amount of time spent worrying; the degree of control one has over one's worrying; and the impact on personal, social, and occupational functioning are key components of the assessment of GAD. Despite these ongoing diagnostic issues, GAD can be a debilitating disorder with serious impact on quality of life (Antai-Otong, 2003; Hoffman, Dukes, & Wittchen, 2008).

GAD is considered the most common of the anxiety disorders, with lifetime prevalence rates of 3% to 4% (Kessler, 2000). Onset of GAD is often early in life and often follows a more chronic course, with changes in severity over time related to life events and environmental stressors. Those with GAD often feel frustrated, disgusted with life, demoralized, and hopeless. Comorbid depression is also common (Ballenger et al., 2001). Indeed, only one third of those with GAD have no comorbid disorder (Kessler). Because comorbid psychiatric diagnoses are common, assessing the true prevalence of this disorder is difficult. However, GAD is common, affecting nearly 4% of the population at any given time. Based on large community-based population studies, the lifetime prevalence rate is nearly 10% (Fifer et al., 1994). Of those presenting at anxiety disorder clinics, 25% have GAD as a primary or comorbid diagnosis (APA, 2000). Thus, assessment of the patient with GAD must include the assessment of mood and somatic symptoms. A standardized questionnaire, such as the Penn State Worry Questionnaire (PSWQ) (Meyer et al., 1990), may help assess the severity of the symptoms and health impacts. Like other anxiety disorders, etiological theories focus on genetic vulnerabilities, epigenetic changes that increase anxiety sensitivity, childhood adversities, environmental stressors, and dysregulations of neurotransmitter systems or the neural circuits that underpin fear and fear conditioning (Cassidy, Lichtenstein-Phelps, Sibrava, Thomas, & Borkovec, 2009; Jetty, Charney, & Goddard, 2001; Scherrer et al., 2000).

Obsessive-Compulsive Disorder

Obsessive-compulsive disorder (OCD) is a psychiatric disorder characterized by severe obsessions and/or compulsions that significantly interfere with normal daily routines. Obsessive or compulsive behaviours are not necessarily signs of a psychiatric disorder if they do not persistently and significantly interfere with the person's ability to function. However, obsessions can consume a person's judgment to the degree that most of his or her day is spent performing actions in an attempt to minimize severe anxiety. Affected patients feel chronically anxious and powerless to control the obsessions and compulsions. The APA (2000) described five diagnostic criteria for OCD:

- **Criterion A.** The presence of obsessions or compulsions. Obsessions are defined as (1) persistent thoughts, images, or impulses that are intrusive and inappropriate, causing marked anxiety, and (2) are not simply excessive fretting over real-life situations; (3) the person tries to ignore or suppress the thoughts or tries to neutralize them by some other thought or action; and (4) the person understands that the thoughts are a product of his or her own mind. Compulsions are defined as (1) repetitive in that the person feels that he or she must perform them because of the thoughts or because of rules that must be rigidly followed and (2) actions performed to reduce stress or to prevent a catastrophe from occurring. The actions and thoughts are not realistically connected and are excessive to the situation.
- **Criterion B.** At some point in the disorder, the patient recognizes that the thoughts and actions are unreasonable or excessive. This criterion does not apply to children.
- **Criterion C.** The presence of the thoughts and rituals causes severe disturbance in daily routines, relationships, or occupational function, and these thoughts and rituals are time-consuming, taking longer than 1 hour a day to complete.
- **Criterion D.** The thoughts or behaviours are not a result of another Axis I disorder.
- **Criterion E.** The thoughts or behaviours are not a result of the presence of a substance or a medical condition.

Many obsessive thoughts and compulsive acts are common in OCD. Checking rituals are common in this disorder. These patients must have objects in a certain order, perform motor activities in a rigid fashion, or arrange things in perfect symmetry. They may take a great deal of time to complete even the simplest task. These individuals tend to experience discontent, rather than anxiety, when things are not symmetrical or perfect. Other patients have magical thinking and perform compulsive rituals to ward off an imagined disaster. They use counting rituals to perform doing-and-undoing rituals (e.g., repeatedly turning on and off the alarm clock) to help them feel that a disaster will not occur. Hoarders feel compelled to check their belongings repeatedly to see that all is accounted for, and they may check the garbage to ensure that nothing of value was discarded.

Some patients have obsessions surrounding aggressive acts of hurting someone or themselves. After hitting a bump in the road, for example, these patients may obsess for hours over whether or not they hit a person. Parents may have recurrent intrusive thoughts that they may hurt their child. Patients with religious obsessions obsess over the meaning of sins and whether they have followed the letter of the law. They tend to be hypermoral and have the need to confess. They may view their obsessions as a form of religious suffering. These patients are often resistant to treatment. Religious obsessions are most common where severe religious restrictions exist. Diagnosis is not made unless the thoughts or rituals clearly exceed cultural or religious norms, occur at inappropriate times as described by members of the same religion or culture, or interfere with social obligations (APA, 2000). Some individuals with OCD have somatic fears and frequently seek medical treatment for physical symptoms, often just to get reassurance. AIDS, cancer, heart attacks, and sexually transmitted diseases are some of the most common obsessional fears.

> **KEY CONCEPT Obsessions** are unwanted, intrusive, and persistent thoughts, impulses, or images that cause anxiety and distress. Obsessions create significant anxiety because they are not under the patient's control and are incongruent with the patient's usual thought patterns.

> **KEY CONCEPT Compulsions** are behaviours that are performed repeatedly, in a ritualistic fashion, with the goal of preventing or relieving anxiety and distress caused by obsessions.

OCD has a 2.5% lifetime prevalence and a 1-year prevalence rate of 0.5% to 2.1% in the adult population. Rates are similar among women and men. First-degree relatives of people with OCD have a higher prevalence rate than the general population. The typical age of onset of OCD is in the early 20s to mid-30s, although symptoms of OCD can begin in childhood. Despite this early onset, it is often 7 to 10 years before individuals seek professional help, due to the shame felt about the nature of their obsessions and compulsions (Hollander, 1997). The most common reasons that individuals with OCD seek professional help include relationship problems, generalized anxiety, alcohol or drug problems, and depression (Nestadt, Bienvenu, Cai, Samuels, & Eaton, 1998). Because children subscribe to myths, superstition, and magical thinking, obsessive and ritualistic behaviours may go unnoticed. Behaviours such as touching every third tree, avoiding cracks in the sidewalk, or consistently verbalizing fears of losing a parent in an accident may have some underlying pathology but are common behaviours in childhood. However, it is increasing concerns about social, academic, and personal impairments that differentiate the common behaviours from OCD. The astute parent may notice that the older child spends great amounts of time on trivial tasks or has falling grades because of poor concentration. Early onset OCD increases the chances of OCD in relatives and predicts poorer treatment outcomes (Busatto et al., 2001). Other predictors of poor outcomes during lifelong treatment include low social functioning and the presence of both obsessions and compulsions (Castle & Groves, 2000; Skoog & Skoog, 1999).

Tourette's syndrome has an interesting relationship with OCD. There are similar alterations in brain functioning, and the two disorders often occur together (Johannes et al., 2003). Other psychiatric disorders co-occur as well. About two thirds of patients with OCD have a comorbid disorder, including depression (Overbeek, Schruers, Vermetten, & Greiz, 2002), social anxiety disorder, and panic disorder (Rasmussen & Eisen, 1990, 1992). Substance use disorders are common, as individuals attempt to self-medicate their anxiety symptoms. A significant number of older depressed patients have OCD (Beekman et al., 2000). In addition, bipolar disorder and cyclothymic disorder may be comorbid with OCD (Kirkby, 2003; Perugi et al., 2002).

Posttraumatic Stress Disorder

Posttraumatic stress disorder (PTSD) affects roughly 8% of the general population, and women are more likely than men to be affected. However, the prevalence of PTSD in clinical populations varies significantly by the type of trauma, ranging from about 20% after motor vehicle crash to more than 80% after a prisoner-of-war experience. PTSD is defined by characteristic symptoms that develop after a traumatic event involving a personal experience of threatened death, injury, or threat to physical integrity. It may also include witnessing such an event happening to another person or learning that a family member or close friend has experienced such an event. Examples of traumatic events are interpersonal trauma (physical and/or sexual assault as a child or an adult), military combat, natural disasters, terrorist attack, being taken hostage, incarceration as a prisoner of war, torture, motor vehicle crash, or being diagnosed with a life-threatening illness.

Individuals with PTSD have three core symptom clusters: reexperiencing, avoidance, and heightened arousal. They reexperience the event through distressing images, thoughts, or perceptions and may have recurrent nightmares. In addition, the patient may experience flashbacks and exhibit extreme stress upon exposure to an event or image that resembles the traumatic event (e.g., fireworks may bring back memories of war). Patients will avoid discussing the event altogether or avoid people and places that remind them of the traumatic event. Heightened arousal is evidenced by difficulty sleeping, irritability, poor concentration, exaggerated startle response, or hypervigilance (APA, 2000).

Risk factors for PTSD include a prior diagnosis of depression or acute stress disorder (Brewin, Andrews, Rose, & Kirk, 1999). Other factors include being female, preexisting personality disorder, the duration and intensity of trauma involved, environmental issues, coping style, low self-esteem, and previous traumatic events.

In considering PTSD that arises as a result of severe collective trauma (e.g., genocide), Canadian nurse Susan Ray (2008) argues that nurses need to understand it as the consequence of a disturbed society rather than as an individual disorder. The dehumanization that occurs, along with attacks on social bonds and values as well as on the individual's personhood, must be recognized.

Acute Stress Disorder

Acute stress disorder (ASD) shares the same three symptom clusters as PTSD but differs in duration (symptoms emerging 2 to 4 days after exposure to a traumatic stressor and lasting up to 1 month) and in the necessity of experiencing dissociative symptoms (numbing, detachment, a reduction of awareness to one's surroundings, derealization, **depersonalization**, or dissociative amnesia). Controversy continues over whether acute stress disorder should be more accurately considered early PTSD and if early dissociation is necessary for diagnosis (Marshall, Spitzer, & Liebowitz, 1999). Both of these disorders are the focus of intense research activity, with leading experts theorizing that these disorders are the result of failed recovery, rather than immediate psychopathological processes. Most individuals will show some level of reexperiencing, avoidance, and hyperarousal in the aftermath of a traumatic event, but they often recover over time.

Although several researchers found that dissociative reactions are associated with more severe and prolonged stress responses and increased risk for PTSD (Classen, Koopman, Hales, & Spiegel, 1998; Grieger et al., 2000; Shalev, Peri, Canetti, & Schreiber, 1996; Yehuda, 2000), others found that dissociation does not add predictive power for the development of PTSD to the overall diagnosis of ASD (Brewin et al., 1999; Harvey & Bryant, 1999b). In a prospective study of 157 victims of violent assaults, Brewin et al. found that ASD and high levels of reexperiencing/arousal symptoms were predictive of later development of PTSD. Harvey and Bryant (1999a) found that in a study of 92 survivors of MVCs, 13% met the criteria for ASD and 21% for subsyndromal ASD. Of the subsyndromal group, 79% satisfied the criteria for all clusters except dissociation. The implication of this is that a significant proportion of acutely traumatized individuals may suffer marked distress without meeting full criteria for ASD and potentially may not receive early intervention when needed (Harvey & Bryant, 1999b). For those who go on to develop stress disorders, recovery processes are often overwhelmed by internal and external factors that lead to persistent and debilitating symptoms.

Social Phobia

Social phobia (social anxiety disorder) involves a persistent fear of social or performance situations in which embarrassment may occur. It is a common anxiety disorder with lifetime prevalence rates of 10% to 13% (Magee, Eaton, Wittchen, McGonagle, & Kessler, 1996), although most who meet criteria do not get diagnosed (Ballenger, 1999). Exposure to a feared social or performance situation nearly always provokes immediate anxiety and may trigger panic attacks. People with social phobias fear that others will scrutinize their behaviour and judge them negatively. They often do not speak up in crowds out of fear of embarrassment. They will go to great lengths to avoid feared situations. If avoidance is not possible, they will suffer through the situation with visible anxiety.

People with social phobia appear to be highly sensitive to disapproval or criticism, tend to evaluate themselves negatively, and have poor self-esteem and a distorted view of personal strengths and weaknesses. They may magnify personal flaws and underrate any talents. They often believe that others would act with more assertiveness in a given social situation. Men and women with social phobia tend to have difficulties with dating and with sexual relationships (Bodinger et al., 2002). Children tend to underachieve in school because of test-taking anxiety. This is an important area that should be assessed in all patients.

Onset is usually in early adolescence. There are two subtypes of this disorder: generalized social phobia is diagnosed when the individual experiences fears related to most social situations, including public performances and social interactions. These individuals are likely to demonstrate deficiencies in social skills, and their phobias interfere with their ability to function. Individuals with specific social phobias fear and avoid only one or two social situations. Classic examples of such situations are eating, writing, or speaking in public or using public bathrooms.

Social phobias, such as panic disorder and specific phobias, are linked to a number of key neurotransmitter systems. Evidence links low dopamine receptor binding to social anxiety disorder (Schneier et al., 2000).

Panic Disorder

Panic is an extreme, overwhelming form of anxiety often experienced when an individual is placed in a real or perceived life-threatening situation. Panic can be normal in response to a serious threat, but abnormal when it becomes more frequent and generalizes to situations that pose no real physical or psychological threat. Some people experience heightened anxiety because they fear experiencing another panic attack. This type of panic interferes with the individual's ability to function in everyday life and is characteristic of panic disorder.

> **KEY CONCEPT Panic** can be a normal but extreme, overwhelming form of anxiety often initiated when an individual is placed in a real or perceived life-threatening situation.

Panic disorder is a chronic condition that has exacerbations and remissions during the course of the disease. Panic disorder typically peaks in the teenage years and then again in the 30s but can surface in childhood or after the fourth decade of life (APA, 2000). Panic disorder can be found in as much as 1.6% of the general population (2.9 million) at any given time, according to the Epidemiological Catchment Area survey. Six-month prevalence rates were reported by an Edmonton group to be 0.4% in males and 1.0% in females (Bland et al., 1988), while others have found lifetime rates to be as high as 6.8% (Wang, Berglund, & Kessler, 2000). Men and women show similar age of onset, but premorbid mood disorders and stressful life events are more common in women (Barzega, Maina, Venturello, & Bogetto, 2001).

Several risk factors have been implicated in the development of panic disorder, including family history, substance and stimulant use or abuse, smoking tobacco, and undertaking severe stressors. In addition to contributing potential genetic predisposition, female gender has been implicated as a risk factor because females have more panic symptoms than do males. People who have several anxiety symptoms and those who experience separation anxiety during childhood often present with panic disorder later in life (Hayward, Killen, & Kraemer, 2000; Slattery et al., 2002). Other disorders that have been shown to precede panic disorder include social anxiety disorder and specific phobias (Barzega et al., 2001). In addition, adolescents with panic disorder may be at higher risk for suicidal thoughts or attempt suicide more often than other adolescents (Valentiner, Gutierrez, & Blacker, 2002).

In addition to comorbid psychiatric disorders being common in those with panic disorder, certain physical health problems are also common. These include vertigo, cardiac disease, gastrointestinal disorders, and asthma. Patients with mitral valve prolapse, migraine headaches, and hypertension may also have an increased incidence of panic disorder. One might ponder whether these medical conditions produce similar somatic sensations to anxiety and over time increase the risk of panic attacks and the development of panic disorder. The population with both physical health problems and panic symptoms reports poorer quality of life than do those without such comorbidity.

Panic disorder is characterized by the appearance of disabling attacks of panic that often lead to other anxiety and mood disorders. Panic disorder can occur with and without agoraphobia. Patients experiencing panic disorder with agoraphobia tend to have more coexisting anxiety disorders, anxiety attacks, and anticipatory anxiety than do patients who have panic disorder without agoraphobia. Women appear more likely to experience panic disorder with agoraphobia and more likely than men to experience panic symptoms after remission (Sheikh, Leskin, & Klein, 2002). Both types include recurrent and unexpected panic attacks followed by 1 month or more of consistent concern about having another attack, worrying about the consequences of having another attack, or changing behaviour because of fear of the attacks (Table 21-2).

Panic Attacks

Panic attacks are sudden, short periods of intense fear or discomfort that are accompanied by significant physical

Table 21.2	Panic Attacks
Discrete period of intense fear or discomfort with four (or more) of the following symptoms that develop abruptly and reach a peak within 10 minutes:	
Palpitations, pounding heart, or accelerated heart rate	Sweating
Sensations of shortness of breath or smothering	Trembling or shaking
Feelings of choking	Nausea or vomiting
Chest pain or discomfort	Chills or hot flushes
Depersonalization (feeling detached from oneself)	Derealization (feeling of unreality)
Paresthesias (numbness or tingling sensations)	Fear of dying
Feeling dizzy, unsteady, light-headed, or faint	Fear of losing control or going crazy

and cognitive symptoms. The physical symptoms are listed in Table 21-2 and reflect cardiorespiratory and gastrointestinal symptoms. Cognitive symptoms include disorganized thinking, irrational fears, depersonalization, and a decreased ability to communicate. Feelings of impending doom or death, fear of going crazy or losing control, and desperation are common.

> ● **CRNENOTE**
>
> Physical symptoms of panic attack are similar to cardiac emergencies. These symptoms are physically taxing and psychologically frightening to patients. Recognition of the seriousness of panic attacks should be communicated to the patient.

A panic attack usually peaks at 10 minutes but the effects can last as long as 30 minutes, followed by a gradual return to normal functioning. Individuals with panic disorder experience recurrent, unexpected panic attacks followed by persistent concern about experiencing subsequent panic attacks. They fear implications of the attacks, and they have behavioural changes related to the attacks (APA, 2000).

Panic attacks cause fear of death because they mimic symptoms of a heart attack. Individuals often seek emergency medical care because they feel as if they are dying, but most will have a negative cardiac workup. People experiencing panic attacks may also believe that the attacks stem from an underlying major medical illness (APA, 2000). Even with sound medical testing and assurance of no underlying disease, these people often remain unconvinced. Panic attacks can occur in individuals first experiencing certain anxiety-provoking medical conditions, such as asthma, or in initial trials of illicit substance use. However, individuals with panic disorder continue to experience panic attacks with or without predisposing conditions (Box 21-1). Panic attacks can be either internally or externally driven (APA). Externally driven panic attacks may result, for example, from actually seeing a feared object. An internally driven panic attack results from an uncomfortable, internal feeling. Sensations of being too hot or cramped in a small room might provoke panic attacks.

Agoraphobia and Other Phobias

Panic attacks can lead to the development of **phobias** or persistent, unrealistic fears of situations, objects, or activities. People with phobias will go to great lengths to avoid the feared objects or situations to deter panic attacks. Box 21-2 presents examples of common phobias. *Agoraphobia*, fear of open spaces, often co-occurs with panic disorder. Agoraphobia can lead to avoidance behaviours. It begins with an intense, irrational fear of being in open spaces, being alone, or being in public places where escape

---

BOX 21.1

Clinical Vignette: Panic Disorder

M, a 22-year-old man, has experienced several life changes, including a recent engagement, loss of his father to cancer and heart disease, graduation from college, and entrance to the workforce as a computer engineer in a large inner-city company. Because of his active lifestyle, his sleep habits have been poor. He frequently uses sleeping aids at night and now drinks a full pot of coffee to start each day. He has started smoking to "relieve the stress." While sitting in heavy traffic on the way to work, he suddenly experienced chest tightness, sweating, shortness of breath, feelings of being "trapped," and foreboding that he was going to die. Fearing a heart attack, he went to an emergency room, where his discomfort subsided within a half hour. After several hours of testing, the doctor informed him that his heart was healthy. During the next few weeks, he experienced several episodes of feeling trapped and slight chest discomfort on his drive to work. He fears future "attacks" while sitting in traffic and while in his crowded office cubicle.

WHAT DO YOU THINK?
- What risk factors does M have that might contribute to the development of panic attacks?
- What lifestyle changes do you think would help M reduce stress?

IN A LIFE

Charles Darwin (1809–1882)
Theory of Evolution

Public Persona

Charles Darwin, credited as the first scientist to gain wide acceptance of the theory of natural selection, might never have published his 1859 seminal work, *Origin of the Species by Means of Natural Selection*, had it not been for his psychiatric illness. Born in England, Charles Darwin, the grandson of a famous poet, inventor, and physician, was expected to accomplish great things. However, his childhood years were troublesome. When he was sent to Cambridge to study medicine, card playing and drinking became his main activities. After meeting a botanist, however, his life changed and he embarked on a 5-year expedition to the Pacific coast of South America.

Personal Realities

Darwin described his sensation of fear, accompanied by troubled beating of the heart, sweat, and trembling of muscles. Thought to have panic disorder, he constantly worried about what he thought he knew until he finally published his ideas on paper. He died in 1882 and was buried in Westminster Abbey.

Source: Darwin, C. (1887). *The life and letters of Charles Darwin*. New York, NY: Appleton & Co.

---

might be difficult or embarrassing. The person fears that if a panic attack occurred, help would not be available, so he or she avoids such situations. Such avoidance interferes with routine functioning and eventually renders the

Acrophobia (fear of heights)
Agoraphobia (fear of open spaces)
Ailurophobia (fear of cats)
Algophobia (fear of pain)
Arachnophobia (fear of spiders)
Brontophobia (fear of thunder)
Claustrophobia (fear of closed spaces)
Cynophobia (fear of dogs)
Entomophobia (fear of insects)
Hematophobia (fear of blood)
Microphobia (fear of germs)
Nyctophobia (fear of night or dark places)
Ophidiophobia (fear of snakes)
Phonophobia (fear of loud noises)
Photophobia (fear of light)
Pyrophobia (fear of fire)
Topophobia (stage fright)
Xenophobia (fear of strangers)
Zoophobia (fear of animal or animals)

person afraid to leave the safety of home. Some affected individuals continue to face feared situations, but with significant trepidation (i.e., going in public only to pay bills, or to take children to school). In many cases, agoraphobia develops quickly after a few panic attacks, but the resulting avoidance behaviours do not decrease the severity of the panic attacks (APA, 2000). Other patients can reduce panic attacks by dodging certain instances that precipitate attacks. Many of these individuals may be able to confront a situation if accompanied by someone else; for example, going out in public may be manageable with a friend.

Specific phobia (formally simple phobia) is a disorder marked by persistent fear of clearly discernible, circumscribed objects or situations, which often leads to avoidance behaviours. The lifetime prevalence rates range from 7% to 11%, and the disorder generally affects women twice as much as men. It has a bimodal distribution, peaking in childhood and then again in the 20s. The focus of the fear in specific phobia may result from the anticipation of being harmed by the phobic object. For example, dogs are feared because of the chance of being bitten or automobiles are feared because of the potential of crashing. The focus of fear may likewise be associated with concerns about losing control, panicking, or fainting on exposure to the phobic object.

Anxiety is usually felt immediately on exposure to the phobic object, and the level of anxiety is usually related to both the proximity of the object and the degree to which escape is possible. For example, anxiety heightens as a cat approaches a person who fears cats and lessens when the cat moves away. At times, the level of anxiety escalates to a full panic attack, particularly when the person must remain in a situation from which escape is deemed to be

impossible. Fear of specific objects is fairly common, and the diagnosis of specific phobia is not made unless the fear significantly interferes with functioning or causes marked distress. Assessment differentiates simple phobia from other diagnoses with overlapping symptoms. Among adult patients who are seen in clinical settings, the most common phobias to least common phobias are situational phobias, natural environment phobias, blood–injection–injury phobia, and animal phobias. The most common phobias among community samples are of heights, mice, spiders, and insects (APA, 2000).

Blood–injection–injury type phobia merits special consideration because the phobia surrounds medical treatments. The physiologic processes that are exhibited during phobic exposure include a strong vasovagal response, which significantly increases blood pressure and pulse, followed by the deceleration of the pulse and lowering of blood pressure in the patient. Monitor closely when giving required injections or medical treatments. About 75% of patients with blood–injection–injury phobia report fainting on exposure. Factors that may predispose individuals to specific phobias may include traumatic events, unexpected panic attacks in the presence of the phobic object or situation, observation of others experiencing a trauma, or a repeated exposure to information warning of dangers, such as parents repeatedly warning young children that dogs bite.

ETIOLOGY OF ANXIETY DISORDERS

Genetic Theories

There are substantial similarities in the etiological theories across many of the anxiety disorders. A meta-analysis of the genetic epidemiology of anxiety disorder found that genes account for 30% to 40% of the risk for panic disorder and that the risk for first-degree relatives was five times that of the general population (Hettema et al., 2001). If the family member manifests panic disorder before 20 years of age, the risk in family members jumps to 20 times that of the general population (APA, 2000). Twin studies have found the occurrence of anxiety disorders to be as much as five times more frequent in monozygotic than in dizygotic twins, suggesting that parenting and other environmental factors cannot wholly account for the development of panic disorder in adolescents. However, social conditioning may play a role in anxiety sensitivity or in overestimating the degree of threat, both of which may increase the risk to develop anxiety disorders. Mundo, Richter, Sam, Macciardi, & Kennedy (2000) discovered a link between the pathogenesis of OCD and the 5-HT$_{1D\beta}$ receptor gene. This discovery may lead to breakthroughs in pharmacologic treatments for OCD.

Neuroanatomic Correlates

Certain neurologic abnormalities have been detected by magnetic resonance imaging with patients with panic disorder. The most common abnormalities are focal areas of abnormal activity in the fear network of the brain. This network includes the central nucleus of the amygdala, the hippocampus, and the periaqueductal gray area in the brain (Gorman, Kent, Sullivan, & Coplan, 2000). The amygdala and the hippocampus are integral parts of memory storage and emotion regulation. Abnormalities in these areas may indicate dysfunctional signaling between the various brain regions.

Interestingly, studies have found a link between infection with β-hemolytic streptococci and the subsequent emergence of OCD symptoms in children (Castle & Groves, 2000; Giedd, Rapaport, Garvey, Perlmutter, & Swedo, 2000). Further structural neuroimaging studies using computed axial tomography and magnetic resonance imaging performed to find total-volume differences in brain structures have shown that a group of children with *Streptococcus*-associated OCD and/or tics have enlarged basal ganglia (caudate, putamen, and globus pallidus) compared to healthy children (Giedd et al.). Basal ganglia structures are important in the control of fine motor movement.

Positron emission tomography and single-photon emission computed tomography reveal differences in cerebral glucose metabolism between patients with OCD and control subjects. Variation in methods of measurement produces some inconsistencies in the research findings. However, the most replicated results demonstrate increased glucose metabolism in the caudate nuclei (part of the basal ganglia), the orbitofrontal gyri (part of the frontal cortex involved in emotion), and the cingulate gyri (considered to be part of the limbic system, involved in connecting memory to emotion). Studies measuring cerebral blood flow and glucose metabolism in patients with OCD during exposure to feared stimuli and during relaxation have further implicated these regions of the brain (Baxter, 1992; Rauch et al., 1994).

Biochemical Theories

Identification of neurotransmitter involvement in panic disorder has evolved from neurochemical studies with panicogenic substances known to produce panic attacks, such as yohimbine, norepinephrine, epinephrine, pentagastrin, sodium lactate, and carbon dioxide (CO_2). In addition, by knowing the pharmacodynamics of medications that reduce panic episodes, investigators have been able to hypothesize which neurotransmitters are involved in panic disorder.

Norepinephrine

Norepinephrine is implicated in anxiety disorders because of its effects on the systems most associated with the physical sensations of anxiety—the cardiovascular, respiratory, and gastrointestinal systems. Cell bodies of norepinephrine neurons in the brain are located in the locus caeruleus, which is one of the internal regulators of numerous biologic rhythms. The cell bodies make extensive projections to the cerebral cortex, cerebellum, limbic system, and spinal cord, as well as to the sympathetic nervous system. Electrical stimulation of the locus caruleus in monkeys increases fear and anxiety. Norepinephrine effects are mediated by two types of receptors, alpha and beta, both of which have important subtypes, which contribute to the complexities of understanding the role of norepinephrine in panic disorder. Some drugs, such as propranolol, act primarily on β-adrenergic receptors, reducing the peripheral symptoms of anxiety, but with limited effectiveness against anxiety or panic symptoms.

Accumulated evidence indicates that a dysregulation of the norepinephrine system may exist in panic disorder. Drugs that increase the activity of the locus caeruleus often are panicogenic in individuals who have panic disorder but not in healthy subjects. For example, yohimbine, an α_2-receptor antagonist, increases the firing rate of norepinephrine neurons, which increases the release of norepinephrine and evokes increasing anxiety symptoms (Sallee, Sethuraman, Sine, & Liu, 2000).

Drugs that inhibit norepinephrine release are thought to be **anxiolytic,** meaning that they diminish anxiety or panic symptoms. Medications such as propranolol and tricyclic antidepressants (TCAs) act on norepinephrine systems. However, only the TCAs have shown efficacy in the treatment of panic disorder.

Serotonin

Serotonin [5-hydroxytryptamine (5-HT)] was indirectly implicated in the etiology of anxiety disorders when it was discovered that drugs that facilitate serotonergic neurotransmission were effective in relieving anxiety and panic symptoms. Selective serotonin reuptake inhibitors (SSRIs) may impede the panic response by decreasing activity in the amygdala and interfering with transmission to extension sites in the hypothalamus (Gorman et al., 2000). These drugs can be activating and may initially increase anxiety symptoms. They produce symptom relief after 2 to 6 weeks of treatment.

Although serotonin may be involved in anxiety disorders, the responsible serotonin circuits and receptor subtypes are unknown. Serotonin systems and their multiple complex interactions with many other neurotransmitter systems make it difficult to identify any primary functional deficits. For example, serotonin and norepinephrine each can affect the release of the other from the nerve terminals, suggesting reciprocal roles in regulating the interaction between these neurotransmitters and their respective receptors.

Gamma-Aminobutyric Acid

Gamma-aminobutyric acid (GABA) is the most abundant inhibitory neurotransmitter in the brain, and very small GABA neurons (interneurons) affect the firing rates of neurons distributed throughout the brain, which explains why GABA has such global effects, such as overall electrical activity, memory processing, anxiety, and the level of consciousness. Thus, depending on dose, the activation of GABA neurons produces anticonvulsant, anxiolytic, or hypnotic actions, but at the same time, it can affect the creation of memory as events happen (anterograde memory). Most of these effects are mediated through the $GABA_A$ receptor complex, a cell membrane ion channel specific to chloride ions. When GABA binds to this receptor, chloride ions flow into the cell and prevent that cell from firing. This receptor complex has binding sites for benzodiazepines, barbiturates, alcohol, and progesterone. These drugs and hormones potentiate GABA effects.

Although drugs that enhance GABA have anxiolytic properties, it has been difficult to tease out any abnormalities in GABA systems. However, newer neuroimaging techniques such as positron emission tomography, single-photon emission computed tomography, magnetic resonance imaging, and magnetic resonance spectroscopy may hold promise for providing more direct information about GABA and its role in anxiety and anxiety disorders.

Corticotropin-Releasing Factor

Corticotropin-releasing factor (CRF) is a neuropeptide that has widespread effects in the brain and in one of the major stress response systems, the hypothalamic–pituitary–adrenal (HPA) axis. CRF receptors are widely distributed in the hypothalamus, as well as the brain regions associated with fear and fear conditioning. Cortisol, the main output of the HPA axis, is significantly elevated during panic attacks (Bandelow et al., 2000). CRF and norepinephrine interact to regulate each other's release from nerve cells.

Cholecystokinin

Cholecystokinin (CCK) is another neuropeptide that has been implicated in the etiology of panic attacks. High concentrations of CCK are found in the cerebral cortex, the amygdala, and the hippocampus—areas implicated in fear and stress responses. Two subtypes of CCK receptors have been identified: CCK-A and CCK-B. CCK-A receptors are predominant in the peripheral systems; CCK-B receptors are widely distributed throughout the brain, particularly in the limbic system and cortex. When administered in challenge tests, CCK induces panic attacks in patients with panic disorder and, to a much lesser degree, in people without panic disorder

(Bradwejn et al., 1992). Although CCK antagonists were developed for the treatment of panic disorder, these compounds did not show sufficient efficacy to be marketed.

Other Neuropeptides

Evidence of altered growth hormone (GH) activity in patients with panic disorder provides additional support for the role of the hypothalamus in panic disorder. In healthy subjects, stimulating α-adrenergic receptors elevates GH. This process is blunted in individuals with panic disorder (Sallee et al., 2000). Another area of research implicates neuroactive steroids, including the various metabolites of progesterone in the development of panic attacks (Strohle et al., 2003). This may contribute to the female gender bias observed in panic disorder.

Psychodynamic Theories

Psychodynamic theories contribute to the understanding of anxiety disorders by explaining the importance of the development of anxiety after separation and loss. Patients with anxiety disorders report greater numbers and severity of recent personal losses at symptom onset than do healthy control subjects. For example, in a study of the background and personality traits of individuals with panic disorder, several commonalities were found, including being fearful or shy as a child; remembering their parents as angry, critical, or frightening; having feelings of discomfort with aggression; having long-term feelings of low self-esteem; and experiencing a stressful life event associated with frustration and resentment that preceded the initial onset of symptoms (Shear, Cooper, Klerman, Busch, & Shapiro, 1993). These researchers proposed the following theory of causation. The child may begin with a neurophysiologic vulnerability that predisposes one to fearfulness. This fearfulness is enhanced by parental behaviours in some way, which results in disturbed parent–child relationships and causes the child to feel conflict about dependence and independence (separating from parents), self-doubt and confusion regarding self-identity, and personal control. These negative feelings of low self-esteem and powerlessness appear to make the individual feel extremely vulnerable to the stress of normal life events, such as going to school, getting married, or becoming a parent. As the person attempts to ignore these negative feelings and seems powerless to control them, he or she continues to experience distress in repeated stressful events. The chronic, intense fear and dread culminate in the first panic attack. However, similar dynamics can also explain the emergence of depression. Factors that determine the specific clinical presentation and health outcomes related to chronic childhood psychological problems remain elusive.

Cognitive-Behavioural Theories

Learning theory underlies most cognitive-behavioural theories of anxiety disorders. Classic conditioning theory suggests that one learns a fear response by linking an adverse or fear-provoking event, such as a car accident, with a previously neutral event, such as crossing a bridge. One becomes conditioned to associate fear with crossing a bridge. Applying this theory to people with panic disorder has limitations. Phobic avoidance, for example, is not always developed secondary to an adverse event.

Further development of this theory led to an understanding of **interoceptive conditioning**, which pairs a somatic discomfort, such as dizziness or palpitations, with an impending panic attack. For example, during a car accident, the individual may experience rapid heartbeat, dizziness, shortness of breath, and panic. Subsequent experiences of dizziness or palpitations, unrelated to an anxiety-provoking situation, incite anxiety and panic. Many cognitive theorists further expound that people with panic disorder may misinterpret mild physical sensations (e.g., sweating, dizziness), causing panic as a result of learned fear (catastrophic interpretation). Some researchers hypothesize that individuals with a low sense of control over their environment or with a particular sensitivity to anxiety are vulnerable to misinterpreting normal stress. Controlled exposure to anxiety-provoking situations and cognitive countering techniques have proven successful in reducing the symptoms of panic.

� PRIORITY CARE ISSUES

Anxiety and depressive disorders are highly associated. Lenze et al. (2000) stated that 9.3% of patients with major depressive disorder have comorbid panic disorder. Increased risk of suicide is more associated with PTSD than any other anxiety disorder; however, multiple health problems (including more than one psychiatric diagnosis) can increase suicide risk.

■ NURSING MANAGEMENT: HUMAN RESPONSE TO PANIC DISORDER

As indicated previously, anxiety disorders are usually treated in outpatient clinics or by private practitioners. Hospitalization is limited to acute exacerbation of anxiety or panic symptoms or comorbid depressive disorder not responsive to antidepressant drug therapy. This section uses panic disorder to outline the nursing care of those with anxiety disorders. Specific differences from the management of panic disorder across the various anxiety disorders will be noted.

Because panic disorder encompasses the physical, psychological, social, and spiritual spheres of the patient's world, the assessment within a bio/psycho/social/spiritual framework is imperative. Physiologic symptoms tend to be the impetus for patients to seek medical assistance. Often, patients are initially seen in emergency rooms, as they seek treatment for their physical symptoms. Biologic, psychological, and social assessments unveil potential contributing factors and identify sources of strength that can guide the nurse to develop an individual action plan.

Biologic Domain

Assessment

Skilful assessment is required to rule out life-threatening causes, including primary or secondary cardiac or neurologic symptoms. Once it is determined that the patient has experienced a panic attack, the nurse should assess for any potential environmental triggers and obtain a detailed history of any previous similar experiences. Questions to ask the patient might include the following:

- What did you experience preceding and during the panic episode, including physical symptoms, feelings, and thoughts?
- When did you begin to feel that way? How long did it last?
- Have you ever experienced some of these symptoms before? If so, under what circumstances?
- Has anyone in your family ever had similar experiences?
- What do you do when you have these experiences that help you to feel safe? Have the feelings and sensations ever gone away on their own?

Substance Use

Assessment for panicogenic substance use, such as sources of caffeine, pseudoephedrine, amphetamines, cocaine, or other stimulants, may rule out contributory issues either related or unrelated to panic disorder. The use of the recreational drug "Ecstasy" has also been linked with panic attacks (REF). Tobacco use can also contribute to the risk for panic symptoms. Many individuals with panic disorder use alcohol or central nervous system (CNS) depressants in an effort to self-medicate anxiety symptoms, and withdrawal from CNS depressants may produce symptoms of panic.

Sleep Patterns

Sleep is often disturbed in patients with panic disorder. In fact, panic attacks can occur during sleep, and the patient may fear sleep for this reason. Nurses should closely assess the impact of sleep disturbance as it can increase the risk of further panic attacks and the development of depression.

Interventions for Biologic Domain

These interventions can assist individuals with either severe anxiety or panic symptoms.

Physical Activity

Active participation in a routine exercise program may help individuals reassess automatic thinking that relates increased heart rate and shortness of breath with a physical crisis. However, drastically changing lifestyle to avoid situations does not aid recovery. Interventions that focus on the physical aspects of anxiety and panic are particularly helpful in reducing the number and severity of the attacks, giving patients an increasing sense of accomplishment and control.

Breathing Control

Hyperventilation is common. Often, people are unaware that they take rapid, shallow breaths when they become anxious. Other common sensations are choking and pressure on the chest, restricting normal breathing.

Teaching patients breathing control can be helpful. Focus on the breathing and help them to identify the rate, pattern, and depth. If the breathing is rapid and shallow, reassure the patient that exercise and breathing practice can help change this breathing pattern. Next, assist the patient in practicing abdominal breathing by performing the following exercises:

- Instruct the patient to breathe deeply by inhaling slowly through the nose. Have him or her place a hand on the abdomen just beneath the rib cage.
- Instruct the patient to observe that when one is breathing deeply, the hand on the abdomen will actually rise.
- After the patient understands this process, ask him or her to inhale slowly through the nose counting to five, pause, and then exhale slowly through pursed lips.
- While the patient exhales, direct the attention to feeling the muscles relax, focusing on "letting go."
- Have the patient repeat the deep abdominal breathing for 10 breaths, pausing between each inhalation and exhalation. Count slowly. If the patient complains of light-headedness, instruct the patient to slow down the rate of his or her deep breathing.
- The patient should stop between each cycle of 10 breaths and monitor normal breathing for 30 seconds.
- This series of 10 slow abdominal breaths, followed by 30 seconds of normal breathing, should be repeated for 3 to 5 minutes.
- Help the patient to establish a time for daily practice of abdominal breathing.

Abdominal breathing may also be used to interrupt an episode of panic as it begins. Once patients have learned to identify their own early signs of panic, they can learn the four-square method of breathing, which helps divert or decrease the severity of the attack. Patients should be instructed as follows:

- Advise the patient to practice during calm periods and to begin by inhaling slowly through the nose, count to four, then hold the breath for a count of four.
- Next, direct the patient to exhale slowly through pursed lips to a count of four and then rest for a count of four (no breath).
- Finally, the patient may take two normal breaths and repeat the sequence.

After patients practice the skill, the nurse should assist patients in identifying early physical cues that will alert them to use this calming technique. Some forms of yoga are especially helpful in teaching breathing relaxation techniques.

Nutritional Planning

Maintaining regular and balanced eating habits reduces the likelihood of hypoglycemic episodes, light-headedness, and fatigue. Patients need to plan to reduce caffeine consumption and then eliminate it from their diet. Many over-the-counter (OTC) remedies are now used to boost energy or increase mental performance, and some of these contain caffeine. The nurse may help the patient develop a reasonable plan to decrease or eliminate all sources of caffeine from his or her diet. The nurse should also assess for other potential sources of stimulants, such as some cold remedies and herbal products, and provide information about substitutes.

Relaxation Techniques

Teaching the patient relaxation techniques is another way to help with panic and anxiety disorders. Some are unaware of the tension in their bodies and first need to learn to monitor their own tension. Isometric exercises and progressive muscle relaxation are helpful methods to learn to differentiate muscle tension from muscle relaxation. This method of relaxation is also helpful when patients have difficulty clearing the mind, focusing, or visualizing a scene, which are often required in other forms of relaxation, such as meditation. Box 21-3 provides one method of progressive muscle relaxation.

SSRI Therapy

Several classes of pharmacologic agents are effective in treating anxiety disorders, including the SSRIs, TCAs, and benzodiazepines. However, the SSRIs are generally considered the first-line treatment of anxiety disorders. Because of side effects and dietary restrictions, monoamine oxidase inhibitor (MAOI) antidepressants generally are used after all other options are exhausted. Open trials (in which the experimental design does not include the researcher being blind to treatment and

BOX 21.3

Implementing Progressive Muscle Relaxation

Choose a quiet, comfortable location where you will not be disturbed for 20–30 minutes. Your position may be lying or sitting, but all parts of your body should be supported, including your head. Wear loose clothing, taking off restrictive items, such as glasses and shoes.

Begin by closing your eyes and clearing your mind. Moving from head to toe, focus on each part of your body and assess the level of tension. Visualize each group of muscles as heavy and relaxed.

Take two or three slow abdominal breaths, pausing briefly between each breath. Imagine the tension flowing from your body.

Each muscle group listed below should be tightened (or tensed isometrically) for 5–10 seconds and then abruptly released; visualize this group of muscles as heavy, limp, and relaxed for 15–20 seconds before tightening the next group of muscles. There are several methods to tighten each muscle group, and suggestions are provided below. Each muscle group may be tightened two to three times until relaxed. Do not overtighten or strain. You should not experience pain.

- Hands (tighten by making fists)

- Biceps (tighten by drawing forearms up and "making a muscle")
- Triceps (extend forearms straight, locking elbows)
- Face (grimace, tightly shutting mouth and eyes; open mouth wide and raise eyebrows)
- Neck (pull head forward to chest and tighten neck muscles)
- Shoulders (raise shoulders toward ears; push shoulders back as if touching them together)
- Chest (take a deep breath and hold for 10 seconds)
- Stomach (suck in your abdominal muscles)
- Buttocks (pull buttocks together)
- Thighs (straighten your legs and squeeze the muscles in thighs and hips)
- Leg calves (pull toes carefully toward you, avoid cramps)
- Feet (curl toes downward and point toes away from your body)

Finally, repeat several deep abdominal breaths and mentally check your body for tension. Rest comfortably for several minutes, breathing normally, and visualize your body as warm and relaxed. Get up slowly when you are finished.

the drug is not compared to placebo) of nefazedone and venlafaxine show specific promise for social phobia (Stein, Fryer, Davidson, Pollack, & Wiita, 1999; Stein, Versiani, Hair, & Kumar, 2002; Van Ameringen, Mancini, Pipe, Campbell, & Oakman, 2002). An exception for the efficacy of psychotropic drugs for an anxiety disorder is in relation to specific phobias. Anxiolytics may give short-term relief of phobic anxiety, but there is no evidence that they affect the course of the disorder. The treatment of choice for specific phobia is exposure therapy (Newman, Erickson, Przeworski, & Dzus, 2003).

Although not all SSRIs have received Health Canada approval for the treatment of panic disorder, some are used as "off-label" treatment of panic attacks. Sertraline (Zoloft), paroxetine (Paxil), and fluoxetine (Prozac) have all proved effective in the treatment of panic disorder in drug trials (Rapaport et al., 2001; Roy-Byrne et al., 2001; Wagstaff, Cheer, Matheson, Ormrod, & Goa, 2002). The initial increase in serotonergic activity from serotonin reuptake blockade may cause temporary increases in panic symptoms and even panic attacks, but this is usually short-lived and can be minimized by lower starting doses (Brauer, Nowicki, Catalano, & Catalano, 2002). Full clinical response is usually seen by 4 to 6 weeks of treatment.

▪ CRNENOTE

Psychopharmacologic treatment is almost always needed. Antidepressants are the medication of choice. Benzodiazepines should only be used for short periods of time. If used for longer periods of time, it is important to taper off benzodiazepines to avoid any rebound anxiety or sleep disturbance.

Administering and Monitoring SSRI

Overall, SSRIs produce fewer side effects than do other drugs, are safer to use, and are not lethal in the event of overdose. They may cause a temporary feeling of overstimulation when initiated, but slow titration can help to alleviate this feeling. Morning dosing decreases interference with sleep, but at higher doses, some patients find the medication sedating.

Paroxetine (Paxil) was the first of the SSRIs to be indicated for anxiety disorders. Dosing begins at 10 mg per day, usually in the morning, and then is increased by 10 mg per week at weekly intervals, not to exceed 60 mg per day. Controlled-release paroxetine (Paxil CR) dosing begins at 12.5 mg per day, increasing by 12.5 mg per day in intervals of not less than 1 week. Maximum dose is 75 mg per day. Sertraline (Zoloft) usually begins at 25 mg per day, increasing after 1 week to 50 mg per day. The maximum dose is 200 mg per day.

Monitoring Side Effects

The most common side effects of the SSRIs are initial dizziness, restlessness and anxiety, and sexual dysfunction. Up to 50% of those on SSRIs can experience some degree of sexual side effects and this must be considered in treatment decisions for panic disorder. The nurse should ensure that the patient is aware of this before the drug is started and should initiate ongoing discussions about any emerging dysfunction during follow-up. Significant weight gain has also been observed in some patients. A withdrawal syndrome has been identified in individuals who suddenly stop taking SSRIs (Finfgeld, 2002). Patient education is an important preventive strategy to minimize withdrawal symptoms.

BOX 21.4

Comparison of the Metabolic Inhibition Profiles and the Elimination Half-Lives of the SSRIs

| DRUG | SPECIFIC CYP ENZYMES | | | | T ½* (IN HOURS) |
	1A2	2C	2D6	3A4	
fluoxetine	NS†	Moderate	Potent	Moderate	25–150 (parent); 180–230 (metabolite)
paroxetine	NS	NS	Potent	NS	10–65
fluvoxamine	Potent	Moderate	NS	Moderate	10–24
sertraline	NS	Moderate	NS	NS	20–36
citalopram	NS	NS	NS	NS	20–48

*T ½ is the time required to eliminate 50% of the drug from the body. T ½ for the metabolite is included for active metabolites.
†Nonsignificant.

Monitoring for Drug Interactions

Although the SSRIs as a class have well-described properties that affect other drugs used at the same time, the relative risk of drug–drug interactions differs among the specific SSRIs. The most common mechanism involved in SSRI–drug interaction is the metabolic inhibition of key liver enzymes responsible for the metabolism of many other drugs. The SSRIs inhibit the metabolism of another drug and thus the level of that other drug would be increased. This increase in drug level would significantly increase the risk of serious side effects, directly affecting adherence to a drug regime. Paroxetine and fluoxetine are the most potent of the SSRIs and thus carry the most risk of drug–drug interactions (see Box 21-4). Common drugs affected by this mechanism include thioridazine, digoxin, phenobarbital, TCAs, phenytoin, theophylline, and warfarin (for a more detailed listing, visit http://www.Drug-Interactions.com). Opposite metabolic interactions can also occur. For example, cimetidine (Tagamet) interferes with the metabolism of paroxetine, which might potentiate toxicity. Other potential drug–drug interactions come from interactions based on pharmacologic actions. For example, SSRIs must be used cautiously with MAOIs as there is a risk of a serious hypertensive crisis. Combinations of SSRI and tryptophan increase the risk of serotonin syndrome, an acute condition characterized by restlessness, blood pressure instability, and varying degrees of disorientation and cognitive impairment. The serotonin syndrome can also arise from combining SSRIs and such recreational drugs as Ecstasy and its analogues.

Teaching Points

Warn patients about using herbal products such as St. John's wort, because the similarity of action can increase the risk of serotonin syndrome. The sedative effects of the medications may impede attention and concentration; thus, sedative SSRIs such as fluvoxamine are given at night. Other SSRIs such as fluoxetine and paroxetine are taken in the morning as they are more stimulating and can interfere with sleep.

Tricyclic Antidepressant Therapy

The TCAs imipramine (Tofranil), nortriptyline (Pamelor), and clomipramine (Anafranil) reduce anxiety and panic symptoms, probably by their dual action on serotonin and norepinephrine receptors. The therapeutic effects of TCAs usually occur after 3 to 4 weeks, but effects have been observed as early as 2 weeks after initiation. These drugs are "off-label" treatments because they are not approved by Health Canada for panic disorder.

Administering and Monitoring TCAs

The TCAs have a relatively long elimination half-life, and complaints of sedation are common. Therefore, single bedtime doses might be most helpful for patients. TCAs are highly bound to plasma proteins and are metabolized in the liver. These medications should be used with extreme caution in patients at risk for suicide. TCAs affect cardiac conduction, and overdoses can be fatal. An electrocardiogram is indicated before initiating the therapy. In cross-tapering to different medications, a sudden discontinuation of TCA use causes cholinergic rebound phenomenon, with flu-like symptoms of nausea, headache, and malaise. Assure patients that these effects do not indicate addiction to the medication.

TCAs may complicate underlying glaucoma, urinary retention, cardiovascular disorders, hepatic diseases, and thyroid dysregulation because of their effects on various other neurotransmitter and hormone systems. They also lower the seizure threshold. Monitor closely if the patient has a seizure disorder. These medications have narrow therapeutic indexes and therefore require monitoring for toxicity at high doses.

Monitoring Side Effects

Adverse effects of TCAs are very common and may compromise patients' willingness to continue using them, but side effects can be reduced by starting with a small dose and increasing slowly. Because patients with panic disorder usually require higher doses of antidepressant medication, anticholinergic side effects (dry mouth and eyes, blurred vision, photophobia, constipation, urinary hesitancy or retention, mydriasis, and tachycardia) are common and may necessitate a change in antidepressant type. Acetylcholine is involved with cognition, and anticholinergic side effects of TCAs may negatively affect cognition in elderly patients. In addition, many TCAs have α-adrenergic receptor effects on the body that lead to orthostatic hypotension, placing elderly individuals at increased risk for falls. Lying and standing blood pressure and pulse should be monitored frequently, especially during periods when the dosage is being increased. Also, observe for signs of dizziness or ataxia. Nortriptyline (Pamelor) has a lower risk for orthostatic hypotension and thus may be indicated if falls present a substantial risk.

The choice to initiate treatment with a TCA rather than an SSRI may be related to cost. TCAs have been on the market for a very long time and thus are very low in price compared to the newer SSRIs (pennies per day compared to dollars per day).

Monitoring for Drug Interactions

TCAs interact with several medications, including MAOIs (severe hypertensive crises), SSRIs, and CNS depressants (enhanced CNS depression). Concomitant treatment with methylphenidate (Ritalin), cimetidine, and oral contraceptives may increase TCA serum levels. Consultation with a psychiatrist is usually warranted if a combination antidepressant therapy is required.

Teaching Points

Instruct the patient to take the medication exactly as prescribed and to be careful with any OTC medications or herbal products. Alcohol should be avoided. Warn the patient of the potential for sedation, especially at the initiation of treatment, and, if appropriate, suggest taking the medication at bedtime. In addition, common and serious side effects of the medications should be discussed along with the specific effects that require immediate attention.

Benzodiazepine Therapy

Specific benzodiazepines have produced antipanic effects, and their therapeutic onset is much faster (hours, not weeks) than that of antidepressants. Therefore, benzodiazepines are tremendously useful in treating intensely distressed patients. Alprazolam (Xanax), lorazepam (Ativan), and clonazepam (Rivotril) are widely used for anxiety disorders. They are well tolerated but carry the risk for withdrawal symptoms upon discontinuation of use.

Administering and Monitoring Benzodiazepines

Treatment may include administering benzodiazepines concurrently with antidepressants for the first 4 weeks, then tapering off the benzodiazepine. This strategy provides rapid symptom relief but avoids the complications of long-term benzodiazepine use. Benzodiazepines with short half-lives do not accumulate in the body, whereas benzodiazepines with half-lives of longer than 24 hours tend to accumulate with chronic treatment, are removed more slowly, and produce less intense symptoms on discontinuation of use (see Chapter 14).

Short-acting benzodiazepines, such as alprazolam and lorazepam, are associated with rebound anxiety, or anxiety that increases after the peak effects of the medication have decreased. Medications with short half-lives should be given in three or four small doses spaced throughout the day, with a higher dose at bedtime to allay the anxiety-related insomnia. Clonazepam, a longer-acting benzodiazepine, requires less frequent dosing and has a lower risk for rebound anxiety. Rebound anxiety and insomnia are also common with the abrupt cessation of benzodiazepine treatment. Symptoms associated with the withdrawal of benzodiazepine therapy are more likely to occur after high doses and long-term therapy. They can also occur after short-term therapy. Withdrawal symptoms manifest in several ways, including psychological (e.g., apprehension, irritability, insomnia, dysphoria), physiologic (e.g., tremor, palpitations, vertigo, sweating, muscle spasm, seizures), and perceptual (e.g., sensory hypersensitivity, depersonalization, feelings of motion, metallic taste).

Because of their depressive CNS effects, benzodiazepines should not be used to treat patients with comorbid sleep apnea. In fact, these drugs may actually decrease the rate and depth of respirations. Exercise caution in elderly patients for these reasons.

Monitoring Side Effects

The side effects of benzodiazepine medications generally include headache, confusion, dizziness, disorientation, sedation, and visual disturbances. Sedation should be monitored after beginning the medication use or increasing the dose. The patient should be cautious about activities that take significant attention and concentration when starting on benzodiazepines.

Monitoring for Drug Interactions

Many benzodiazepines have active metabolites, so the pharmacologic effects can last for very long periods of time. The longer-acting drugs accumulate in fat stores, which means that women (who have higher percentage of body fat) and obese patients can continue to have drug effects long after the drug is discontinued. Drugs that interact with benzodiazepines include TCAs and digoxin; interaction may result in increased serum TCA or digoxin levels. Histamine-2 blockers (cimetidine) used with benzodiazepines may potentiate sedative effects. Monitor closely for effectiveness in patients who smoke; cigarette smoking may increase the clearance of benzodiazepines.

Teaching Points

Warn patients to avoid alcohol because of the additive effects on CNS depression. In addition, warn them not to engage in activities that require strict attention and concentration until the sedative effects of the medication are known.

Psychological Domain

Assessment

A complete psychological assessment is necessary to determine patterns of panic attacks; characteristic symptoms in attacks; and the patient's emotional, cognitive, and behavioural responses (see Chapter 11). A comprehensive assessment includes overall mental status, suicidal tendencies and thoughts, cognitive thought patterns, avoidance behaviour patterns, and any comorbid depression symptoms. The patient's perceptions regarding his or her symptoms are discussed, as well as present and past coping strategies.

Self-Report Scales

Self-evaluation is difficult in panic disorder. Often, specific triggers are no longer present, and the patient lives in fear of another panic attack with little sense of being able to control the attacks. Several tools are available to characterize and rate the patient's state of anxiety. Examples of these symptom and behavioural

---

BOX 21.5

Rating Scales for Assessment of Panic Disorder and Anxiety Disorders

PANIC SYMPTOMS
Panic-Associated Symptom Scale (PASS; Argyle et al., 1991)
Acute Panic Inventory (Dillon, Gorman, Liebowitz, Fyer, & Klein, 1987)
National Institute of Mental Health Panic Questionnaire (NIMH PQ; Scupi, Maser, & Uhde, 1992)

COGNITIONS
Anxiety Sensitivity Index (Reiss, Peterson, & Gursky, 1986)
Agoraphobia Cognitions Questionnaire (Chambless, Caputo, Bright, & Gallagher, 1984)
Body Sensations Questionnaire (Chambless et al., 1984)

PHOBIAS
Mobility Inventory for Agoraphobia (Chambless, Caputo, Jasin, Gracely, & Williams, 1985)
Fear Questionnaire (Marks & Matthews, 1979)

ANXIETY
State-Trait Anxiety Inventory (STAI; Spielberger, Gorsuch, & Luchene, 1976)
Penn State Worry Questionnaire (PSWQ; Meyer, Miller, Metzger, & Borkovec, 1990)
Beck Anxiety Inventory (Beck, Epstein, Brown, & Steer, 1988)

---

rating scales are provided in Box 21-5. All of these tools are self-report measures and, as such, are limited by the individual's self-awareness and openness. However, the Hamilton Rating Scale for Anxiety (HAM-A), provided in Table 21-3, is an example of a scale rated by the clinician (Hamilton, 1959). This 14-item scale reflects both psychological and somatic aspects of anxiety.

Mental Status Examination

During the mental status examination, individuals with panic disorder may exhibit anxiety symptoms, including restlessness, irritability, poor concentration, and apprehensive behaviour. Assess by direct questioning if the patient is experiencing suicidal thoughts, especially if the person is abusing substances or is taking antidepressant medications.

Assessment of Cognitive Thought Patterns

Catastrophic misinterpretations of trivial physical symptoms can trigger panic symptoms. Once identified, these thoughts should serve as a basis for individualizing patient education to counter such false beliefs. Table 21-4 presents an example of a scale to assess catastrophic misinterpretations of the symptoms of panic. Several studies have found that individuals who feel a sense of control have less severe panic attacks. Individuals who fear loss of control during a panic attack often make the following type of statements:

- "I feel trapped."
- "I'm afraid others will know, or I'll hurt someone."
- "I feel alone. I can't help myself."
- "I'm losing control."

Such individuals also tend to show low self-esteem, feelings of helplessness, demoralization, and overwhelming fears of experiencing panic attacks. They may have difficulty with assertiveness or expressing feelings.

Interventions for Psychological Domain

Often, anxiety disorders require both pharmacotherapy and psychotherapeutic interventions. The outpatient nurse can assist the patient in identifying triggers to anxiety and countering these triggers with individualized psychological measures. Distraction techniques, positive self-talk, and psychotherapy (e.g., cognitive-behavioural therapy [CBT], panic control treatment, exposure therapy, implosion therapy) can be useful.

Peplau (1989) devised general guidelines for nursing interventions that might be successful in treating patients with anxiety. These interventions help the patient attend to and react to input other than the subjective experience of anxiety. They are designed to help the patient focus on other stimuli and cope with anxiety in any form (Table 21-5). A comparison of effective and

Table 21.3	Hamilton Rating Scale for Anxiety

Max Hamilton designed this scale to help clinicians gather information about anxiety states. The symptom inventory provides scaled information that classifies anxiety behaviour and assists the clinician in targeting behaviours and achieving outcome measures.
Provide a rating for each indicator based on the following scale:

0 = None   1 = Mild   2 = Moderate
3 = Severe   4 = Severe, grossly disabling

Item	Symptoms	Rating
Anxious mood	Worries, anticipation of the worst, fearful anticipation, irritability	
Tension	Feelings of tension, fatigability, startle response, moved to tears easily, trembling, feelings of restlessness, inability to relax	
Fear	Of dark, strangers, being left alone, animals, traffic, crowds	
Insomnia	Difficulty in falling asleep, broken sleep, unsatisfying sleep and fatigue on waking, dreams, nightmares, night terrors	
Intellectual (cognitive)	Difficulty concentrating, poor memory	
Depressed mood	Loss of interest, lack of pleasure in hobbies, depression, early waking, diurnal swings	
Somatic (sensory)	Tinnitus, blurring of vision, hot and cold flushes, feelings of weakness, picking sensation	
Somatic (muscular)	Pains and aches, twitching, stiffness, myoclonic jerks, grinding of teeth, unsteady voice, increased muscular tone	
Cardiovascular symptoms	Tachycardia, palpitations, pain in chest, throbbing of vessels, fainting feelings, missing beat	
Respiratory symptoms	Pressure or constriction in chest, choking feelings, sighing, dyspnea	
Gastrointestinal symptoms	Difficulty in swallowing, wind, abdominal pain, burning sensation, abdominal fullness, nausea, vomiting, borborygmi, looseness of bowels, loss of weight, constipation	
Genitourinary symptoms	Frequency of micturition, urgency of micturition, amenorrhea, menorrhagic, development of frigidity, premature ejaculation, loss of libido, impotence	
Autonomic symptoms	Dry mouth, flushing, pallor, tendency to sweat, giddiness, tension headache, raising of hair	
Behaviour at interview	Fidgeting, restlessness or pacing, tremor of hands, furrowed brow, strained face, sighing or rapid respiration, facial pallor, swallowing, belching, brisk tendon jerks, dilated pupils, exophthalmos	

From Hamilton, M. (1959). The assessment of anxiety states by rating. *British Journal of Medical Psychology, 32,* 54.

Table 21.4	Panic Attack Cognitions Questionnaire

Rate each of the following thoughts according to the degree to which you believe each thought contributes to your panic attack.
1 = Not at all   3 = Quite a lot
2 = Somewhat   4 = Very much

1. I'm going to die.	1	2	3	4
2. I'm going insane.	1	2	3	4
3. I'm losing control.	1	2	3	4
4. This will never end.	1	2	3	4
5. I'm really scared.	1	2	3	4
6. I'm having a heart attack.	1	2	3	4
7. I'm going to pass out.	1	2	3	4
8. I don't know what people will think.	1	2	3	4
9. I won't be able to get out of here.	1	2	3	4
10. I don't understand what is happening to me.	1	2	3	4
11. People will think I am crazy.	1	2	3	4
12. I'll always be this way.	1	2	3	4
13. I am going to throw up.	1	2	3	4
14. I must have a brain tumour.	1	2	3	4
15. I'll choke to death.	1	2	3	4
16. I'm going to act foolish.	1	2	3	4
17. I'm going blind.	1	2	3	4
18. I'll hurt someone.	1	2	3	4
19. I'm going to have a stroke.	1	2	3	4
20. I'm going to scream.	1	2	3	4
21. I'm going to babble or talk funny.	1	2	3	4
22. I'll be paralyzed by fear.	1	2	3	4
23. Something is physically wrong with me.	1	2	3	4
24. I won't be able to breathe.	1	2	3	4
25. Something terrible will happen.	1	2	3	4
26. I'm going to make a scene.	1	2	3	4

Adapted from Clum, G. A. (1990). Panic attack cognitions questionnaire. *Coping with panic: A drug-free approach to dealing with anxiety attacks.* Pacific Grove. CA: Brooks/Cole.

Table 21.5	Nursing Interventions Based on Degrees of Anxiety
Degree of Anxiety	**Nursing Interventions**
Mild	Learning is possible. The nurse assists the patient to use the energy that anxiety provides to encourage learning.
Moderate	The nurse needs to check his or her own anxiety so that the patient does not empathize with it. Encourage the patient to talk: to focus on one experience, to describe it fully, then to formulate the patient's generalizations about that experience.
Severe	Learning is less possible. Allow relief behaviours to be used but do not ask about them. Encourage the patient to talk: ventilation of random ideas is likely to reduce anxiety to a moderate level. When this is observed by the nurse, proceed as above.
Panic	Learning is impossible. The nurse needs to stay with the patient. Allow pacing and walk with the patient. No content inputs to the patient's thinking should be made by the nurse. (They burden the patient, who will distort them.) Pick up on what the patient says, for example, Pt: "What's happening to me—how did I get here?" N: "Say what you notice." Short phrases by the nurse—direct, to the point of the patient's comment, and investigative—match the current attention span of the patient in panic and therefore are more likely to be heard, grasped, and acted on, with the patient's responses gradually reducing the anxiety in a helpful way. Do not touch the patient; patients experiencing panic are very concerned about survival, are experiencing grave threat to self, and usually distort intentions of all invasions of their personal space.

Adapted from Peplau, H. (1989). Theoretical constructs: Anxiety, self, and hallucinations. In A. O'Toole & S. Welt (Eds.), *Interpersonal theory in nursing practice: Selected works of Hildegard E. Peplau.* New York, NY: Springer.

ineffective dialogue with a person with an anxiety disorder can be found in Box 21-6.

Distraction

Once patients can identify the early symptoms of panic, they may learn to implement **distraction** behaviours that take the focus off the physical sensations. Some distraction activities include initiating a conversation with a nearby person and engaging in a physical activity (e.g., walking, gardening, house cleaning). Performing simple repetitive activities such as snapping a rubber band against the wrist, counting backward from 100 by threes, and counting objects along the roadway might deter an attack.

Positive Self-Talk

During states of increased anxiety and panic, individuals can learn to counter fearful or negative thoughts by using planned and rehearsed positive coping statements, called positive self-talk. "This is only anxiety, and it will pass," "I can handle these symptoms," and "I'll get through this" are examples of positive self-talk. These types of positive statements can give the individual a focal point and reduce fear when panic symptoms begin. Handheld cards that carry positive statements can be carried in a purse or wallet so that the person can retrieve them quickly when panic symptoms are felt.

Psychotherapies for Anxiety Disorders

Cognitive-behavioural therapy is a highly effective tool for treating severe anxiety or panic symptoms. It has been considered the first-line treatment for panic and other anxiety disorders and is often used in conjunction with medications, including the SSRIs, in treating panic disorder (Kampman, Keijsers, Hoogduin, & Hendriks,

2002). The goals of CBT include helping the patient to manage his or her anxiety and correcting anxiety-provoking thoughts through interventions, including cognitive restructuring, breathing training, and psychoeducation.

Panic control treatment involves an intentional exposure (through exercise) to panic-invoking sensations such as dizziness, hyperventilation, tightness in chest, and sweating. Identified patterns become targets for treatment. Patients are taught to use breathing training and cognitive restructuring to manage their responses and are instructed to practice these techniques between therapy sessions to adapt the skills to other situations.

Exposure therapy is the treatment of choice for agoraphobia, specific phobias, and OCD. The patient is repeatedly exposed to real or simulated anxiety-provoking situations until he or she becomes desensitized and anxiety subsides.

Systematic desensitization, another exposure method used to desensitize patients, exposes the patient to a hierarchy of feared situations that the patient has rated from least to most feared. The patient is taught to use muscle relaxation as levels of anxiety increase through multisituational exposure. Planning and implementing exposure therapy requires special training. Because of the multitude of outpatients in treatment for agoraphobia, exposure therapy would be a useful tool for home health psychiatric nurses. Outcomes of home-based exposure treatment are similar to clinic-based treatment outcomes.

Implosive therapy is a provocative technique useful in treating agoraphobia in which the therapist identifies phobic stimuli for the patient and then presents highly anxiety-provoking imagery to the patient, describing the feared scene as dramatically and vividly as possible. **Flooding** is a technique used to desensitize the patient

BOX 21.6

Therapeutic Dialogue: Panic Disorder With Agoraphobia

Mark, a 55-year-old Caucasian man, was admitted 4 days ago to the psychiatric unit with exacerbation of anxiety symptoms and panic attacks during the last 3 weeks. He has a 30-year history of uncontrolled anxiety that is refractory to medications and psychotherapies. On admission, he stated that he feels suicidal at times because he thinks that his life is not within his control. He feels embarrassed, angry, and "trapped" by his disorder. During the past 24 hours, Mark is seen crying at times; he also isolates himself in his room. Michelle, Mark's nurse, enters his room to make a supportive contact and to assess his current mental status.

INEFFECTIVE APPROACH

Nurse: Oh... Why are you crying?

Patient: (Looks up, gives a nervous chuckle) Obviously, because I'm upset. I am tired of living this way. I just want to be normal again. I can't even remember what that feels like.

Nurse: You look normal to me. Everyone has bad days. It'll pass.

Patient: I've felt this way longer than you've been alive. I've tried everything and nothing works.

Nurse: You're not the first depressed person that I've taken care of. You just need to go to groups and stay out of your room more. You'll start feeling better.

Patient: (Angrily) Oh, it's just that easy. You have no idea what I'm going through! You don't know me! You're just a kid.

Nurse: I can help you if you help yourself. A group starts in 5 minutes, and I'd like to see you there.

Patient: I'm not going to no damn group! I want to be alone so I can think!

Nurse: (Looks about anxiously) Maybe I should come back after you've calmed down a little.

EFFECTIVE APPROACH

Nurse: Mark, I noticed that you are staying in your room more today. What's troubling you?

Patient: (Looks up) I feel like I've lost complete control of my life. I'm so anxious and nothing helps. I'm tired of it.

Nurse: I see. That must be difficult. Can you tell me more about what you are feeling right now?

Patient: I feel like I'm going crazy. I worry all the time about having panic attacks. They make me scared I'm going to die. Sometimes I think I'd be better off dead.

Nurse: (Remains silent, continues to give eye contact)

Patient: Do you know what it's like to be a prisoner to your emotions? I can't even go out of the house sometimes and when I do, it's terrifying. I don't know what to think anymore.

Nurse: Mark, you have lived with this disorder for a long time. You say that the medications do not work to your liking, but what has helped you in the past?

Patient: Well, I learned in relaxation group that panic symptoms are probably caused by chemicals in my brain that are not working correctly. I learned that medications can help, but they don't work well for me. I tried an exposure plan and relaxation techniques to deal with my fears of leaving the house and my chronic anxiety. That did help some, but it's scary to do.

Nurse: It sounds like you have learned much about your illness, one that can be treated, so that you don't always have to feel this way.

Patient: This is easier to say right now when I'm here and can get help if I need it. It's hard to remember this when I'm in the middle of a panic attack and think I'm dying.

Nurse: It's harder when you're alone?

Patient: Much harder! And I'm alone so much of the time.

Nurse: Let's talk about some ways you can manage your panics when you're alone. Tell me some of the techniques you've learned.

CRITICAL THINKING CHALLENGE

- What tone is established by the nurse's opening question in the first scenario?
- Which therapeutic communication techniques did the nurse use in the second scenario to avoid the pitfalls encountered in the first scenario?
- What information was uncovered in the second scenario that was not touched on in the first?
- What predictions can you make about the interpersonal relationship likely to develop between the nurse and the patient in each scenario?

---

to the fear associated with a particular anxiety-provoking stimulus. Desensitizing is done by presenting feared objects or situations repeatedly without session breaks until the anxiety dissipates. For example, a patient with ophidiophobia might be presented with a real snake repeatedly until his or her anxiety decreases.

Psychoeducation programs help to educate patients and families about the symptoms of panic. Individuals with panic disorder legitimately fear going crazy, losing control, or dying because of their physical symptoms. Attempting to convince a patient that such fears are groundless only heightens anxiety and impedes communication. Information and physical evidence, such as electrocardiogram results and laboratory test results, should be presented in a caring and open manner that demonstrates acceptance and understanding of the patient's situation.

Box 21-7 suggests topics for individual or small-group discussion. It is especially important to cover such topics as the differences between panic attacks and heart attacks, the difference between panic disorder and other psychiatric disorders, and the effectiveness of various treatment methods.

Psychoeducation Checklist

When caring for the patient with anxiety disorders, be sure to include the following topic areas in the teaching plan:

- Psychopharmacologic agents (anxiolytics or antidepressants) if ordered, including drug action, dosage, frequency, and possible adverse effects
- Breathing control measures
- Potential dietary triggers
- Exercise
- Progressive muscle relaxation
- Distraction behaviours
- Relevant psychotherapies and where they are available
- Time- and specific stress-management strategies
- Positive coping strategies

• CRNENOTE

CBT is the first-line psychotherapy for panic disorder, giving patients a sense of control over the recurring threats of panic and obsessions.

Social Domain

Individuals with anxiety disorders often deteriorate socially as the disorder takes its toll on relationships with family and friends. If the disorder becomes severe enough, the person may become completely isolated. Therefore, it is an important area for assessment and active intervention if necessary.

Assessment

During the assessment, the nurse needs to assess the patient's understanding of how the anxiety or panic symptoms and associated avoidance behaviours have affected his or her life along with that of the family. Pertinent questions include the following:

- How has the disorder affected your family's social life?
- What limitations related to travel has the disorder placed on you or your family?w
- What coping strategies have you used to manage the symptoms?
- How has the disorder affected your family members or others? (Fig. 21-1)

Cultural Factors

Cultural competence calls for the understanding of cultural knowledge, cultural awareness, cultural assessment skills, and cultural practice. Therefore, cultural differences must be considered in the assessment of panic disorder. Different cultures interpret sensations, feelings, or understandings differently. For example, symptoms of anxiety might be seen as witchcraft or magic in some cultures (APA, 2000). Several cultures do not have a word to describe "anxiety" or "anxious" and instead may use words or meanings to suggest physical complaints. In addition, showing anxiety may be a sign of weakness in some cultures (Chen, Reich, & Chung, 2002). Many Asian OTC herbal remedies contain substances that may induce panic by increasing the heart rate, basal metabolic rate, blood pressure, and sweating (Chen et al.). Diet pills and ginseng are two examples.

Interventions for Social Domain

Individuals with panic disorder, especially those with significant anxiety sensitivity, may need assistance in reevaluating their lifestyle. Time management can be a useful tool. In the workplace or at home, underestimating the time needed to complete a chore or being overly involved in several activities at once increases stress and anxiety. Procrastination, lack of assertiveness, and difficulties with prioritizing or delegating tasks intensify these problems.

Writing a list of chores to be completed and estimating the time needed to complete them provide concrete feedback to the individual. Crossing out each activity as it is completed helps the patient to regain a sense of control and accomplishment. Large tasks should be broken into a series of smaller tasks to minimize stress and maximize a sense of achievement. Rest, relaxation, and family time—frequently omitted from the daily schedule—must be included.

Family Response to Disorder

Families afflicted with panic disorder have difficulty with overall communication. Parents with agoraphobia may become discouraged and self-critical regarding their child-rearing abilities, which may cause their children to be overly dependent. Parents with panic disorder may inadvertently cause excessive fears, phobias, or excessive worry in their children. Individuals will need a tremendous amount of support and encouragement from significant others.

Pharmacologic treatment for anxiety disorders also affects the family in other ways. Medications used to treat these disorders readily cross the placenta and are excreted in breast milk. Open discussions regarding the benefits of a healthy mother and available options for women who wish to breast-feed and the recognition of a woman's right to participate in the decision-making process are all important in postpartum panic disorder. Pregnancy may actually protect against certain anxiety disorders, but postpartum onset of such disorders is not uncommon.

FIGURE 21.1 Bio/psycho/social/spiritual interventions for patients with panic disorder.

Spiritual Domain

Anxiety can be understood as basic to the human condition. Existentialist thinkers (see Box 21-8) argue that, because we humans are aware of our own mortality, the apprehension that death will end our existence fills us with foreboding. This **existential anxiety** must be accepted and faced or it can subvert our everyday life. We can feel alienated and estranged (not at home) in the world. We look to find meaning in our lives, a raison d'étre. Existentialists note that, as neither nature nor culture can do this for us, individual humans are, in a sense, self-making. Viktor Frankl (1992), in *Man's Search for Meaning*, described the wish of every human as being to have a meaningful life (see Chapter 8 for logotherapy).

Paul Tillich (1952), the author of *The Courage to Be* and a theistic existentialist, finds that existential anxiety involves three areas of apprehension: fate and death (the absolute threat to self), emptiness and meaninglessness (worry that there is no ultimate meaning), and guilt and condemnation (perceived threats to one's identity). Being human involves confronting and reconciling such anxiety.

The importance of understanding the relation between existential anxiety and clinical anxiety is being explored by researchers. The Existential Anxiety Scale (EAS) has been developed, for instance, based on Tillich's theory (Weems, Costa, Dehon, & Berman, 2004). Early results

BOX 21.8

Some "Existentialist" Thinkers and an Example of Their Work

Søren Kierkegaard	*Either Or: A Fragment of a Life* (1843/1944)
Friedrich Nietzsche	*Thus Spoke Zarathustra* (1883/1985)
Martin Heidegger	*Being and Time* (1927/1962)
Karl Jaspers	*On My Philosophy* (1941/1955)
Gabriel Marcel	*The Mystery of Being* (1951)
Jean-Paul Sartre	*Being and Nothingness* (1943/1956)
Simone de Beauvoir	*The Second Sex* (1949/1953)
Henrik Ibsen	*A Doll's House* (1879/1889)
Albert Camus	*The Myth of Sisyphus* (1942/1955)
Dostoevsky	*Notes from the Underground* (1864/1918)
Samuel Beckett	*Waiting for Godot* (1953/1955)
Eugène Ionesco	*The Chairs* (1952/1958)

suggest that existential anxiety, as measured by the EAS, is common and associated with symptoms of anxiety and depression (Weems et al., 2004). A critical review of the literature by Koslander, Barbosa da Silva, and Roxberg (2009) concluded that "it is evident that addressing patients' existential and spiritual needs helps them improve mentally" (p. 40). They argue that an existential perspective should be an element of mental health care.

A spiritual-based approach to PTSD in combat veterans has been studied (intervention versus control) by Bormann, Thorp, Wetherell, and Golshan (2008). Their group intervention involved using mantra (sacred name) repetition (e.g., "Jesus, Jesus," "Om Mani Padme Hum," or "Rama Rama") as a focusing strategy to interrupt "fight or flight" responses in stressful situations. Using this intervention, PTSD symptom severity and psychological distress were reduced. Quality of life was increased. Overall, it is increasingly recognized that a holistic approach to people with anxiety disorders, one that includes the spiritual domain, is necessary.

▆◀ EVALUATION AND TREATMENT OUTCOMES

Patients can be assisted to keep a daily log of the severity of anxiety and the frequency, duration, and severity of panic episodes. This log will be a basic tool for monitoring progress as symptoms decrease. A number of self-help books have been written and can provide a rich source of reinforcement of simple interventions that can attenuate the intensity and frequency of panic symptoms. Rating scales may also be helpful to monitor changes in misinterpretations or other symptoms related to panic. Medications alone provide significant short-term improvement for many individuals, but a long-term combination of psychosocial and pharmacologic treatment is usually necessary.

Although many researchers consider panic disorder a chronic, long-term condition, the positive results from outcome studies should be shared with patients to provide encouragement and optimism that patients can learn to manage these symptoms. Outcome studies have demonstrated success with panic control treatment, CBT, exposure therapy, and various medications specific to certain symptoms. Figure 21-2 illustrates a number of examples of bio/psycho/social/spiritual treatment outcomes for individuals with panic disorder.

▆◀ CONTINUUM OF CARE

As with any disorder, the continuum of patient care across multiple settings is crucial. Patients are treated in the least restrictive environment that will meet their safety needs. As the patient progresses through treatment, the environment of care changes from an emergency or inpatient setting to outpatient clinics or individual therapy sessions.

Inpatient-Focused Care

Inpatient settings provide control for the individual with comorbid depression, increased risk of suicide, or poor treatment response to typical treatment strategies.

FIGURE 21.2 Bio/psycho/social/spiritual outcomes for patients with panic disorder.

Emergency Care!

Because individuals with panic disorder are likely to first present for treatment in an emergency room or primary care setting, nurses working in these settings should be involved in early recognition and referral. Consultation with a psychiatrist or mental health professional by the primary care physician can decrease both costs and overall patient symptoms (Katon, Roy-Byrne, Russo, & Cowley, 2002). Unnecessary emergency department visits cause soaring health care costs. Several interventions may be useful in reducing the number of emergency room visits related to panic symptoms. Psychiatric consultation and nursing education can be provided in the emergency department to explore other avenues of treatment. Remembering that the patient experiencing a panic attack is in crisis, nurses can take several measures to help alleviate symptoms, including the following:

- Stay with the patient and maintain a calm demeanour. (Anxiety often produces more anxiety, and a calm presence will help calm the patient.)
- Reassure the patient that you will not leave, that this episode will pass, and that he or she is in a safe place. (The patient often fears dying and cannot see beyond the panic attack.)
- Give clear, concise directions, using short sentences. Do not use medical jargon.
- Walk or pace with the patient to an environment with minimal stimulation. (The patient in panic has excessive energy.)
- Administer PRN anxiolytic medications as ordered and appropriate. (Pharmacotherapy is effective in treating acute panic.)

After the panic attack has resolved, allow the patient to vent his or her feelings. This often helps the patient in clarifying his or her feelings.

Family Interventions

In addition to learning the symptoms of panic disorder, nurses should have information sheets or pamphlets available concerning the disorder and any medications prescribed. Parents, especially single parents, will need assistance in child rearing and may benefit from services designed to provide some respite. Moreover, the entire family will need support in adjusting to the disorder. A referral for family therapy may be indicated. Involving the entire family in the therapy process is imperative. Families experience the symptoms, treatments, clinical setbacks, and recovery from chronic mental illnesses as a unit. Misunderstandings, misconceptions, false information, and stigma of mental illness, singly or collectively, impede recovery efforts.

Community Treatment

Most individuals with panic disorder will be treated on an outpatient basis. Referral lists of community resources and support groups are useful in this setting. Nurses can be directly involved in treatment, conducting psychoeducation groups on relaxation and breathing techniques, symptom management, and anger management. Advanced practice nurses conduct CBT and individual and family psychotherapies. In addition, medication monitoring groups reemphasize the role of the medications, monitor for side effects, and enhance treatment compliance overall (see Nursing Care Plan 21-1).

■■■ ASSESSMENT AND TREATMENT ISSUES SPECIFIC TO OBSESSIVE-COMPULSIVE DISORDER

Patients with OCD can be difficult to treat because of their symptoms and the pathology of the disease. The obsessions and compulsions consistently interfere with recovery efforts during the treatment course. Most patients with OCD are treated in specific outpatient programs and in private physician practice, but short-term hospitalization is often used for comorbid depression and for treatment refractory symptoms. It is very important that all staff members be consistent in their expectations and acceptance of the patient's behaviours to keep these patients from becoming frustrated or confused regarding expectations during treatment (Box 21-9).

Individuals with OCD do not consider their compulsions pleasurable. Often, they recognize them as odd and may initially try to resist them. Resistance eventually fails, and patients incorporate repetitive behaviours into daily routines, performing activities in a specific, ritual order. If this sequence is disturbed, the person experiences extreme anxiety until the process can be repeated in the correct sequence. Interpersonal relationships suffer, and the patient may actively isolate himself or herself. Indeed, individuals with OCD are more likely to be young, separated or divorced, and unemployed.

Assessment

Patients with OCD do not have a higher prevalence of physical disease. However, they may complain of multiple physical symptoms. With late-onset OCD (after 35 years of age) and with symptoms in children that occur after a febrile illness, cerebral pathology should be excluded. Each patient with OCD should be assessed for dermatologic lesions caused by repetitive hand washing, excessive cleaning with caustic agents, or bathing. Osteoarthritic joint damage secondary to cleaning rituals may be observed.

The nurse should assess the type and severity of the patient's obsessions and compulsions. Most individuals will

Nursing Care Plan 21.1

A Patient With Panic Disorder

Bill is a 65-year-old, unmarried man who began having his first panic attacks after he retired from a post office position 2 years ago. He has been able to live alone until recently, when his daughter became concerned that he was isolating himself and refused to drive, to pay bills, or to go to the grocery store for food. He admitted to being fearful of leaving because of extreme nervousness and fear of a panic attack. His daughter convinced him to seek help, and he is now in a day treatment program at a local facility. He is able to attend the program most days.

Settings: Day Treatment Program, Adult Psychiatric Services

Baseline Assessment: Bill averages three or four panic attacks per week. His mental status is normal, with no cognitive impairment. Mini-mental status examination is within normal limits. He has depressive symptoms but does not meet the criteria for a mood disorder. He misses his job and feels as if part of his identity is lost. Vital signs are normal. He has a known 10-year history of hypertension, with a heart attack at the age of 57 years. He would like to "get rid of the feeling of nervousness" and be able to enjoy life like he did before retirement.

Associated Psychiatric Diagnosis	Medications
Axis I: Panic disorder with agoraphobia	Paroxetine CR (Paxil) 12.5 mg qd
Axis II: None	Lisinopril (Zestril) 20 mg daily
Axis III: A history of hypertension	Lorazepam (Ativan) 1 mg every 6 hours
Axis IV: Social problems (unable to leave home)	PRN for extreme anxiety
Educational problems (failing in school)	
GAF = Current 60	
Potential 90	

Care Plan for Panic Symptoms

Defining Characteristics	Related Factors
Trembling, increased pulse	Impending panic attacks
Fearful, irritable, scared, worried	Panic attacks
Apprehensive	

Outcomes

Initial	Long-term
Develop skills to decrease the impact of panic attack.	Carry out normal daily living and social activities outside of the house

Interventions

Interventions	Rationale	Ongoing Assessment
Meet daily with Bill to assess if he has had a panic attack within the last 24 hours.	Asking Bill to monitor panic attacks will provide data regarding potential antecedents to attacks.	Determine whether Bill has had a panic attack.
Using a calm, reassuring approach, encourage verbalization of feelings, perceptions, and fears. Identify periods of time when anxiety level is at its highest.	Discussing the experience of anxiety will help the patient notice when his anxiety increases.	Explore the antecedents and determine whether he was able to practice techniques from education programs.
Teach Bill how to perform relaxation techniques.	Having strategies to deal with impending panic attack will decrease the intensity of the experience.	Observe effectiveness of his technique and changes in anxiety/panic episodes.

Continued

Nursing Care Plan 21.1 (Continued)

Interventions

Interventions	Rationale	Ongoing Assessment
Teach Bill about the actions and side effects of paroxetine. Explain the purposes of each of the medications and track the use of PRN medications. Also, monitor for the use of alcohol and herbal supplements.	Panic attacks are neurobiologic occurrences that respond to medications.	Determine whether panic attacks decrease over time and whether there are side effects. Determine his commitment to relieving his panic attacks.

Evaluation

Outcomes	Revised Outcomes	Interventions
Bill's panic attacks decreased to once a week. Attended day treatment program every day. Able to go to grocery store.	Increase social activity outside of house.	Meet with Bill twice a week to monitor progress. Continue to reinforce the use of strategies in managing anticipatory anxiety.

BOX 21.9

Clinical Vignette: Obsessive-Compulsive Disorder

Robert, a 32-year-old man, is a new patient at a local psychiatric unit. He admitted himself to have his medicines evaluated because his obsessive thoughts and depression have worsened since his recent divorce. While in the hospital, he has quickly become viewed as a "problem patient" because he hoards linens and demands a new bar of soap for each of his five daily showers. He is compelled to open and close his door five times when he leaves or enters his room but does not know why. This behaviour has led to arguments with his roommate. In an effort to "help him," the staff locked his bathroom door to prevent him from showering so frequently. He tried to enter his bathroom to shower and panicked when the staff refused to allow him to shower, telling him "You can live without it." After receiving PRN medication for extreme anxiety, Robert signed out of the hospital against medical advice because of embarrassment and anger toward the nursing staff.

WHAT DO YOU THINK?
- How could the staff have handled the situation differently so as to not disrupt Robert's or the unit's clinical care?
- What nursing interventions might be appropriate in providing Robert's care?

---

appear neatly dressed and groomed, cooperative, and eager to answer questions. Orientation and memory are not usually impaired, but patients may be distracted by obsessional thoughts. Individuals with severe symptoms may be preoccupied with fears or with discussing their obsessions, but in most instances, direct questions must be asked to reveal symptoms. For example, the nurse may begin indirectly by asking how long it takes the individual to dress in the morning or leave the house, but usually follow-up questions are needed, such as: Do you find yourself frequently returning to the house to make sure that you have turned off the lights or the stove, even when you know that you have already checked this? Does this happen every day? Are you ever late for work or for important appointments?

Identifying the degree to which the OCD symptoms interfere with the patient's daily functioning is important. Several rating scales can be used to identify symptoms and monitor improvement. Examples of these scales are provided in Box 21-10. The Yale-Brown Obsessive Compulsive Scale (Y-BOCS) is a popular, clinician-rated 16-item scale that obtains separate subtotals for the severity of obsessions and compulsions. The Maudsley Obsessive-Compulsive Inventory is a 30-item, true–false, self-assessment tool that may help the individual to recognize individual symptoms.

Nurses must consider sociocultural factors when evaluating OCD. At times, cultural or religious beliefs may be misunderstood and mistaken for obsessions or compulsions. Shame and embarrassment over the irrational thoughts and behaviours often lead to social isolation and relational difficulties. The time demands related to the compulsions often lead to decreased occupational success. Thus, the assessment of current level of functioning in social, occupational, and personal spheres is important.

Family Response to Disorder

Those with more severe symptoms are more likely to be more impaired in social skills and have more difficulties with intimacy and consequently are less likely to marry. Some studies have also shown higher divorce rates for individuals with OCD (Grabe et al., 2000). They also have higher rates of celibacy, possibly because they fear being dirty or becoming contaminated.

OCD often diminishes the quality of family relationships. Individuals with this disorder may ask family members to become involved in their rituals of checking or providing repeated reassurance (Koran, 2000). Those with OCD can become very angry and frustrated with family members for failing to comply with their requests for help with rituals. This can result in verbal and even physical altercations. Many family members find themselves modifying routines to suit a patient's symptoms and report this to be at least moderately distressing for them (Calvocoressi et al., 1999). The most troublesome symptoms of OCD for families to cope with include the patients' ruminations, long-standing unemployment, rituals, noncompliance with medication, depression, withdrawal from social and family contact, lack of motivation, and excessive arguing (Cooper, 1996). Spouses report a variety of issues such as sexual difficulties, overwhelming feelings of frustration, anger, guilt and fatigue, and disrupted family and social life. Other relatives reported moderate to severe burden in coping with an individual with OCD. They stated that they had difficulty going on holidays, had poor social relationships, and neglected their hobbies due to their relative's illness (Magliano, Tosini, Guarneri, Marasco, & Catapano, 1996).

Treatment

Clomipramine (a TCA) and venlafaxine (a selective serotonin and norepinephrine reuptake inhibitor) have been compared for the treatment of OCD. One preliminary study shows that venlafaxine may be as efficacious as clomipramine but with less harsh side effects (Albert, Aguglia, Maina, & Bogetto, 2002). Although extremely rare, psychosurgery has been used to treat extremely severe OCD that has not responded to prolonged and intensive drug treatment, behavioural therapy, or a combination of the two. Modern stereotactic surgical techniques that produce lesions of the cingulum (a bundle of connective pathways between the two hemispheres) or the anterior limb of the internal capsule (a region near the thalamus and part of the circuit connecting to the cortex) may bring about substantial clinical benefit in some patients without causing significant morbidity (Kim et al., 2003). Other treatment options include radiotherapy and deep brain stimulation in which electrical current is applied through an electrode inserted into the brain (Nuttin, Cosyn, Demeulemeester, Gybels, & Meyerson, 1999).

For the patient with cleaning or hand-washing compulsions, attention to skin condition is necessary. Encourage the patient to use tepid water when washing and hand cream after washing. Remove harsh, abrasive soaps and replace with moisturizing soaps. The treatment team would work with the patient to decrease the frequency of washing by structuring time schedules and time-limited washing.

Specific Interventions for OCD

Response Prevention

An effective behavioural intervention for patients with OCD who perform rituals is exposure with response prevention. The patient is exposed to situations or objects that are known to induce anxiety but is asked to refrain from performing the ritualistic behaviours. One goal of this procedure is to help the patient understand that resisting the rituals while exposed to the object of anxiety is less stressful and time-consuming than performing the rituals. Another goal is to confound the expectation of distressing outcomes and eventually extinguish the compulsive behaviours. Most patients improve with exposure and response prevention, but few become completely symptom free.

Thought Stopping

Thought stopping is used with patients who have obsessional thoughts. The patient is taught to interrupt obsessional thoughts by saying "Stop!" either aloud or subvocally. This activity interrupts and delays the uncontrollable spiral of obsessional thoughts. Research supporting this technique is scant; however, practitioners have found it useful in multimodal treatment with exposure and response prevention, relaxation, and cognitive restructuring.

Cognitive Restructuring

Cognitive restructuring is a method of teaching the patient to restructure dysfunctional thought processes by defining and testing them (Beck, Emery, & Greenberg, 1985). Its goal is to alter the patient's immediate, dysfunctional appraisal of a situation and perception of long-term consequences. The patient is taught to monitor automatic thoughts, then to recognize the connection between thoughts, emotional responses, and behaviours. The distorted thoughts are examined and tested by for-or-against evidence presented by the therapist, which helps the patient to realistically assess the likelihood that the feared event will happen if the compulsive behaviour is not performed. The patient begins to analyze his or her thoughts as incongruent with reality. For example, even if the alarm clock is not checked 30 times before going to bed, it will still go off in the morning, and the patient will not be disciplined for tardiness at work. Maybe it needs to be checked only once or twice (see Chapter 15).

Cue Cards

Cue cards are tools used to help the patient restructure thought patterns. They contain statements that are

BOX 21.11

Examples of Cue Card Statements

It's the OCD, not me.
These are only OC thoughts; OC thoughts don't mean action; I will not act on the thoughts.
My anxiety level goes up but will always go down. I never sat with the anxiety long enough to see that it would not harm me.
Trust myself.
I did it right the first time.
Checking the locks again won't keep me safe. I really am safe in the world.

positively oriented and pertain to the patient's specific obsessions and compulsions. Cue cards use information from the patient's symptom hierarchy, an organizational system that breaks down the obsessions and compulsions from least to most anxiety provoking. These cards can help reinforce the belief that the patient is safe and can tolerate the anxiety caused by delaying or controlling compulsive rituals. Box 21-11 provides examples of cue cards.

Interventions for Social Domain

- For the hospitalized patient, unit routines must be carefully and clearly explained to decrease the fear of the unknown. Initially, providing a private room may decrease the fear and anxiety related to explaining one's behaviour to other patients.
- Help the patient choose relaxation or recreational activities that can be interrupted and returned to, so as to minimize frustration.
- Assist the patient in arranging a schedule of activities that incorporates some private time but also integrates the patient into normal unit activities.

Family Interventions

The families of patients with OCD will need to be educated about the etiology of the disorder. Understanding the biologic basis of the disorder should decrease some of the stigma and embarrassment they may feel about the bizarre nature of the patient's obsessions and compulsions. Education about both biologic and psychological treatment approaches should be provided. Family assistance in monitoring symptom remission and medication side effects is invaluable. Family members can also assist the patient with behavioural and cognitive interventions.

Community Treatment

Partial hospitalization programs and day treatment programs care for most patients with OCD. They allow patients to maintain significant independence, while beginning medications and behavioural therapies. Specific day treatment psychotherapy programs for OCD are available in some larger urban centres. Specific outpatient clinics may also be available. Self-help groups and self-help books can also help patients keep their symptoms under control.

Evaluation and Treatment Outcomes

Several methods can be used to measure the response to treatment, including changes in Y-BOCS scores or other rating scales, self-reports regarding decreases in the frequency and duration of rituals, increasing sense of self-efficacy, and the ability to complete the activities of daily living in a timely manner. The patient should be able to participate in family and social activities with minimal anxiety. Both the patient and the family should also have knowledge about OCD and any additional sources of information and support in their community.

ASSESSMENT AND TREATMENT ISSUES SPECIFIC TO GENERALIZED ANXIETY DISORDER

Assessment

In addition to GAD being associated with increasing age and being female, other correlates have been identified. These include being previously married, being unemployed, and working within the home, suggesting that psychosocial and environmental factors are involved in the development of GAD. Thus, a detailed psychosocial history is important. Chronic sleep disturbance is a common symptom for individuals with GAD, so the patient's sleep pattern should be assessed closely.

Intervention

Interventions for GAD are aimed at decreasing both the fundamental anxiety symptoms and any related depression symptoms. Until very recently, benzodiazepines were widely used in the treatment of GAD (Martin et al., 2007). However, due to the chronic nature of GAD and the risks related to the long-term use of benzodiazepines, this class of anxiolytics is no longer considered a first-line treatment (Sheehan, 1999). Rather, SSRIs or selective norepinephrine and serotonin reuptake inhibitors have become mainstays in the pharmacologic treatment of GAD (Rickels & Rynn, 2002; Sheehan). The most proven psychological therapy used for GAD is CBT. Alcohol should be avoided because it disturbs the sleep cycle. Good sleep hygiene is important. Avoiding such things as alcohol and coffee (even tea for those very sensitive to caffeine) in the evening, eating late in the evening, working on difficult work-related or personal issues in the evening, and initiating evening discussion about sensitive issues with family members all may decrease sleep disturbance. Having bedtime routines that include a warm bath, quiet reading, and relaxation techniques all promote sleep.

SPECIFIC ASSESSMENT AND TREATMENT ISSUES RELATED TO ACUTE STRESS DISORDER AND POSTTRAUMATIC STRESS DISORDER

Assessment

A major risk factor related to developing ASD and going on to develop PTSD is having experienced previous serious stressors or traumatic events. Thus, it is very important to garner information about the past contexts of patients' lives and about the previous experiences that the individuals feel strongly affected their health. What may appear an exaggerated response to a relatively small incident may actually be related to being triggered by past memories and emotional responses. Common tools to assess for past stressful life events include the Trauma Event Inventory (Bremner, Vermetten, & Mazure, 2000), the Adverse Childhood Events Survey (Dube et al., 2003), and the Childhood Trauma Questionnaire (Bernstein, Ahluvalia, Pogge, & Handelsman, 1997).

There are also a number of standardized questionnaires that have been developed to assess the presence and severity of posttraumatic symptoms. These include the Acute Stress Disorder Scale (Bryant, 1999), the Clinician Administered PTSD Scale (CAPS; Blake et al., 1995), and the Posttraumatic Symptom Scale (Foa & Tolin, 2000). The use of standardized questionnaires and surveys should be based on the characteristics of the agency and the specific population. Standardized data can serve important roles in funding and ongoing program evaluation and development.

Treatment

There are no treatment guidelines for the treatment of ASD. Controversy exists around the efficacy of critical incident debriefing as a general response to traumatic events. While some studies have shown positive results, others have shown either no efficacy in attenuating the risk of ASD or PTSD (Arendt & Elklit, 2001; Kagee, 2002) or demonstrated worse outcomes for stress-related disorders (Greenberg, 2001; Summerfield, 1995). Reassurance that acute symptoms are very common (normalizing the patient experiences and sensations) and that for many individuals the acute symptoms will fade with time may be all that is needed in the immediate aftermath of a traumatic event.

Unlike ASD, clinical treatment guidelines have been established for PTSD. They include pharmacologic therapies, such as antidepressants (TCAs and SSRIs) and mood stabilizers (carbamazepine and valproate). Minipress, an antihypertensive agent, has been found to decrease the recurrent nightmares in patients with PTSD (Raskind et al., 2002). This is an area for future research. Most individuals with PTSD benefit from a combination of pharmacotherapy and specific psychotherapies, such as CBT and prolonged exposure techniques (Foa, 1997).

SUMMARY OF KEY POINTS

☐ Anxiety-related disorders are the most common of all psychiatric disorders and comprise a wide range of disorders. The anxiety disorders do display important similarities in symptoms (e.g., recurring severe anxiety, anxiety sensitivity), longitudinal course (chronic course with exacerbations and remissions), risk factors, etiological factors, pharmacologic strategies, and nonpharmacologic interventions.

☐ Those experiencing anxiety disorders have high levels of physical and emotional symptoms and often experience dual diagnoses with other anxiety disorders, substance use disorder, or depression. These disorders often significantly impair individuals' ability to function socially, occupationally, and personally.

☐ Treatment approaches for all anxiety-related disorders are somewhat similar, including pharmacotherapies, psychological treatments, or often a combination of both.

☐ Current research points to a combination of biologic, psychologic, social, and spiritual factors that cause persistent anxiety. Other research demonstrates that there are also personality traits that predispose individuals to anxiety disorders, including low self-esteem, external locus of control, some negative family influences, and some traumatic or stressful precipitating event. These components combine to yield a true bio/psycho/social/spiritual theory of causation.

☐ Nurses at the generalist level use interventions from each of the dimensions—biologic, psychological, social, and spiritual. Approaching these patients with knowledge of the disorder, understanding, and calm is crucial. Nurses can be instrumental in crisis intervention, medication management, and psychoeducation. Psychoeducation is crucial in the management of anxiety disorders and includes methods to help patients control and cope with the anxiety reactions (e.g., control of breathing, stress reduction, relaxation techniques), education regarding medication side effects and management, and education of family members to understand these disorders.

CRITICAL THINKING CHALLENGES

1 How does patient culture affect the assessment of anxiety?

2 How might one differentiate shyness from social anxiety disorder?

3 How might the etiology of depression and anxiety be similar, as antidepressant medications are used to treat both?

4 What are some of the barriers in assessing pathologic anxiety in children? Are anxiety disorders underdiagnosed or overdiagnosed in children? Explain.

5 What role might parents, aside from genetics, play in contributing to the development of anxiety disorders in their offspring?

6 What are the risks and benefits of treating anxiety disorders with benzodiazepine medications in individuals with substance abuse?

7 Pregnancy appears to protect against the development of some anxiety disorders, and postpartum onset of anxiety disorders is not uncommon. What bio/psycho/social/spiritual dynamics may be involved?

WEB LINKS

www.adaa.org This is the site of the Anxiety Disorders Association of America (ADAA), a national nonprofit organization dedicated to the prevention, treatment, and cure of anxiety disorders and to improving the lives of all people who suffer from them.

www.nimh.nih.gov/anxiety/anxietymenu.cfm This is the National Institute of Mental Health's anxiety disorder website. An anxiety disorders education program is available.

MOVIES, NOVELS, AND BIOGRAPHIES

Shake Hands with the Devil: Journey of Roméo Dallaire: 2007. In this award-winning documentary, Lt. General Roméo Dallaire relates his experiences in Rwanda, Central Africa, during a time of genocide and his experiences with PTSD following his return to Canada (see In a Life sidebar).

VIEWING POINTS: Identify the symptoms of PTSD as described by General Dallaire. What do you think are the barriers to recovery from PTSD that may still exist for Canadian soldiers?

As Good As It Gets: 1997. Novelist Melvin Udall, played by Jack Nicholson, lives in his own world of obsessive-compulsive behaviour patterns, avoiding cracks in sidewalks and rigidly adhering to a regimen of daily breakfasts in the café where single mom Carol Connelly, played by Helen Hunt, works. Udall's world is changed when he unwillingly becomes a sitter for his next-door neighbour's dog.

VIEWING POINTS: Identify the behaviours that indicate that Udall has an anxiety disorder. Observe feelings that are generated in you by Udall's behaviour. How are Udall's friends able to tolerate his behaviour?

REFERENCES

Albert, U., Aguglia, E., Maina, G., & Bogetto, F. (2002). Venlafaxine versus clomipramine in the treatment of obsessive-compulsive disorder: A preliminary single-blind, 12 week, controlled study. *Journal of Clinical Psychiatry, 63*(11), 1004–1009.

American Psychiatric Association. (2000). *Diagnostic and statistical manual of mental disorders* (4th ed., Text revision). Washington, DC: Author.

Antai-Otong, D. (2003). Current treatment of generalized anxiety disorder. *Journal of Psychosocial Nursing & Mental Health Service, 41*(12), 20–29.

Arendt, M. & Elklit, A. (2001). Effectiveness of psychological debriefing. *Acta Psychiatric Scandinavia, 104*(6), 423–437.

Argyle, N., Deltito, J., Allerup, P., Maier, W., Albus, M., Nutzinger, D., et al. (1991). The Panic-Associated Symptom Scale: Measuring the severity of panic disorder. *Acta Psychiatrica Scandinavica, 83*, 20–26.

Ballenger, J. C. (1999). Current treatments of the anxiety disorders in adults. *Biological Psychiatry, 46*(11), 1579–1594.

Ballenger, J. C., Davidson, J. R., Lecrubier, Y., Nutt, D. J., Borkovec, T. D., Rickels K. et al. (2001). Consensus statement on generalized anxiety disorder from the International Consensus Group on Depression and Anxiety. *Journal of Clinical Psychiatry, 62* (Suppl 11), 53–58.

Bandelow, B., Wedekind, D., Pauls, J., Brooks, A., Hajak, G., & Ruther, E. (2000). Salivary cortisol in panic attacks. *American Journal of Psychiatry, 157*, 454–456.

Barzega, G., Maina, G., Venturello, S., & Bogetto, F. (2001). Gender-related differences in the onset of panic disorder. *Acta Psychiatrica Scandinavica, 103*(3), 189–195.

Baxter, L. (1992). Neuroimaging studies of obsessive compulsive disorder. *Psychiatric Clinics of North America, 15*(4), 871–883.

Beck, A., Emery, C., & Greenberg, R. L. (1985). *Anxiety disorders and phobias: A cognitive perspective*. New York, NY: Basic Books.

Beck, A., Epstein, N., Brown, G., & Steer, R. (1988). An inventory for measuring clinical anxiety: The Beck Anxiety Inventory. *Journal of Consulting and Clinical Psychology, 56*, 893–897.

Beekman, A., de Beurs, E., von Balkom, A., Deeg, D., van Dyck, R., & van Tilburg, W. (2000). Anxiety and depression in later life: Co-occurrence and communality of risk factors. *American Journal of Psychiatry, 157*, 89–95.

Bernstein, D. P., Ahluvalia, T., Pogge, D., & Handelsman, L. (1997). Validity of the Childhood Trauma Questionnaire in an adolescent psychiatric population. *Journal of the American Academy of Child and Adolescent Psychiatry, 36*, 340–346.

Blake, D. D., Weathers, F. W., Nagy, L. M., Kaloupek, D. G., Gusman, F. D., Charney, D. S., et al. (1995). The development of a Clinician-Administered PTSD Scale. *Journal of Traumatic Stress, 8*(1), 75–90.

Bland, R. C., Newman, S. C., & Orn, H. (1988). Period prevalence of psychiatric disorders in Edmonton. *Acta Psychiatrica Scandinavica, 338*(Suppl.), 33–42.

Bodinger, L., Hermesh, H., Aizenberg, D., Valevski, A., Marom, S., Shiloh, R., et al. (2002). Sexual function and behaviour in social phobia. *Journal of Clinical Psychiatry, 63*(10), 874–879.

Bormann, J., Thorp, S., Wetherell, J., & Golshan, S. (2008). A spiritually based group intervention for combat veterans with posttraumatic stress disorder. *Journal of Holistic Nursing, 26*(2), 109–116.

Bradwejn, J., Koszycki, D., du Tertre, A., Bourin, M., Palmour, R., & Ervin, F. (1992). The cholecystokinin hypothesis of panic and anxiety disorders: A review. *Journal of Psychopharmacology, 6*, 345–351.

Brauer, H., Nowicki, P., Catalano, G., & Catalano, M. (2002). Panic attacks associated with citalopram. *Southern Medical Journal, 95*(9), 1088–1089.

Bremner, J. D. Vermetten, E., & Mazure, C. M. (2000). Development and preliminary psychometric properties of an instrument for the measurement of childhood trauma: the Early Trauma Inventory. *Depression and Anxiety, 12*(1), 1–12.

Brewin, C., Andrews, B., Rose, S., & Kirk, M. (1999). Acute stress disorder and posttraumatic stress disorder in victims of violent crime. *American Journal of Psychiatry, 156*(3), 360–366.

Bryant, R. A. (1999). The acute stress disorder scale: A tool for predicting posttraumatic stress disorder. *Australian Journal of Emergency Management, 14*, 13–15.

Busatto, G., Buchpiguel, C. A., Zamignani, D. R., Garrido, G. E., Glabus, M. F., Rosario-Campos, M. C., et al. (2001). Regional cerebral blood flow abnormalities in early-onset obsessive-compulsive disorder: An exploratory SPECT study. *Journal of the American Academy of Child and Adolescent Psychiatry, 40*(3), 347–354.

Calvocoressi, L., Mazure, C. M., Kasl, S. V., Skolnick, J., Fisk, D., Vegso, S. J., et al. (1999). Family accommodation of obsessive-compulsive symptoms: Instrument development and assessment of family behavior. *Journal of Nervouse and Mental Disorders, 187*, 636–642.

Cassidy, J., Lichtenstein-Phelps, J., Sibrava, N. J., Thomas, C. L. Jr., & Borkovec, T. D. (2009). Generalized anxiety disorder: connections with self-reported attachment. *Journal of Behavior Therapy and Experimental Psychiatry, 40*(1), 23–38.

Castellanos, D., & Hunter, T. (2000). Anxiety disorders in children and adolescents. *Southern Medical Journal, 92*(10), 946–954.

Castle, D., & Groves, A. (2000). The internal and external boundaries of obsessive-compulsive disorder. *Australian and New Zealand Journal of Psychiatry, 34*, 249–255.

CBC Digital Archives. (2000). *The ghosts of Rwanda.* Retrieved November 26, 2009, from http://archives.cbc.ca/war_conflict/peacekeeping/topics/1686-11622/

CBC News Online. (2003). *Indepth: Romeo Dallaire.* Retrieved November 26, 2009, from http://www.cbc.ca/news/background/dallaire/

Chambless, D. L., Caputo, G. C., Bright, P., & Gallagher, R. (1984). Assessment of fear in agoraphobics: The Body Sensations Questionnaire and the Agoraphobic Cognitions Questionnaire. *Journal of Consulting and Clinical Psychology, 52*, 1090–1097.

Chambless, D. L., Caputo, G. C., Jasin, S. E., Gracely, E. J., & Williams, C. (1985). The Mobility Inventory for Agoraphobia. *Behaviour Research and Therapy, 23*, 35–44.

Chen, J-P., Reich, L., & Chung, H. (2002). Anxiety disorders. *Western Journal of Medicine, 176*(4), 249–253.

Classen, C., Koopman, C., Hales, R., & Spiegel, D. (1998). Acute stress disorder as a predictor of posttraumatic stress symptoms. *The American Journal of Psychiatry, 155*(5), 620–624.

Clum, G. A. (1990). Panic attack cognitions questionnaire. In *Coping with panic: A drug-free approach to dealing with anxiety attacks.* Pacific Grove, CA: Brooks/Cole.

Cooper, J. (1970). The Leyton Obsessional Inventory. *Psychiatric Medicine, 1*, 48.

Cooper, M. (1996). Obsessive-compulsive disorder: Effects on family members. *Orthopsychiatry, 66*, 296–304.

Darwin, C. (1887). *The life and letters of Charles Darwin.* New York, NY: Appleton & Co.

Dillon, D. J., Gorman, J. M., Liebowitz, M. R., Fyer, A. J., & Klein, D. F. (1987). Measurement of lactate-induced panic and anxiety. *Psychiatry Research, 20*, 97–105.

Dube, S. R., Felitti, V. J., Dong, M., Chapman, D. P., Giles, W. H., & Anda, R. F. (2003). Childhood abuse, neglect, and household dysfunction and the risk of illicit drug use: The adverse childhood experiences study. *Pediatrics, 111*(3), 564–572.

Enoch, M. A., Xu, K., Ferro, E., Harris, C. R., & Goldman, D. (2003). Genetic origins of anxiety in women: A role for a functional catechol-O-methyltransferase polymorphism. *Psychiatric Genetics, 13*(1), 33–41.

Fifer, S. K., Mathias, S. D., Patrick, D. L., Mazonson, P. D., Lubeck, D. P., & Buesching, D. P. (1994). Untreated anxiety among adult primary care patients in a Halth Maintenance Organization. *Archives of General Psychiatry, 51*, 740–750.

Finfgeld, D. L. (2002). Selective serotonin reuptake inhibitor: Discontinuation syndrome. *Journal of Psychosocial Nursing and Mental Health Services, 40*(12), 14–18.

Foa, E. B. (1997). Psychological processes related to recovery from a trauma and an effective treatment for PTSD. *Annals of the New York Academy of Science, 821*, 410–424.

Foa, E. B. & Tolin, D. F. (2000). Comparison of the PTSD Symptom Scale-Interview Version and the Clinician-Administered PTSD scale. *Journal of Traumatic Stress, 13*(2), 181–191.

Frankl, V. (1992). *Man's search for meaning: An introduction to logotherapy* (4th ed.). Boston, MA: Beacon Press.

Friedman, S., Smith, L., Fogel, D., Paradis, C., Viswanathan, R., Ackerman, R., et al. (2002). The incidence and influence of early traumatic life events in patients with panic disorder: A comparison with other psychiatric outpatients. *Journal of Anxiety Disorders, 16*(3), 259–272.

Giedd, J., Rapaport, J., Garvey, M., Perlmutter, S., & Swedo, S. (2000). MRI assessment of children with obsessive compulsive disorder or tics associated with streptococcal infection. *American Journal of Psychiatry, 157*(2), 281–283.

Goodman, W., Price, L., Rasmussen, S., Mazure, C., Fleischmann, R. L., Hill, C. L., (1989). The Yale-Brown Obsessive Compulsive Scale (Y-BOCS): Part 1. Development, use and reliability. *Archives of General Psychiatry, 46*, 1006–1011.

Gorman, J., Kent, J., Sullivan, G., & Coplan, J. (2000). Neuroanatomical hypothesis of panic disorder, revised. *American Journal of Psychiatry, 157*(4), 493–505.

Grabe, H. J., Meyer, C., Hapke, U., Rumpf, H-J., Freyberger, H. J., Dilling, H., et al. (2000). Prevalence, quality of life and psychosocial function in obsessive-compulsive disorder and subclinical obsessive-compulsive disorder in northern Germany. *European Archives of Psychiatry & Clinical Neuroscience, 250*, 262–268.

Greenberg, N. (2001). A critical review of psychological debriefing: the management of psychological health after traumatic experiences. *Journal of the Royal Naval Medical Service, 87*(3), 158–161.

Grieger, T. A., Staab, J. P., Cardeña, E., McCarroll, J. E., Brandt, G. T., Fullerton, C. S., et al. (2000). Acute stress disorder and subsequent posttraumatic stress disorder in a group of exposed disaster workers. *Depression and Anxiety, 11*(4), 183–184.

Hamilton, M. (1959). The assessment of anxiety states by rating. *British Journal of Medical Psychology, 32*, 54.

Harvey, A. G., & Bryant, R. A. (1999a). Predictors of acute stress following motor vehicle accidents. *Journal of Traumatic Stress, 12*(3), 519–525.

Harvey, A. G., & Bryant, R. A., (1999b). Acute stress disorder across trauma popultions. *The Journal of Nervous and Mental Disease, 187*(7), 443–446.

Hayward, C., Killen, J., & Kraemer, H. (2000). Predictors of panic attacks in adolescents. *Journal of the American Academy of Child and Adolescent Psychiatry, 39*(2), 207–214.

Heer, J. (2004, April). Romeo Dallaire: Haunted by genocide. *Boston Globe, Ideas.* Retrieved November 25, 2009, from http://www.jeetheer.com/politics/dallaire.htm

Hettema, J. M., Neale, M. C., & Kendler, K. S. (2001). A review and meta-analysis of the genetic epidemiology of anxiety disorders. *American Journal of Psychiatry, 158*(10), 1568–1578.

Hoffman, D. L., Dukes, E. M., & Wittchen, H. U. (2008). Human and economic burden of generalized anxiety disorder. *Depression and Anxiety, 25*(1), 72–90.

Hollander, E. (1997). Obsessive-compulsive disorder: The hidden epidemic. *Journal of Clinical Psychiatry, 58*, 3–6.

Jetty, P. V., Charney, D. S., & Goddard, A. W. (2001). Neurobiology of generalized anxiety disorder. *Psychiatric Clinics of North America, 24*(1), 75–97.

Johannes, S., Wieringa, B. M., Nager, W., Rada, D., Muller-Vahl, K. R., Emrish, H. M., et al. (2003). Tourette syndrome and obsessive-compulsive disorder: Event-related brain potentials show similar mechanisms of frontal inhibition but dissimilar target evaluation processes. *Behaviour Neurology, 14*(1–2), 9–17.

Kagee, A. (2002). Concerns about the effectiveness of critical incident stress debriefing in ameliorating stress reactions. *Critical Care, 6*(1), 88.

Kampman, M., Keijsers, G., Hoogduin, C., & Hendriks, G. (2002). A randomized, double-blind, placebo-controlled study of the effects of adjunctive paroxetine in panic disorder patients unsuccessfully treated with cognitive-behavioural therapy alone. *Journal of Clinical Psychiatry, 63*(9), 772–777.

Katon, W., Roy-Byrne, P., Russo, J., & Cowley, D. (2002). Cost-effectiveness and cost offset of a collaborative care intervention for primary care patients with panic disorder. *Archives of General Psychiatry, 59*(12), 1098–1104.

Kessler, R. C. (2000). The epidemiology of pure and comorbid generalized anxiety disorder: a review and evaluation of recent research. *Acta Psychiatrica Scandinavica, Suppl.* (406), 7–13.

Kim, C. H., Chang, J. W., Koo, M. S., Kim, J. W., Suh, H. S., Park, I. H., et al. (2003). Anterior cingulotomy for refractory obsessive-compulsive disorder. *Acta Psychiatrica Scandinavica, 107*(4), 241–243.

Kirkby, K. (2003). Obsessive-compulsive disorder: Towards better understanding and outcomes. *Current Opinion in Psychiatry, 16*(1), 49–55.

Koran, L. M. (2000). Quality of life in obsessive-compulsive disorder. *Psychiatric Clinics of North America, 23*, 509–517.

Koslander, T., Barbosa da Silva, A., & Roxberg, A. (2009). Existential and spiritual needs in mental health care: An ethical and holistic perspective. *Journal of Holistic Nursing, 27*(1), 34–42.

Lenze, E., Mulsant, B., Shear, M., Schulberg, H., Dew, M. A., Begley, A., et al. (2000). Comorbid anxiety disorders in depressed elderly patients. *American Journal of Psychiatry, 157*(5), 722–728.

Magee, W. J., Eaton, W. W., Wittchen, H. U. McGonagle, K. A., & Kesler, R. C. (1996). Agoraphobia, simple phobia and social phobia in the national Comorbidity Survey. *Archives of General Psychiatry, 53*, 159–168.

Magliano, L., Tosini, P., Guarneri, M., Marasco, C., & Catapano, F. (1996). Burden on the families of patients with obsessive-compulsive disorder: A pilot study. *European Psychiatry, 11*(4), 192–197.

Marks, I. M., & Matthews, A. M. (1979). Brief standard self-rating for phobic patients. *Behaviour Research and Therapy, 17*, 263–267.

Martin, J. L., Sainz-Pardo, M., Furukawa, T. A., Martín-Sánchez, E., Seoane, T., & Galán, C. (2007). Benzodiazepines in generalized anxiety disorder: Heterogeneity of outcomes based on a systematic review and meta-analysis of clinical trials. *Journal of Psychopharmacology, 21*(7), 774–782.

Marshall, R., Schneier, F., Lin, S. H., Simpson, H. B., Vermes, D., & Liebowitz, M. (2000). Childhood trauma and dissociative symptoms in panic disorder. *American Journal of Psychiatry, 157*(3), 451–453.

Marshall, R. D., Spitzer, R., & Liebowitz, M. R. (1999). Review and critique of the new DSM-IV diagnoses of acute stress disorder. *The American Journal of Psychiatry, 156*(11), 1677–1685.

McEwen, B. (2005). Stressed or stressed out: What is the difference? *Journal of Psychiatry and Neuroscience, 30*, 315–318.

Melke, J., Landen, M., Baghei, F., Rosmond, R., Holm, G., Bjorntorp, P., et al. (2001). Serotonin transporter gene polymorphisms are associated with anxiety-related personality traits in women. *American Journal of Medical Genetics, 105*(5), 458–463.

Meyer, T., Miller, M., Metzger, R., & Borkovec, T. (1990). Development and validation of the Penn State Worry Questionnaire. *Behaviour Research and Therapy, 28*(6), 487–495.

Mundo, E., Richter, M., Sam, F., Macciardi, F., & Kennedy, J. (2000). Is the 5-HT (1D beta) receptor gene implicated in the pathogenesis of obsessive-compulsive disorder? *American Journal of Psychiatry, 157*(7), 1160–1161.

Nestadt, G., Bienvenu, O. J., Cai, G., Samuels, J., & Eaton, W. W. (1998). Incidence of obsessive-compulsive disorder in adults. *The Journal of Nervous and Mental Disorder, 186*(7), 401–406.

Newman, M., Erickson, T., Przeworski, A., & Dzus, E. (2003). Self-help and minimal contact therapies for anxiety disorders: Is human contact necessary for therapeutic efficacy? *Journal of Clinical Psychology, 59*(3), 251–274.

Newman, S. C., Bland, R. C., & Orn, H. T. (1998). The prevalence of mental disorders in the elderly in Edmonton: A community survey using GMS-AGE-CAT. Geriatric Mental State-Automated Geriatric Examination for Computer Assisted Taxonomy. *The Canadian Journal of Psychiatry, 43*(9), 910–914.

Nuttin, B., Cosyn, P., Demeulemeester, H., Gybels, J., & Meyerson, B. (1999). Electrical stimulation in anterior limbs of internal capsules in patients with obsessive-compulsive disorder. *Lancet, 354*(9189), 1526.

Overbeek, T., Schruers, K., Vermetten, E., & Greiz, E. (2002). Comorbidity of obsessive-compulsive disorder and depression: Prevalence, symptom severity, and treatment effect. *Journal of Clinical Psychiatry, 63*(12), 1106–1112.

Peplau, H. (1989). Theoretic constructs: Anxiety, self, and hallucinations. In A. O'Toole, & S. Welt (Eds.), *Interpersonal theory in nursing practice: Selected works of Hildegard E. Peplau.* New York, NY: Springer.

Perugi, G., Toni, C., Frare, F., Travierso, M., Hantouche, E., & Akiskal, H. (2002). Obsessive-compulsive-bipolar comorbidity: A systematic exploration of clinical features and treatment outcome. *Journal of Clinical Psychiatry, 63*(12), 1129–1134.

Rachman, S., & Hodgson, R. (1980). *Obsessions and compulsions.* New York, NY: Prentice-Hall.

Rapaport, M. H., Wolkow, R., Rubin, A., Hackett, E., Pollack, M., & Ota, K. U. (2001). Sertraline treatment of panic disorder: Results of a long-term study. *Acta Psychiatrica Scandinavica, 104*(4), 289–298.

Raskind, M., Thompson, C., Petrie, E., Dobie, D., Rein, R., Hoff, D., et al. (2002). Prazosin reduces nightmares in combat veterans with posttraumatic stress disorder. *Journal of Clinical Psychiatry, 63*(7), 565–568.

Rasmussen, S. A., & Eisen, J. L. (1990). Epidemiology of obsessive-compulsive disorder. *Journal of Clinical Psychiatry, 51*, 10–13.

Rasmussen, S. A., & Eisen, J. L. (1992). The epidemiology and clinical features of obsessive-compulsive disorder. *Psychiatric Clinics of North America, 15*, 743–758.

Rauch, S., Jenike, M., Alpert, N., Baer, L., Breiter, H., Savage, C. R., et al. (1994). Regional cerebral blood flow measured during symptom provocation in obsessive-compulsive disorder using oxygen 15-labeled carbon dioxide and positron emission tomography. *Archives of General Psychiatry, 51*, 62–70.

Ray, S. (2008). Trauma from a global perspective. *Issues in Mental Health Nursing, 29*, 63–72.

Regier, D. A., Rae, D. S., Narrow, W. E., Kaelber, C. T., & Schatzberg A. F. (1998). Prevalence of anxiety disorders and their comorbidity with mood and addictive disorders. *British Journal of Psychiatry, 34*(Suppl.), 24–28.

Reiss, S., Peterson, R. A., & Gursky, D. M. (1986). Anxiety sensitivity, anxiety frequency, and the prediction of fearfulness. *Behaviour Research and Therapy, 24*, 1–8.

Rickels, K., & Rynn, M. (2002). Pharmacotherapy of generalized anxiety disorder. *Journal of Clinical Psychiatry, 63* (Suppl 14), 9–16.

Roy-Byrne, P. P., Clary, C. M., Miceli, R. J., Colucci, S. V., Xu, Y., & Grundzinski, A. N. (2001). The effect of selective serotonin reuptake inhibitor treatment of panic disorder on emergency room and laboratory resource utilization. *Journal of Clinical Psychiatry, 62*(9), 678–682.

Sallee, F., Sethuraman, G., Sine, L., & Liu, H. (2000). Yohimbine challenge in children with anxiety disorders. *American Journal of Psychiatry, 157*, 1236–1242.

Sareen, J., & Stein., M. (2000). A review of the epidemiology and approaches to the treatment of social anxiety disorder. *Drugs, 59*(3), 497–509.

Scherrer, J. F., True, W. R., Xian, H., Lyons, M. J., Eisen, S. A., Goldberg, J., et al. (2000). Evidence for genetic influences common and specific to symptoms of generalized anxiety and panic. *Journal of Affective Disorders, 57*(1–3), 25–35.

Schneier, F., Liebowitz, M., Abi-Dargham, A., Zea-Ponce, Y., Lin, S., & Laruelle, M. (2000). Low dopamine D2 receptor binding potential in social phobia. *American Journal of Psychiatry, 157*(3), 457–459.

Scupi, B. S., Maser, J. D., & Uhde, T. W. (1992). The National Institute of Mental Health Panic Questionnaire: An instrument for assessing clinical characteristics of panic disorder. *Journal of Nervous and Mental Disease, 180*, 566–572.

Shalev, A. Y., Peri, T., Canetti, L., & Schreiber, S. (1996). Predictors of PTSD in injured trauma survivors: A prospective study. *The American Journal of Psychiatry, 153*(2), 219–225.

Shear, M. K., Cooper, A. M., Klerman, G. L., Busch, F. N., & Shapiro, T. (1993). A psychodynamic model of panic disorder. *American Journal of Psychiatry, 150*, 859–866.

Sheehan, D. V. (1999). Enlafaxine extended release (XR) in the treatment of generalized anxiety disorder. *Journal of Clinical Psychiatry, 60* (Suppl, 22), 23–28.

Sheikh, J. I., Leskin, G. A., & Klein, D. F. (2002). Gender differences in panic disorder: Findings from the National Comorbidity Survey. *American Journal of Psychiatry, 159*(8), 1438.

Skoog, G., & Skoog, I. (1999). A 40-year follow-up of patients with obsessive-compulsive disorder. *Archives of General Psychiatry, 56*, 121–127.

Slattery, M., Klein, D., Mannuzza, S., Moulton, J., Pine, D., & Klein, R. (2002). Relationship between separation anxiety disorder, parental panic disorder, and atopic disorders in children: a controlled high-risk study (Statistical data included). *Journal of the American Academy of Child and Adolescent Psychiatry, 41*(8), 947–954.

Spielberger, C. D., Gorsuch, R. L., & Luchene, R. E. (1976). *Manual for the State-Trait Anxiety Inventory.* Palo Alto, CA: Consulting Psychologists Press.

Statistics Canada. (2003). *Canadian community health survey: Mental health and well-being.* Retrieved November 26, 2009, from http://www.statcan.gc.ca/pub/82-617-x/index-eng.htm

Stein, D., Versiani, M., Hair, T., & Kumar, R. (2002). Efficacy of paroxetine for relapse prevention in social anxiety disorder: A 24-week study. *Archives in General Psychiatry, 59*(12), 1111–1118.

Stein, M., Fryer, A., Davidson, J., Pollack, M., & Wiita, B. (1999). Fluvoxamine treatment of social phobia (social anxiety disorder): A double-blind, placebo-controlled trial. *American Journal of Psychiatry, 156*(5), 756–760.

Strohle, A., Romeo, E., Di Michele, F., Pasini, A., Hermann, B., Gajewsky, G., et al. (2003). Induced panic attacks shift gamma-aminobutyric acid type A receptor modulatory neuroactive steroid composition in patients with panic disorder: Preliminary results. *Archives in General Psychiatry, 60*(2), 161–168.

Summerfield, D. (1995). Debriefing after psychological trauma: Inappropriate exporting of western culture may cause additional harm. *British Medical Journal, 311*(7003), 509.

Tillich, P. (1952). *The courage to be.* New Haven, CT: Yale University Press.

Valentiner, D., Gutierrez, P., & Blacker, D. (2002). Anxiety measures and their relationship to adolescent suicidal ideation and behaviour. *Journal of Anxiety Disorders, 16*(1), 11–32.

Van Ameringen, M., Mancini, C., Pipe, B., Campbell, M., & Oakman, J. (2002). Topiramate treatment for SSRI-induced weight gain in anxiety disorders. *Journal of Clinical Psychiatry, 63*(11), 981–984.

Wagstaff, A. F., Cheer, S. M., Matheson, A. F., Ormrod, D., & Goa, K. L. (2002). Spotlight on paroxetine in psychiatric disorders in adults. *CNS Drugs, 16*(6), 425–434.

Wang, P., Berglund, P., & Kessler, R. (2000). Recent care of common mental disorders in the United States: Prevalence and conformance with evidenced-based recommendations. *Journal of General Internal Medicine, 15*, 284–292.

Weems, C., Costa, N., Dehon, C., & Berman, S. (2004). Paul Tillich's theory of existential anxiety: A preliminary conceptual and empirical examination. *Anxiety, Stress, and Coping, 17*(4), 383–399.

Woodward, L. (2001). Life course outcomes of young people with anxiety disorders in adolescence. *Journal of the American Academy of Child and Adolescent Psychiatry, 40*(9), 1086–1093.

Yehuda, R. (2000). Biology of posttraumatic stress disorder. *Journal of Clinical Psychiatry, 61*(Suppl 7), 14–21.

CHAPTER 22

Somatoform and Related Disorders

L. Elizabeth Hood

Adapted from the chapter "Somatoform and Related Disorders" by Mary Ann Boyd

LEARNING OBJECTIVES

After studying this chapter, you will be able to:

- Explain the concept of somatization and its occurrence in people with mental health problems.
- Discuss epidemiologic factors related to somatic problems.
- Compare the etiologic theories of somatization disorder from a bio/psycho/social/spiritual perspective.
- Contrast the major differences between somatoform and factitious disorders.
- Discuss human responses to somatization disorder.
- Apply the elements of nursing management to a patient with somatization disorder.

KEY CONCEPT

- somatization

KEY TERMS

- alexithymia • factitious disorders • malingering • pseudologia fantastica
- pseudoneurologic symptoms • psychosomatic • somatization
disorder • somatoform disorders

---

*T*he connection between the mind and the body has been hypothesized and described for centuries. The term **psychosomatic** describes conditions in which a psychological state contributes to the development of physical illness. For example, the connection between stress and heart disease is well documented and serves as the rationale for stress management interventions for heart attack victims. The term *somatization* is used when unexplained physical symptoms are present that are related to psychological distress. This chapter explores the concept of somatization and explains the care of patients whose psychiatric disorder has as its primary characteristic the manifestation of unexplained physical symptoms related to psychological distress.

KEY CONCEPT Somatization is the term used when unexplained physical symptoms are present that are related to psychological distress.

Although somatization is common in many psychiatric disorders, including depression, anxiety, and psychosis, it is the primary symptom of somatoform and factitious disorders. A **somatoform disorder** is one in which the patient experiences physical symptoms as a result of psychological stress. The prevalence of somatoform disorders in general practice ranges from 16% to 21%, often occurring comorbidly with anxiety or depressive disorders (De Waal, Arnold, Eekhof, & Van Hemert, 2004). A **factitious disorder** is one in which the patient self-inflicts injury, as a result of psychological stress, in order to seek medical treatment. The major difference between the two diagnostic categories is that in the somatoform disorders, the physical symptoms are not deliberately produced by the patient. Controversy also exists over diagnostic validity and the use of exclusionary criteria (organic disease) over positive criteria (observable behaviour) and overlap between anxiety and mood disorders for classification of the somatoform disorders (Lowe et al., 2008). Currently, the somatoform disorders are clustered into six different clinical syndromes:

1. Somatization disorder
2. Undifferentiated somatoform disorder
3. Conversion disorder
4. Pain disorder
5. Hypochondriasis
6. Body dysmorphic disorder (BDD)

The factitious disorders include factitious disorder and factitious disorder not specified. This chapter presents the nursing care of patients experiencing somatoform disorders and factitious disorders. *Somatization disorder* is explained in detail because symptoms of all the other somatoform disorders are present.

Somatization

Anyone who feels the pain of a sore throat or the ache of influenza has a somatic symptom (from *soma*, meaning body), but it is not considered to be somatization unless the physical symptoms are an expression of emotional stress. Previously known as "hysteria" or "Briquet's syndrome," the cluster of symptoms associated with dysfunctional preoccupation with physical malady is now called somatization disorder (Mai, 2004). There may or may not be an identifiable physiologic cause of the medical problems, but chronic stress is obvious. With somatization, physical sensations are amplified, and the individual seeks medical care for the symptoms. People who somatize view their personal problems in physical terms rather than psychosocial terms. For example, a woman quits her job complaining of being chronically tired instead of recognizing that she is emotionally stressed from a coworker's constant harassment. These individuals internalize stress or cope with life problems by expressing their anxiety, stress, and frustration through their own physical symptoms.

■■■ CULTURAL DIFFERENCES IN SOMATIZATION

A high correlation exists between somatization and ethnicity (Kirmayer & Young, 1998). Because norms, values, and expectations about illness are culturally based, physical sensations are experienced according to culturally defined expectations. In cultures in which the expression of physical discomfort is more acceptable than that of psychological distress, the disruption of basic bodily functions, such as digestive or menstrual cycles, sleep, physical balance, and orientation, is commonly the focus of patient concern, instead of problems with interpersonal relationships, economic crises, the death of a spouse, adjustment to marriage, or the inability to become pregnant.

■■■ GENDER AND SOMATIZATION

Females experience somatization disorder at a rate ten to one higher than males (Yates, 2008). Although the actual somatic experience appears to be different in men than in women (Kroenke & Spitzer, 1998), one group of researchers showed that women were more likely to be diversified somatizers, who have frequent, brief sickness with a variety of complaints. Men were more likely to be asthenic somatizers, with fewer diverse complaints but more chronically disabled by fatigue, weakness, or common minor illnesses.

Somatization Disorder

Somatization disorder is a chronic relapsing condition characterized by multiple physical symptoms that typically develop during times of emotional distress. The disorder can change with time and can vary from person to person (American Psychiatric Association [APA], 2000).

The APA defines somatization disorder as "a polysymptomatic disorder that begins before age 30 years, extends over a period of several years, and is characterized by a combination of pain, gastrointestinal, sexual, and psychoneurological symptoms" (APA, p. 485).

■■■ CLINICAL COURSE

In somatization disorder, patients have recurring, multiple, and clinically significant somatic problems that involve several body systems. Other somatoform disorders are characterized by only one set of complaints, such as conversion disorder (see later discussion) or pain disorder. Physical problems in somatization disorder cut across all body systems, such as gastrointestinal (nausea, vomiting, diarrhea), neurologic (headache, backache), or musculoskeletal (aching legs). The physical illness may last 6 to 9 months. These individuals perceive themselves as being "sicker than the sick" and report all aspects of their health as poor. They are often disabled and cannot work. They quickly become frustrated with their primary health care providers, who do not seem to appreciate the seriousness of their symptoms and are unable to verify a particular problem that accounts for their extreme discomfort.

Table 22.1   Key Diagnostic Characteristics of Somatization Disorder 300.81

DSM IV

Diagnostic Criteria and Target Symptoms	Associated Findings
• History of many physical complaints beginning before age 30 and occurring over a period of several years • Complaints requiring treatment or causing significant impairment in social, occupational, or other important areas of functioning • History of pain related to at least four different sites or functions, such as head, abdomen, back, joints, extremities, chest, rectum, during menstruation, during sexual intercourse, or during urination • History of at least two gastrointestinal symptoms, such as nausea, bloating, vomiting (other than during pregnancy), diarrhea, or intolerance of several different foods • History of at least one sexual or reproductive symptom, such as sexual indifference, erectile or ejaculatory dysfunction, irregular menses, excessive menstrual bleeding, vomiting throughout pregnancy • History of one pseudoneurologic symptom or deficit suggesting a neurologic condition not limited to pain, such as conversion symptoms (impaired coordination or balance, paralysis or localized weakness, difficulty swallowing or lump in throat, aphonia, urinary retention, hallucinations, loss of touch or pain sensation, double vision, blindness, deafness, seizures) or dissociative symptoms, for example, amnesia or loss of consciousness (other than fainting) • Symptoms cannot be explained by a known general medical condition or direct effects of a substance • Symptoms unexplainable or excessive • When a general medical condition exists, the physical complaints or resulting impairments are in excess of what would be expected from the history, physical examination, or laboratory findings • Symptoms are not intentionally produced or feigned	*Associated Behavioural Findings* • Colourful, exaggerated complaints lacking specific factual information • Inconsistent history • Treatment sought from several physicians with numerous medical examinations, diagnostic procedures, surgeries, and hospitalizations • Anxiety and depressed mood • Impulsive with antisocial behaviour, suicide threats and attempts, and marital discord *Associated Physical Findings* • Absence of objective findings to fully explain subjective complaints • Possible diagnosis of functional disorders, such as irritable bowel syndrome

Consequently, they "provider-shop," moving from one to another until they find one who will give them new medication, hospitalize them, or perform surgery. Characteristically, these individuals undergo multiple surgeries. People with somatization disorder sometimes evoke negative subjective responses in health care providers who need to be aware of such responses and be able to deal with them in a constructive way. This may include discussing their feelings with a clinical supervisor.

CRNENOTE

Individuals with somatoform disorders will seek health care from multiple providers but often avoid mental health specialists.

Because a psychiatric diagnosis of somatization disorder is made only after numerous unexplained physical problems, psychiatric and mental health (PMH) nurses do not usually care for these individuals early in the disorder; rather, these patients are more likely to have been encountered early on by nurses in primary care and medical-surgical settings.

DIAGNOSTIC CRITERIA

The diagnosis is made when there is a pattern of multiple, recurring, and "significant" somatic complaints. Table 22-1 lists the key diagnostic criteria and target symptoms of somatization disorder. A significant complaint is one that received medical treatment or for which the symptoms cause impairment in social, occupational, or other areas of functioning (APA, 2000).

SOMATIZATION DISORDER IN SPECIAL POPULATIONS

Evidence suggests that this disorder occurs in all populations and cultures. However, the type and frequency of somatic symptoms may differ across cultures.

Children

Although many children experience unexplained medical symptoms, somatization disorder is not usually diagnosed until adolescence. Menstrual difficulties may be one of the first symptoms. More research is needed to identify risk factors and treatment outcomes (Lieb, Pfister, Mastaler, & Wittchen, 2000).

Older Adults

While somatization disorder occurs in the older adult, new onset of somatic symptoms in late life warrants a thorough investigation for hidden medical or psychiatric disorders (Yates, 2008). Subjective lack of well-being (never feeling good), rather than objective health measures, may be an indicator of somatization (Schneider et al., 2003). In the older adult, somatic symptoms can represent many things, such as depression or bereavement. Recognizing the complexity of physical manifestations and assessing the symptom pattern are important.

▰◖ EPIDEMIOLOGY

The estimated prevalence of somatization disorder ranges from 0.2% (males) to 2% (females) of the general population (APA, 2000; Grabe et al., 2003; Noyes et al., 2006). Because these individuals see themselves as medically sick and may never see a mental health provider, these estimates may underrepresent the true prevalence. Some estimates are as high as 11% of the population. Thus, in many people, somatization disorder is unrecognized, undiagnosed, and mismanaged in primary care settings (Yates, 2008).

Age of Onset

Somatization disorder, by definition, begins before the age of 30 years, usually during adolescence. The individual may not receive a diagnosis until later, but one unexplained somatic symptom must be present before 30 years. This disorder typically has its onset in childhood or adolescence and is remarkably stable, lasting many years into adulthood (Lieb et al., 2002; Mullick, 2002). Patients who begin to have symptoms after 30 years will not likely meet the criteria for somatization disorder in the *Diagnostic and Statistical Manual of Mental Disorders*, 4th ed., Text Revision (*DSM-IV-TR*; APA, 2000). Instead, a diagnosable medical problem will more likely be revealed (Gureje, Simon, Ustun, & Goldberg, 1997).

Gender, Ethnic, and Cultural Differences

Somatization disorder occurs primarily in women, particularly those in lower socioeconomic status and with high emotional distress (Ladwig, Marten-Mittag, Erazo, & Gundel, 2001). The prevalence in men in the United States and Canada is less than 0.2%. Reports of greater prevalence, for example, among Mexican Americans (Mai, 2004), southeast Asians, and male Canadian immigrants from Vietnam (Kirmayer & Young, 1998), suggest that cultural factors contribute to the appearance of the disorder.

Comorbidity

Somatization disorder frequently coexists with other psychiatric disorders, most commonly depression. Others include panic disorder, mania, phobic disorder, obsessive-compulsive disorder, psychotic disorders, and personality disorders (Garyfallos et al., 1999). Nurses rarely see patients who have only somatization disorder.

Ultimately, numerous unexplained medical problems also coexist with this disorder because many patients have received medical and surgical treatments, often unnecessarily, and are plagued with side effects. A disproportionately high number of women who eventually receive diagnoses of somatization disorder have been treated for irritable bowel syndrome, polycystic ovary disease, and chronic pain. It is estimated that as many as 94% of people with irritable bowel syndrome have psychiatric disorders, especially major depression, anxiety, and somatization disorder (Whitehead, Palsson, & Jones, 2002). Many also have had non–cancer-related hysterectomies. Even after the patient is treated by mental health providers and develops some understanding of the disorder, the physical problems do not disappear.

▰◖ ETIOLOGY

The cause of somatization disorder is unknown. The following are theories regarding the development of the disorder.

Biologic Theories
Neuropathologic Theory

The neuropathology of somatization disorder is unknown. Evidence suggests decreased activity in certain brain areas, such as the caudate nuclei, left putamen, and right precentral gyrus (Garcia-Campayo, Sanz-Carrillo, Baringo, & Ceballos, 2001; Hakala et al., 2002). These findings indicate that hypometabolism may be associated with somatization disorder.

Genetic

Although somatization disorder has been shown to run in families, the exact transmission mechanism is unclear. Strong evidence suggests an increased risk for somatization disorder in first-degree relatives, indicating a familial or genetic effect (APA, 2000). Because many women with somatization disorder live in chaotic families, environmental influence could explain the high prevalence in first-degree relatives. Males in these families show high risk for antisocial personality disorder and substance abuse (Cloninger, Reich, & Guze, 1995).

Biochemical Changes

Research is as yet insufficient to identify specific biochemical changes that would lead to somatization disorder. However, because these patients experience other psychiatric problems, such as depression or panic, clearly many neurobiologic changes occur. Women with this disorder often have numerous menstrual problems and often undergo hysterectomies. Because of these symptoms, studies are needed to determine the involvement of the hypothalamic–pituitary–gonadal axis, which regulates estrogen and testosterone secretion.

Psychological Theories

Somatization has been explained as a form of social or emotional communication, meaning the bodily symptoms express an emotion that cannot be verbalized. The adolescent who experiences severe abdominal pain after her parents' argument or the wife who receives nurturing from her husband only when she has back pain are two examples of how the body expresses emotions. From this perspective, somatization may be a way of maintaining relationships. Following this line of reasoning, as an individual's physical problems become a way of controlling relationships, so somatization becomes a learned behaviour pattern. With time, physical symptoms develop automatically in response to perceived threats. Finally, somatization disorder develops when somatizing becomes a way of life. Although there is little research, as yet, on the childhood adversities of individuals with somatization disorder, the possible association between childhood trauma and somatization is being explored as an etiological factor (Spitzer, Barnow, Gau, Freyberger, & Grabe, 2008).

Social Theories

While somatization disorder occurs everywhere, the symptoms may vary between cultures. In addition, the conceptualization of somatization disorder is primarily Western.

BOX 22.1

Somatization in Chinese Culture

In Chinese tradition, the health of the individual reflects a balance between positive and negative forces within the body: five elements at work in nature and in the body control conditions (fire, water, wood, earth, metal); five viscera (liver, heart, spleen, kidneys, lungs); five emotions (anger, joy, worry, sorrow, fear); and five climatic conditions (wind, heat, humidity, dryness, cold). All illness is explained by imbalances among these elements. Because emotion is related to the circulation of vital air within the body, anger is believed to result from an adverse current of vital air to the liver. Emotional outbursts are seen as results of imbalances among the natural elements, rather than results of the person's behaviour.

The stigma of mental illness in the Chinese culture is so great that it can have an adverse effect on a family for many generations. If problems can be attributed to natural causes, the individual and family are less responsible, and stigma is minimized. The Chinese have a culturally acceptable term for symptoms of mental distress—the closest translation of which would be *neurasthenia*—which comprises somatic complaints of headaches, insomnia, dizziness, aches and pains, poor memory, anxiety, weakness, and loss of energy.

In non-Western societies, where the mind–body distinction is not made and symptoms have different meanings and explanations, these physical manifestations are not labelled as a psychiatric disorder (Box 22-1). For example, within Chinese culture as well as in Latin American countries, depression is more likely described with somatic symptoms, such as headaches, gastrointestinal disturbances, or complaints of "nerves," rather than with the sadness or guilt associated with major depression (Jorge, 2003; Yick, Shibusawa, & Agbayani-Siewert, 2003).

■ RISK FACTORS

Somatization disorder tends to run in families, and children of mothers with multiple unexplained somatic complaints are themselves more likely to have somatic problems. Adults are at higher risk for unexplained medical symptoms if they experienced unexplained symptoms as children or if, around the age of 15, their parents were in poor health (Hotopf, Mayou, Wadsworth, & Wessely, 1999). Female gender, substance use, and anxiety disorder seem to be risk factors, and women with somatization disorder appear more likely to have been sexually abused as children than those with other psychiatric conditions, such as mood disorders (Lieb et al., 2002). Individuals with depression are especially likely to experience somatization (Gureje & Simon, 1999).

INTERDISCIPLINARY TREATMENT

The care of patients with somatization disorder involves three approaches:

- Providing long-term general management of the chronic condition
- Conservatively treating symptoms of comorbid psychiatric and physical problems
- Providing care in special settings, including group treatment

The cornerstone of management is trust. Ideally, the patient sees only one health care provider at regularly scheduled visits. During each primary care visit, the provider should conduct a partial physical examination of the organ system in which the patient has complaints. Physical symptoms are to be treated conservatively using the least intrusive approach. In the mental health setting, the use of cognitive-behaviour therapy (CBT) produced significant clinical benefits beyond other current treatment methods (Allen, Woolfolk, Escobar, Gara, & Hamer, 2006), such as antidepressants or supportive psychotherapy (Mai, 2004). In a review of 31 clinical trials, patients treated with CBT showed more improvement than control subjects did in 71% of the studies. Benefits were observed whether or not psychological distress was ameliorated (Kroenke & Swindle, 2000).

NURSING MANAGEMENT: HUMAN RESPONSE TO DISORDER

Somatization is the primary response to this disorder. The defining characteristics, depicted in the bio/psycho/social/spiritual model (Fig. 22-1), are so well integrated that separating the psychological and social dimensions is difficult. The most common characteristics include the following:

- Reporting the same symptoms repeatedly
- Receiving support from the environment that otherwise might not be forthcoming (e.g., gaining a spouse's attention because of severe back pain)
- Expressing concern about the physical problems inconsistent with the severity of the illness (being "sicker than the sick")

FIGURE 22.1 Bio/psycho/social/spiritual characteristics of patients with somatization disorder.

BOX 22.2

Health Attitude Survey

On a scale of 1–5, please indicate the extent to which you agree (5) or disagree (1).

DISSATISFACTION WITH CARE

1. I have been satisfied with the medical care I have received. (R)
2. Doctors have done the best they could to diagnose and treat my health problems. (R)
3. Doctors have taken my health problems seriously.
4. My health problems have been thoroughly evaluated. (R)
5. Doctors do not seem to know much about the health problems I have had.
6. My health problems have been completely explained. (R)
7. Doctors seem to think I am exaggerating my health problems.
8. My response to treatment has not been satisfactory.
9. My response to treatment is usually excellent. (R)

FRUSTRATION WITH ILL HEALTH

10. I am tired of feeling sick and would like to get to the bottom of my health problems.
11. I have felt ill for quite a while now.
12. I am going to keep searching for an answer to my health problems.
13. I do not think there is anything seriously wrong with my body. (R)

HIGH UTILIZATION OF CARE

14. I have seen many different doctors over the years.
15. I have taken a lot of medicine recently.
16. I do not go to the doctor often. (R)
17. I have had relatively good health over the years.

EXCESSIVE HEALTH WORRY

18. I sometimes worry too much about my health.
19. I often fear the worst when I develop symptoms.
20. I have trouble getting my mind off my health.

PSYCHOLOGICAL DISTRESS

21. Sometimes I feel depressed and cannot seem to shake it off.
22. I have sought help for emotional or stress-related problems.
23. It is easy to relax and stay calm. (R)
24. I believe the stress I am under may be affecting my health.

DISCORDANT COMMUNICATION OF DISTRESS

25. Some people think that I am capable of more work than I feel able to do.
26. Some people think that I have been sick just to gain attention.
27. It is difficult for me to find the right words for my feelings.

(R) indicates items reversed for scoring purposes. Scoring—The higher the score, the more likely somatization is a problem.

From Noyes, R. Jr., Langbehn, D., Happel, R., Sieren, L., & Muller, B. (1999). Health attitude survey: A scale for assessing somatizing patients. *Psychosomatics, 40*(6), 470–478.

Biologic Domain

During the assessment interview, allow enough time for the patient to explain all medical problems; a hurried assessment interview blocks communication.

Assessment

Past medical treatment will have been ineffective because it did not address the underlying psychiatric disorder. However, PMH nurses typically see these patients for coexistent problems related to the psychiatric disorder, such as depression, rather than for the somatization disorder itself. While taking the patient's history, the nurse will discover that the individual has had medical problems or multiple surgeries and realize that somatization disorder is a strong possibility. If the patient has not already received a diagnosis of somatization disorder, the nurse should screen for it by determining the presence of the most commonly reported problems associated with this disorder, which include dysmenorrhea, lump in throat, vomiting, shortness of breath, burning in sex organs, painful extremities, and amnesia. If the patient has these symptoms, he or she should be seen by a mental health provider qualified to make the diagnosis. Box 22-2 presents the Health Attitude Survey, which can be used as a screening test for somatization.

Review of Systems

Although these patients' symptoms have usually received considerable attention from the medical community, a careful review of systems is important because the appearance of physical problems is usually related to psychosocial problems. Even as the nurse continues to see the patient for mental health problems, an ongoing awareness of biologic symptoms is important, particularly because these symptoms are de-emphasized in the overall management.

Pain is the most common problem in people with this disorder. Because the pain is usually related to symptoms of all the major body systems, it is unlikely that a somatic intervention such as an analgesic will be effective on a long-term basis. The nurse must remember that although there is no medical explanation for the pain, the patient's pain is real and has serious psychosocial implications. A careful assessment should include the following questions:

- What is the pain like?
- What is the extent of the pain?
- What helps the pain get better?
- When is the pain at its worst?
- What has worked in the past to relieve the pain?

Physical Functioning

The actual physical functioning of these individuals is often marginal. They usually have problems with sleep, fatigue, activity, and sexual functioning. Assessment of these areas will generate data to be used in establishing a nursing diagnosis. The amount and quality of sleep are important, as are the times when the individual sleeps. For example, an individual may sleep a total of 6 hours each diurnal cycle, but only from 2 to 6 AM, plus an afternoon nap.

Fatigue is a constant problem, and a variety of physical problems interfere with normal activity. These patients report overwhelming lack of energy, which makes maintaining usual routines or accomplishing daily tasks impossible. Fatigue is accompanied by the inability to concentrate on simple functions, leading to decreased performance and disinterest in surroundings. Patients tend to be lethargic and listless and often have little energy (Box 22-3).

Female patients with this disorder usually have had multiple gynecologic problems. The reason is not known, but symptoms of dysmenorrhea, painful intercourse, and pain in the sex organs suggest involvement of the hypothalamic–pituitary–gonadal axis. Physiologic indicators, such as those produced by laboratory tests, are not available. However, a careful assessment of the patient's menstrual history, gynecologic problems, and sexual functioning is important. The physical manifestations of somatization disorder often lead to altered sexual behaviour.

Pharmacologic Assessment

A psychopharmacologic assessment of these patients is challenging. Patients with somatization disorder frequently provider-shop, perhaps seeing seven or eight different providers within a year. Because they often receive medications from each provider, they are usually taking a large number of drugs. They tend to protect their sources and may not truthfully identify the actual number of medications they are ingesting. A thorough pharmacologic best possible medication history (BPMH) and assessment of all current home medications is needed not only because of the number of medications but also because these individuals frequently have unusual side effects. Moreover, because of their somatic sensitivity, they often overreact to medication.

Patients with somatization disorder spend much of their life trying to find out what is wrong with them. When one provider after another finds little or no explanation for their symptoms, they may become anxious. To alleviate their anxiety, they either self-medicate with over-the-counter medications and substances of abuse (e.g., alcohol, marijuana) or find a provider who prescribes an anxiolytic. Because the anxiety of their disorder cannot be treated within a few weeks with an anxiolytic, they become dependent on medication that should not have been prescribed in the first place.

BOX 22.3

Clinical Vignette: Somatization Disorder and Stress

Ms. J, age 42 years, has been coming to the mental health clinic for 2 years for her nerves. She has seen only the physician for medication but now has been referred to the nurse's new stress management group because she is experiencing side effects of all the medications that have been tried. The psychiatrist has diagnosed somatization disorder and wants her to learn to manage her "nerves" without medication.

At the first meeting with the nurse, Ms. J was preoccupied with chest pain and bloating that had lasted for the past 6 months. Her chest pain is constant and sharp at times. The pain does not prevent her from going to her job as a waitress but does interfere with meal preparation at night for her family and her ability to have sexual intercourse. She has numerous other physical problems, including allergies to certain perfumes, dysmenorrhea, ovarian polycystic disease (ovarian cysts), chronic urinary tract infections, and rashes.

She is constantly fatigued and has frequent leg cramps. She states that she is too tired to fix dinner for her family. On days off from work, she takes a nap in the afternoon, sleeping until evening. She is unable to fall asleep at night.

She believes that she will soon have to have her gallbladder removed because of occasional referred pain to her back and nausea that occurs a couple hours after eating. She is not enthusiastic about a stress management group and does not believe that it will help her problems; however, she has agreed to consider it, while insisting that the psychiatrist continue prescribing diazepam (Valium).

WHAT DO YOU THINK?

- How would you prioritize Ms. J's physical symptoms?
- What strategies would you use in the group to help Ms. J explore the roots of her stress and fatigue?

Although anxiolytics have a place in therapeutics, most are addictive and therefore not recommended for long-term use. They also tend to complicate the treatment of somatoform disorders. Unfortunately, by the time a patient with a somatoform disorder sees a mental health provider, he or she has often already begun taking one of the benzodiazepines. Indeed, the reason a patient agrees to see a mental health provider is often that the primary health provider has refused to continue prescribing an anxiolytic until the patient has undergone psychiatric evaluation.

Nursing Diagnoses for the Biologic Domain

Because somatization disorder is a chronic illness, a patient could receive almost any one of the nursing diagnoses at some point in life. At least one nursing diagnosis likely will be related to the individual's physical state. Fatigue, pain, and disturbed sleep patterns are usually supported by the assessment data. The challenge in devising outcomes for these problems is to avoid focusing on the biologic aspects and instead help the patient overcome the fatigue, pain, or sleep problem through bio/psycho/social/spiritual approaches.

Interventions for the Biologic Domain

Nursing interventions that focus on the biologic dimension become especially important because medical treatment must be conservative, and aggressive pharmacologic treatment must be avoided. Each time a nurse sees the patient, time spent on the physical complaints should be limited. The goal is to help the person better understand the meaning behind the physical manifestations of the somatization disorder. Several biologic interventions, including pain management, activity enhancement, nutrition regulation, relaxation, and pharmacologic interventions may also be useful in caring for patients with somatization disorder.

Pain Management

Pain is a primary issue, but a single approach to its management rarely works. After a careful assessment of the pain, the nurse should develop nonpharmacologic strategies to reduce it (see Caudill-Slosberg, 2002). If gastrointestinal pain is frequent, for example, eating and bowel habits should be explored and modified. For back pain, exercises and consultation from a physical therapist may be useful. And while headaches are particularly challenging, self-monitoring and tracking them engage the patient in the therapeutic process and help to identify psychosocial triggers.

Activity Enhancement

Helping the patient establish a daily activity routine, especially during times when the patient does not work, may alleviate some of the difficulty with sleeping. Encouraging good sleep hygiene with established patterns and times for sleeping and waking is especially helpful. Although patients typically use various reasons to avoid activity, regular exercise is important to improve the overall physical state. The nurse needs to work with the patient to foster adequate movement for healthier living.

Nutrition Regulation

Patients with somatization disorder often have gastrointestinal problems including special nutritional needs. The nurse should discuss with the patient the nutritional value of foods. Because these individuals often take medications that lead to weight gain, weight control strategies may be discussed (see Chapter 13). Overweight individuals should be given suggestions for healthy, low-calorie foods. Patients should be taught about balancing dietary intake with activity levels to increase their awareness of food choices.

Relaxation

Patients taking anxiolytic medication for stress reduction can also be taught relaxation techniques. The challenge is to help a patient develop strategies for routine practice and evaluation of effect. The nurse may consider a variety of techniques, including simple relaxation techniques, distraction, and guided imagery (see Chapter 13).

Psychopharmacologic Interventions

No particular medication is recommended for somatization disorder. However, psychiatric symptoms of comorbid disorders, such as depression and anxiety, may be treated pharmacologically as appropriate. Patients with somatization disorder often suffer from depression. And while depressed mood itself is not an indication to initiate antidepressant treatment, if the mood persists and insomnia, decreased appetite, decreased libido, and anhedonia are also present, aggressive psychopharmacologic management is indicated (Fallon et al., 2003). A wide variety of drugs is available, including the selective serotonin reuptake inhibitors (SSRIs), tricyclic antidepressants (TCAs), and monoamine oxidase inhibitors (MAOIs; see Chapters 14 and 20). Patients with somatization disorder usually take several different antidepressants throughout the course of the disorder. Evidence that the depressive symptoms are cleared should be sought before discontinuing use of the medication (see Box 22-4).

BOX 22.4

Drug Profile: Phenelzine (Nardil)

DRUG CLASS: Monoamine oxidase (MAO) inhibitor

RECEPTOR AFFINITY: Inhibits MAO, an enzyme responsible for breaking down biogenic amines, such as epinephrine, norepinephrine, and serotonin, allowing them to accumulate in neuronal storage sites throughout the central and peripheral nervous systems.

INDICATIONS: Treatment of depression characterized as "atypical, nonendogenous," or "neurotic" or of depression that is nonresponsive to other antidepressant therapy or when other antidepressant therapy is contraindicated.

ROUTE AND DOSAGE: Available as 15-mg tablets.

Adults: Initially, 15 mg PO tid, increasing to at least 60 mg/day at a fairly rapid pace consistent with patient tolerance. Therapy at 60 mg/day may be necessary for at least 4 weeks before response occurs. After maximum benefit is achieved, dosage is reduced gradually over several weeks. Maintenance dose may be 15 mg/day or every other day.

Geriatric: Adjust dosage accordingly because patients older than 60 years of age are more prone to develop adverse effects.

Pediatric: Not recommended for children younger than 16 years of age.

HALF-LIFE (PEAK EFFECTS): Unknown (48–96 hours).

SELECTED ADVERSE REACTIONS: Dizziness, vertigo, headache, overactivity, hyperreflexia, tremors, muscle twitching, mania, hypomania, jitteriness, confusion, memory impairment, insomnia, weakness, fatigue, overstimulation, restlessness, increased anxiety, agitation, blurred vision, sweating, constipation, diarrhea, nausea, abdominal pain, edema, dry mouth, anorexia, weight changes, hypertensive crisis, orthostatic hypotension, and disturbed cardiac rate and rhythm.

WARNINGS: Contraindicated in patients with pheochromocytoma, congestive heart failure, hepatic dysfunction, severe renal impairment, cardiovascular disease, history of headache, and myelography within previous 24 hours or scheduled within next 48 hours. Use cautiously in patients with seizure disorders, hyperthyroidism, pregnancy, or lactation, and those scheduled for elective surgery. Possible hypertensive crisis, coma, and severe convulsions may occur if administered with TCAs; possible hypertensive crisis when taken with foods containing tyramine. Increased risk for adverse interaction is possible when given with meperidine. Additive hypoglycemic effect can occur when taken with insulin and oral sulfonylureas.

SPECIFIC PATIENT/FAMILY EDUCATION:
- Take drug exactly as prescribed; do not stop taking abruptly or without consulting your health care provider.
- Avoid consuming any foods containing tyramine while taking this drug and for 2 weeks afterward.
- Avoid alcohol, sleep-inducing drugs, over-the-counter drugs such as cold and hay fever remedies, and appetite suppressants—all of which may cause serious or life-threatening problems.
- Report any signs and symptoms of adverse reactions.
- Maintain appointments for follow-up blood tests.
- Report any complaints of unusual or severe headache or yellowing of eyes or skin.
- Avoid driving a car or performing any activities that require alertness.
- Change position slowly when going from a lying to sitting or standing position to minimize dizziness or weakness.

Phenelzine (Nardil) is one of the MAOIs found effective in treating not just depression (see Chapters 14 and 20) but also the chronic pain and headaches common in people with somatization disorder. Food–drug interactions are the most serious side effects of MAOIs; while taking such agents, patients should avoid foods high in tyramine (see Chapter 14).

Anxiety associated with a somatization disorder is more difficult than depression to treat pharmacologically. Nonpharmacologic approaches such as biofeedback or relaxation are preferred. Benzodiazepines should be avoided because of the psychological dependence associated with these medications. Buspirone (BuSpar), a nonbenzodiazepine, does not lead to tolerance or withdrawal and, although not as potent as benzodiazepines, may be useful for relief of anxiety.

Monitoring Medications, Interactions, and Side Effects

In somatization disorder, patients are usually treated in the community, where they often engage in self-medication. Once the nurse completes a BPMH of all current home medicinal substances, including self-prescribed and over-the-counter remedies, vitamins and herbal supplements, etc., the information should be documented and reported to the rest of the interdisciplinary team. The nurse questions and listens carefully to determine the full scope of medications, how they are used, and effects that the patient attributes to each substance. Using the BPMH, an evaluation of possible drug–drug interactions needs to be completed by the prescriber through a medication reconciliation process. The nurse needs to work with the patient, pharmacist, and physician to support the patient in maintaining a safe and effective pharmacotherapeutic regime. Individuals with somatization disorder often have idiosyncratic reactions to their medications. Side effects should be assessed, but the patient should be encouraged to compare the benefits of the medication with any problems related to side effects.

In working with patients with somatization disorder, the nurse must always be on the lookout for drug–drug interactions. Medications patients are taking for physical problems could interact with psychiatric medications. Patients may be taking alternative medicines, such as herbal supplements, and these also need to be evaluated for possible adverse interactions (Garcia-Campayo & Sanz-Carrillo, 2000). The patient should be encouraged to use the same pharmacy to fill all prescriptions so that possible reactions can be checked.

Psychological Domain

The cognitive functioning of individuals with somatization disorder is usually within normal limits. Often, what is most noticeable about their mental status is their flamboyant appearance and exaggerated speech. They are often dressed in attention-getting clothes, with bright colours, flashy shoes, or an outrageous hairstyle. Their language is colourful and can be entertaining. However, these individuals seem preoccupied with personal illnesses and may even keep a record of symptoms. They constantly focus on bodily functions, and "living with diseases" truly becomes a way of life.

Individuals with somatization disorder usually have intense emotional reactions to life stressors. They often have a series of personal crises beginning at an early age. Typically, a new symptom or medical problem develops during times of emotional stress. It is critical that the physical assessment data be linked to psychological and social events. A history of major psychological events should be compared with the chronology of physical problems. Special attention should be paid to any history of sexual abuse or trauma in the patient's younger years. Early sexual abuse also may interfere with esteem, belonging, and sexual fulfillment in adulthood.

The individual's mood is usually labile, often shifting from extremely excited to depressed. Response to physical symptoms is often exaggerated, such as interpreting a simple cold as pneumonia or a brief chest pain as a heart attack. Family members may not believe the physical symptoms are real, instead viewing them as attention-seeking behaviour, since the symptoms often do improve when the patient receives attention. For example, a woman who has been in bed for 3 weeks with severe back pain may suddenly feel much better once her children visit her.

There is emerging evidence that some people with somatic symptoms have **alexithymia**, which is a difficulty identifying and expressing feelings in words (De Gucht & Heiser, 2003; Mai, 2004). Researchers in Toronto studying alexithymia in patients with somatoform pain disorder found that they were more descriptive of the location and severity of pain (Cox, Kuch, Parker, Shulman, & Evans, 1994). Research continues into illness patterns in people who have difficulty identifying and expressing emotion (Kojima, Senda, Nagaya, Tokudome, & Furukawa, 2003; Porcelli et al., 2003).

> **CRNENOTE**
>
> Encourage patients with somatoform disorder to discuss and explore psychosocial and spiritual issues as well as their physical problems.

Assessment

While gathering information from the biologic domain, the nurse concurrently assesses mental status in the psychological domain. Components include appearance, psychomotor behaviour, mood, affect, perception, thought content and process, sensorium, insight, and judgment (see Chapter 11).

Nursing Diagnoses for the Psychological Domain

Nursing diagnoses related to the psychological domain and typical of people with somatization disorder include anxiety, ineffective sexuality patterns, impaired social interactions, ineffective coping, and ineffective therapeutic regimen management.

Interventions for the Psychological Domain

The choice of psychological intervention depends on the specific problem the patient is experiencing. CBT, which helps the patient identify, connect, and change feelings, thoughts, and behaviour, is the most effective treatment for somatization disorder (Mai, 2004). Supportive psychotherapy, counselling, and patient education are also useful strategies. The most important and ongoing intervention is the development and maintenance of a therapeutic relationship.

Development of a Therapeutic Relationship

The most difficult yet crucial aspect of nursing care is developing a sound, person-centred, positive, and helping nurse–patient relationship. Without it, the nurse is just one more provider who fails to meet the patient's needs and expectations. Developing this relationship requires time and patience. Therapeutic communication techniques are used to help the patient explore underlying psychosocial and spiritual problems related to the physical manifestations of the disorder (see Box 22-5).

BOX 22.5

Therapeutic Dialogue: **Establishing a Relationship**

INEFFECTIVE APPROACH

Nurse: Good morning, Ms. C.

Patient: I'm in so much pain. Take that breakfast away.

Nurse: You don't want your breakfast?

Patient: Can't you see? I hurt! When I hurt, I can't eat!

Nurse: If you don't eat now, you probably won't be able to have anything until lunch.

Patient: Who cares. I have no intention of being here at lunchtime. I don't belong here.

Nurse: Ms. C, I don't think that your doctor would have admitted you unless there is a problem. I would like to talk to you about why you are here.

Patient: Nurse, I'm just here. It's none of your business.

Nurse: Oh.

Patient: Please leave me alone.

Nurse: Sure, I will see you later.

EFFECTIVE APPROACH

Nurse: Good morning, Ms. C.

Patient: I'm in so much pain. Take that breakfast away.

Nurse: (Silently removes the tray, pulls up a chair, and sits down.)

Patient: My back hurts.

Nurse: Oh, when did the back pain start?

Patient: Last night. It's this bed. I couldn't get comfortable.

Nurse: These beds can be pretty uncomfortable.

Patient: My back pain is shooting down my leg.

Nurse: Does anything help it?

Patient: Sometimes if I straighten out my leg it helps.

Nurse: Can I help you straighten out your leg?

Patient: Oh, it's OK. The pain is going away. What did you say your name is?

Nurse: I'm Susan Miller, your nurse while you are here.

Patient: I won't be here long. I don't belong in a psychiatric unit.

Nurse: While you are here, I would like to spend time with you.

Patient: OK, but you understand, I do not have any psychiatric problems.

Nurse: We can talk about whatever you want. But, since you want to get out of here, we might want to focus on what it will take to get you ready for discharge.

CRITICAL THINKING CHALLENGE

• What communication mistakes did the nurse in the first scenario make?

• What communication strategies helped the patient feel comfortable with the nurse in the second scenario? How is the second scenario different from the first?

During periods when symptoms of other psychiatric disorders surface, additional therapeutic interventions may be needed (see Chapter 9). For example, the occurrence of depression requires additional supportive or cognitive approaches.

Counselling

Counselling, with a focus on problem solving, is needed from time to time. These patients have chaotic lives and need support through a multitude of crises. Although they sometimes appear flamboyant and self-assured, their constant complaints may irritate others. The consequences of their impaired social interactions must be examined within a counselling framework. The nurse helps the patient identify stressors, explore related thoughts and feelings, and develop positive coping responses to an often chaotic lifestyle.

Patient Education: Health Teaching

Health teaching is useful throughout the nurse–patient relationship. These patients have many questions about illnesses, symptoms, and treatments. Emphasis should be upon positive health care practices rather than the effects of serious illness. Because of problems in managing medications and treatment, the therapeutic regimen needs constant monitoring; this provides ample opportunity for teaching. One area that might require special health teaching is impaired sexuality. Because of their history of physical problems related to the reproductive tract, patients may have difficulty carrying out normal sexual activity, such as intercourse, reaching orgasm, and so forth. Basic teaching about normal sexual function is often needed (see Box 22-6).

Social Domain

People with somatization disorder spend excessive time seeking medical care and attending to their multiple illnesses. Because they believe themselves to be very sick, they also believe that they are disabled and cannot work; thus, most are unemployed. So while these individuals are rarely satisfied with health care providers who can find no basis for a medical diagnosis, their

Psychoeducation Checklist: Somatization Disorder

When caring for the patient with somatization disorder, be sure to include the following topic areas in the teaching plan:

- Psychopharmacologic agents (anxiolytics) if ordered, including drug, action, dosage, frequency, and possible adverse effects
- Nonpharmacologic pain relief measures
- Exercise
- Nutrition
- Social interaction
- Appropriate health care practices
- Problem solving
- Relaxation and anxiety-reduction techniques
- Sexual functioning

social network may consist more of these providers than of their peers. Identifying a support network requires sorting out health care providers from their family and friends.

Assessment

It is important to identify both beneficial and harmful relationships within the patient's family. Family members may become weary of the patient's constant physical complaints. In assessing relations, however, it is important that other members with social problems and psychiatric disorders be identified, as the individual suffering from somatization disorder tends to live in a chaotic family with multiple problems. For instance, women may be married to abusive men with antisocial personality disorders, and alcoholism is common.

Symptoms of somatization disorder may disrupt the family's social life. A change in routine or a major life event often precipitates a symptom's appearance. For example, a patient planning a vacation with the family may decide at the last minute that she cannot go because her back pain has returned and she will be unable to sit in the car. Such family disruptions are common.

Nursing Diagnoses for the Social Domain

Some of the nursing diagnoses related to the social domain that are typical of people with somatization disorder include risk for caregiver role strain, ineffective community coping, disabled family coping, and social isolation.

Interventions for the Social Domain

Patients with somatic disorders are usually isolated from family and community. Strengthening relationships and encouraging social activity often become the focus of nursing care. The nurse should help the patient identify individuals with whom contact is desired, encourage him or her to reinitiate a relationship, and ask for a commitment to contact them. The nurse should counsel the patient about talking too much about his or her symptoms with these individuals and emphasize that medical information should be shared with the nurse.

Group Interventions

Although these patients may not be good candidates for insight group psychotherapy, they do benefit from cognitive-behavioural groups that focus on developing coping skills for everyday life (Lidbeck, 2003). Because most of the patients are women, participation in groups that address feminist issues should be encouraged, which may help to strengthen their assertiveness skills and improve their generally low self-esteem (Fig. 22-2).

When leading a group that has members with somatization disorder, redirection can keep the group from giving too much attention to a person's illness. However, these individuals need reassurance and support while in a group. They may insist that they do not fit in with or belong in the group; in reality, they are feeling insecure and threatened in the situation. The group leader needs to show patience and understanding in order to engage the individual effectively in meaningful group interaction.

Family Interventions

The results of a family assessment often reveal a need for education about the disorder, helpful strategies for dealing with the patient's multiple complaints, and, usually, help in developing more effective communication patterns. Because of the chaotic nature of their families and the lack of healthy problem solving, physical, psychological, or sexual abuse may be evident (see Chapter 37).

Spiritual Domain

Encompassing the bio/psycho/social domains, the spiritual domain pertains to the way people with a somatization disorder connect experiences, make meaning of their illness, and find purpose in life. Patients with this disorder are preoccupied with physical concerns and often are out of balance in terms of

Spiritual
1. Listen sensitively
2. Support connection with others
3. Support hope

Biologic
1. Establish pain management program; include nonpharmacologic pain relief measures
2. Set up daily routine for patient
3. Encourage regular exercise
4. Monitor nutritional intake
5. Emphasize positive health care practices
6. Administer medications

Social
1. Involve in problem-solving groups
2. Assist with developing skills for everyday life
3. Encourage use of resources for support and information
4. Promote social interaction outside the home

Psychological
1. Establish trusting relationship
2. Identify stressors and positive coping strategies
3. Assist with identifying personal strengths
4. Reinforce anxiety-reduction strategies
5. Focus on problem-solving strategies
6. Use relaxation techniques

FIGURE 22.2 Bio/psycho/social/spiritual interventions for patients with somatization disorder.

their psychological, social, and spiritual needs. They may feel at odds with the prescribed therapeutic regimen and may show frustration or anger toward themselves or others. They may feel abandoned or punished by a sacred power greater than themselves, to whom they would otherwise turn. This higher, sacred power may be known to them as God, the Creator, or Allah, for example, or not named out of respect, depending on their religion, or by a term individually chosen such as "the Universe."

Assessment

To assess the spiritual domain, nurses inquire about status, meaning, ambiguity, and hope using questions such as: What has happened? What is being ill like for you? What does being ill mean in your life? Personal strengths are assessed with questions such as: What brings joy and peace to you? How has your illness influenced the way you understand the world? Do you have spiritual beliefs that have been affected by your illness experience? Questions to elicit information about connections with self, others, and a higher power include: How are you right now? What sustains or heals your spirit? Who is significant to you? How do you feel connected to the world and events around you?

Are there spiritual acts, such as prayer, that you find helpful? (Burkhardt & Nagai-Jacobson, 2008)

Nursing Diagnoses for the Spiritual Domain

Nursing diagnoses related to the spiritual domain and typical of people with somatization disorder include hopelessness, spiritual distress, and potential for enhanced spiritual well-being. These are comparable to the *DSM-IV-TR* diagnosis of *spiritual problem*.

Interventions for the Spiritual Domain

Individuals with somatic disorders often have low self-esteem and sometimes feel estranged from others. For individuals who belong to a religious group, this can include estrangement from their faith communities. Nurses intervene by creating a safe and caring environment to help the person explore deep questions related to connection, meaning, and purpose. Trust, rapport, and a mutual plan for care are developed with the use of presence, empathy, and sensitivity. Based on the person's assessed needs, nurses may also facilitate religious practices, assist with life review or reminiscence therapy, or make a referral to a spiritual care expert (Taylor, 2002).

FIGURE 22.3 Bio/psycho/social/spiritual outcomes for patients with somatization disorder.

EVALUATION AND TREATMENT OUTCOMES

The outcomes for patients with somatization disorder must be realistic and formulated with the patient. Because this is a lifelong disorder, small successes should be expected. Specific outcomes should be identified. Over time, there should be a gradual reduction in the number of health care providers the individual contacts and gradual improvement in the ability to cope with stresses (Fig. 22-3).

CONTINUUM OF CARE

For individuals experiencing somatization disorder, mental health services ranging from inpatient care to health promotion may occur in various health care settings over the course of life.

Inpatient Care

Ideally, individuals with somatization disorder will spend minimal time in the hospital. Inpatient stays occur when their comorbid psychiatric disorders become symptomatic. In order to provide consistency of care while in inpatient care, the patient should be the responsibility of one primary nurse who provides or oversees all the nursing care. The inpatient nurse must establish a relationship with the patient (and family) and consult other nursing staff members about this disorder.

Emergency Care!

The emergencies these individuals experience may be physical (e.g., chest pain, back pain, gastrointestinal symptoms) or stress responses related to a psychosocial crisis. Occasionally, these individuals become suicidal and require an intensive level of care. Generally speaking, nonpharmacologic interventions should be tried first, with a very conservative use of antianxiety medications.

Community Treatment

Individuals with somatization disorder can spend a lifetime in the health care system and still have little continuity of care. Switching from provider to provider is detrimental to their long-term care. Most are outpatients. When they are hospitalized, it is usually for evaluation of physical problems. When their comorbid psychiatric disorders, such as depression, become symptomatic, these patients may also be hospitalized for a short time (see Nursing Care Plan 22-1).

Nursing Care Plan 22.1

The Patient With Somatization Disorder

SC is a 48-year-old woman who is making her weekly visit to her primary care physician for unexplained multiple somatic problems. This week, her concern is recurring abdominal pain that fits no symptom pattern. Upon physical examination, a cause of her abdominal pain could not be found. She is requesting a refill of alprazolam (Xanax), which is the only medication that relieves her pain. She is in the process of applying for disability income because of being completely disabled by neck and shoulder pain. The physician and office staff avoid her whenever possible. The physician will not refill the prescription until SC is evaluated by the consulting mental health team that provides weekly evaluations and services.

Setting: Primary Care Office

Baseline Assessment: SC is a 48-year-old obese Caucasian woman who appears very angry. She resents being forced to see a psychiatric clinician for the only medication that works to alleviate her pain. She denies any psychiatric problems or emotional distress. She is wearing a short, black top and too tight slacks. Her hair is in curlers; she says that it is too much trouble to comb her hair. Cognitive aspects of mental status appear normal, but she admits to being slightly depressed and takes the alprazolam for her nerves. She says she has nothing to live for but denies any thoughts of suicide. She is dependent on her children for everything and feels very guilty about it. She spends most of her waking hours going to various doctors and taking combinations of medications to relieve her pains. She has no friends or nonfamily social contacts.

Associated Psychiatric Diagnosis	Medications
Axis I: R/O depression	Premarin, 1.2 mg qd
Axis II: Somatization disorder	Alprazolam (Xanax), 25 mg tid
Axis III: S/P hysterectomy	Ranitidine HCL (Zantac), 150 mg with meals
S/P gastric bypass	Simethicone, 1,235 mg qid with meals
S/P carpel tunnel release	Calcium carbonate, 1,200 mg qd
Chronic shoulder, neck pain, vertigo	Multiple vitamin, qd
Axis IV: Social problems (father died 6 months ago,	Zolpidem tartrate (Ambien), 10 mg at hs PRN
divorced 9 months)	Ibuprofen, 600 mg q4h PRN pain
Economic problems (small pension)	Maalox, PRN
Occupational problems (potential disability)	Preparation H suppositories
GAF = Current, 60	
Potential, 75	

Nursing Diagnosis 1: Chronic Low Self-Esteem

Defining Characteristics	Related Factors
Self-negating verbalizations (long-standing)	Feeling unimportant to family
Hesitant to try new things	Feeling rejected by ex-husband
Expresses guilt	Constant physical problems interfering with normal social
Evaluates self as being unable to deal with events	activities

Outcomes

Initial	Long-term
Identify need to increase self-esteem.	Participate in individual or group therapy for esteem building.

Interventions

Interventions	Rationale	Ongoing Assessment
Establish rapport with the patient.	Individuals with low self-esteem feel vulnerable and may be reluctant to discuss true feelings.	Ask the patient for her perceptions of care and the helping relationship.

Continued

Nursing Care Plan 22.1 (*Continued*)

Interventions

Interventions	Rationale	Ongoing Assessment
Encourage the patient to spend time dressing and grooming appropriately.	Confidence and self-esteem improve when a person looks well groomed.	Monitor responses.
Encourage the patient to discuss various somatic problems, as well as psychological and interpersonal issues.	Patients with somatization disorder need time to express their physical problems. It helps them feel valued. The best way to build a relationship is to acknowledge physical symptoms.	Monitor time that the patient spends explaining physical symptoms.
Explore opportunities for SC to meet other people with similar, nonmedical interests.	Focusing SC on meeting others will improve the possibilities of increasing contacts.	Observe willingness to identify other interests besides physical problems.

Evaluation

Outcomes	Revised Outcomes	Interventions
SC admitted to having low self-esteem but was very reluctant to consider meeting new people.	Focus on building self-esteem.	Identify activities that will enhance self-esteem.

Nursing Diagnosis 2: Ineffective Therapeutic Regimen Management

Defining Characteristics	Related Factors
Choices of daily living ineffective for meeting health care goal Verbalizes difficulty with prescribed regimens	Inappropriate use of benzodiazepines for nerves

Outcomes

Initial	Long-term
Openly discuss the use of medications.	Use nonpharmacologic means for stress reduction.

Interventions

Interventions	Rationale	Ongoing Assessment
Clarify the frequency and purpose of taking alprazolam.	Unsupervised polypharmacy is very common with these patients. Further clarification is usually needed.	Carefully track self-report of medication use; determine whether the patient is disclosing the use of all medications.
Educate the patient about the effects of combining medications, emphasizing negative effects.	Education about combining medication is the beginning of helping the patient become effective in medication regimen.	Observe the patient's ability and willingness to consider negative effects.
Explore ways to gradually reduce number of medications, including other means of managing physical symptoms.	Help the patient to identify appropriate ways and means to manage health care regimens.	Evaluate the patient's ability to problem solve.

Evaluation

Outcomes	Revised Outcomes	Interventions
Patient disclosed the use of medications but was unwilling to consider changing ineffective use of medication.	Identify next step if primary care physician does not refill prescription.	Discuss the possibility of not being able to obtain alprazolam. Refer the patient to mental health clinic for further evaluation.

■◗ MENTAL HEALTH PROMOTION

Patients with somatization disorder are encouraged to focus on staying healthy rather than on the symptoms of their illness. For these individuals, approaching the topic of health promotion usually has to be within the context of preventing further problems. Setting aside time for themselves and identifying activities that meet their psychological and spiritual needs, such as connecting with their faith group, are important in maintaining a healthy balance.

Other Somatoform Disorders

The other somatoform disorders have many symptoms that are similar to those of somatization disorder but are often not debilitating. The following discussion summarizes other somatoform disorders and highlights the primary focus of nursing management.

■◗ UNDIFFERENTIATED SOMATOFORM DISORDER

Patients who complain of only one type of physical problem, lasting at least 6 months without adequate explanation, may be diagnosed with undifferentiated somatoform disorder. This disorder is different from somatization disorder in that prior to 30 years of age, these patients do not have multiple, unexplained physical problems; rather, they may have just one. Fatigue, loss of appetite, and gastrointestinal or genitourinary problems are the most common complaints. This disorder is most frequently seen in women of lower socioeconomic status. The course of the disorder is unpredictable, and another mental or physical disorder is often diagnosed. Nursing care for this disorder is similar to that for somatization disorder.

■◗ CONVERSION DISORDER

In conversion disorder, the somatic symptoms pertain specifically to neurologic conditions affecting voluntary motor or sensory function, called **pseudoneurologic symptoms**. Patients with conversion disorder present with symptoms of impaired coordination or balance, paralysis, aphonia (inability to produce sound), difficulty swallowing or a sensation of a lump in the throat, and urinary retention. They also may have loss of sensation, vision problems, blindness, deafness, and hallucinations. In some instances, they may have seizures (APA, 2000). These symptoms do not follow neurologic paths but rather follow the individual's conceptualization of

the problem. If only the pseudoneurologic symptoms are present, the patient receives a diagnosis of conversion disorder. The nurse must understand that the physical sensation is real for the patient. There is evidence of a relationship between childhood trauma (e.g., sexual abuse) and conversion disorder (Roelofs, Keijsers, Hoogduin, Naring, & Moene, 2002). In approaching this patient, the nurse treats the conversion symptom as a real symptom that may have distressing psychological aspects. The nurse intervenes by acknowledging the pain and helps the patient deal with it. As trust develops within the nurse–patient relationship, the nurse can help the patient develop approaches to solving everyday problems.

■◗ PAIN DISORDER

In pain disorder, pain severe enough for the patient to seek medical attention interferes with social and occupational functioning. The onset of the pain is associated with psychological factors, such as a traumatic or humiliating experience (e.g., combat-related posttraumatic stress disorder; O'Toole, Marshall, Schureck, & Dobson, 1998). Because of the pain, the individual cannot return to work or school. Unemployment, disability, and family problems frequently follow. Pain disorder is believed to be relatively common. From 10% to 15% of adults in the United States within a given year are disabled by back pain (APA, 2000). Pain disorder may occur at any age. Women experience headaches and musculoskeletal pain more often than do men. Acute pain tends to resolve within a short time; chronic pain may persist for many years. Pain medication should be prescribed conservatively. If mood disorders are also present, mood stabilizers not only treat the depression but also may treat the pain (Maurer, Volz, & Sauer, 1999). Nursing care focuses on helping patients identify strategies to relieve pain (Caudill-Slosberg, 2002) and to examine stressors in their lives.

■◗ HYPOCHONDRIASIS

The difference between hypochondriasis and the other somatoform disorders is that patients with hypochondriasis are preoccupied with their fears about developing a serious illness based on their misinterpretation of body sensations. In hypochondriasis, the fear of having an illness continues despite medical reassurance and interferes with psychosocial functioning. These individuals spend time and money on repeated examinations looking for feared illnesses. For example, an occasional cough or the appearance of a small sore results in the person making an appointment with an oncologist. Hypochondriasis sometimes appears if the patient had a serious childhood illness or if a family member has a serious illness. The prevalence of hypochondriasis in general medical practice is estimated to be between 2% and 7% (APA, 2000). These patients are most likely seen in medical-surgical settings, unless they have a coexisting psychiatric disorder.

Several interventions have been effective in reducing patients' fears of experiencing serious illnesses. CBT, stress management, and group interventions lead to a decrease in intensity and increase in control of symptoms (Fava, Grandi, Rafanelli, Fabbri, & Cazzaro, 2000; Walker, Vincent, Furer, Cox, & Kjemisted, 1999). It is unknown whether the positive outcomes result from the intervention itself or from the symptom validation and increased attention given to the patient. However, based on these studies, nursing management should include

listening to the patient's report of symptoms and fears, validating it by acknowledging that the fears may be real, asking the patient to monitor symptoms in a journal, and encouraging the patient to bring the journal to the next visit. By actually seeing the symptom pattern, the nurse can continue assessment and help the patient better understand the significance and implications of symptoms. The outcome of this approach should be a decrease in fear and better control of the symptoms.

■ BODY DYSMORPHIC DISORDER

Patients with BDD focus on real (but slight) or imagined defects in appearance, such as a large nose, thinning hair, or small genitals. Preoccupation with the defect causes significant distress and interferes with their ability to function socially. They feel so self-conscious that they avoid work or public situations. Some fear that their "ugly" body part will malfunction. This disorder occurs equally in men and women, but few epidemiologic data are available. In anxiety disorders and depression, BDD is estimated to occur in 5% to 40% of patients (APA, 2000). BDD may be present in 25% of patients with anorexia nervosa (Rabe-Jablonska & Tomasz, 2000). In patients receiving dermatology care and cosmetic surgery, the estimate is 6% to 15% (Phillips, Dufresne, Wilkel, & Vittorio, 2000; Uzun et al., 2003).

BDD usually begins in adolescence and continues throughout adulthood. Individuals with BDD are not usually seen in psychiatric settings unless they have a coexisting psychiatric disorder or a family member insists on psychiatric attention. BDD is an extremely debilitating disorder and can significantly impair an individual's quality of life (Box 22-7). The obvious nursing diagnosis

---

IN A LIFE

Emily Carr (1871–1945)
Canadian Painter and Writer

Public Persona

Emily Carr was an accomplished artist and writer best known for her vivid depictions of Native culture and Canadian West Coast nature. Influenced by early educational sojourns in San Francisco, England, and France and later encouraged by the important artists known as the Group of Seven, Carr developed her unique impressionistic style in both painting and writing. Embellished with dramatizations and idealism, works like *Growing Pains* autobiographically depict the struggle of her life. Raised in a strict Victorian home, Carr has been described as rebellious, yet overweight, irritable, and socially insecure.

Personal Realities

Carr's career was interrupted many times with bouts of poor health. Just more than 100 years ago, Carr was treated in an English sanatorium. Many of the symptoms she described were representatives of what today is called hypochondriasis, clinical depression, and/or conversion disorder.

BOX 22.7

Clinical Vignette: Body Dysmorphic Disorder

K, a 16-year-old girl, has believed for about 6 months that her pubic bone is becoming increasingly dislocated and prominent. She believes that everyone stares at and talks about it. She does not remember a particular event related to the appearance of the symptom but is absolutely convinced that she can be helped only by a surgical correction of her pubic bone.

She was treated recently for anorexia nervosa with marginal success. Although her weight is nearly normal, she continues to be preoccupied with the looks of her body. She spends almost the entire day in her bedroom, wearing excessively large pajamas, and she refuses to leave the house. Once or twice a day, she lowers herself to the ground

and measures, with her fingers, the distance between her pelvic girdle and the ground in order to check the position of the pubic bone.

In desperation, her parents called the clinic for help. The family was referred to a home health agency and a psychiatric home health nurse who arranged for an assessment visit.

WHAT DO YOU THINK?
- How should the nurse approach K? Should an assessment begin immediately?
- From the vignette, identify nursing diagnoses, outcomes, and interventions.

Adapted from Sobanski, E., & Schmidt, M. H. (2000). 'Everybody looks at my pubic bone'—A case report of an adolescent patient with body dysmorphic disorder. *Acta Psychiatrica Scandinavica, 101*, 80–82.

is impaired body image. While developing a therapeutic relationship, the nurse should respect these patients' preoccupations and avoid challenging their beliefs. However, the nurse should also assess the extent of preoccupation with the body part. If the patient is actually disfigured, the preoccupation may take on a phobic quality (Newell, 1999). If so, referral to a mental health specialist should be considered. The generalist nurse can help the patient by developing interventions for other nursing diagnoses that may be present, such as social isolation, low self-esteem, and ineffective coping. These patients will often be treated with an antidepressant (Phillips & Najjar, 2003).

Factitious Disorders

The other type of psychiatric disorder characterized by somatization is *factitious disorder*. Patients with this disorder intentionally cause an illness or injury to receive the attention of health care workers. These individuals are motivated solely by the desire to become a patient and develop a dependent relationship with a health care provider. There are two classes of factitious disorders: factitious disorder and factitious disorder, not otherwise specified.

▰▰◣ FACTITIOUS DISORDER

Although feigned illnesses have been described for centuries, it was not until 1951 that the term *Münchausen's syndrome* was used to describe the most severe form of this disorder, which was characterized by fabricating a physical illness, having recurrent hospitalizations, and going from one provider to another (Asher, 1951). Today, this disorder is called factitious disorder and is differentiated from **malingering,** in which the individual who intentionally produces illness symptoms is motivated by another specific self-serving goal, such as being classified as disabled or avoiding work.

Unlike people with borderline personality disorder, who typically injure themselves overtly and readily admit to self-harm, patients with factitious disorder injure themselves covertly. The illnesses are produced in such a manner that the health care provider is tricked into believing that a true physical or psychiatric disorder is present. The *DSM-IV-TR* identifies three subtypes of factitious disorder: (1) one that has predominantly psychological symptoms; (2) one that has predominately physical symptoms (Münchausen's syndrome); and (3) one that has a combination of physical and psychological manifestations, with neither one predominating (APA, 2000).

The self-produced physical symptoms appear as medical illnesses and cut across all body systems. They include seizure disorders, wound-healing disorders, the abscess processes (introduction of infectious material below the skin surface), and feigned fever (rubbing the thermometer). In one study of 42 children and adolescents who falsify chronic illness, most patients were female, and the most commonly reported falsified or induced conditions were fevers, ketoacidosis, purpura, and infections (Libow, 2000).

These patients are extremely creative in simulating illnesses, and they tell fascinating but false stories of personal triumph. These tales are referred to as **pseudologia fantastica** and are a core symptom of the disorder. Pseudologia fantastica are stories that are not entirely improbable and often contain a matrix of truth and falsehood. These patients falsify blood, urine, and other samples by contaminating them with protein or fecal material. They self-inject anticoagulants to receive diagnoses of "bleeding of undetermined origin" or ingest thyroid hormones to produce thyrotoxicosis. They also inflict injury on themselves by inserting objects or feces into open wounds or body orifices, such as the urinary tract. They produce their own surgical scars, especially abdominal, and when treated surgically, they delay wound healing through scratching, rubbing, or manipulating the wound and introducing bacteria into the wound. These patients put themselves in life-threatening situations through actions such as ingesting allergens known to produce an anaphylactic reaction.

Patients who feign primarily psychological symptoms appear much less commonly than those who feign physical signs and symptoms (Sadock & Sadock, 2007). Psychological symptoms appear as psychotic symptoms such as hallucinations and delusions, cognitive deficits such as memory loss, dissociative symptoms such as amnesia, and conversion symptoms such as pseudoblindness or pseudoparalysis. These individuals often appear psychotic, depressed, or suicidal after an unconfirmed tragedy. When questioned about details, they become defensive and uncooperative. Sometimes, these individuals have a combination of both physical and psychiatric symptoms.

Epidemiology

The prevalence of factitious disorder is difficult to determine because its secretive nature interferes with traditional epidemiological research methods (Krahn, Li, & O'Connor, 2003). Prevalence estimates range widely from 0.0001% to 15% but, as reported in a German study (Fliege et al., 2007), it is most commonly considered to represent findings in about 1% of psychiatric consultations in general hospitals (APA, 2000). Eight percent of psychiatric patients (mostly women with a mean age of 36.2) in one Spanish hospital showed factitious psychological symptoms (Catalina, Gómez Macias, & deCos, 2008). The most frequent factitious psychological symptom reported was worsening of symptoms at the time of discharge planning. Once thought to occur predominantly in men, this disorder is now reported predominantly in women. No genetic pattern has been identified, but it does seem to run in families. Many of these people have comorbid psychiatric disorders, such as mood disorders, personality disorders, and substance-related disorders (Sadock & Sadock, 2007).

Etiology

The etiology of factitious disorder is believed to have a psychodynamic basis. The theory is that these individuals, who were often abused as children, received nurturance only during times of illness; thus, they try to recreate illness or injury in a desperate attempt to receive love and attention. During the actual self-injury, the individual is reported to be in a trance-like, dissociative state. Many patients report having had an intimate relationship with a health care provider, either as a child or as an adult, and then experiencing rejection when the relationship ended. The self-injury and subsequent attention are the individual's attempts to reenact those experiences and gain control over the situation and the other person. Patients often exhibit aggression after being discovered, allowing them to express revenge on their perceived tormenter (Feldman, 2004).

These patients are usually discovered in medical-surgical settings. They are hostile and distance themselves from others. Their network is void of friends and family and usually consists only of health care providers, who change at regular intervals. In factitious disorder, the patients fabricate a detailed and exaggerated medical history. When the interventions do not work and the fabrication is discovered, the health care team may feel manipulated and angry. When the patient is confronted with the evidence, he or she becomes enraged and often leaves that health care situation, only to enter another. Eventually, the person is referred for mental health treatment. The course of the disorder usually consists of intermittent episodes (APA, 2000).

■ NURSING MANAGEMENT: HUMAN RESPONSE TO DISORDER

The overall goal of treatment is for the patient to replace the dysfunctional, attention-seeking behaviours with positive behaviours. To begin treatment, the patient must acknowledge the deception, but confrontation does not appear to lead to acknowledgment (Krahn et al., 2003). The mental health team has to accept and value the patient as a human being who needs help. As the pattern of self-injury is well established and meets overwhelming psychological needs, giving up the behaviours is difficult. The treatment is long-term psychotherapy. The generalist PMH nurse will most likely care for the patient during or after periods of feigned illness. More is known about the treatment of individuals with factitious physical disorders than of those with psychological disorders.

Assessment

A nursing assessment should focus on obtaining a history of medical and psychological illnesses. Physical disabilities should be identified. Early childhood experiences, particularly instances of abuse, neglect, or abandonment, should be identified in order to understand the underlying psychological dynamics of the individual and the role of self-injury. Family assessment is important; relationships become strained as family members become aware of this disorder's self-inflicted nature.

Nursing Diagnoses

The nursing diagnoses could include almost any diagnosis, such as risk for trauma, risk for self-mutilation, ineffective individual coping, or low self-esteem.

Desired outcomes include decreased self-injurious behaviour and increased positive coping behaviours. Any nursing intervention must be implemented within the context of a strong nurse–patient relationship (Moffatt, 2000).

Nursing Interventions

Nurses must continually examine their own feelings about these patients. The fabrications and deceits may provoke anger and a sense of betrayal in the nurse. To be effective with these patients, the nurse must be aware of these feelings and resolve them by developing a better understanding of the underlying psychodynamic issues. Therapeutic confrontation in the context of a helping relationship can be effective if the patient feels supported and accepted and if there is clear communication between the patient, the mental health care team, and family members. All care should be centralized within one facility, and the patient should see providers regularly, even when not in active crisis. Offering the patient a face-saving way of giving up the factitious disorder is often crucial. The treatment goal is recovery not confession. Behavioural techniques that shape new behaviours help the patient move toward a new life.

The goal is for care to be given within the context of one system. A team that knows the patient, agrees on a treatment approach, and follows through is crucial to the patient's eventual recovery. For this to happen, the medical, psychiatric, inpatient, and outpatient teams need to communicate with each other on a regular basis. Family members must also be aware of the need for consistent treatment.

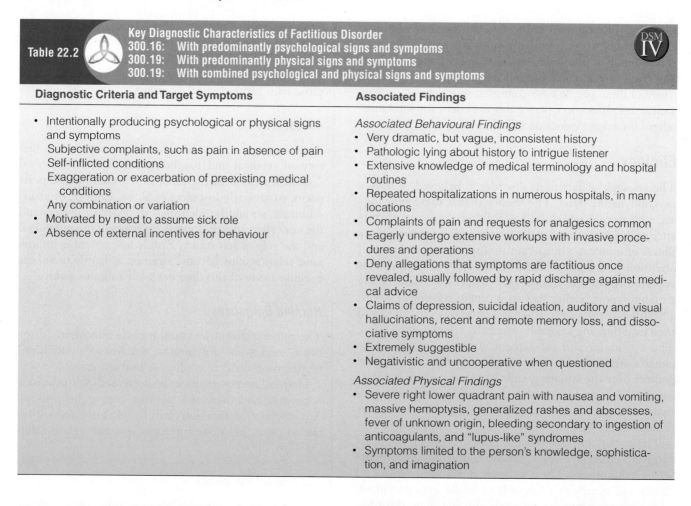

Table 22.2	Key Diagnostic Characteristics of Factitious Disorder	
	300.16: With predominantly psychological signs and symptoms	DSM IV
	300.19: With predominantly physical signs and symptoms	
	300.19: With combined psychological and physical signs and symptoms	

Diagnostic Criteria and Target Symptoms	Associated Findings

<ul><li>Intentionally producing psychological or physical signs and symptoms
  Subjective complaints, such as pain in absence of pain
  Self-inflicted conditions
  Exaggeration or exacerbation of preexisting medical conditions
  Any combination or variation</li><li>Motivated by need to assume sick role</li><li>Absence of external incentives for behaviour</li></ul>
	Associated Behavioural Findings
	<ul><li>Very dramatic, but vague, inconsistent history</li><li>Pathologic lying about history to intrigue listener</li><li>Extensive knowledge of medical terminology and hospital routines</li><li>Repeated hospitalizations in numerous hospitals, in many locations</li><li>Complaints of pain and requests for analgesics common</li><li>Eagerly undergo extensive workups with invasive procedures and operations</li><li>Deny allegations that symptoms are factitious once revealed, usually followed by rapid discharge against medical advice</li><li>Claims of depression, suicidal ideation, auditory and visual hallucinations, recent and remote memory loss, and dissociative symptoms</li><li>Extremely suggestible</li><li>Negativistic and uncooperative when questioned</li></ul>*Associated Physical Findings*
	<ul><li>Severe right lower quadrant pain with nausea and vomiting, massive hemoptysis, generalized rashes and abscesses, fever of unknown origin, bleeding secondary to ingestion of anticoagulants, and "lupus-like" syndromes</li><li>Symptoms limited to the person's knowledge, sophistication, and imagination</li></ul>

FACTITIOUS DISORDER, NOT OTHERWISE SPECIFIED

The diagnosis of factitious disorder not otherwise specified is reserved for people who do not quite meet all the diagnostic criteria of factitious disorder (Table 22-2). Within the category of factitious disorder not otherwise specified, the *DSM-IV-TR* includes a rare but dramatic disorder, factitious disorder by proxy, or *Münchausen's by proxy*, which involves a person's inflicting injury on another—usually a mother on her own child—hoping thereby to gain the attention of a health care provider. These actions include inducing seizures, poisoning, or smothering. This most severe form of child abuse is usually identified in the emergency room or by critical care nurses (Hughes & Corbo-Richert, 1999). The mother rarely admits to injuring the child and thus is not amenable to treatment; the child is removed from the mother's care. This form of child abuse is distinguished from other forms by the routine, unwitting involvement of health care workers, who subject the child to physical harm and emotional distress through tests, procedures, and medication trials. Some researchers suspect that children who are abused in this way may later experience factitious disorder (Libow, 2000).

SUMMARY OF KEY POINTS

▢   Somatization is psychological stress that is manifested in physical symptoms and is the chief characteristic of somatoform disorders and factitious disorders. The difference between these two types of disorders is that in somatoform disorders, the individuals experience unexplained physical symptoms but do not self-inflict injuries, whereas in factitious disorders, individuals self-inflict injuries to gain medical attention.

▢   Somatization is affected by sociocultural and gender factors. It occurs more frequently in women than in men; in those less educated; in those living in urban areas; and in those who are older, separated, widowed, or divorced.

▢   The somatoform disorders are clustered into six different clinical syndromes: (1) somatization disorder, (2) undifferentiated somatoform disorder, (3) conversion disorder, (4) pain disorder, (5) hypochondriasis, and (6) BDD. The person with somatization disorder suffers multiple physical problems and symptoms, in contrast to those with other clinical subtypes in which one major symptom recurs.

■ Somatization disorder, which occurs primarily in women and is the most complex of the somatoform disorders, is a chronic relapsing condition characterized by multiple physical symptoms that develop during times of emotional distress.

■ Factitious disorders include two subtypes: (1) factitious disorder and (2) factitious disorder, not otherwise specified. In factitious disorder, the patient fabricates physical or psychological symptoms (or both) in order to appear sick. Factitious disorder, not otherwise specified includes factitious disorder by proxy, the intentional production of symptoms in others, usually in children by their mothers.

■ Identifying and diagnosing somatoform and factitious disorders is very complex because patients with these disorders refuse to accept any psychiatric basis for their problems and often go for years moving from one health care provider to another, seeking medical attention but avoiding psychiatric assessment.

■ These patients are often seen on the medical-surgical units of hospitals and can go years without receiving a correct diagnosis. In most cases, they eventually receive mental health treatment because of comorbid conditions, such as depression and panic.

■ The development of the nurse–patient relationship is crucial to assessing these patients and identifying appropriate nursing diagnoses and interventions. Because these patients deny any psychiatric basis for their problem and continue to focus on their symptoms having a medical basis, the nurse must take a nonjudgmental, open approach that acknowledges the symptoms while helping the patient explore and understand his or her behaviour and focus on new ways of coping with stress.

■ Health teaching is important in helping the individual develop positive lifestyle changes in place of somatization responses. Identifying personal strengths and supporting the development of positive skills improve self-esteem and personal confidence. Teaching the use of biofeedback and relaxation provides the patient with positive coping skills.

CRITICAL THINKING CHALLENGES

1 A depressed young white woman is admitted to a psychiatric unit in a state of agitation. She reports extreme abdominal pain. Her admitting provider tells you that she has a classic case of somatization disorder and to de-emphasize her physical symptoms. Under no circumstances is she to have any pain medication. Conceptualize how to approach, assess, and intervene with this patient.

2 Compare and contrast somatoform disorders with factitious disorders.

3 Develop a motivation continuum of "self-injury" for patients with borderline personality disorder, somatization disorder, factitious disorder, and factitious disorder by proxy.

4 Develop a teaching plan for an individual who has a long history of somatization disorder but who recently received a diagnosis of breast cancer. How will the patient be able to differentiate the physical symptoms of somatization disorder from those associated with the treatment of her breast cancer?

5 A woman of Chinese origin was admitted for panic attacks and numerous somatic problems, ranging from dysmenorrhea to painful joints. Results of all medical examinations have been negative. She truly believes that her panic attacks are caused by a weak heart. What approaches should the nurse use in providing culturally sensitive nursing care?

6 A person experiencing depression with somatic features is started on a regimen of Nardil, 15 mg tid. She believes that she is allergic to most foods but insists on having wine in the evenings because it helps digest her food. Develop a teaching plan that provides the knowledge that she needs to prevent a hypertensive crisis caused by excessive tyramine but that is sensitive to the patient's food preferences.

WEB LINKS

www.intelihealth.com InteliHealth provides health information. Somatization disorder can be found through a search on this Aetna website.

www.mental-health-matters.com/disorders This is the site of Mental Health Matters, a website for consumers and professionals, which describes several psychiatric disorders, including somatization disorder.

MOVIES, NOVELS, AND BIOGRAPHIES

The Piano: 1992. This is a thought-provoking account of the life of an English colonial settler who encounters isolation, repression, exploitation, and abuse. The traumatic origin and functional limitations indicative of conversion disorder are poignantly depicted in this movie. Experiencing nonorganic habitual dysphonia (mutism), the main character asserts and expresses herself with others mainly through music. Somatoform and related disorders are rarely clearly depicted in films. The Piano exemplifies the functional physical, interpersonal, and occupational effects of symptoms associated with conversion disorder.

VIEWING POINTS: Identify the symptoms and related behaviour associated with somatoform disorder. Consider the effects of emotional and physical trauma.

REFERENCES

Allen, L. A., Woolfolk, R. L., Escobar, J. I., Gara, M. A., & Hamer, R. M. (2006). Cognitive-behavioral therapy for somatization disorder. *Archives of Internal Medicine, 166*, 1512–1518.

American Psychiatric Association. (2000). *Diagnostic and statistical manual of mental disorders* (4th ed., Text revision). Washington, DC: Author.

Asher, R. (1951). Münchausen's syndrome. *Lancet, 1*, 339–341.

Burkhardt, M. A., & Nagai-Jacobson, M. G. (2008). Spirituality and health. In B. M. Dossey & L. Keegan. *Holistic nursing: A handbook for practice* (5th ed., pp. 617–645). Toronto, ON: Jones and Bartlett Publishers.

Catalina, M. L., Gómez Macias, V., & de Cos, A. (2008). Prevalence of factitious disorder with psychological symptoms in hospitalized patients. *Actas Espaniolas de Psiquiatria, 36*(6), 345–349.

Caudill-Slosberg, M. A. (2002). *Managing pain before it manages you* (rev. ed.). New York, NY: Guilford Press.

Cloninger, R. C, Reich, T., & Guze, S. (1995). The multifactorial model of disease transmission: III. Familial relations between sociopathy and hysteria (Briquet's syndrome). *British Journal of Psychiatry, 127*, 23–32.

Cox, B. J., Kuch, K., Parker, J. D., Shulman, I. D., & Evans, R. J. (1994). Alexithymia in somatoform disorder patients with chronic pain. *Journal of Psychosomatic Research, 38*(6), 523–527.

De Gucht, V., & Heiser, W. (2003). Alexithymia and somatization: A quantitative review of the literature. *Journal of Psychosomatic Research, 54*, 425–434.

De Waal, M. W. M., Arnold, I. A., Eekhof, J. A. H., & Van Hermert, A. M. (2004). Somatoform disorders in general practice. *British Journal of Psychiatry, 184*, 470–476.

Fallon, B. A., Qureshi, A. I., Schneier, F. R., Sanchez-Lacay, A., Vermes, D., Feinstein, R., et al. (2003). An open trial of fluvoxamine for hypochondriasis. *Psychosomatics, 44*(4), 298–303.

Fava, G., Grandi, S., Rafanelli, C., Fabbri, S., & Cazzaro, M. (2000). Explanatory therapy in hypochondriasis. *Journal of Clinical Psychiatry, 61*(4), 317–322.

Feldman, M. D. (2004). *Playing sick? Untangling the web of Munchausen syndrome, Munchausen by proxy, malingering factitious disorders.* Philadelphia, PA: Brunner Routledge, Taylor & Francis.

Fliege, H., Grimm, M. A., Eckhardt-Henn, A., Gieler, U., Martin, K., & Klapp, B. F. (2007). Frequency of ICD-10 factitious disorder: Survey of senior hospital consultants and physicians in private practice. *Psychosomatics, 48*, 60–64.

Garcia-Campayo, J., & Sanz-Carrillo, C. (2000). The use of alternative medicines by somatoform disorder patients in Spain. *British Journal of General Practice, 50*(455), 487–488.

Garcia-Campayo, J., Sanz-Carrillo, C., Baringo, T., & Ceballos, C. (2001). A SPECT scan in somatization disorder patients: An exploratory study of eleven cases. *Australian and New Zealand Journal of Psychiatry, 35*(3), 359–363.

Garyfallos, G., Adamopoulou, A., Karastergiou, A., Voikli, M., Ikonomidis, N., Donias, S., et al. (1999). Somatoform disorders: Comorbidity with other DSM-III-R psychiatric diagnoses in Greece. *Comprehensive Psychiatry, 40*(4), 299–307.

Grabe, H. J., Meyer, C., Hapke, U., Rumpf, H. J., Freyberger, H. J., Dilling, H., et al. (2003). Specific somatoform disorder in the general population. *Psychosomatics, 44*(4), 304–311.

Gureje, O., & Simon, G. E. (1999). The natural history of somatization in primary care. *Psychological Medicine, 29*(3), 669–676.

Gureje, O., Simon, G. E., Ustun, T. B., & Goldberg, D. P. (1997). Somatization in cross-cultural perspective: A World Health Organization study in primary care. *American Journal of Psychiatry, 154*(7), 989–995.

Hakala, M., Karlsson, H., Ruotsalainen, U., Koponen, S., Bergman, J., Stenman, H., et al. (2002). Severe somatization in women is associated with altered cerebral glucose metabolism. *Psychological Medicine, 32*(8), 1379–1385.

Hotopf, M., Mayou, R., Wadsworth, M., & Wessely, S. (1999). Childhood risk factors for adults with medically unexplained symptoms: Results from a national birth cohort study. *American Journal of Psychiatry, 156*(11), 1796–1800.

Hughes, L. M., & Corbo-Richert, B. (1999). Munchausen syndrome by proxy: Literature review and implications for critical care nurses. *Critical Care Nurse, 19*(3), 71–78.

Jorge, J. R. (2003). Depression in Brazil and other Latin American countries. *Seishin Shinkeigaku Zasshi, 105*(1), 9–16.

Kirmayer, L. J., & Young, A. (1998). Culture and somatization: Clinical, epidemiological correlates. *Psychosomatic Medicine, 60*, 420–430.

Kojima, M., Senda, Y., Nagaya, T., Tokudome, S., & Furukawa, T. A. (2003). Alexithymia, depression and social support among Japanese workers. *Psychotherapy and Psychosomatics, 72*(6), 307–314.

Krahn, L. E., Li, H., & O'Connor, M. K. (2003). Patients who strive to be ill: Factitious disorder with physical symptoms. *American Journal of Psychiatry, 160*(6), 1163–1168.

Kroenke, K., & Spitzer, R. (1998). Gender differences in the reporting of physical and somatoform symptoms. *Psychosomatic Medicine, 60*, 150–155.

Kroenke, K., & Swindle, R. (2000). Cognitive-behavioral therapy for somatization and symptom syndromes: A critical review of controlled clinical trials. *Psychotherapy Psychosomatics, 69*(4), 205–215.

Ladwig, K. H., Marten-Mittag, B., Erazo, N., & Gundel, H. (2001). Identifying somatization disorder in a population-based health examination survey: Psychosocial burden and gender differences. *Psychosomatics, 42*(6), 511–518.

Libow, J. A. (2000). Child and adolescent illness falsification. *Pediatrics, 105*(2), 336–342.

Lidbeck, M. (2003). Group therapy for somatization disorders in primary care: Maintenance of treatment goals of short cognitive-behavioural treatment one-and-a-half-year follow-up. *Acta Psychiatrica Scandinavica, 107*(5), 449–456.

Lieb, R., Pfister, H., Mastaler, M., & Wittchen, H. U. (2000). Somatoform syndromes and disorders in a representative population sample of adolescents and young adults: Prevalence, comorbidity and impairments. *Acta Psychiatrica Scandinavica, 101*(3), 194–208.

Lieb, R., Zimmermann, P., Friis, R. H., Hofler, M., Tholen, S., & Wittchen, H. U. (2002). The natural course of DSM-IV somatoform disorders and syndromes among adolescents and young adults: A prospective-longitudinal community study. *European Psychiatry, 17*(6), 321–331.

Lowe, B., Mundt, C., Herzog, W., Brunner, R., Backenstrass, M., Kronmuller, K., et al. (2008). Validity of current somatoform disorder diagnoses: Perspectives for classification in DSM-V and ICD-11. *Psychopatology, 41*, 4–9.

Mai, F. (2004). Somatization disorder: A practical review. *Canadian Journal of Psychiatry, 49*, 652–662.

Maurer, I., Volz, H. P., & Sauer, H. (1999). Gabapentin leads to remission of somatoform pain disorder with major depression. *Pharmacopsychiatry, 32*(6), 255–257.

Moffatt, C. (2000). Self-inflicted wounding: Identification, assessment and management. *British Journal of Community Nursing, 5*(1), 34–40.

Mullick, M. S. (2002). Somatoform disorders in children and adolescents. *Bangladesh Medical Research Council Bulletin, 28*(3), 112–122.

Newell, R. J. (1999). Altered body image: A fear-avoidance model of psychosocial difficulties following disfigurement. *Journal of Advanced Nursing, 30*(5), 1230–1238.

Noyes, R. Jr., Langbehn, D., Happel, R., Sieren, L., & Muller, B. (1999). Health Attitude Survey: A scale for assessing somatizing patients. *Psychosomatics, 40*(6), 470–478.

Noyes, R., Stuart, S., Watson, D. B., & Langbehn, D. R. (2006). Distinguishing between hypochondriasis and somatization disorder: A review of the existing literature. *Psychotherapy and Psychosomatics, 75*(5), 270–281.

O'Toole, B. I., Marshall, R. P., Schureck, R. J., & Dobson, M. (1998). Post-traumatic stress disorder and comorbidity in Australian Vietnam veterans: Risk factors, chronicity and combat. *Australian and New Zealand Journal of Psychiatry, 32*(1), 32–42.

Phillips, K. A., & Najjar, F. (2003). An open-label study of citalopram in body dysmorphic disorder. *Journal of Clinical Psychiatry, 64*(6), 715–720.

Phillips, K. A., Dufresne, R. J., Wilkel, C. S., & Vittorio, C. C. (2000). Rate of body dysmorphic disorder in dermatology patients. *Journal of American Academy of Dermatology, 42*(3), 436–441.

Porcelli, P., Bagby, R. M., Taylor, G. J., DeCarne, M., Leandro, G., & Todarello, O. (2003). Alexithymia as predictor of treatment outcome in patients with functional gastrointestinal disorders. *Psychosomatic Medicine, 65*(5), 911–918.

Rabe-Jablonska, J. J., & Tomasz, M. (2000). The links between body dysmorphic disorder and eating disorders. *European Psychiatry, 15*(5), 302–305.

Roelofs, K., Keijsers, G. P., Hoogduin, K. A., Naring, G. W., & Moene, F. C. (2002). Childhood abuse in patients with conversion disorders. *American Journal of Psychiatry, 159*(11), 1908–1913.

Sadock, B. J., & Sadock, V. A. (2007). *Kaplan & Sadock's Synopsis of psychiatry: Behavioral sciences/clinical psychiatry* (10th ed., pp. 658–664). Baltimore, MD: Lippincott Williams and Wilkins.

Schneider, G., Wachter, M., Driesch, G., Kruse, A., Nehen, H. G., & Heuft, G. (2003). Subjective body complaint as an indicator of somatization in elderly patients. *Psychosomatics, 44*(2), 91–99.

Sobanski, E., & Schmidt, M. H. (2000). 'Everybody looks at my pubic bone'—A case report of an adolescent patient with body dysmorphic disorder. *Acta Psychiatrica Scandinavica, 101*, 80–82.

Spitzer, C., Barnow, S., Gau, K., Freyberger, H. J., & Grabe, H. (2008). Childhood maltreatment in patients with somatization disorder. *Australian and New Zealand Journal of Psychiatry, 42*(4), 335–341.

Taylor, E. J. (2002). *Spiritual care: Nursing theory, research, and practice.* Upper Saddle River, NJ: Prentice Hall.

Uzun, O., Basoglu, C., Akar, A., Cansever, A., Ozsahin, A., Cetil, M., et al. (2003). Body dysmorphic disorder in patients with acne. *Comprehensive Psychiatry, 44*(5), 415–419.

Walker, J., Vincent, N., Furer, P., Cox, B., & Kjemisted, K. (1999). Treatment preference in hypochondriasis. *Journal of Behavior Therapy & Experimental Psychiatry, 30*(4), 251–258.

Whitehead, W. E., Palsson, O., & Jones, K. R. (2002). Systematic review of the comorbidity of irritable bowel syndrome with other disorders: What are the causes and implications? *Gastroenterology, 122*(4), 1140–1156.

Yates, W. R. (2008). Somatoform disorders. Accessed February 20, 2009, from http://www.emedicine.medscape.com/article/294908

Yick, A. G., Shibusawa, T., & Agbayani-Siewert, P. (2003). Partner violence, depression, and practice implications with families of Chinese descent. *Journal of Cultural Diversity, 10*(3), 96–104.

CHAPTER 23

Eating Disorders

Kathryn Weaver

Adapted from the chapter "Eating Disorders" by Jane H. White

KEY CONCEPTS

- body dissatisfaction
- body image distortion/disturbed body experience
- dietary restraint
- drive for thinness
- enmeshment
- interoceptive awareness
- sexuality fears

LEARNING OBJECTIVES

After studying this chapter, you will be able to:

- Distinguish the signs and symptoms of anorexia nervosa, bulimia nervosa, and binge eating disorder.
- Describe biological, psychological, and social etiologic theories of anorexia nervosa, bulimia nervosa, and binge eating disorder within the broader spiritual dimension.
- Explain the importance of body image, body dissatisfaction, and gender identity in developmental theories that explain etiology of eating disorders.
- Appreciate the role obesity plays in the development of anorexia nervosa and bulimia nervosa and as a consequence of binge eating disorder.
- Describe the neurobiology and neurochemistry in anorexia nervosa, bulimia nervosa, and binge eating disorder.
- Explain the impact of sociocultural norms on the development of eating disorders.
- Describe the risk factors and protective factors associated with the development of eating disorders.
- Formulate nursing diagnoses for individuals with eating disorders.
- Identify and describe nursing interventions for individuals with anorexia nervosa, bulimia nervosa, and binge eating disorder.
- Analyze special concerns within the nurse–client relationship for the nursing care of individuals with eating disorders.
- Identify strategies for the prevention and early detection of eating disorders.

KEY TERMS

- anorexia nervosa • binge eating • binge eating disorder • body image
- bulimia nervosa • cue elimination • self-monitoring

*A*lthough eating disorders are now in the national news, particularly when they affect a celebrity, the first Canadian publication about eating disorders was a clinical case report in the *Maritime Medical News* of April 1895 by a New Brunswick physician, Peter Inches who described a 17-year-old with low weight, loss of menses, and "almost complete refusal of food of any kind" (p. 74). His report was for the most part ignored. Today, however, the fact that an increasing number of individuals, families, and communities are affected by eating disorders means there is a concominant increased focus on anorexia, **bulimia nervosa** (BN), and obesity, their identification and treatment.

This chapter focuses on **anorexia nervosa** (AN), BN, and **binge eating disorder** (BED). In addition, the role obesity plays both in the development of eating disorders and as a consequence of BED is considered. Symptoms of all these disorders, such as dieting, binge eating, weight fluctuations, and preoccupation with weight and shape, overlap significantly. Thus, these symptoms may be viewed holistically within the "Loonie Theory" (Anorexics and Bulimics Anonymous, 2002, p. 37), named after the Canadian one-dollar coin (embossed with a loon) that pictures all the eating disorders as one entity. On one side of the coin is the intense restriction of AN. On the other side is the overeating of BED that some consider compulsive eating. The edge of the coin is BN, wherein individuals binge eat, experience the terror of getting fat, and then purge to regain a sense of control over their weight. Individuals do not rigidly adhere to one position on the loonie, but may experiment with flipping the coin; for instance, they may move from AN to the other side of BED or to the edges of BN. Many who express symptoms primarily of BN attempt to control bingeing and purging through AN, believing they are cured when they succeed for a time. They may also cycle back and forth from AN to BN to BED.

The Loonie theory helps illustrate the complexity of eating disorders as a number of individuals with AN may have bulimic symptoms, and those with BN have anorexic symptoms. For this reason, the types of anorexia, such as the purging type, and the types of bulimia, such as the restricting type, are differentiated based on the predominant symptom the individual shows to manipulate food and weight. Eating disorders differ in definition, clinical course, etiologies, and interventions, and are considered separately in this chapter. Yet, because their risk factors

and prevention strategies are similar, they are discussed together under one heading.

Anorexia Nervosa

▬◖ CLINICAL COURSE

The onset of AN is usually in early adolescence. The onset can be slow, and serious dieting can be present long before an emaciated body—the result of starvation—is noticed. This discovery often prompts the diagnosis of full- or partial-syndrome eating disorder. Partial syndrome (subclinical) is described as *Eating Disorders Not Otherwise Specified* (EDNOS) in the American Psychiatric Association (APA) *Diagnostic and Statistical Manual of Mental Disorders*, 4th ed., Text revision (*DSM-IV-TR*) (2000). The difference between full and partial syndromes are quantitative, not qualitative (Park & Beaudet, 2007; Sancho, Arija, & Canals, 2008). Full-syndrome eating disorders must fully meet stringent medical diagnostic criteria; partial syndrome cases, in which most but not all of the symptoms are present, have a higher incidence. Many affected individuals may not receive appropriate diagnosis and early treatment of their symptoms until they progress to full syndrome (see Fig. 23-1). In some cases, they receive no treatment. Although usually associated with adolescents and younger persons, the risk of eating disorders goes across the lifespan. In a nationally representative sample of Canadian women aged 50 years and older, 2.6% who were 50 to 64 years old and 1.8% over 65 years of age reported eating disorder symptomatology (Gadalla, 2008).

The long-term outcome of AN has improved during the past 15 to 20 years because awareness has increased early detection. AN can be regarded as a chronic condition, with relapses characterized by significant weight loss, and yet, eating disorders are considered by many clinicians to be curable (Anderson, 2001) with full recovery possible (Weaver, Wuest, & Ciliska, 2005). Nonetheless, reporting conclusive outcomes for AN is difficult because of the variety of definitions used to determine recovery. Conclusions from a review of 119 outcome studies revealed that 47% of individuals recovered (Steinhausen, 2002). In these and other more recent studies, approximately one third of individuals go on to experience BN (Eddy et al., 2008). A 20-year study of the AN client population in British Columbia supports prior reports that AN has the highest mortality rate of any psychiatric disorder in young females (Birmingham, Su, Hlynsky, Goldner, & Gao, 2005). For adults, a longer duration of treatment predicts positive outcome (Fichter & Quadflieg, 1999; Steinhausen, 2002); predictors of weight maintenance in adolescents are high motivation to introduce any change which

---

IN A LIFE GETTING THE MESSAGE OUT

Sara Thornton: Facing the Sunshine
A Canadian Survivor

Sarah Jane Thornton grew up in a middle class neighbourhood where she encountered sexual abuse from the age of 5 until she was 12 years old. By the time she reached high school, she had turned to alcohol, drugs, and promiscuity to cope. At age 16, she moved to the other side of the country in the hopes of leaving her problems behind. Working in a bar, wearing a bikini, and selling beer, she became preoccupied with body image. She began to systematically eat less and exercise more as the problems she thought she had left behind crept back into her life. She was hospitalized for 2 years after a suicide attempt at age 21, able to gradually get her eating disorder under control with the help of psychotherapy, along with writing a book about her life and her own inner strength. Sara is featured in the film *Through True Eyes: Process of Recovery from Eating Disorders* (Atlantic Mediaworks, 2007). Today, she balances motherhood and academia in New Brunswick, Canada, sharing her experiences and struggles to help others find inspiration in overcoming eating disorders.

Source: Thornton, S. J. (personal communication, October 30, 2008); Thornton, S. J. (2007). *Facing the sunshine: A young woman's emergence from the shadows of sexual abuse and anorexia.* Salem, NH: Soaring Wings.

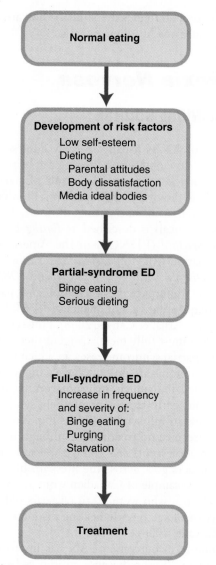

FIGURE 23.1 Continuum of dieting disorders with ED symptoms.

leads to improvement in the disorder and less depressive symptomatology (Castro-Fornieles et al., 2007). Poor outcome has been related to an initial minimum weight, less weight gain, the presence of purging (vomiting and laxative misuse), a later age of onset, substance abuse, the development of mood and anxiety disorders, and other psychological symptoms including depression (Berkman, Lohr, & Bulik, 2007; Steinhausen, Grigoriou-Serbanescu, Boyadjieva, Neumarker, & Metzke, 2008).

■■■ DIAGNOSTIC CRITERIA

The diagnostic criteria for AN have been refined in each edition of the *DSM-IV-TR* (APA, 2000). For example, the amount of weight loss or lack of weight gain required for the diagnosis of AN has changed over time. In the third edition of the *DSM* (APA, 1987), a weight 75% of

that appropriate to age and height is required, whereas in the *DSM-IV-TR* (2000), a weight 85% of the appropriate weight is specified. It is important to note that the *DSM-IV-TR* still requires amenorrhea as a criterion (see Table 23-1), thereby excluding men from the diagnosis of AN. The World Health Organization diagnostic criteria (1993) more inclusively require a widespread endocrine disorder manifest as amenorrhea in women and as a loss of sexual interest and potency in men.

AN is categorized into two major types: (a) restricting and (b) binge–purge. The purging associated with this type of AN occurs when the individual perceives having eaten too much (even if only a normal or small-sized meal or snack was eaten). Many of the clinical features associated with AN result from malnutrition or semistarvation. For example, classic research on volunteers who have been semistarved and observations of prisoners of war and conscientious objectors have demonstrated that these states of starvation are characterized by symptoms of food preoccupation, binge eating, depression, obsession, and apathy. Drastic measures to resist perceived "overeating" persist long after the semistarvation experience, even when food is plentiful. Many somatic systems are compromised in individuals with eating disorders. Table 23-2 presents the medical complications, signs, and symptoms of eating disorders that result from starving or binge eating and purging.

Originally, the central feature of AN was thought to be a distorted **body image** (Bruch, 1973). Body image refers to a mental picture of one's own body. Body image disturbance occurs when there is extreme discrepancy between one's own mental picture of his or her body and the perception of the outside world. For adolescents, body image has a complex psychological impact on overall self-concept and is a crucial factor in determining how adolescents both interact with others and expect society to respond to them. Individuals with AN may have body image distortion in that they may "see" themselves as obese and undesirable, even when emaciated. However, AN is not always associated with **body image distortion** (Andersen & Yager, 2005). Rather, individuals with AN may suffer from *disturbed body experience*, which contributes to body dissatisfaction. They "see that they are thin," but they may cling to slenderness as "protection against a body that they loathe" (Massey-Stokes, 2001, p. 292), and maintaining the image of seeing themselves as overweight justifies subsequent restrictive behaviours.

> **KEY CONCEPT** **Body image distortion** occurs when the individual perceives his or her body disparately from how the world or society views it.

Essential to the diagnosis of AN are self-induced starvation behaviours, relentless *drive for thinness* or a morbid fear of becoming fat, and signs and symptoms resulting from the starvation. Individuals with AN see themselves as

Table 23.1 Key Diagnostic Characteristics for Anorexia Nervosa	DSM IV

Diagnostic Criteria	Target Symptoms and Associated Findings
• Refusal to maintain body weight at or above a minimally normal weight for age and height • Intense fear of gaining weight or becoming fat, even though underweight • Disturbance in the way the person experiences body shape or weight • Undue influence of body weight or shape on self-evaluation or denial of seriousness of current low body weight • Absence of at least three consecutive menstrual cycles (in postmenarcheal females) • Restricting type: not regularly engaged in binge eating or purging behaviour (such as self-induced vomiting or misuse of laxatives, diuretics, or enemas) • Binge eating and purging type: regularly engaging in binge eating or purging behaviour	• Depressive symptoms such as depressed mood, social withdrawal, irritability, insomnia, and diminished interest in sex • Obsessive-compulsive features related and unrelated to food • Preoccupation with thought of food • Concerns about eating in public • Feelings of ineffectiveness • Strong need to control one's environment • Inflexible thinking • Limited social spontaneity and overly restrained initiative and emotional expression *Associated Physical Examination Findings* • Complaints of constipation and abdominal pain • Cold intolerance • Lethargy and excess energy • Emaciation • Significant hypotension, hypothermia, and skin dryness • Bradycardia and possible peripheral edema • Hypertrophy of salivary glands, particularly the parotid gland • Dental enamel erosion related to induced vomiting • Scars or calluses on dorsum of hand from contact with teeth for inducing vomiting *Associated Laboratory Findings* • Leukopenia and mild anemia • Elevated blood urea nitrogen • Hypercholesterolemia • Elevated liver function studies • Electrolyte imbalances, metabolic alkalosis, or metabolic acidosis • Low normal serum thyroxine levels; decreased serum triiodothyronine levels • Low serum estrogen levels • Sinus bradycardia • Metabolic encephalopathy • Significantly reduced resting energy expenditure • Increased ventricular/brain ratio secondary to starvation

fat, fear becoming fatter, and are "driven" to work toward "undoing" this fear. They ignore body signals or cues, such as hunger and weakness, and concentrate all efforts on controlling food intake. Their entire mental focus narrows to only one goal: weight loss. Typical thought patterns are "If I gain a kilo, I'll keep gaining." Such all-or-nothing thinking keeps these individuals on rigid regimens for weight loss. Thus, the behaviour of individuals with AN becomes organized around food-related activities, such as preparing food, counting calories, and reading cookbooks. Much behaviour concerning what, when, and how they eat is ritualistic. Food combinations and the order in which foods may be eaten and under which circumstances the foods can be eaten seem bizarre to healthier people. One individual, for example, would eat only green apples, carrying a green apple with her to all meals outside of her home, and consuming it only if it were cut into smaller than bite-sized pieces (Thornton, 2008, personal communication). Box 23-1 lists the common psychological characteristics.

BOX 23.1

Psychological Characteristics Related to Eating Disorders

Anorexia Nervosa
  Decreased interoceptive
     awareness
  Sexuality conflict/fears
  Maturity fears
  Ritualistic behaviours
  Perfectionism
  Dietary restraint

Bulimia Nervosa
  Impulsivity
  Boundary problems
  Limit-setting difficulties
  Dietary restraint

Binge Eating Disorder
  Negative mood

Self-deprecation
Social insecurity

Anorexia, Bulimia Nervosa, and Binge Eating Disorder
  Difficulty expressing
     anger
  Low self-esteem
  Body dissatisfaction
  Powerlessness
  Ineffectiveness
  Obsessiveness
  Compulsiveness
  Nonassertiveness
  Cognitive distortions

Table 23.2   Complications of Eating Disorders

Body System	Symptoms
From Starvation to Weight Loss	
Musculoskeletal	Loss of muscle mass and loss of fat (emaciation)
	Osteopenia (*bone mineral* deficiency) and less frequently, osteoporosis
Metabolic	Hypothyroidism (symptoms include lack of energy, weakness, intolerance to cold, and bradycardia)
Cardiac	Hypoglycemia and decreased insulin sensitivity
Gastrointestinal	Bradycardia, hypotension, loss of cardiac muscle, small heart, cardiac arrhythmias including atrial and ventricular premature contractions, prolonged QT interval, ventricular tachycardia, and sudden death
Reproductive	Delayed gastric emptying, bloating, constipation, abdominal pain, gas, and diarrhea
	Amenorrhea, low levels of luteinizing hormone and follicle-stimulating hormone, and irregular periods
Dermatologic	Dry, cracking skin and brittle nails due to dehydration, lanugo (fine babylike hair over body), edema, and acrocyanosis (bluish hands and feet); hair thinning
	Leukopenia, anemia, thrombocytopenia, hypercholesterolemia, and hypercarotenemia
Hematologic	Abnormal taste sensation (possible zinc deficiency)
Neuropsychiatric	Neurologic deficits in cognitive processing of new information; decreased total brain volume; increased brain ventricular size
	Apathetic depression, mild organic mental symptoms, sleep disturbances, and fatigue
Related to Purging (Vomiting and Laxative Abuse)	
Metabolic	Electrolyte abnormalities, particularly hypokalemia and hypochloremic alkalosis; hypomagnesemia; increased blood urea nitrogen
Gastrointestinal	Salivary gland and pancreatic inflammation and enlargement with increase in serum amylase; esophageal and gastric erosion (esophagitis); dysfunctional bowel with haustral dilation; superior mesenteric artery syndrome
Dental	Erosion of dental enamel (perimolysis), particularly frontal teeth with decreased decay
Neuropsychiatric	Seizures (related to large fluid shifts and electrolyte disturbances), mild neuropathies, fatigue, weakness, and mild organic mental symptoms
Cardiac	Ipecac cardiomyopathy arrhythmias
Binge Eating to Weight Gain	
Gastrointestinal	Heartburn; abdominal discomfort; bloating; gastric rupture; symptoms of fullness may interrupt sleep
Metabolic	Gall bladder disease; type 2 diabetes
Cardiac	Hypertension and hypercholestremia
Musculoskeletal	Arthritis
Respiratory	Shortness of breath; asthma; sleep apnea; snoring

KEY CONCEPT   Drive for thinness is an intense physical and emotional process that overrides all physiologic body cues.

Because individuals with AN feel inadequate, many fear emotional maturation and the unknown challenges the next developmental stages would bring. For some, remaining physically small is believed to symbolize remaining childlike. Weight loss becomes a way for them to experience some sense of control and to combat feelings of inadequacy and ineffectiveness. Every lost kilogram is viewed as a success, and weight loss often confers a feeling of virtuousness. Perfectionism is an important characteristic (Nilsson, Sundbom, & Hagglof, 2008; Pike et al., 2008).

Individuals with AN may avoid conflict, have difficulty expressing negative emotions, especially anger (Miotto, Pollini, Restaneo, Favaretto, & Preti, 2008), and an overwhelming sense of guilt. In addition, they may have difficulty defining feelings because they are confused about or unsure of emotions and visceral cues, such as hunger; therefore, their responses to cues are inaccurate and inappropriate. Often they cannot name the feelings they are experiencing. This uncertainty and confusion is called a lack of *interoceptive awareness*, and it is thought to be partially responsible for developing and maintaining this disorder and some instances of BN. Because of the ritualistic behaviours, all-encompassing focus on food and weight, and feelings of inadequacy that accompany AN, social contacts are gradually reduced and the person becomes isolated. With more severe weight loss come other symptoms, such as apathy, depression, and even mistrust of others.

> ☘ **KEY CONCEPT Interoceptive awareness** is a term used to describe the sensory response to emotional and visceral cues, such as hunger.

■◗ EPIDEMIOLOGY

Almost one in five Canadian women is concerned about her weight (Park & Beaudet, 2007). Findings from an Ontario study revealed 0.66% of women and 0.16% of men aged 15 to 64 had full-syndrome AN; an additional 1.15% of women and 0.76% of men had partial-syndrome AN (Woodside et al., 2001). The lifetime prevalence of AN is reported to be 0.5% to 1%, with a similar prevalence found in most Western countries. AN appears to be more prevalent within ethnic minorities and in other countries than previously recognized or reported. Cultural change itself may be associated with increased vulnerability to eating disorders, especially when values about physical aesthetics are involved (Lam, Lee, Fung, Ho, & Lee, 2009; Miller & Pumariega, 2001). For example, eating disorder symptommatology has increased among Chinese women exposed to Western views of ideal body types (Lee & Lee, 2000).

Age of Onset

The age of onset is typically between 14 and 16 years. Adolescents are vulnerable because of stressors associated with their development, especially concerns about body image, autonomy, and peer pressure, and their susceptibility to such influences as the media, which extols an ideal body type and discusses dieting and exercise as ways to achieve success, popularity, and power. Unhealthy dieting behaviours are prevalent in Canadian girls as young as 10 years of age (McVey, Tweed, & Blackmore, 2004) and in boys at 13 years (Jonat & Birmingham, 2004).

Gender Differences

In clinical settings, females are 10 times more likely to have AN than males. This disparity has been attributed to society's influence on females to achieve an ideal body type. Box 23-2 highlights some of the findings about eating disorders in males.

Ethnic and Cultural Differences

Contextual variables that may influence eating disorders include level of acculturation, socioeconomic status, peer socialization, family structure, and immigration.

BOX 23.2

Boys and Men With Eating Disorders

Eating disorders have been present in males for as long as in females. Morton described the first case of loss of appetite in the absence of medical disease in an adolescent male (Silverman, 1990). More recently, Health Canada (2003) reported a ratio of male to female cases of approximately 1:5 in a survey of more than 30,000 people conducted in 2001 and 2002. Eating disorders in men and boys are becoming more prevalent.

Woodside (2004, p. 86) questions "Why are fewer affected men identified in formal treatment settings?" He argues that young men may tend to dismiss symptoms or attribute them to other causes (e.g., poor eating habits) because of societal expectations that persons with eating disorders are female. Feminist writer Soran (2006) further asserts that men and boys are apt to suffer in silence and isolation and be insufficiently treated because eating disorders continue to be viewed as "female" problems. However, this picture may change as media messages increasingly target boys and men in emphasizing dieting and encouraging such surgical options as pectoral or calf implants to achieve the ideal male physique (Hatmaker, 2005).

Men are more likely to have a later onset than women, at about age 20.5 years. Boys and men involved in an occupation or a sport in which weight control influences performance, such as wrestling (Braun, Sunday, Huang, & Halmi, 1999) and body building (Goldfield, Blouin, & Woodside, 2006), reported high rates of weight and shape preoccupation, intensive body modification practices, binge eating, and BN. In studies comparing men and women on personality characteristics, men had lower drive for thinness and body dissatisfaction scores (Joiner, Katz, & Heatherton, 2000) and were less at risk for perfectionism, harm avoidance, and reward dependence (Woodside et al., 2004).

In an older investigation, predictors of binge eating were different for men compared with women. Anger and depression preceded binges in men, whereas dieting failure was the most significant predictor of a binge in women (Costanzo, Musante, Friedman, Kern, & Tomlinson, 1999). Men and women did not differ with regard to comorbid conditions, such as depression and substance abuse. In the first study to examine the relationship between childhood sexual abuse and eating disorders in gay and bisexual men, Feldman and Meyer (2007) found that a history of childhood sexual abuse was related to bulimia but not AN. Although prior studies indicate that values and expectations concerning physical appearance in the gay community exert pressure on men to conform, Felman and Meyer suggest that men may engage in disordered eating to cope with histories of sexual abuse.

The influence of ethnic group has been identified as a significant contributing factor in eating disorder development in Canada. Female Canadian Jewish adolescents have reported more eating disordered behaviours and attitudes compared with their non-Jewish counterparts (Pinhas, Heinmaa, Bryden, Bradley, & Toner, 2008). Eating disorders also tend to be more common in young people who have recently immigrated, even when eating disorders are not common in their country of origin (Reijonen, Prat, Patel, & Greydanus, 2003). McDonald and Kennedy (2005) found that immigrants are substantially less likely to be obese or overweight upon arrival to Canada and that excess weight gain with additional years in Canada is influenced by the extent to which immigrants interact with members of their ethnic group residing in the same area. Immigrants of Chinese ethnicity exhibited the lowest rates of being overweight and obese, and this did not increase over time because local Chinese-Canadian communities are sufficiently well established to reduce acculturation lifestyle choices.

Familial Predisposition

First-degree relatives of people with AN have higher rates of this disorder. Rates of partial syndrome cases among female family members of individuals with AN are even higher (Strober, Freeman, Lampert, Diamond, & Kaye, 2000; Woodside, Field, Garfinkel, & Heinmaa, 1998). Female relatives also have high rates of depression, leading researchers to hypothesize that a shared genetic factor may influence the development of both disorders.

Comorbidity

Comorbid major depression and dysthymia are common in AN (Jordan et al., 2008), as are obsessive-compulsive disorder (OCD) and anxiety disorders such as phobias and panic disorder (Swinbourne & Touyz, 2007). Often OCD symptoms predate the AN diagnosis by about 5 years, leading many researchers to consider OCD a causative or risk factor for AN (Anderluk, Tchanturia, Rabe-Hesketh, & Treasure, 2003; Milos, Spindler, Ruggiero, Klaghofer, & Schnyder, 2002). Cluster C personality disorders are also associated (Kaye, Klump, Frank, & Strober, 2000) with AN. Comorbid conditions may resolve when AN has been treated successfully. In other cases, symptoms of a premorbid condition, such as OCD, remain even though an individual has recovered. This finding has influenced many experts to believe that certain characteristics of AN, such as perfectionism and preoccupation with symmetry or specific object placement, are trait, rather than state, characteristics and may actually influence the development of the disorder.

ETIOLOGY

Some of the risk factors and the etiologic factors for eating disorders overlap. For example, dieting is a risk factor for the development of AN, but it is also a biologic etiologic factor, and in its most serious form—starving—it is also a symptom. It is helpful to view the overlap of risk factors, causes, and symptoms along a continuum from less to more severe (see Fig. 23-1). Most experts agree that eating disorders are multidimensional and multidetermined. Figure 23-2 depicts the etiologic factors for AN within their larger spiritual dimension.

Biologic Theories

Most of what is known about the etiology of AN is focused on psychological factors with little conclusive evidence regarding biologic theories of causation. Part of this difficulty stems from the many comorbid conditions, such as depression and OCD, associated with the diagnosis of AN, which some researchers view as having a shared etiology. In addition, many of the biologic changes noted in AN have been determined to be the result of starvation and are considered state, rather than trait or causative, factors. Little evidence exists to substantiate that dysregulations in appetite-satiety systems cause AN, as some have suggested. Appetite dysregulation is best viewed as the end product or result of an interaction between the environment and physiology. The bio/psycho/social/spiritual model of this interaction best explains the etiology (see Fig. 23-2).

Neuropathologic Theories

Magnetic resonance imaging and computed tomography disclose changes in the brain (e.g., cerebral ventricular enlargement, dilation of the third and lateral ventricles, and enlargement of the cortical sulci and the interhemispheric fusion) of individuals with AN who have significant weight loss. This neuropathy and the deficits in white matter reverse with weight gain. Yet, grey matter changes resulting from starvation may not fully return to normal after months of weight restoration (Muhlau et al., 2007). To date, evidence supports that brain structure changes follow rather than cause AN.

Genetic Theories

Genetic research on eating disorders is only beginning. The existence of comorbid conditions makes it difficult to determine the influence of genetics on AN. Separating genetic influences from environmental influences when twins share a similar family environment is difficult, but investigators reviewing data from twin studies have

FIGURE 23.2 Bio/psycho/social/spiritual etiologies for patients with AN and OCD.

demonstrated that the concordance rate for monozygotic twins is higher (44%) than for dizygotic twins (12.5%). Thus, a genetic factor may be involved in the etiology of AN (Bulik, Sullivan, Wade, & Kendler, 2000).

Biochemical Theories

Studies of neuroendocrine, neuropeptide, vasopressin, oxytocin, and neurotransmitter functioning indicate that these systems may be related to maintaining AN. Endogenous opioids may contribute to the eventual denial of hunger in clients with the disorder, and this is supported in some studies reporting weight gain after receiving opiate antagonists. Thyroid function is also decreased. However, these neurotransmitter and neuroendocrine abnormalities, such as blunted serotonergic function in low-weight patients, must be viewed with caution as causative factors because these disturbances are state related and tend to normalize after symptom remission and weight gain (Bailer & Kaye, 2003). In these individuals, effects on central serotonergic function may result from starvation, rather than trigger it (Ward, Tiller, Treasure, & Russell, 2000). Based on the best evidence, these biochemical changes may be viewed as indicating vulnerability in some individuals who under certain psychological and environmental conditions, such as cultural pressures, starve themselves (Klump, Bulik, Kaye, Treasure, & Tyson, 2009).

Psychological Theories

The most widely accepted theory of AN is psychodynamic. In this theory, key tasks of separation-individuation and autonomy are interrupted. Struggles around identity and role, body image formation, and *sexuality fears* predominate. During early adolescence, when individuals begin to establish their independence and autonomy, some girls may feel inadequate or ineffective. Dieting and weight control may be viewed as a means to defend against these feelings. In later adolescence, when separation-individuation is a developmental task, similar conflicts arise when an adolescent is ill prepared for this stage and feels inadequate and ineffective in going forward emotionally. Because AN is usually diagnosed between 14 and 18 years of age, developmental struggles of adolescence have long been an acceptable theory of causation (Bruch, 1973).

Gender identity has been hypothesized to explain the significant difference between the numbers of females and males who experience AN and BN. Studies have shown that girls and boys do not differ dramatically in self-esteem until just before adolescence. At the time self-doubt increases in girls, pubertal weight gain can also occur, resulting in a more rounded, mature female shape. These normal developmental occurrences can add to confusion about identity. Such confusion and self-doubt are further promoted by conflicting messages that girls receive from society about their roles in life. Girls may interpret expectations about how they should look, what roles they should perform, and what they should achieve in society as pressures to achieve "all." They often try to please others to avoid conflicts around perceived expectations. According to Martin (2007), the body becomes the "perfect battleground for perfect-girl tendencies because it is tangible, measurable, obvious. It takes four long years to see 'summa cum laude' etched across our college diplomas, but stepping on a scale can instantly tell us whether we have succeeded or failed" (p. 18). Girls strive for perfection on the scale because they think it is a more attainable goal than being perfect in every other aspect of their lives and they believe it is the one thing they can completely control. High personal standards expressed in an absolute and competitive way (e.g., "I feel I must be the best, or not do anything at all") and expressing more perceived benefits of thinness (e.g., increased popularity) were prominent in 14- to 21-year-old girls with disordered eating (Gustafsson, Edlund, Kjellin, & Norring, 2008). Feminists have focused on this role pressure to partly explain the significant increase in eating disorders and the greater prevalence in females. Box 23-3 outlines some feminist assumptions regarding role, feminism, and eating disorder development.

KEY CONCEPT **Sexuality fears** are often underlying issues for patients with AN. Starvation is viewed as a response to these fears.

AN usually develops during adolescence, when dating begins. Female adolescents usually experience dating as more stressful than males do because intimacy is more important to females and they tend to attribute the failure of a relationship to an inadequacy in themselves (Streigel-Moore, 1993). During the past decade, females have become involved sexually at increasingly younger ages. Although they are often ill prepared, they can experience a great deal of pressure from peers to do so. Female adolescents in early stages of AN express negative attitudes to sexuality and dating (Ruuska, Kaltiala-Heino, Koivisto, & Rantanen, 2003). Bruch (1973) has described self-starvation as the female adolescent's response to her fear of adult sexuality. Sexual anxieties may promote binge eating as well.

Social Theories

The media, the fashion industry, and peer pressure are significant social influences in the development of eating

BOX 23.3
Feminist Ideology and Eating Disorders

Since the 1970s, proponents of the feminist cultural model of eating disorders have advanced a position to explain the higher prevalence of these disorders in women. Feminists believe there is a struggle women have today similar to ones they believe women have had in history. They believe that during the Victorian era, "hysteria," a well-known emotional illness, developed as a result of oppression when women were not allowed to express their feelings and opinions and were "silenced" by a male-dominated society. Feminist scholars claim that women today are socialized to avoid self-expression in the face of conflict, seek attachment through putting others first, judge self by external standards, and present an outward compliant self while the inner self grows angry. They believe that the development of an eating disorder is a reaction against these expectations and norms of society (Gutwill, 1994).

Feminists have taken issue with what they call the biomedical model of explanation for the development of eating disorders, seeing it as limiting and patriarchal. It is the recovery of society that must take place to decrease the prevalence of eating disorders. Feminists believe that this will occur only when women are emancipated, given a voice, and socialized differently. They call for more research in which women are coresearchers as well as "subjects," helping to provide the investigators with their own stories and perspectives.

disorders. Magazines and television shows depict young girls and adolescents, with thin and often emaciated bodies, as glamorous to young women (Ahzern, Bennett, & Hetherington, 2008). Women already practicing dietary restraint were found to eat less after watching slim models on television (Anschutz, Van Strien, & Engels, 2008). Two of the most common adolescent dieting methods—restricting calories and taking diet pills—have been shown to be influenced by women's beauty and fashion magazines (Thomsen, Weber, & Brown, 2002). For younger girls, dolls such as Barbie have been found to negatively influence their views of normal body types (Dittmar, Halliwell, & Ive, 2006) (see Box 23-4).

KEY CONCEPT With **body dissatisfaction**, the body becomes overvalued as a way of determining one's worth. Body dissatisfaction has been related to low self-esteem, depression, dieting, bingeing, and purging.

Comparing one's own body to the bodies of models may produce significant *body dissatisfaction*, a key characteristic associated with dieting, low self-esteem, and development of an eating disorder. Images from television and fashion magazines are particularly powerful for young girls and adolescents struggling with the tasks of identity

BOX 23.4

Research for Best Practice: Does Barbie Make Girls Want to Be Thin?

From Dittmar, H., Halliwell, E., & Ive, S. (2006). Does Barbie make girls want to be thin? The effect of experimental exposure to images of dolls on the body image of 5- to 8- year-old girls. Developmental Psychology, 42, 283–292.

THE PURPOSE: Barbie is the best-selling fashion doll in the world with most 3- to 10-year-olds owning at least one Barbie doll. However, Barbie's body proportions are unrealistic and unattainable (e.g., Barbie's proportions require adult heights of 6'2" [1.88 m] to 7'5" [2.26 m] with a waist 39% smaller than that of individuals with AN). A great deal of research has demonstrated that thin, ideal models of beauty lead to increased body dissatisfaction among adult women. This study was designed to examine the effects of exposure to Barbie doll stimuli for younger girls aged 5–8 years.

METHODS: A story was read aloud while girls looked at images of Barbie dolls, Emme dolls (based on full-figured models), or neutral (control) images. Body image concerns were assessed through an evaluative measure of body esteem and pictorial measures of body shape, from which girls chose figures that represented their actual body shape, the shape they desired to be, and their ideal shape as an adult woman.

FINDINGS: The researchers found that girls exposed to Barbie reported lower body esteem and greater desire for a thinner body shape than girls in the other exposure conditions. However, the Barbie doll effect was age-related in that the detrimental effect was evident already for girls ranging from age 5½–6½ years but was more pronounced among 6½–7½ year-olds. An unanticipated finding was that older girls (over 7 years old) reported a greater desire to be thin when they become adults, after exposure to Emme dolls (compared with neutral control images).

IMPLICATIONS FOR NURSING: This research provides an understanding that early exposure to dolls epitomizing an unrealistically thin body ideal may damage girls' body image, contributing to an increased risk of disordered eating and weight cycling. Our present educational programs tend to target older girls often during adolescence, while the findings from this study demonstrate the need to target younger girls and to emphasize nonappearance-related sources of self-esteem. Nurses can assist parents in choosing appropriate models of dolls for younger children.

---

and body image formation (Andrist, 2003). Body dissatisfaction resulting from perceiving one's own body as falling short of an ideal, may include dissatisfaction about one's weight, shape, size, or even a certain body part. Adolescents, including those not overweight, may act to overcome this dissatisfaction through dieting and overexercising. In those who have other risk factors and are thus more vulnerable, eating disorder symptoms may develop. The perception of oneself as overweight when at acceptable weight for height is not exclusive to adolescents. In analyzing data from the 2000/2001 Canadian Community Health Survey, Gucciardi, Wang, Badiani, and Stewart (2007) found the prevalence of distorted weight perception was 23.6% for women between the ages of 20 and 60 years and 7.8% for men with the probability of distorted perception significantly increased with age.

Family Responses

Early family theories and studies have classically labelled the family of the individual with AN as *enmeshed*, overprotective, rigid, and unable to resolve conflicts. In an enmeshed family, boundaries that define individual autonomy are weak: One member may relay communication from another to a third; excessive togetherness may intrude on privacy (Minuchin, Rossman, & Baker, 1978). In a study of 30 mother and daughter dyads, Ogden and Steward (2000) found high body dissatisfaction and dietary restraint for daughters when both mothers and

daughters believed that boundaries between each other were unclear and that they should live up to each other's expectations.

KEY CONCEPT Enmeshment refers to an extreme form of intensity in family interactions.

Overprotectiveness is defined as a high degree of concern for one another. Parental overprotectiveness may hinder the child's development of autonomy and competence (Minuchin et al., 1978). *Rigidity* refers to families that are heavily committed to maintain the status quo and that find change difficult. Conflict is avoided, and a strong moral code or religious orientation is usually the rationale. Family focus on appearance has an influence on young women, particularly those who are easily made anxious (Davis, Shister, Blackmore, & Fox, 2004). Once an eating disorder has developed, the intrinsic characteristics of the disorder itself mitigate the effect of family concern (Senra, Sanchez-Cao, Seoane, & Leung, 2008).

Spiritual Theories

Core struggles in eating disorders are spiritual in nature. Spirituality involves developing a sense of life meaning and purpose that includes experiences such as compassion, loving, accepting love, being able to feel hope, receiving inspiration, feeling enlightened, personal fulfillment, and being honest and congruent (Berrett, Hardman, O'Grady, & Scott Richards, 2007; Pilch, 1988). A 23-year-old former client described, to Richards, Smith, Berrett, O'Grady, and Bartz (2007), feeling "unlovable. I could not give love, for I was incapable. I lost my self-respect and went against all I believed to be true. It was a downward spiral that almost led to my death" (p. 174). Indeed, individuals tend to lose the ability to affirm their self-worth and identity, defining themselves as the eating disorder and feeling distant and disconnected from family and friends (Weaver et al., 2005). Consideration of these spiritual constructs prevents the reduction of the eating disorder to a constellation of disease symptoms.

Historically, eating disorder psychopathology has been postulated among 14th century fasting saints (Bell, 1985). For example, Catherine of Sienna (1347–1380) who fasted as part of extreme asceticism demonstrated profound preoccupation with eating and drinking that seems not unlike modern individuals with restricting AN (Reda & Sacco, 2001). Eating practices continue to be associated with strong memories and emotions, in particular guilt, shame, well-being and self-worth, and with religious expression (Dell & Josephson, 2007; Marsden, Karagianni, & Morgan, 2007). Garrett (1996) has interpreted AN as attempting to transform oneself through self-control and isolation into a more worthy person to society, and recovery as reconnecting with self, others and nature after having been strengthened through suffering.

In sum, these findings indicate no one predominant etiologic factor for AN. Rather, biopsychosocial and spiritual factors converge to contribute to its development.

■ RISK FACTORS

Risk factors for developing eating disorders are well known. Similar factors put in individuals at risk for AN, BN, and BED. Risk factors are classified in the same way as the etiologic categories: biologic, psychological, social, and spiritual (Fig. 23-3).

Biologic

Biological risk factors include dieting, altered metabolic rate, and a history of overweight or obesity. Dieting despite weight loss and an increase in basal metabolic rate are the most studied biologic risk factors. Individuals diet because of body dissatisfaction, a need for control, an actual weight gain, and the fear of weight gain. Girls at risk for developing AN may begin to diet in response to a prepubertal weight increase. For individuals at risk for BN, dietary restraint leads to binge eating, purging ensues because of fear of becoming fat, and further dieting occurs in response to the binge eating and its associated negative affect. Those who develop obesity may have a history of

"yo-yo" dieting also known as weight cycling, which has impaired their metabolic response (the amount of calories burned daily) so that over time their dieting efforts become ineffective as the cycle of gaining weight back and attempting to lose the weight recurs (Grubbs, 1993).

High-level exercise and compulsive physical activity can precipitate and maintain such eating disorder symptoms as obsession with food, poor concentration, and binge eating (Davis et al., 1997). A personal history of overweight or obesity was reported by women recovering from AN (Weaver et al., 2005) and individuals with BED (Streigel-Moore et al., 2007).

Psychological

Results of numerous studies have shown that low self-esteem, body dissatisfaction, and feelings of ineffectiveness also put individuals at risk for an eating disorder. Women with AN specifically reported lower self-esteem (Vince & Walker, 2008) and significantly higher rates of negative affectivity, perfectionism and family discord, and higher parental demands than women with other psychiatric disorders (Pike et al., 2008). The role of weight and shape concerns was most salient in the year preceding the onset of AN. Recent research on these factors has demonstrated that resilience or protective factors, such as academic achievement and positive self-esteem, can mediate these risk factors and prevent development of an eating disorder (Croll, Neumark-Sztainer, Story, & Ireland, 2002).

Women with AN may go on to experience binge eating and purging (White, 2000). This relationship has been explained as incomplete recovery that eventually turns into purging when restricting food intake is no longer effective. Factors found to influence crossover from AN to BN include low self-directedness and perceived parental criticism (Tozzi et al., 2005).

Childhood sexual abuse has been suggested as a risk factor for eating disorders. Gay and bisexual men with a history of childhood sexual abuse were found more likely to experience eating disorders compared with men who do not have a history of sexual abuse (Feldman & Meyer, 2007). Increasingly, researchers report childhood sexual abuse as a risk factor for the development of full and partial BN not necessarily mediated by dietary restriction (Leonard, Steiger, & Kao, 2003; Sanci et al., 2008). As well, middle school girls who were teased about their appearance or overweight by older siblings demonstrated significantly higher levels of body dissatisfaction, thin idealization, dietary restriction, bulimic behaviours and depression, and lower levels of self-esteem than girls who were not teased (Keery, Boutelle, van den Berg, & Thompson, 2005). In comparing the rates and parameters of abuse in women with AN and borderline personality disorder (BPD), Laporte and Guttman (2001) found that women with AN experienced less multiple abuse at an

FIGURE 23.3 Bio/psycho/social/spiritual risk factors for eating disorders.

older age than those with personality disorder. Nonetheless, sexual or physical abuse occurred in one fifth and verbal abuse in one third of the women with AN of the latter study and sexual abuse alone in 6% of the former study. Therefore, inquiring about history of sexual, physical, and verbal victimization in assessing a person with an eating disorder is necessary to identify deleterious effects that can be addressed in the treatment.

Researchers have found a relationship between stress and binge eating (Harrington, Crowther, Henrickson, & Mickelson, 2006; Johnson & Wardle, 2005). Women with BN report a higher incidence of stressful life events than women with other eating disorders (Vince & Walker, 2008), and the recent findings of Streigel-Moore et al. (2007) suggest that elevated levels of perceived stress prior to the age of 14 may precede the onset of BEDs.

Sociocultural

The media, the fashion industry, and the society's focus on the ideal body type are social risk factors for eating disorders. In addition, peer pressure and attitudes influence eating behaviours. Some adolescents have reported that dieting, binge eating, and purging were learned behaviours, resulting from peer pressure and a need to conform. Through meta-analysis of 232 studies, Vince and Walker (2008) found a strong association between disordered eating and being teased about weight and shape by family and friends. Specifically, Binford, Mussell, Peterson, Crow, and Mitchell (2004) found those with early onset BED reported a higher frequency of being teased about their weight.

Individuals with eating disorders are more likely to perceive their families as having excessive appearance and achievement concerns and to be more critical of the family's functioning than their parents (Vandereyken, 2002). Parental attitudes about weight have been found to influence body dissatisfaction and dieting; parental comments about weight or shape, or even parents' worrying about their own weight, can influence adolescents in much the same way as the media does (Smolak, Levine, & Schermer, 1999). May, Kim, McHale, and Crouter (2006) found that daughters' weight concerns increased from age 11 to 16 and then declined, whereas sons' concerns declined beginning at age 11. Increases in daughters' weight concerns were linked to increases in conflict with mothers and fathers and decreases in maternal intimacy and knowledge. Declines in sons' weight concerns were associated with decline in conflict with fathers.

In other studies, low levels of paternal affection, communication, and time spent with daughters and sons during their childhood were associated with high rates of eating and weight problems and eating disorders during their adolescence or early adulthood (Dallos & Denford, 2008; Johnson, Cohen, Kasen, & Brook, 2002). A childhood history of family discord and high parental demands are considered risk factors for BED (Striegel-Moore et al., 2007).

Athletes are at greater risk for developing eating disorders because lower body weights give a definite competitive advantage. The actual performance demands of a sport and the sports environment itself can intensify body and weight related concerns because of such factors as pressure from coaches and parents, social comparisons with teammates, team weigh-ins, physique-revealing uniforms, and judging criteria (Greenleaf, Petrie, Carter, & Reel, 2009). Elite athletes training for national and international competition and those competing in leanness (versus non-leanness) sports are particularly at risk (Greenleaf et al.; Hagmar, Hirschberg, Berglund, & Berglund, 2008). Excessive exercise and perfectionism are thought to precipitate symptoms (Davis, Katzman, &

Kirsch, 1999). Ballet dancers are at high risk because of the need to maintain a particular appearance; male as well as female athletes are at risk for developing eating disorders (see Box 23-5). In particular, boys and men involved in sports that necessitate weight restrictions such as wrestling, body building, rowing, ski jumping, and swimming are at risk (Hatmaker, 2005).

Spiritual

Eating in response to emotional cues such as boredom, loneliness, and anxiety—rather than hunger—may arise from unmet basic needs, including the need for belongingness and self-esteem. Such emotional eating is considered a risk factor in eating disorders. Indeed lower levels of spiritual well-being correlated with higher levels of emotional eating among female college students (Hawks, Goudy, & Gast, 2003).

■ INTERDISCIPLINARY TREATMENT

Treatment of the patient with AN focuses on initiating nutritional rehabilitation, resolving conflicts around body image disturbance, increasing effective coping, addressing

---

BOX 23.5

Research for Best Practice: Females and Athletics

From Buchholz, A., Mack, H., McVey, G., Feder, S., & Barrowman, N. (2008). BodySense: An evaluation of a positive body image intervention on sport climate for female athletes. Eating Disorders, 16, 308–321.

THE QUESTION: Many investigations have highlighted that young female athletes in competitive sports settings are more at risk for eating disorders. Indeed, there is a growing body of research on the female athlete triad (amenorrhea, osteoporosis, and disordered eating), especially because of the dramatic increase in women participating in organized sports during the past 30 years. This triad is caused by an imbalance between energy intake and expenditure, and is associated with health complications. The goal of this study was to evaluate the effectiveness of an interdisciplinary prevention program to reduce pressures to be thin in sport and promote positive body image and eating behaviours.

METHODS: Participants were competitive female gymnasts (aged 11–18 years), parents and coaches from seven Ontario gymnastic clubs randomly selected into intervention or control groups. The intervention program "BodySense" provided education in areas such as eating attitudes and beliefs, unique body size, resisting pressures to diet, assertiveness, and stress management. Measures of perceived pressure to be thin, self-efficacy over dieting pressures, awareness and internalization of societal pressure to be thin,

body esteem, and eating attitudes and behaviours were completed pre and post intervention.

FINDINGS: Coaches, parents, and athletes perceived significant pressure to be thin in the sport environment. Participation in the BodySense program resulted in athletes perceiving a reduction in pressure, from their sports clubs, to be thin although no changes were found in body esteem, eating attitudes and behaviours, self-efficacy over dieting pressures, or awareness and internalization of sociocultural attitudes toward appearance. More than half of the athletes and coaches reported that having a lower body weight was helpful toward athletic success, and approximately one third of both athletes and coaches acknowledged normal female pubescent development as a disadvantage to gymnasts. Parental measures were analyzed for mothers, as very few fathers completed questionnaires at both time intervals.

IMPLICATIONS FOR NURSING: Assessing high-risk groups such as young female athletes for environmental pressures that contribute to the development of eating disorders is important in working in the community and for school health nurses. Because the findings suggest that symptoms of the female athlete triad may be normalized and thus ignored by athletes and coaches alike, involvement of parents, judges, and sports administrators and associations is essential to prevention efforts to modify the sport climate messages perceived by athletes.

Table 23.3	Criteria for Hospitalization of Patients With Eating Disorders
Medical	**Psychiatric**
• Weight loss <75% below ideal • Heart rate for adults and adolescents <40 beats/min; children <20 beats/min • Temperature, <36°C • Blood pressure <90/60 mm Hg; children, <80/50 mm Hg • Glucose <60 mg/dL • Serum potassium <3 mEq/L • Severe dehydration • Electrolyte imbalance	• Risk for suicide • Severe depression • Failure to comply with treatment • Inadequate response to treatment at another level of care (outpatient)

Adapted from American Psychiatric Association (APA). (2006a). *Practice guideline for the treatment of patients with eating disorders* (3rd ed.). Washington, DC: Author. Available at the American Psychiatric Association Web site.

the underlying conflicts related to maturity fears and role conflict, and assisting the family with healthy functioning and communication. Several methods are used to accomplish these goals, and when selecting the type of treatment (i.e., inpatient, day hospitalization, or outpatient), clinicians use both standardized criteria and personal clinical judgment (Schwartz, Mansbach, Marion, Katzman, & Forman, 2008). The criteria for hospital admission are outlined in Table 23-3. Typically, the medical complications presented in Table 23-2 and suicidality influence the decision to hospitalize an individual with an eating disorder.

In most instances, to restore weight an individual with AN may be admitted to a specialized eating disorder unit or program, or to a general psychiatric medical or pediatric unit. All members of the team participate in a weight-gain protocol. Dietitians plan this weight-increasing program; physicians, nurses, psychologists, and social workers monitor the refeeding process and its effects and establish the intensive therapies that must be instituted after the refeeding phase. Individuals with AN are often intelligent, engaging, and (with the exception of their emaciated state) appear nonimpaired. Thus, they may be erroneously perceived as less sick (Wolfe & Gimby, 2003). It is therefore important to remember the high rates of mortality and medical complications among individuals with eating disorders. If their somatic systems are seriously compromised, a medical unit might be the choice for the initial intensive refeeding phase. These individuals must be monitored closely because at the time of admission they are severely malnourished (see Table 23-2).

The intensive therapies needed to help patients with their underlying issues (e.g., body dissatisfaction and low self-esteem) and families with communication usually begin after refeeding because concentration is usually

impaired in the severely undernourished individual with anorexia. During this phase of treatment, a privilege-earning program is often implemented in which privileges, such as having visitors and receiving passes to go outside the hospital, are earned based on weight gain. After an acceptable weight (at least 85% of ideal) is established, the patient may be discharged to a partial hospitalization program or an intensive outpatient program. Art therapy and psychodrama have been demonstrated to be more effective than traditional group therapy for adolescents with eating disorders, especially during the acute phases, when the concentration required for verbal therapy may be impaired (Diamond-Raab & Orrell-Valente, 2002). Family therapy typically begins while the individual is still hospitalized.

■ PHARMACOLOGIC INTERVENTIONS

Many experts claim that the symptoms of AN, such as body distortion and hyperkinesis, are primarily the result of starvation, which causes changes in brain chemistry. Thus, restoring weight influences symptom remission more than psychopharmacology. In fact, it is generally held that the core symptoms of AN are refractory to psychotropic medications; however, these medications are useful in treating comorbid psychiatric conditions and preventing relapses (Rossi et al., 2007). The use of tricyclic antidepressants is discouraged, as this may increase susceptibility to hypotension and cardiac arrhythmias (Kaplan & Noble, 2007). Research has demonstrated that selective serotonin reuptake inhibitors (SSRIs) are not effective for individuals who are in the acute phase of AN (Strober, Pataki, Freeman, & DeAntonio, 1999), possibly because their low body weights cause low protein stores, and protein is needed for SSRI metabolism. However, some clinical experts have found that the SSRIs can be effective later, during outpatient treatment and after weight restoration. Symptoms such as obsessiveness, ritualistic behaviours, and perfectionism can remit with these medications. SSRIs must be used with caution, and the client's weight must be constantly monitored because, during the initiation phase, some of the SSRIs may cause weight loss. Butroprion is contraindicated because of increased risk of seizures (Kaplan & Noble). Recently, olanzapine has been used for severe AN, resulting in weight gain, less resistance to treatment, and reduced agitation (Jensen & Mejlhede, 2000; LaVia, Grey, & Kaye, 2000). The use of this drug and others in this category is currently being investigated in ongoing randomized control trials.

There is no evidence to support the efficacy of mood stabilizers (e.g., lithium) for treating AN, and these medications must be used only with extreme caution in clients with dehydration and compromised renal function (Kaplan & Noble, 2007). Investigation of prokinetic agents to alleviate GI complaints associated with refeeding (e.g., bloating, early satiety) resulted in removal of Prepulside (cisipride) from the market because of potentially fatal cardiac effects (Meyer et al., 2003). Estrogen replacement therapy in the form of oral contraceptive pills has not been found effective in preventing osteopenia/osteoporosis in AN (American Psychiatric Association, 2006a, 2006b). Many clinicians believe using hormone replacement provides false reassurance to those with AN. Given the concerns with pharmacological interventions, Rossi and colleagues (2007) recommend the careful assessment of medical complications of starvation which may impede catabolism and excretion of various agents and the use of such agents only within the context of client support based on nutritional and psychotherapeutic approaches.

■ PRIORITY CARE ISSUES

Mortality with AN is estimated at approximately 10% occurring within 7 to 10 years of diagnosis (Birmingham et al., 2005; Sullivan, 2002). Death may occur due to suicide, infection, or effects of starvation including cardiac arrhythmias. Some studies report mortality rates for women with AN aged 15 to 24 years as 12 times higher than the mortality rates from all other causes for age-matched community-comparison groups of women and as two times higher than for other female psychiatric populations (Eckert, Halmi, Marchi, Grove, & Crosby, 1995; Sullivan, 1995). Factors that correlate with death are illness of long duration, bingeing and purging, and comorbid illnesses (Herzog et al., 2000). Substance abuse, particularly severe alcohol use, predicts mortality (Keel, Dorer, Eddy, Charatan, & Herzog, 2003; Korndorfer et al., 2003).

Another issue to consider with this population is stigma. Many young girls with AN are avoided, especially in their emaciated state. Research shows that peers do not know how to approach those with AN who appear both frightening and fragile (Gowers & Shore, 1999), and that men expressed strong uncomfortable feelings about dating a woman with an eating disorder (Sobol & Bursztyn, 1998). A university study found prejudice and discrimination as evidenced by greater reported discomfort interacting on a personal basis with persons with AN compared to those with depression and mononucleosis (Stewart, Schiavo, Herzog, & Franko, 2008). Stigma toward those with AN may impede seeking treatment.

■ NURSING MANAGEMENT: HUMAN RESPONSE TO ANOREXIA NERVOSA DISORDER

Establishing a therapeutic relationship with individuals with AN may be difficult initially because they may be suspicious and mistrustful. They often express

---

BOX 23.6

Therapeutic Dialogue: The Client With an Eating Disorder

INEFFECTIVE APPROACH

Nurse: You haven't eaten your lunch yet.

Client: I can't. I'm already fat.

Nurse: Look at you, you're skin and bones.

Client: I'll eat when I go out this afternoon on pass.

Nurse: You can't go on pass. You have to start realizing that you are sick. Because you can't take care of yourself, we are in charge.

Client: You're trying to control me.

Nurse: We are trying to be responsible.

Client: I won't eat!

Nurse: We have set up punishments for not eating.

Client: Then I won't go out! At least I won't get fatter.

EFFECTIVE APPROACH

Nurse: You haven't eaten your lunch.

Client: I can't. I'm already fat.

Nurse: You're uncomfortable with how you see yourself and with eating?

Client: I'll eat when I go out on pass.

Nurse: You and I, and the other members of your treatment team wrote your behavioural plan together. You know then that you will not be able to go out because your pass is dependent on eating both breakfast and lunch.

Client: You're trying to control me.

Nurse: The plan is to help you learn to take control over the eating disorder. It sure does mean a lot of hard work for you. How can I help you now with this meal?

Client: What if I eat half?

Nurse: No, you must eat all of it. Why don't I sit here while you eat? Eating is scary for you. We can talk about other choices you have on the unit; tonight, you can choose the movie or board games.

Client: Okay, at least I have some choices.

CRITICAL THINKING CHALLENGE

- What effect did the first interaction have on the client's behaviour? Why?
- In the second interaction, what theories and interventions regarding eating disorders did the nurse use in her approach to the client?

fear of adults, especially health care professionals, whom they believe want to "make them fat." By the time they are hospitalized, mistrust can almost reach a state of paranoia. Because of their low body weight and starvation, they are often impatient and irritable. A firm, accepting, and patient approach is important. Providing a rationale for all interventions helps build trust, as does a consistently nonreactive approach. Power struggles over eating are common, and remaining nonreactive is a challenge. In avoiding such power struggles, the nurse should monitor his or her own feelings of frustration and need for control (see Box 23-6).

Nursing management involves bio/psycho/social/spiritual assessment and interventions (see Nursing Care Plan 23-1).

Biologic Domain

Assessment

A thorough evaluation of the client's body systems is important because many systems can be compromised by starvation. A careful history from both the individual with AN and the family, including the length and duration of symptoms, such as avoiding meals and

---

Nursing Care Plan 23.1

Nursing Care Plan for a Patient With AN

JS is a 16-year-old female adolescent who appears much younger. She is 165 cm (5'5") tall and weighs 42 kg (92 pounds). She has been treated unsuccessfully in an outpatient clinic and now is being admitted to stabilize her weight. She does not believe that she is too thin and resents being hospitalized. Her hospitalization was precipitated by being asked to leave the gymnastics team because of her low body weight.

Setting: Inpatient Psychiatric Unit

Baseline Assessment: JS appears frail, pale, and dressed in oversized clothes. She is tearful, and states that she is depressed and angry and that she has no friends, adding "Why would anyone want to bother with a nothing like me? I am everyone's worst nightmare!" Physical examination results include bradycardia with pulse = 48, hypotension (88/58), constipation, amenorrhea, dry skin patches, cold intolerance, BMI = 15.3, dehydration, and temperature elevation, 99°F. Laboratory results include hypokalemia (K⁺ = 3.5), leukopenia (WBCs < 5,000), elevated BUN, abnormal thyroid functioning, and bone density of one standard deviation below mean age-adjusted scores.

Associated Psychiatric Diagnosis	Medications

Axis I: Anorexia nervosa
        Binge-eating/purging type
Axis II: None
Axis III: None
Axis IV: Social support (social withdrawal)
        GAF = Current 55
        Potential 75
	Fluoxetine (Prozac), 20 mg in AM

Nursing Diagnosis 1: Spiritual Distress Related to Loss of Relationship With Self and Others

Defining Characteristics	Related Factors
Questions or expresses inner conflict about the meaning or purpose of her illness, her life, or life in general Expresses or evidences guilt, injustice, hopelessness, despair, and/or abandonment. Withdrawal from, or loss of, relationships Refers to self as "bad," "sinful," or "unlovable"	"Why would anyone want to bother with a nothing like me?" Tearful, feels depressed and angry. Says she has no friends I am everyone's worst nightmare!"

Continued

Nursing Care Plan 23.1 *(Continued)*

Nursing Diagnosis 2: Imbalanced Nutrition: Less Than Body Requirements

Defining Characteristics	Related Factors
Unable to increase food intake Weight more than 20% below ideal weight	Believes she cannot eat most foods Purges by vomiting "occasionally" Exercises 3–4 hours daily Sleep pattern disturbed by exercise

Outcomes

Initial	Long-term
Maintains daily intake of 1,500 cal Eliminates exercising while in hospital Ceases purging for 1 week	Gains 0.5–1.5 kg (1–3 pounds) per week until weight is at least 85% of ideal weight. Develops strategies to maintain weight.

Interventions

Interventions	Rationale	Ongoing Assessment
Encourage JS to verbalize feelings such as anxiety related to food and weight gain—develop a therapeutic relationship.	Through a relationship and examining her feelings, she may be more likely to cooperate with nutritional regimen.	Determine anxiety level when discussing food and weight gain.
Monitor meals and snacks, record the amount eaten.	Severe anorexia is life threatening. Aggressive interventions are needed to ensure adequate intake.	Assess JS's ability to complete meals on time and without supplements.
Do not substitute other foods for food on meal trays. Limit caffeine intake to one cup coffee or soda daily.	People with anorexia usually "play games" with food. By prohibiting substitution, a more positive approach is encouraged. Caffeine is an appetite suppressant and has a diuretic effect.	Support JS in following her nutritional regimen.
Monitor JS' behaviour 1 hour after meals for purging. Weigh her daily in hospital gown after she has voided. Monitor vital signs daily, electrolytes. Provide psychoeducational intervention. Teach risks of osteopenia and role of fat-soluble vitamins.	Physical signs of impending complications include evidence of purging, decreasing body weight, hypotension, hyperthermia, and hypokalemia. Increase awareness.	Monitor vital signs, weight, and electrolytes, especially potassium. Observe comprehension of material. Repeat teaching after refeeding if concentration was initially impaired.

Evaluation

Outcomes	Revised Outcomes	Interventions
JS gains 2 kg (5 pounds) at the end of 1½ weeks. Has been cooperative with meal regimen. She has begun to acknowledge the seriousness of her illness and the life-threatening aspects of severe dieting and purging.	Ceases binge–purge episodes for 1 week. Continues to increase her weight 0.5–1.5 kg/week (1–3 pounds/week). Establish and maintain regular, adequate nutritional eating habits.	Daily weights while on unsupervised meals. Praise her for her successes. Arrange for discharge to outpatient clinic or day hospital program. Participation in relapse-prevention classes.

Nursing Diagnosis 3: Disturbed Body Image/Body Experience

Defining Characteristics	Related Factors
Verbalizes that she is too fat Perceives herself as unattractive Hides body in large, baggy clothing	Inaccurate perceptions of physical appearance secondary to anorexia nervosa Believes that "one can never be too rich or too thin" Equates physical fitness and attractiveness with thinness

Continued

Nursing Care Plan 23.1 (Continued)

Outcomes

Initial	Long-term
Verbalizes feelings related to changing body shape and weight Identifies beliefs about controlling body size	Acknowledges negative consequences of too little fat on body Identifies positive aspects of her body and its ability to function

Interventions

Interventions	Rationale	Ongoing Assessment
Explore JS's beliefs and feelings about body. Maintain a nonjudgmental approach.	To help JS gain a more positive body image, an understanding of her own views is important.	Monitor for statements that identify perceptions of her body. Is her view *distorted* or *dissatisfied*?
Assist JS in identifying positive physical characteristics.	In anorexia, the body is viewed negatively. By focusing on parts of the body that are positive, such as eyes or hands, JS can begin to experience a positive image of her body.	Observe for her reaction to her body. Which areas are viewed positively? Observe for negative statements related to body size and self-esteem.
Clarify JS's views about an ideal body.	Many societal cues idealize an unrealistically thin female body.	Monitor for statements indicating external pressures to lose weight, experiences of teasing about body changes, or evidence of sexual abuse from others.
Provide education related to normal growth of women's bodies and the protective role of fat.	Providing education will help in reinforcing a broader view of the importance of a healthy body.	Assess willingness to learn information

Evaluation

Outcomes	Revised Outcomes	Interventions
JS revealed that she believes that she is too fat but does have positive physical traits—her eyes. She believes that those who are overweight have lost control of their lives. She knows some models who are 6′ and weigh barely 45 kg (100 pounds).	JS accepts alternative beliefs related to her own body.	Gradually, focus on other positive physical aspects of JS's body. Discuss grooming that encourages a more attractive look. Challenge her beliefs about body weights of models.
Willing to read information about normal body functioning.	JS accepts a new view of body functioning as a complex phenomenon.	Discuss the biologic aspect of the development of body weight. Emphasize multiple factors that determine body weight.

Outcomes

Initial	Long-term
Begins to expresses inner distress in acceptable ways (e.g., talking, journaling art work)	Spiritual Health as evidenced by: Using a type of spiritual experience/expression that provides her comfort Connecting with others to share thoughts, feelings, and beliefs

Interventions

Interventions	Rationale	Ongoing Assessment
Model self-awareness and acceptance without harsh self-judgment.	JS will not trust a nurse who does not demonstrate self-comfort.	Ask: How do you feel about the changes in your life that have come about because of the eating disorder?

Continued

Nursing Care Plan 23.1 (Continued)

Interventions

Interventions	Rationale	Ongoing Assessment
Create an accepting, nonjudgmental atmosphere. Spend nontask time with JS.	Establishes rapport and the therapeutic relationship, which promotes communication and open expression. Being with the person who is suffering gives meaning to his or her experience.	Assess her ability to see and affirm her self-worth and identity. Does she define herself as the eating disorder? Is she feeling distant and disconnected from family and friends? Does she know what she does and does not have control over? Does she accept her human limitations within the context of any traumatic experiences?
Be open to and encourage JS to experience and verbalize feelings, perceptions, and fears	Helps her access potential healing resources to well-being. Releasing emotions can provide energy and freedom.	
Encourage her to identify values that guide her everyday behaviour and her actions in times of crisis, loss, and tragedy.	Helps her clarify values and beliefs by reflecting on past behaviours. Experience is a major source for values development.	
Observe and listen empathetically to her communication.	Listening to the "unacceptable" helps the process of finding meaning, healing, growth, and reentering life with a renewed sense of purpose and connection to others and self.	
Help JS tell her story about the eating disorder and any painful traumatic experiences in descriptive rather than evaluative terms.	Storytelling minimizes self-judgment and allows emergence of patterns that aid understanding.	
Help JS develop a healthy, positive outlook through such things as letter writing, meditation, and/or imagery.	Helps her access potential healing resources to enhance well-being and reduce negative affectivity.	
Offer patience, repetition, and reassurance over an extended period of time.	Consistency and ongoing support can help her reconnect with herself and others.	

Evaluation

Outcomes	Revised Outcomes	Interventions
She has begun to acknowledge the meaning of the eating disorder in her life and the life-threatening aspects of severe dieting and purging.	Establish and maintain appropriate self-care strategies that include adequate nutrition and eating practices, and self-development.	Participation in comprehensive and individualized treatment program.

overexercising, is necessary to assess altered nutrition. The longer the duration of these behaviours typically means more difficult and prolonged recovery periods.

· CRNENOTE

Eating disorders are serious psychiatric disorders that threaten life. Careful assessment and referral for treatment are important nursing interventions.

The individual's body mass index (BMI) is calculated by dividing weight in kilograms squared by height in meters. BMI is thought to reflect weight more accurately than weight alone. A healthy BMI is between about 19 and 25. Currently, criteria for discharge require patients to be at least 85% of ideal weight according to height and weight tables or to have a BMI of approximately 17.

Nursing Diagnoses for Biologic Domain

A primary nursing diagnosis is Imbalanced Nutrition: Less Than Body Requirements.

Interventions for Biologic Domain

Refeeding is the chief intervention during the hospital or initial stage of treatment (Fig. 23-4). The nurse will encounter resistance to weight gain and refusal to eat and must monitor and record all intake carefully as part

Spiritual

1. Model self awareness and acceptance
2. Suspend negative judgment
3. Encourage description of eating disorder experiences
4. Encourage expression of life history
5. Activities to promote reflection and awareness
6. Peer debriefing of countertransference experiences

Biologic

1. Assess and monitor somatic symptoms
2. Weigh daily
3. Record all intake
4. Supervise bathroom if purging
5. Establish normal sleep routine
6. Administer medication for depression
7. Monitor exercise

Social

1. Be supportive but firm with family
2. Include family in therapies and teaching
3. Suggest resources for information and support
4. Assist teachers with discharge plans and re-entry into classroom

Psychological

1. Establish trust
2. Use diary self-monitoring to help identify emotions
3. Correct cognitive distortions
4. Encourage movement–dance therapies
5. Assist with realistic goal setting
6. Provide education to clarify misconceptions

FIGURE 23.4 Bio/psycho/social/spiritual interventions for individuals with AN.

of the weight gain protocol. The refeeding protocol typically starts with 1,500 cal per day and is increased slowly until about 3,500 cal per day is consumed in several meals. The usual plan for individuals with very low weights is a weight gain of between 0.5 and 1.0 kg (1 and 2 pounds) a week.

Weight-increasing protocols usually take the form of a behavioural plan, using positive reinforcements (i.e., outings or passes) and negative reinforcements (i.e., returning to bed rest) to encourage weight gain. The reinforcements are incremental and based on progress. For example, phone calls, walks around the unit, and walks outside the hospital occur before the day passes and before the weekend passes. These protocols provide ready-made, consistent responses to food-refusal behaviours, and should be carried out in a caring and supportive context. When all staff members agree on a clear protocol for behaviours related to eating and weight gain, reactivity of the staff to the individual with AN is greatly reduced. During the implementation of negative reinforcements, the individual must be helped to see that these actions are not punitive. On rare occasions when the individual is unable to recognize or accept the eating disorder as harmful, nasogastric tube feedings may be necessary.

Menses history also must be assessed. Most individuals with AN have reached menarche but have experienced amenorrhea for some months because of starvation. A return to regular menses signifies substantial body

fat restoration. Sleep disturbance is also common, and these individuals are viewed as hyperkinetic. They sleep little, but usually awaken in an energized state. A structured, healthy sleep routine must be established immediately to conserve energy and calorie expenditure. To further conserve energy, individuals are often relegated to bed rest until a certain amount of weight is regained. Exercise is generally not permitted during refeeding and only with caution, after this phase. Inpatients must be closely supervised because they are often found exercising in their rooms, running in places, and doing calisthenics.

Psychological Domain

Assessment

The psychological symptoms that individuals with anorexia experience are listed in Box 23-1. The classic symptoms—fear of weight gain, unrealistic expectations and thinking, and ritualistic behaviours—are easily noted during a clinical interview. Conflicts, such as sexuality fears and feelings of ineffectiveness, often underlie this disorder but may not be apparent during the interview. However, a variety of instruments are available to clinicians and researchers for determining the presence and severity of symptoms. Box 23-7 lists well-known instruments used to assess psychological symptoms associated with eating disorders. The Eating Attitude Test

BOX 23.7

Assessment Instruments

1. Tests for Disordered Eating (Symptoms)

Compulsive Eating Scale
Dunn, P. K., & Ondercin, P. (1981). Personality variables related to compulsive eating in college women. *Journal of Clinical Psychology, 31*, 43–49.

Eating Attitude Tests
Garner, D. M., & Garfinkel, P. E. (1979). The Eating Attitude Test: An index of the symptoms of anorexia nervosa. *Psychological Medicine, 9*, 273–279.
Garner, D. M., Olmsted, M. P., Bohr, Y., & Garfinkel, P. E. (1982). The Eating Attitude Test: Psychometric features and clinical correlates. *Psychological Medicine, 12*, 871–878.

Children's Eating Attitude Test (CHEAT)
Maloney, M., McGuire, J., & Daniels, S. R. (1988). Reliability testing of a children's version of the Eating Attitude Test. *Journal of the American Academy of Child and Adolescent Psychiatry, 27*, 541–543.

Eating Disorder Examination-Questionnaire (EDE-Q)
Carolyn Black, Rutgers University Eating Disorders Clinic, 41C Gordon Road, Piscataway, NJ 08854

Eating Disorder Inventory-2 (EDI-2) and EDI-2 Symptom Checklist (EDI-2-SC)
Garner, D. M. (1991a). *Eating disorder inventory—2 professional manual*. Odessa, FL: Psychological Assessment Resources.
Garner, D. M. (1991b). *Eating disorder inventory—C*. Lutz, FL: Psychological Assessment Resources.

Eating Habits Questionnaire (Restraint Scale)
Herman, C. P., & Mack, D. (1975). Restrained and unrestrained eating. *Journal of Personality, 43*, 647–660.

Yale-Brown-Cornell Eating Disorder Scale (YBC-EDS)
Mazure, C. M., Halmi, K. A., Sunday, S. R., Romano, S. J., & Einhorn, A. M. (1994). Yale-Brown-Cornell Eating Disorder Scale: Development, use, reliability, and validity. *Journal of Psychiatric Research, 28*, 425–445.

2. Tests of Body Dissatisfaction/Body Image

Body Shape Questionnaire (BSQ)
Cooper, P., Taylor, M., Cooper, Z., & Fairburn, C. (1987). The development and validation of the BSQ. *International Journal of Eating Disorders, 6*, 485–494.

Colour-a-Person Test
Wooley, S. C., & Kearney-Cooke, A. (1986). Intensive treatment of bulimia and body image disturbance. In K. D. Brownell & J. P. Foreyt (Eds.), *Handbook of eating disorders: Physiology, psychology and treatment of obesity, anorexia, and bulimia* (pp. 476–502). New York, NY: Basic Books.

3. Tests of Emotional and Cognitive Components

Cognitive Behavioural Dieting Scale
Martz, D. M., Sturgis, E. T., & Gustafson, S. B. (1996). Development and preliminary validation of the Cognitive Behavioral Dieting Scale. *International Journal of Eating Disorders, 19*, 297–309.

Emotional Eating Scale
Arrow, B., Kenardy, J., & Agras, W. S. (1995). The emotional eating scale: The development of a measure to assess coping with negative affect by eating. *Internationl Journal of Eating Disorders, 18*, 79–90.

4. Risk Factors Identification

The McKnight Risk Factor Survey
Shisslak, et al. (1999). Development and evaluation of the McKnight Risk Factor Survey for assessing potential risk and protective factors for disordered eating in preadolescent and adolescent girls. *International Journal of Eating Disorders, 25*, 195–214 (Versions available for younger and older children).

---

is frequently used in community and clinical samples (Box 23-8). There is an abbreviated 26-item version of this test, EAT26, and also a child version, the CHEAT. The results of these paper-and-pencil tests can help identify the most significant symptoms for an individual and indicate a focus for interventions, especially therapy.

Nursing Diagnosis for Psychological Domain

Two common nursing diagnoses in AN are Anxiety and Disturbed Body Image.

Interventions for Psychological Domain

For interoceptive awareness problems (inability to experience visceral cues and emotions), the nurse can encourage keeping a journal. Most of these individuals use a somatic complaint such as "I feel bloated" or "I'm fat" to replace a negative emotion such as guilt or anger.

Although these complaints may be related to refeeding, they often are part of body dissatisfaction. A qualitative study of the bodily experiences of women with eating difficulties found that shame of one's body was a major theme (Rørtveit, Åström, & Severinsson, 2009). A clinical implication of this research is that nurses need to make it possible for women to speak about such feelings. Help individuals to identify feelings by having them write a description of the "fat feeling" and list possible underlying emotions and troublesome situations next to this description.

Understanding Feelings

Identifying feelings, such as anxiety and fear, and especially negative emotions, such as anger, is the first step in helping individuals decrease conflict avoidance and develop effective strategies for managing these feelings. Do not attempt to change distorted body image by

BOX 23.8

Eating Attitude Test

Please place an (x) under the column that applies best to each of the numbered statements. All the results will be strictly confidential. Most of the questions relate to food or eating, although other types of questions have been included. Please answer each question carefully. Thank you.

	Always	Very Often	Often	Sometimes	Rarely	Never
1. Like eating with other people	—	—	—	—	—	×
2. Prepare food for others but do not eat what I cook	×	—	—	—	—	—
3. Become anxious before eating	×	—	—	—	—	—
4. Am terrified about being overweight	×	—	—	—	—	—
5. Avoid eating when I am hungry	×	—	—	—	—	—
6. Find myself preoccupied with food	×	—	—	—	—	—
7. Have gone on binge eating in which I feel that I may not be able to stop	×	—	—	—	—	—
8. Cut my food into small pieces	×	—	—	—	—	—
9. Am aware of the calorie content of foods that I eat	×	—	—	—	—	—
10. Particularly avoid foods with a high carbohydrate content (e.g., bread, potatoes, rice)	×	—	—	—	—	—
11. Feel bloated after meals	×	—	—	—	—	—
12. Feel that others would prefer that I ate more	×	—	—	—	—	—
13. Vomit after I have eaten	×	—	—	—	—	—
14. Feel extremely guilty after eating	×	—	—	—	—	—
15. Am preoccupied with a desire to be thinner	×	—	—	—	—	—
16. Exercise strenuously to burn off calories	×	—	—	—	—	—
17. Weigh myself several times a day	×	—	—	—	—	—
18. Like my clothes to fit tightly	—	—	—	—	—	×
19. Enjoy eating meat	—	—	—	—	—	×
20. Wake up early in the morning	×	—	—	—	—	—
21. Eat the same food day after day	×	—	—	—	—	—
22. Think about burning up calories when I exercise	×	—	—	—	—	—
23. Have regular menstrual periods	—	—	—	—	—	×
24. Am aware that other people think I am too thin	×	—	—	—	—	—
25. Am preoccupied with the thought of having fat in my body	×	—	—	—	—	—
26. Take longer than others to eat	×	—	—	—	—	—
27. Enjoy eating at restaurants	—	—	—	—	—	×
28. Take laxatives	×	—	—	—	—	—
29. Avoid foods with sugar in them	×	—	—	—	—	—
30. Eat diet foods	×	—	—	—	—	—
31. Feel that food controls my life	×	—	—	—	—	—
32. Display self-control around food	×	—	—	—	—	—
33. Feel that others pressure me to eat	×	—	—	—	—	—
34. Give too much time and thought to food	×	—	—	—	—	—
35. Suffer from constipation	—	×	—	—	—	—
36. Feel uncomfortable after eating sweets	×	—	—	—	—	—
37. Engage in dieting behaviour	×	—	—	—	—	—
38. Like my stomach to be empty	×	—	—	—	—	—
39. Enjoy trying new rich foods	—	—	—	—	—	×
40. Have the impulse to vomit after meals	×	—	—	—	—	—

Scoring: The patient is given the questionnaire without the X's, just blank. Three points are assigned to endorsements that coincide with the X's; the adjacent alternatives are weighted as two points and one point. A total score of more than 30 indicates significant concerns with eating behaviour.

From Garner, D., & Garfinkel, P. (1979). The Eating Attitude Test: An index of the symptoms of anorexia nervosa. *Psychological Medicine, 9*, 273–279.

merely pointing out that the individual is actually too thin. This symptom is often the last to resolve itself, and some individuals may take years to see their bodies realistically. However, individuals can continue to fear becoming fat but not be driven to act on the distortion by starving. The fear of becoming fat eventually lessens with time.

The nurse can help individuals with eating disorders restructure the way they view the world, especially relative to food, eating, weight, and shape. Faulty ways of viewing these situations result in ineffective coping. Table 23-4 lists some cognitive distortions commonly experienced by individuals with eating disorders and some typical restructuring responses that challenge the distortion, which the nurse can present as more realistic ways of perceiving situations. Other therapies, such as movement and dance therapy, can help the individual experience pleasure from his or her body, although dance should be used cautiously during refeeding because of energy-expenditure concerns. Imagery and relaxation are often used to overcome distortions and to decrease anxiety.

While in the hospital, individuals usually are evaluated for discharge to day hospitalization or outpatient therapy, depending on the resources available, the extent of family support, and comorbidity. In both instances, the individual and family participate in a combination of individual and family therapy.

Psychotherapy

Interpersonal therapy (IPT) is a type of treatment that focuses on uncovering and resolving the developmental and psychological issues underlying the disorder. Role transitions, control, and ineffective feelings typically are the focus (McIntosh et al., 2005). Cognitive therapy may also be incorporated to continue to address and change distortions about food and interactions with others (Wilson et al., 1999). A third treatment option, nonspecific supportive clinical management, includes education, care, support, and fostering a therapeutic relationship that promotes adherence to treatment through use of praise, reassurance, and advice. Nonspecific supportive clinical management emphasizes the resumption of normal eating and the restoration of weight, providing verbal and written information on weight maintenance strategies, energy requirements, and relearning to eat normally. Other therapy content is dictated by the client.

Patient Education

When weight is restored and concentration is improved, individuals with AN can maximally benefit from psychoeducation. Although these individuals have much knowledge about food and calories, they also have misinformation that needs clarifying. For example, they are often unclear about the role of "fats" in a healthy diet and try to be as "fat free" as possible. A thorough assessment of their knowledge is important because they may seem to be "walking calorie books" with little information on the importance of including all nutrients in a healthy diet.

> **· CRNENOTE**
>
> **CRNENOTE** Setting realistic eating goals is one of the most helpful interventions for individuals with eating disorders. Because those with AN are often perfectionistic, they often set unrealistic goals.

Table 23.4	Cognitive Distortions Typical of Patients With Eating Disorders, With Restructuring Statements
Distortion	**Clarification or Restructuring**
Dichotomous or all-or-nothing thinking "I've gained 1 kilo (2 pounds), so I'll be up by 50 kilos (100 pounds) soon."	"You have never gained 50 kilos (100 pounds), but I understand that gaining 1 kilo (2 pounds) is scary."
Magnification "I binged last night, so I can't go out with anyone."	"Feeling bad and guilty about a binge are difficult feelings, but you are in treatment and you have been monitoring and changing your eating."
Selective abstraction "I can only be happy 5 kilos (10 pounds) lighter."	"When you were 5 kilos (10 pounds) lighter, you were hospitalized. You can choose to be happy about many things in your life."
Overgeneralization "I didn't eat anything yesterday and did okay, so I don't think *not* eating for a week or two will harm me."	"Any starvation harms the body, whether or not outward signs were apparent to you. The more you starve, the more problems your body will encounter."
Catastrophizing "I purged last night for the first time in 4 months—I'll never recover."	"Recovery includes ups and downs, and it is expected you will still have some mild but infrequent symptoms."

BOX 23.9

Psychoeducation Checklist: Anorexia Nervosa

When caring for the patient with AN, be sure to include the following topic areas in the teaching plan:

- Psychopharmacologic agents, if used, including drug, action, dosage, frequency, and possible adverse effects
- Nutrition and eating patterns
- Effect of restrictive eating or dieting
- Weight monitoring
- Safety and comfort measures
- Avoidance of triggers
- Self-monitoring techniques
- Trust
- Realistic goal setting
- Resources

Teaching Points

One of the most helpful skills the nurse can teach is to set realistic goals around food and other activities. Because of perfectionism, individuals with AN often set unrealistic goals and end up frustrated. The nurse can help them consider essential topic areas pertinent to their recovery (see Box 23-9) and support them to formulate smaller, more realistic, attainable goals.

Social Domain

Nursing Diagnosis for Social Domain

Ineffective Coping is a predominant nursing diagnosis with regard to the social domain.

Interventions for Social Domain

Younger individuals with AN may have lost some school time because of hospitalization. Integrating back into a school and classroom setting is difficult for most. Shame and guilt about having an eating disorder and being hospitalized must be addressed. Because these clients typically have isolated themselves before hospitalization and treatment, renewing friendships and relationships with peers may provoke anxiety. Involving school nurses and teachers in the reentry process may help.

Family and friends may not know how to use helpful collaborative approaches. Their own emotional reactions (e.g., anger, distress, anxiety, guilt, and fear) prevent them from expressing themselves as intended. When they believe their role is to "fix" the eating disorder, they may say things that are not helpful (Brown & Geller, 2006). Families and friends often need direction. Box 23-10 provides a list of general strategies and suggested readings that may assist them.

Because family members experience significant distress, extensive treatment and follow-up is required.

BOX 23.10

What Family and Friends Can Do to Help Those With Eating Disorders

- Tell the person you are concerned, you care, and you would like to help. Suggest that the person seek professional help from a physician or therapist.
- If the person refuses to seek professional help, encourage reaching out to an adult, such as a teacher, school nurse, or counsellor.
- Do not discuss weight, the number of calories being consumed, or particular eating habits. Do try to talk about things other than food, weight, counting calories, and exercise.
- Avoid making comments about a person's appearance. Concern about weight loss may be interpreted as a compliment; comments regarding weight gain may be felt as criticism.
- It will not help to become involved in a power struggle. You cannot force the person to eat.
- You can offer support. Ultimately, however, the responsibility and the decision to accept help and to change rest with the person.
- Read and educate yourself regarding these disorders.

Burden, conflict regarding the seriousness of the AN and caregiving role, attitudes and actions of others, stigma directed toward the family, and social support influence family functioning (Dimitropoulos, Carter, Schachter, & Woodside, 2008). Skilled therapists are able to help family members with their feelings, increase effective communication, decrease protectiveness, and resolve guilt. In therapy with the whole family and the person with AN, a therapist, psychologist, advanced practice nurse, or social worker meet regularly with them, at least once a week. This method has been demonstrated to be more effective than family therapy that does not include the individual with AN (Eisler et al., 2000) or individual therapy on its own (Robin et al., 1999). The family therapy focuses on such issues as separation-individuation, autonomy, ineffective communication, and practical issues, such as how parents can help their daughters or sons to effectively monitor food intake. Many family theorists believe that eating disorders develop because of family dysfunction and therefore have some unrealized meaning for each family. For example, the individual may be attempting to keep a splitting, divorcing, or estranged family together with the eating disorder. In other instances, parents may be trying to prevent a daughter from separating and individuating because they are emotionally unprepared for this process. The development of an eating disorder may be a reaction to these situations. Therapy helps to uncover these meanings and to improve effective, supportive parenting.

Often siblings become resentful of the attention the individual with an eating disorder gets from the parents. Having siblings attend family sessions to discuss these

BOX 23.11

Spirituality of the Nurse: Beginning the Journey

BODY IMAGE

Mirror mirror on the wall
You're really not that fair at all
You make me look like someone big
When really I'm a lean thin twig
This person standing looking in
Should take some time and draw her twin
Apprize herself and look inside
And find the girl she tries to hide
The one who can help her see the light
With all the strength and love to fight
Bring her out and show us all
And she will help you stand up tall
Look in the mirror, just one more glance
I bet she's telling you to take that stance
Say it loud and say it free
I love me just for who I see

By Nicole Boutilier,
*University of New Brunswick,
Canada*

In the fall of my last year of a Nursing degree I participated in a community clinical to experience how female students on campus coped with eating issues. The most valuable preparational learning activity was to create artwork that would elicit a feeling when viewed and reflect the ideals of appropriate, acceptable support. My topic was body image, and this was fate and irony playing out in my world because I have always been plagued with having the worst body image of myself! In composing an original poem, my fears, the insecurities, the lies I tell myself, the media's influence, and my family's role, all came into play. I realized that I had extended my understanding into knowing how a person with an eating issue might be feeling. I learned that we do things because our mind tricks us into thinking that we will not be what we think people want us to be. Big, small, fat, anorexic, short, tall … we cannot ever measure up to what society wants and thinks we should be. As we allow this problem to worsen, we lose sight of reality and things start to spiral out of control. Only those around us can see the monsters we are becoming when we ignore the little voice inside telling us not to listen to fashion and media ideals and peer pressure. I focused on the need to get back the person who became lost in the process of conforming to the expected norms. In doing so, I realized that food was not a factor in my struggle to be smaller but, rather, that my coping with stress and everyday struggles played havoc with my body and self esteem. I think somewhere in the back of my mind that I was aware of this before joining the clinic; but it hit home to me then that we are all suffering needlessly on our own. Fashion has set the norm, size zero being the most sought after size by the youth today. Girls try to be super thin, unaware of the problems this brings. It is time to take a stand and show the media that we are not going to put up with their harmful norms.

feelings and the effect the illness has had on them is helpful. Further research is needed to explore social support to individuals with eating disorders and to identify helpful approaches that would enable nurses and other caregivers reduce the occurrence of unhelpful interactions.

Spiritual Domain

In order to form a therapeutic alliance with an individual struggling with AN, the nurse must first make meaning of personal experiences with eating issues and self-preservation strategies. The nurse cannot effectively model self-awareness and acceptance to others without having engaged in this critical self-development. In Box 23-11, a senior student nurse describes her reflective, creative journey of becoming an authentic change agent in her own life, as she prepared to work with persons confronting eating issues. In identifying values and pressures guiding her own behaviour and actions, the student nurse was able to suspend negative judgment and to identify the points of interest with future clients.

The crux of the spiritual interventions is establishing trust, rapport, and consistency; supporting; and enabling the client to give voice and subsequently meaning to her or his experience through telling the history and story of the eating disorder experience. The nurse helps the patient recognize patterns and identify and clarify values. Encouraging activities that promote reflection and self-awareness helps the client access potential solutions to well-being and reduces depression, anxiety, relationship distress, social role conflict, and eating disorder symptoms (Scott Richards, Berrett, Hardman, & Eggett, 2006). In interacting with an individual whose body has served as a container for pain, suffering, and disgust and has subsequently starved, stuffed, or purged, the nurse may encounter body countertranference or the phenomenon of experiencing a similar type of discomfort in the nurse's own body (Orbach, 2004). The nurse must be attuned to these body sensations, expect this phenomenon to occur and use the information generated to further explore the client's body image and affectivity. Without awareness and self-monitoring, the nurse may communicate any personal body discomfort to the client. Individual or group peer debriefing sessions are also helpful to manage such countertransference.

■ EVALUATION AND TREATMENT OUTCOMES

Several factors influence the outcome of treatment for AN. Particularly, long duration of symptoms and low weight at treatment onset predict poor outcomes, whereas family

BOX 23.12

Research for Best Practice: Understanding Recovery from Eating Disorders

From Patching, J., & Lawler, J. (2009). Understanding women's experiences of developing an eating disorder and recovering: a life-history approach. Nursing Inquiry, 16, 10–21.

BACKGROUND: Dominant conceptualizations of eating disorders tend to place a preexisting template on cause and effect leading to cure/treatment. Exploring and understanding eating disorders in the framework of the lived experience may develop a more holistic understanding of the conditions.

PURPOSE: To explore the lived experience of developing, living, and recovering from an eating disorder as a complete experience.

METHOD: Life-history interviews were used with 20 women who had recovered from AN, BN, or both and who had remained healthy. The interviews focused on the women's narratives and experience rather than a diagnostic therapeutic model.

FINDINGS: Three themes of control, connectedness, and conflict emerged as significant. The development of the eating disorder was attributed to a lack of control, a sense of nonconnectedness to family and peers and extreme conflict with significant others. Recovery occurred when the women reengaged with life, developed skills necessary for conflict resolution and rediscovered their sense of self.

IMPLICATIONS FOR NURSING: Rather than viewing the development of and recovery from an eating disorder as separate and discrete events, the data from the interviews suggest they are better viewed as one entity—that is, the journey of an individual attempting to discover and develop her sense of self. Understanding the eating disorder as a symptom of deeper issues rather than a condition in and of itself will help nurses assess, interview, and evaluate individual responses. Addressing the deeper issue, when the individual is 'ready' to make that choice, may lead to recovery.

support and involvement generally improve outcomes. Comorbid conditions and their severity will also influence recovery. Individuals are discharged from the hospital at weights somewhat below what is considered ideal before restoration of healthy eating and changes in maladaptive thinking have occurred. Recovery is a complex process of self-development over time (see Box 23-12). Individuals in the process of recovering may continue to restrict foods and have cognitive distortions in the initial phases of recovery (Weaver et al., 2005). Without intensive ongoing outpatient treatment, including nutritional counselling and support, they are unlikely to recover fully. Distorted thinking and eating patterns can set the stage for a relapse and later for the possible development of other eating disorders. Many of the instruments used to assess eating disorder symptoms (see Box 23-7) can be used throughout the individual's treatment to evaluate attitudes and thinking processes that continue to prevent full recovery. Nurses are ideally positioned within hospital and community health treatment settings to help individuals with AN facilitate their recovery.

◼◼◼ CONTINUUM OF CARE

Hospitalization

AN its acute stage requires hospitalization.

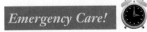

Emergency Care!

Death may result from cardiac problems associated with starvation and suicide. However, emergency care is not usually needed for individuals with AN. Family members

and peers usually notice the weight loss and emaciation before the individual's systems are compromised to the degree that they require emergency treatment. If systems are compromised enough to warrant emergency treatment, or the individual is suicidal, she or he usually is admitted immediately for inpatient care.

Family therapy, initiated in the hospital, is continued more intensively after discharge (see Chapter 17).

Outpatient Treatment

After refeeding, treatment of AN may take place on an outpatient basis and involve continued individual and family therapy, nutrition counselling to reinforce healthy eating patterns and attitudes, and physician visits to monitor weight and evaluate somatic recovery. Support groups, often suggested, should not be substituted for therapy. In fact, some self-directed support groups that lack professional leadership can actually delay or prevent needed professional treatment. The role of support groups to maintain recovery requires further study.

Bulimia Nervosa

Until about 30 years ago, BN was thought to be a subtype of AN. However, findings from extensive investigations have identified its characteristics as a separate entity that is now actually more prevalent than AN. Individuals with BN are usually older at onset than are those with AN. The disorder generally is not as life threatening as AN. The usual treatment is outpatient therapy. Outcomes are better for BN than for AN, and mortality rates are lower.

CLINICAL COURSE

There are few outward signs associated with BN. Individuals binge and purge in secret and are typically of normal weight; therefore, BN does not come to the attention of parents and peers as quickly as AN. Treatment consequently can be delayed for years as individuals attempt on their own to get their eating under control. Once treatment is undertaken and completed, they are capable of full recovery, except in cases in which personality disorders and comorbid serious depression are also present.

Individuals with BN may present as overwhelmed and overly committed and have difficulty with setting limits and establishing appropriate boundaries. They have many rules regarding food and food restriction, and they feel ashamed, guilty, and disgusted about binge eating and purging. They may also be impulsive in other areas of their lives, such as spending.

DIAGNOSTIC CRITERIA

The key characteristics for the diagnosis of BN appear in Table 23-5 (also see Box 23-1). There are two types of BN: purging type and restricting type. Individuals with the restricting type are similar to those with AN. However, in BN, restricting is followed by binge eating, which is then followed by another period of restricting. In the purging type, binge eating is followed by purging. The difference between purging in the individual with AN and purging in the individual with BN is the severe weight loss and amenorrhea that accompanies AN. BN involves engaging in recurrent episodes of binge eating and compensatory purging in the form of vomiting; using laxatives, diuretics, or emetics; or nonpurging compensatory behaviours, such as fasting or overexercising in order to avoid weight gain. These episodes must occur at least twice a week for a period of at least 3 months in order to meet the *DSM-IV-TR* criteria (APA, 2000). People with BN may binge and purge a number of times a day.

Binge eating is defined as rapid, episodic, impulsive, and uncontrollable ingestion of a large amount of food during a short period of time, usually 1 to 2 hours. Eating is followed by feelings of guilt, remorse, and often self-contempt, leading to purging. To assuage the out-of-control feeling, severe dieting referred to as *dietary restraint* is instituted, precipitating the next binge. The restrictions are viewed as "rules," such as no sweets or no fats. Each binge seems to influence stricter rules about what cannot be consumed, leading to more frequent binge eating and subsequent guilt, self-loathing, purging,

Table 23.5 ☘ Key Diagnostic Characteristics for Bulimia Nervosa

Diagnostic Criteria	Target Symptoms and Associated Findings
• Recurrent episodes of binge eating • Characterized by both of the following: eating in a discrete period of time an amount larger than most people would eat during a similar period of time and under similar circumstances; sense of lack of control over eating during the episode • Recurrent inappropriate compensatory behaviour to; prevent weight gain, such as self-induced vomiting, misuse of laxatives, diuretics, enemas, or other medications; fasting; or excessive exercise • Binge eating and inappropriate compensatory behaviours occurring on average at least twice a week for 3 months • Associated Physical Examination Findings • Self-evaluation unduly influenced by body shape and weight • Not occurring exclusively during episodes of anorexia nervosa • Purging type: regular engagement in self-induced vomiting or misuse of diuretics, laxatives, or enemas • Nonpurging type: use of other inappropriate compensatory behaviours, such as fasting or excessive exercise without regular engagement in self-induced vomiting, or misuse of laxatives, diuretics, or enemas	• Usually within normal weight range, possible overweight or underweight • Restriction of total calorie consumption between binges, selecting low-calorie foods while avoiding foods perceived to be fattening or likely to trigger a binge • Increased frequency of depressive symptoms and anxiety symptoms • Possible substance abuse or dependence involving alcohol or stimulants *Associate Physical Examination* • Loss of dental enamel • Chipped, ragged, or moth-eaten teeth appearance • Increased incidence of dental caries • Scars on the dorsum of hand from manually inducing vomiting • Cardiac and skeletal myopathies from use of syrup of ipecac for vomiting • Menstrual irregularities • Dependence on laxatives • Esophageal tears *Associate Laboratory Findings* • Fluid and electrolyte abnormalities • Metabolic alkalosis (from vomiting) or metabolic acidosis (from diarrhea) • Mildly elevated serum amylase levels

or *dietary restraint* (Fig. 23-5). This cycle has prompted clinicians to focus the treatment on interventions related to dietary restraint or purging behaviours. Bohon, Stice, and Burton (2009) found dietary restraint and compensatory symptoms negatively correlated with the length of time to remission, and this suggests that when dietary restraint is resolved, or purging is prevented, binge eating is decreased.

> **KEY CONCEPT   Dietary restraint** was originally described to explain the differences between the eating patterns of obese individuals and those of normal-weight people (Herman & Mack, 1973). The concept has since evolved into the development of the widely used Three Factor Questionnaire now called the Eating Inventory (Stunkard & Messick, 1985, 1988).

As shown in Figure 23-5, dietary restriction contributes to overeating and bingeing. Restriction may operate in a straightforward fashion by instigating a drive toward repletion. It may also alter one's perceptual reactivation to attractive food cues, making them more irresistible. Restriction may make dieters more prone to feel distress over their dietary "failures," especially if dieting has become a way to overcome body dissatisfaction, and to compensate for distress through binge eating. Whether the eating is influenced by hunger, the attraction of forbidden foods, or internal needs to assuage failure, there is significant evidence that restraining one's intake is a precondition for subsequent overeating.

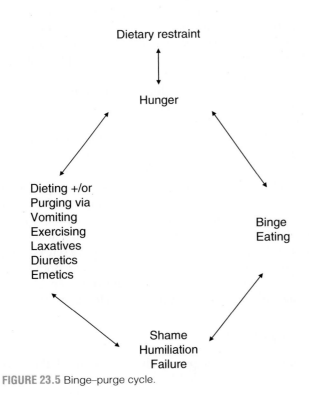

FIGURE 23.5 Binge–purge cycle.

BULIMIA NERVOSA IN SPECIAL POPULATIONS

BN occurs in all age groups. It is not as common in children as in adolescents and adults; children appear more likely to have BED (APA, 2000; Johnston, 2004). This finding has only recently been reported, and more data are needed to substantiate the theory.

EPIDEMIOLOGY

Lifetime prevalence of BN is reported to be 3% to 8%, depending on whether clinical or community populations are sampled. Stricter criteria are used when clinical groups are studied, making the prevalence rate lower. An Ontario study found that 0.13% of men and 1.46% of women had full-syndrome BN, with an additional 0.95% of men and 1.70% of women having partial-syndrome BN (Woodside et al., 2001). The occurrence is more common than that of AN (Gauvin, Steiger, & Brodeur, 2009).

Age of Onset

Typically, the age of onset for BN is later than that for AN, occurring in late adolescence or early adulthood, and may coincide with a developmental transition (e.g., leaving home to attend university) or psychosocial stress (Yager & Powers, 2007).

Gender Differences

In the community setting, a ratio of three to five females to one male experience BN (Health Canada, 2003; Woodside et al., 2001) (see Box 23-2).

Ethnic and Cultural Differences

BN is related to culture in the same way as AN. In Western cultures and those becoming westernized in their norms, the focus on achieving a thin ideal body underlies the dieting and dietary restraint that set up the trajectory toward a diagnosable eating disorder. Hispanic and white women have higher reported rates than do Asian and African Americans. There is a paucity of research exploring ethnic and culture differences among Canadian women.

Familial Differences

There is some support for a familial link for BN. First-degree relatives of women with BN are more likely to have eating disorders than control subjects and women with other psychiatric disorders (Yager & Powers, 2007).

Comorbidity

The most common comorbid conditions are substance misuse, depression, and OCD. In a recent study, women continued having OCD after remission of their bulimic symptoms, suggesting that some comorbid conditions are trait-related and may actually have a role in precipitating the disorder (Morgan, Wolfe, Metzger, & Jimersonm, 2007). Cluster B, Axis II disorders, such as BPD, are also identified frequently with BN. Bulimic clients with BPD have reported stronger feelings of ineffectiveness and more problems with interoceptive awareness than bulimic clients without BPD (Zeeck et al., 2007). Many women with BN have had AN previously.

ETIOLOGY

Some of the predisposing or risk factors for BN overlap with theories of causality (see Fig. 23-2). For example, dieting puts an individual at risk for the development of BN. The dieting can turn into dietary restraint, which leads to binge eating and purging. However, not all individuals who diet experience BN. The interplay of other risk factors (e.g., body dissatisfaction and separation-individuation issues) most likely explains the development of this disorder.

Biologic Theories

Some progress has been made in understanding the biologic causes of BN. Dieting, one of the most important factors, occurs in girls as young as 7 years of age. Canadian children in grades three and four have said they would rather lose a parent, get cancer, or live through nuclear war than be fat (National Eating Disorder Information Centre, 1998). Dieting is believed to affect the neurotransmitters, including serotonin, which are involved in the appetite, satiety, and eating patterns of BN. Levels of cholecystokinin, a hormone associated with satiation, are thought to be low in some individuals with BN (Aja, 2006). As in AN, overexercising has also contributed to some of the symptoms of BN, especially in individuals with the restricting type.

Neuropathologic

The changes in the brain are the result rather than the cause of eating dysregulation. As with AN, these changes resolve when symptoms such as dietary restraint, binge eating, and purging remit.

Genetic

A specific gene responsible for BN has not been identified. Recently, twin studies have been reviewed to determine the role genetics might play in the development of BN.

Whereas it has been widely recognized that environment also plays a role, genetic influences outweighed environmental ones (Bulik, 2005). Findings are treated with caution because sorting out environmental and genetic influences is difficult when twins live in the same environment.

Biochemical

The most frequently studied biochemical theory in BN relates to lowered brain serotonin neurotransmission. People with BN are believed to have altered modulation of central serotonin neuronal systems (Kaye et al., 2000). Studies have looked to tryptophan, an amino acid and serotonin precursor, to explain this mechanism. Findings have demonstrated that women with BN experience symptoms of depressed mood, a desire to binge, and an increase in weight and shape concerns when tryptophan is depleted (Smith, Fairburn, & Cowen, 1999; Wolfe et al., 2000). Chronic depletion of tryptophan is considered one of the major mechanisms whereby persistent dieting can lead to eating disorder development in vulnerable individuals.

Psychological and Social Theories

Psychological factors in the etiology of BN have been studied extensively, and most experts believe that these factors converge with environmental or sociocultural factors within individuals with a biologic predisposition, causing symptoms to develop. As with AN, psychoanalytic developmental theories that explain separation-individuation are important in causality. Because the age of onset for BN is late adolescence/early adulthood, going away to college, for example, may represent the first physical separation for some adolescents who are unprepared for the emotional separation. In addition, an inability to set limits and develop healthy boundaries leads to a sense of being overwhelmed and "drained." In most instances, women with BN are not assertive and have difficulty saying no, fearing that they will not be liked. Overwhelming feelings often lead to binge eating, either to avoid or to distract oneself from feelings such as resentment, or binge eating can serve to assuage emptiness, filling up a "drained" self with food. Engaging in binge eating can leave the individual feeling out of control, lowering self-esteem and efficacy. To try to regain control and improve self-esteem, the individual may resume the cycle of dieting. Both binge eating and purging may serve as regulation strategies for coping with negative affect (Polivy & Hermann, 1993).

Cognitive Theory

Cognitive theory helps explain the distorted thinking present in people with BN. This explanation is similar for depression, in which a particular thought pattern is learned (see Chapter 15 for an explanation of cognitive theory). Many experts view BN as a disorder of thinking, in that distortions are the basis of behaviours such as binge eating and purging. Psychological triggering mechanism models explain that cues such as stress, negative emotions, and environment (e.g., the presence of attractive food) play a role in etiology. However, these cognitive and triggering theories are viewed as an explanation for maintaining the binge eating once it has been established, rather than an explanation of causality.

The same sociocultural factors that underlie AN play a significant role in the development of BN.

Family

The families of individuals who experience BN have been primarily studied from the perspectives of researchers and clinicians, and are reported to be chaotic, with few rules and unclear boundaries. The perspectives of the families themselves have received little research attention. A review of recent studies showed a strong relationship of BN with poor caregiver relationships (Vince & Walker, 2008). As with AN, theories of causation do not individually explain the development of BN. Rather, the convergence of many factors at a vulnerable stage of individual development helps explain causality.

■ RISK FACTORS

The risk or predisposing factors for BN are included in Figure 23-3.

■ INTERDISCIPLINARY TREATMENT

Individuals with BN benefit from a comprehensive multifaceted treatment approach. The goals for the treatment focus on stabilizing and then normalizing eating, which means stopping the binge–purge cycle; restructuring dysfunctional thought patterns and attitudes, especially about eating, weight, and shape; teaching healthy boundary setting; and resolving conflicts about separation-individuation. The treatment usually takes place in an outpatient setting, except when the client is suicidal or when past outpatient treatment has failed (Table 23-3).

Therapy for BN focuses on psychological issues, such as boundary setting and separation-individuation conflicts and on changing problematic behaviours and dysfunctional thinking. Intensive psychotherapy and pharmacologic interventions are necessary in treating binge eating and purging. Nutrition counselling helps stabilize and normalize eating. Support groups are also involved. Family therapy is not usually a part of the treatment because

many people with BN live on college campuses away from home or are older and on their own. Usually, the treatment becomes less intensive as symptoms remit.

■ PRIORITY CARE ISSUES

Given the comorbid conditions of depression and BPD, some individuals with BN may become suicidal. They are also often at risk for self-mutilation. Because they display high levels of impulsivity, shoplifting, and overspending, financial and legal difficulties have been associated with BN.

■ NURSING MANAGEMENT: HUMAN RESPONSE TO BULIMIA NERVOSA DISORDER

The primary nursing diagnoses for patients with BN are Imbalanced Nutrition: Less Than or More Than Body Requirements, Powerlessness, Anxiety, and Ineffective Coping.

Therapeutic Relationship

Individuals with BN experience shame and guilt, have an intense need to please and be liked, and may approach the nurse–client relationship in a superficial manner. They are too ashamed to discuss their symptoms but do not want to disappoint others, so they may discuss more social or unrelated issues in an attempt to engage the nurse. A nonjudgmental approach stressing the importance of the relationship and outlining its purpose is important from the outset. Explaining the nature of the relationship and the goals of therapy will help clarify the boundaries (see Chapter 9).

Biologic Domain

Despite that most individuals with BN maintain normal weights, the physical ramifications of this disorder may parallel those of AN or obesity. Clients who purge risk fluid and electrolyte abnormalities; hypokalemia contributes to muscle weakness and fatigability, cardiac arrhythmias, palpitations, and cardiac conduction defects. Neuropsychiatric disturbances, such as poor concentration and attention, and sleep disturbances are common.

BOX 23.13

Drug Profile: *Fluoxetine Hydrochloride (Prozac)*

DRUG CLASS: Selective serotonin reuptake inhibitor

RECEPTOR AFFINITY: Inhibits central nervous system neuronal uptake of serotonin with little effect on norepinephrine; thought to antagonize muscarinic, histaminergic, and α-adrenergic receptors.

INDICATIONS: Treatment of depressive disorders, most effective in major depression, obesity, bulimia, and OCD

ROUTES AND DOSAGE: Available in 10- and 20-mg pulvules and 20 mg/5 mL oral solution

Adults: 20 mg/day in the morning, not to exceed 80 mg/day. Full antidepressant effect may not be seen for up to 4 weeks. If no improvement, dosage is increased after several weeks. Dosages 20 mg/day are administered twice daily. For eating disorders: typically 40 mg to 60 mg/day recommended.

Geriatric: Administer at lower or less-frequent doses; monitor responses to guide dosage.

Children: Safety and efficacy have not been established.

HALF-LIFE (PEAK EFFECT): 2–3 days (6–8 hours)

SELECTED ADVERSE REACTIONS: Headache, nervousness, insomnia, drowsiness, anxiety, tremors, dizziness, light-headedness, nausea, vomiting, diarrhea, dry mouth, anorexia, dyspepsia, constipation, taste changes, upper respiratory infections, pharyngitis, painful menstruation, sexual dysfunction, urinary frequency, sweating, rash, pruritus, weight loss, asthenia, and fever.

WARNINGS: Avoid use in pregnancy and while breast-feeding. Use with caution in patients with impaired hepatic or renal function and diabetes mellitus. Possible risk for toxicity if taken with tricyclic antidepressants.

SPECIAL PATIENT AND FAMILY EDUCATION:
- Be aware that the drug may take up to 4 weeks to get full antidepressant effect.
- Take the drug in the morning or in divided doses, if necessary.
- Report any adverse reactions.
- Avoid driving a car or performing hazardous activities because the drug may cause drowsiness or dizziness.
- Eat small, frequent meals to help with complaints of nausea and vomiting.

Assessment

The nurse should assess current eating patterns, determine the number of times a day the individual binges and purges, and note dietary restraint practices. Sleep patterns and exercise habits are also important.

Nursing Diagnoses for Biologic Domain

Imbalanced Nutrition: Less Than/More Than Body Requirements and Disturbed Sleep Pattern are typical nursing diagnoses for the biologic domain.

Interventions for Biologic Domain

If the client is admitted to the hospital, meals and all food intake must be strictly monitored to normalize eating. Bathroom visits should also be supervised to prevent purging. Outpatients are asked to record their intake, binges, and purges to form a foundation for changing behaviours with psychotherapy. Because individuals with BN have chaotic lifestyles and are often overcommitted, sleep may be a low priority. Sleep-deprived individuals may assume that food would be helpful, and they begin to eat, triggering a binge. To encourage regular sleep patterns, individuals should go to bed and rise at about the same time every day.

Pharmacologic Interventions

Whereas pharmacologic intervention is effective for symptom remission in BN, experts agree that the combination of cognitive-behavioural therapy (CBT) and medication has had the best results (Hall, Friedman, & Leach, 2008). Fluoxetine (Prozac) has been the most studied for BN in clinical trials (see Box 23-13). Effective doses are usually 60 mg per day, a higher dosage than that used to treat depression. Sertraline (Zoloft) has also been used effectively. These medications, prescribed for binge eating and purging, are effective even when depression is not present (Trunko & Kaye, 2008). Weight is monitored as decreased appetite and weight loss are common during the first few weeks of administration. It is also important to monitor the intake of medication for possible purging after administration. The effect of the medication depends on the time taken for its absorption.

Teaching Points

Individuals should be instructed to take medication as prescribed. SSRIs should be taken in the morning because they can cause insomnia. Individuals should be informed that any weight loss they initially experience is temporary and is usually regained after a few weeks, when the medication dosage has stabilized.

Psychosocial Domain

Assessment

Psychological assessment focuses on cognitive distortions—cues or stimuli that lead to dysfunctional behaviour affecting symptom development—and knowledge deficits. The psychological characteristics typical of individuals with BN are presented in Box 23-1. Examples of cognitive distortions present in BN are given in Table 23-4. These thought patterns form the basis for "rules" and lead the way to destructive eating patterns. During routine history taking, individuals may relate many of these distortions. Situations that produce feelings of being overwhelmed and powerless need to be explored, as does the individual's ability to set boundaries, control impulsivity, and maintain quality relationships. These underlying issues may precipitate binge eating. Several assessment tools are available to gauge such characteristics as body dissatisfaction and impulsivity (see Box 23-7). Body dissatisfaction should be openly explored. Mood is evaluated because many people with BN also have depression.

Nursing Diagnoses for Psychosocial Domain

Deficient Knowledge and Disturbed Thought Processes are among the common diagnoses for the psychosocial domain.

Interventions for Psychosocial Domain

Studies comparing various psychotherapy methods have demonstrated that CBT produces the best results (Hay, Bacaltchuk, & Stefano, 2004/2009; Shapiro et al., 2007) and that the combination of CBT and pharmacologic interventions is best for decreasing binge eating and vomiting (Shapiro et al.). CBT is usually conducted in a group, with one or two sessions a week. IPT has had positive outcomes but may take longer to change binge eating and purging symptoms. Behavioural therapy alone has not been as effective as CBT. While binge eating may persist, little work can be done on underlying interpersonal issues, such as boundary setting, because the client feels out of control with eating. Therefore, cognitive therapy is begun first, to address the distorted thinking processes influencing dietary restraint, binge eating, and purging. Decreasing these symptoms will eliminate the out-of-control feelings.

Because CBT requires a specialist's care, current treatment research explores the use of self-help models, including manuals that can be combined with psychopharmacology (Sysko & Walsh, 2008). This research has found little evidence for the specific efficacy of self-help in comparison to other treatments, and recommends additional studies of self-help to determine the specific utility of such help interventions for BN.

Behavioural Techniques

The behavioural techniques, such as **cue elimination** and response prevention, require self-monitoring to individualize the therapy. **Self-monitoring** is accomplished using a diary, in which the individual records

binges, purges, precipitating emotions, and environmental cues. Emotional and environmental cues are identified, and alternative responses are formulated, tried, and reinforced. When a cue or stimulus leads to a dysfunctional or unhealthy response, the response can be eliminated, or an alternate, healthier response to the cue can be substituted, tried, and then reinforced. Figure 23-6 gives two examples of behavioural interventions. In example 1, for the individual with AN, the response is modified or altered to a healthier one; in example 2, for the individual with BN, the cue is changed to produce a different, healthier response. Other techniques, such as postponing binges and purges through distraction, a technique to interrupt the cycle, are also effective.

Psychoeducation

In addition to cognitive and behavioural techniques, educational strategies are also incorporated.

Teaching Points

Psychoeducation for individuals with BN focuses on setting boundaries and healthy limits, developing assertiveness, learning nutritional concepts related to

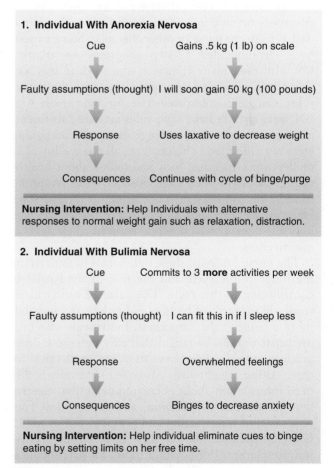

FIGURE 23.6 Examples of the relationship of cues, thoughts, and responses: behavioural interventions.

healthy eating, discussing societal definitions of beauty, and clarifying misconceptions about food (Hendricks & Thompson, 2005; White, 1999). Rules that result from dichotomous thinking also must be addressed because of their role in dietary restraint and resulting binge eating.

Family Assessment and Intervention

Families caring for members with BN report experiencing intense emotions, including guilt, feelings of helplessness, anger, fear, and self-blame (Perkins, Winn, Murray, Murphy, & Schmidt, 2004). Winn and colleagues (2007) found that family caregivers of adolescents with BN may experience negative caregiving experiences including stigma and problems with services. The nurse must explore with families the negative impact of giving care to assess its physical and psychosocial toll and to evaluate coping capacity. A number of strategies that families apply to manage the difficulties associated with the eating disorder are thinking positively, using humour, maintaining their own interests, and actively obtaining information (Perkins et al.).

Group Therapy

Group therapy is cost-effective and increases learning effectively because individuals learn from each other as well as from the nurse or other therapist. Some experts have recommended 12-step programs for treating BN. However, many clinicians who work in this specialty have noted that these programs, with their strict rules, can be counterproductive for individuals with BN, who already have rigid rules and are "abstinent" in many ways that lead to binge eating. Broad parameters regarding food choices (e.g., all foods allowed in moderation), together with knowledge about healthy eating, should be encouraged instead. After symptoms subside, individuals can concentrate on interpersonal issues in therapy, such as feelings of inadequacy and low self-esteem, which often underlie their lack of assertiveness.

The nurse can assist these individuals to understand the binge–purge cycle and the role of rigid rules in contributing to this cycle. The value of eating meals regularly to ward off hunger and reduce the possibility of a binge is also important. Individuals who misuse laxatives must be taught that although these drugs produce water-weight loss, they are ineffective for true, lasting weight loss. Moreover, individuals also need information about potassium depletion, electrolyte imbalances, dehydration, and the medical consequences of binge eating and purging. For example, laxative-dependent bowel may result from laxative misuse (Garner, 1997). Other topics for psychoeducation are included in Box 23-14.

BOX 23.14

Psychoeducation Checklist: Bulimia Nervosa

When caring for the individual with BN, be sure to include the following topic areas in the teaching plan:

- Psychopharmacologic agents, if used, including drug, action, dosage, frequency, and possible adverse effects
- Binge–purge cycle and effects on body
- Nutrition and eating patterns
- Hydration
- Avoidance of cues
- Cognitive distortions
- Limit setting
- Appropriate boundary setting
- Assertiveness
- Resources
- Self-monitoring and behavioural interventions
- Realistic goal setting

Spiritual Domain

Assessment

The role of spirituality in the life of an individual with BN can be assessed through their expressions of loss and powerlessness, self-care, quality of relationships, history of conflicts and painful traumatic experiences, attitudes about food and overeating, and self-judgment. The nurse must strive to see the person beyond the dieting behaviour.

Nursing Diagnoses for Spiritual Domain

Loss and Powerlessness are among the common diagnoses for the spiritual domain.

Interventions for Spiritual Domain

The nurse encourages clients to express feelings of loss and powerlessness without negative self-judgment (Berrett et al., 2007). Clients will benefit from exploring what they do and do not have control over and to accept their human limitations. Those who binge eat and purge can learn to delay these behaviours through engaging in activities such as journal writing, affirming positive self-worth, meditation, and imagery. These strategies may also help deal with comorbid depression and anxiety. Nurses can create the context for clients with BN to build support that includes support from self and others.

■ EVALUATION AND TREATMENT OUTCOMES

Individuals with BN have better recovery outcomes than do those with AN. Outcomes have improved since the early 1990s, partially because of earlier detection, research on treatments that are most effective, and neuropharmacologic research and advances. Approximately 55% to 70% of individuals with BN achieve full recovery within 5 to 12 years (Hay & Bacaltchuk, 2007; Keski-Rahkonen et al., 2009), although one third of those who recover experience relapse (Yager & Powers, 2007). Good outcome has been associated with a shorter duration of illness: receiving treatment within the first few years of illness is associated with an 80% recovery rate (Reas, Williamson, Martin, & Zucker, 2000); early response to treatment is considered the most consistent posttreatment predictor of a better outcome (Hay & Bacaltchuk). Factors associated with poor outcome include comorbid depression or personality disorder, substance misuse, premorbid and paternal obesity, low motivation for change, and weak impulse control (Berkman et al., 2007; Hay & Bacaltchuk).

▆▆▆ CONTINUUM OF CARE

Although individuals with BN are less likely than those with AN to require hospitalization, those with extreme dehydration and electrolyte imbalance, depression and suicidality, or symptoms that have not remitted with outpatient treatment, need hospitalization. However, most treatment takes place in outpatient settings. After treatment, referrals to recovery groups and support groups are important to prevent relapse.

Binge Eating Disorder

BED, introduced into the *DSM-IV* as a provisional diagnosis in 2004, is more prevalent than both AN and BN, and is not uncommon in men. It is associated with high comorbidity, obesity, psychosocial impairment, and poor overall health. When diagnosed, the usual treatment is outpatient therapy.

▆▆▆ CLINICAL COURSE

Individuals with BED binge eat in the same way as those with BN but do not compensate for binges through purging or other behaviours. Box 23-15 describes the current understanding about BED. Individuals describe eating without awareness of doing so or with awareness that the binge eating is abnormal, verbalizing the need to eat "until it's all gone" and that "Sometimes it's hard to stop" (Lyons, 1998, p. 1162).

Outward signs associated with BED may include overweight, obesity, and associated consequences such as gall bladder disease and arthritis. Through these manifestations, BED may come to the attention of family and peers.

BOX 23.15
Binge Eating Disorder

BED, still in the research stage to refine its characteristics for inclusion in the *DSM-IV-TR* (APA, 2000) as a separate entity, is estimated to affect 3%–4% of the population. The criteria for BED consist of binge eating, which includes both the ingestion of a large amount of food in a short period of time and a sense of loss of control during the binge; distress regarding the binge; eating until uncomfortably full; and feelings of guilt or depression following the binge. Purging does not occur with BED, and this helps differentiate it from BN. In addition, investigators have shown that individuals with BED have lower dietary restraint and are higher in weight, even though many are not obese, than those with BN. It has been estimated that 10%–30% of obese individuals have BED. Some women with BN have reported that they binged without purging for several years before developing BN at as young as age 10 years (Bulik et al., 1998).

CBT has not been as effective for BED as it is for BN. Investigations have shown that sibutramin and topiramate have been effective in reducing binges, decreasing binge eating and appetite. Sibutramin (serotonin-norepinephrine reuptake inhibitor) has resulted in weight loss of up to 10% of initial body weight (Yager, 2008). Topiramate (antiepileptic agent) has demonstrated efficacy in the treatment of BED-related obesity (McElroy et al., 2003; Wilding, Van Gaal, Rissanen, Vercruysse, & Fitchet, 2004). Orlistat inhibits gastrointestinal lipase, an enzyme that breaks down triglycerides in the intestine so that triglycerides from the diet are prevented from being hydrolyzed into absorbable free fatty acids and are excreted undigested, thus preventing approximately 30% of dietary fat from being absorbed (Thomson, 2006).

Treatment can be delayed for years as individuals attempt on their own or with commercial weight loss programs to control their eating. Outcomes have not been extensively studied; poor prognosis is expected given the difficulty individuals experience in attempting to achieve and maintain weight loss, and in cases in which mood and anxiety disorders are also present.

Individuals with BED may miss work, school, or social activities to binge eat. Obese people with BED often are extremely distressed by their binge eating, feel bad about themselves, and are preoccupied with their appearance. Most feel ashamed, may avoid social gatherings, and try to hide their problem. Often they are so successful that close family members and friends do not know that they binge eat.

▆▆▆ DIAGNOSTIC CRITERIA

The key characteristics for the diagnosis of BED appear in Table 23-6 (also see Box 23-15). Persistent overeating, feelings of loss of control, and marked distress occur. Binge eating is influenced by such cues as dietary

Table 23.6 Key Diagnostic Characteristics for Binge Eating Disorder	
Diagnostic Criteria	**Target Symptoms and Associated Findings**
• Recurrent episodes of binge eating • The bingeeating episodes are associated with at least three of the following: 1. eating much more rapidly than normal 2. eating until feeling uncomfortably full 3. eating large amounts of food when not feeling physically hungry 4. eating alone because of being embarrassed by how much one is eating 5. feeling disgusted with oneself, depressed, or very guilty after overeating • Marked distress regarding binge eating • The binge eating occurs, on average, at least 2 days a week for 6 months. • The binge eating is not associated with the regular use of inappropriate compensatory behaviours (e.g., purging, fasting, excessive exercise) and does not occur exclusively during the course of anorexia nervosa or bulimia nervosa.	• Usually leads to overweight and less often to obesity • Individuals tend to binge on foods that are chocolate, high fat, sweet, or salty. • Depression and anxiety contribute to body dissatisfaction. • Those who binge eat frequently use dieting and join fitness programs to control resultant weight gain (Lyons, 1998; Williamson, 1990). These behaviours are not excessive as they are with BN–purging type.

restraint, hunger, and negative affective states. Although obesity affects approximately 65% of clients with BED and increases progressively over time (Yager, 2008), overweight and obesity are not diagnostic criteria.

According to the *DSM-IV* (2000), the frequency criterion for binge eating with BED is the same as with BN. One difference between BED and BN is that BED binge eating episodes may last the entire day rather than occur in a discrete period of time, whereas binge eating episode with purging BN is terminated by vomiting or laxative misuse (Mitchell, Devlin, De Zwaan, Crow, & Peterson, 2008). A difference between BED and nonpurging BN is that BED binge eating is more apt to preceed rather than follow dieting behaviour.

BINGE EATING DISORDER IN SPECIAL POPULATIONS

BED affects 20% to 30% of those attending university or medical centre weight reduction programs. Children appear more likely to have BED than BN (APA, 2000). BED is more prevalent in certain clinical populations, including diabetes (Yager & Powers, 2007).

EPIDEMIOLOGY

BED in individuals with type 2 diabetes is more common than AN or BN. Lifetime prevalence in community populations is estimated to be 3.5% among women and 2% among men (Hudson, Hiripi, Pope, & Kessler, 2007).

Age of Onset

Binge eating occurs in young children. Lamerz et al. (2005) found that 2% of parents of 1,979 German children aged 5 to 6 years reported their child's binge eating episodes and a significant relationship between binge eating and obesity. In this and other studies, dieting behaviour was neither prominent nor preceded the onset of binge eating (Bindford, Mussell, Peterson, Crow, & Mitchell, 2004; Grilo & Masheb, 2000). Using the data from the Canadian Community Health Survey in 2002, women aged 15 years or older, identified as being concerned about their weight, were younger and more likely to be overweight or obese than nonweight concerned women (Park & Beaudet, 2008).

Gender Differences

A ratio of 1.5 females to 1 male experience BED.

Ethnic and Cultural Differences

There does not appear to be a significant difference in the prevalence of BED by ethnicity. BED is considered as common among American black women as among white women (Mitchell et al., 2008). Other races have not been studied.

Familial Differences

Approximately 20% of relatives of individuals with BED experience BED while 10% of relatives do not. First-degree relatives report significantly higher lifetime rates of anxiety disorders, mood disorders (in particular, bipolar I or II disorder, and any depressive disorder) and eating disorders than the first-degree relatives of those without BED (Hudson et al., 2006; Lilenfeld, Ringham, Kalarchian, & Marcus, 2008). Elevated lifetime rates of any substance use disorder and dysthymic disorder were more prevalent among female relatives of women with BED when compared with those of women without BED.

Comorbidity

The most common comorbid conditions are mood and anxiety disorders. Grilo, White, and Masheb (2009) found, overall, 74% of inpatients with BED had at least one additional lifetime psychiatric disorder and 43% had at least one current psychiatric disorder. Mood (in particular depression) and anxiety (in particular panic attacks) were the most common lifetime and current comorbidity; substance use disorders were infrequent.

Complications

Medical complications of BED include obesity, diabetes, hypertension, high cholesterol, gallbladder disease, kidney disease and/or failure, heart disease, arthritis, certain types of cancer, bone deterioration, menstrual irregularities, ovarian abnormalities, complications of pregnancy, depression, anxiety, and suicidal thoughts. Obese individuals with BED may also experience the consequences of stigma such as increased risk of depression, economic hardship, isolation, and social withdrawal. These stigmatized individuals have negative body image, poorer psychosocial functioning, and higher incidence of binge eating. Similarly, in a community sample of 1st year university students, women who gained weight experienced greater body dissatisfaction and drive for thinness compared to those who lost or maintained weight (Provencher et al., 2009). A source of stigma may be the causal beliefs that both the public (Potestio, McLaren, Vollman, & Doyle-Baker, 2008) and health professionals (Vallis, Currie, Laylor, & Ransom, 2007) hold about the etiology of obesity, causing obese individuals to be seen as less attractive and to blame for their weight and any weight loss failures. In another study of the public's beliefs about the nature and treatment of BED, Mond and Hay (2008) found that (a) BED was perceived by the general public as a problem of low-self esteem or depression, (b) medication and therapy were not highly regarded, and (c) primary care practitioners were favoured over mental health specialists as treatment providers. Such attitudes and beliefs influence how individuals with BED engage in help-seeking behaviours and because of these biases, obese persons with BED may be at greater risk for receiving compromised treatment (Bannon, Hunter-Reel, Wilson, & Karlin, 2009).

ETIOLOGY

Research of the etiology of BED is limited. Preliminary studies suggest overweight and obesity are risk factors. However, other studies that have found a moderate heritability for BED (e.g., Bulik, 2005) argue against the notion that obesity causes binge eating or vice versa. It is postulated that binge eating functions to modulate negative emotional states.

Biologic Theories

The main difference between BED and the other eating disorders is that individuals with BED exhibit lower eating restraint (Wilfrey, Schwartz, Spurrell, & Fairburn, 2000). No subjective differences in ratings of hunger and satiety between those with BED and obese controls were found when instructed to binge eat, and visual cues of the amount consumed and control of meal size were eliminated (Samuels, Zimmerli, Devlin, Kissileff, & Walsh, 2009).

Genetic

A genetic component is believed to influence risk. Heritability estimates for BED are 41% (Reichborn-Kjennerud, Bulik, Tambs, & Harris, 2004).

Psychological and Social Theories

Negative mood precedes binge eating and deterioration of mood follows binge eating, and this suggests that affect regulation difficulties are likely lead to binge eating and that binge eating may not be effective for regulating overall mood (Hilbert & Tuschen-Caffier, 2007). Nonetheless, some individuals describe experiences of dissociation and "numbing out" while binge eating (Yager & Powers, 2007, p. 23). Obese individuals with BED are more likely to request for professional psychological help than obese nonbinge eaters. Their greater sense of social insecurity and the impairment in interpersonal relationships associated with overweight condition may contribute to this issue, and the intrinsic feeling of ineffectiveness and self-deprecation maintained by social stigmatization promotes the vicious circle leading to binge eating through negative feedback on self-esteem.

Cognitive Theory

Increasing evidence indicates that dysfunctional attitudes regarding eating, weight, and shape are as central to BED as to AN and BN (Ramacciotti et al., 2008). Indeed, the majority of individuals seeking treatment for BED reported regularly pinching the areas of their bodies to check for fatness and avoiding clothing that enhanced body awareness (Reas, Grilo, Masheb, & Wilson, 2005). Extreme concern with weight and shape, in combination with low self-esteem, may lead some people to adopt, or think they should adopt, rigid dietary rules and restrict eating in unrealistic ways. This propensity for setting unrealistic aims in regard to body appearance and food intake, unsuccessful striving to meet them, and equating lack of complete achievement with abject failure can be the seed for the disruption of eating behaviour. Dietary restraint (discussed in BN) is thought to decrease energy and increase hunger and craving, leading to binge eating behaviours. *Disinhibition* occurs once the "diet" is broken: the individual will no longer maintain control, and compensating through overeating occurs (Dolan & Ford, 1991). Because of the inflexibility of these eating schemes, any minor transgression can lead to an all-or-nothing reaction, such that all attempts to control eating are abandoned, resulting in a binge. The tendency to evaluate self-worth in terms of weight and shape and a dichotomous (black-and-white) thinking style, together with having unrealistic weight goals, low self-efficacy, poor coping, or problem-solving skills, have been identified as significant psychological predictors of weight regain in obesity (Ramacciotti et al., 2008).

Spiritual Underpinnings

Dieting, central to the thinness ideal, detracts from underlying reasons for eating without being hungry. Such reasons include "neglect, lack of trust, lack of love, sexual abuse, physical abuse, unexpressed rage, grief, being the object of discrimination, and protection from getting hurt again" (Roth, 1992, p. 4). It is difficult to express these needs and individuals. When dieting results in binge eating and individuals plan for a binge, they often hide their food and eating from others, thus increasing their sense of disconnection from self and others.

■ RISK FACTORS

The risk or predisposing factors for BED are included in Figure 23-3.

■ INTERDISCIPLINARY TREATMENT

The treatment methods for BED in current use include CBT, interpersonal psychotherapy, medications, self-help support groups, and commercial weight loss and exercise programs. Surgical interventions are recommended for morbidly obese (BMI > 40) adult clients for whom other weight loss attempts have failed (Lau, 2007). Individual or group CBT has been found to reduce binge eating with abstinence for 4 months following treatment, but it did not result in weight loss (Brownley, Berkman, Sedway, Lohr, & Bulik, 2007). Medications may contribute to the treatment of BED. Both clients and treatment providers have identified that improving self-esteem, improving body experience, and learning problem solving skills are core to recovery (Vanderlinden, Buis, Pieters, & Probst, 2006).

As with the treatment of AN and BN, a comprehensive interdisciplinary approach is needed. The treatment goals focus on reducing binge eating, effecting and maintaining weight loss if overweight or obese, restructuring dysfunctional thinking about food and appearance, alleviating comorbid depression and anxiety, and addressing harassment. Treatment occurs in an outpatient setting, except for the rare time the client is hospitalized for bariatric surgery.

Nutrition counselling is an important treatment component focusing on portion size and control, the role of emotions on eating behaviours, healthy food and nutrient choices, self-monitoring, and strategies to delay binge eating. The therapy focuses on changing problematic behaviours and dysfunctional thinking using CBT and addressing underlying issues, such as low self-esteem, lack of assertiveness, and harassment. Clients may also access commercial weight loss and fitness programs as well as self-help support groups. Alternative therapies such as relaxation and yoga, monitored by holistic health professionals, also may be helpful.

■ PRIORITY CARE ISSUES

Comorbid obesity, overweight, depression, and anxiety can contribute to cardiac and other health crises. The risk of type 2 diabetes is significant in the presence of obesity.

■ NURSING MANAGEMENT: HUMAN RESPONSE TO BINGE EATING DISORDER

The primary nursing diagnoses for patients with BED may include Imbalanced Nutrition: More Than Body Requirements, Impaired Physical Mobility, Activity Intolerance, Anxiety, Ineffective Coping, and Ineffective Health Maintenance. The nurse establishes a therapeutic relationship and through this connection helps monitor the client's self-care abilities including dietary intake and activity, teaches and models effective problem solving, and makes nutritional recommendations, taking into account the client's individual needs.

Therapeutic Relationship

Individuals with BED may experience a great deal of shame and guilt in response to negative judgments of their eating behaviours, overweight, and obesity. They often are reluctant to participate in formal fitness programs for fear of being ridiculed. They may opt out of such programs when they believe they have nothing in common with other group members. Often those who have BED suffer with the disorder for years, feeling very lonely. The nurse builds a relationship of trust through modelling self-acceptance, nonjudgmental approach, and discussing the role of the nurse–client relationship in regard to the goals of therapy (see Chapter 9).

Biologic Domain

Most individuals with BED become overweight or obese. The medical consequences of cardiovascular disease, diabetes, and arthritis as well as other health threats are considered in all aspects of the nursing process.

Assessment

The nurse should assess current binge eating patterns and associated symptoms. In a population-based survey of 4,096 community residents, where 6.1% reported BED symptoms, BED was independently associated with acid regurgitation, heartburn, dysphagia, bloating, upper abdominal pain, diarrhea, urgency, constipation, and feeling of anal blockage. These symptoms may interfere with sleep (Lyons, 1998). Two implications from this work are that clients presenting with GI symptoms be questioned regarding BED, and clients presenting with BED be screened for GI symptoms. Psychosocial-spiritual assessment is also warranted given the likelihood of comorbid depression, anxiety, and stigmatization.

Nursing Diagnoses for Biologic Domain

Imbalanced Nutrition: More Than Body Requirements, Impaired Physical Mobility, and Activity Intolerance are examples of nursing diagnoses for the biologic domain.

Interventions for Biologic Domain

Clients are asked to record their intake, binges, and feelings associated with food and eating to form a foundation for changing behaviours with CBT. As noted above, symptoms of gastric distress should be assessed. Clients should be monitored for associated complications such as diabetes, cardiovascular disease, and arthritis. Physical mobility, activity, and sleep patterns are evaluated.

Pharmacologic Interventions

Sibutramine, topiramate, and orlistat are currently used in the long-term treatment of obesity. Other medications, usually SSRIs, may treat anxiety and depression symptomatology. Prozac is often used to reduce binge eating (see Box 23-13).

Teaching Points

Individuals taking the aforementioned weight loss agents should be informed that weight will be regained if the medication is stopped unless lifestyle interventions which include physical activity and stress management are incorporated. Those taking orlistat should be instructed to expect looser greasy stools. The instructions for SSRI use are contained in Chapter 14.

Psychosocial Domain

Assessment

Psychological assessment for the individual with BED is similar to that for the individual with BN, requiring identification of cognitive distortions and knowledge deficits. Dissociation is evaluated given the self-reports of binge eating to "numb out." Symptoms of anxiety and mood disorders are explored in-depth (see Chapters 20 and 21).

Nursing Diagnoses for Psychosocial Domain

Common diagnoses for the psychosocial domain include Anxiety, Ineffective Coping, Deficient Knowledge, and Social Isolation.

Interventions for Psychosocial Domain

Behavioural interventions, including CBT, are moderately effective for treating BED (Brownley et al., 2007). Clients are taught the techniques to monitor and change their eating habits, as well as to change the way they respond to difficult and stressful situations. CBT was found to decrease the number of binge days, the number of binge episodes, and psychological features of BED such as hunger and disinhibition.

Family

Individuals with binge eating consider family support of the utmost importance (Lyons, 1998). However, there is little research into family needs, and families may need support themselves.

Psychoeducation

The nurse can assist the individual with BED to eat appropriately portioned meals regularly to reduce hunger and binge eating. Individuals also need information about the medical consequences of binge eating. Other topics for psychoeducation are included in Box 23-16.

BOX 23.16

Psychoeducation Checklist: Binge Eating Disorder

When caring for the individual with BED, consider the following topics:

- Health and lifestyle.
- How weight reduction can be attained.
- Applied knowledge about food and healthy eating.
- Principles of dieting.
- The importance of being present of one's body and choices.
- Relaxation techniques.
- Stress management.
- The importance of physical activity.
- Strength training; instruction and practical exercises.
- Accessing resources; computers as an aid in eating well and achieving nutritional goals.
- Planning for holidays.

Teaching Points

Keeping in mind that many BED clients are overweight or obese and may have experienced harassment, psychoeducation focuses on principles of dieting, lifestyle changes to maintain weight loss, the importance of being cognizant of one's body, relaxation techniques, strength training, and how to deal with stress. Studies report a high attrition rate for psychoeducational programs (e.g., Stahre, Tärnell, Håkanson, & Hällström, 2007). Therefore, attending to client emotional comfort, briefing, and debriefing must be considered.

Spiritual Domain

Assessment

The nurse assesses the client's lifestyle choices, watchful of expressions of self-judgment and self-acceptance, enabling the client to describe any painful traumatic experiences with harassment and discrimination as well as associated feelings and responses. The nurse listens to stories of exclusion and development interruption in obese BED clients who were denied opportunities for multidimensional growth through extracurricular activities such as shopping for clothing, party invitations, and participating in recreational/sporting events.

Nursing Diagnoses for Spiritual Domain

Potential diagnoses for the spiritual domain include Ineffective Protection: Reduced Quality of Life and Impaired Self-Identity. The individual with BED who may binge eat in response to various biopsychosocial experiences, environmental cues, trauma and nonevents, struggles to protect himself or herself from such underlying issues as isolation and discrimination, filling himself or herself with food without awareness of deeper unmet identity needs.

Interventions for Spiritual Domain

Give BED clients the opportunities to discuss their experiences of stress, relationship conflict, and trauma. Support them to narrate themes of disappointment and pain in response to stigma. Through the safety of the nurse–client relationship, they can develop their capacity to reconnect with themselves, with others, and, when appropriate, the larger universal life force. The nurse may anticipate the need to provide anticipatory guidance for individuals to catch up missed developmental milestones such as dating and intimacy (Ciliska, 1990). Helping them attend to their growth and well-being during the course of treatment may help reduce depression and anxiety, relationship distress, social role conflict, and eating disorder symptoms. (Scott Richards et al., 2006).

■ EVALUATION AND TREATMENT OUTCOMES

Those with BED may find it harder than other people to continue weight loss treatment (Yager, 2008). In addition, they may be more likely to regain weight quickly. These are some of the reasons that people with BED may require the treatment that focuses on their binge eating before they try to lose weight. Even those who are not overweight are frequently distressed by their binge eating and may benefit from treatment.

Studies of the natural course of BED reveal that at 12- to 13-year follow-up approximately 8% to 10% were still affected by BED while 67% to 69% no longer met the *DSM-IV* criteria for an eating disorder (Fichter, Quadflieg, & Hedlund, 2008; Wade, Bergin, Tiggemann, Bulik, & Fairburn, 2006). Studies comparing various methods have found that medication and behavioural interventions were moderately effective while self-help and other interventions were not (Brownley et al., 2007).

■ CONTINUUM OF CARE

Individuals do not require hospitalization for BED. However, the consequence of obesity may involve hospitalization for surgical intervention such as gastric bypass or gastric banding surgery (Hydock, 2005). The treatment may take place over many years (see Chapter 4).

PREVENTION OF EATING DISORDERS

Eating disorders are among the most preventable mental disorders. National eating disorder awareness and advocacy groups work toward educating the general public, those at risk, and those who work with groups at risk, such as teachers and coaches. They also monitor the media and work to remove unhealthy advertisements and articles that appear in magazines appealing to vulnerable individuals. A list of online resources and some programs and their purposes is found in the Web Links section at the end of this chapter.

Prevention and early detection strategies for parents and schoolteachers are often the focus of school nurses and community mental health nurses. Specific strategies to promote positive body image in young children include a children's picture book called *Shapesville* which was found to increase the appearance satisfaction and awareness of healthy eating in 5- to 9-year-old girls (Dohnt & Tiggemann, 2008) and a peer program whereby older students (4th to 7th grade) were taught to teach younger (kindergarten—3rd grade) buddies about nutrition, physical activity, and healthy body image (Stock et al., 2007). Successful overweight and obesity prevention programs are delivered in school settings with program leaders having access to specialist support (Kirk, Bornstein, Navarro, & Swanson, 2009). For example, a school intervention program targeting children in grades 4 to 6 over a 2-year period and including components of nutrition education, nutrition policy, social marketing, and parent outreach resulted in a 50% reduction in the incidence of overweight (Foster et al., 2008). The researchers recommended further research focus (a) on school environment (e.g., physical education classes) and environment beyond schools (e.g., corner stores, fast food outlets, homes) and (b) with younger ages given the high prevalence of children expressing body dissatisfaction in grades 4 to 6 and the rising Canadian obesity epidemic.

Other strategies for parents and children appear in Table 23-7 and are based on research of risk factors and protective factors. These protective factors, such as confidence and healthy competition in athletics, have been shown to prevent the development of an eating disorder for individuals at risk (Taylor et al., 1998). Dieting, low self-esteem, and body dissatisfaction are examples of risk factors underlying the development of eating disorders that can be reversed with early identification and intervention.

Society has begun to engage in an effort to help young individuals resist developing eating disorders. Many of the Web links listed at the end of this chapter have online help and resources for young individuals, families, teachers, and health care professionals.

Table 23.7 Prevention Strategies for Parents and Children

Parents Education	Children Education
Real versus ideal weight	Peer pressure regarding eating and weight
Influence of attitudes, behaviours, and teasing	Menses, puberty, and normal weight gain
Ways to increase self-esteem	Strategies for obesity
Role of media: TV and magazines	Ways to develop or improve self-esteem
Signs and symptoms	Body image traps: media and retail clothing
Interventions for obesity	Adapting and coping with problems
Boys at risk also	Reporting friends with signs of eating disorders
Observe for rituals	**Screening** for risk factors
Supervision of eating and exercise	**Assessment** for treatment
	Follow-up: monitor for relapse

SUMMARY OF KEY POINTS

☐ AN, BN, and BED have some common symptoms but are classified as discrete disorders in the *DSM-IV-TR*.

☐ Eating disorders are best viewed along a continuum that includes subclinical or partial-syndrome disorders; because these disorders occur more frequently than full syndromes, they are often overlooked but, once identified, can be prevented from worsening.

☐ Similar factors predispose individuals to the development of AN, BN, and BED, and these factors represent a bio/psycho/social/spiritual model of risk and threaten spiritual health and well-being. These disorders are preventable, and identifying risk factors assists with prevention strategies.

☐ Etiologic factors contribute in combination to the development of eating disorders; no one factor provides an explanation.

☐ Mood and anxiety disorders are significantly more frequent in individuals with eating disorders than the general community.

☐ All of the eating disorders have physical, emotional, social, and spiritual consequences that threaten health, well-being, and even life.

☐ Treatment of AN almost always includes hospitalization for refeeding; BN and BED are treated primarily on an outpatient basis.

☐ For individuals with BN, CBT improves symptoms sooner than does IPT, and CBT is most effective when combined with medication. For individuals with anorexia, family therapy plus individual IPT are the most effective. Research on best practice for BED is in its infancy.

☐ Pharmacotherapy can be effective for BN but less so for AN, especially during acute malnourishment.

☐ Individuals with eating disorders require responsive treatment addressing both specific (e.g., eating behaviour) and nonspecific (e.g., underlying) vulnerabilities.

☐ The outcomes for BN are better than those for AN and BED. The type and severity of comorbid conditions and the length of the illness influence outcomes.

CRITICAL THINKING CHALLENGES

1 Discuss the potential difficulties and risks in attempting to treat a client with AN in an outpatient setting.

2 A client in the clinic is examined for BN and is prescribed fluoxetine. She reports great success immediately and attributes this to the weight lost. What are your concerns and interventions?

3 The nurse caring for an overweight BED client is obese himself. How can nurses be supported to examine personal attitudes, biases, and experiences with weight gain and loss? What are the dangers of not engaging in this type of self-development?

4 Parents are often in need of support and suggestions for how to help prevent eating disorders. Develop a teaching program and include the topics and rationale for the suggestions chosen.

5 Identify the important nursing management components of a refeeding program for a hospitalized individual with AN.

6 Bulimia nervosa is often described as a closet disorder with secretive binge eating and purging. Identify the signs and symptoms of each system involved for someone with this disorder.

7 Amid extensive health policy and programming to address global obesity, how do nurses best advocate for the needs of individuals and families affected by anorexia and BN?

8 Positive outcomes for the recovery of BED, BN, and AN are dependent on many factors. Identify the factors that promote positive outcomes and those related to poorer outcomes and prognosis.

WEB LINKS

www.nedic.ca National Eating Disorder Information Centre (NEDIC), CW 1-211, 200 Elizabeth Street, Toronto, ON, M5G 2C4. This site provides information and resources for individuals, families, friends, and teachers on eating disorders and weight preoccupation. It offers an information and support telephone line at (416) 340–4156.

www.bana.ca Bulimia Anorexia Nervosa Association (BANA), University of Windsor, Windsor ON. The BANA site has information on specialized treatment

education, support services for individuals affected directly and indirectly by eating disorders, and prevention of eating disorders, negative body image, and low self-esteem.

www.sheenasplace.org Sheena's Place, 87 Spadina Road, Toronto, ON M5R 2T1. This site describes Sheena's Place, Canada's first community-based centre to offer services at no cost to people affected by severe eating and body image issues. The site provides information and support to parents, siblings, friends, spouses, partners, teachers, and other care providers.

www.something-fishy.org A website about Eating Disorders that is dedicated to raising awareness, emphasizing that Eating Disorders are NOT about food and weight; they are just the symptoms of something deeper going on, inside.

www.disorderedeating.ca The Eating Disorder Resource Centre of British Columbia provides educational, referral and research services to people struggling with disordered eating, their support networks, community-based organizations, students, educators, and professionals.

kidshelp.sympatico.ca (1-800-668-6868) This Kids Help Phone site offers a toll-free, national telephone counselling service for Canadian children and youth experiencing violence, alcohol or drug abuse, issues related to suicide, or suffering from an eating disorder. It features tips for parents and others.

MOVIES, NOVELS, AND BIOGRAPHIES

Through True Eyes: Process of Recovery from Eating Disorders: **2007.** This 23-minute documentary based on the research of Dr. Kate Weaver (University of New Brunswick, Canada) portrays the stories of three women who have successfully battled eating disorders. The stories describe how trauma and life pressures can lead to a sense of having no control, and how eating disorders compensate with a sense of artificial control.

VIEWING POINTS: Consider the thought processes of those struggling with ED. Do you think that it was right that two of the women with AN received medical care against their will? Are you able to identify from the women's stories that denial by friends, family, and even naïve health care practitioners evokes a sense of loneliness and isolation?

Killing Us Softly 3: Advertising's Image of Women: **2000.** This 32-minute documentary illustrates and critiques over 160 ads and TV commercials that portray women in narrowly defined and marginalized ways. Themes include body image, objectification of women, trivialization of women's power, sexuality, pornography, and violence. Although the film is mainly about women, it suggests the effects of a media culture that limits men's emotion.

VIEWING POINTS: Corporations and their advertisers use images of girls and women to sell products. How does this contribute to eating disorders? What is the possible impact on older women and women considered overweight who do not measure up to media images of beauty? Do advertisers have a responsibility to society regarding the attitudes that their images support?

Slim Hopes: Advertising & the Obsession with Thinness: **1995.** This award-winning short film deconstructs the way female bodies are depicted in advertising images and the negative effects of these images on women's health. There are six themes entitled: Impossible beauty, Waif look, Constructed bodies, Food & sex, Food & control, Weight loss industry, and Freeing imaginations.

VIEWING POINTS: The thin ideal for women portrayed in the media fosters body dissatisfaction because it is unobtainable by most women. What are the costs of this dissatisfaction to health and society? What cultural expectations for women and for men underlie the media messages? What effect do the media messages and associated expectations have on how boys and men view and relate to girls and women, and to themselves? What is the effect on how girls and women view and relate to boys and men, and to themselves? What can nurses do to help clients resist these harmful media messages? What can nurses do to help themselves?

REFERENCES

Ahzern, A. L., Bennett, K. M., and Hetherington, M. M. (2008). Internalization of the ultra-thin ideal: Positive implicit associations with underweight fashion models are associated with drive for thinness in young women. *Eating Disorders, 16,* 294–307.

Aja, S. (2006). Serotonin-3 receptors in gastric mechanisms of cholecystokinin-induced satiety. *American Journal of Physiological Regulatory Integrative Comprehensive Physiology, 291*(1), R112–R114.

American Psychiatric Association. (1987). *Diagnostic and statistical manual of mental disorders (DSM-III)* (3rd ed.). Washington, DC: Author.

American Psychiatric Association. (2000). *Diagnostic and statistical manual of mental disorders* (4th ed., Text revision). Washington, DC: Author.

American Psychiatric Association. (2006a). *Practice guideline for the treatment of patients with eating disorders* (3rd ed.). Washington (DC): Author. Available from the American Psychiatric Association Web site.

American Psychiatric Association. (2006b). *American Psychiatric Association practice guidelines for the treatment of psychiatric disorders.* Washington, DC: Author.

Anderluk, M. B., Tchanturia, K., Rabe-Hesketh, S., & Treasure, J. (2003). Childhood obsessive-compulsive personality traits in adult women with eating disorders: Defining a broader eating disorder phenotype. *American Journal of Psychiatry, 160*(2), 242–247.

Anderson, A. (2001). Progress in eating disorder research. *American Journal of Psychiatry, 158,* 515–517.

Andersen, A., & Yager, J. (2005). Eating disorders. In B. J. Saddock & V. A. Saddock (Eds.), *Kaplan & Saddock's comprehensive textbook of psychiatry* (8th ed., pp. 2002–2021). Philadelphia, PA: Lippincott Williams & Wilkins.

Andrist, L. (2003). Media images, body dissatisfaction, and disordered eating in adolescent women. *American Journal of Maternal/Child Nursing, 28*(2), 119–123.

Anorexics and Bulimics Anonymous. (2002). *The Loonie Theory.* In *The fellowship details its program of recovery for anorexia and bulimia* (pp. 37–44). Edmonton, AB: Author.

Anschutz, D. J., Van Strien, T., & Engels, R. C. M. E. (2008). Exposure to slim images in mass media: Television commercials as reminders of restriction in restrained eaters. *Health Psychology, 27,* 401–408.

Arrow, B., Kenardy, J., & Agras, W. S. (1995). The emotional eating scale: The development of a measure to assess coping with negative affect by eating. *Internationl Journal of Eating Disorders, 18,* 79–90.

Bailer, U. F., & Kaye, W. H. (2003). A review of neuropeptide and neuroendocrine dysregulation in anorexia and bulimia nervosa. *Current Drug Targets CNS Neuronal Disorders, 2*(1), 53–59.

Bannon, K. L., Hunter-Reel, D., Wilson, T., & Karlin, R. A. (2009). The effects of causal beliefs and binge eating on the stigmatization of obesity. *International Journal of Eating Disorders, 42,* 118–124.

Bell, R. M. (1985). *Holy anorexia.* Chicago, IL: University of Chicago Press.

Berkman, N. D., Lohr, K. N., & Bulik, C. M. (2007). Outcomes of eating disorders: A systematic review of the literature. *International Journal of Eating Disorders, 40,* 293–309.

Berrett, M. E., Hardman, R. K., O'Grady, K., & Scott Richards, P. (2007). The Role of Spirituality in the Treatment of Trauma and Eating Disorders: Recommendations for Clinical Practice. *Eating Disorders, 15,* 373–389.

Binford, R. B., Mussell, M. P., Peterson, C. B., Crow, S. J., & Mitchell, J. E. (2004). Relation of binge eating age of onset to functional aspects of binge eating in binge eating disorder. *International Journal of Eating Disorders, 35,* 286–292.

Birmingham, C. L., Su, J., Hlynsky, J. A., Goldner, E. M., & Gao, M. (2005). The mortality rate from anorexia nervosa. *International journal of Eating Disorders, 38,* 143–146.

Bohon, C., Stice, E., & Burton, E. (2009). Maintenance factors for persistence of bulimic pathology: a prospective natural history study. *International Journal of Eating Disorders, 42,* 173–178.

Braun, D. L., Sunday, S. R., Huang, A., & Halmi, K. A. (1999). More males seek treatment for eating disorders. *International Journal of Eating Disorders, 25*(4), 415–424.

Brown, K. E., & Geller, J. (2006). Supporting friends and family members with eating disorders: discrepancies between intentions and reality. *Eating Disorders, 14,* 215–228.

Brownley, K. A., Berkman, N. D., Sedway, J. A., Lohr, K. N., & Bulik, C. M. (2007). Binge eating disorder treatment: A systematic review of randomized controlled trials. *International Journal of Eating Disorders, 40,* 337–348.

Bruch, H. (1973). *Eating disorders: Obesity, anorexia nervosa and the person within.* New York, NY: Basic Books.

Buchholz, A., Mack, H., McVey, G., Feder, S., & Barrowman, N. (2008). BodySense: An evaluation of a positive body image intervention on sport climate for female athletes. *Eating Disorders, 16,* 308–321.

Bulik, C. M. (2005). Exploring the gene-environment nexus in eating disorders. *Journal of Psychiatry & Neuroscience, 30,* 335–339.

Bulik, C. M., Sullivan, P., Wade, T., & Kendler, K. (2000). Twin studies of eating disorders: A review. *International Journal of Eating Disorders, 27,* 1–20.

Castro-Fornieles, J., Casula, V., Saura, B. Martinez, E., Lazaro, L., Vila, M., et al. (2007). Predictors of weight maintenance after hospital discharge in adolescent anorexia nervosa. *International Journal of Eating Disorders, 40,* 129–136.

Ciliska, D. (1990). *Beyond dieting: Psychoeducational interventions for chronically obese women.* Brunner/Mazzel Eating Disorders Monograph Series, 5. New York: Taylor & Francis.

Cooper, P., Taylor, M., Cooper, Z., & Fairburn, C. (1987). The development and validation of the BSQ. *International Journal of Eating Disorders, 6,* 485–494.

Costanzo, P. R., Musante, G. J., Friedman, K. E., Kern, L. S., & Tomlinson, K. (1999). The gender specificity of emotional, situational, and behavioral indicators of binge eating in a diet-seeking obese population. *International Journal of Eating Disorders, 26*(2), 205–210.

Croll, J., Neumark-Sztainer, D., Story, M., & Ireland, M. (2002). Prevalence and risk and protective factors related to disordered eating behaviors among adolescents: Relationship to gender and ethnicity. *Journal of Adolescent Health, 13*(2), 166–175.

Dallos, R., & Denford, S. (2008). A qualitative exploration of relationship and attachment themes in families with an eating disorder. *Clinical Child Psychology & Psychiatry, 13,* 305–322.

Davis, C., Katzman, D. K., & Kirsch, C. (1999). Compulsive physical activity with anorexia nervosa: A psycho-behavioural spiral of pathology. *Journal of Nervous and Mental Diseases, 187*(6), 336–342.

Davis, C., Katzman, D. K., Kaptein, S., Kirsh, C., Brewer, H., Kalmbach, K., et al. (1997). The prevalence of high-level exercise in the eating disorders: Etiological implications. *Comprehensive Psychiatry, 38*(6), 321–326.

Davis, C., Shuster, B., Blackmore, E., & Fox, J. (2004). Looking good—family focus on appearance and the risk for eating disorders. *International Journal of Eating Disorders, 35*, 136–144.

Dell, M. L., & Josephson, A. M. (2007). Religious and spiritual factors in childhood and adolescent eating disorders and obesity. *Southern Medical Association, 100*, 628–632.

Diamond-Raab, L., & Orrell-Valente, J. K. (2002) Art therapy, psychodrama and verbal therapy: An integrative model of group therapy in the treatment of adolescents with anorexia nervosa and bulimia nervosa. *Child and Adolescent Psychiatric Clinics of North America, 11*(2), 343–364.

Dimitropoulos, G., Carter, J., Schachter, R., & Woodside, D. B. (2008). Predictors of family functioning in carers of individuals with anorexia nervosa. *International Journal of Eating Disorders, 41*, 739–747.

Dittmar, H., Halliwell, E., & Ive, S. (2006). Does Barbie make girls want to be thin? The effect of experimental exposure to images of dolls on the body image of 5- to 8- year-old girls. *Developmental Psychology, 42*, 283–292.

Dohnt, H., & Tiggermann, M. (2008). Promoting positive body image in young girls: An evaluation of 'Shapesville.' *European Eating Disorder Review, 16*, 222–233.

Dolan, B. & Ford, K. (1991). Binge eating and dietary restraint: A cross-cultural analysis. *International Journal of Eating Disorders, 10*, 345–353.

Dunn, P. K., & Ondercin, P. (1981). Personality variables related to compulsive eating in college women. *Journal of Clinical Psychology, 31*, 43–49.

Eckert, E. D., Halmi, K. A., Marchi, P., Grove, W., & Crosby, R. (1995). Ten-year follow-up of anorexia nervosa: Clinical course and outcome. *Psychological Medicine, 25*, 143–156.

Eddy, K. T., Dorer, D. J., Franko, D. L., Tahilani, K., Thompson-Brenner, H., & Herzog, D. B. (2008). Diagnostic crossover in anorexia nervosa and bulimia nervosa: Implications for DSM-V. *American Journal of Psychiatry, 165*, 245–250.

Eisler, I., Dare, C., Hodes, M., Russell, G., Dodge, E., & LeGrange, D. (2000). Family therapy for adolescent anorexia nervosa: The results of a controlled comparison of two family interventions. *Journal of Child Psychology and Psychiatry, 41*, 727–736.

Feldman, M. B., & Meyer, I. H. (2007). Childhood abuse and eating disorders in gay and bisexual men. *International Journal of Eating Disorders, 40*, 418–423.

Fichter, M. M., & Quadflieg, N. (1999). Six-year course and outcome of anorexia nervosa. *International Journal of Eating Disorders, 26*(4), 359–385.

Fichter, M. M., Quadflieg, N., & Hedlund, S. (2008). Long-term course of binge eating disorder and bulimia nervosa: Relevance for nosology and diagnostic criteria. *International Journal of Eating Disorders, 41*, 577–586.

Foster, G. D., Sherman, S., Borradaile, K. E., Grundy, K. M., Vander Veur, S. S., & Nachmani, et al. (2008). A policy-based school intervention to prevent overweight and obesity. *Pediatrics, 121*, 794–802.

Gadalla, T. M. (2008). Eating disorders and associated psychiatric comorbidity in elderly Canadian women. *Archives of Womens Mental Health, 11*, 577–362.

Garner, D. (1997). Psychoeducational principles in treatment. In D. M. Garner & P. E. Garfinkel (Eds.), *Handbook of treatment for eating disorders* (2nd ed., pp. 145–177). New York, NY: Guilford Press.

Garner, D. M. (1991a). *Eating disorder inventory—2 professional manual.* Odessa, FL: Psychological Assessment Resources.

Garner, D. M. (1991b). *Eating disorder inventory—C.* Lutz, FL: Psychological Assessment Resources.

Garner, D. M., & Garfinkel, P. E. (1979). The Eating Attitude Test: An index of the symptoms of anorexia nervosa. *Psychosomatic Medicine, 10*, 647–656.

Garner, D. M., Olmsted, M. P., Bohr, Y., & Garfinkel, P. E. (1982). The Eating Attitude Test: Psychometric features and clinical correlates. *Psychological Medicine, 12*, 871–878.

Garrett, C. J. (1996). Recovery from anorexia nervosa: A Durkheimian interpretation. *Social Science Medicine, 10*, 1489–1506.

Gauvin, L., Steiger, H., & Brodeur, J-M. (2009). Eating-disorder symptoms and syndromes in a sample of urban-dwelling Canadian women: Contributions toward a population health perspective. *International Journal of Eating Disorders, 42*, 158–165.

Goldfield, G. S., Blouin, A. G., & Woodside, D. B. (2006). Body image, binge eating, and bulimia nervosa in male bodybuilders. *Canadian Journal of Psychiatry, 51*, 160–168.

Grilo, C. M., & Masheb, R. M. (2000). Onset of dieting *vs* binge eating in outpatients with binge eating disorder. *International Journal of Obesity, 24*, 404–409.

Grilo, C. M., White, M. A., & Masheb, R. M. (2009). DSM-IV psychiatric disorder comorbidity and its correlates in binge eating disorder. *International Journal of Eating Disorders, 42*, 228–234.

Greenleaf, C., Petrie, T. A., Carter, J., & Reel, J. J. (2009). Female collegiate athletes: prevalence of eating disorders and disordered eating behaviors. *Journal of American College Health, 57*, 489–495.

Grubbs, L. (1993). The critical role of exercise in weight control. *Nurse Practitioner, 18*(4), 20–29.

Gowers, S. G., & Shore, A. (1999). The stigma of eating disorders. *International Journal of Clinical Practice, 53*(5), 386–388.

Gucciardi, E., Wang, S. C., Badiani, T., & Stewart, D. E. (2007). Beyond adolescence: Exploring Canadian women and men's perception of overweight. *Women's Health Issues, 17*, 374–382.

Gustafsson, S. A., Edlund, B., Kjellin, L., & Norring, C. (2008). Personal standards, self-evaluation and perceived benefits of thinness in girls and young women with disturbed eating. *European Eating Disorders Review, 16*, 463–471.

Gutwill, S. (1994). Women's eating problems: Social context and the internalization of culture. In C. Bloom, L. Zaphiropdous, A. Gitter, S. Gutwill, & L. Kogel (Eds.), *Eating problems: A feminist psychoanalytic treatment model* (pp. 1–27). New York, NY: Basic Books.

Hagmar, M., Hirschberg, A. L., Berglund, L., & Berglund, B. (2008). Special attention to the weight-control strategies employed by Olympic athletes striving for leanness is required. *Clinical Journal of Sport Medicine, 18*, 5–9.

Hall, M. N., Friedman, R. J., II, & Leach, L. (2008). Treatment of Bulimia Nervosa. *American Family Physician, 77*(11), 1588, 1592. Retrieved April 11, 2009, from ProQuest Nursing & Allied Health Source database. (Document ID: 1486040891).

Harrington, E. F., Crowther, J. H., Payne Henrickson, H. C., & Mickelson, K. D. (2006). The relationships among trauma, stress, relationships, and binge eating. *Culture Diversity Ethnic Minority Psychology, 12*, 212–229.

Hatmaker, G. (2005). Boys with eating disorders. *Journal of School Nursing, 21*, 329–332.

Hawks, S. R., Gougy, M. B., & Gast, J. A. (2003). Emotional eating and spiritual well-being: A possible connection? *American Journal of Health Education, 34*, 30–33.

Hay, P. J., & Bacaltchuk, J. (2007). Bulimia Nervosa. *American Family Physician, 75*, 1699–1702.

Hay, P. P. J., Bacaltchuk. J., & Stefano, S. (2004/2009). Psychotherapy for bulimia nervosa and binging. *Cochrane Database of Systematic Reviews 2004*, Issue 3. Art. No.: CD000562. DOI: 10.1002/14651858.CD000562.pub2. Re-published online with edits: 21 January 2009 in Issue 1, 2009.

Health Canada. (2003). *Canadian community health survey.* Ottawa, ON: Statistics Canada.

Hendricks, P. S., & Thompson, J. K. (2005). An integration of cognitive-behavioral therapy and interpersonal psychotherapy for bulimia nervosa: a case study using the case formulation method. *International Journal of Eating Disorders, 37*, 171–174.

Herman, C. P., & Mack, D. (1975). Restrained and unrestrained eating. *Journal of Personality, 43*, 647–660.

Herzog, D. B., Greenwood, D. N., Dorer, D. J., Flores, A. T., Ekebald, E. R., Richards, A., et al. (2000). Mortality in eating disorders: A descriptive study. *International Journal of Eating Disorders, 28*, 20–26.

Hilbert, A., & Tuschen-Caffier, B. (2007). Maintenance of Binge Eating through Negative Mood: A Naturalistic Comparison of Binge Eating Disorder and Bulimia Nervosa. *International Journal of Eating Disorders, 40*, 521–530.

Hudson, J. I., Lalonde, J. K., Berry, J. M., Pindyck, L. J., Bulik, C. M., Crow, S. J., et al. (2006). Binge-eating disorder as a distinct familial phenotype in obese individuals, *Archives of General Psychiatry, 63*, 313–319.

Hudson, J. I., Hiripi, E., Pope, H. G., & Kessler, R. C. (2007). The prevalence and correlates of eating disorders in the national comorbidity survey replication. *Biological Psychiatry, 61*, 348–358.

Hydock, C. M. (2005). A brief overview of bariatric surgical procedures currently being used to treat the obese patient. *Critical Care Nursing Quarterly, 28*, 217–226.

Inches, P. R. (1895). Anorexia nervosa. *Maritime Medical News, 7*, 73–75.

Jensen, V. S., & Mejlhede, A. (2000). Anorexia nervosa treatment with olanzapine. *British Journal of Psychiatry, 177*(2), 87.

Johnson, F., & Wardle, J. (2005). Dietary restraint, body dissatisfaction, and psychological distress: A prospective study. *Journal of Abnormal Psychology, 114*, 119–125

Johnson, J. G., Cohen, P., Kasen, S., & Brook, J. S. (2002). Childhood adversities associated with risk for eating disorders or weight problems during adolescence or early adulthood. *American Journal of Psychiatry, 159*, 394–400.

Johnston, J. M. (2004). Over and above. Eating disorders and childhood obesity: Who are the real gluttons? *Canadian Medical Association Journal, 171*, 1459–1460.

Joiner, T. E., Katz, J., & Heatherton, T. F. (2000). Personality factors differentiate late adolescent females and males with chronic bulimic symptoms. *International Journal of Eating Disorders, 27*, 191–197.

Jonat, L. M., & Birmingham, C. L. (2004). Disordered eating attitudes and behaviours in the high-school students of a rural Canadian community. *Eating & Weight Disorders, 9*(4), 306–308.

Jordan, J., Joyce, P. R., Carter, F. A., Horn, J., McIntosh, V. V., Luty, S. E., et al. (2008). Specific and nonspecific comorbidity in anorexia nervosa. *International Journal of Eating Disorders, 41*, 47–56.

Kaplan, A. S., & Noble, S. (2007). Pharmacological approaches to the outpatient treatment of anorexia nervosa. In J. Yager & P. S. Powers (eds.), *Clinical manual of eating disorders* (pp. 138–142). Washington, DC: APA.

Kaye, W. H., Gendall, K. A., Fernstrom, M. H., Fernstrom, J. D., McConana, C. W., & Weltzin, T. E. (2000). Effects of acute tryptophan depletion on mood in bulimia nervosa. *Biological Psychiatry, 47*(2), 151–157.

Kaye, W. H., Klump, K. L., Frank, G. K., & Strober, M. (2000). Anorexia and bulimia. *Annual Review of Medicine, 51*, 299–313.

Keel, P. K., Dorer, D. J., Eddy, K. T., Charatan, D. L., & Herzog, D. B. (2003). Predictors of mortality in eating disorders. *Archives of General Psychiatry, 60*, 179–183.

Keery, H., Boutelle, K., van den Berg, P., & Thompson, K. (2005). The impact of appearance-related teasing by family members. *Journal of Adolescent Health, 37*, 120–127.

Keski-Rahkonen, A., Hoek, H., Linna, M., Raevuori, A., Sihvola, E., Bulik, C., et al. (2009). Incidence and outcomes of bulimia nervosa: a nationwide population-based study. *Psychological Medicine, 39*, 823–31.

Kirk, S., Bornstein, P., Navarro, E., & Swanson, E. (2009). *Effective non-clinical interventions to prevent and treat childhood overweight and obesity in Newfoundland and Labrador.* St. John's, NL: Newfoundland and Labrador Centre for Applied Health Research, Memorial University.

Klump, K. L. Bulik, C. M., Kaye, W. H., Treasure, J., & Tyson, E. (2009). Academy for eating disorders position paper: Eating disorders are serious mental illnesses. *International Journal of Eating Disorders, 42*, 97–103.

Korndorfer, S. R., Lucas, A. R., Suman, V. J., et al. (2003). Long-term survival of patients with anorexia nervosa: A population based study in Rochester, MN. *Mayo Clinic Proceedings, 78*(3), 278–284.

Lam, T. H., Lee, S. W., Fung, S., Ho, S. Y., Lee, P. W. H., & Stewart, S. M. (2009). Sociocultural influences on body dissatisfaction and dieting in Hong Kong girls. *European Eating Disorders Review, 17*, 152–160.

Lamerz, A., Kuepper-Nybelen, J., Wehle, C., Bruning, N., Trost-Brinkhues, G., Brenner, H., et al. (2005). Social class, parental education, and obesity prevalence in a study of six-year-old children in Germany. *International Journal of Obesity, 29*, 373–380.

Laporte, L., & Guttman, H. (2001). Abusive relationships in families of women with borderline personality disorder, anorexia nervosa and a control group. *Journal of Nervous and Mental Disease, 180*, 522–531.

Lau, D. C. W. (2007). Synopsis of the 2006 Canadian clinical practice guidelines on the management and prevention of obesity in adults and children. *Canadian Medical Association Journal, 176*, 1103–1106.

LaVia, M. C., Grey, M., & Kaye, W. H. (2000). Case reports of olanzapine treatment of anorexia nervosa. *International Journal of Eating Disorders, 27*, 363–366.

Lee, S., & Lee, A. M. (2000). Disordered eating in three communities of China: A comparative study of female high school students in Hong Kong, Shenzhen, and rural Hunan. *International Journal of Eating Disorders, 27*, 317–327.

Leonard, S., Steiger, H., & Kao, A. (2003). Childhood and adulthood abuse in bulimic and nonbulimic women: Prevalences and psychological correlates. *International Journal of Eating Disorders, 33*, 397–405.

Lilenfeld, L. R., Ringham, R., Kalarchian, M. A., & Marcus, M. (2008). A family history study of binge-eating disorder. *Comprehensive Psychiatry, 49*, 247–254.

Lyons, M. (1998). The phenomenon of compulsive overeating in a selected group of professional women. *Journal of Advanced Nursing, 27*, 1158–1164.

Maloney, M., McGuire, J., & Daniels, S. R. (1988). Reliability testing of a children's version of the Eating Attitude Test. *Journal of the American Academy of Child and Adolescent Psychiatry, 27*, 541–543.

Marsden, P., Karagianni, E., & Morgan, J. F. (2007). Spirituality and clinical care in eating disorders: A qualitative study. *International Journal of Eating Disorders, 40*, 7–12.

Martin, C. E. (2007). *Perfect girls, starving daughters: How the quest for perfection is harming young women.* New York, NY: Berkley.

Martz, D. M., Sturgis, E. T., & Gustafson, S. B. (1996). Development and preliminary validation of the Cognitive Behavioral Dieting Scale. *International Journal of Eating Disorders, 19*, 297–309.

Massey-Stokes, M. (2001). Communication, expressing feelings, and creative problem solving. In J. J. Robert-McComb (Ed.), *Eating disorders in women and children: Prevention, stress management, and treatment* (pp. 291–307). Boca Raton, FL: CRC Press.

May, A. L., Kim, J-Y., McHale, S., & Crouter, A. C. (2006). Parent-adolescent relationships and the development of weight concerns from early to late adolescence. *International Journal of Eating, 39*(8), 729–740.

Mazure, C. M., Halmi, K. A., Sunday, S. R., Romano, S. J., & Einhorn, A. M. (1994). Yale-Brown-Cornell Eating Disorder Scale: Development, use, reliability, and validity. *Journal of Psychiatric Research, 28*, 425–445.

McDonald, J. T., & Kennedy, S. (2005). Is immigration to Canada associated with unhealthy weight gain? Overweight and obesity among Canada's immigrants. *Social Science & Medicine, 61*, 2469–2481.

McElroy, S. L., Arnold, L. M., Shapira, N. A. Keck Jr., P. E., Rosenthal, N. R., Karim, M. R., et al. (2003). Topiramate in the treatment of binge eating disorder associated with obesity: A randomized, placebo-controlled trial. *American Journal of Psychiatry, 160*, 255–61.

McIntosh, V., Jordan, J., Carter, F. A., Luty, S. E., McKenzie, J. M., Bulik, C. M., et al. (2005). Three Psychotherapies for Anorexia Nervosa: A Randomized, Controlled Trial. *American Journal of Psychiatry, 162*, 741–747.

McVey, G., Tweed, S., & Blackmore, E. (2004). Dieting among preadolescent and young adolescent females. *Canadian Medical Association Journal, 170*, 1559–1561.

Meyer, J. S., Mehdirad, A., Salem, B. I., Jamry, W. A., Kulikowska, A., & Kulikowski, P. (2003). Sudden arrhythmia death syndrome: Importance of the long QT syndrome. *American Family Physician, 68*, 483–488, 417–419, 561.

Miller, M. N., & Pumariega, A. J. (2001). Culture and eating disorders: A historical and cross-cultural review. *Psychiatry, 64*(2), 93–110.

Milos, G., Spindler, A., Ruggiero, G., Klaghofer, R., & Schnyder, V. (2002). Comorbidity of obsessive-compulsive disorders and duration of eating disorders. *International Journal of Eating Disorders, 36*(3), 284–289.

Minuchin, S., Rossman, B. L., & Baker, L. (1978). *Psychosomatic families.* Cambridge, MA: Harvard University Press.

Miotto, P., Pollini, B., Restaneo, A., Favaretto, G., & Preti, A. (2008). Aggressiveness, anger, and hostility in eating disorders. *Comprehensive Psychiatry, 49*, 364–373.

Mitchell, J. E., Devlin, M. J., De Zwaan, M., Crow, S. J., & Peterson, C. B. (2008). *Binge-eating disorder: clinical foundations and treatment.* New York: Guilford.

Mond, J., & Hay, P. J. (2008). Public perceptions of binge eating and its treatment. *The International Journal of Eating Disorders, 41*, 419–426.

Morgan, J. C., Wolfe, B. E., Metzger, E. D., & Jimerson, D. C. (2007). Obsessive-compulsive characteristics in women who have recovered from bulimia nervosa. *International Journal of Eating Disorders, 40*, 381–385.

Muhlau, M., Gaser, C., Ilg, R., Conrad, B., Leibl, C., Cebulla, M. H., et al. (2007). Gray matter decreases of the anterior cingulate cortex in anorexia nervosa. *American Journal of Psychiatry, 164*, 1850–1857.

National Eating Disorder Information Centre. (1998). *Canadian children in grade three and four say they'd rather lose a parent, get cancer, or live through nuclear war than be fat* [Online.] Retrieved from *http://www.nedic.ca/*

Nilsson, K., Sundbom, E., & Hagglof, B. (2008). A longitudinal study of perfectionism in adolescent onset anorexia nervosa-restricting type. *European Eating Disorder Review, 16*, 386–394.

Ogden, J., & Steward, J. (2000). The role of the mother–daughter relationship in explaining weight concern. *International Journal of Eating Disorders, 28*(11), 78–83.

Orbach, S. (2004). What can we learn from the therapist's body? *Attachment & Human Development, 6,* 141–150.

Park, J., & Beaudet, M. P. (2007). Eating attitudes and their correlates among Canadian women concerned about their weight. *European Eating Disorders Review, 15,* 311–320.

Patching, J., & Lawler, J. (2009). Understanding women's experiences of developing an eating disorder and recovering: A life-history approach. *Nursing Inquiry, 16,* 10–21.

Perkins, S., Winn, S., Murray, J., Murphy, R., & Schmidt, U. (2004). A qualitative study of the experiences of caring for a person with bulimia nervosa. Part 1: The emotional impact of caring. *International Journal of Eating Disorders, 36*(3), 256–268.

Pike, K. M., Hilbert, A., Wilfley, D. E., Fairburn, C. G., Dohm, F.-A., Walsh, B. T., & Striegel-Moore, R. (2008). Toward an understanding of risk factors for anorexia nervosa: A case-control study. *Psychological Medicine, 38,* 1443–1453.

Pilch, J. L. (1988). Wellness spirituality. *Health Values, 12*(3), 28–31.

Pinhas, L., Heinmaa, M., Bryden, P., Bradley, S., & Toner, B. (2008). Disordered eating in Jewish adolescent girls. *Canadian Journal of Psychiatry, 53,* 601–608.

Polivy, J., & Herman, C. P. (1993). Etiology of binge eating: Psychological mechanisms. In C. G. Fairburn & G. T. Wilson (Eds.), *Binge eating: Nature, assessment and treatment* (pp. 173–205). New York, NY: Guilford.

Potestio, M. L., McLaren, L., Robinson Vollman, A., & Doyle-Baker, P. K. (2008). Childhood obesity: perceptions held by the public in Calgary, Canada. *Canadian Journal of Public Health. Revue Canadienne de Sante Publique, 99*(2), 86–90.

Ramacciotti, C. D., Coli, E., Bondi, E., Burgalassi, A., Massimetti, G., & Dell'Osso, L. (2008). Shared psychopathology in obese subjects with and without binge-eating disorder. *International Journal of Eating Disorders, 41,* 643–649.

Provencher, V., Polivy, J., Wintre, M. G., Pratt, M. W., Pancer, S. M., Birnie-Lefcovitch, S., & Adams, G. R. (2009). Who gains or who loses weight? Psychosocial factors among first-year university students. *Physiology & Behavior, 96*(1), 135–141.

Reas, D. L., Williamson, D. A., Martin, C. K., & Zucker, N. L. (2000). Duration of illness predicts outcome for bulimia nervosa: A long term follow up study. *International Journal of Eating Disorders, 27,* 428–434.

Reas, D. L., Grilo, C. M., Masheb, R. M., & Wilson, G. T. (2005). Body checking and avoidance in overweight patients with binge eating disorder. *International Journal of Eating Disorders, 37,* 342–346.

Reda, M., & Sacco, G. (2001). Anorexia and the holiness of Saint Catherine of Siena. *Journal of Criminal Justice and Popular Culture* (G. Newman, Trans.), *8*(1), 37–47.

Reichborn-Kjennerud, T., Bulik, C., Tambs, K., & Harris, J. (2004). Genetic and environmental influences on binge eating in the absence of compensatory behaviours: A population-based twin study. *International Journal of Eating Disorders, 36,* 307–314.

Reijonen, J. H., Prat, H. D., Patel, D. R., & Greydanus, D. E. (2003). Eating disorders in the adolescent population: An overview. *Journal of Adolescent Research, 18,* 209–222.

Richards, P. S., Smith, M. H., Berrett, M. E., O'Grady, K., & Bartz, J. D. (2007). A theist spiritual treatment for women with eating disorders. *Journal of Clinical Psychology, 65,* 172–184.

Rørtveit, K., Åström, S., & Severinsson, E. (2009). The feeling of being trapped in and ashamed of one's own body. *International Journal of Mental Health Nursing, 18,* 91–99.

Rossi, G., Balottin, U., Rossi, M., Chiappedi, M., Fazzi, E., & Lanzi, G. (2007). Pharmacological treatment of anorexia nervosa: a retrospective study in preadolescents and adolescents. *Clinical Pediatrics, 46*(9), 806–811.

Roth, G. (1992). *When food is love: Exploring the relationship between eating and intimacy.* New York: Plume.

Ruuska, J., Kaltiala-Heino, R., Koivisto, A-M., & Rantanen, P. (2003). Puberty, sexual development and eating disorders in adolescent outpatients. *European Child & Adolescent Psychology, 12,* 214–220.

Samuels, F., Zimmerli, E. J., Devlin, M. J., Kissileff, H. R., & Walsh, B. T. (2009). The development of hunger and fullness during a laboratory meal in patients with binge eating disorder. *International Journal of Eating Disorders, 42,* 125–129.

Sancho, C., Arija, M. V., & Canals, J., (2008). Personality in non-clinical adolescents with eating disorders. *European Eating Disorders Review, 16,* 133–138.

Sanci, L., Coffey, C., Olsson, C., Reid, S., Carlin, J. B., & Patton, G. (2008). Chilhood sexual abuse and eating disorders in females: Findings from the Victoria adolescent health cohort study. *Archives of Pediatric and Adolescent Medicine, 162,* 261–267.

Schwartz, B. I., Mansbach, J. M., Marion, J. G., Katzman, D. K., & Forman, S. F. (2008). Variations in admission practices for adolescents with anorexia nervosa: A North American sample. *Journal of Adolescent Health, 43,* 425–431.

Scott Richards, P., Berrett, M. E., & Hardman, R. K., & Eggett, D. L. (2006). Comparative efficacy of spirituality, cognitive, and emotional support groups for treating eating disorder inpatients. *Eating Disorders, 14,* 401–415.

Senra, C., Sanchez-Cao, E., Seoane, G., & Leung, Y. K. (2008). Evolution of self-concept deficits in patients with eating disorders: The role of family cocern about weight and appearance. *European Eating Disorders Review, 15,* 131–138.

Shapiro, J. R., Berkman, N. D., Brownley, K. A., Sedway, J. A., Lohr, K. N., & Bulik, C. M. (2007). Bulimia nervosa treatment: a systematic review of randomized controlled trials. *International Journal of Eating Disorders, 40,* 321–336.

Shisslak, C., Renger, R., Sharpe, T., Crago, M., McKnight, K. M., Gray, N., et al. (1999). Development and evaluation of the McKnight Risk Factor Survey for assessing potential risk and protective factors for disordered eating in preadolescent and adolescent girls. *International Journal of Eating Disorders, 25,* 195–214.

Smith, K. A., Fairburn, C. G., & Cowen, P. J. (1999). Symptomatic relapse in bulimia nervosa following acute tryptophan depletion. *Archives of General Psychiatry, 56*(2), 171–176.

Smolak, L., Levine, M.P., & Schermer, F. (1999). Parental input and weight concerns among elementary school children. *International Journal of Eating Disorders, 25,* 263–271.

Sobol, J., & Bursztyn, M. (1998). Dating people with anorexia nervosa and bulimia nervosa: Attitudes and beliefs of university students. *Women & Health, 27*(3), 73–85.

Soran, C. (2006). What about the boys? Addressing issues of masculinity within male anorexia nervosa in a feminist therapeutic environment. *International Journal of Men's Health, 5,* 251–267.

Stahre, L., Tärnell, B., Håkanson, C., & Hällström, T. (2007). A randomized controlled trial of two weight-reducing short-term group treatment programs for obesity with an 18-month follow-up. *International Journal of Behavioral Medicine, 14,* 48–55.

Steinhausen, H-C. (2002). The outcome of anorexia nervosa in the 20th century. *American Journal of Psychiatry, 159,* 1284–1293.

Steinhausen, H-C., Grigoroiu-Serbanescu, M., Boyadjieva, S., Neumarker, K-J., & Metzke. C. W. (2008). Course and predictors of rehospitalization in adolescent anorexia nervosa in a multisite study. *International Journal of eating disorders, 41,* 29–36.

Stewart, M-C., Schiavo, R. S., Herzog, D. B., & Franko, D. L. (2008). Stereotypes, prejudice and discrimination of women with anorexia nervosa. *European Eating Disorders Review, 16,* 311–318.

Stock, S., Miranda, C., Evans, S., Plessis, S., Ridley, J., & Yeh, S. (2007). Healthy buddies: A novel, peer-led health promotion program for the prevention of obesity and eating disorders in children in elementary school. *Pediatrics, 120,* 1059–1068.

Streigel-Moore, R. (1993). Etiology of binge eating: A developmental perspective. In C. G. Fairburn & G. T. Wilson (Eds.), *Binge eating, nature, assessment and treatment* (pp. 144–172). New York, NY: Guilford.

Striegel-Moore, R. H., Dohm, F-A., Kraemer, H. C., Schreiber, G. B., Taylor, C. B., & Daniels, S. R. (2007). Risk Factors for binge-eating disorders: An exploratory study. *International Journal of Eating Disorders, 40,* 481–487.

Strober, M., Freeman, R., Lampert, C., Diamond, J., & Kaye, W. H. (2000). Controlled family study of anorexia nervosa and bulimia nervosa: Evidence of shared liability and transmission of partial syndromes. *American Journal of Psychiatry, 157*(3), 393–401.

Strober, M., Pataki, C., Freeman, R., & DeAntonio, M. (1999). No effect of adjunctive fluoxetine on eating behavior or weight phobia during the inpatient treatment of anorexia nervosa: An historical case controlled study. *Journal of Child and Adolescent Psychopharmacology, 9*(3), 195–201.

Stunkard, A. J., & Messick, S. (1985). The Three-Factor Eating Questionnaire to measure dietary restraint and hunger. *Journal of Psychosomatic Research, 29,* 71–83.

Stunkard, A. J., & Messick, S. (1988). *Eating Inventory manual.* San Antonio, TX: The Psychological Corporation.

Sullivan, P. (1995). Mortality in anorexia nervosa. *American Journal of Psychiatry, 152,* 1073–1074.

Sullivan, P. (2002). Course and outcome of anorexia nervosa and bulimia nervosa. In C. D. Fairburn, & K. D. Brownell (Eds.), *Eating disorders and obesity* (2nd ed., pp. 226–232). New York: Guilford.

Swinbourne, J. N., & Touyz, S. W. (2007). The co-morbidity of eating disorders and anxiety disorders: A review. *Europrean eating Disorders Review, 15,* 253–274.

Sysko, R., & Walsh, B. T. (2008). A critical evaluation of the efficacy of self-help interventions for the treatment of bulimia nervosa and binge-eating disorder. *International Journal of Eating Disorders, 41*(2), 97–112.

Taylor, C. B., Sharpe, T., Shisslak, C., Bryson, S., Estes, L. S., Gray, N., et al. (1998). Factors associated with weight loss in adolescent girls. *International Journal of Eating Disorders, 24,* 31–42.

Thomsen, S. R., Weber, M. M., & Brown, L. B. (2002). The relationship between reading beauty and fashion magazines and the use of pathogenic dieting methods among adolescent females. *Adolescence, 37*(145), 1–18.

Thomson, P. D. R. (2006). *2006 Physicians' Desk Reference.* Available at: www.pdr.net

Thornton, S. J. (2007). Facing the sunshine: A young woman's emergence from the shadows of sexual abuse and anorexia. Salem, NH: Soaring Wings.

Tozzi, F., Thornton, L. M., Klump, K. L., Fichter, M. M., Halmi, K. A., Kaplan, A. S., et al. (2005). Symptom fluctuation in eating disorders: Correlates of diagnostic crossover. *American Journal of Psychiatry, 162,* 732–740.

Trunko, M. E., & Kaye, W. H. (2008). Pharmacological treatment of bulimia nervosa. *Psychiatric Times, 25*(6), 52, 56–58.

Vallis, T. M., Currie, B., Laylor, D., & Ransom, T. (2007). Healthcare professional bias against the obese: How do we know if we have a problem? *Canadian Journal of Diabetes, 31,* 365–370.

Vandereyken, W. (2002). Families of patients with eating disorders. In C. G. Fairburn & K. D. Brownell (Eds.), *Eating disorders and obesity* (2nd ed., pp. 215–220). New York, NY: Guilford.

Vanderlinden, J., Buis, H., Pieters, G., & Probst, M. (2006). Which elements in the treatment of eating disorders are necessary 'ingredients' in the recovery process? – A comparison between the patient's and therapist's view. *European Eating Disorders Review, 15,* 357–365.

Vince, E., & Walker, I. (2008, August). A set of meta-analytic studies on the factors associated with disordered eating. *Internet Journal of Mental Health, 5*(1), 2–2. Retrieved April 2, 2009, from CINAHL database.

Wade, T. D., Bergin, J. L., Tiggemann, M., Bulik, C. M., & Fairburn, C. G. (2006). Prevalence and long-term course of lifetime eating disorders in an adult Australian twin cohort. *Australian and New Zealand Journal of Psychiatry, 40* (2), 121–128.

Ward, A., Tiller, J., Treasure, J., & Russell, G. (2000). Eating disorders: Psyche or soma. *International Journal of Eating Disorders, 27,* 279–287.

Weaver, K. D., Wuest, J., & Ciliska, D. (2005). Understanding women's journey of recovering from anorexia nervosa. *Qualitative Health Research, 15*(2), 188–206.

White, J. H. (1999). The development and clinical testing of an outpatient program for women with bulimia nervosa. *Archives of Psychiatric Nursing, 13*(4), 179–191.

White, J. H. (2000). Symptom development in bulimia nervosa: A comparison of women with and without a history of anorexia nervosa. *Archives of Psychiatric Nursing, 14*(2), 81–92.

Wilding. J., Van Gaal, L., Rissanen, A., Vercruysse, F., & Fitchet, M. (2004). A randomized double-blind placebo-controlled study of the long-term efficacy and safety of topiramate in the treatment of obese subjects. *International Journal of Obesity Related Metabolic Disorders, 28,* 1399–1410.

Wilfrey, D. E., Schwartz, M. B., Spurrell, E. B., & Fairburn, C.G. (2000). Using the eating disorder examination to identify the specific psychopathology of binge eating disorder. *International Journal of Eating Disorders, 27,* 259–269.

Wilson, G. T., Loeb, K. L., Walsh, B. T., Labouvie, E., Petkova, E., Liu, X., et al. (1999). Psychological versus pharmacological treatments of bulimia nervosa: Predictors and processes of change. *Journal of Consulting and Clinical Psychology, 67*(4), 451–459.

Winn, S., Perkins, S., Walwyn, R., Schmidt, U., Eisler, I., Treasure, J., et al. (2007). Predictors of mental health problems and negative caregiving experiences in carers of adolescents with bulimia. *International Journal of Eating Disorders, 40,* 171–178.

Wolfe, B. E., & Gimby, L. B. (2003). Caring for the hospitalized patient with an eating disorder. *Nursing Clinics of North America, 38,* 75–99.

Wolfe, B. E., Metzger, E. D., Levine, J. M., Finkelstein, D. M., Cooper, T. B., & Jimerson, D. C. (2000). Serotonin function following remission from bulimia nervosa. *Neuropsychopharmacology, 22*(3), 257–263.

Woodside, D. B., Bulik, C. M., Thornton, L., Klump, K. L., Tozzi, F., Fichter, M. M., et al. (2004). Personality in men with eating disorders. *Journal of Psychosomatic Research, 57,* 273–278.

Woodside, D. B., Field, L. L., Garfinkel, P., & Heinmaa, M. (1998). Specificity of eating disorders diagnoses in families of probands with anorexia nervosa and bulimia nervosa. *Comprehensive Psychiatry, 39*(5), 261–264.

Woodside, B., Garfinkel, P., Lin, E., Goering, P., Kaplan, A., Goldbloom, D. S., et al. (2001). Comparisons of men with full or partial eating disorders, men without eating disorders, and women with eating disorders in the community. *American Journal of Psychiatry, 158*(4), 570–574.

World Health Organization. (1993). *The ICD-10 classification of mental and behavioural disorders: Diagnostic criteria for research.* Geneva, Switzerland: Author.

Yager, J. (2008). Binge eating disorder: The search for better treatments. *American Journal of Psychiatry, 165,* 4–6.

Yager, J., & Powers, P. S. (2007). *Clinical manual of eating disorders.* Arlington, VA: APA.

Zeeck A., Birindelli, E., Sandholz, A., Joos, A., Herzog, T., & Hartmann, A. (2007). Symptom severity and treatment course of bulimic patients with and without a borderline personality disorder. *European Eating Disorders Review, 15,* 430–438.

CHAPTER 24

Substance-Related Disorders

Diane Kunyk and Charl Els

Adapted from the chapter "Substance Use Disorders" by
Barbara G. Falz, Richard V. Wing, and Jean Robinson Hughes

LEARNING OBJECTIVES

After studying this chapter, you will be able to:

- Conceptualize "addiction" as a prevalent, chronic, relapsing, and treatable medical disorder.
- Describe the features of the bio/psycho/social/spiritual and the public health models for understanding addiction in Canadian settings.
- Describe the principles of safe and effective treatment of substance-related disorders.
- Outline the essential components of a comprehensive assessment, matching patients with appropriate multi-modal treatment interventions, as well as monitoring progress and effectiveness of treatment.
- Formulate an individualized nursing care plan.

KEY CONCEPTS

- addiction
- motivation for change

KEY TERMS

- alcohol • ambivalence • amphetamines • caffeine • cannabis • cocaine
- concurrent mental disorders • craving • delirium tremens • denial
- detoxification • hallucinogens • harm reduction • inhalants • intoxication
- methadone maintenance • motivational interviewing • multi-modal
- nicotine/tobacco • opioids • phencyclidine • relapse • remission
- sedatives/hypnotics/anxiolytics • substance abuse and dependence
- substance-induced disorders • substance-related disorders • tolerance
- therapeutic alliance • twelve-step facilitation • withdrawal

*A*ddiction is recognized by the major disease classification systems as a bona fide, chronic, and relapsing medical condition (American Psychiatric Association [APA], 2000; WHO, 2007). Advances in brain imaging and other research have demonstrated that repeated exposure to alcohol, tobacco, and/or other drugs (ATOD) over time may alter brain structure, chemistry, and function in susceptible individuals, leading to a potential loss of control over their use of ATOD, and continued use despite harm. This conceptualization,

along with emerging theories and understandings, have made advances in addiction treatment possible, providing increasingly optimistic outcomes for those affected with the disease.

Addiction affects people regardless of their age, gender, sexual orientation, socio-economic status, education, culture, or occupation. It is estimated to cost the Canadian economy almost $40 billion annually in health care costs and loss of productivity, a burden greater than the economic impact of all other mental illnesses combined (Rehm et al., 2006). Addiction is considered a leading occupation health issue, ranking second as the cause of disability, and affecting individuals predominantly in their prime working years. Since addiction is the most common of all mental conditions, proven to be the leading preventable cause of death and disease globally, and the single greatest contributor to excess health care spending, it has been argued that addiction is the most important illness of our time (Els, 2007).

> **KEY CONCEPT** **Addiction**, a chronic, relapsing, and treatable medical condition, is the leading preventable cause of death and disease.

Yet addiction is often neglected, and remains largely undertreated in Canadian society. There are massive barriers (e.g., stigma and resources) for persons with addiction to overcome in order to access the treatment they need, and these systemic barriers are considered as intractable as the disease of addiction itself. Nurses encounter addicted patients in their everyday practice, and are favourably situated to help individuals affected by the disease. With the necessary knowledge, skills, and attitudes conducive to health promotion, nurses are able to safely and effectively manage this disorder, and thereby reduce this care deficit.

This chapter reviews the categories of **substance-related disorders (SRD)**, current theories regarding the etiology of substance use disorders (abuse and dependence), and evidence-based treatment interventions. The role of the nurse is discussed in terms of early identification, assessment, and intervention planning with the purpose of helping to meet the needs of individuals and their family, and to satisfy the ethical duty of patient advocacy. Selected topics of interest, including tobacco dependence in the mentally ill population and nurses with substance use disorders, are also explored.

DIAGNOSTIC CRITERIA

Addiction is a chronic, relapsing brain disorder that results from the prolonged effects of exposure of the brain to drugs (or substances or chemicals). Behavioural and social-context aspects are considered important components of the illness. Addiction reflects pervasive changes in brain function at structural (molecular and cellular) and functional levels. It develops in an individual who may be considered potentially "vulnerable" (on biological, psychological, social, or spiritual levels), and the result of chronic exposure leads to neuro-adaptation in the brain rendering the user incapable of maintaining abstinence or control over use. The manifestation of addiction includes (a) the continued use of a substance

despite harm (or negative consequences), (b) tolerance, withdrawal, and loss of control over the use of the substance, and (c) large amounts of time spent acquiring or recovering from the effects of the substance(s) used (Leshner, 1997). In every day use, however, the term addiction has been applied to the repeated use of a multitude of things, from heroin to video games (Beckson, 2003).

The APA's (2000) *Diagnostic and Statistical Manual of Mental Disorders*, 4th ed., Text revision (*DSM-IV-TR*) does not refer to the term "addiction." Rather the classification of SRD refers to disorders related to taking of drugs of abuse, to the side effects of medications, as well as to toxin exposure, and includes two categories: **substance use disorders** (substance dependence and substance abuse) and **substance-induced disorders** (substance intoxication, substance withdrawal, substance-induced delirium, substance-induced persisting dementia, substance-induced persisting amnesia, substance-induced psychotic disorder, substance-induced mood disorder, substance-induced anxiety disorder, substance-induced sexual dysfunction, and substance-induced sleep disorder). There are 11 classes (some broader than others) of heterogenous substances referred to in this classification system, including **alcohol**, **amphetamine** (and similarly acting substances and sympathomimetics), **caffeine**, **cannabis** (marijuana), **cocaine**, **hallucinogens**, **inhalants**, **nicotine** (tobacco), **opioids**, **phencyclidine** ([PCP], and ketamine), **sedative**, **hypnotic**, or **anxiolytic-related drugs**. The association between SRD and each class of substance is outlined in Table 24-1.

Substance dependence refers to the continued use of a substance despite significant substance-related problems and a pattern of repeated self-administration that can result in tolerance, withdrawal, and compulsive drug-taking behaviour. **Craving**, defined as a strong desire to use the substance, is experienced by most individuals. Substance dependence as characterized by a maladaptive pattern of substance use, leading to clinically significant impairment or distress, and manifested by three (or more) of the following occurring at any time in the same 12-month period:

- **Tolerance** as defined by either of the a need for markedly increased amounts of the substance to achieve intoxication or desired effect, or markedly diminished effect with continued use of the same amount of the substance,
- **Withdrawal** as manifested by the characteristic withdrawal syndrome for the substance, or by the ingestion of the same (or a closely related) to relieve or avoid withdrawal symptoms,
- Taking of the substance in larger amounts, or over a longer period, than was intended,

Table 24.1 Association between Substance-Related Disorders and Classes of Substances

	Depen-dence	Abuse	Intoxi-cation	With-drawal	Intoxi-cation Delirium	With-drawal Delirium	Dementia	Amnestic Disorder	Psychotic Disorders	Mood Disorders	Anxiety Disorders	Sexual Dysfunction	Sleep Disorders
Alcohol	X	X	X	X	I	W	P	P	I/W	I/W	I/W	I	I/W
Amphetamines	X	X	X	X	I				I	I/W	I	I	I/W
Caffeine			X								I		I
Cannabis	X	X	X		I				I		I		
Cocaine	X	X	X	X	I				I	I/W	I/W	I	I/W
Hallucinogens	X	X	X		I				I*	I	I		
Inhalants	X	X	X		I		P		I	I	I		
Nicotine	X			X									
Opioids	X	X	X	X	I				I	I		I	I/W
Phencyclidine	X	X	X		I				I	I	I		
Sedatives, hypnotics, or anxiolytics	X	X	X	X	I	W	P	P	I/W	I/W	W	I	I/W
Polysubstance	X												
Other	X	X	X	X	I	W	P	P	I/W	I/W	I/W	I	I/W

Note: X, I, W, I/W, or P indicates that the category is recognized in *DSM-IV-TR*. In addition, I indicates that the specifier With Onset During Intoxication may be noted for the category (except for Intoxication Delirium); W indicates that the specifier With Onset During Withdrawal may be noted for the category (except for Withdrawal Delirium); and I/W indicates that either With Onset During Intoxication or With Onset Withdrawal may be noted for the category. P indicates that the disease is persisting.

*Also Hallucinogen Persisting Perception Disorder (Flashbacks).

Reprinted with permission from the *Diagnostic and Statistical Manual of Mental Disorders* (4th ed., Text revision). Copyright 2000. American Psychiatric Association.

- A persistent desire or unsuccessful efforts to cut down or control substance use,
- Spending a great deal of time in activities to obtain the substance, use the substance, or recover from its effects,
- A reduction or abstinence of important social, occupational, or recreational activities because of substance use, and
- Continued substance use despite the knowledge of having a persistent or recurrent physical or psychological problem that is likely to have been caused or exacerbated by the substance.

The more prevalent disorder of **substance abuse** refers to a maladaptive use of chemical substance(s) leading to clinically significant outcomes or distress (e.g., recurrent legal problems, failure to perform at work/home/school, and physically hazardous behaviour). The criteria do *not* include tolerance, withdrawal, or a pattern of compulsive use. Instead *it includes* the harmful consequences of repeated use. It is pre-empted by the diagnosis of substance dependence at any point in the individual's life, and for that specific class (or classes) of substances. Substance abuse is manifested by one (or more) of the following occurring within a 12-month period:

- Recurrent substance use resulting in a failure to fulfill major role obligations at work, school, or home (e.g., repeated absences or poor work performance related to substance use; suspensions from school; neglect of children),
- Recurrent substance use in situations in which it is physically hazardous (e.g., driving an automobile impaired by substance use),
- Recurrent substance-related legal problems (e.g., arrests for substance-related disorderly conduct), and
- Continued substance use despite having persistent or recurrent social or interpersonal problems caused or exacerbated by the effects of the substance (e.g., arguments with spouse about consequences of intoxication).

The substance-induced disorder of **intoxication** is described as the development of a reversible substance-specific syndrome due to the recent ingestion of (or exposure to) a substance. The maladaptive behaviours associated with intoxication (e.g., belligerence, mood lability, cognitive impairment, impaired judgment, impaired social, or occupational functioning) are due to the direct physiological effects of the substance on the central nervous system (CNS). These behaviours place the individual at significant risk for adverse effects (e.g., accidents, general medical complications, disruption in social and family relationships, vocational or financial difficulties, and legal problems).

Substance withdrawal is the development of a substance-specific maladaptive behavioural change that is due to the cessation, or reduction, of heavy and prolonged substance use. This may cause clinically significant distress or impairment in social, occupational, or other important areas of functioning and, as a result, most individuals will experience craving to re-administer the substance to reduce the discomforting symptoms. Some withdrawal syndromes are life-threatening, others are simply uncomfortable, and some are even less pronounced.

Clinical Course

Addiction is a *chronic* disease, and a mental disorder, that threatens the health and wellbeing of affected individuals. There is considerable heterogeneity among people with substance use disorders but periods of sustained use are often interrupted by periods of partial or complete **remission** (a period when the symptoms of the disease are abated). In some individuals, dependence on a single substance may lead to the use of, and dependence on, another substance. When addiction is neglected and remains untreated, the disease typically progresses in severity, and may even result in premature death (Kleber et al., 2006).

Addiction is widely considered to be amenable to treatment. The outcomes to evidence-based interventions are similar to other chronic disease conditions including hypertension, asthma, and Type 2 diabetes (McLellan, Lewis, O'Brien, & Kleber, 2000). Most persons who struggle with addiction will have one or more **relapses** (the return to substance use after a drug-free period) during their ongoing process of recovery. Some of the most commonly cited precursors to relapse include substance-related reminder cues (e.g., sights, sounds, smells, or thoughts), negative mood states, positive mood states, and sampling the drug itself, even in small doses (Hoffman & Froemke, 2007).

■ EPIDEMIOLOGY

Epidemiological data on alcohol, tobacco, and other drugs come from several sources. Surveys, such as the Canadian Community Health Survey: Mental Health and Well-Being (CCHS) and the National Population Health Survey (NPHS), examine prevalence in selected populations during a given time period or for a period of years. The Canadian Tobacco Use Monitoring Survey (CTUMS) tracks changes in smoking prevalence by province-sex-age groups (15 years of age and older) on a semi-annual basis. The Canadian Community Epidemiology Network on Drug Use (CCENDU) serves as a surveillance system and provides comparative data about the nature, extent, and consequences of harmful use or abuse of substances. In addition, given that many of the national surveys do not identify Aboriginal people who are living in mainstream Canada or include those living in designated communities (on reserves), the National Native Addictions Partnership Foundation's Treatment Activity Reporting System (TARS) has been created to track substance use among these populations. The following epidemiological data are from these sources unless otherwise noted.

The rates of use of tobacco products (leading to nicotine dependence) have steadily decreased in Canada since their peak in the early 1960s. However, smoking remains the single most preventable cause of death in Canada, responsible for approximately 37,000 deaths from direct causes, and a further 1,100 to 7,800 deaths related to second hand smoke. Most people initiate their use of tobacco products between the ages of 11 and 15, and for this reason tobacco dependence is aptly described as a pediatric disease that continues into adulthood in most cases. Despite the serious health risks, approximately 18% of Canadians smoke with the highest proportion of smokers in the 20 to 24 age grouping (28%). Over 70% of smokers want to quit, almost half have tried to quit at least once in the past year, and fully one third of current smokers report that they want to quit in the next month (Leatherdale & Shields, 2009).

There is substantive variability in the reported prevalence use rates of alcohol and other drugs related to methodologic (e.g., definition of terms) and cultural (e.g., legal status of the substance) differences (Somers, Goldner, Waraich, & Hsu, 2004). Keeping these limitations in mind, estimates show that in 2002 about 2.6% of the household population aged 15 years or older were dependent on alcohol, and 0.8% were dependent on illicit drugs. Of those who drank during the previous year, 17% (13.6% of all Canadians) were considered high-risk drinkers (25% men, 9% women). Both binge drinking (60%) and heavy illicit drug use (37%) occurred most frequently during the early adult years (20 to 24 years of age). Current figures show that approximately 6,700 Canadians die each year from alcohol use (mostly from accidents and suicides), and another 86,000 are hospitalized. Both the prevalence of past-year drinking, and the proportion of heavy drinking, has increased in the last decade for both men and women. Furthermore, the lifetime use of most illicit drugs by both men and women has more than doubled in these 10 years.

Gender Differences

Men (47%) generally engage in heavy drinking more frequently than women (24%), and are also more likely to be dependent on alcohol (3.9% versus 1.1%) and drugs (1.1% versus 0.5%). In addition, male tobacco smokers continue to outnumber women at every age but the difference is marginal among teens. More men have tried cannabis (50.1% versus 39.2%), or another illicit drug other than cannabis (21.1% versus 12.2%) at least once in their lifetime. Men have also experienced more harm from their own alcohol use when compared with women (30.2% versus 18.4%).

Women, however, outnumber men in the frequency of harmful use of prescribed psychoactive medications. Drug and alcohol use patterns also vary within women according to certain demographic factors (age, education, marital status, employment, race, and ethnicity), and her partner's substance use pattern (Gomberg, 1999). These patterns can result in numerous health effects such as the following:

- Physical health problems (tend to be more severe and immediate)
- Reproductive problems (disruptions in menstrual cycle, fetal development, child birth, menopause, and sexual responsiveness and dysfunction)
- Associated mental health disorders (anxiety, depression, phobias, panic, and eating disorders)
- Increased risk for suicide ideation and completion.

Age Differences

In general, for both men and women, frequency of drinking increases with age, income, and education just as smoking and illicit drug use decreases across these variables.

Youth

It is difficult to define what constitutes a substance use problem among youth when some involvement with alcohol, tobacco, and other drugs is considered statistically and culturally normative in Canada. Attitudes have grown increasingly tolerant of youth experimentation, and harmful use has increased (e.g., multiple substances, larger amount consumed, and more frequent use). An increasing number of youth are drinking at an early age (two thirds of students in grades 7 to 9 have consumed alcohol). Current patterns show that the prevalence of drug use increases with age throughout adolescence, and only about one third to one fourth of youth (12 to 19 years of age) do not use drugs.

Second to caffeine, alcohol remains the most commonly used substance (peaking in use at ages 18 to 19), followed by tobacco and cannabis, and 3% to 10% of mainstream youth engage in the nonmedical use of inhalants, stimulants, cocaine, tranquilizers, and barbiturates. Among those youth who engage in illegal substance use, about one third report problematic use (e.g., attending school or playing a sport while high, or using drugs in the morning). This risk is related to increases in physical injury, property damage, or engaging in unprotected sexual activity. Indeed, about one in four youth aged 15 to 19 years reports some type of harm connected to their drinking—more than double the rate for the population as a whole (Johnston, O'Malley, & Bachman, 2000).

Older Adults

Older adults are more susceptible to the effects of alcohol than younger adults because of the physiologic changes associated with aging: an increase in the percentage of body fat, a reduction in lean body mass, and a reduction in the total volume of water in the body (less body water to dilute the alcohol). No more than one drink a day for both men and women older than 65 years is recommended but approximately 11% of men and 9% of women older than 75 years exceed these recommendations (Adams, Barry, & Fleming, 1996). Prescription drug use is more prevalent among those older than 64 years than among younger adults, and approximately 18% of older women and 14% of senior men commonly use three or more prescription drugs (compared with 2% of younger women and 8% of younger men).

Adding to the challenge of substance use is the evidence that older adults are less likely than younger adults to perceive their drug use as problematic (Nemes et al., 2004). This may be because of the effects of harmful use patterns, which vary somewhat for older adults, are often misattributed to aging: confusion, forgetfulness, anxiety, depression, sleep problems, injury from falls, reduction in the effectiveness of medications, conflict or withdrawal from family and friends, and improper eating habits accompanied by weight loss. A number of older adults who have coped well in the past using positive strategies find themselves using substances in later years to manage the loss, or the overwhelming caregiving responsibilities, of their partners (Fleming et al., 1999).

The Societal Costs of Substance Abuse

Alcohol, tobacco, and other drug use exact a heavy toll on the health of individuals and communities. Addiction is a leading cause of morbidity and mortality in Canada, accounting for 21% of total mortality, 23% of total potential years of life lost, 8% of total hospitalizations, and 10% of hospitalization days due to any cause (Single, Robson, Rehm, & Xie, 1999). The costs incurred to Canadian society were estimated at nearly $40 billion in 2002 when health care (e.g., hospitalization, treatment services), the workplace (e.g., employee assistance programs, drug testing), transfer payments (e.g., social welfare, workers' compensation), crime and law enforcement (e.g., police, courts), and lost productivity (e.g., reduced output, sick time) were considered (Rehm et al., 2006).

The ensuing substance use problems associated with, or stemming from, perinatal and childhood exposure to ATOD are also profound. The evidence that being impaired while engaged in activities of significant responsibility (work, school, or taking care of children) is a common occurrence reported by adults (26%) who are dependent on alcohol, and highlights the pervasive nature of this problem. The rise in violence associated with the sale and distribution of illicit drugs in neighbourhoods and schools jeopardizes the health and well-being of communities. At the same time, the criminalization of illicit drug users under current drug control legislation in Canada contradicts the objectives of public health and may even contribute to the drug-related problems (prevention of infectious disease transmission among illicit drug users) that harm reduction tries to alleviate (Fischer, 2005).

■ ETIOLOGICAL THEORIES

The **bio/psycho/social/spiritual** model conceptualizes addiction as a disorder with multi-factorial pathogenesis, predisposing, precipitating, and modulating factors that encompasses the body, the mind (psyche), the spirit, as well as social and environmental influences in studying the disease and formulating treatment (West, 2006). It is vital to understand that this disease typically develops, and comes to expression, in behavioural ways with varying degrees of embedded biological, psychological, social, and spiritual aspects, that cannot be explained in isolation or with one reductionist theory alone. Environmental or conditioned cues, of which there may be tens of thousands that individuals associate with their drug use, also become a part of the addiction, all within a complex environment where economic, political, and other dynamic factors may influence the course of the disease.

Biological

There is large body of evidence examining the influence of addictive substances on the brain, including sophisticated brain-imaging techniques that demonstrate structural and functional changes in the addicted brain. The addicted brain has been demonstrated to be different from the non-addicted brain, and this is manifested by changes in gene expression, receptor availability, metabolic activity, and responsiveness to environmental cues (Leshner, 1997). These pervasive changes in brain function may persist long after the individual stops taking the drug on molecular, cellular, structural, and functional levels. These demonstrated changes to brain structure and function form the foundation and evidence for addiction to be classified as a "disease of the brain" and a true psychiatric disorder.

The use of addictive substances has been found to increase extracellular levels of dopamine. This dopamine-related "high" becomes the reinforcement mechanism in the brain. The brain, in essence, remembers this pleasure and wants it repeated. But the neurochemical status in the brain readjusts to these increased levels of dopamine as being the "normal" neurochemical state; the user then requires increased amounts of substances to produce the same dopamine-related effects (Goldstein & Volkow, 2002). This need for increased amounts of a substance to achieve (or obtain) the same results (effects) is termed tolerance, and is considered one of the hallmark features of addiction. Often, cravings to use ATOD dominate the thoughts, and affect mood and behaviour, of the addicted individual. Just as food is linked to daily survival, once the brain has become addicted to a substance, it takes on the same level of salience or significance to the level of "life-sustaining." The substance is no longer sought only for pleasure but for the need to relieve distress or to relieve withdrawal. Eventually, the drive to obtain and use the drug is perceived to be all that matters, despite devastating consequences.

Psychological Theories

The psychological theories refer to the relative contribution that psychological factors have in the initiation and maintenance of the substance-related disorders. These theories suggest that some individuals are born with certain temperaments and subsequently develop particular personality traits, vulnerabilities, or even personality disorders that may make them more susceptible to SRD. Although commonly referred to as a risk factor, the concept of an "addictive personality" has not been adequately conceptualized or validated. Psychosocial needs common to those who become addicted include the need to feel self-worth, to have control over the environment, to feel intimate contact with others, to accomplish something valuable, and to eliminate pain or other powerful negative feelings. Six other identified psychodynamic issues postulated to lead to substance abuse are the following: excessive dependency needs, need for success or power, inability to adequately care for self, gender identity problems, inability to cope with overwhelming painful feelings, and dysfunctional family dynamics.

Behavioural Theories

Many investigators have turned their attention to the behavioural characteristics of childhood and adolescence that might predispose a person to substance abuse. Some have postulated that conduct problems of childhood, such as deviance, misbehaviour, and aggression, might be important behavioural risk factors for later substance abuse, particularly for boys. A few studies demonstrate a strong connection between childhood conduct problems, hyperactivity, impulsivity, and future substance abuse. A history of general deviance or maladaptive social patterns in the form of interface with the law (or criminal justice system), or long-standing behavioural problems has been linked to risk for developing drug dependence.

Social Theories

Much research has focussed on sociological factors, peer drug use and affiliation with peers as determinants of teenage alcohol, tobacco, and other drug involvement. Peer interaction is a crucial influencing factor in determining adolescents' exposure to alcohol, tobacco, and drugs. The proportion of users versus non-users (peer), and peers' perceptions of alcohol use as being a useful way of reducing tension and other alleged positive attributes contribute to their increased use. Specific neighbourhood characteristics may also be factors suggesting an increased risk for drug abuse, including high population density, physical deterioration, high levels of crime, and illegal drug trafficking (Hesselbrock, Hesselbrock, & Epstein, 1999).

Spiritual Theories

Spirituality (which is not to be confused with religion) has a close and intimate relationship with the field of addiction care; individuals who have recovered from addiction often mention spiritual experiences or motivation as a major contributory factor. Spirituality can be defined as the relationship between an individual and the sacred, perhaps represented by a transcendent higher being (or higher power) or force (or mind of the universe). This relationship is personal to the individual and does not require affiliation with any organized religion; religion is *not* necessary for an individual to develop his or her spirituality (see Chapter 6). The Twelve Steps of Alcoholics Anonymous (AA; refer to Box 24-1), empirically derived by a group of persons living with chronic alcoholism, references "a power greater than us," "God," "Higher Power," and "a spiritual experience." Working the Twelve Steps (or **twelve-step facilitation** [TSF]) is not considered to be practicing a religion because of the following:

- Major religions that have examined the Twelve Steps have come to the conclusion that they do not conflict with their beliefs,
- AA, considered the "prototype" of TSF, has spread around the world, including non-Christian countries,
- Joining AA does not require learning any theology, creed, or catechism.
- The requirement of AA membership (access to meetings and fellowship) is simply the "desire to quit drinking."

BOX 24.1

The Twelve Steps of Alcoholics Anonymous

1. We admitted we were powerless over alcohol—that our lives had become unmanageable.
2. Came to believe that a Power greater than ourselves could restore us to sanity.
3. Made a decision to turn our will and our lives over to the care of God *as we understood Him.*
4. Made a searching and fearless moral inventory of ourselves.
5. Admitted to God, to ourselves, and to another human being the exact nature of our wrongs.
6. Were entirely ready to have God remove all these defects of character.
7. Humbly asked Him to remove our shortcomings.
8. Made a list of all persons we had harmed, and became willing to make amends to them all.
9. Made direct amends to such people wherever possible, except when to do so would injure them or others.
10. Continued to take personal inventory and, when we were wrong, promptly admitted it.
11. Sought through prayer and meditation to improve our conscious contact with God as we understood Him, praying only for knowledge of His will for us and the power to carry that out.
12. Having had a spiritual awakening as a result of these steps, we tried to carry this message to alcoholics and to practice these principles in all our affairs.

Source: The Twelve Steps are reprinted with permission of Alcoholics Anonymous World Services, Inc. (AAWS) Permission to reprint the Twelve Steps does not mean that AAWS has reviewed or approved the contents of this publication, or that AAWS necessarily agrees with the views expressed herein. A.A. is a program of recovery from alcoholism *only*—use of the Twelve Steps in connection with programs and activities which are patterned after A.A., but which address other problems, or in any other non-A.A. context, does not imply otherwise.

IN A LIFE

Jann Arden (1962–)
Vocalist, songwriter, author, producer, actress

Public Persona

Jann Arden has received 19 Juno Award nominations and has won eight of these including songwriter of the year in 1995 and 2002, as well as female artist of the year in 1995 and 2001. She has also won awards at the MuchMusic Video Awards, the Prairie Music Awards, the Western Canadian Music Awards, and at the ARIA Awards. Seventeen of her singles have achieved Top Ten status, and she has released 10 albums. In 2007, Arden was inducted into the Canadian Association of Broadcasters Hall of Fame and was the winner of the International Achievement Awards at the 2007 Western Canadian Music Awards. She has written two books of personal reflections and poetry, and a monthly advice column in *Elle Canada* magazine. Jann Arden is well known for her comedic talents and in 2003, she starred in her own Canadian TV reality show called The Arden Diner. She has published two books (the first book climbed to three on Canada's Globe and Mail non-fiction Bestseller list), performed in "The Vagina Dialogues," and made a number of charity appearances, including one in Africa for World Vision.

Personal Realities

Born in a small town in Alberta, Arden has travelled a circuitous road to success. She spent most of the 1980s playing in bars and busking until she was assaulted and robbed of the $4 she earned for the day. Alcohol was her close companion while she worked through a string of jobs including ball washing at a golf course and a deckhand on a salmon boat. Upon reflection, she notes that alcohol held her back. Arden told *Chatelaine* that she quit drinking on "January 20, 1989. You don't forget the date." She is now reported to abstain from alcohol, nicotine, and even caffeine.

Source: http://www.jannarden.com, Chatelaine, October 1995.

As addiction has a spiritual component, the nurse may have the implied mandate to inquire about spirituality, and to offer appropriate referral to spiritual counselling. The nurse may support, at the patient's direction, spiritual and/or religious activities.

Public Health Model

The *public health model* (also called epidemiological homeostasis) is about the interaction between the host, agent, vector, and environment. This provides a framework that incorporates the biological, psychological, social, and spiritual theories as they pertain to addiction in a manner that can demonstrate their relationships. It is within these relationships that interventions can be designed to reduce the spread of the disease of addiction. The clinical understanding of dependence is based on examining the interaction between the affected individual (*the host*) and the substance of abuse (*the agent*). This domain includes the psychopharmacology of the substance of abuse, and the biological, psychological, and spiritual components of the individual. Here is where phenomena such as tolerance, withdrawal, and family history may be examined.

Many clinical tools, as well as most approaches to controlling addiction at the public health level, depend on additional aspects of this disease, and incorporate some of the social theoretical components. One of these includes consideration of the *vector* and, in the case of the spread of the disease of addiction, these include the suppliers and "pushers" involved in the manufacture and/or distribution of addictive substances. The tobacco industry, for example, is the vector of the disease of tobacco

BOX 24.2

Application of the Public Health Model to the Situation of Tobacco in Health Care Settings

THE SITUATION: For decades, the use of tobacco products has been tolerated; sometimes even in health care settings. This *environment* has been culpable to the spread of the disease of tobacco dependence through measures including allowing smoking in designated areas or rooms, selling tobacco products on site, and allowing smoking in visible areas. In this setting, the *hosts* (tobacco consumers) have been accommodated for their addiction. Furthermore, some patients, employees, physicians and volunteers have become *incidental hosts* through their exposure to second-hand smoke during the course of care delivery. The vector of the disease in this situation is tobacco industry who, in efforts to increase sales, has heavily marketed their product and sometimes funded health professionals and health facilities as a measure to gain credibility. Nurses (along with other health care professionals) have, at times, been a *secondary vector* in the hospital situation by storing, dispensing, lighting, and even rolling cigarettes, selling and gifting tobacco, supervising smoking, scheduled activities around "smoke breaks," and there are even reports of nurses smoking with patients as a measure to establish therapeutic relationships. There is anecdotal evidence of patients who are former smokers who relapse as a response to the smell of tobacco on nurses' clothing or breath.

INTERVENTION: The placement of this situation into the Public Health Model allows for the development of a comprehensive tobacco control policy to limit the spread of the disease. Elements include the following:
- The closure of all designated smoking rooms and areas indoors,
- Prevent nicotine withdrawal in patients through appropriate pharmacotherapy,
- Eliminating tobacco sales on site,
- Reject funding and any other form of relationship with the tobacco industry,
- Designating all outdoor areas as smoke-free including parking areas,
- Supporting nurses and other health employees to quit smoking with comprehensive and ongoing workplace wellness programs.

Source: Kunyk, D., Els, C., Predy, G., & Haase, M. (2007). Development and introduction of a comprehensive tobacco control policy in a Canadian regional health authority. *Preventing Chronic Disease: Public Health Research, Practice, and Policy, 4*(2), 1–8.

dependence, and profits through the making and selling of tobacco, marketing its product through advertising and promotions, and by lobbying government for favoured treatment. Secondary vectors, such as convenience stores or newspapers who print advertisements of addictive substances, may also promote the disease of addiction. Nurses (e.g., in psychiatric settings) facilitating tobacco use (e.g., by dispensing tobacco to patients) may also be considered secondary vectors in spreading the disease. Examining the concept of the vector opens possibilities of controlling the spread of addiction to include effective interventions such as restrictions on advertising, de-normalization, and advocating for corporate responsibility.

The other major, core elements in the public health model are the cultural, political, economic, legal, and historical settings in which the agent, the host, and the vector interact. These unique and varied settings comprise the *environment*. Understanding the large and small environments in which the vector-agent-host interactions occur and tailoring approached appropriate to them is as essential for effective treatment and prevention of addiction as is tailoring nursing care to the patient (host). The National Anti-Drug Strategy as well as taxation on alcohol and tobacco are examples of interventions that may positively change the environment to positively impact addiction. An advantage to the public health model is its ability to consider intervention at both the individual (e.g., clinical) and environmental (e.g., legislation and social marketing) levels. By placing treatment and prevention strategies in the model, it allows the nurse to better understand how their work fits into the larger picture and how they can best contribute beyond their day-to-day practice. An application of the public health model to the situation of tobacco in health care settings may be found in Box 24-2.

CLASSES OF SUBSTANCES

The following section will review the 11 major substances/categories classifications: alcohol, amphetamine, caffeine, cannabis, cocaine, hallucinogens, inhalants, nicotine, opioids, PCP, as well as sedative/hypnotic drugs and anxiolytics. A description of each substance, its biological action, and salient effects will be addressed. As a supplement, Table 24-2 summarizes the frequently encountered non-psychiatric symptoms, Table 24-3 refers to the frequently encountered psychiatric effects, and Table 24-4 addresses the frequently encountered withdrawal symptoms to abused substances.

Alcohol

Alcohol is produced by fermenting (for beer and wine) and distilling (for rum, whiskey, vodka, and other "hard liquor" forms). Historically, this psychoactive substance's use dates back to at least 8000 BC, and is only second to

Table 24.2 Frequently Observed *Intoxication* Symptoms, Non-Psychiatric (other) by Class of Substance of Abuse

Class of Substance	GIT							Ophthalmic						Other						
	Appetite	Chills, Sweating	Diarrhea	Dry mouth	Nasal congestion	Nausea Vomiting	Weight loss	Colour vision (brighter and richer)	Conjunctivitis	Nystagmus	Ptosis (bilateral)	Pupillary constriction or dilation	Wernecke's syndrome—ocular manifestations	Dyspnea	Hyperthermia	Hypoglycemia	Joint aches	Muscle weakness	Rhabdomyolysis	Sleep architecture (decreased rapid eye movements)
Alcohol										+			+ =			+ =				+ =
Amphetamines	↓	+				+	+					↑		+			+	+		
Caffeine																				
Cannabis	↑			+				+	+			↑								
Cocaine	↓	+			+ =	+	+					↑		+				+		
Hallucinogens		+										↑								
Inhalants																				
Nicotine /Tobacco		+ =	+ =			+ =														+ =
Opioids	↓	+				+					+	↓↑								
PCP/Phencyclidine						+				+					+				+	
Sedative, hypnotic, anxiolytic-related drugs	↑ =			+ =		+ =				+				+ =	+ =		+ =			+ =

Continued

Table 24.2 Frequently Observed *Intoxication* Symptoms, Non-Psychiatric (other) by Class of Substance of Abuse (*Continued*)

Class of Substance	CNS															CVS				
	Amnesia	Ataxia, Dysarthria, Disorientation	Delirium	Drowsiness, stupor, coma	Dyskinesia, Dystonia	Gait (unsteady)	Incoordination	Numbness, Reduced response to pain, Muscle rigidity	Psychomotor agitation or rigidity	Seizures	Slurred speech, Impaired attention or memory	Transient Ischemic Attacks Non-hemorrhagic infarctions	Tremor	Ataxia, Dysarthria, Hyperacusis	Wernicke's syndrome	Bradycardia	Chest pain, arrhythmias	Hypertension / Hypotension	Palpitations	Tachycardia
Alcohol	+ =	+ =	+	+		+	+		+ =		+				+ =					
Amphetamines			+	+	+				+	+						+	+	↕		+
Caffeine							+													
Cannabis			+ =																	+
Cocaine			+	+	+				+	+		+ =				+	+	↕		+
Hallucinogens							+						+						+	+
Inhalants																				
Nicotine /Tobacco			+ =															= ←		+ =
Opioids				+				+	+		+					+ =		←		
PCP/Phencyclidine		+ =						+	+ =	+				+				←		+
Sedative, hypnotic, anxiolytic-related drugs	+ =	+ =	+ =	+		+	+				+							→ =		

+ = Present symptom (included in *DSM-IV-TR*)
= Frequently observed symptom (not included in *DSM-IV-TR*)

Sources:
American Psychiatric Association (APA). (2000). *The diagnostic and statistical manual of mental disorders* (4th ed., Text revision). Washington, DC: Author.
Shiloh, R., Nutt, D., Weizman, A. (2000). *Atlas of Psychiatric Pharmacotherapy.* Rev. ed. London: Martin Dunitz.

Table 24.3 Frequently Observed *Intoxication* Symptoms, Psychiatric, by Class of Substance of Abuse

Class of Substance	Affective					Psychotic											Anxiety			Other						
	Affective blunting	Dysphoria	Euphoria	Manic-like state	Mood lability	Depersonalization	Formication	Hallucinations[1]	Ideas of reference	Impulsiveness, Unpredictability	Inappropriate behaviour[2]	Impaired judgment	Paranoid delusions or ideations	Distorted space/time perceptions	Stereotyped behaviour	Synesthesias	Anxiety (Non-specific)	Panic-like attacks	Phobias	Belligerence, Assaultiveness	Flashbacks	Hypervigilance	Impaired social, occupational functioning	Interpersonal sensitivity	Psychomotor agitation/retardation	Tension, Anger
Alcohol		+ =		+ =	+						+	+					+ =	+ =	+ =				+			
Amphetamines	+		+					+	+ =			+	+ =		+		+					+	+	+	+	
Caffeine																										
Cannabis		+ =	+	+ =		+ =		+				+	+ =	+			+	+ =			+ =		+	+		
Cocaine	+	+	+				+ =	+				+	+ =		+		+					+	+			
Hallucinogens								+				+				+	+	+ =			+		+	+	+	
Inhalants												+											+			
Nicotine/Tobacco																										
Opioids		+	+					+				+											+		+	
PCP/Phencyclidine				+ =		+ =		+		+		+		+ =						+			+		+[3]	
Sedative, hypnotic, anxiolytic-related drugs					+						+	+											+			

+ Present symptom (included in *DSM-IV-TR*)
= Frequently observed symptom (not included in *DSM-IV-TR*)
[1] Non-specific auditory, visual or tactile
[2] Sexual or aggressive
[3] Only psychomotor agitation is part of *DSM-IV-TR* criteria

Table 24.4	Frequently Observed *Symptoms of Withdrawal*, by Class of Substance of Abuse													
Class of Substance	*DSM-IV-TR* Symptoms of Withdrawal													
	Anxiety	Appetite	Autonomic activity[1]	Cognitive	Depressed / dysphoric mood	Fatigue	Fever	GIT	Grand Mal Seizures	Hand Tremor	Hallucinations	Psychomotor activity[2]	Sleep impact[3]	Other
Alcohol	+		⇧[4]					+[5]	+	+	+[6]	A	⇩	
Amphetamines		⇧			+	+						⇧/⇩	⇧/⇩[7]	
Caffeine[8]														
Cannabis														
Cocaine		⇧			+	+						⇧/⇩	⇧/⇩[7]	
Hallucinogens[8]														
Inhalants[8]														
Nicotine / Tobacco	+	⇧[9]	+[10]	+[11]	+								⇩	+[12,13]
Opioids					+		+	+[5,14]					⇩	+[15,16,17,18]
PCP/Phencyclidine[8]														
Sedative, hypnotic, anxiolytic-related drugs	+		⇧					+[5]	+	+	+[6]	⇧	⇩	

+ Present symptom (included in *DSM-IV-TR*)

[1] Autonomic activity: Hyperactivity (⇧), Hypoactivity (⇩)

[2] Psychomotor Activity: Agitation (⇧) or Depression (⇩)

[3] Sleep disturbance: Insomnia (⇩), Hypersomnia (⇧)

[4] Sweating or pulse rate >100

[5] Nausea and vomiting

[6] Hallucinations: Visual (V), Tactile (T), Auditory (A); or Illusions

[7] With vivid, unpleasant dreams

[8] Withdrawal symptoms not recognized in *DSM-IV-TR*

[9] Increased appetite or weight gain

[10] Decreased heart rate

[11] Difficulties concentrating

[12] Irritability, frustration, anger

[13] Restlessness

[14] Diarrhea

[15] Yawning

[16] Pupillary dilatation, piloerection, or sweating

[17] Muscle aches

[18] Lacrimation or rhinorrhea

Sources:
American Psychiatric Association (APA). (2000). *The diagnostic and statistical manual of mental disorders* (4th ed., Text revision). Washington, DC: Author.
Shiloh, R., Nutt, D., Weizman, A. (2000). *Atlas of psychiatric pharmacotherapy*. Rev. ed. London: Martin Dunitz.

caffeine in the prevalence of use. Alcohol (or ethanol) is a widely used addictive and sedative drug, second only to tobacco in its contribution to death, disease, disability, and excess health care spending in Canada. The majority of Canadians consuming alcohol on a regular basis are neither addicted (physiologically or psychologically) to it nor are they abusing it. For some individuals "moderate consumption" of alcohol may have health benefits, and for subsets of the population, safe drinking limits exist (up to nine standard drinks per week for [non-pregnant] females, and up to 14 drinks per week for males; Brands, Kahan, Selby, & Wilson, 2000). As a precautionary measure, for persons with psychiatric illness, those on psychotropic medications, or those with a history of addiction, the concept of "safe drinking limits" does not generally apply. Alcohol consumption is measured in terms of the numbers of "standard drink," each of which contains 13.6 g of alcohol. Different beverages contain different concentrations, and conversion into a "standard drink" is described as the following:

- 43 mL (1.5 oz) spirit (40% alcohol), or
- 142 mL (5 oz) table wine (12% alcohol), or
- 341 mL (12 oz) regular beer (5% alcohol), or
- 85 mL (3 oz) fortified wine (18% alcohol).

Alcohol is water-soluble and, after oral ingestion, it is rapidly and efficiently absorbed from the stomach, small intestine, and colon into the bloodstream. It then crosses the blood–brain barrier and produces a dose-dependent sedative effect by depressing the CNS impacting on a variety of neurotransmitters. It produces a general increase in the fluidity of membranes in the CNS, making these more permeable to potassium (K^+) and chloride (Cl^-) and closing sodium (Na^+) and calcium (Ca^{++}) channels. Alcohol may lead to respiratory depression, and the CNS and respiratory effects can be cumulative when combined with other CNS and respiratory depressants, for example, barbiturates, benzodiazepines, sedating psychotropic medications, and opioids. Alcohol reaches all tissues in the body, and in pregnant women it also crosses the placenta to reach the fetus, where it is especially harmful to the developing brain in utero.

The metabolism of alcohol is linear, and the average healthy adult can metabolize one "standard drink" per hour. Alcohol is metabolized (oxidation) in the liver by alcohol-dehydrogenase and other enzymes, producing acetaldehyde, which is toxic, but which is metabolized by aldehyde dehydrogenase. The inhibition of aldehyde dedydrogenase enzyme (which metabolizes acetaldehyde) can cause an accumulation of acetaldehyde, leading to symptoms of toxicity. A small quantity of alcohol is also excreted through the lungs.

The odour of alcohol is not a reliable indicator of intoxication or impairment. The level of impairment resulting from the use of alcohol is determined by measuring breath or blood alcohol levels (BAL), and the level at which a person is considered to be legally impaired varies with jurisdiction and country. There are blood alcohol content/concentration (BAC) limits for the operation of a vehicle, for instance 0.05% in some Canadian provinces, and 0.08% in others. However, within the criminal code of Canada, the operator of a vehicle could be charged for impaired driving without necessarily reaching the legal alcohol limit.

The physiological effects of alcohol are dependent on a multitude of physiological factors that include, among many others, dose, genetic factors, the level of tolerance, gender, body mass, body fat, liver mass, metabolic rate. The acute effects of alcohol are usually characterized by a feeling of warmth, relaxation, mild sedation and a sense of social disinhibition. In alcohol naïve individuals, a blood alcohol concentration of 160 mg% is associated with obvious intoxication symptoms, which may not be evident in persons who have developed tolerance on physiological or behavioural level. In progressively higher concentrations, there is a greater depressant effect on inhibition and behavioural control, producing heightened emotions, emotional lability (or mood swings), impulsivity, impaired motor and cognitive functioning (including impairment in memory, concentration, attention span, and judgment). In increasingly higher concentrations, it also leads to more severe impairment of motor functions and speech, black-outs, confusion, delirium, respiratory failure, stupor, coma (at about 400 to 560 mg%), and death. Although sedating, alcohol impairs the quality of sleep by disturbing the normal sleep architecture.

Alcohol use is also associated with worsening of certain psychiatric conditions and symptoms, and may increase risk of depression, suicide, homicide, and the risk of harm to self or others. Alcohol also induces the liver enzyme system that leads to more rapid metabolism of therapeutic (and other) compounds, with an anticipated potential for lower therapeutic effects. Excessive or long-term use of alcohol can adversely affect any or all body systems, and some of which could be serious, disabling, and irreversible even if alcohol use is discontinued. These include varying degrees of cognitive impairment, amnestic disorder, dementia, and other neurological complications, for example, neuropathies, cerebellar degeneration, and brain atrophy. In the category of alcohol-induced cognitive disorders, there are the conditions of Wernicke's syndrome and Korsakoff's syndrome. The former develops as a result of thiamine deficiency, and manifests with oculomotor dysfunction, ataxia, and confusion, while the latter is characterized by both retrograde and anterograde amnesia with confabulation as a key feature.

Reduction of consumption, or abstinence, in some individuals may lead to withdrawal symptoms, which may even progress into life-threatening complications. Symptoms of withdrawal typically start hours after the last drink, and may include nausea and vomiting, tactile disturbances, tremor, auditory disturbances, paroxysmal sweats, visual disturbances, anxiety, headaches (or sensations of fullness in the head), agitation, and disturbances in orientation and clouding of the sensorium. It may also include autonomic disturbances, for example, blood pressure increases, tachycardia, diaphoresis, and in severe cases withdrawal may progress to seizures (tonic-clonic), delirium (**delirium tremens**), or death. The level of withdrawal is used to determine the most appropriate dose of pharmacotherapy-assisted symptom-triggered **detoxification** management, and is measured by conducting a brief rating scale, the Clinical Institute Withdrawal Assessment for Alcohol (CIWA-R; Revised, Clinical Institute of Alcohol Withdrawal for Alcohol, Addiction Research Foundation, or Centre for Addiction and Mental Health [CAMH]) found in Appendix G.

Amphetamines (or Amphetamine-like substances)

Amphetamine class drugs include methamphetamine, amphetamine, dextroamphetamine, methylphenidate, as well as selected diet medications (anorexants and selected anti-obesity drugs). The street names include "speed," "crystal," "jib," "ice," "crank," "bennies," "meth," and "uppers," (and many other names) and the amphetamine class drugs can be taken orally, snorted, smoked, or injected.

These drugs act like adrenaline (sympathomimetic), and are stimulating to the CNS and peripheral nervous system. This leads to increased catecholamine release, inhibition of reuptake, and may further act as mono-amine oxidase inhibitors. They are used to treat attention-deficit hyperactivity disorder in children, narcolepsy, depression, and obesity (on a short-term basis). Some people engage in the harmful use of these drugs to achieve the effects of alertness, increased concentration, a sense of increased energy, euphoria, and appetite suppression. There are also drugs from other classes which may mimic the stimulant effects of the amphetamines (e.g., caffeine, cocaine, and ephedrine, phentermine, and mazindol). Depending on the level of purity, the effects of amphetamines typically last for about 6 to 8 hours when injected or taken orally, and longer if smoked. Due to questionable purity, amphetamines may also indirectly act as catecholamine agonists, and cause the release of newly synthesized norepinephrine. Like cocaine, they block the reuptake of norepinephrine and dopamine, but these do not affect the serotonergic system as strongly. They also affect the peripheral nervous system but are typically unpredictable.

Some individuals may engage in inappropriate use (or diversion) of amphetamines, even when appropriately prescribed and dispensed. Inappropriate use also leads to desired effects of alertness, increased concentration, a sense of increased energy, euphoria, and appetite

suppression to lose weight but often leads to problems as a result of misuse, or the setting in which it was obtained or used.

Although the amphetamines are often thought of as aphrodisiacs, they may have the opposite effect. They also act on the peripheral system as powerful sympathomimetics (substances mimicking the effects of the sympathetic nervous system) stimulating both α and β receptors, leading to flushing, excitement, tachycardia, arrhythmias, chest pain, hypertension, and peripheral hyperthermia (Weaver & Schnoll, 1999). The effects of amphetamine use and the clinical course of an overdose are similar to those of cocaine.

Caffeine

Caffeine is the world's most popular psychoactive substance, and the most widely used drug. It is a mild CNS stimulant that is isolated from coffee beans, tea plants, cocao pods, guarana plants, and kola nuts. It is found in many drinks (e.g., coffee, tea, cocoa, soft drinks, and "energy drinks"), and chocolate, and in many over-the-counter medications (e.g., analgesics, stimulants, appetite suppressants, and cold relief preparations). A typical cup of brewed coffee contains 100 mg caffeine, but the content may vary greatly depending on the type of product or beverage.

Caffeine exerts stimulating effects on both mental and motor performance, and is subjectively viewed as beneficial by some in alleviating mood. It does, however, cause or exacerbate tremors; impair motor performance; lead to anxiety, dysphoria, and insomnia. When used in high doses over the course of time, it can be associated with unpleasant withdrawal symptoms when abruptly tapered or discontinued.

Caffeine expectedly curbs fatigue and increases mental acuity. Higher doses increase the heart rate; stimulate respiratory, vasomotor, and vagal centres and cardiac muscles, resulting in increased heart contractibility, dilate pulmonary and coronary blood vessels; and constrict blood flow to the cerebral vascular system. Modest consumption of caffeine, in otherwise healthy persons, is not associated with adverse health consequences but increasing evidence suggests the existence of the syndrome of dependence with the chronic use of caffeine. The theoretical and potentially lethal dose of caffeine is estimated as 5,000 mg, or the equivalent of 40 cups of coffee, if consumed over a very brief period of time.

Cannabis (Marijuana)

Cannabis has been cultivated from the plant *Cannabis sativa*, for centuries, and it is the most commonly used illicit drug in Canada. Although occasionally classified as a hallucinogenic drug, its effects are less intense than that of other hallucinogens. Cannabis delivers numerous fat-soluble cannabinoids (the main active component of the plant) to the brain where its active ingredient, D-9-tetrahydrocannabinol (9-Δ-THC or THC), acts as an agonist at the cannabinoid CB_1-receptors, and also exerts an effect on the μ-opioid receptor. It can be ingested orally, smoked, or vaporized, and has many street names including "grass," "weed," "pot," "dope," "hash," and "herb." Cannabis is often used with alcohol (which reinforces cannabis' effects), tobacco, and other drugs. Depending on the dose and route of administration, the effects begin shortly after administration (when smoked), and typically last from 1 to 3 hours (or longer when swallowed).

The body will store cannabinoids for weeks in deposits of fat tissue and in the brain, and its slow release causes urine drug screens to remain positive for several weeks after last use in persons chronically using heavy doses. Cannabis' effects include relaxation, euphoria, at times dyscoria (abnormal pupillary reaction or shape), distortion of senses, conjunctival injection, spatial misperception, time distortion (time standing still), tachycardia, hypotension, and increased appetite/food cravings ("the munchies"). In the short term, it can result in motor impairment, loss of coordination, balance, and slowing of reaction time. This translates into the potential for significant impairment in the ability to safely operate machinery or a vehicle, and studies show that approximately 4% to 14% of drivers who sustained injury or died in traffic accidents tested positive for THC (Ramaekers, Berghaus, van Laar, & Drummer, 2004). When smoked, cannabis delivers to the body similar toxic chemicals to tobacco, and exposure during pregnancy may result in cognitive problems in offspring.

Long-term use may impair consolidation of memory, recall ability, and impair cognition, hence interfering with academic functioning. Weight gain can also occur as a result of chronic appetite stimulation. Persons consuming high potency cannabis, or heavy doses, may develop psychotic symptoms, and the use of cannabis is recognized as an independent risk factor in the development of schizophrenia and psychosis. A controversial syndrome possibly associated with chronic, heavy cannabis use is that of lower ambition, decreased volition, and poor scholastic and academic performance called the "amotivational syndrome."

Cannabinoids are also synthetically produced and commercially available for the treatment of selected medical conditions/symptoms (e.g., appetite stimulation related to medical illness in HIV/AIDS, remedy pain, multiple sclerosis, and for the treatment of nausea). Only under very specific and regulated circumstances, individuals who qualify may access the drug through the federal Medical Marijuana Access Regulations. Unless the particular individual has a legal exemption, it is illegal to possess, cultivate, or sell cannabis in Canada.

Cocaine

Cocaine ("coke," "blow," "snow," "crack," and other street names) is a powerful and highly addictive stimulant, which is either snorted (powder), smoked (crack), or injected. Cocaine, also a local anesthetic, is isolated from the *Erythroxylum coca* plant, native to South America. The leaves are refined into cocaine hydrochloride, a crystalline form (white powder appearance), while the smokable form, called *free-base* cocaine, is created by chemical alteration. Cocaine is highly addictive, and is often co-administered with other addictive chemicals like alcohol or tobacco. *Crack cocaine*, often called "crack" or "rock," is a form of free-base cocaine produced by mixing the crystal with water and baking soda or sodium bicarbonate and boiling it until a solid precipitant remains. The crystalline substance is then broken into pieces ("cracked") and smoked in cigarettes or water pipes. This ultra-potent form of chemically altered cocaine produces a rapid high and an intense euphoria, followed by an even more dramatic crash-phase. It is considered extremely addictive because of the intense and rapid onset of euphoric effects, and the relative access cost (or street price per "hit") is lower than for other cocaine forms.

When snorted, injected, or smoked, cocaine rapidly crosses the blood–brain barrier and peak intoxication occurs within seconds after intravenous injection or crack smoking. Injecting releases the drug directly into the bloodstream and heightens the intensity of its effects. Smoking entails the inhalation of cocaine vapour or smoke into the lungs, where absorption into the bloodstream is as rapid as by injection (National Institute on Drug Abuse [NIDA], 2009). Dopamine and dopamine metabolite levels are depleted by prolonged cocaine use, leading to increased prolactin levels. Cocaine use causes tachycardia, hypertension, dilated pupils, and rises in body temperature. It may contribute to seizures, myocardial infarcts, cerebrovascular accidents, and crosses the placenta. Cocaine used with alcohol leads to the formation of a unique metabolite, which is especially cardiotoxic.

Shortly after cocaine is snorted or injected, the individual experiences a sudden burst of alertness and energy ("cocaine rush"), euphoria, increased feelings of self-confidence, being in control, and sociability, which last 10 to 20 minutes when smoked, and 60 to 90 minutes when powder is snorted. There is an increase in sense awareness (e.g., sexuality is heightened, sound, touch, and sight are more acute). There is also a decreased need for sleep and a lowering of appetite. Along with this, anxiety and restlessness as well as agitation may occur. With the use of higher doses, there may also occur panic, mania, psychosis (hallucinations, disorganization, and delusions), erratic and bizarre behaviours, potentially leading up to violence and potential risk of harm. The use of cocaine in an individual with a vulnerability to depression, mania, or psychosis may experience exacerbation of symptoms of related psychiatric conditions.

The high is followed by a significant and intense depressive phase (let-down effect or "cocaine crash") in which the subject feels irritable, depressed, tired, and displays increased appetite and powerful cravings for the drug. The individual may desperately seek cocaine or even other drugs, to self-medicate some of the unpleasant side-effects of the crash phase. Similar to the severe anxiety, restlessness and agitation of intoxication, these symptoms may also appear during withdrawal. These, along with drug-seeking behaviour, may last for weeks, contributing to the extremely high relapse rates observed in these persons.

Hallucinogens

The hallucinogens (the "psychedelics") refer to a class of drugs that are sometimes used in religious/spiritual settings, and may be termed "entheogens." There are more than 100 different hallucinogens with substantially different molecular structures and unique features. These drugs have salient effects in changing the senses (e.g., visual, auditory, gustatory, tactile, and olfactory), and may induce euphoria or dysphoria, altered body image, distorted sensory perceptions, confusion, incoordination, and impaired judgment and memory. In severe cases, individuals have reported paranoia, depersonalization, illusions, delusions, and hallucinations. Several of these drugs are used alone or in conjunction with alcohol, tobacco, and other street drugs, predominantly in settings of nightclubs, bars, and rave scenes and have colloquially become known as "club drugs."

Most hallucinogens belong to one of six categories:

1. The indolealkylamines: LSD/D-lysergic acid diethylamide, LSA/D-lysergic amide (morning glory seeds), Psilocybin (magic mushrooms), Psilocin and DMT (dimethyltryptamine or the "spirit molecule")
2. Phenylethylamines: Mescaline (from cactus plant) and Designer drugs including: MDMA (3,4-methlyendioxymethamphetamine), or Ecstasy (XTC), MDA (methlyendioxyamphetamine), TMA (trimethoxyamphetamine), STP (2,5-domethoxy-4-methylamphetamine), PMA (paramethoxyamphetamine)
3. Arylcycloalkylamines (PCP and ketamine)
4. Cannabinoids (THC)
5. Anticholinergics
6. Diterpene salvinorin-A (*Salvia divinorum*)

Hallucinogens typically affect the autonomic and regulatory nervous systems first, increasing heart rate and body temperature, and slightly elevating blood pressure. The individual may experience dry mouth, dizziness, and subjective feelings of being hot or cold. Intense mood and sexual behaviour changes may occur; and the subject may feel unusually close to others or distant and isolated.

Methamphetamine (MDMA) causes serotonin to be released from neurons in greater amounts than usual, activating serotonin receptors. Further, MDMA causes excess dopamine release from neurons, and there are suggestions that it can damage and destroy serotonin-containing neurons. Also, MDMA can cause hallucinations, confusion, depression, sleep problems, drug craving, severe anxiety, and paranoia and, in high doses, MDMA can cause a sharp increase in body temperature (malignant hyperthermia), leading to muscle breakdown (myolysis), kidney failure, cardiovascular collapse, and death.

Phencyclidine (PCP or "angel dust"), not a true hallucinogen, can affect many neurotransmitter systems; it interferes with the functioning of the glutamate but also enhances dopamine release. At low to moderate doses, PCP causes altered perception of body image but rarely produces visual hallucinations. PCP can also cause effects that mimic the primary symptoms of schizophrenia, such as delusions and mental turmoil. People who use PCP for long periods of time have memory loss and speech difficulties.

Ketamine is an anesthetic drug, leading to dissociation. Although ketamine (street name: Special-K) is classified as a "club drug," it follows the characteristics of PCP, albeit less potent on an equivalent mass basis, and possesses properties overlapping with the *DSM-IV-TR* class of hallucinogens. Ketamine has legitimate medical utility in both human and veterinary medicine, with specific value in emergency medicine. The only known and documented source of illicit sales is through the manufacturing pharmaceutical industry linked to third world settings or "war-time medicine." In illicit settings it is often injected, insufflated (i.e., blown into a body cavity), smoked, or taken orally, and it has a similar physical appearance to cocaine (pure). Ketamine has been reported as the selected drug of choice in "date rape" cases.

The mechanism of action on the brain is similar for both PCP and ketamine, namely to block a specific subset of protein molecules, called NMDA (*N*-methyl-D-aspartic acid) receptors, involved in memory functions of the brain. With this NMDA antagonism, ketamine typically induces a state of sensory deprivation and dissociation by blocking signals from the senses and certain brain parts to the conscious mind, and interfering with memory and other cognitive functions. Upon administration, a state of acute mental decompensation can occur, characterized by diminished ability to think and carry on daily activities, and typically includes loss of memory (both long term and short term). A sense of detachment from the external world, or from their own body, occurs and in this dissociative states certain thoughts, emotions, sensations, and/or memories may not be integrated in the usual fashion when compared to a drug-free state. In sufficient doses the appearance of disorganization can occur, and there can also follow the appearance of stupor.

Inhalants

Inhalants refer to a group of chemical vapours or gasses, including organic solvents, or *volatile substances*, that are inhaled (breathed in), causing a high. These substances are not intended for human consumption, and although the effects may vary, several are considered CNS depressants. Inhalants typically are used by younger individuals; in lower socio-economic settings, are often universally available and accessible, as well as generally affordable. The relative ease of access, and local custom, are factors in promoting their use, and inhalant, particularly solvent use, is a particular challenge in the Aboriginal communities of Canada. The inhalants are divided into four classes, but there are hundreds of different chemicals belonging to this class of abused substances:

1. Volatile solvents (benzene, toluene, xylene, acetone, hexane, felt-tip markers, hobby glue, airplane glue, polyvinyl chloride cement, rubber cement, dry cleaning fluid, spot removers, degreasers, computer cleaners, paint and nail polish removers, paint thinners, correction fluids, lighter fluid)
2. Aerosols or spray cans (whipped cream and cooking oil sprays, hair spray, fluorocarbon, butane, [pressurized liquids or gases], asthma sprays, deodorants, air fresheners)
3. Gases (oxide [laughing gas], chloroform, halothane, ether, butane, propane, enflurane, isoflurane, ethyl chloride)
4. Nitrites (amyl, butyl, isopropyl nitrite)

As a class, the inhalants are known to cause euphoria, sedation, emotional lability, and/or impaired judgment. In some cases, intoxication can result in respiratory depression, stupor, and coma. Most inhalants are common household products that give off mind-altering chemical fumes when sniffed. The chemical structure of the various types of inhalants is diverse, making it difficult to generalize about their effects. However, serious health consequences may ensue, including hearing loss, damage to the liver, kidney, lungs, and heart, as well as bone marrow suppression. The vaporous fumes can alter brain chemistry and may permanently damage the brain and CNS. Magnetic resonance imaging scans of users demonstrate severe changes in cerebral white matter (NIDA, 2005b), including atrophy, and a fetal solvent syndrome has been described. The nitrates are associated with unsafe sexual practices with an increased risk of contracting HIV and hepatitis. Associated with nitrous oxide may be frostbite, anoxia, nerve damage, and loss of motor control. The inhalants are considered to be potentially addictive.

Nicotine (Tobacco)

If tobacco was introduced to the market today, it could not become a legal product because of its lethality. Tobacco smoke contains over 4,000 chemicals, of which there are at least 172 toxic substances, 33 hazardous air pollutants, 47 chemicals restricted as hazardous waste, and 67 known human or animal carcinogens (Repace, 2006). These exist whether tobacco smoke is inhaled in the act of smoking, or inhaled by non-smokers out of the air indoors or outdoors. Nicotine is an addictive chemical found within the tobacco plant, has both stimulant and depressant effects, and is considered as the fundamental chemical "driver" of the process of addiction in the brain. The use of tobacco products without nicotine would not be addictive but, paradoxically, nicotine is not the harmful chemical found within tobacco products and pharmaceutical grade nicotine is generally considered safe. It is the tar, other chemicals, additives, and substances in tobacco products that threaten health.

Tobacco is most commonly consumed by smoking cigarettes but it is also smoked as cigars, pipes, or bidis (small hand-rolled cigarettes), chewed as chewing tobacco, sniffed as dry snuff or held inside the lip or cheek as wet snuff. Following inhalation, nicotine is rapidly delivered via the arterial system to the brain where it binds primarily to $\alpha_4\beta_2$ nicotinic receptors (natural ligands—a molecule, or group of molecules that binds to another to form a larger complex—for acetylcholine), which are central to the initiation and maintenance of nicotine addiction. When chronically stimulated by nicotine, up-regulation and desensitization of these receptors follow. The stimulation of these nicotinic receptors ultimately results in the release of dopamine in the "pleasure centre" of the brain. The reward pathway also becomes desensitized as a result of chronic exposure to nicotine and represents a second major maladaptive change in brain function that follows tobacco administration.

A cigarette provides approximately 10 puffs, and a person who smokes 20 cigarettes/day (one pack) is taking 200 doses of nicotine daily. No other drug, even cocaine, is dosed that frequently, and conditioned cues to smoke become established. As a result, desiring a cigarette becomes associated with everyday events such as getting up in the morning, drinking coffee or alcohol, taking a break, and having a conversation. The quantity and power of this conditioning is unique to cigarette smoking, and it is one of the reasons that smoking is so difficult to quit. Signs of tobacco dependence include the urge to smoke within minutes of waking, smoking at regular intervals throughout the day, and continuing to smoke despite wanting to quit. People who are dependent may become tolerant to the desired effects and may no longer experience pleasure from smoking but continue to smoke in order to avoid nicotine withdrawal.

Symptoms of nicotine withdrawal vary but may include cravings, irritability, restlessness, difficulty concentrating, depression, frustration, anxiety, insomnia, fatigue, and increased appetite. Most symptoms reach maximum intensity at 24 to 48 hours, and are relieved within a few weeks, but some individuals may be unable to concentrate and have strong cravings to smoke for weeks or months after quitting smoking. The tobacco plant contains a class of chemicals, the β-carbolines, which are monoamine oxidase inhibitors (like certain antidepressants). Quitting smoking also stops the ingestion of this naturally found antidepressant and, for this reason, depressive symptoms may be triggered in some individuals who are quitting smoking.

The use of tobacco products remains the most important preventable cause of death and disease, and is projected to kill one billion deaths internationally during the 21st century. Tobacco is a risk factor for six of the eight leading causes of death, is responsible for 1 out of every 10 deaths of adults globally, and 45% of smokers will die of a tobacco-induced disorder (Lerman, Patterson, & Berrettini, 2005). Cigarettes are a highly lucrative sales item and this has shaped the tobacco industry's rejection of evidence that supports the lethal consequences of tobacco addiction but also necessitates their need to find "replacements" for their sick and dying customers from markets including youth, woman, and third world countries.

Opioids

The opioids represent a broad category of psychoactive drugs, consisting of both licit and illicit drugs, that act by attaching to the endogenous opioid receptors in the brain. They are typically used as antitussives (cough suppressants), analgesics, and to treat pulmonary edema. Heroin is processed from morphine, a naturally occurring substance extracted from the seed pod of certain varieties of the poppy plant. It is illegal, highly addictive, and represents the most commonly abused and most rapidly acting of the opioids. It is typically sold as a white or brownish powder or as the black sticky substance known as "black tar heroin." On the streets, it is frequently "cut" with other substances such as sugar, starch, powdered milk, quinine, strychnine, or other poisons. It can be sniffed, snorted, and smoked but is most frequently injected, which poses risks for the transmission of HIV and other diseases from the sharing of needles or other injection equipment.

The opioid family of drugs are available on the street ("horse," "greys," "oxy's," "demonol," "dilly," "smack," "H," "speedball," "junk," etc.) and include the following:

1. Pure opioid agonists that include
   a. Naturally occurring alkaloids: (opium), morphine, codeine,
   b. Semi-synthetic drugs (e.g., heroin [diacetylmorphine]), and
   c. Synthetic drugs (e.g., oxycodone, methadone, fentanyl, meperidine, hydrocodone, propoxyphene, tramadol)

2. Mixed agonist-antagonists (e.g., pentazocine, butorphanol)
3. Partial agonists: buprenorphine (combined with naloxone).

Opioids cause CNS depression, sleep or stupor, and analgesia, and possess strong reinforcing properties that can quickly trigger addiction when used improperly. Opiates elicit their effects by binding to opioid receptors that are widely distributed throughout the brain and body. The effect produced by activated receptors in the brain correlates with the area of the brain involved. Two important effects produced by opioids are pleasure (or reward) and pain relief (analgesia). The brain itself also produces substances known as endorphins that activate the opiate receptors. Research indicates that endorphins are involved in many functions, including respiration, nausea, vomiting, pain modulation, and hormonal regulation (NIDA, 2005a).

Opioids may cause tolerance and physical dependence (sometimes rapidly), which appear to be specific for each receptor subtype. The use of opioids may in the early stages be associated with euphoria in some cases. Tolerance develops particularly to the analgesic, respiratory depression, and sedative actions of the opioids. The common physical effects associated with the use of the opioids include sweating, nausea, constipation (which can progress to narcotic bowel syndrome), and dose-dependent sedation, fatigue, confusion, cognitive impairment, respiratory depression, as well as reproductive and endocrine effects (e.g., suppression of testosterone in men and menstrual irregularities in women). In some cases, the opioids are used concurrently with other sedative drugs (e.g., benzodiazepines, alcohol, barbiturates, or sedating antidepressants). In these cases, the risk of CNS and respiratory depression may be especially salient thus warranting an even higher level of vigilance in their assessment and management. There is further a phenomenon called medication-induced headaches, for example, with the chronic use of analgesics, where the analgesic drug is causally linked to the exacerbation of the headache, and improvement is noticed when the analgesic is discontinued.

Even when following a regime as prescribed by a physician, individuals may become addicted to opioids, especially when injudiciously prescribed. Inquiry into the patterns of abuse of opioids should occur if persons report or are found to be "double-doctoring," "borrowing pain killers from others," buying black market opioids, when individuals run out of their medication early, or when triplicate prescriptions are reported to be lost or stolen. When use of the drug is discontinued, or rapidly tapered after a period of continuous use, a rebound hyperexcitability withdrawal syndrome may occur. Withdrawal may be associated with severe cravings and mimics a "bad case of the flu," involving both the respiratory and gastrointestinal (GI) systems. It may include symptoms of anxiety, dysphoria, nausea, vomiting, muscle aches, lacrimation or rhinorrhea, papillary dilatation, piloerection, sweating, diarrhea, yawning, fever, and insomnia. These withdrawal symptoms are not typically life threatening, but can be particularly uncomfortable, and may lead to significant distress. Medically ill, pregnant, very young and very old individuals at risk of opioid withdrawal may be more prone to developing medical complications during withdrawal from opioids or combination drugs.

Sedative, Hypnotic, and Anxiolytic-Related Drugs

Sedative, hypnotic, and anxiolytic-related (antianxiety) agents are synthetic medications that are sedating, induce sleep, and reduce anxiety. Barbiturates were the first class of drugs used to treat sleep disturbances and anxiety, and have largely been replaced by benzodiazepines because of their comparative safety with regard to potential toxicity and addictive qualities. Benzodiazepine is often used to sedate individuals pre-operatively, to treat seizures and alcohol withdrawal, and as muscle relaxants. They are manufactured in laboratories of pharmaceutical companies, and their street names include "benzos," "tranks," and "downers."

There are in excess of 50 different benzodiazepines (e.g., diazepam, oxazepam, temazepam, lorazepam) available on the global markets but only a few are available in Canada. Benzodiazepines modulate γ-aminobutyric acid (GABA) transmission and interact with specific receptor sites in the brain. GABA is the most abundant inhibitory neurotransmitter in the brain. Benzodiazepines, by displacing an endogenous binding inhibitor, increase GABA's affinity for its receptor and thus enhance GABA function. Benzodiazepines act in a manner similar to alcohol and other sedative hypnotics, making neuronal membranes more permeable to K^+ and Cl^- and closing Na^+ and Ca^{++} channels, causing CNS depression.

Flunitrazepam also belongs to the benzodiazepine family, and it is illegal to possess, traffic, import, or produce in Canada. Also known as "roofies," "roachies," "La Roche," "rope," "rophies," and "ruffies," flunitrazepam is referred to as a "date rape" drug. It comes as a white tablet, scored on one side, and turns liquids bright blue when dissolved. It is rarely taken on its own; rather it is usually taken to increase the effect of other drugs, especially alcohol, marijuana or heroin. It is also taken to decrease the after effects of other drugs such as cocaine, ecstasy, or amphetamines. The most extreme and immediate dangers of flunitrazepam are caused by its intoxicating and sedating effects.

Although not a benzodiazepine, *GHB* (γ-hydroxybutyrate) is another drug in the sedative-hypnotic class. Like flunitrazepam, it is a potent CNS depressant that is illegal to possess, traffic, import, or produce in Canada.

Its street names include "G," "liquid ecstasy," "liquid x," "grievous bodily harm." In its liquid form, GHB looks like water (but could be straw coloured), has almost no smell (if pure), and is almost tasteless (if pure) or has a slightly salty or solvent taste that can be easily masked. It is also available as a white powder or capsule, or can be sold in liquid vials, or produced from its precursors obtained through the internet. It has gained popularity as a "club drug" for its euphoric and sedative effects, is used by some body builders, and has also been used to facilitate sexual assault ("date rape"). At a low dose, the effect is similar to the influence of alcohol but there is only a slight difference between a dose that produces the desired effects and a dose that puts the user at risk. Since it is illegal, there are no controls over the strength and purity of the drugs produced, and there are risks of toxic effects, overdose, and even death. The withdrawal syndrome is especially troublesome and may lead to severe medical complications.

The abuse of sedative, hypnotic, and anxiolytic-related agents is common and complex, especially among people who abuse other drugs to enhance their effects (e.g., opioids and alcohol) or to ease the agitation of drugs that have stimulant effects, such as ecstasy or cocaine. This is extremely dangerous and can put individuals at risk for overdose, causing coma or death. The combination of benzodiazepines and alcohol also complicates withdrawal treatment because the individual may seem to improve after the alcohol withdrawal syndrome subsides, only to have similar symptoms emerge as the benzodiazepine withdrawal syndrome appears. The severity of symptoms during benzodiazepine withdrawal depends on the duration and dosage of regular use; symptoms include the following:

- Anxiety rebound—tension, agitation, tremulousness, insomnia, anorexia.
- Autonomic rebound—hypertension, tachycardia, sweating, hyperpyrexia.
- Sensory excitement—paresthesias, photophobia, hyperacusis (sensitivity to sound), illusions.
- Motor excitation—hyperreflexia, tremors, myoclonus, fasciculation (visible muscle contraction), myalgia, muscle weakness, tonic–clonic convulsions.
- Cognitive excitement—nightmares, delirium, depersonalization, hallucinations.

Process Addictions

A range of other compulsive behaviours have been postulated to form part of the addiction-related disorder spectrum. These include "sex addiction," "exercise addiction," "video gaming addiction," "gambling addiction" (which is classified as an impulse control disorder), and others. The *DSM-IV-TR* (APA, 2000) diagnostic indicators for persistent and recurrent maladaptive gambling

BOX 24.3

Principles of Addiction Treatment

1. Addiction is a complex but treatable disease that affects brain function and behaviour. Drugs of abuse alter the brain's structure and function, resulting in changes that persist long after drug use has ceased. This may explain why drug abusers are at risk for relapse even after long periods of abstinence and despite the potentially devastating consequences.

2. No single treatment is appropriate for everyone. Matching treatment settings, interventions, and services to an individual's particular problems and needs is critical to his or her ultimate success in returning to productive functioning in the family, workplace, and society.

3. Treatment needs to be readily available. Because drug-addicted individuals may be uncertain about entering treatment, taking advantage of available services the moment people are ready for treatment is critical. Potential patients can be lost if treatment is not immediately available or readily accessible. As with other chronic diseases, the earlier treatment is offered in the disease process, the greater the likelihood of positive outcomes.

4. Effective treatment attends to multiple needs of the individual, not just his or her drug abuse. To be effective, treatment must address the individual's drug abuse and any associated medical, psychological, social, vocational, and legal problems. It is also important that treatment be appropriate to the individual's age, gender, ethnicity, and culture.

5. Remaining in treatment for an adequate period of time is critical. The appropriate duration for an individual depends on the type and degree of his or her problems and needs. Research indicates that most addicted individuals need at least 3 months in treatment to significantly reduce or stop their drug use and that the best outcomes occur with longer durations of treatment. Recovery from drug addiction is a longterm process and frequently requires multiple episodes of treatment. As with other chronic illnesses, relapses to drug abuse can occur and should signal a need for treatment to be reinstated or adjusted. Because individuals often leave treatment prematurely, programs should include strategies to engage and keep patients in treatment.

6. Counselling—individual and/or group—and other behavioural therapies are the most commonly used forms of drug abuse treatment. Behavioural therapies vary in their focus and may involve addressing a patient's motivation to change, providing incentives for abstinence, building skills to resist drug use, replacing drug-using activities with constructive and rewarding activities, improving problem solving skills, and facilitating better interpersonal relationships. Also, participation in group therapy and other peer support programs during and following treatment can help maintain abstinence.

7. Medications are an important element of treatment for many patients, especially when combined with counselling and other behavioural therapies. For example, methadone and buprenorphine are effective in helping individuals addicted to heroin or other opioids stabilize their lives and reduce their illicit drug use. Naltrexone is also an effective medication for some opioid-addicted individuals and some patients with alcohol dependence. Other medications for alcohol dependence include acamprosate, disulfiram, and topiramate. For persons addicted to nicotine, a nicotine replacement product (such as patches, gum, or lozenges) or an oral medication (such as bupropion or varenicline) can be an effective component of treatment when part of a comprehensive behavioural treatment program.

8. An individual's treatment and services plan must be assessed continually and modified as necessary to ensure that it meets his or her changing needs. A patient may require varying combinations of services and treatment components during the course of treatment and recovery. In addition to counselling or psychotherapy, a patient may require medication, medical services, family therapy, parenting instruction, vocational rehabilitation, and/or social and legal services. For many patients, a continuing care approach provides the best results, with the treatment intensity varying according to a person's changing needs.

9. Many drug-addicted individuals also have other mental disorders. Because drug abuse and addiction—both of which are mental disorders—often co-occur with other mental illnesses, patients presenting with one condition should be assessed for the other(s). And when these problems co-occur, treatment should address both (or all), including the use of medications as appropriate.

10. Medically assisted detoxification is only the first stage of addiction treatment and by itself does little to change long-term drug abuse. Although medically assisted detoxification can safely manage the acute physical symptoms of withdrawal and, for some, can pave the way for effective long-term addiction treatment, detoxification alone is rarely sufficient to help addicted individuals achieve long-term abstinence. Thus, patients should be encouraged to continue drug treatment following detoxification. Motivational enhancement and incentive strategies, begun at initial patient intake, can improve treatment engagement.

11. Treatment does not need to be voluntary to be effective. Sanctions or enticements from family, employment settings, and/or the criminal justice system can significantly increase treatment entry, retention rates, and the ultimate success of drug treatment interventions.

12. Drug use during treatment must be monitored continuously, as lapses during treatment do occur. Knowing their drug use is being monitored can be a powerful incentive for patients and can help them withstand urges to use drugs. Monitoring also provides an early indication of a return to drug use, signaling a possible need to adjust an individual's treatment plan to better meet his or her needs.

13. Treatment programs should assess patients for the presence of HIV/AIDS, hepatitis B and C, tuberculosis, and other infectious diseases as well as provide targeted risk-reduction counselling to help patients modify or change behaviours that place them at risk of contracting or spreading infectious diseases. Typically, drug abuse treatment addresses some of the drug-related behaviours that put people at risk of infectious diseases. Targeted counselling specifically focused on reducing infectious disease risk can help patients further reduce or avoid substance-related and other high-risk behaviours. Counselling can also help those who are already infected to manage their illness. Moreover, engaging in substance abuse treatment can facilitate adherence to other medical treatments. Patients may be reluctant to accept screening for HIV (and other infectious diseases); therefore, it is incumbent upon treatment providers to encourage and support HIV screening and inform patients that highly active antiretroviral therapy (HAART) has proven effective in combating HIV, including among drug-abusing populations.

From The United States Government's National Institute on Drug Abuse (revised April 2009). Available at: http://www.drugabuse.gov/PODAT/PODATIndex.html

behaviour are five (or more) of the following in the same 12-month period:

- is preoccupied with gambling (e.g., preoccupied with reliving past gambling experiences, handicapping or planning the next venture, or thinking of ways to get money with which to gamble),
- needs to gamble with increasing amounts of money in order to achieve the desired excitement,
- has repeated unsuccessful efforts to control, cut back, or stop gambling,
- is restless or irritable when attempting to cut down or stop gambling,
- gambles as a way of escaping from problems or of relieving a dysphoric mood (e.g., feelings of helplessness, guilt, anxiety, depression),
- after losing money gambling, often returns another day to get even ("chasing" one's losses),
- lies to family members, therapist, or others to conceal the extent of involvement with gambling,
- has committed illegal acts such as forgery, fraud, theft, or embezzlement to finance gambling,
- has jeopardized or lost a significant relationship, job, or educational or career opportunity because of gambling,
- relies on others to provide money to relieve a desperate financial situation caused by gambling, or
- the gambling behaviour is not better accounted for by a manic episode.

More research is needed for the process addictions and related conditions to reach the necessary internal consistency of criteria, or the diagnostic stability for inclusion in the categories of addictions, or in the DSM classification system, which would then have to be expanded beyond the current designation of "substance-related disorders."

▨ INTERDISCIPLINARY TREATMENT RECOMMENDATIONS FOR PATIENTS WITH SRD

The National Institute on Drug Abuse (NIDA) updated their seminal document titled: *"Principles of Drug Addiction Treatment"* in 2009 to reflect the most up-to-date treatment concepts and recommendations (Box 24-3). These principles are intended to address addiction to alcohol, tobacco, and other drugs and are based on the existing body of scientific evidence. They provide a critical starting point for any discussion about treatment for addiction.

Goals of Addiction Treatment

Safe and effective treatment for individuals with SRD requires the completion of a comprehensive assessment,

---

BOX 24.4

Goals of Addiction Treatment

The *goals* of addiction treatment include the following:
- Treatment retention.
- Reduction in severity and frequency of substance use episodes.
- Reducing harm caused by substances, with the ultimate goal of total abstinence.
- Management of comorbid psychiatric and medical conditions.
- Improving the patient's quality of life.
- Improving all areas of life affected by addiction (e.g., employment, interpersonal relationships, interface with the law/criminal justice system, physical health).
- Improving all levels of adaptive functioning.
- Preventing relapse to substance use.

---

matching treatment to include the evidence-based modalities available for the particular disorder and comorbidities, as well as follow-up on a longitudinal basis. Treatment should be culturally sensitive and appropriate, taking into account the specific needs and preferences of the patient. Issues related to gay, lesbian, and transgender individuals, pregnant women, ethnic minorities, gender-related variables, age, and medical needs are to be considered as well in the treatment provision. See Box 24-4 for specific goals of addiction treatment.

The **multi-modal** treatment of addiction recognizes the chronic and relapsing nature of this medical condition, and therefore conceptualizes recovery as a "process" and not an event. Treatment typically involves a combination of psychosocial interventions as well as pharmacotherapy where (and if) available for a particular condition. A longitudinal approach to management of this chronic disease (like with other chronic medical conditions) is ideal and, in general, the iterative goals of treatment are first to engage, to assess, to motivate, and help to retain the patient in a safe and effective evidence-based treatment setting. Treatment retention and adherence to mutually agreed-upon goals generally maximizes the potential benefits of treatment and improves outcomes.

Treatment further seeks to help educate patients, their family members, caregivers, and significant others (e.g., spouse, partner) about addiction as a disease, its causes, consequences, longitudinal approaches to, and the options for interdisciplinary treatment. In some cases and situations, **harm reduction** may be an interim step toward abstinence, and these philosophies are not mutually exclusive. Understanding the complementary nature of this approach is vital, and this may mean using a harm reduction approach under certain circumstances and thereby initially working toward reducing harm as a first step toward abstinence.

The **therapeutic alliance** (or the "helping alliance" between the nurse and the patient) is a *key ingredient* that is vital for treatment success. This therapeutic alliance builds a foundation of trust and non-judgment, provides hope for recovery, and begins at the very first meeting with the patient. Nurses should aim to establish rapport and create a positive alliance with the patient, which is the trusting relationship within which change can be negotiated. This generally facilitates treatment, improves adherence with treatment, and ultimately improves outcomes.

In order to establish a therapeutic alliance, the nurse should try to minimize or avoid premature and inappropriate confrontations, judgment, negative interactions, advice without permission, and other approaches not congruent with motivation-based techniques. Some health professionals may experience an element of negative bias and stereotyping of people, perhaps stemming from their own particular background, psychodynamics, or their own losses or experiences with addiction. For the ethical professional, it is important to make the effort of processing any unresolved conflicts and losses in her/his own life and to successfully work through any related issues. The evidence clearly suggests that confrontational style is generally not helpful for addiction treatment, and can lead to the patient being more defensive, displaying increased levels of **denial**, decreased levels of treatment acceptance, and even disengagement in treatment. Among the most important and valuable skills and attitudes, translating into treatment success for the patient, is the nurse's appropriate empathy, boundary setting, confidence, instillation of hope, and the provision of support and encouragement.

Multi-Dimensional Assessment

Assessment serves as an early mechanism to engage, motivate, and retain the patient in treatment, and to assess for any imminent risk of harm. It further aims to guide ongoing management, and allows for the measurement of progress and outcomes. Assessment involves an evaluation of the following domains, including:

- Substance use description, including:
  - Onset of use or change of pattern of use.
  - Quantity per day or per week.
  - Frequency of use, and periods of abstinence.
  - Route of use (e.g., injection, smoke, snort, oral ingestion).
  - Prior treatment received (e.g., 12 steps, residential care).
  - Sources of substances (e.g., black market, double doctoring, borrowing others' medication).

- A comprehensive psychiatric assessment, including obtaining a family and social history. Assessment should incorporate details of any emotional and behavioural condition, or complications (psychiatric, emotional, behavioural status, including any potential for imminent and substantial risk of harm to self or to others, e.g., risk of suicide or risk of aggression, including homicide).
- A comprehensive physical assessment, including screening for infectious diseases (e.g., HIV, STDs, TB, hepatitis). The assessment of biomedical conditions and complications, associated with substance use, forms part of this domain. The assessment should further focus on the risk for acute intoxication and/or withdrawal potential in the patient.
- Collateral information from others (with necessary consent).
- Qualitative and quantitative screening for substance use, using toxicology testing/drug screens (in urine, saliva, blood, hair, or relevant matrices), as well as laboratory testing, for example, liver function testing.
- Inquiry about the patient's preferences for treatment. The patient's level of treatment acceptance and elements of resistance should be explored.
  - Assessment of risk for relapse (relapse potential) and recovery environment.
  - The use of structured rating scales to help quantify clinical features and provide baseline for serial monitoring of progress.

Principles of Matching Treatment

As an overarching principle, treatment should be offered on the least restrictive level of care that is proven to be safe and likely to be effective. Patients are matched to the most appropriate level of care, based on availability, along with the assessment of their condition and comorbidities, with respect to the individuals' preference. Refer to Box 24-5 for a variety of levels of care that have been described by the American Society of Addiction Medicine (ASAM).

Harm Reduction

Countless examples of harm reduction exist, with varying levels of evidence to support its benefit and the most appropriate application in the context of SRD. Harm reduction, a community health intervention designed to reduce the consequences of substance use to the individual, the family, and society, has replaced a moral or criminal approach to drug use and addiction (Canadian Centre on Substance Abuse [CCSA], 2005). The purpose of this approach is to *reduce the risk* for adverse consequences arising from substance use, while recognizing that abstinence is ideal, and works with the individual regardless of his or her commitment to reduce use. Harm reduction forms part of a continuum of care, and should not be viewed as exclusive

---

BOX 24.5

Levels of Substance-Abuse Care

LEVEL I: Outpatient treatment
This represents an organized non-residential treatment service, or office-based outpatient practice, with provision of professionally directed ATOD treatment. This treatment typically includes scheduled sessions (fewer than 9 hours/week), and may include individual therapy and/or group therapy, with or without participation in self-help groups such as Alcoholic Anonymous.

LEVEL II: Intensive outpatient treatment (including partial hospitalization)
On this level, there is provision of a structured program of ATOD treatment service components to patients, with a minimum of 9 treatment hours per week. This includes full spectrum day or evening treatment programs but participants continue to live at home or in special residences.

LEVEL III: Medically monitored intensive inpatient treatment (residential)
This is a residential setting and represents organized addiction services including a formal regimen of around-the-clock professionally directed evaluation, care, and treatment in an inpatient (or residential) setting. This includes 24-hour

observation, monitoring, and treatment where needed, and direct nursing supervision of care is available.

LEVEL IV: Medically managed intensive inpatient treatment
This is the most intensive level of care, and represents 24-hour medically directed evaluation, care, and treatment in an acute care inpatient (e.g., psychiatric) setting. Patients suffering from severe withdrawal syndromes (e.g., withdrawal delirium or delirium tremens), or those with significant medical, emotional, or behavioural problems (e.g., associated with severe and persistent mental illness such as bipolar disorder, schizophrenia, borderline personality, severe depression, or those with psychosis or suicidality), that require the level of intensity of medical and nursing services offered on this level, are also considered eligible for this inpatient level of care. Persons who have a substance overdose, and who cannot be safely managed in the emergency department, may also be best matched to this level of care. Individuals who have failed on a less restrictive level of care, and whose ongoing substance use poses a risk of harm to their physical or mental health, may also be offered more intensive levels of care.

---

of the overarching goal of abstinence. Fischer (2005, p. 13) suggests five general principles of harm reduction:

- Harm reduction focuses on the consequences of substance use, not on the use itself, requiring decisions about which harms to be targeted and in what order based on what is known about patient's welfare, public health, and the severity of the problem.
- Harm reduction focuses on the pragmatic and effective minimization of use-related harms.
- Meaningful and realistic efforts must be made to actively understand and consider the social and environmental context in which substance use occurs.
- Education, knowledge, and informed decision making by substance users and potential users are key pillars of harm reduction.
- Misinformed or ineffective interventions or policy can be considered sources of substance-related harms, and must also be targeted for harm reduction interventions.

As an example, interventions for alcohol-related harm reduction include education about the safe use of alcohol, provision of food at bars to reduce the incidence of rapid intoxication, and encouragement of the use of a "designated driver."

Psychosocial Interventions

Effective psychosocial treatment exists for the addictive disorders, and includes the following:

- Motivational interviewing
- Cognitive-behavioural therapy

- Behavioural therapies
  - Contingency management
  - Community reinforcement
  - Cue exposure and relaxation training
  - Aversion therapy
- Self-help groups and 12-Step facilitation
- Relapse prevention
- Psychodynamic and interpersonal therapy
- Group therapy and family therapy
- Brief therapies
- Self-guided therapies
- Hypnotherapy

Motivational Interviewing

Motivational Interviewing (MI) is a directive, patient-centred style of counselling that helps patients to explore and resolve their ambivalence (the presence of both positive and negative feelings) about changing (Miller & Rollnick, 2002). It has wide application in practice for behavioural change, not only for the field of addiction. It is based, in part, on stages of change as delineated in Box 24-6. Some of the techniques in MI involve listening reflectively, eliciting motivational statements, and examining ambivalence. Those using this form of counselling avoid non-therapeutic responses such as directing and giving advice without patient permission, threatening with consequences, being coercive, and inappropriately raising concern without permission because these place the patient in an unhelpful, passive role. This model allows for the process of change to be viewed along a

BOX 24.6

Stages of Change

This model provides a framework for a "staged" approach to interventions for substance use. It recognizes that quitting is not typically a singular event but rather a dynamic process. Five stages have been identified, and guide the appropriate intervention for the individual at that time. These stages include the following:

1. **Precontemplation:** In this first stage, the user has no intention to quit in the next 6 months. An appropriate intervention for the nurse is to encourage consideration of the benefits and risks of continued use.
2. **Contemplation:** An individual in the contemplation stage is aware that a problem exists and is seriously thinking about quitting at some point but has not yet made a plan to do so. At this stage, the nurse, for example, may assist by reinforcing reasons for change, and exploring new ones.
3. **Preparation:** At this stage, the individual has made a decision to quit within the next 30 days and prepares to do so. An example of appropriate nursing intervention is identify barriers to stopping and elicit solutions.
4. **Action:** The individual has quit within the past 6 months and is actively applying cessation skills. An appropriate nursing intervention is to ask how the individual is doing and advise regarding relapse prevention.
5. **Maintenance:** The individual has quit for more than 6 months. The nurse may ask how the patient is doing regarding risk situations and relapses, and offer encouragement.

Many individuals will cycle through the Stages of Changes a number of times. Each attempt to quit provides new opportunities to learn new skills and techniques that will help in the next attempt.

Source: Prochaska, J., Diclemente, C., & Norcross, J. (1992). In search of how people change: Applications to addictive behaviors. *American Psychologist, 47*(9), 1102–1114.

---

continuum, and where concrete steps can be taken to help individuals increase readiness for changing behaviour.

MI involves at least two processes: increasing preferred behaviours and decreasing non-preferred behaviours. Ambivalence is an expected part of the process of change, and resistance to change is to be expected. In the efforts to help patients move through the stages of change, from pre-contemplation through to contemplation, preparation, action, and maintenance, two critical components emerge that are iteratively assessed for their influence. These are *conviction* (importance) and *confidence*. Strategies for increasing the patient's conviction include asking questions regarding the relative importance of changing behaviour; examining the risks and benefits of the particular behaviour and of changing; exploring concerns about behaviour; having the "hypothetical look over the fence," and exploring possible next steps. Enhancing confidence also includes brainstorming solutions, focusing on successful past efforts, and serial reassessment and repetition of the process. Building motivation for change is conducted by asking open-ended questions, listening reflectively, issuing affirming and summarizing statements, but also eliciting self-motivational statements from the patient. These include problem recognition, expression of concern, the intention to change, and a sense of optimism. Refer to Box 24-7 for principles of MI.

Some of the signals of successful MI are the following: you are speaking slowly, the patient is doing much more of the talking than you, the patient is actively talking about behaviour change, and finally, you are listening very carefully, and gently directing the interview at appropriate moments. The acronym FRAMES (*f*eedback, *r*esponsibility, *a*dvice, *m*enu, *e*mpathy, *s*elf-efficacy) was coined by

Miller and Sanchez in 1994 to summarize elements of brief interventions with patients using MI (refer to Box 24-8).

CRNENOTE

MI approaches help patients recognize ambivalence, identify barriers, and develop health-behaviour change strategies.

Cognitive-Behavioural Therapy

Cognitive approaches to addiction hypothesize that if an individual can change the way he or she thinks about a situation, both the emotional reaction to it and the behavioural response will change. Psychoeducational materials, groups, and one-on-one interactions with nurses also impart information to reduce knowledge deficits related to alcohol, tobacco, and other drug dependence. For additional discussion on cognitive-behavioural therapy, refer to Chapter 15.

Twelve-Step Facilitation

TSF emphasizes the conceptualization of substance dependence as an incurable, progressive disease that has spiritual, cognitive, and behavioural components. AA was the first twelve-step self-help group and started in the mid-1930s by Bill W. and a physician. The AA movement is now a worldwide fellowship of people with problems (current or past) related to alcohol, who provide support, individually and at meetings, to others who seek help. The only criterion for entry into AA is the "desire to quit drinking." Many treatment programs discuss concepts from AA, hold

---

BOX 24.7

The Principles of Motivational Enhancement

1. **Avoid arguing:** Generally, the more the therapist tells a patient "You can't do this," the more likely he or she will respond, if unconsciously, with "I will." Resistance to change is influenced by how the therapist responds to the patient's ambivalence.
2. **Express empathy:** The attitude underlying empathy might also be called acceptance, and it is not the same as approval of harmful behaviour, but rather an unconditional acceptance of where the patient is at in terms of the behaviour. Through skilful reflective listening the therapist can seek to understand the patient's feelings and perspectives without judging, criticizing, or blaming. Paradoxically, this kind of acceptance of people as they are, appears to free them to change, whereas insistence on change and non-acceptance of "where they are at" in the process of change, can have the effect of keeping people as they are. It is not helpful to view the patient as "problematic," "pathological," "unwilling to change," or "incapable of change," rather, the patient's situation is understood as one of being "stuck."
3. **Develop discrepancy:** Motivation for change is created when people perceive a discrepancy between their present behaviour and important personal goals. Thus, MI aims at developing discrepancy until it overrides attachment to the present behaviour. This is accomplished without coercion. It is the patient who gives voice to concerns and intentions to change.
4. **Roll with resistance:** When encountering resistance, the therapist acknowledges ambivalence as natural. The patient is invited to consider new information and perspectives. The responsibility for change is repeatedly handed back to the patient, but with the offer of help and support. It is not the therapist's role to generate all the solutions, or to tell the patient what to do. Directive approaches may elicit "Yes, but..." responses from the patient, with little or no change following, and often a disengagement and dropping out of treatment.
5. **Support self-efficacy:** This refers to the reinforcement of the patient's belief in his or her ability to carry out and succeed. Change is a step-wise approach, and each small step along the journey should be reinforced and supported. The therapist's expectations about a patient's chances for recovery can have a powerful impact on outcome.

BOX 24.8

F.R.A.M.E.S: Effective Elements of Brief Intervention

FEEDBACK
Provide patients with personal feedback regarding their individual status, such as personal alcohol and other drug consumption relative to norms, information about elevated liver enzyme values, and so forth.

RESPONSIBILITY
Emphasize the individual's freedom of choice and personal responsibility for change. General themes are as follows:

1. It's up to you; you're free to decide to change or not.
2. No one else can decide for you or force you to change.
3. You're the one who has to do it if it's going to happen.

ADVICE
Include a clear recommendation or advice on the need for change, typically in a supportive and concerned, rather than in a judgmental, manner.

MENU
Provide a menu of treatment options, from which patients may pick those that seem more suitable or appealing.

EMPATHIC COUNSELLING
Show warmth, support, respect, and understanding in communication with patients.

SELF-EFFICACY
Reinforce self-efficacy, or an optimistic feeling that he or she can change.

meetings at treatment facilities, and encourage patients to attend community meetings when appropriate. They also encourage continuing use of AA and other self-help groups as part of an ongoing plan for continued abstinence. Khantzian and Mack (1994) identified the therapeutic elements of AA including the following:

- Instilling hope through meeting others who are no longer drinking,
- Encouraging honesty, openness, and a willingness to listen to others,
- Emphasizing shared experiences and the development of a friendship network of sober individuals,
- Focusing on abstinence and the loss of control over the ability to drink,
- Fostering reliance on others, not on isolation and attempts to control drinking by the use of willpower, and
- Adding a spiritual dimension that turns away from ego defence mechanisms such as denial and avoidance toward a better quality of life and the capacity to love and help others.

TSF firmly endorses the need for abstinence, and are considered by members as lifelong programs of recovery, with success attained one day at a time. The importance of recognizing and relying on a "higher power" or a power greater than the individual is a central element of these programs. Members of self-help groups can attend meetings on a self-determined or prescribed schedule which, if necessary, could be every day or even twice a day. Periods associated with high risk of relapse (e.g., holidays, weekends, family functions) are particularly appropriate times for attending meetings. A sponsor who is compatible with the patient can be particularly supportive and offer guidance through the recovery process, particularly during periods of high stress or increased craving.

There are now more than 60 different TSF fellowships available world-wide including AA, NA, DRA, CA, SA, SSA, among others. They do not solicit members, engage in political or religious activities, make medical or psychiatric diagnoses, engage in education about addiction to the general population, or provide mental health, vocational, or legal counselling. Although many have reported benefits from AA-related programs, exactly how effective they are compared with other treatments and how they work have yet to be shown (Brown & Graves, 2005). There is some evidence to suggest that there is a positive correlation between AA attendance (and active participation during meetings) and reduced alcohol consumption, improved psychological functioning, and better social supports. Additionally, treatment programs that include TSF have, in general, more positive outcomes than those who do not. Inclusion in TSF is considered a routine part of addiction treatment in most settings. However, an individual's refusal to participate in a self-help group is non-synonymous with his or her resistance to treatment in general. Self-help groups are not beneficial for all people, and some persons may not embrace the spiritual dimension of the program. Alternative programs for sobriety, although not as widely available, have been developed to address this problem, such as Women for Sobriety and Secular Organizations for Sobriety.

Group Therapy

An integral and valuable component of the treatment regimen for many with a substance use disorder is group therapy, and advantages of this approach include the following:

- The presence of others with an addiction may provide comfort,
- Other group members who are further along in their recovery may act as role models,
- Group members may offer a wide menu of coping strategies,
- Some members may act as "buddies" outside of the group setting, and
- The public nature of group settings can act as a deterrent for relapse. It has been noted that individuals recovering from substance use disorders may be highly skilled at detecting each other's concealed substance use or early relapse.

The efficacy of group therapy is similar to individual therapy, and it can be a successful component of a combined treatment program. For more detailed information about group therapy, refer to Chapter 16.

Family Therapy

Long-term family therapy is often beneficial after the initial stages of detoxification and stabilization. Behavioural couples therapy for people with alcoholism can improve family functioning, reduce stressors, smooth marital adjustment, and lessen domestic violence and verbal conflict (O'Farrell, 1999). Families can often unwittingly support addiction by, for instance, continuing to supply money to the individual, allowing adult children to live at home while continuing their substance use, and "bailing out" individuals from legal and other difficulties that result from substance use. Family therapy can bring these behaviours to light and assist family members to set limits on their further support. More detailed information is available in Chapter 17.

■ INTEGRATING PHARMACOTHERAPY AND PSYCHOSOCIAL INTERVENTIONS

Pharmacotherapy, where available and appropriate, is routinely combined with psychosocial treatment (which includes TSF), and is not recommended for use in isolation of psychosocial interventions. Medications for SRD are generally utilized to treat intoxication, withdrawal, to reduce the reinforcing effects of drugs, to prevent relapse, and to treat comorbid medical or psychiatric conditions. For most of the disorders there is not sufficient evidence for the use of pharmacotherapy, but for the disorders related to alcohol, tobacco, and opioids, the empirical evidence supports the use of pharmacotherapy. These are incorporated in the following sections.

Treatment of Tobacco Addiction

In a Cochrane review of nursing interventions for smoking cessation, Rice and Stead (2004) concluded that smoking cessation and/or counselling given by nurses can be effective. They identified that the nursing challenge is the incorporation of smoking behavioural monitoring and smoking cessation interventions as part of their daily practice. All patients can be asked about their tobacco use and given advice and/or counselling to quit along with reinforcement and follow-up. To dramatically enhance the likelihood of a successful quit attempt, clinical findings support the offer, and provision, of simple and strategic behavioural counselling and pharmacotherapy to every person interested in quitting. Those who are not ready to make an attempt at cessation should be offered empathetic counselling designed to permit a reassessment of their reasons for continued smoking and an invitation to seek assistance with cessation at any time. Several levels of evidence support the use of the following modalities:

Psychosocial interventions

Psychosocial interventions, such as group, individual, telephone, office, or web-based counselling, should be routinely offered in combination with medication for increased successful cessation rates. The provision of simple advice regarding the avoidance of high risk relapse situations, recognition of settings or circumstances where smoking has been particularly common, management of acute cravings, and development of smoke free guidelines for home and vehicles are all important in accentuating the likelihood of cessation success. Although the evidence suggests that interventions are effective across a broad range of populations, tailored interventions may be advised for selected sub-populations (e.g., individuals with mentally illness, pregnant smokers, smokeless tobacco users, and minority groups).

Pharmacological interventions

Nicotine replacement therapy (NRT) is available in four forms: transdermal patch, chewing "gum," inhaler/vaporizer, and lozenge. Individuals who smoke seek to maintain a certain individualized level of nicotine and when their nicotine levels fall, distinct and significant discomfort usually occurs (withdrawal symptoms). NRT stimulates nicotine receptors and extinguishes withdrawal symptoms, and its appropriate use typically doubles success rates of quit attempts. Combinations of NRT (e.g., patch and inhaler concurrently) have the advantage of allowing the smoker to titrate their nicotine intake to meet their unique needs, and are associated with increased levels of success.

Bupropion is an anti-depressant that was serendipitously found to be effective in tobacco cessation. Bupropion inhibits the reuptake of dopamine in the reward centres of the brain, as well as norepinephrine, a chemical associated with withdrawal symptoms. Its use has been shown to double success rates in those attempting to quit smoking.

Varenicline, a third-generation smoking cessation pharmacotherapy, directly and distinctly binds to $\alpha 4\beta 2$ nicotinic receptors. These receptor sites are completely blocked but only partially stimulated reducing the transmission of neurological impulses and causing a reduced amount of dopamine to be released in the reward centres of the brain. Consequently, the smoker experiences little to no withdrawal symptoms, and no pleasurable sensation if a cigarette is smoked. Varenicline has been shown to be the most superior pharmacotherapy for cessation when compared with NRT and bupropion, with an odds ratio of quitting of approximately 3:1. Current evidence suggests that varenicline is not associated with a higher rate of neuropsychiatric adverse effects than placebo or bupropion, with the exception of insomnia. Quitting smoking can, however, lead to exacerbation of a pre-existing mood disorder, anxiety, depression, agitation, irritability, and even a potential for increased risk of harm.

A recent change in the U.S. labelling of varenicline and bupropion was made that was based on post-marketing reports as opposed to systematic trial evidence. The purpose of the warning was to heighten the level of awareness of adverse events and to mitigate potential risks in patients taking either varenicline and bupropion. It notest the potential risk of serious mental health events including changes in behaviour, depressed mood, hostility, and suicidal thoughts when taking either bupropion or varenicline. Risks while taking either of these medications to must always be weighed against the significant health benefits of quitting smoking, and the awareness that this symptomology may also be expressed in response to tobacco cessation.

The scientific evidence does not support the use of alternative tobacco-based nicotine delivery systems (e.g., smokeless tobacco) as a smoking cessation aid. Despite claims by the tobacco industry to the contrary, these are not considered a "harm reduction" measure, and may in actuality discourage or postpone cessation efforts in smokers who would otherwise have quit, or may induce another form of tobacco dependency with associated health consequences such as pancreatic cancer.

Clinical Guidelines for Tobacco Dependence Treatment

Clinical Practice Guidelines that can serve as a suitable template for the delivery of smoking cessation treatments by nurses can be found in Box 24-9.

Treatment of Alcohol-Related Disorders

The treatment of alcohol-related disorders consists of achieving safe withdrawal from the substance, followed by psychosocial interventions and the option of pharmacotherapy. Management of intoxication and withdrawal (Box 24-10) may require a safe environment, and hospitalization may be indicated if there is a history of seizures, delirium, or comorbid medical or psychiatric conditions. The use of symptom-guided withdrawal protocols is considered most favourable. Standardized doses of benzodiazepines are provided based on an evaluation of the level of withdrawal (as determined by the CIWA score in Appendix G). Medication administered early

BOX 24.9

The 5 A Approach to Tobacco Addiction Treatment

A1 = Ask—Systematically identify all tobacco users at every visit.

A2 = Advise—In a clear, strong, and personalized fashion all tobacco users should be strongly advised to quit.

A3 = Assess—Every tobacco user's willingness to make a quit attempt should be assessed.

A4 = Assist—Help the patient set a quit date, advise the patient to tell family and friends about quitting and to remove tobacco products from the home/work environment, and anticipate challenges in the weeks to come. Also offer the combination of pharmacotherapy and psychosocial interventions.

A5 = Arrange follow-up—Ensure follow-up contact and approach the treatment in a longitudinal fashion.

Source: Fiore et al. (2008). *Treating tobacco use and dependence: 2008 update.* Clinical Practice Guideline. Rockville, MC: U.S. Department of health and Human Services. Public Health Service.

BOX 24.10

Clinical Features of Alcohol Withdrawal

MINOR WITHDRAWAL: Patients are anxious, and may experience nausea and vomiting, coarse tremor, sweating, tachycardia, and hypertension. Symptoms typically appear 6–12 hours after the last drink, or shortly after the BAL reach zero, and are usually resolved within 48–72 hours.

INTERMEDIATE WITHDRAWAL: Patients experience the symptoms of minor withdrawal in addition to seizures, dysrythmias, and/or hallucinosis. Within 12–72 hours after cessation of drinking, grand mal and non-focal seizures typically occur. Dysrythmias range in severity from occasional ectopic beats to atrial fibrillation and supraventricular or ventricular tachycardia. Patients are aware of the unreal nature of their auditory or visual hallucinations and remain oriented and alert.

MAJOR WITHDRAWAL (DELIRIUM TREMENS): Patients experience severe agitation, gross tremulousness, marked psychomotor and autonomic hyperactivity, global confusion, disorientation and auditory, visual or tactile hallucinations. They tend to occur 5 or 6 days after severe, untreated withdrawal. Symptoms fluctuate and are often more severe at night. These may include severe diaphoresis and vomiting, tachycardia, hypertension, and fever. Sudden death can occur.

Source: Brands, B., Kahan, M., Selby, P., & Wilson, L. (2000). *Medical management of alcohol and drug-related problems: A physician's manual* (2nd ed.) Toronto, ON: Centre for Addiction and Mental Health.

in the course of withdrawal (and in sufficient dosages) can prevent the development of delirium tremens. Poor nutrition and vitamin deficiencies are often symptoms of alcohol dependence. Thiamine (vitamin B_1) may be needed when a patient is in withdrawal to decrease ataxia and other symptoms of deficiency. It is usually given orally, 100 mg four times daily, but can be given intramuscularly or by intravenous infusion with glucose. Folic acid deficiency is corrected with administration of 1 mg orally, four times daily. Magnesium deficiency also is found in those with long-term alcohol dependence. Magnesium sulfate, which enhances the body's response to thiamine and reduces seizures, is given as a prophylactic for patients with histories of withdrawal seizures. The usual dose is 1 g intramuscularly, four times daily for 2 days. Along with the use of benzodiazepines, multivitamins and thiamine, fluid balance should be monitored, and supportive treatment provided.

Following detoxification, there are several medication options that exists to support the treatment of alcohol dependence. These include the following:

- *Disulfiram*, a medication that blocks the effects of aldehyde dehydrogenase and leads to a severely unpleasant reaction (including flushing, nausea, vomiting, and diarrhoea) when the person consumes alcohol. It is suitable only for reliable and motivated patients. This is not a treatment for alcoholism, but rather an adjunct therapy that deters drinking while the individual learns new coping skills and alters abuse behaviours through other treatment approaches. Disulfiram's potential adverse effects include hepatotoxicity and neuropathy which, along with potentially severe interactions with alcohol, limit its widespread use (O'Connor & Schottenfeld, 1998).

- *Naltrexone*, originally used as a treatment for opioid-related disorders, targets alcohol's effects on the brain, and requires relatively normal liver functions. The use of this opioid antagonist medication patient cannot be in conjunction with any opioid medication as it will trigger an opioid withdrawal syndrome. It is further contra-indicated in pregnancy and suicidal patients. Naltrexone may be particularly useful in patients who continue to drink heavily (McCaul, Wand, Eissenberg, Rohde, & Cheskin, 2000). Targeted use of naltrexone also may be effective for decreasing alcohol consumption levels among problem drinkers who do not suffer from alcoholism.

- *Acamprosate* has the ability to curb cravings for alcohol and may be an effective adjunct treatment in motivated persons who are also receiving psychosocial interventions.

Psychosocial interventions, as described earlier, should be offered at all stages of treatment in combination with pharmacotherapy, and at the appropriate level of care. The suggestion to include attendance at AA is routinely offered. The outcome monitoring for alcohol addiction treatment includes reporting on sobriety and abstinence. Serial monitoring of liver function tests and Early

Detection of Alcohol Consumption (EDAC) testing can provide valuable information on the course of the condition and success of treatment, and supplement the self-reported abstinence and sobriety.

Treatment of Cannabis-Related Disorders

The mainstay for the treatment of the cannabis-related disorders is psychosocial treatment. This includes motivational enhancement, psychodynamic and interpersonal therapy, and relapse prevention. There is no medication proven to be superior to placebo in the treatment of this condition.

Treatment of Cocaine-Related Disorders

Withdrawal from cocaine is usually relatively uncomplicated. It is complicated by the exceptionally high risk of relapse, and the challenge is often to establish a recovery environment in which risk to relapse is minimized. Cocaine detoxification is not typically associated with medical complications, and usually requires only supportive care. However, if a patient develops psychotic symptoms (e.g., hallucinations, delusions, or paranoia) during intoxication phases, specific treatments to remedy this may be required, such as the use of atypical antipsychotics.

When an individual steadily uses increasing doses of cocaine, the associated restlessness and anxiety may proceed to overstimulation and agitation, followed by convulsions and CNS depression. In lethal overdose, death generally results from respiratory failure. A toxic psychosis is also possible, and may be accompanied by physical signs of CNS stimulation (tachycardia, hypertension, cardiac arrhythmias, sweating, hyperpyrexia, and convulsions). The management of the medical complications of an overdose or intoxication may require hospitalization.

Long-term cocaine use depletes norepinephrine and, when the drug is discontinued, results in a "crash" causing the user to sleep 12 to 18 hours. Upon awakening, withdrawal symptoms may occur that are characterized by sleep disturbances with rebound REM sleep, anergia (lack of energy), decreased libido, depression with possible suicidality, anhedonia, poor concentration, and cocaine craving. Depression typically resolves, and unless an underlying major depressive disorder is demonstrated, the use of antidepressants is not indicated.

When cocaine is used with alcohol, a potentially dangerous interaction may develop. Taken in combination, the two drugs are converted by the body to cocaethylene, which has a longer duration of action in the brain and is more cardiotoxic than either drug alone. Notably, this mixture of cocaine and alcohol is the most common two-drug combination that results in drug-related death (NIDA, 2009).

Treating cocaine addiction is complex and involves assessing the psychobiological, social, and pharmacologic aspects of abuse. Psychosocial interventions form the mainstay of treatment for cocaine addiction treatment, and residential care may be required in cases where relapse risk cannot be adequately managed on an outpatient basis. Stabilization of the patient's recovery environment is pivotal in achieving lasting abstinence from cocaine, and inclusion in a TSF programs is recommended (e.g., Narcotics Anonymous). Patients using cocaine should be advised to abstain from alcohol as well, and if applicable, offered opportunities to quit smoking. To date, there is no medication proven to be superior to placebo in regards to cocaine addiction treatment. However, there are promising options, for example, topiramate, disulfiram, or modafinil, which may be considered in cases where psychosocial treatment alone has failed to yield optimal results.

Treatment of Opioid-Related Disorders

Opioid intoxication typically does not require treatment except in cases where CNS or respiratory depression is a risk, or where it is combined with other depressants (e.g., alcohol, barbiturates, or benzodiazepines). The use of an opioid-receptor blocker, for example, naloxone or naltrexone may be indicated in such cases, along with supportive treatment and monitoring of vital signs.

Detoxification management is usually not associated with medical complications, and serves only as the first stage of ongoing treatment for addiction to opioids. Detoxification is conducted with the use of medication options, for example, methadone, buprenorphine (combined with naloxone in Canada), or by using a tapering regime of the existing opioid. Clonidine is also useful in curbing withdrawal symptoms during abrupt discontinuation of opioids, and can be combined with naltrexone. Care must be taken to avoid the development of orthostatic hypotension during detoxification using clonidine.

For the treatment of opioid addiction in individuals who have not achieved abstinence through psychosocial interventions, there are three options available in Canada: Methadone, Buprenorphine (with naloxone), and Naltrexone. For the first two options, the prescribing physician is required to have completed special training and to have been granted exemption and be registered at the provincial professional regulatory body.

Treatment of Amphetamine-Related Disorders

Amphetamine withdrawal symptoms are not as pronounced as those of cocaine withdrawal, and are treated similarly. Evidence in support of treatment for addiction using pharmacologic agents is limited, and is similar to that used for cocaine.

Treatment of Caffeine-Related Disorders

Caffeine withdrawal symptoms may include headache, insomnia, abnormal dreams, drowsiness, fatigue, impaired psychomotor performance, difficulty concentrating, craving, yawning, and nausea. Heavy consumers of caffeine who drastically and rapidly reduce or discontinue consumption may be at risk for withdrawal. Preferentially, caffeine should be reduced gradually in those considered to be consuming in excess, and this may occur over the course of days or weeks. Those deemed physiologically dependent may benefit from additional support. Psychoeducation can help individuals learn about the caffeine contents of beverages and medication providing the ability to gradually switch to decaffeinated beverages, and withdrawal symptoms can be managed individually.

■ IMPLEMENTING NURSING INTERVENTIONS

There is no standardized treatment program that will work for every substance-dependent individual because they differ greatly with respect to severity of the disorder and the biologic, psychological, social, and spiritual features

of their dependence. Often several approaches can work together whereas others may be deemed inappropriate. Treatment programs usually combine many different interventions to provide a comprehensive approach based on the individual's needs. Nursing interventions vary depending on the nature of the current problems, the status and severity of the illness, and the individual's situation. For an individual who is being detoxified, physical interventions (e.g., monitoring vital signs and neurologic functioning) are necessary. When the substance use disorder is secondary to other physical or psychiatric problems, education of individuals and their family may be a priority. See Nursing Care Plan 24-1 as an example.

KEY CONCEPT Enhancing **motivation for change** involves recognizing a problem, searching for a way to change, and then beginning and sustaining the change strategy (Miller, 1995). Ambivalence about substance use is normal and can be resolved by working with patients' own concerns about their use of alcohol and other drugs. Motivation is fluid and can be modified. Counselling is patient-centred, empathic, and built on reflective listening (Brown & Graves, 2005). The patient is accepted and viewed as having the resources and motivation for change; the counsellor's task is to foster that motivation. Experiences such as increased distress levels, critical life events, a period of evaluation or appraisal of one's life, recognizing negative consequences of use, and positive and negative external incentives for change can all influence a patient's commitment to change (U.S. DHHS, 1999).

■ SPECIAL POPULATIONS

Individuals With Concurrent Disorders

Many substance-dependent people have **concurrent mental disorders**. Also known as dual disorders, dual diagnosis, and comorbid substance abuse disorders and mental disorders (Centre for Addiction and Mental Health, 2005), concurrent mental disorder can be defined as the coexistence of at least one mental disorder and at least one substance of abuse or dependence, as defined by the *DSM-IV-TR*. Some disorders are, in part, a by-product of long-term substance dependence; others predispose the individual to alcohol, tobacco or other drug use. For example, alcohol dependence is 21 times more likely to occur among people with antisocial personality disorders and four times more likely among people with schizophrenia; and among those treated for alcohol-related disorders, up to 70% to 80% may have a mental disorder (Health Canada, 2002a). Nurses should be aware that individuals with substance dependence often have anxiety disorders, phobias, or obsessive-compulsive

Nursing Care Plan 24.1

Patient With Alcoholism

Jonas G. is a 55-year-old mechanic with a 25-year history of alcohol dependence. He is the youngest of three children born of "blue-collar" parents who valued hard work. His mother is still living with his older sister, but his father died of cirrhosis, a complication of years of alcohol abuse. Jonas has two children who are married with children, living in other provinces. He rarely sees them. He has been drinking as much as 2 L of vodka per day for 3 years since sustaining a work-related back injury. He has a history of binge drinking on weekends. He began smoking in his early teens and continues to smoke a pack a day of cigarettes.

Recently, his wife moved out of the house after 28 years of marriage. An argument about his "drinking" (alcohol consumption) ended in a physical fight. She had to be treated in the emergency room for a broken arm. Their relationship had progressively deteriorated over the years. Jonas was sexually impotent due to excessive drinking and heavy smoking, and she had moved into the spare bedroom. He was admitted to the hospital through the emergency department 2 weeks after his wife left him, with a gash above his right eye from a fall he sustained while intoxicated. His wife returned to care for him.

Jonas began to have symptoms of alcohol withdrawal and became anxious shortly after admission. He requested hospital admission for alcohol detoxification and was transferred to a detoxification and brief treatment unit.

Setting: Inpatient Detoxification Unit, Psychiatric Hospital

Baseline Assessment: First admission, last drink and cigarette at 7 PM. Admission vital signs: T 99.2°F, HR 98, R 20, BP 140/88 on admission to the ER. He has a history of withdrawal seizures and hallucinations (likely delirium tremens during past withdrawal). He had a BAL of 0.15 mg%, becoming increasingly anxious and restless over the next hour. His CIWA score was 17, and he was given diazepam, 20 mg PO, as ordered, at that time. Decision to conduct CIWA 4-hourly.

Five hours after admission, vital signs were T 99.8°F, HR 110, R 22, BP 152/100. He continued to be anxious and was tremulous, diaphoretic, and nauseous. CIWA Score had increased to 22, and diazepam 20 mg PO stat was given. The decision was made to conduct CIWA scores hourly. The next CIWA score was 15, and 4 hours later it was 10.

Associated Psychiatric Diagnosis	Medications
Axis I: Alcohol dependence	Deferred until detoxification is complete, after which consideration will be given to acamprosate, naltrexone, or disulfiram.
Alcohol withdrawal	Thiamine Folic acid Multivitamins Diazepam, 20 mg stat, followed by CIWA score, based on elevated BP, HR, and tremors Haloperidol, 5.0 mg IM PRN, for hallucinations or agitation
Nicotine (tobacco) withdrawal	Transdermal nicotine patch 21 mg QD PRN Nicotine inhaler 10 mg, puff on cartridge for 45 minutes, as directed PRN
Nicotine dependence	Deferred, but continuation of Nicotine replacement is offered post detoxification.
Axis II: None	See above.
Axis III: Unspecified back injury Alcohol withdrawal	
Axis IV: Social problems (social withdrawal); occupational problems (work-related injury)	
Axis V: GAF = Current 60; Potential 75	

Nursing Diagnosis 1: Risk Related to Alcohol Withdrawal

Defining Characteristics	Related Factors
Altered vital signs Altered cerebral function secondary to alcohol withdrawal Altered mood states	Withdrawal is common among patients consuming more than 40 drinks/week, or in those with other risk factors. Symptoms of detoxification include fever, high blood pressure, tachycardia, tremor or sweating, confusion, and dehydration. Level of consciousness, orientation, perceptual disturbances (hallucinations or illusions), mood and thought processes including suicide ideation and cognitive deficits.

Continued

Nursing Care Plan 24.1 (Continued)

Outcomes

Initial	Discharge
1. Detoxification from alcohol will be monitored, based on CIWA Score, and management implemented to treat symptoms and to prevent complications.	2. Bridging from in-patient from Level IV care for detoxification to a regime that is acceptable to JG and keeps him engaged in ongoing treatment.

Interventions

Interventions	Rationale	Ongoing Assessment
Welcome to treatment and assure Jonas that he is in a safe place. Inform of what he may expect during withdrawal. Start with engagement for treatment.	Begin to establish relationship, a therapeutic alliance, with the patient.	See Box 24-8
Monitor vital signs, orientation, and identify stage of alcohol withdrawal and severity of symptoms.	The more severe the reactions, the more likely that anxiety, disorientation, confusion, and restlessness increase.	Administer (symptom-triggered, CIWA) Diazepam (for elevated BP, HR, and tremors) and Haloperidol (for hallucinations or tremors) prn and report symptoms.
Institute seizure precautions (bed in low position, padded side rails).	Withdrawal seizures usually occur within 48 hours after last drink.	Monitor for seizure activity.
Orient patient to surroundings and call light, maintain consistent physical environment.	Disorientation often occurs as BAL drops. These symptoms can last several days.	Determine Jonas' level of orientation to surroundings, and whether he can use call light.
Avoid sudden moves, loud noises, discussion of patient at bedside, and lighting that casts shadows downward.	Decreased environmental stimulation helps calm the patient, which in turn promotes optimal CNS responses.	Observe reactions to loud noises and monitor room environment.

Evaluation

Outcomes (at 3 days)	Revised Outcomes	Interventions
Orientated, hydrated and no seizure activity.	Engage in the development of a recovery plan.	Continue to monitor for any signs of disorientation.

Nursing Diagnosis 2: Discomfort Related to Nicotine Withdrawal

Defining Characteristics	Related Factors
Symptoms of nicotine withdrawal include irritability, restlessness, anxiety, insomnia and fatigue.	Discomfort related to nicotine withdrawal may be difficult to distinguish from alcohol withdrawal.

Outcomes

Initial	Discharge
1. Will be comfortable without smoking during hospitalization period	2. Will be provided additional resources and supports to extend tobacco abstinence into a cessation attempt, if desired.

Interventions

Intervention	Rationale	Ongoing Assessment
Explain that the hospital has a non-smoking policy. This is to protect patients, visitors, and staff from the harmful effects of second-hand smoke. The purpose of the policy is not to "force" Jonas to quit smoking, or to "make his life difficult."	There are direct causes and linkages between exposure to second-hand smoke and serious health effects among non-smokers.	Monitor Jonas' level of comfort and assess for break through cravings. Assess for sleep disruption; if present, may remove patch at bedtime.

Continued

Nursing Care Plan 24.1 (Continued)

Interventions

Intervention	Rationale	Ongoing Assessment
Discuss prevention of discomfort related to nicotine withdrawal. Assess whether Jonas' wife is a current smoker and the influence this may have on Jonas' ability to abstain. Offer a 21 mg transdermal nicotine patch qd to prevent withdrawal. This can be combined with other forms of NRT.	The blood level of nicotine begins to drop immediately following smoking a cigarette. Smell off of clothing, and cigarette products, may provide potent cues to smoke. The higher dose 21 mg nicotine patch, recommended for pack per day smoker, may not be of sufficient dosage to prevent breakthrough cravings. Side effects may include sleep disruption.	

Evaluation

Outcomes (Day 2)	Revised Outcomes	Interventions
Refused nicotine patch, and becomes increasingly anxious to leave the unit to smoke.	Remain abstinent and engaged in the treatment regimen on the unit.	Offer prn nicotine inhaler to provide some immediate relief, and re-offer nicotine patch for longer term effects.

and affective disorders, such as major depression and dysthymia (Fu et al., 2002). Other coexisting mental disorders include personality disorders and attention-deficit hyperactivity disorder (Rosenthal & Westreich, 1999). These are discussed in detail in Chapters 25 and 28. Nurses need to remember that individuals do not compartmentalize their problems, so health professionals should not either.

Mental Illness and Tobacco Use

There is a longstanding and robust historical relationship between people with mental illness and the use of tobacco products. When compared with the general population, the mentally ill are two to three times more likely to smoke and are less likely to quit (Lasser et al., 2000). Up to 90% of persons with schizophrenia are smokers (Williams & Ziedonis, 2004), and those with mental illness smoke almost one-half of all cigarettes smoked in North America (Lasser et al.). Financially deprived and socially disenfranchised persons may "pick butts" because they cannot afford cigarettes which exposes them to communicable diseases and to the higher tar content found in tobacco closer to the cigarette butt. Persons living with mental illness have higher rates of cardiovascular and respiratory morbidity, type 2 diabetes, and are more likely to die of tobacco related illness than from any other cause. The health benefits of smoking cessation are undisputed, but some mentally ill smokers may be discouraged from quitting out of fear of a disorder relapse. There is

no evidence to suggest that standard tobacco-cessation interventions cannot be effective for persons with mental illness or addiction (Els & Kunyk, 2008).

Aboriginal Populations

Although accurate and complete data are limited regarding the prevalence of alcohol and drug consumption among the Aboriginal communities, there is a consensus that they suffer significantly higher rates of addiction when compared with the general Canadian population (Kirby & Keon, 2004). Further, the rates of fetal alcohol syndrome (FAS; and its effects) are higher among the Aboriginal community. Experts agree that although the causes of the addiction problems in Aboriginal and non-Aboriginal communities may be similar, Aboriginal communities have added cultural factors that affect individual decision making. Addiction has been implicated as both the cause and effect of the relatively poor health of Canada's Aboriginal people since their contact began with Europeans (National Native Addictions Partnership Foundation, 2000). As their once powerful role in the economic exchange systems of early Canada was displaced through economic developments, the Aboriginal people lost their traditional economies and became particularly vulnerable to the health and social problems characteristic of economically marginalized members of all industrialized societies—crippling alcohol, tobacco, and harmful substance use patterns (solvents, street drugs, prescription drugs).

Although improving, the overall health of Aboriginal people in Canada is significantly poorer than that of the rest of Canadians. Aboriginal people are more likely than non-Aboriginal people to be hospitalized, four times more likely to be injured or poisoned, nearly twice as likely to die, and six to eight times more likely to complete suicide—due to related impairments from alcohol or other psychoactive drugs (Single, Robson, & Scott, 1997). In addition, substance abuse plays a significant role in criminal behaviour both in terms of incarceration (more than 75% of Aboriginals in jail have alcohol problems) and homicide (10 times higher than the non-Aboriginal population; Health Canada, 1999b). Although alcohol remains the primary substance of choice for 58% of Aboriginal substance users, about 20% of users choose other drugs (from which they are three times more likely to die than non-Aboriginals). When compared with the general population, Aboriginals are significantly more likely to use multiple drugs (46% of substance users in treatment centres in Saskatchewan).

Pregnancy and Substance Use

Drug and alcohol use during pregnancy can have serious detrimental effects on the course of pregnancy, as well as on the physiologic status of the fetus and newborn. According to the Public Health Agency of Canada (1998), the national rate of FAS (a specific cluster of anomalies associated with the use of alcohol during pregnancy) has been estimated to be 1 to 2 per 1,000 live births. The CCSA has estimated the lifetime costs associated with the care of an individual with FAS (extra health care, education, and social services) to be about $1.4 million. Although the severity of problems and complications often depends on the amount of substance abuse during pregnancy, studies show that any amount of substance use during pregnancy puts the newborn at much higher risk for developmental, neurologic, and behavioural problems.

For pregnant women who are substance dependent, social and emotional pressures and concerns associated with their treatment are heightened because treatment affects the well-being of their children. The nurse should be aware of special social, emotional, and legal issues involving treatment of chemically dependent pregnant women, and be sensitive to their special needs. For example, they may fear that, by seeking prenatal care, their drug use will be detected by urine toxicology tests and cause them to lose custody of their children. Marion (1995) suggested a comprehensive approach to treatment in the perinatal period, including prenatal and perinatal care; pharmacologic interventions, such as **methadone maintenance** programs; life skills training, such as relapse prevention and social skills training; mother–infant development assessment; and early childhood development programs and social work services, as required.

HIV/AIDS and Substance Use

Intravenous drug users may be considered particularly at risk for HIV/AIDS infection because some share hypodermic needles, syringes, and other supplies used to inject drugs. Some individuals who abuse drugs and alcohol may be at high risk for sexual transmission of HIV/AIDS because they may fail to use adequate precautions and preventive methods while intoxicated or may engage in risky sexual encounters to obtain money or drugs.

The dual diagnosis of a substance use disorder and HIV/AIDS infection requires extremely careful assessment and intervention planning. Continued alcohol and drug use can interfere with the medical treatment of HIV/AIDS; for example, alcohol, marijuana, cocaine, and amphetamines are immunosuppressants that further impair the seriously compromised immune system of a individuals with HIV/AIDS. Addicted persons infected with HIV/AIDS may have difficulty adhering to medication schedules, and some would not benefit fully from antiviral medications because of this. Other complicating factors include the financial, social, and emotional stressors (including stigma) experienced by addicts and people with alcoholism who must also cope with the devastating diagnosis of HIV/AIDS disease.

Addiction treatment programs have an important role for individuals with HIV/AIDS disease, substance dependence, and concurrent mental health problems. Because the issues facing these individuals are so complex, planning treatment and priority setting are essential. Addiction treatment is nearly always necessary for the addicted individual to follow with other HIV/AIDS-related health and mental health interventions. Thus, at the initial diagnosis of HIV/AIDS infection, substance dependence issues need to be evaluated and addressed.

Children and Youth

Not all young people who experiment with substances proceed to levels that bring health problems. Some use certain substances for recreational purposes, whereas others use them for self medication (e.g., emotional distress or insomnia). Recurrent problems related to substances, such as difficulties with family or friends and school attendance, most commonly arise as a result of increased frequency of use (Bonomo & Proimos, 2005).

In general, the younger a person starts using ATOD, the more likely they are to progress and exceed occasional illicit experimentation and to move into frequent abuse, with a higher chance of developing addiction. This is because drug use during times of critical brain development may cause permanent changes in the way the brain works and responds to rewards and consequences. Those who start drinking before age 15 are four times more likely to develop alcohol dependence than if they wait to start until the age of 21, regardless of any additional or environmental factors that may be present. The serious risks of substances to youth are physical (e.g., liver and heart damage, impaired brain function, impaired reproductive organ development), psychological (e.g., depression, sleep disorders, conduct disorders) and social (e.g., academic performance, relationships with family/friends, and increased exposure to risk situations; Hoffman & Froemke, 2007).

Alcohol and tobacco are the most commonly used substances by young people and result in 95% of the morbidity and mortality related to substance use in this age grouping. Despite the public and political concerns about the use of illicit drugs, such drugs are much less commonly used than alcohol and tobacco, although they may pose more serious immediate health risks. About 90% of people with substance abuse or dependence disorders started using under the age of 18 and half of these started under the age of 15 (Bonomo & Proimos, 2005).

It is important to address a developing substance abuse problem in young people as early as possible, with a recognition that they are different from adults in many ways: their unique developmental (e.g., difficulty comprehending future consequences) and psychiatric issues, differences in values and belief systems, and environmental considerations (such as strong peer influence). Family involvement plays a critical role in an adolescent's treatment and recovery (Hoffman & Froemke, 2007).

The Nurse With a Substance-Related Disorder

Nurses, along with most other professions and occupations, may also develop SRD. During a 30-day period, about 1.2% of the Canadian workforce experiences a substance abuse disorder, and a further 0.8% has a comorbid mental disorder (Dewa, Lesage, Goering, & Caveen, 2004). Substance abuse in the workplace affects performance (in judgment, alertness, perception, motor coordination, and emotional state) and is a major cause of unemployment, absenteeism, and workplace accidents. The recognition of addiction as a treatable medical illness (as opposed to a lifestyle choice) places a "duty to accommodate" on the employer, and this is increasingly reflected in employee assistance programs. For further information, see Chapter 5.

Rather than being protected by the special knowledge, skills, or insights nurses may have due to their education or professional experiences, some researchers consider nurses to be at particular risk for substance use disorders because of high job strain, disruption, and fatigue related to shift work, ease of access to medications in the workplace, and their knowledge of the benefits of medications (Lillibridge, Cox, & Cross, 2002; Trinkoff, Zhou, Storr, & Soeken, 2000). The evidence suggests that the prevalence of SRD among nurses may be similar to, or greater than, the general population (Smardon, 1998).

When nurses abuse or become dependent on substances, more than their own health and welfare is placed at risk. There are also patient safety concerns because of the risk associated impaired nursing practice and, when drugs are accessed from the workplace, patients may be under-medicated and suffer as a consequence. It may even place the safety of other health professionals at risk. To reduce this risk, and improve the recovery of the impaired nurse, the focus of the profession must be on prevention, early identification, multi-modal treatment, and return to practice with long-term supports.

Unfortunately the issue of substance use disorders amongst nurses is extremely sensitive, and difficult for the profession to address. Historically, nurses have concealed their addiction because of their fear of professional, employer, peer, and legal reprisals (Heise, 2003). The impaired nurse may not be able to recognize their illness and to seek help, and this inability places some responsibility on others to intervene. Perhaps one of the more difficult challenges nurses may have involves addressing a nurse colleague whom they suspect has an addiction and is practicing while impaired. Nurses have a responsibility in this situation to ensure patient safety, and to assist their nurse-colleague in accessing appropriate care and supports (e.g., confidential employee assistance programs are available in many workplaces throughout Canada), with the goal of successful return to practice. Reducing the stigma associated with substance use by nurses is critical so that nurses can help one another recognize the problem and seek treatment for it. Refer to Box 24-11 for the Canadian Nurses Association Position Statement on "problematic substance" use by nurses.

THE NURSE AS HEALTH ADVOCATE

The Code of Ethics for Registered Nurses (Canadian Nurses Association [CNA], 2008) serves as a foundation for nurses' ethical practice, and this includes endeavours that nurses may undertake to address social inequities. Nurses are expected to uphold principles of justice by safeguarding human rights, equity and fairness and by promoting the public good. Individuals with addiction are among the more marginalized and impoverished members of Canadian society. The challenges associated

BOX 24.11

Canadian Nurses Association Position Statement (2009)

The CNA acknowledges that "problematic substance" use by nurses is a serious and complex issue because it is a direct threat to the delivery of safe, competent, compassionate and ethical nursing care insofar as it can impair the nurse's cognitive and motor functions and interfere with judgment and decision-making. The CNA believes that the protection of the public from any possible harm caused by an incapacitated nurse is paramount in addressing problematic substance use by nurses. Stakeholder roles in addressing the problem include those of the:

- Individual nurse with a substance-related disorder, who is accountable to for his/her fitness to practice according to the values and responsibilities according to the Code of Ethics and Standards of Practice. The features of addiction, including denial and craving, may make this difficult

and the nurse may require the involvement and support of other stakeholders.

- Nurse colleagues, who are required to be attentive to signs that a colleague is unable, for whatever reason, to perform his or her duties, and to intervene compassionately. This duty is grounded in professional ethics and standards, as well as legal requirements.
- Nursing profession, is responsible to protect the public by ensuring that nurses are capable of providing safe, competent, compassionate, and ethical care. It also has a collective responsibility for emphasizing prevention, rehabilitation, and re-entry into the workplace, and this may include defining and advocating for health work environments as well as availability of effective, accessible treatment and rehabilitation programs.

Source: Canadian Nurses Association. (2009). *Position statement: Problematic substance use by nurses.* Available at: http://www.cna-aiic.ca/CNA/issues/position/protection/default_e.aspx

---

with their illness are often exacerbated by the experience of stigma, placing an additional burden for overcoming barriers to accessing care. Stigma includes having fixed ideas and judgments—such as thinking that people with substance use and mental health problems are not normal; that they caused their own problems; or that they can simply get over their problems if they want to do so. In its eighth Annual National Report Card on Health Care (2008), the Canadian Medical Association reported on the perception of mental illness and addiction among Canadians. Their survey findings indicated that only about half of Canadians say drug addiction (51%) and alcoholism (49%) are either serious illnesses or mental illnesses. Only 21% of Canadians would socialize with a co-worker who has either an alcohol or drug addiction. The stigma and shame associated with drug and alcohol dependence can, in effect, isolate those with addiction from the rest of society.

The use of alcohol, tobacco, and other drugs threatens to affect the overall welfare of our nation and our health care system. Nurses are well positioned on the frontlines of the health care system to be provided opportunities to understand the needs and vulnerabilities of those with substance use disorders, to be aware of available services and resources, and to note the existing deficits. It is well within the role of the nurse to seek opportunities to reduce the stigma and misunderstanding associated with addiction, as well as to collaborate and advocate for broader societal changes through policy, legislation, and other mechanisms to improve conditions for preventing and treating addiction at a population level. In these times of health care reform, nurses may have to proactively advocate for health-care systems that ensure accessibility, universality, and comprehensiveness of services in order to meet the needs of individuals with addictions and their families.

SUMMARY OF KEY POINTS

☐ Addiction is recognized by the major global disease classification systems as a chronic medical disorder characterized by periods of remission and relapse. Drugs of abuse alter the brain's structure and function, resulting in changes that persist long after drug use has ceased. Addiction is amenable to evidence-based treatment but remains largely untreated.

☐ The *DSM-IV-TR* classification of SRD includes substance use disorders (including substance dependence and substance abuse) and substance-induced disorders (including substance intoxication and substance withdrawal). These are classified according to the substances of alcohol, amphetamines and other stimulants, cannabis (marijuana), caffeine, cocaine, hallucinogens, inhalants, nicotine, opioids, PCP, and sedative-hypnotics and anxiolytics.

☐ The bio/psycho/social/spiritual model conceptualizes addiction as a disorder with multifactorial pathogenesis, including predisposing, precipitating, and modulating factors, that encompasses the body, the mind (psyche), the spirit, as well as social and environmental influences.

☐ Accurate and comprehensive assessment is crucial in planning addiction treatment interventions. Assessment should consider all substances for pattern of use, including factors of tolerance; withdrawal symptoms; consequences of use; loss of control over amount, frequency, or duration of use; desire or efforts to cease or control use; social, vocational, and recreational activities affected by use; and history of previous addiction treatment. It also includes investigating family and social support systems. Treatment plans must be assessed continually and modified as necessary to ensure that they meet the changing needs of the patient.

◻ Medically assisted and symptom-triggered detoxification is only the first stage of addiction treatment. By itself detoxification does little to change long-term drug abuse.

◻ In some individuals, the reduction of consumption, or abstinence, of alcohol may lead to withdrawal symptoms which may progress into life-threatening complications. Symptoms of alcohol withdrawal may include nausea and vomiting, tactile disturbances, tremor, auditory disturbances, paroxysmal sweats, visual disturbances, anxiety, headaches (or sensations of fullness in the head), agitation, and disturbances in orientation and clouding of the sensorium. It may also include autonomic disturbances, for example, blood pressure increases, tachycardia, diaphoresis, and in the most severe cases withdrawal may progress to seizures (tonic-clonic), delirium (delirium tremens), or death.

◻ The use of tobacco products remains the leading preventable cause of death and disease globally. Tobacco addiction is vastly undertreated; most individuals who smoke want to quit but few are helped in doing so. Nurses can effectively intervene and, as a minimum, should incorporate the 5As (Ask, Advise, Assess, Assist, and Arrange follow-up) into their daily practice. Uptake of smokeless tobacco is not considered a treatment for smoking cessation.

◻ The purpose of harm reduction is to reduce the risk for adverse consequences arising from substance use, and works with the individual to achieve this goal regardless of his or her commitment to reduce use. Harm reduction forms only one part of a continuum of care, and is not viewed as exclusive of the overarching goal of abstinence.

◻ MI helps to explore and resolve ambivalence by examining the conviction (importance) and the confidence in the process to change. Therapeutic approaches include avoiding arguing, expressing empathy, developing discrepancy, rolling with resistance, and supporting self-efficacy, and the purpose of using these are to motivate patients, resolve ambivalence, and to help patients change health-related behaviours.

◻ Many individuals with substance use disorders also have other mental disorders, and patients presenting with one condition should be assessed for others. When these conditions co-occur, treatment should address both (or all) at the same time (integrated or parallel treatment).

◻ Stigma can be a massive barrier for individuals with substance use disorders, and the nurse is well placed to reduce this stigma and misunderstanding. It is within the nursing role to collaborate and advocate for broader societal changes through policy, legislation, and other mechanisms to improve conditions for preventing and treating addiction.

CRITICAL THINKING CHALLENGES

1 What is your understanding of the etiology of addiction? Based on this understanding, what would be your priorities for patient education?

2 Jeff H., a 35-year-old cocaine-dependent patient, has recently entered a rehabilitation program. What goals do you believe would be realistic to achieve by the end of his projected 30-day inpatient stay?

3 You are working in an orthopaedic unit, and Mary L. has been admitted for treatment for a fractured femur. She has been drinking recently and has a BAL of 0.08%. What further information in the following areas would you need to plan her care?
   a. Medical
   b. Alcohol, tobacco, and other drug use related
   c. Other psychosocial issues

4 Medical use of marijuana has been approved in Canada. How would you explain its availability and use to a patient inquiry? What do you think are the advantages and disadvantages of this public policy?

5 Hannah K. presented with suicide ideation at the emergency department. When you see her she appears agitated and restless, and expresses a desire to leave the emergency department despite the fact she has not yet been seen by a physician. You note that she smokes, and has been waiting at the hospital to be assessed for almost 7 hours. What steps can you take to alleviate her nicotine withdrawal?

6 John M. has sought treatment for depression and job stress. He came to your psychiatric assessment unit smelling of alcohol. He believes that he does not have a drinking problem but a job problem. What interventions would you use for possible alcohol abuse or dependence?

7 Sylvia G. has been using heroin intravenously heavily for 2 years. She has come into the hospital with an abscess on her leg. What symptoms would you expect to observe as she experiences withdrawal from opiates? What medications would likely be used to ease these symptoms?

8 After Sylvia G. is free of withdrawal symptoms, she expresses interest in obtaining drug treatment. What are her options? How would you describe them to her?

9 Raymond L. has been treated for hypertension at your clinic. You notice that he complains of peripheral neuropathy and has an unsteady gait. What other medical signs would corroborate alcoholism?

10 Andre P. is being treated for cocaine dependence in a residential treatment facility. He asks you whether or not he should try to quit smoking at the same time. How do you respond?

WEB LINKS

www.aa.org   This is the official site for the program of Alcoholics Anonymous. Information about this program and about alcoholism is available.

www.al-anon.org   The purpose of Al-Anon is to help families and friends of people with alcoholism recover from the effects of living with the problem drinking of a relative or friend.

www.alcoholreports.blogspot.com   This is an international website dedicated to proving current information on news, reports, publications, and peer-reviewed research articles concerning alcoholism and alcohol-related problems.

www.camh.net   The Centre for Addiction and Mental Health (CAMH) is Canada's leading addiction and mental health teaching hospital.

www.can-adaptt.net   The Canadian Action Network for the Advancement, Dissemination and Adoption of Practice-Informed Tobacco Treatment (CAN-ADAPTT) is a Practice-based Research Network committed to facilitating research and knowledge exchange among those who are in positions to help smokers make changes to their behaviour.

www.ccsa.ca   The Canadian Centre on Substance Abuse is a national agency that promotes informed debate on substance abuse; disseminates information on the nature, extent, and consequences of substance abuse; and supports and assists organizations involved in substance abuse treatment, prevention, and educational programming.

www.cfdp.ca   The Canadian Foundation for Drug Policy is a non-profit organization that recommends effective and humane drug laws and policies in Canada.

www.health.org   The website of the National Clearinghouse for Alcohol and drug information and PREVline includes a catalogue of publications that discuss relevant treatment issues and research findings. It is possible to search several databases using this site.

www.nhic.org   The National Health Information Center (NHIC) is consumer focussed and has the ability to conduct searches for health-related topics, including alcoholism and addiction issues.

www.hhs.gov   The U.S. Department of Health and Human Services (DHHS) website contains foundational reports and best practice guidelines.

www.phac-aspc.gc.ca   Canada's Drug Strategy Division is the focal point within the federal government for harm reduction, prevention, and health promotion/population health initiatives concerning alcohol and other drugs issues.

www.rnao.org   The Registered Nurses of Ontario have developed nursing best practice guidelines for integrating smoking cessation into daily nursing practice

as well as for supporting patients on methadone maintenance treatment.

www.well.com/user/woa   Web of Addictions. This site contains fact sheets and in-depth information on special topics, links to resources, and ways to contact various groups and get help with addictions.

www.samhsa.gov   The website of the Substance Abuse and Mental Health Services Administration is a federal government site with funding, research, consumer information, and resources.

MOVIES, NOVELS, AND BIOGRAPHIES

Nurse Jackie: 2009. This dark comedy series is about an emergency room nurse addicted to medications (related to chronic pain from a back injury) and enabled by the hospital pharmacist. In this production by Showtime, the title character is portrayed as a "competent and compassionate nurse" but one who also violates the nurses' code of ethics.

VIEWING POINTS: What do you think your responsibilities would be if you were a colleague of Nurse Jackie? What are some of the ethical considerations in this situation? What support would you expect from your nurses association and from your employer?

Rachel Getting Married: 2009. This movie tells the story about young woman, Kym, who is released from rehabilitation for a few days to attend her sister's wedding. The home environment can be challenging for a recovering addict, and this is heightened by the emotions surrounding a wedding. Kym has been treated a number of times since her teen years, and the tenuous nature of recovery is portrayed including the mistrust of family members, and Kym herself, of her current abstinence.

VIEWING POINTS: How would you describe to others the distinction between detoxification and treatment? What does this film say to you about recovery as a process or an event? How could a recovering addict prepare for returning to the home situation?

Why can't they just stop? Addiction. New knowledge. New treatments. New Hope: 2007. This award winning HBO documentary addresses different aspects of addiction in order to shed light on the most current, promising developments in the field. Through personal stories from affected individuals and their families who struggle to help them find treatment, common misconceptions are replaced by insight into addiction's complexity.

VIEWING POINTS: How would you respond to someone asking why an individual just can't stop their use of substances? What is your personal position on the issue? How do you think your position will influence your nursing care?

REFERENCES AND SUGGESTED READINGS

Alcoholic Anonymous. (2004). *Alcoholics anonymous*. Online 4th ed., Retrieved July 26, 2009, from http://www.aa.org/bigbookonline

American Psychiatric Association. (2000). *The diagnostic and statistical manual of mental disorders* (4th ed., Text revision). Washington, DC: Author.

Blow, F. C., Walton, M. A., Barry, K. L., Coyne, J. C., Mudd, S. A., & Copeland, L. A. (2000). The relationship between alcohol problems and health functioning of older adults in primary care settings. *Journal of the American Geriatrics Society, 48*(7), 769–774.

Bonomo, Y., & Proimos, H. (2005). Substance misuse: Alcohol, tobacco, inhalants, and other drugs. *British Medical Journal, 330,* 777–781.

Brady, K. T., Myrick, H., & Malcolm, R. (1999). Sedative-hypnotic and anxiolytic agents. Specific drugs of abuse: Pharmacological and clinical aspects. In B. S. McCrady & E. E. Epstein (Eds.), *Addictions: A comprehensive guide book* (pp. 98–102). New York, NY: Oxford University Press.

Brands, B., Kahan, M., Selby, P., & Wilson, L. (2000). *Medical management of alcohol and drug-related problems: A physician's manual* (2nd ed.). Toronto, ON: Centre for Addiction and Mental Health.

Brown, T., & Graves, G. (2005). Availability and use of evidence-based treatment. In *Substance abuse in Canada: Current challenges and choices* (pp. 23–29). Ottawa, ON: Canadian Centre on Substance Abuse.

Canadian Centre on Substance Abuse. (2000). *Straight facts about drugs and drug abuse*. Ottawa, ON: Author. Available at: http://www.ccsa.ca

Canadian Centre on Substance Abuse. (2004). *Canadian addiction survey: A national survey of Canadian's use of alcohol and other drugs. Focus on gender*. Ottawa, ON: Author.

Canadian Centre on Substance Abuse. (2005). *Substance abuse in Canada: Current challenges and choices 2005*. Ottawa, ON: Author.

Canadian Centre on Substance Abuse. (2007). *A national survey of Canadians' use of alcohol and other drugs: Prevalence of use and related harms: Detailed report*. Ottawa, ON: Author.

Canadian Centre of Substance Abuse. (2008). *The essentials of… Seniors and substance abuse*. Ottawa, ON: Author.

Canadian Community Health Survey (CCHS). (2005). *Mental health and wellbeing*. Ottawa, ON: Statistics Canada. Available at: http://www. statcan.ca

Canadian Nurses Association. (2008). *Code of Ethics for Registered Nurses*. Available at: http://www.cna-aiic.ca/CNA/practice/ethics/code/default_e. aspx

Canadian Nurses Association. (2009). *Position statement: Problematic substance use by nurses*. Available at: http://www.cna-aiic.ca/CNA/issues/position/protection/default_e.aspx

Carroll, K. M. (1998). *A cognitive-behavioral approach: Treating cocaine addiction* (pp. 8–14). Rockville, MD: National Institute on Drug Abuse.

Centre for Addiction and Mental Health. (2005). *Information about concurrent disorders*. Updated January 14, 2005.

Chapman, S. (2007). *Public health advocacy and tobacco control: Making smoking history*. Oxford, UK: Blackwell.

Coambs, R. B., & McAndrews, M. P. (1994). The effects of psychoactive substances on workplace performance. In S. Macdonald & P. Roman (Eds.), *Drug testing in the workplace: Research advances in alcohol and drug problems* (Vol. 2, pp. 77–96). New York, NY: Plenum Press.

DeLima, M. S., de Olivera Soceres, B. G., Reisser, A. A., & Farrell, M. (2002). Pharmacological treatment of cocaine dependence: A systematic review. *Addiction, 97*(8), 931–949.

Dewa, C., Lesage, A., Goering, P., & Caveen, M. (2004). Nature and prevalence of mental illness in the workplace. *Health Papers, 5*(2), Special Issue.

Dunst, C. J., Trivette, C. M., & Deal, A. G. (1994). *Supporting and strengthening families: Methods, strategies and practices*. Cambridge, MA: Brookline Books.

Els, C. (2007). Addiction is a mental disorder, best managed in a (public) mental health setting – but our system is failing us. *Canadian Journal of Psychiatry, 52*(3), 167–169.

Els, C., & Kunyk, D. (2008). Management of tobacco addiction in patients with mental illness. *Smoking Cessation Rounds, 2*(2), 1–6.

Faltz, B. (contributing author). (1993). *Women and HIV: Train the trainer program*. San Francisco, CA: California Nurses Association.

Fingerhood, M. (2000). Substance abuse in older people. *Journal of the American Geriatric Society, 48*(8), 985–995.

Finkelstein, N. (1993). Treatment programming for alcohol and drug-dependent pregnant women. *International Journal of Addictions, 28*(13), 1275–1309.

Fiore, M., Jaén, C., Baker, T., Bailey, W. C., Benowitz, N., Curry, S. J., et al. (2008). *Treating tobacco use and dependence: 2008 Update*. Clinical Practice Guideline. Rockville, MC: U.S. Department of Health and Human Services. Public Health Service.

Fischer, B. (2005). Harm reduction. In *Substance abuse in Canada: Current challenges and choices* (pp. 11–15). Ottawa, ON: Canadian Centre on Substance Abuse.

Fu, Q., Heath, A., Bucholz, K. K., Nelson, E., Goldberg, J., Lyons, M. J., et al. (2002). Shared genetic risk of major depression, alcohol dependence, and marijuana dependence: Contribution of antisocial personality disorder in men. *Archives of General Psychiatry, 59*(12), 1125–1132.

Galanter, M., & Kleber, H. (1999). *Textbook of substance abuse treatment*. (2nd ed). Washington, DC: The American Psychiatric Press.

Gomberg, E. S. (1999). Women. In B. S. McCrady & E. E. Epstein (Eds.), *Addictions: A comprehensive guide* (pp. 527–541). New York, NY: Oxford University Press.

Gottlieb, L. N., & Rowat, K. (1987). The McGill model of nursing: A practice-derived model. *Advances in Nursing Science, 9,* 51–61.

Government of Canada. (2008). *Canada's drug strategy*. Ottawa, ON: Interdepartmental Working Group on Substance Abuse, Minister of Public Works and Government Services Canada. Cat. H39–440/1998E. Available at: http://www.hc-sc.gc.ca

Graham, A., Schultz, T., Mayo-Smith, M., Ries, R., & Wilford, B. (Eds.). (2003). *Principles of addiction medicine* (3rd ed.). Chevy Chase, MD: American Society of Addiction Medicine.

Health Canada. (1996). *Exploring the links between substance use and mental health: Section I. A discussion paper. Section II. A round table*. Canada's Drug Strategy. Cat. No. H39–360/1–1996E. Ottawa, ON: Author.

Health Canada. (1999a). *A second diagnostic on the health of First Nations and Inuit people in Canada: November, 1999*. Ottawa, ON: Author.

Health Canada. (1999b). *Literature review: Evaluation strategies in Aboriginal substance abuse programs. A discussion*. First Nations and Inuit Health Branch (FNIHB), Ottawa, ON: Author.

Health Canada. (2001a). *Best practices: Treatment and Rehabilitation for women with substance use disorders*. Cat. No. H49–153/2001E. Ottawa, ON: Author.

Health Canada. (2001b). *Preventing substance use problems among young people: A compendium of best practices*. Cat. No. H39–580/2001E. Ottawa, ON: Author.

Health Canada. (2002c). *A report on mental illnesses in Canada*. Cat. 0–662–32817–5. Ottawa, ON: Author.

Health Canada. (2003a). *Medical marijuana*. Ottawa, ON: Author. Available at: http://www.hc-sc.gc.ca

Health Canada. (2003b). *Best practices: Treatment and rehabilitation for seniors with substance use problems*. Cat. H46–2/03–295E. Ottawa, ON: Author. Available at: http://www.hc-sc.gc.ca

Health Canada. (2006). *Summary of results of the 2004–05 youth smoking survey*. Ottawa, ON: Health Canada. Retrieved September, 2006, from http://www.hc-sc.gc.ca

Health Canada. (2008). *Canadian addiction survey (CAS): Focus on Gender*. Cat.: H128–1/07–519E. Ottawa, ON: Author.

Health Canada. (2009). *Canadian tobacco use monitoring survey (CTUMS): Summary of results for the first half of 2008 (February to June)*. Ottawa, ON: Health Canada. Retrieved July 20, 2009, from http://www.hc-sc.gc.ca

Heise, B. (2003). The historical contact of addiction in the nursing profession: 1850–1982. *Journal of Addictions Nursing, 14,* 117–124.

Hesselbrock, M. N., Hesselbrock, V. M., & Epstein, E. E. (1999). Theories of alcohol and other drug use disorders. In B. S. McCrady & E. E. Epstein (Eds.), *Addictions: A comprehensive guide* (pp. 50–71). New York, NY: Oxford University Press.

Hoffman, J., & Froemke, S. (Producer). (2007). *Why can't they just stop? Addiction. New knowledge. New treatments. New Hope*. HBO Documentary Films, Robert Wood Johnson Foundation, NIDA, NIAAA. HBO & HBO Video.

Janssen, P. A., Demorest, L. C., & Whynot, E. M. (2005). Acupuncture for substance abuse treatment in the downtown eastside of Vancouver. *Journal of Urban Health, 82*(2), 285–295.

Johnston, L. D., O'Malley, P., & Bachman, J. G. (2000). *Monitoring the future: National survey results on adolescent drug use. Overview of key findings, 1999*. Rockville, MD: U.S. Department of Health and Human Services.

Kenna, G. A. (2004). Alcohol use by healthcare professionals. *Drug and Alcohol Dependence, 75*(1), 107–116.

Kirby, M. (2006). *Out of the shadows at last: Transforming mental health, mental illness and addiction services in Canada*. Ottawa, ON: Standing Senate Committee on Social Affairs, Science and Technology. Retrieved

March 13, 2008, from http://www.parl.gc.ca/39/1/parlbus/commbus/sen-ate/com-e/soci-e/rep-e/rep02may06-e.htm

Kleber, H., Weiss, R., Anton, R., George, T., Greenfield, S., Kosten, T., et al. (2006). *Practice guidelines for the treatment of patients with Substance Use Disorders* (2nd ed.). Arlington, VA: American Psychiatric Association

Kunyk, D., Els, C., Predy, G., & Haase, M. (2007). Development and intro-duction of a comprehensive tobacco control policy in a Canadian regional health authority. *Preventing Chronic Disease: Public Health Research, Practice, and Policy, 4*(2), 1–8.

Larimer, M. E. (1998). Harm reduction for alcohol problems: Expanding access to and acceptability of prevention and treatment services. In G. A. Marlatt (Ed.), *Harm reduction: Pragmatic strategies for managing high-risk behaviors* (pp. 69–121). New York, NY: Guilford Press.

Lasser, K., Boyd, J., Woolhandler, S., Himmelstein, D., McCornick, D., & Bor, D. (2000). Smoking and mental illness – a population-based preva-lence study. *Journal of the American Medical Association, 284*(20), 2606–2610.

Laundergan, J. C., & Williams, T. (1993). The Hazelden residential fam-ily program: A combined systems and disease model approach. In T. J. O'Farrell (Ed.), *Treating alcohol problems: Marital and family interventions* (pp. 145–169). New York, NY: Guilford Press.

Leatherdale, S., & Shields, M (2009). Smoking cessation: Intentions, attemps and techniques. *Statistics Canada Heatlh Reports.* Accessed July 20, 2009, from http://www.statcan.gc.ca/pub/82-003-x/2009003/article/10904-eng.htm

Lerman, D., Patterson, F., & Berrettini, W. (2005). Treating tobacco depen-dence: state of the science and new direction. *Journal of Clinical Oncology, 23*, 311–323.

Leshner, A. (1997). Addiction is a brain disease, and it matters. *Science, 278*(3), 45–47.

Lillibridge, J., Cox, M., & Cross, W. (2002). Uncovering the secret: giv-ing voice to the experiences of nurses who misuse substances. *Journal of Advanced Nursing, 39*(3), 219–229.

Lowinson, J., Ruiz, P., Millman, R., & Landrod, J. (Eds.). (2005). *Substance abuse: A comprehensive textbook* (4th ed.). Philadelphia, PA: Lippincott Williams & Wilkins.

Ludwig, M. A., Marecki, M., Wooldridge, P. J., & Sherman, L. M. (1996). Neonatal nurses' knowledge of and attitudes toward caring for cocaine exposed infants and their mothers. *Journal of Perinatal and Neonatal Nurs-ing, 9*(4), 81–95.

MacKay, R. C., Hughes, J. R., & Carver, E. J. (1990). *Empathy in the helping relationship.* New York, NY: Springer Publishing.

Marion, I. J. (1995). *Pregnant substance abusing women* (pp. 2–11). Rockville, MD: U.S. Department of Health and Human Services.

Markey, B. T., & Stone, J. B. (1997). An alcohol and drug education program for nurses. *AORN Journal, 66*(5), 845–853.

Martin, J. K., Kraft, J. M., & Roman, P. M. (1994). Extent and impact of alcohol and drug use problems in the workplace: A review of the empiri-cal evidence. In S. Macdonald & P. Roman (Eds.), *Drug testing in the workplace: Research advances in alcohol and drug problems* (Vol. 2, pp. 3–31). New York, NY: Plenum Press.

McCaul, M. E., Wand, G. S., Eissenberg, T., Rohde, C. A., & Cheskin, L. J. (2000). Naltrexone alters subjective and psychomotor responses to alcohol in heavy drinking subjects. *Neuropsychopharmacology, 22*(5), 480–492.

McLellan, A. T., Lewis, D., O'Brien, C., & Kleber, H. (2000). Drug depen-dence, a chronic medical illness: Implications for treatment, insurance, and outcomes evaluation. *Journal of the American Medical Association, 284*(13), 1689-1695.

Miller, W. R. (1995). Increasing motivation for change. In R. K. Hester & W. R. Miller (Eds.), *Handbook of alcoholism treatment approaches: Effective alternatives* (2nd ed., pp. 89–104). Boston, MA: Allyn & Brown.

Miller, W. R., & Rollnick, S. (2002). *Motivational interviewing: Preparing people for change.* New York: Guilford Press.

Miller, W. R., & Sanchez, V. C. (1994). Motivating young adults for treatment and lifestyle change. In G. Howard & P. E. Nathan (Eds.), *Alcohol use and misuse by young adults.* Notre Dame, IN: University of Notre Dame Press.

Monahan, G. (2003). Drug use/misuse among health professionals. *Substance Use and Misuse, 38*, 1871–1881.

Nace, E. P. (1997). Alcoholics Anonymous. In J. H. Lowinson, P. Ruiz, R. B. Millman, & J. G. Langrod (Eds.), *Substance abuse: A comprehensive textbook* (3rd ed., pp. 383–390). Baltimore, MD: Williams & Wilkins.

Nagy, P. D. (1994). *Intensive outpatient treatment for alcohol and other drug abuse* (p. 21). Rockville, MD: U.S. Department of Health and Human Services.

National Institute on Alcohol Abuse and Alcoholism (NIAAA). (2002). Alcohol and minorities: An update. *Alcohol Alert, 55.* Available at: http://www.niaaa.nih.902

National Institute on Drug Abuse (NIDA). (2005a). *Research Report: Heroin: Abuse and Addiction.* NIH Publication Number 05-4165. Bethesda, MD: Author.

National Institute on Drug Abuse (NIDA). (2005b). *Research Report Series: Inhalant Abuse.* Publication Number 05-3818. Bethesda, MD: Author.

National Institute on Drug Abuse (NIDA). (2008). *Principles of drug addiction treatment: A research-based guide* (pp. 1–3). Rockville, MD: Author.

National Institute on Drug Abuse (NIDA). (2009). Research Report: *Cocaine: Abuse and Addiction.* NIH Publication Number 09-4166. Bethesda, MD: Author.

National Native Addictions Partnership Foundation (NNADAP). (2000). *NNADAP Renewal Framework: For implementing the strategic recommenda-tions of the 1998, General review of the National Native Alcohol and Drug Abuse Program.* Draft working paper, prepared for the Framework Sub-committee of the NNADAP. December 2000.

National Native Addictions Partnership Foundation's Treatment Activity Reporting System (TARS). Database for health-related information on Aboriginal Canadians.

National Population Survey. Statistics Canada. Ottawa. Collects cross-sec-tional as well as longitudinal data designed to enhance the understanding of the processes affecting health.

Nemes, S., Rao, P. A., Zeiler, C., Munly, K., Holtz, K. D., & Hoffman, J. (2004). Computerized screening of substance abuse problems in a primary care setting: Older vs. younger adults. *American Journal of Drug and Alcohol Abuse, 30*(3), 627–642.

O'Connor, P. G., & Schottenfeld, R. S. (1998). Departments of Internal Medicine and Psychiatry Medical Progress: Patients with alcohol prob-lems. *New England Journal of Medicine, 338*(9), 592–602.

O'Farrell, J. (1999). Alcoholism treatment and the family: Do family and individual treatments for alcoholic adults have preventative effects for children? *Journal of Studies on Alcohol, 13*, 125–129.

Pandina, R., & Hendren, R. (1999). Other drugs of abuse: Inhalants, designer drugs, and steroids. Specific drugs of abuse: Pharmacological and clinical aspects. In B. S. McCrady & E. E. Epstein (Eds.), *Addictions: A comprehen-sive guide book* (p. 173). New York, NY: Oxford University Press.

Public Health Agency of Canada. (1998). *Alcohol and pregnancy.* The Canadian Perinatal Surveillance System. Last updated 2003. Available at: http://www.fas-saf.com

Ramaekers, J. G., Berghaus, G., van Laar, M., Drummer, O. H. (2004). Dose related risk of motor vehicle crashes after cannabis use. *Drug Alcohol Review, 23*(3):319–344.

Rehm, J., Ballunas, D., Brochu, S., Fischer, B., Gnam, W., Patra, J., et al. (2006). *The costs of substance abuse in Canada.* Ottawa, ON: Canadian Centre on Substance Abuse.

Repace, J. (2006). Exposure to second hand smoke. In W. R. Otts, A. C. Steinman, & L. A. Wallace (Eds.), *Exposure analysis* (pp. 201–231). Ann Arbor, MI: CRC Press.

Rice, V., & Stead, L. (2004). *Nursing interventions for smoking cessation* (Cochrane Review). Cochrane Library, Issue 1.

Rosenthal, R. N., & Westreich, L. (1999). Treatment of persons with dual diagnoses of substance use disorder and other psychological problems. In B. S. McCrady & E. E. Epstein (Eds.), *Addictions: A comprehensive guide* (pp. 439–476). New York, NY: Oxford University Press.

SAMHSA. (2000). *National household survey on drug abuse.* Office of Applied Studies. Retrieved June 2003, from, http://www.samhsa.gov

Selwyn, P. A., & Merino, F. L. (1997). Medical complications and treatment. In J. H. Lowinson, P. Ruiz, R. B. Millman, & J. G. Langrod (Eds.), *Sub-stance abuse: A comprehensive textbook* (3rd ed., pp. 597–619). Baltimore, MD: Williams & Wilkins.

Single, E. (2005). New directions in alcohol policy. In *Substance abuse in Canada: Current challenges and choices* (pp. 5–9). Ottawa, ON: Canadian Centre on Substance Abuse.

Single, E., Rehm, J., Robson, L., & Truong, M. (2000). The relative risks and etiologic fractions of different causes of death and disease attributable to alcohol, tobacco and illicit drug use in Canada. *Canadian Medical Asso-ciation Journal, 162*(12), 1669–1675.

Single, E., Robson, L., & Scott, K. (1997). *Morbidity and mortality related to alcohol, tobacco, and illicit drug use among indigenous people in Canada.* Ottawa, ON: Canadian Centre on Substance Abuse.

Smardon, M. (1998). An integrative review of substance abuse among nurses from 1981–1997. *The Online Journal of Knowledge Synthesis for Nursing, 5*(1).

Somers, J., Goldner, E., Waraich, P., & Hsu, L. (2004). Prevalence studies of substance-related disorders: A systematic review of the literature. *Canadian Journal of Psychiatry, 49*, 373–384.

Stanton, M. D., & Heath, A. W. (1997). Family and marital therapy. In J. H. Lowinson, P. Ruiz, R. B. Millman, & J. G. Langrod (Eds.), *Substance abuse: A comprehensive textbook* (3rd ed., pp. 448–453). Baltimore, MD: Williams & Wilkins.

Statistics Canada. (2002). *Statistical snapshots of Canada's seniors*. Available at: http://www.hc.sc.ga

Statistics Canada. (2003). *2001 Census: Analysis series. Aboriginal peoples of Canada: A demographic profile*. Ottawa, ON: Minister of Industry.

Statistics Canada. (2004). *Health reports: How healthy are Canadians?* Ottawa, ON: Author. Available at: http://www.hc-sc.gc.ca

Storr, C., Trinkoff, A., & Anthony, J. (1999). Job strain and non-medical drug use. *Drug and Alcohol Dependence, 55*, 45–51.

Sullivan, J., Sykora, K., Schneiderman, J., Narajo, C., & Sellters, E. (1989). Assessment of Alcohol Withdrawa: The revised clinical institute withdrawal assessment for alcohol scale (CIWA-Ar). *Addiction, 84*(11), 1353–1357.

Thomas, G. (2005, June). *Addiction and treatment centres in Canada: An environmental scan*. Ottawa, ON: Canadian Centre on Substance Abuse.

Trinkoff, A. M., Zhou, Q., Storr, C. L., & Soeken, K. L. (2000). Workplace access, negative proscriptors, job strain, and substance use in registered nurses. *Nursing Research, 49*(2), 83–90.

U.S. Department of Health and Human Services (DHHS). (1999). *Enhancing motivation for change in substance abuse treatment*. Washington, DC: Author.

U.S. Department of Health and Human Services (DHHS). (2000). *Substance abuse treatment for persons with HIV/AIDS* (pp. 70–71). Washington, DC: Author.

Volkow, N. (2001). Drug abuse and mental illness: Progress in understanding comorbidity. *American Journal of Psychiatry, 158*(8), 1181–1182.

West, R. (2006). *Theory of addiction*. Oxford, UK: Blackwell Publishing/Addiction Press.

Williams, J., & Ziedonis, D. (2004). Addressing tobacco among individuals with a mental illness or an addiction. *Addictive Behavior, 29*(6), 1067–1083.

World Health Organization. (2007). *International statistical classification of disease and related health problems* (10th ed.). Geneva, Switzerland: Author.

World Health Organization. (2009, May). *Call for pictorial warnings on tobacco packs: Media release*. Geneva, Switzerland: Author. Available at: http://www.who.int/mediacentre/news/releases/2009/no_tobacco_day_20090529/en/index.html

Personality and Impulse-Control Disorders

Stephen VanSlyke

Adapted from the chapter "Personality and Impulse-Control Disorders" by Mary Ann Boyd and Barbara J. Limandri

KEY CONCEPTS

- personality
- personality disorder
- personality traits

LEARNING OBJECTIVES

After studying this chapter, you will be able to:

- Identify the common features of personality disorders.
- Distinguish between the concepts of personality and personality disorder.
- Analyze the prevailing biologic, psychological, and social theories explaining the development of personality disorders.
- Discuss the epidemiology of each personality disorder.
- Distinguish among the three clusters of personality disorders.
- Formulate nursing diagnoses and plan interventions for clients with specific personality disorders.
- Compare the psychoanalytic explanation of the borderline personality disorder with the biosocial theory.
- Apply the nursing process to individuals with a diagnosis of borderline personality disorder.
- Analyze special concerns within the nurse–client relationship common to treating those with personality disorders.
- Compare and contrast the impulse-control disorders.

KEY TERMS

• adaptive inflexibility • affective instability • attachment • cognitive schema • communication triad • dialectical behaviour therapy (DBT) • dichotomous thinking • dissociation • emotional dysregulation • emotional vulnerability • emotions • identity diffusion • impulsivity • inhibited grieving • invalidating environment • kleptomania • parasuicidal behaviour • projective identification • psychopathy • pyromania • self-identity • separation-individuation • skills groups • splitting • temperament • tenuous stability • thought stopping • trichotillomania • vicious circles of behaviour

The concept of personality seems deceivingly simple but is very complex. Historically, the term *personality* was derived from the Greek *persona*, the theatrical mask used by dramatic players. Originally, the term had the connotation of a projected pretence or allusion. With time, the connotation changed from being an external surface representation to the internal traits of the individual.

KEY CONCEPT Personality is a complex pattern of characteristics, largely outside the person's awareness, that compose the individual's distinctive pattern of perceiving, feeling, thinking, coping, and behaving. The personality emerges from a complicated interaction of biologic dispositions, psychological experiences, and environmental situations.

Today, personality is conceptualized as a complex pattern of psychological characteristics that are not easily altered and that are largely outside the person's awareness. These characteristics or traits include the individual's specific style of perceiving, thinking, and feeling about self, others, and the environment. These styles or traits are similar across many different social or personal situations and are expressed in almost every facet of functioning. Intrinsic and pervasive, they emerge from a complicated interaction of biologic dispositions, psychological experiences, and environmental situations that ultimately make up the individual's distinctive personality (Millon, Millon, Meagher, Grossman, & Ramnath, 2004). Psychologists are exploring whether there are basic or primary personality traits (Rushton & Irwing, 2008). The Big Five or five-factor model names these traits as **O**penness (to experience), **C**onscientiousness, **E**xtraversion, **A**greeableness, and **N**euroticism (emotional instability). (Hint: Use the mnemonic **OCEAN** to remember them.)

KEY CONCEPT Personality traits are prominent aspects of personality that are exhibited in a wide range of important social and personal contexts (American Psychiatric Association [APA], 2000, p. 770).

Personality Disorders

No sharp division exists between normal and abnormal personality functioning. Instead, personalities are viewed on a continuum from normal at one end to abnormal at the other. Many of the same processes involved in the development of a "normal" personality are responsible for the development of a personality disorder.

IN A LIFE

Ferdinand Waldo Demara (1921–1982)
The Great Impostor

Public Persona

Ferdinand Waldo Demara spent much of his adult life using forged, stolen, or nonexistent credentials to gain employment in numerous and varied vocations. He became most famous for his masquerade as a commissioned Surgeon-Lieutenant in the Royal Canadian Navy in 1951, having stolen the identity of the Canadian physician Dr. Joseph Cyr. Demara was apparently competent in his role as a physician, relying on medical texts and a medical assistant. Demara had similar success in other branches of the military, as a psychologist in a college, as a prison warden, and as a well-respected school teacher.

Personal Realities

Demara's life was patterned by the establishment of personal connections with individuals (often in the context of a religious order), theft of this person's identity, and subsequent employment using these false credentials. Once caught, he would disappear, only to reappear claiming a new identity. It was a sense of emptiness and boredom that would kindle Demara's dreams and his need to act as an impostor to fulfill his seemingly well-intentioned passions.

Source: Crichton, R. (1959). *The great impostor.* New York, NY: Random House.

KEY CONCEPT A **personality disorder** is an enduring pattern of inner experience and behaviour that deviates markedly from the expectations of the individual's culture, is pervasive and inflexible, has an onset in adolescence or early adulthood, is stable with time, and leads to distress or impairment (APA, 2000, p. 685).

Personality disorders are classified under Axis II of the *Diagnostic and Statistical Manual of Mental Disorders*, 4th ed., Text Revision (*DSM-IV-TR*) multiaxial system for diagnoses, separate from the other mental disorders presented thus far, which are classified under Axis I (APA, 2000). Separate classification under Axis II was intended to focus attention on the manifestations of behavioural patterns that might be overlooked in light of the more pronounced disorders of Axis I; it does not imply difference in pathogenesis or treatment interventions. Frequently, an Axis II diagnosis coexists with an Axis I diagnosis, in which case, the Axis II diagnosis may serve as the background through which the person experiences the other diagnosis. For example, a person who has a dependent personality disorder might also have symptoms of generalized anxiety disorder when faced with demands to function autonomously. The co-occurrence of personality disorders with other health concerns has contributed to recommendations for change in the diagnostic classification of personality disorders in the *DSM-V* (O'Donohue, Fowler, & Lilienfeld, 2007; Widiger & Samuel, 2005).

Ten personality disorders are recognized as psychiatric diagnoses and are organized into three clusters based on the dimensions of *odd-eccentric*, *dramatic-emotional*, and *anxious-fearful* behaviours or symptoms. Cluster A consists of the disorders that most broadly characterize odd and eccentric misfit disorders, including paranoid personality disorder, schizoid personality disorder, and schizotypal personality disorder. People with cluster B disorders show great **impulsivity** (acting without considering the consequences of the act or alternate actions) and emotionality; these disorders consist of borderline personality disorder (BPD), antisocial personality disorder (APD), histrionic personality disorder, and narcissistic personality disorder. Dramatic and erratic behaviour best characterizes people with cluster B disorders. Cluster C disorders feature a predominant sense of anxiety and fearfulness and include avoidant personality disorder, dependent personality disorder, and obsessive-compulsive personality disorder.

BPD is highlighted in this chapter because it is severely incapacitating and difficult to treat. APD is also emphasized. Symptoms associated with both of these disorders often provoke negative reactions on the part of the clinician, which interferes with the clinician's ability to provide effective care. Impulse-control disorders are summarized at the end of the chapter. These disorders commonly coexist with other mental disorders.

PERSONALITY DISORDER VERSUS PERSONALITY TRAITS

To receive a diagnosis of a personality disorder, an individual must demonstrate the criteria behaviours persistently and to such an extent that they impair the ability to function socially and occupationally. In some people, the underlying feelings and behaviours may be intermittent and interfere interpersonally without obvious impairment. Instead of having a personality disorder, the individual is said to have traits of the disorder, which also can be noted under Axis II without a formal diagnosis. Students learning about personality disorders and traits for the first time probably will question whether these personality patterns are truly mental disorders. These questions are shared by much of the general public. Even within the psychiatric community, there is much debate regarding the status of personality disorders. Students may also feel frustrated in caring for individuals with these disorders or traits because sometimes problems may seem to be patterns of behaviours over which the individual could gain control and because the client may seem otherwise emotionally healthy. Unfortunately, that is not the case. These patterns of thinking and behaviour are not easily changed,

and these individuals need a great amount of help and understanding from mental health providers. Changing lifelong personality patterns is difficult and requires much understanding and support.

COMMON FEATURES AND DIAGNOSTIC CRITERIA

The personality disorder diagnosis is based on the manifestation of abnormal, inflexible behaviour patterns of long duration, traced to adolescence or early adulthood. These behaviours are pervasive across a broad range of personal and social situations and cause significant distress or impairment to social or occupational functioning. These abnormal behaviour patterns must deviate markedly from the expectations of the individual's culture and must manifest in two or more of the following areas: cognition, or ways of perceiving and interpreting self, other people, and events; affectivity, or the range, intensity, lability, and appropriateness of emotional responses; interpersonal functioning; and impulse control. For immigrants who may be having difficulty learning new acceptable social and cultural behaviour patterns and adjusting to a new culture, the diagnosis of a personality disorder may be delayed beyond this difficult adjustment period.

Maladaptive Cognitive Schema

Cognitive schemas are patterns of thoughts that determine how a person interprets events. Each person's cognitive schemas screen, code, and evaluate the incoming stimuli. In personality disorders, maladaptive cognitive schemas cause the misinterpretation of other people's actions or reactions and of events that result in dysfunctional ways of responding. For example, if a person thinks that no one can be trusted, an innocent, friendly gesture can be interpreted as a suspicious behaviour, provoking a hostile response, instead of a reciprocal friendly greeting.

Affectivity and Emotional Instability

Emotions are psychophysiologic reactions that define a person's mood and can be categorized as negative (e.g., anger, fright, anxiety, guilt, shame, sadness, envy, jealousy, disgust), positive (e.g., happiness, pride, relief, love), and neutral (e.g., hope, compassion, empathy, sympathy, contentment). Emotions can affect one's ability to learn and function by affecting one's memory and how one accesses and stores information. Emotional arousal, particularly increased negative emotional arousal characteristic of people with personality disorders, can decrease one's ability to remember new information and accurately perceive the environment (Herpertz, Kunnert, Schwenger, & Sass, 1999; Hurlemann, Hawellek, Maier, & Dolan, 2007).

Impaired Self-Identity and Interpersonal Functioning

Self-identity is central to the normal development of one's personality. Self-identity includes an integration of social and occupational roles and affiliations, self-attributed personality traits, attitudes about gender roles, beliefs about sexuality and intimacy, long-term goals, political ideologies, and religious beliefs. Without an adequately formed identity, an individual's goal-directed behaviour is impaired, and interpersonal relationships are disrupted. Each individual's abilities, limitations, and goals are shaped by one's identity. In personality disorders, self-identity is often disturbed or absent.

Impulsivity and Destructive Behaviour

People with personality disorders often come to the attention of the mental health clinician because their impulsive behaviour results in negative consequences to others or themselves. They seem unable to consider the consequences of their actions before acting on their impulses. For example, an individual may feel rage toward another and lack skills to resist the impulse to attack that person physically, even though this action may be punished.

▰▰ SEVERITY OF DISORDER

Three generally agreed-on essential and interdependent criteria are used for determining the severity of personality pathology: tenuous stability, adaptive inflexibility, and a tendency to become trapped in rigid and inflexible patterns of behaviour that are self-defeating.

Tenuous Stability

Tenuous stability refers to fragile personality patterns that lack resiliency under subjective stress. These individuals may have exaggerated emotional reactions to stressful situations and cannot cope emotionally with normal stressful situations. They do not easily learn coping skills and may be overwhelmed when new difficulties arise.

Adaptive Inflexibility

Adaptive inflexibility describes rigidity in interactions with others, achievement of goals, and coping with stress. In the normal course of daily living, people learn when to take the initiative and modify environmental factors, as well as when to adapt to a given situation. They learn to be flexible in interactions with other people and their environment. Socially appropriate reactions that are proportional to the situation are the norm. Personalities become pathologic when individuals cannot adapt effectively to new circumstances and, instead, begin arranging their lives to avoid stressful situations. Their view of the world and expectations of people within it are inflexible. Consequently, there are no opportunities to learn and practice new coping skills.

Tendency to Become Trapped

The tendency to become trapped in rigid and inflexible patterns of behaviour creates **vicious circles of behaviour** that are self-defeating. These individuals become so rigid and inflexible in their interactions and role functioning that they generate and perpetuate dilemmas, provoke new predicaments, and set into motion self-defeating sequences with others. They restrict opportunities for new learning, misconstrue benign events, and provoke reactions in others that reactivate earlier problems (Millon et al., 2004). For example, a normal reaction of feeling angry at receiving a parking ticket usually subsides, and the person decides either to pay the fine or to appeal the case in court. The person with a personality disorder may get angry about receiving the ticket, but the anger controls his actions. For example, he may lash out verbally at the police officer who gave the ticket and get another citation, or when appearing in court, he may scream at the judge in the courtroom and end up receiving a more severe sentence such as having to serve time in jail. What begins as a normal stressful daily life event becomes a series of disastrous interpersonal conflicts and ends in a bad situation for the person with the personality disorder. Modulating emotions and behaviours requires psychoneurologic resources and learned coping skills. The individual with a normal reaction of anger may count to 10 before responding to the ticket or commiserate with a companion. However, the person with a personality disorder lacks cognitive modulation of the emotion and may intimidate others with an irrational angry outburst.

Cluster A Disorders: Odd-Eccentric

▰▰ PARANOID PERSONALITY DISORDER: SUSPICIOUS PATTERN

The most prominent features of paranoid personality disorder are mistrust of others and the desire to avoid relationships in which one is not in control or loses power. These individuals are suspicious, guarded, and hostile. They are consistently mistrustful of others' motives, even relatives and close friends. Actions of others are often misinterpreted as deception, deprecation, and betrayal, especially regarding fidelity or trustworthiness of a spouse or friend (Millon et al., 2004). Minor innocuous incidents are often misinterpreted as having sinister or hidden meaning, and suspicions are magnified into major distortions of reality. People with paranoid personalities are unforgiving and hold grudges; their typical emotional responses are anger and hostility. They distance themselves from others and are outwardly argumentative and abrasive; internally, they may hold private hopes of being understood and feel powerless, fearful, and vulnerable (Hayward, 2007; Links & Stockwell, 2004).

Other hallmark features of paranoid personality disorder are persistent ideas of self-importance and the tendency to be rigid and controlled. These people are blind to their own unattractive behaviours and characteristics; they often are hypercritical and attribute these traits to others. Their outward demeanour often seems cold, sullen, and humourless. They want to appear controlled and objective, yet often they react emotionally, displaying signs of nervousness, anger, envy, and jealousy. Orderly by nature, they are hypervigilant to any environmental changes that may loosen their control on the world. Because people with this disorder are extremely sensitive about appearing "strange" or "bizarre," they will not seek mental health care until they decompensate into a psychosis (Table 25-1).

Epidemiology

Canadian prevalence data are lacking for paranoid personality disorder as well as for other types of personality disorders (Health Canada, 2002). In the United States, the prevalence of paranoid personality disorder is reported to be between 0.5% and 2.5% in the general population. In inpatient settings, 10% to 30% of clients have this disorder, and in outpatient settings, 2% to 10% have the disorder (APA, 2000). Axis I disorders, such as generalized anxiety disorder, mood disorders, and schizophrenia, can coexist with paranoid personality disorder, but minor Axis I symptoms usually are not seen. Other Axis II disorders can also coexist, such as narcissistic, avoidant, and obsessive-compulsive personality disorders (Millon et al., 2004).

Etiology

The etiologic factors of paranoid personality disorder are unclear. Experts speculate that there may be a genetic predisposition for an irregular maturation. An underlying excess in limbic and sympathetic system reactivity or a neurochemical acceleration of synaptic transmission may exist. These dysfunctions can give rise to the hypersensitivity, cognitive autism, and social isolation that characterize these clients. As children, these individuals tend to be active and intrusive, difficult to manage, hyperactive, and irritable, and they have frequent temper outbursts.

Nursing Management

Nurses are most likely to see these clients for other health problems but will formulate nursing diagnoses based on the client's underlying suspiciousness (Ward, 2004). An assessment of these individuals will reveal disturbed or illogical thoughts that demonstrate the misinterpretation of environmental stimuli. For example, a man was convinced that his wife was having an affair with the neighbour because his wife and the neighbour left their homes for work at the same time each morning. Although the man's beliefs were illogical, he never once considered that he was wrong. He frequently followed them but never caught them together. He continued to believe that they were having an affair. The nursing diagnosis of disturbed thought processes is usually supported by the assessment data.

Because of their inability to develop relationships, these individuals are often socially isolated and lack social support systems. Yet, the nursing diagnosis of social isolation is not appropriate for the person with paranoid personality disorder because the person does not meet the defining characteristics of feelings of aloneness, rejection, desire for contact with people, and insecurity in social situations.

Nursing interventions based on the establishment of a nurse–client relationship are difficult to implement because of the person's mistrust. If a trusting relationship is established, the nurse helps the individual identify problematic areas, such as getting along with others or keeping a job. Through therapeutic techniques such as acceptance, confrontation, and reflection, the nurse and the client examine a problematic area to gain another view of the situation. Changing thought patterns takes time. Client outcomes are evaluated in terms of small changes in thinking and behaviour.

Because paranoid personality disorder has extreme anxiety at its root, there is likely to be disruption in the dopaminergic tracts between the limbic and the cortical areas (Pezze & Feldon, 2004). Therefore, serotonin-dopamine antagonists such as risperidone (Risperdal), olanzapine (Zyprexa), or quetiapine (Seroquel) may be prescribed. The nurse needs to explain how these drugs work to elicit adherence.

▉◖ SCHIZOID PERSONALITY DISORDER: ASOCIAL PATTERN

People with schizoid personality disorder are expressively impassive and interpersonally unengaged (Millon et al., 2004). They tend to be unable to experience the

| Table 25.1 | A Summary of Diagnostic Characteristics of Cluster A Disorders | |

Diagnostic Criteria and Target Symptoms

Paranoid Personality Disorder 301.0
- Pervasive distrust and suspiciousness of others interpreted as malevolent (often with little or no justification or evidence to support it)
- Assumption of exploitation, harm, or deception; feelings that others are plotting against him or her with possible sudden attacks (associated with feelings of deep or irreversible injury) at any time for no reason
- Preoccupation with doubts of loyalty or untrustworthiness of friends and associates; deviation from doubts viewed as support for assumptions
- Reluctance to confide in others or become close in fear that information will be used against him or her
- Interpretation of hidden meanings into remarks or events, believing them to be demeaning and threatening
- Holding of grudges with unwillingness to forgive; minor intrusions arouse major hostility, persisting for long periods of time
- Quick to react and counterattack to perceived insults—possible pathologic jealousy with recurrent suspiciousness about the fidelity of spouse or sexual partner
- Not occurring exclusively during the course of another psychiatric disorder; not a direct physiologic effect of a general medical condition

Schizoid Personality Disorder 301.20
- Pervasive pattern of detachment from social relating
- Restricted range for emotional expression
- Lacking desire for intimacy
- Indifference to opportunities for close relationships
- Little satisfaction from being part of family or social group
- Preference for alone time rather than being with others; choosing solitary activities or hobbies
- Little, if any, interest in having sexual experiences with others
- Reduced pleasure from sensory, bodily, or interpersonal experiences
- No close friends or relatives
- Indifference to approval or criticism from others
- Emotional coldness, detachment, or flattened activity
- Not occurring exclusively during the course of another psychiatric disorder; not a direct physiologic effect of a general medical condition

Schizotypal Personality Disorder 301.22
- Pervasive pattern of social and interpersonal deficits evidenced by acute discomfort, reduced capacity for close relationships, cognitive and perceptual distortions, and eccentric behaviour
- Ideas of reference
- Odd beliefs or magical thinking influencing behaviour, such as superstitions, and preoccupation with paranormal phenomena, special powers, etc.
- Perceptual alterations
- Odd thinking and speech
- Suspiciousness or paranoid ideation
- Stiff, inappropriate, or constricted interactions
- Odd or eccentric behaviour or appearance
- Few close friends or confidants (other than the first-degree relatives)
- Anxiety in social situations, especially unfamiliar ones; no decrease in anxiety with increasing familiarity
- Not occurring exclusively during the course of another psychiatric disorder

joyful and pleasurable aspects of life. They are introverted and reclusive, and clinically they appear distant, aloof, apathetic, and emotionally detached. They have difficulties making friends, seem uninterested in social activities, and appear to gain little satisfaction in personal relationships. In fact, they appear to be incapable of forming social relationships. Interests are directed at objects, things, and abstractions. As children, they engage primarily in solitary activities, such as stamp collecting, computer games, electronic equipment, or academic pursuits such as mathematics or engineering. In addition, there seems to be a cognitive deficit characterized by obscure thought processes, particularly about social matters. Communication with others is confused and lacks focus. These individuals reveal minimum introspection and self-awareness, and interpersonal experiences are described in a very mechanical way (see Table 25-1).

Epidemiology

Schizoid personality disorder is rarely diagnosed in clinical settings (Lenzenweger & Clarkin, 2005). It is estimated that the prevalence of schizoid personality disorder ranges from 0% to 8%, with a median prevalence of 1.7% (Torgersen, Kringlen, & Cramer, 2001). In the homeless mentally ill population, the incidence of traits is estimated at 14% (Rouff, 2000). The most prevalent comorbid disorder is avoidant personality disorder, which occurs in 5% of the cases. Dependent and obsessive-compulsive disorders (OCDs) may coexist with schizoid personality disorder (Torgersen et al.).

Etiology

The etiologic processes are speculative. There may be defects in either the limbic or the reticular regions of the brain that may result in the development of the schizoid pattern (Millon et al., 2004). The defects of this personality disorder may stem from an adrenergic–cholinergic imbalance in which the parasympathetic division of the autonomic nervous system is functionally dominant. Excesses or deficiencies in acetylcholine and norepinephrine may result in the proliferation and scattering of neural impulses that may be responsible for the cognitive "slippage" or affective deficits.

Nursing Management

Impaired social interactions and chronic low self-esteem are typical diagnoses of individuals with schizoid personality disorder. Major treatment goals are to enhance the experience of pleasure, prevent social isolation, and increase emotional responsiveness to others. Because these individuals often lack customary social skills, social skills training is useful in enhancing their ability to relate in interpersonal situations. The primary focus is to increase the person's ability to feel pleasure. The nurse balances interventions between encouraging enough social activity that prevents the individual from retreating to a fantasy world and too much social activity that becomes intolerable.

The nurse may find working with these individuals unrewarding and become frustrated, feel helpless, or feel bored during the interactions. It is difficult to establish a therapeutic relationship with these individuals because they tend to shy away from interactions. The evaluation of outcomes should be in terms of increasing the client's feelings of satisfaction with solitary activities.

■ SCHIZOTYPAL PERSONALITY DISORDER: ECCENTRIC PATTERN

People with the schizotypal personality disorder are characterized by a pattern of social and interpersonal deficits. They are void of any close friends other than the first-degree relatives. They have odd beliefs about their world that are inconsistent with their cultural norms. Ideas of reference (incorrect interpretations of events as having special, personal meaning) are often present, as are unusual perceptual delusions and odd, circumstantial, and metaphorical thinking and speech. Their mood is constricted or inappropriate, and they have excessive social anxieties of a paranoid character that do not diminish with familiarity. Their appearance and behaviour are characterized as odd, eccentric, or peculiar. They usually exhibit an avoidant behaviour pattern (see Table 25-1).

If these individuals do become psychotic, they seem totally disoriented and confused. Many will exhibit posturing, grimacing, inappropriate giggling, and peculiar mannerisms. Speech tends to ramble. Fantasy, hallucinations, and bizarre, fragmented delusions may be present. Regressive acts such as soiling and wetting the bed may occur. These individuals may consume food in an infantile or ravenous manner. Symptoms mirror but fall short of features that would justify the diagnosis of schizophrenia. The person's tendency is to remain socially isolated, dependent on family members or institutions. These individuals avoid social interaction that can keep them functional, and well-intentioned relatives or institutional staff will protect them, reinforcing their dependency. People with this disorder are particularly prone to experiencing disorganized schizophrenia.

Epidemiology

The prevalence of schizotypal personality disorder is estimated to range from 0.6% to 5.1%, with a median rate of about 3% of the nonclinical population. In a clinical sample of psychiatric clients, the prevalence ranged from 2.0% to 64%, with a median prevalence of 17.5% (Torgersen et al., 2001). This wide variation in prevalence rates may reflect the controversy surrounding the classification of schizotypal disorder as a separate personality disorder, instead of a component of schizophrenia.

Etiology

The etiology of schizotypal personality disorder is unknown. The neurodevelopmental explanation posits that schizotypy can be explained by insults to the nervous system, such as oxygen deprivation, at critical developmental periods. There is speculation that this disorder is part of a continuum of schizophrenia-related disorders and is really closely related to chronic schizophrenia (Matta et al., 2000). When the genetics of personality disorders are considered, there is evidence of a link between schizotypal personality disorder and schizophrenia (Matta et al.). Additional research is needed to determine whether this disorder is a milder form of schizophrenia.

People with schizotypal personality disorder have widespread cognitive deficits involving the left hemisphere more than the right and impaired cholinergic responsivity. Therefore, they have difficulty with short-term memory and verbal learning (Cadenhead, Perry, Shafer, & Braff, 1999; Voglmaier et al., 2000). They also exhibit visual, perceptual, and working memory deficits (Farmer et al., 2000).

Nursing Management

Depending on the amount of decompensation (deterioration of functioning and exacerbation of symptoms), the assessment of a client with a schizotypal personality disorder can generate a range of nursing diagnoses. If a person has severe symptoms, such as delusional thinking or perceptual disturbances, the nursing diagnoses are similar to those for a person with schizophrenia (see Chapter 18). If symptoms are mild, the typical nursing diagnoses include social isolation, ineffective coping, low self-esteem, and impaired social interactions.

People with schizotypal personality disorder need help in increasing their sense of self-worth and recognizing their positive attributes. They can benefit from interventions such as social skills training and environmental management that increases their psychosocial functioning. Their odd, eccentric thoughts and behaviours alienate them from others. Reinforcing and modelling socially appropriate dress and behaviour can improve their overall appearance and ability to relate in the environment (Hayward, 2007). Because they have a hard time generalizing from one situation to another, attention to cognitive skills is important (Waldeck & Miller, 2000).

▰◗ CONTINUUM OF CARE

People with cluster A personality disorders are rarely seen in mental health treatment because they seldom admit to mental health problems. They can improve their quality of life through psychotherapy, but their suspiciousness, lack of trust, and impaired social interactions make it difficult to establish a therapeutic relationship (Hayward, 2007). They do not usually seek treatment unless more serious symptoms appear, such as depression or anxiety. Medications are not generally used unless there is coexisting anxiety or depression. Even individuals with schizotypal personality disorder have a relatively stable course. Few actually experience schizophrenia or another psychotic disorder (APA, 2000). They seek health care for other problems and come to the attention of mental health professionals when their odd behaviour interferes with their daily activities. At these times, brief interventions are needed, such as self-care assistance, reality orientation, and role enhancement (Bulechek, Butcher, & McCloskey Dochterman, 2008).

Nursing care is often provided in a home or primary care setting, with the personality disorder being secondary to the purpose of the care. This means that nurses are focusing on other aspects of client care and may miss the underlying psychiatric disorder. A psychiatric nursing consult may be needed for these individuals to help identify the disorder.

▪ CRNENOTE

Nurses will care for individuals who have a personality disorder in contexts other than mental health settings and in situations in which the personality disorder is not the focus of care. While the disorder may not be identified, the client may have been unhelpfully labelled as "difficult."

Cluster B Disorders: Dramatic-Emotional

▰◗ BORDERLINE PERSONALITY DISORDER: UNSTABLE PATTERN

Clinical Course of Disorder

In 1938, the term *borderline* was first used to refer to a group of disorders that did not quite fit the definition of either neurosis or psychosis (Stern, 1938). The term evolved from the psychoanalytic conceptualization of the disorder as a dysfunctional personality structure. In 1980, BPD was formally recognized as a distinct disorder in the *DSM-III*. In the *DSM-IV-TR*, BPD is defined as "a pervasive pattern of instability of interpersonal relationships, self-image, and affects, and marked impulsivity that begins by early adulthood and is present in a variety of contexts" (APA, 2000, p. 706). Given that people diagnosed with BPD appear very different from one another, consideration is being given to the creation of three primary subgroups—depressed, impulsive, and psychotic—to further delineate this diagnosis (Dean, 2006). Table 25-2 outlines the diagnostic characteristics of BPD.

People with BPD have problems in regulating their moods, developing a sense of self, maintaining interpersonal relationships, maintaining reality-based cognitive processes, and avoiding impulsive or destructive behaviour. They appear more competent than they actually are and often set unrealistically high expectations for themselves. When these expectations are not met, they experience intense shame, self-hate, and self-directed anger. Their lives are like soap operas—one crisis after another. Some of the crises are caused by the individual's dysfunctional lifestyle or inadequate social milieu, but many are caused by fate—the death of a spouse or a diagnosis of

Table 25.2	A Summary of Diagnostic Characteristics of Borderline Personality Disorder 301.83	

Diagnostic Criteria and Target Symptoms	Associated Behavioural Findings
• Pervasive pattern of unstable interpersonal relationships, self-image, and affects • Frantic efforts to avoid real or imagined abandonment • Pattern of unstable and intense interpersonal relationships (alternating between the extremes of idealization and devaluation) • Identity disturbance (markedly and persistently unstable self-image or sense of self) • Impulsivity in at least two areas that are potentially self-damaging (spending, sex, substance abuse, reckless driving, or binge eating) • Recurrent suicidal behaviour, gestures, or threats; or self-mutilating behaviour • Affective instability due to a marked reactivity of mood (intense episodes lasting a few hours and only rarely more than a few days) • Chronic feelings of emptiness • Inappropriate, intense anger or difficulty controlling anger • Transient, stress-related paranoid ideation or severe dissociative symptoms • Beginning by early adulthood and presenting in a variety of contexts	• Pattern of undermining self at the moment a goal is to be realized • Possible psychotic-like symptoms during times of stress • Recurrent job losses, interrupted education, and broken marriages • History of physical and sexual abuse, neglect, hostile conflict, and early parental loss or separation

an illness. They react emotionally with minimal coping skills. The intensity of their dysregulation often frightens themselves and others. Friends, family members, and coworkers limit their contact with them, which furthers their sense of aloneness, abandonment, and self-hatred. It also diminishes opportunities for learning self-corrective measures.

Affective Instability

Affective instability (rapid and extreme shift in mood) is a core characteristic of BPD and is evidenced by erratic emotional responses to situations and intense sensitivity to criticism or perceived slights. For example, a person may greet a casual acquaintance with intense affection, yet later be aloof with the same acquaintance. Friends describe individuals with BPD as moody, irresponsible, or intense. These individuals fail to recognize their own emotional responses, thoughts, beliefs, and behaviours. Clinically, when a stressful situation is encountered, these individuals react with shifts in emotions. They seem to have a limited ability to develop emotional buffers to stressful situations. Regulating anger, anxiety, and sadness is particularly problematic. Difficulty with the intensity and regulation of emotion negatively affects their social behaviours and relationships, including relations with health professionals (Holm & Severinsson, 2008). These affective symptoms

have been shown to be long-lasting components of the disorder (Zanarini et al., 2007).

Identity Disturbances

Identity diffusion occurs when a person lacks aspects of personal identity or when personal identity is poorly developed (Erikson, 1968). Four factors of identity are most commonly disturbed: role absorption (narrowly defining self within a single role), painful incoherence (distressed sense of internal disharmony), inconsistency (lack of coherence in thoughts, feelings, and actions), and lack of commitment (Wilkinson-Ryan & Westen, 2000). Other factors of the personality identity (e.g., religious ideologies, moral value systems, sexual attitudes) appear to be less important in identity diffusion. Clinically, these clients appear to have no sense of their own identity and direction; this becomes a source of great distress to these individuals and is often manifested by chronic feelings of emptiness and boredom. It is not unusual for people with BPD to direct their actions in accord with the wishes of other people. For example, one woman with BPD describes herself:

> I am a singer because my mother wanted me to be. I live in the city because my manager thought that I should. I become whatever anyone tells me to be. Whenever someone recommends a song, I wonder why I didn't think of that. My boyfriend tells me what to wear.

Unstable Interpersonal Relationships

People with BPD have an extreme fear of abandonment as well as a history of unstable, insecure attachments (Meyer & Pilkonis, 2005). This abandonment likely stems from ambivalent early childhood attachment and invalidations within the early parent–child bond (Yen et al., 2002). Most never experienced a consistently secure, nurturing relationship and are constantly seeking reassurance and validation. In an attempt to meet their interpersonal needs, they idealize others and establish intense relationships that violate others' interpersonal boundaries, which leads to rejection (Bartholomew & Horowitz, 1991). When these relationships do not live up to their expectations, they devalue the person. Continually disappointed in relationships, these individuals, who already are intensely emotional and have a poor sense of self, feel estranged from others and feel inadequate in the face of perceived social standards. Intense shame and self-hate follow. These feelings often result in self-injurious behaviours, such as cutting the wrist, self-inflicted burns, or head banging.

In social situations, people with BPD use elaborate strategies to structure interactions. That is, they restrict their relationships to ones in which they feel in control. They distance themselves from groups when feeling anxious (which is most of the time) and rarely use their social support system. Even if they are married or have a supportive extended family, they are reluctant to share their feelings (Krause, Mendelson, & Lynch, 2003). They do not want to burden anyone; they fear rejection and also assume that people are tired of hearing them repeat the same issues (Miller, 1994).

A controversial area of BPD is separating early childhood abuse and trauma from pathologic development. In fact, people with confirmed childhood abuse and neglect histories showed a fourfold likelihood of having a personality disorder (Johnson, Cohen, Brown, Smailes, & Bernstein, 1999). Although trauma and abuse do not seem to cause BPD, they may sufficiently disturb identity and affect regulation to contribute to disordered personality development (Grover et al., 2007; Zanarini et al., 1997).

Cognitive Dysfunctions

People with BPD have dichotomous thinking. Cognitively, they evaluate experiences, people, and objects in terms of mutually exclusive categories (e.g., good or bad, success or failure, trustworthy or deceitful), which informs extreme interpretations of events that would normally be viewed as including both positive and negative aspects. There are also times when their thinking becomes disorganized. Irrelevant, bizarre notions and vague or scattered thought connections are sometimes present, as well as delusions and hallucinations.

Another cognitive dysfunction common in BPD is **dissociation**, in which thoughts and ideas can be split off from consciousness (Martin, 2007). Dissociation can be conceptualized as lying on a continuum from minor dissociations of daily life, such as daydreaming, to a breakdown in the usually integrated functions of consciousness, memory, perception of self or the environment, and sensory-motor behaviours. For example, in driving familiar roads, people often get lost in their thoughts or dissociate and suddenly do not remember what happened during that part of the trip. Environmental stimuli are ignored, and there are changes in the perception of reality. The individual is physically present but mentally in another place. Dissociation serves a useful purpose; in the case of driving a familiar road, dissociation alleviates the boredom of driving. It is also a coping strategy for avoiding disturbing events. In dissociating, the person does not have to be aware of or remember traumatic events. There is a strong correlation between dissociation and self-injurious behaviour (Zanarini, Ruser, Frankenburg, & Hennen, 2000).

Dysfunctional Behaviours

Impaired Problem Solving

In BPD, there is often a failure to engage in active problem solving. Instead, problem solving is attempted by soliciting help from others in a helpless, hopeless manner (Linehan, 1993a). Suggestions are rarely taken.

Impulsivity

Impulsivity is also characteristic of people with BPD. Because impulse-driven people have difficulty delaying gratification or thinking through the consequences before acting on their feelings, their actions are often unpredictable. Essentially, they act in the moment and clean up the mess afterward. Gambling, spending money irresponsibly, binge eating, engaging in unsafe sex, and abusing substances are typical of these individuals. They can also be physically or verbally aggressive. Job losses, interrupted education, and unsuccessful relationships are common.

Self-Injurious Behaviours

The turmoil and unsuccessful interpersonal relationships and the social experiences associated with BPD may lead the person to undermine himself or herself when a goal is about to be reached. The most serious consequences are suicide attempts or **parasuicidal behaviours** (deliberate self-injury with an intent to harm oneself). For example, in a study of a burn unit from 1980 to 1991, a total of 31 individuals were admitted with self-inflicted burns. Sixteen of the clients had inflicted nonlethal injuries and the other 15 lethal injuries (Tuohig, Saffle, Sullivan, Morris, & Lento, 1995). The prevalence of self-injurious behaviour is estimated to be 43% to 67% of people with BPD (Soloff, Lis, Kelly, Cornelius, & Ulrich, 2004). Self-injurious behaviour can be compulsive, episodic, or repetitive and is more likely to occur when the individual with BPD is depressed; has highly unstable interpersonal relationships, especially problems with intimacy and sociability; and is paranoid, hypervigilant (alert, watchful), and resentful (Paris, 2007; Yeomans, Hull, & Clarkin, 1994). Some well-known self-injurious behaviours follow:

- *Compulsive self-injurious behaviours* occur many times daily and are repetitive and ritualistic. For example, hair pulling, which can be a separate disorder (**trichotillomania**) or a behaviour of other personality disorders, involves pulling out hair, especially from the scalp, eyebrows, and eyelashes. Hair is plucked, examined, and sometimes eaten. Hair-pulling sessions may take several hours (Boughn, 2005). Most hair pullers do not seek help unless the symptoms are severe, and then they usually consult dermatologists or family practitioners.

- *Episodic self-injurious behaviours* occur every so often. These are especially common in people with BPD and develop into habitual coping behavioural patterns during periods when stress (progressive tension manifested by feelings of anger, depression, or anxiety) rises to an intolerable level. The individual reports being numb or empty and ends this dissociated state with a self-injurious behaviour that elicits feeling. One half to two thirds of people with BPD with self-injurious behaviours experience little or no associated pain (Links, Heslegrave, & van Reekum, 1998); rather, endogenous endorphins (opioids) are released, which dampen pain perception and activate the brain's pleasure centre. In addition, tension is relieved and a sense of calmness or even pleasure may follow. These feelings are believed to be reinforcing, and the person learns to relieve stress and anxiety by self-mutilation. The individuals harm themselves to feel better, get rapid relief from distressing thoughts and emotions, and gain a sense of control.

- *Repetitive self-mutilation* occurs when occasional self-injury turns into an overwhelming preoccupation. These people develop an identity as a "cutter" or "burner," for example, and describe themselves as being addicted to their self-harm. In an interpretive phenomenological study of people with BPD, Nehls (1999) described the emotional conflict these individuals experience when their perceived efforts to comfort themselves are interpreted by others as manipulation, resulting in their being denied care. Sometimes clients and nurses determine the risk for suicide by whether the intended outcome of a parasuicidal episode is death or injury. The underlying assumption is that those who

attempt to kill themselves are at higher risk than those who self-injure. In reality, there should be no distinction between self-damaging behaviours and suicide attempts. All self-injurious behaviours should be considered potentially life threatening and taken seriously.

BORDERLINE PERSONALITY DISORDER IN SPECIAL POPULATIONS

Many children and adolescents show symptoms similar to those of BPD, such as moodiness, self-destruction, impulsiveness, lack of temper control, and rejection sensitivity. If a family member has BPD, the adolescent should be carefully assessed for this disorder. Because symptoms of BPD begin in adolescence, it makes sense that some of the children and adolescents would meet the criteria for BPD, even though it is not diagnosed before young adulthood. More likely, there are personality traits, such as impulsivity and mood instability, in many adolescents that should be recognized and treated whether or not BPD actually develops.

Epidemiology

The estimated prevalence of BPD in the general population ranges from 0.3% to 2.0%, with a median rate of 1.6%. In clinical populations, BPD is the most frequently diagnosed personality disorder; its prevalence ranges from 11% to 70%, with a median of 31%. The average prevalence among outpatients is 8% to 27%, and among inpatients, 15% to 51% (Lenzenweger & Clarkin, 2005; Lyons, 1995; Widiger & Weissman, 1991). More than three fourths (77%) of the individuals with diagnoses of BPD are young women (mean age, mid-20s; Lyons, 1995). One explanation for this is that it is more socially acceptable for women than men to seek help from the health care system. Another reason is that childhood sexual abuse, which more commonly affects girls, is one of the strongest risk factors for BPD. Others think that gender bias in diagnosing may have a role (Grilo, 2002).

Ample clinical reports show the coexistence of personality disorders with Axis I disorders, but epidemiologic research is scant. BPD is associated with mood, substance abuse, eating, dissociative, and anxiety disorders (Farabaugh et al., 2005; Johnson, Sheahan, & Chard, 2003; Teplin, O'Connell, Daiter, & Varenbut, 2004).

Risk Factors

Various studies show that physical abuse and sexual abuse appear to be significant risk factors for BPD: 55% to 80% of individuals with BPD have reported a history of childhood sexual abuse and/or physical abuse (Jordan, 2004). Other earlier studies cite parental loss and separation (Zweig-Frank, Paris, & Guzder, 1994a, 1994b). Clearly, more studies are needed to identify risk factors for the development of BPD.

Etiology

What causes BPD remains largely unknown. Little evidence supports a biologic cause. Theories of psychological and social causes are more prolific.

Biologic Theories

There is no consensus regarding a biologic etiology of BPD, and no studies to date show a genetic component. The underlying assumption is that personality disorders develop within the context of the normal personality. Some argue that personality and Axis I disorders actually exist on a continuum and that personality traits and mood episodes are derived from the same underlying neurotransmitter dysfunctions and genetic constitution. These genetically determined traits become the organizing principle for the entire personality. Magnetic resonance imaging studies of 21 female clients with both BPD and posttraumatic stress disorder, compared with a matched healthy control sample, showed that women with BPD had a 16% smaller amygdala than did the healthy control subjects (Driessen et al., 2000). These findings are consistent with the neurologic effects of prolonged exposure to cortisol. Patterns of impaired executive functioning in people with BPD have been identified, leading to speculation about the extent neural pathways contribute to suicidal behaviour (LeGris & van Reekum, 2006).

Biologic abnormalities are associated with three BPD characteristics: affective instability; transient psychotic episodes; and impulsive, aggressive, and suicidal behaviour. Impulsivity and emotional instability are unusually intense in these individuals, and these traits are known to be inheritable. Associated brain dysfunction occurs in the limbic system and the frontal lobe and increases the behaviours of impulsiveness, parasuicide, and mood disturbance. A decrease in serotonin activity and an increase in α_2-noradrenergic receptor sites may be related to the irritability and impulsiveness common in people with this disorder (Coccaro, Kavoussi, Hauger, Cooper, & Ferris, 1998; Oquendo & Mann, 2000).

It has also been hypothesized that an increase in dopamine may be responsible for transient psychotic states. These dysfunctions could be caused by a number of events, including trauma, epilepsy, and attention deficit hyperactivity disorder (ADHD; Greene & Ugarriza, 1995; van Reekum, 1993). People with BPD manifest psychotic-like symptoms, including paranoid thinking, dissociation, depersonalization, and derealization. These symptoms seem to be associated with intense anxiety. There is some evidence that these symptoms are associated with excessive dopaminergic activity (Skodol et al., 2002).

Psychological Theories

Psychoanalytic Theories

The psychoanalytic views of BPD focus on two important psychoanalytic concepts: separation-individuation and projective identification. A person with BPD has not achieved the normal and healthy developmental stage of **separation-individuation**, during which a child develops a sense of self, a permanent sense of significant others (object constancy), and integration of seeing both bad and good components of self (Mahler, Pine, & Bergman, 1975). Margaret Klein and Otto Kernberg both contributed to Object Relations Theory. The theory explains how the objects (real and internalized relationships with significant people) contribute to personality and are expressed through defences and interpersonal interactions (Clarkin, Yeomans, & Kernberg, 2006; Magnavita, 2004). Those with BPD lack the ability to separate from the primary caregiver and develop a separate and distinct personality or self-identity. Psychoanalytic theory suggests that these separation difficulties occur because the primary caregivers' behaviours have been inconsistent or insensitive to the needs of the child. The child develops ambivalent feelings regarding interpersonal relationships and therefore has no basis for establishing trusting and secure relationships in the future. Children experience feelings of intense fear and anger in separating themselves from others. This problem continues into adulthood, and they continue to experience difficulties in maintaining personal boundaries and in interpersonal interactions and relationships. Often, these individuals falsely attribute to others their own unacceptable feelings, impulses, or thoughts, termed **projective identification**. Projective identification is believed to play an important role in the development of BPD and is a defence mechanism by which people with BPD protect their fragile self-image. For example, when overwhelmed by anxiety or anger at being disregarded by another, they defend against the intensity of these feelings by unconsciously blaming others for what happens to them. They project their feelings onto a significant other with the unconscious hope that the other knows how to deal with it. Projective identification becomes a defensive way of interacting with the world, which leads to more rejection.

Maladaptive Cognitive Processes

Cognitive schemas are important in understanding BPD (and APD as well). Individuals with personality disorders

Table 25.3	Maladaptive Schemas
Domain	**Schemas With Definitions**
I. Disconnection and rejection	1. *Abandonment/instability* Important people will not be there 2. *Mistrust/abuse* Other people will use the client for own selfish ends 3. *Emotional deprivation* Emotional connection will not be fulfilled 4. *Defectiveness/scheme* One is flawed, bad, or worthless 5. *Social isolation/alienation* Being different from or not fitting in
II. Impaired autonomy and performance	1. *Dependence/incompetence* Belief that one is unable to function on one's own 2. *Vulnerability to harm and illness* Fear that disaster is about to strike 3. *Enmeshment/undeveloped self* Excessive emotional involvement at the expense of normal social development 4. *Failure* Belief that one has failed
III. Impaired limits	1. *Entitlement/grandiosity* Belief that one is superior to other; entitled to special rights 2. *Insufficient self-control/self-discipline* Difficulty or refusal to exercise sufficient self-control
IV. Other directedness	1. *Subjugation* Excessive surrendering of control to others because of feeling coerced 2. *Self-sacrifice* Excessive focus on voluntarily meeting the needs of others at the expense of one's own gratification 3. *Approval seeking/recognition seeking* Excessive emphasis on gaining approval, recognition, or attention
V. Overvigilance and inhibition	1. *Negativity/pessimism* Lifelong focus on the negative aspects of life 2. *Emotional inhibition* Excessive inhibition of spontaneous action, feeling, or communication 3. *Unrelenting standard/hypercriticalness* Belief that one must meet very high standards; perfectionistic, rigid 4. *Punitiveness* Belief that people should be harshly punished

Young, J. E. (1999). *Cognitive therapy for personality disorders: A schema-focused approach.* Sarasota, FL: Professional Resource Press.

develop maladaptive schemas leading them to misinterpret environmental stimuli continuously, which in turn leads to rigid and inflexible behaviour patterns in response to new situations and people. Because those with BPD have been conditioned to anticipate rejection and disappointment in the past, they become entrenched in a pattern of fear and anxiety regarding encountering new people or situations. They have fears that a disaster is going to strike any minute. Early in life, individuals with BPD and other personality disorders develop maladaptive schemas or dysfunctional ways of interpreting people and events. Table 25-3 explains 18 major maladaptive schemas at work in those with personality disorders. The work of cognitive therapists is to challenge these distortions in thinking patterns and replace them with realistic ones.

Biosocial Theories

The biosocial learning theory was developed by Theodore Millon, who viewed BPD as a distinct disorder that develops as a result of both biologic and psychological factors (Millon & Davis, 1999). While he supported the biologic determination of personality, he believed that a child's interaction with the environment and learning and experience could greatly affect his or her biologic predisposition. He argued that each individual possesses a biologically based pattern of sensitivities and behavioural dispositions that shapes his or her experiences, including active-passive behaviour or a tendency to take initiative versus reacting to events, sensitivity to pleasure or pain, and sensitivity behaviour to self and others. Millon believed that BPD is a particular cycloid personality pattern representing a moderately dysfunctional dependent or ambivalent orientation, often expressed in intense endogenous moods, described as patterns of recurring dejection and apathy interspersed with spells of anger, anxiety, or euphoria.

A further elaboration of Millon's multidimensional model incorporates biologic explanations into the behaviour. Cloninger, Bayon, and Svrakic (1998) described personality disorder behaviours based on temperament and character dimensions derived from a factor analysis design. Cluster A disorders are associated with low-reward dependence and social attachment mediated by norepinephrine and serotonin. Cluster B disorders are associated with high novelty seeking mediated by dopamine. Novelty-seeking behaviour includes exhilaration, exploration, impulsivity, extravagance, and irritability. Cluster C disorders are associated with high harm avoidance mediated by γ-aminobutyric acid (GABA) and serotonin.

The current biosocial theory of BPD proposed by Marsha Linehan and colleagues at the University of Washington is similar to Millon's theory, with a focus on the interaction of both biologic and social learning influences. Her primary focus is on the particular behavioural patterns observed in BPD, including emotional vulnerability, self-invalidation, unrelenting crises, inhibited grieving, active passivity, and apparent competence (Linehan, 1993a; Box 25-1).

This biosocial viewpoint presents BPD as a multifaceted problem, a combination of a person's innate **emotional vulnerability** and his or her inability to control that emotion in social interactions (**emotional dysregulation**) and the environment (Linehan, 1993a). The emotional dysregulation and aggressive impulsivity entail both social learning and biologic regulation. Much of the neurobiologic research is directed at neurotransmitter functions involving serotonin, norepinephrine, dopamine, acetylcholine, GABA,

and vasopressin (Coccaro et al., 1998; Silk, 2000). In fact, restoring balance in these systems permits more consistent neural firing between the limbic system and the frontal and prefrontal cortex. When these pathways are functional, the person has a greater capacity to think about his or her emotions and modulate behaviours more responsibly.

The biosocial viewpoint supports the notion that the ability to control one's emotion is in part a learning process, learned from one's private experiences and encounters with the social environment. BPD is believed to develop when these emotionally vulnerable individuals interact with an **invalidating environment**, a social situation that negates the individual's private emotional responses and communication. In other words, when the person's core emotional responses and communications are continuously dismissed, trivialized, devalued, punished, and discredited (invalidated) by others whom the person respects or values, the person receives confused messages about expressing his or her own feelings.

A minor example of invalidating environment or response follows: The parents of Emily, a 4-year-old girl, tell her that the family is going to grandmother's house for a family meal. The child responds, "I am not going to Gramma's. I hate Stevie (cousin)." The parents reply, "You don't hate Stevie. He is a wonderful child. He is your cousin, and only a spoiled, selfish little girl would say such a thing." The parents have devalued Emily's feelings and discredited her comments, thereby invalidating her feelings and sense of personal worth.

The most severe form of invalidation occurs in situations of child sexual abuse. Often, the abusing adult has told the child that this is a "special secret" between them, that the child should feel guilty if he or she tells anyone, and that telling someone would end their trust and special relationship. The child experiences feelings of fear, pain,

---

BOX 25.1

Behavioural Patterns in BPD

1. *Emotional vulnerability.* Person experiences a pattern of pervasive difficulties in regulating negative emotions, including a high sensitivity to negative emotional stimuli, high emotional intensity, and slow return to emotional baseline.

2. *Self-invalidation.* Person fails to recognize one's own emotional responses, thoughts, beliefs, and behaviours and sets unrealistically high standards and expectations for self. May include intense shame, self-hate, and self-directed anger. Person has no personal awareness and tends to blame social environment for unrealistic expectations and demands.

3. *Unrelenting crises.* Person experiences a pattern of frequent, stressful, negative environmental events, disruptions, and roadblocks—some caused by the individual's dysfunctional lifestyle, others by an inadequate social

milieu, and many by fate or chance.

4. *Inhibited grieving.* Person tries to inhibit and overcontrol negative emotional responses, especially those associated with grief and loss, including sadness, anger, guilt, shame, anxiety, and panic.

5. *Active passivity.* Person fails to engage actively in solving own life problems but will actively seek problem solving from others in the environment; learned helplessness, hopelessness.

6. *Apparent competence.* Tendency for the individual to appear deceptively more competent than he or she actually is; usually due to failure of competencies to generalize across expected moods, situations, and time, and failure to display adequate nonverbal cues of emotional distress.

From Linehan, M. (1993a). *Cognitive-behavioral treatment of borderline personality disorder* (p. 10). New York, NY: Guilford Press.

and sadness, yet this trusted adult continuously dismisses the child's true feelings and tells the child what he or she should feel. Children often learn to endure sexual abuse for years, suppressing their true feelings. In disclosing the secret to a nonoffending adult, the child risks not being believed or attended to, and possible punishment.

In reality, all children, not just those who are emotionally vulnerable, learn to trust their own feelings and learn when and how to express them by interacting with their environments, including parents, families, friends, and social situations. If they constantly meet with an invalidating environment, they cannot learn to trust their own feelings—when to be angry, sad, or happy—or how to regulate their emotions. They become emotionally dysregulated. This emotional dysregulation leads to further difficulties in identity disturbances, interpersonal relationships, and the development of impulsive, parasuicidal behaviours.

Interdisciplinary Treatment

BPD is a very complex disorder that requires the whole mental health care team. The symptoms of the disorder usually require a variety of medications, including mood stabilizers, antidepressants, and anxiolytics; careful medication monitoring is necessary. Psychotherapy is needed to help the individual manage the dysfunctional moods, impulsive behaviours, and self-injurious behaviours. Specially trained therapists who are comfortable with the many demands of these clients are needed. These therapists represent a variety of mental health disciplines, including psychology, social work, and advanced practice nursing. This can be a lifelong disorder requiring ongoing treatment as the individual copes with multiple interpersonal crises.

Dialectical Behaviour Therapy

Dialectical behaviour therapy (DBT), developed by Linehan, is an important biosocial approach to treatment that combines numerous cognitive and behaviour therapy strategies. For DBT to be effective, the therapists and coaches must work with clients as partners and be willing to focus on many interconnected behaviours (e.g., parasuicidal and substance abuse) and not a single diagnosis. It requires clients to understand their disorder by actively participating in formulating treatment goals by collecting data about their own behaviours, identifying treatment targets in individual therapy, and working with the therapists in changing these target behaviours. The core treatment procedures include problem solving, exposure techniques (gradual exposure to cues that set off aversive emotions), skill training, contingency management (reinforcement of positive behaviour), and cognitive modification. **Skills groups** are an integral part of DBT and are taught in group settings in which members practice emotional regulation, interpersonal effectiveness, core mindfulness skills, and distress tolerance.

Emotional regulation skills are taught to manage intense, labile moods. They involve helping the client label and analyze the context of the emotion and develop strategies to reduce emotional vulnerability. Teaching individuals to observe and describe emotions without judging them or blocking them helps clients experience emotions without stimulating secondary feelings that cause more distress. For example, describing the emotion of anger without judging it as being "bad" can eliminate feelings of guilt that lead to self-injury.

Interpersonal effectiveness skills include the development of assertiveness and problem-solving skills within an interpersonal context. Clients are given strategies to meet their goals in a particular situation, while at the same time maintaining relationships with others and their self-respect.

Mindfulness skills are the psychological and behavioural versions of meditation skills usually taught in Eastern spiritual practice and are used to help the person improve observation, description, and participation skills by learning to focus the mind and awareness on the current moment's activity in a nonjudgmental and effective manner.

Distress tolerance skills involve helping the individual tolerate and accept distress as a part of normal life. Self-management skills focus on helping clients learn how to control, manage, or change behaviours, thoughts, or emotional responses to events (Linehan, 1993a; van den Bosch, Verheul, Schippers, & van den Brink, 2002).

The DBT model has been the most researched of any single treatment strategy and consistently demonstrates clinical effectiveness. When used on an inpatient basis, it requires total staff commitment and reinforcement and has shown significant improvement in depression, anxiety, and dissociation symptoms and a highly significant decrease in parasuicidal behaviour (Bohus et al., 2000). DBT is more often incorporated into a long-term outpatient treatment approach because the greatest effectiveness occurs when skills are reinforced over time and practiced in a variety of daily living settings (Feigenbaum, 2007). Members of the treatment team must maintain a positive approach and assume a skills-coaching role with clients. Probably the most significant interference in treatment with people with BPD is a pessimistic and oppositional attitude of health care professionals (Horsfall, 1999; Nehls, 1998, 1999).

Family Response to Disorder

Individuals with BPD are typically part of a chaotic family system, but they usually add to the chaos (Gerull, Meares, Stevenson, Korner, & Newman, 2008). Their family often feels captive to these individuals. Family members are afraid to disagree with them or refuse to meet their multiple needs, fearing that self-destructive behaviours will follow. During the course of the disorder, family members often get "burned out" and withdraw from the individual, only adding to the person's fear of abandonment (Hoffman, Fruzzetti, & Buteau, 2007). Variations in DBT treatment including the involvement of family and others have emerged in the literature (Black, Blum, Pfohl, & John, 2004; Van Wel et al., 2006).

■ NURSING MANAGEMENT: HUMAN RESPONSE TO BPD

People with BPD are unstable in a variety of areas, including mood, interpersonal relationships, self-esteem, and self-identity, and they often exhibit behavioural and cognitive dysregulations. These manifest in a number of ways, the most prominent of which are listed in Box 25-2. These people may have problems in daily living—maintaining intimate relationships, keeping a job, and living within the law (Box 25-3).

They may enter the mental health system early (young adulthood or before), but because of their chaotic lifestyle, they typically do not receive consistent treatment. They drop in and out of treatment as it suits their mood and usually do not remain with one clinician for long-term treatment. People with BPD usually seek help from health care workers because of consequences of their numerous life crises, medical conditions, or other psychiatric disorders (e.g., depression) or for physical treatment of self-injury. Thus, other problems usually may need attention before the client's underlying

---

BOX 25.2

Response Patterns of Individuals With BPD

Affective (mood) dysregulation
Mood lability
Problems with anger
Interpersonal dysregulation
Chaotic relationships
Fears of abandonment
Self-dysregulation
Identity disturbance or difficulties with sense of self
Sense of emptiness
Behavioural dysregulation
Parasuicidal behaviour or threats
Impulsive behaviour
Cognitive dysregulation
Dissociative responses
Paranoid ideation

Courtesy of M. Linehan, Department of Psychology, Box 351525, University of Washington, Seattle, WA 98195–1525.

BOX 25.3

Clinical Vignette: Borderline Personality Disorder

JS is a 22-year-old single woman who was recently fired from her job as a data entry clerk. She is living with her mother and stepfather, who brought her to the emergency room after finding her crouched in a foetal position in the bathroom, her wrists bleeding. She seemed to be in a daze. This is her first psychiatric admission, although her mother and stepfather have suspected that she has "needed help" for a long time. In high school, she received brief treatment for a potential eating disorder. She remains very thin but is able to eat at least one meal per day. During periods of stress, however, she will go for days without eating.

JS is the second of three children. Her parents divorced when she was 3 years old. She has not seen her father since he left. Although she has pleasant memories of her father, her mother has told her that he beat JS and her sisters when he was drinking. When JS was 6 years old, her older sister died following an automobile accident. JS was in the car but was uninjured. As a child, JS was seen as a potential singing star. Her natural musical talent attracted her teachers' support, which encouraged her to develop her talent. She received singing lessons and entered provincial competitions in high school. Although she enjoyed the attention, she was never really comfortable in the limelight and felt "guilty" about having a talent that she sometimes resented. She was able to make friends but found that she was unable to keep them. They described her as "too intense" and emotional. She had one boyfriend in high school, but she was very uncomfortable with any physical closeness. After ending the relationship with the boyfriend, she concentrated on dieting to have a "perfect body." When her dieting attracted her parents' attention, she vowed to eat just enough to keep them "off her back about it." She spent much of her leisure time with her grandmother. She attended university briefly but was unable to concentrate. It was during her time at university and after her grandmother's death that JS began cutting her wrists during periods of stress. It seemed to calm her.

After leaving university, JS returned home. She had several jobs and short-lived friendships. She was usually fired from her job because of "moodiness," and it would take her several months before she would again find another. She would spend days in her room listening to music. Her recent episode followed being fired from work and spending 3 days in her bedroom.

WHAT DO YOU THINK?
• How would you describe JS's mood?
• Are JS's losses (father, sister) really severe enough to affect her ability to relate to others now? Do the losses seem to relate to the self-injury?
• What behaviours indicate that there are problems with self-esteem and self-identity?

personality disorder can be addressed. Sometimes, the nurse will not know that the person has BPD. However, during an assessment, it becomes clear that these individuals let things bother them more than do others or have an inflexible view of the world. They also seem to have great difficulty changing behaviour, no matter the consequences. Because they see the world differently from the average person, they have difficulty in successfully relating to other people and living a satisfying life.

Biologic Domain

Biologic Assessment

People with BPD are usually able to maintain personal hygiene and physical functioning. Because of the comorbidity of BPD and eating disorders and substance abuse, a nutritional assessment may be needed. The assessment should also include the use of caffeinated beverages, such as coffee, tea, and soft drinks, and alcohol. With individuals who engage in binging or purging, an assessment should include examining the teeth for pitting and discolouration, as well as the hands and fingers for redness and calluses caused by inducing vomiting. The client should be queried about physiologic responses of emotion. Sleep patterns also should be assessed because sleep alterations may suggest coexisting depression or mania.

Physical Indicators of Self-Injurious Behaviours

Clients with BPD should be assessed for self-injurious behaviours or suicide attempts. It is important to ask the individual about specific self-abusive behaviours, such as cutting, scratching, or overdosing. He or she may wear long sleeves to hide an injury on the arms. Specifically asking about thoughts of hurting oneself when experiencing a major upset provides an opportunity for prevention and for coaching the client toward alternative self-soothing measures.

Pharmacologic Assessment

Clients with BPD may be taking several medications. For example, one person may be taking a small dose of an antipsychotic and a mood stabilizer. Another may be taking a selective serotonin reuptake inhibitor (SSRI) and an anxiolytic. Initially, individuals may be reluctant to disclose all the medications they are taking because, for many, there has been a period of trial and error. They are fearful of having medication taken away from them. The development of rapport with special attention to a nonjudgmental approach is especially important when eliciting current medication practices. The effectiveness of the medication in relieving the target

symptom needs to be determined. The use of alcohol and street drugs should be carefully assessed to determine drug interactions.

Nursing Diagnoses for the Biologic Domain

Nursing diagnoses focusing on the biologic domain include disturbed sleep pattern, imbalanced nutrition, self-mutilation or risk for self-mutilation, and ineffective therapeutic regimen management.

Interventions for the Biologic Domain

The interventions for the biologic domain may address a whole spectrum of problems. Usually, the individuals are managing hydration, self-care, and pain well. This section focuses on those areas most likely to be problematic.

Sleep Enhancement

The facilitation of regular sleep–wake cycles may be needed because of disturbed sleep patterns. Conservative approaches should be exhausted before recommending medication. Establishing a regular bedtime routine, monitoring bedtime snacks and drinks, and avoiding foods and drinks that interfere with sleep should be tried. If relaxation exercises are used, they should be adapted to the tolerance of the individual. Moderate exercises (e.g., brisk walking) 3 to 4 hours before bedtime activate both serotonin and endorphins, thereby enhancing calmness and a sense of well-being before bedtime. For individuals who have difficulty falling asleep and experience interrupted sleep, it helps to establish some basic sleeping routines. The bedroom should be reserved for only two activities: sleeping and sex. Therefore, the client should remove the television, computer, and exercise equipment from the bedroom. If the individual is not asleep within 15 minutes, he or she should get out of bed and go to another room to read, watch television, or listen to soft music. The client should return to bed when sleepy. If the person is not asleep in 15 minutes, the same process should be repeated.

Special consideration must be made for individuals who have been physically and sexually abused and who may be unable to put themselves in a vulnerable position (e.g., lying down in a room with other people or closing their eyes). These clients may need additional safeguards to help them sleep, such as a night light or repositioning of furniture to afford easy exit.

Nutritional Balance

The nutritional status of the person with BPD can quickly become a priority, particularly if the individual has coexisting eating disorders or substance abuse. Eating is often a response to stress, and clients can quickly become overweight. This is especially a problem when the individual has also been taking medications that can promote weight gain, such as antipsychotics, antidepressants, or mood stabilizers. Helping the client to learn the basics of nutrition, make reasonable choices, and develop other coping strategies is a useful intervention. If individuals are engaging in purging or severe dieting practices, teaching them about the dangers of both of these practices is important (see Chapter 23). Referral to an eating disorders specialist may be needed.

Prevention and Treatment of Self-Injury

Clients with BPD are usually admitted to the inpatient setting because of threats of self-injury. Observing for antecedents of self-injurious behaviour and intervening before an episode is an important safety intervention. Clients can learn to identify situations leading to self-destructive behaviour and develop preventive strategies. Because individuals with BPD are impulsive and may respond to stress by harming themselves, observation of the person's interactions and assessment of mood, level of distress, and agitation are important in determining the threat of self-injury.

Remembering that self-injury is an effort to self-soothe by activating endogenous endorphins, the nurse can assist the individual to find more productive and enduring ways to find comfort. Linehan (1993b) suggests using a self-soothing exercise and focusing on each of the five senses:

- Vision (e.g., go outside and look at the stars or flowers or autumn leaves)
- Hearing (e.g., listen to beautiful or invigorating music or the sounds of nature)
- Smell (e.g., light a scented candle, boil a cinnamon stick in water)
- Taste (e.g., drink a soothing, warm, nonalcoholic beverage)
- Touch (e.g., take a hot bubble bath, pet your dog or cat, get a massage)

For clients who injure themselves repeatedly to experience an emotional release after the injury, medication that blocks the endogenous opioids system or reward system may help control the behaviour. Preliminary studies show that naltrexone (ReVia) has reduced the incidence of self-injurious behaviour. It has been used to treat dissociative symptoms with some success (Bohus et al., 1999), as have low doses of serotonin-dopamine antagonists, such as clozapine, olanzapine, and risperidone (McDougle, Kresch, & Posey, 2000).

Pharmacologic Interventions

Less medication is better for people with BPD. No specific drug is available for the treatment of BPD. Individuals should take medications only for target symptoms for a short time (e.g., an antidepressant for a bout with depression) because they may be taking many medications, particularly if they have a comorbid disorder, such as a mood disorder or substance abuse. Pharmacotherapy is used to control emotional dysregulation, impulsive aggression, cognitive disturbances, and anxiety as an adjunct to psychotherapy (Cardish, 2007).

Controlling Emotional Dysregulation

Target symptoms of emotional dysregulation include instability of mood, marked shifts from or to depression, stress-related and transient mood crashes, rejection sensitivity, and inappropriate and intense outbursts of anger. Because decreased central serotonin neurotransmission has been implicated in the emotional dysregulation and impulsive-aggressive behaviours, the SSRIs have been tried with some efficacy. An improvement in depressed mood and lability, rejection sensitivity, impulsive behaviour, self-injury, psychosis, and hostility has been shown with fluoxetine (Prozac) in BPD. SSRIs and serotonin-norepinephrine reuptake inhibitors have been most extensively studied and used clinically to treat depression, aggression, and emotional dysregulation. Sertraline (Zoloft), paroxetine (Paxil), and citalopram (Celexa) are most often used, and venlafaxine (Effexor) and mirtazapine (Remeron) have been similarly effective, especially with attentional disturbance and agitation symptoms (Stahl & Grady, 2005).

Reducing Impulsivity

Impulsivity, anger outbursts, and mood lability may be treated effectively with the newer GABA-ergic anticonvulsants such as lamotrigine (Lamictal), gabapentin (Neurontin), and topiramate (Topamax; Coccaro, 1998; Pinto & Akiskal, 1998). These appear to act by regulating neural firing in the mesolimbic area. Carbamazepine (Tegretol) and lithium have also been used, but these have a less favourable side-effect profile. Divalproex is still the most frequently used drug for impulsivity and aggression (Hollander et al., 2003; Kavoussi & Coccaro, 1998).

Managing Transient Psychotic Episodes

Antipsychotic medications may be useful when the client demonstrates thought disorganization, misinterpretation of reality, and high levels of emotional instability. Low doses of antipsychotics are most often used (Soloff, 2000).

Decreasing Anxiety

If an individual is experiencing anxiety, a nonbenzodiazepine such as buspirone (Bu-Spar) may be used

BOX 25.4

Drug Profile: Buspirone (Buspar)

DRUG CLASS: Antianxiety agent

RECEPTOR AFFINITY: Binds to serotonin receptors and acts as an agonist to 5-HT$_{1B}$. Clinical significance unclear. Exact mechanism of action unknown.

INDICATIONS: Management of anxiety disorders or short-term relief of symptoms of anxiety.

ROUTES AND DOSAGE: Available in 10-mg tablets.

Adults: Initially, 15 mg/day (5 mg tid). Increased by 5 mg/day at intervals of 2–3 day to achieve optimal therapeutic response. Not to exceed 60 mg/day.

Children: Safety and efficacy younger than 18 years of age not established.

HALF-LIFE (PEAK EFFECT): 3–11 hours (40–90 minutes).

SELECT ADVERSE REACTIONS: Dizziness, headache, nervousness, insomnia, light-headedness, nausea, dry mouth, vomiting, gastric distress, diarrhea, tachycardia, and palpitations.

WARNING: Contraindicated in clients with hypersensitivity to buspirone, marked liver or renal impairment, and during lactation. Alcohol and other CNS depressants can cause increased sedation. Decreased effects seen if given with fluoxetine.

SPECIFIC CLIENT/FAMILY EDUCATION:
- Take the drug exactly as prescribed; may take with foods or meals if gastrointestinal upset occurs.
- Avoid alcohol and other CNS depressants.
- Notify the prescriber before taking any over-the-counter or prescription medications.
- Avoid driving or performing hazardous activities that require alertness and concentration.
- Use ice chips or sugarless candies to alleviate dry mouth.
- Notify the prescriber of any abnormal involuntary movements of facial or neck muscles, abnormal posture, or yellowing of the skin or eyes.
- Continue medical follow-up and do not abruptly discontinue its use.

(Box 25-4). Buspirone appears to be an ideal antianxiety drug. Unlike the benzodiazepines, it does not have the sedation, ataxia, tolerance, and withdrawal effects and does not lead to abuse. However, buspirone takes longer to act than do the benzodiazepines. If a client has been taking benzodiazepines for years, buspirone may not lead to much improvement. When switching from a benzodiazepine to buspirone, the withdrawal symptoms may be unpleasant (or even dangerous), and buspirone will not have any effect on the distress. Because buspirone is a serotonin (5-HT$_{1A}$) agonist, its use with an SSRI enhances the benefits of both drugs to reduce anxiety and depression symptoms (Stahl & Grady, 2005) but exposes the client to serotonin syndrome risk.

More often, people with BPD find buspirone ineffective if their type of anxiety is intense and accompanied by agitation and aggression. Because this anxiety seems to be mediated by serotonergic connections in the prefrontal cortex and anterior cingulum, SSRIs at higher doses than those used for depression are more effective (Best, Williams, & Coccaro, 2002; Gurvits, Koenigsberg, & Siever, 2000).

Monitoring and Administering Medications

In inpatient settings, it is relatively easy to control medications; in other settings, clients must be aware that it is their responsibility to take their medications and monitor the number and type of drugs being taken. Individuals who rely on medications to help them deal with stress or those who are periodically suicidal are at high risk for abuse of medications. Those who have unusual side effects are at high risk for nonadherence. The nurse determines whether the individual is actually taking the medication, whether the medication is being taken as prescribed, the effect on target symptoms, and the use of any over-the-counter drugs (e.g., antihistamines or sleeping pills).

However, the client cannot rely just on the medication. Assuming responsibility for taking the medication regularly, understanding the effects of the medication, and augmenting the medication with other strategies is the most effective approach. The nurse helps the individual assume this responsibility and provides guidance that supports self-efficacy and competence. It is also important for the nurse to emphasize that the medications provide the physiologic balance, but it is the client's effort and skills that provide the social and behavioural balance. Stressing this may help the individual to not overinvest in the medication and feel more confident of her or his own skills.

Side-Effect Monitoring and Management

Individuals with BPD appear to be sensitive to many medications, and they often dose the medication according to their understanding of the side effects. Listen carefully to the person's description of the side effects. Any unusual side effects should be accurately documented and reported to the prescriber.

Teaching Points

Clients should be educated about the medications and their interactions with other drugs and substances.

Interventions include teaching individuals about the medication and how and where it acts in the brain and body, helping establish a routine for taking prescribed medication, reporting side effects, and facilitating the development of positive coping strategies to deal with daily stresses, rather than relying on medications. Eliciting the client's partnership in care improves adherence and, thereby, outcomes.

Psychological Domain

Psychological Assessment

People with BPD have usually experienced significant losses in their lives that shape their view of the world. They experience **inhibited grieving**, "a pattern of repetitive, significant trauma and loss, together with an inability to fully experience and personally integrate or resolve these events" (Linehan, 1993a, p. 89). They have unresolved grief that can last for years and avoid situations that evoke those feelings of separation and loss. During the assessment, the nurse can identify the losses (real or perceived) and explore the client's experience during these losses, paying particular attention to whether the individual has reached resolution. A history of physical or sexual abuse and an early separation from significant caregivers may provide important clues to the severity of the disturbances.

Mood fluctuations are common and can be assessed by any number of the depression and anxiety screening scales, or by asking the following questions:

- What things or events bother you and make you feel happy, sad, and angry?
- Do these things or events trouble you more than they trouble other people?
- Do friends and family tell you that you are moody?
- Do you get angry easily?
- Do you have trouble with your temper?
- Do you think you were born with these feelings, or did something happen to make you feel this way?

Appearance and activity level generally reflect the person's mood and psychomotor activity. Many of those with BPD have been physically or sexually abused and thus should be assessed for depression. A disheveled appearance can reflect depression or an agitated state. When feeling good, these individuals can be very engaging; they tend to be dramatic in their style of dress and attract attention, such as by wearing an unusual hairstyle or heavy makeup. Because physical appearance reflects identity, clients may experiment with their appearance and seek affirmation and acceptance from others. Body piercing, tattoos, and other adornments provide a mechanism to define self.

Impulsivity

Impulsivity can be identified by asking the client if he or she does things impulsively or on the spur of the moment (e.g., "Have there been times when you were hurt by your actions or were sorry later that you acted in the way you did?"). Direct questions about gambling, choices in sexual partners, sexual activities, fights, arguments, arrests, and alcohol drinking habits can also help in identifying areas of impulsive behaviour.

From a neurophysiologic perspective, impulsively acting before thinking seems to be mediated by rapid nerve firing in the mesolimbic area. This activates psychomotor responses before pathways reach the prefrontal cortex (Best et al., 2002). Teaching the client strategies to slow down automatic responses (e.g., deep breathing, counting to 10) allows time to think before acting.

Cognitive Disturbances

The mental status examination of those with BPD usually reveals normal thought processes that are not disorganized or confused, except during periods of stress. Those with BPD usually exhibit **dichotomous thinking**, or a tendency to view things as absolute—either black or white, good or bad—with no perception of compromise. Dichotomous thinking can be assessed by asking clients how they view other people. Evidence of dichotomous thinking is indicated with responses of "good" or "bad," "wonderful" or "terrible." A therapeutic approach that focuses on understanding during the early stages of treatment and then, as treatment continues, increasingly moves the client to deconstruct unhelpful object relations attributions is recommended (Gregory, 2007).

Dissociation and Transient Psychotic Episodes

There may be periods of dissociation and transient psychotic episodes. Dissociation can be assessed by asking if there is ever a time when the person does not remember events or has the feeling of being separate from his or her body. Some individuals refer to this as "spacing out." By asking specific information about how often, how long, and when dissociation first was used, the nurse can get an idea of how important dissociation is as a coping skill. It is important to ask the person what is happening in the environment when dissociation occurs. Frequent dissociation indicates a highly habitual coping mechanism that will be difficult to change. Because transient psychotic states occur, it is also important to elicit data regarding the presence of hallucinations or delusions along with their frequency and circumstances.

Risk Assessment: Suicide or Self-Injury

It is critical that individuals with BPD be assessed for suicidal and self-damaging behaviours, including alcohol and drug abuse. (Suicide assessment is discussed in Chapter 38.) An assessment should include direct questions, asking if the person thinks about or engages in self-injurious behaviours. If so, the nurse should continue to explore the behaviours: what is done, how it is done, its frequency, and the circumstances surrounding the self-injurious behaviour. It is helpful to explain briefly to the client that sometimes people cut, scratch, or pick at themselves as a way of bringing some relief and comfort. Although the behaviour brings temporary relief, it also places the person at risk for infection. Approaching the assessment in this way conveys a sense of understanding and is more likely to invite the individual to disclose honestly.

Nursing Diagnoses for the Psychological Domain

One of the first diagnoses to consider is the risk for self-mutilation because protection of the individual from self-injury is always a priority. If cognitive changes are present (dissociation and transient psychosis), two other diagnoses may be appropriate: disturbed thought process and ineffective coping. The disturbed thought process diagnosis is used if dissociative and psychotic episodes actually interfere with daily living. For example, a secretary could not complete processing letters because she was unable to differentiate whether the voices on the dictating machine were being transmitted by the machine or by her hallucinations. The nurse helped her learn to differentiate the hallucinations from dictation. The client learned to take her headset off, take a deep breath, and listen to her external environment. When she recognized "the voice" as her partner criticizing her, she was able to use her cognitive reframing strategies to refocus on reality.

If the individual copes with stressful situations by dissociating or hallucinating, the diagnosis of ineffective coping is used. The outcome in this instance would be the substitution of positive coping skills for the dissociations or hallucinations.

Other nursing diagnoses that are typically supported by assessment data include personal identity disturbance, anxiety, grieving, low self-esteem, powerlessness, posttrauma response, defensive coping, and spiritual distress. The identification of outcomes depends on the nursing diagnoses (Fig. 25-1).

FIGURE 25.1 Bio/psycho/social/spiritual outcomes for individuals with BPD.

Interventions for the Psychological Domain

The challenge of working with people with BPD is engaging the individual in a therapeutic relationship that will survive its emotional ups and downs. The client needs to understand that the nurse is there to coach her or him to develop self-modulation skills. A relationship based on mutual respect and consistency is crucial for helping the person with those skills. Self-awareness skills, along with access to supervision and collaboration, are needed by the nurse. Because individuals with BPD are frequently hospitalized, even nurses in acute care settings have an opportunity to develop a long-term relationship (Fig. 25-2). A challenge that may face nurses within this nurse–client relationship is a maladaptive coping behaviour that persons with BPD may use called **splitting**. Splitting is a primitive defence mechanism involving the compartmentalization of opposite and conflicting affect states (Campbell, 2004). A developmental task of childhood is to learn how to understand the world (including self and others) in a complex way, rather than as all one way or all another, such as seeing a particular person as being all good or all bad. In other words, the task is to see "shades of grey," not just "black and white." The person with BPD, perhaps because of severe abuse in childhood, may not have successfully achieved this developmental task. The use of splitting as a defence can create difficult problems for them in maintaining relationships. It can have chaotic effects on the relationships of those around them. Nurses and other staff members may find themselves in conflict with each other when working with people with BPD (Bland, Tudor, & Whitehouse, 2007). It is important that members of the care team are particularly aware of their professional interactions and respond appropriately as team members. Understanding relationship dynamics, while not simply blaming discord within the team on a client with BPD, is what is called for.

Generalist psychiatric and mental health (PMH) nurses do not function as the client's primary therapists, but they do need to establish a therapeutic relationship that strengthens the client's coping skills and self-esteem and supports individual psychotherapy. The therapeutic relationship helps the client to experience a model of healthy interaction with consistency, limit setting, caring, and respect for others (both self-respect and respect for the person). Individuals who have low self-esteem need help in recognizing genuine respect from others and reciprocating with respect for others. In the therapeutic relationship, the nurse models self-respect by observing personal limits, being assertive, and clearly communicating expectations. Consistency is critical in building self-esteem.

FIGURE 25.2 Bio/psycho/social/spiritual interventions for individuals with BPD.

Abandonment and Intimacy Fears

A key to helping individuals with BPD is recognizing their fears of both abandonment and intimacy. Informing the client of the length of the relationship as much as possible allows the individual to engage in and prepare for termination with the least pain of abandonment. If the client's hospitalization is time limited, the nurse overtly acknowledges the limit and reminds the person with each contact how many sessions remain (Box 25-5).

In day treatment and outpatient settings, the duration of treatment may be indeterminate, but the nurse may not be available that entire time. The termination process cannot be casual; this would stimulate abandonment fears. However, some clients end prematurely when the nurse informs them of the impending end as a way to leave before being rejected. Anticipating premature closure, the nurse explores with the individual anticipated feelings, including the wish to run away. After careful planning, the nurse anticipates, in advance, the client's feelings, discusses how to cope with them, reviews the progress the individual has made, and summarizes what the person has learned from the relationship that can be generalized to future encounters.

Establishing Personal Boundaries and Limitations

Personal boundaries are highly context specific; for example, stroking the hair of a stranger on the bus would be inappropriate, but stroking the hair and face of one's intimate partner while sitting together would be appropriate. Our personal physical space needs (boundaries) are distinct from behavioural and emotional limits we have. These concepts apply both to the client and the nurse. Furthermore, limits may be temporary (e.g., "I can't talk with you right now, but after the change of shift, I can be available for 30 minutes.").

Testing limits is a natural way of identifying where the boundaries are and how strong they are. Therefore, it is necessary to state clearly the enduring limits (e.g., the written rules or contract) and the consequences of violating them. The limits must then be consistently maintained. Clarifying limits requires making explicit what is usually implicit. Despite the clinical setting (e.g., hospital, day treatment setting, outpatient clinic), the nurse must clearly state the day, time, and duration of each contact with the client and remain consistent in those expectations. This may mean having a standing appointment in day treatment or a mental

---

BOX 25.5

Therapeutic Dialogue: *Borderline Personality Disorder*

INEFFECTIVE APPROACH

Client: Hey, you know what? You are my favorite nurse. That night nurse sure doesn't understand me the way you do.

Nurse: Oh, I'm glad you are comfortable with me. Which night nurse?

Client: You know, Sue.

Nurse: Did you have problems with her?

Client: She is terrible. She sleeps all night or she is on the telephone.

Nurse: Oh, that doesn't sound very professional to me. Anything else?

Client: Yeah, she said that you didn't know what you were doing. She said that you couldn't nurse your way out of a paper bag (smiling).

Nurse: She did, did she. (Getting angry.) She should talk.

Client: Well, I gotta go to group. Where will you be? I feel so much better if I know where you are. I don't know how I can possibly be discharged tomorrow.

EFFECTIVE APPROACH

Client: Hey, you know what? You are my favorite nurse. That night nurse sure doesn't understand me the way you do.

Nurse: I really like you, Sara. Tomorrow you will be discharged, and I'm glad that you will be able to return home. (The nurse avoided responding to "favorite nurse"

statement. Redirected the interaction to impending discharge.)

Client: That night nurse slept all night.

Nurse: What was your night like? (Redirecting the interaction to Sara's experience.)

Client: It was terrible. Couldn't sleep all night. I'm not sure that I'm ready to go home.

Nurse: Oh, so you are not quite sure about discharge? (Reflection.)

Client: I get so, so lonely. Then, I want to hurt myself.

Nurse: Lonely feelings have started that chain of events that led to cutting, haven't they? (Validation.)

Client: Yes, I'm very scared. I haven't cut myself for 1 week now.

Nurse: Do you have a plan for dealing with your lonely feelings when they occur?

Client: I'm supposed to start thinking about something that is pleasant—like spring flowers in the meadow.

Nurse: Does that work for you?

Client: Yes, sometimes.

CRITICAL THINKING QUESTIONS

- How did the nurse in the first scenario get sidetracked?
- How was the nurse in the second scenario able to keep the client focused on herself and her impending discharge?

health clinic or noting the time during each shift that the nurse will talk individually with the hospitalized client. The nurse should refrain from offering personal information, which is frequently confusing to the person with BPD. At times, the person may present in a somewhat arrogant and entitled way. It is important for the nurse to recognize such a presentation as reflective of internal confusion and dissonance. Responding in a very neutral manner avoids confrontation and a power struggle, which might also unwittingly reinforce the client's internal sense of inferiority.

Some additional strategies for establishing the boundaries of the relationship include the following:

- Documenting in the client chart the agreed-on appointment expectations
- Sharing the treatment plan with the client
- Confronting violations of the agreement in a nonpunitive way
- Discussing the purpose of limits in the therapeutic relationship and applicability to other relationships

When individuals violate boundaries, it is important to respond right away but without taking the behaviour personally. For example, if a client is flirtatious, simply say something like, "I feel uncomfortable with your overly friendly behaviour. It seems out of place since we have a professional relationship. That would be more fitting for an intimate relationship, which we do not and will not have."

Management of Dissociative States

The desired outcome for someone who dissociates is to reduce or eliminate the dissociative experiences. The natural tendency is to want to "fix it." Unfortunately, there are limited medications for dissociation, but because the SSRIs, dopamine antagonists, and serotonin-dopamine antagonists affect other target symptoms, the dissociative experiences decrease. Because dissociation occurs during periods of stress, the best approach is to help the individual develop other strategies to deal with stress.

The nurse can teach the client how to identify when he or she is dissociating and then to use some grounding strategies in the moment. Basic to grounding is planting both feet firmly on the floor or ground, then taking a deep abdominal breath to the count of 4, holding it to the count of 4, exhaling to the count of 4, and then holding it to the count of 4. This is called the four-square method of breathing. The benefit of this approach is to bring about a deep, slow breath that activates the calming mechanisms of the parasympathetic system.

After the grounding exercise, the client uses one or more senses to make contact with the environment, such as touching the fabric of a nearby chair or listening to the traffic noise. As the client improves in self-esteem and the ability to relate to others, the frequency of dissociation should decrease.

Behavioural Interventions

The goal of behavioural interventions is to replace dysfunctional behaviours with positive ones. The nurse has an important role in helping individuals control emotions and behaviours by acknowledging and validating desired behaviours and by ignoring or confronting undesired behaviours. Clients often test the nurse for a response, and nurses must decide how to respond to particular behaviours. This can be tricky because even negative responses can be viewed as positive reinforcement for the client. In some instances, if the behaviour is irritating but not harmful or demeaning, it is best to ignore rather than focus on it. However, grossly inappropriate and disrespectful behaviours require confrontation. If a client throws a glass of water on an assistant because the client is angry at the treatment team for refusing to increase her hospital privileges, an appropriate intervention would include confronting the individual with her behaviour and issuing the consequences, such as losing her privileges and apologizing to the assistant.

However, this incident can be used to help the individual understand why such behaviour is inappropriate and how it can be changed. The nurse should explore with the client what happened, what events led up to the behaviour, what were the consequences, and what feelings were aroused. Advanced practice nurses or other therapists will explore the origins of the client's behaviours and responses, but the generalist nurse needs to help the person explore ways to change behaviours involved in the current situation. The laboriousness of this analytical process may be a sufficient incentive for the client to abandon the dysfunctional behaviour.

Emotional Regulation

A major goal of cognitive therapeutic interventions is emotional regulation—recognizing and controlling the expression of feelings. Clients often fail even to recognize their feelings; instead, they respond quickly without thinking about the consequences. Remember, the time needed for taking action is shorter than the time needed for thinking before acting. Pausing makes up for the momentary lag between the limbic and autonomic response and the prefrontal response.

The nurse can help the client identify feelings and gain control over expressions such as anger, disappointment, or frustration. The goal is for individuals to tolerate their feelings without feeling compelled to act out those feelings on another person or on themselves.

A helpful technique for managing feelings is known as the **communication triad**. The triad provides a specific syntax and order for clients to identify and express their feelings and seek relief. The "sentence" consists of three parts:

- An "I" statement to identify the prevailing feeling
- A nonjudgmental statement of the emotional trigger
- What the individual would like differently or what would restore comfort to the situation

The nurse must emphasize with clients that they begin with the "I" statement and the identification of feelings, although many want to begin with the condition. If the person begins with the condition, the statement becomes accusatory and likely to evoke defensiveness (e.g., "When you interrupt me, I get mad."). Beginning with "I" allows the client to identify and express the feeling first and take full ownership. For example, the individual who is angry with another client in the group might say, "Joe, I feel angry ('I' statement with ownership of feeling) when you interrupt me (the trigger or conditions of the emotion), and I would like you to apologize and try not to do that with me (what the individual wants and the remedy)." This simple skill is easy to teach, is easy to reinforce and to encourage others to reinforce, and is a surprisingly effective way of moderating the emotional tone.

Another element of emotional regulation is learning to delay gratification. When clients want something that is not immediately available, the nurse can teach individuals to distract themselves, find alternate ways of meeting the need, and think about what would happen if they have to wait to meet the need.

The practice of **thought stopping** might also help the person to control the inappropriate expression of feelings. In thought stopping, the client identifies what feelings and thoughts exist together. For example, when the person is ruminating about a perceived hurt, the individual might say "Stop that" (referring to the ruminative thought) and engage in a distracting activity. Three activities associated with thought stopping are effective:

- Taking a quick deep breath when the behaviour is noted (this also stimulates relaxation)
- Visualizing a stop sign or saying "stop" when possible (this allows the person to hear externally and internally)
- Deliberately replacing the undesired behaviour with a positive alternative (e.g., instead of ruminating about an angry situation, thinking about a neutral or positive self-affirmation)

The sequencing and combining of the steps puts the person back in control.

Challenging Dysfunctional Thinking

The nurse can often challenge the individual's dysfunctional ways of thinking and challenge the person to think about the event in a different way. When a client engages in catastrophic thinking, the nurse can challenge by asking, "What is the worst that could happen?" and "How likely would that be to occur?" Or, in dichotomous thinking, when the client fixates on one extreme perception or alternates between the extremes only, the nurse can ask the person to think about any examples of exceptions to the extreme. The point of the challenge is not to debate or argue with the individual but to provide different perspectives to consider. Encouraging clients to keep journals of real interactions to process with the nurse or therapist is another effective way of testing the reality of their thinking and anticipations, affording more choices and flexibility (Box 25-6).

In problem solving, the nurse might encourage the individual to debate both sides of the problem and then search for common ground. Practicing communication and negotiation skills through role playing helps the client make mistakes and correct them without harm to her or his self-esteem. The nurse also encourages clients to use these skills in their everyday lives and report back on the results, asking individuals how they feel applying the skills and how doing so affects their self-perceptions. Success, even partial success, builds a sense of competence and self-esteem (Box 25-7).

BOX 25.6

Challenging Dysfunctional Thinking

Ms. S had worked for the same company for 20 years with a good job record. Following an accident, she made some minor mistakes in her work that she quickly corrected. She informed her company's nurse that her work was "really slipping" and that she was fearful of her coworkers' disapproval and getting fired from her job. The nurse asked her to keep a journal of coworkers' comments for the next week. At the next visit, the following dialogue occurred:

Nurse: I noticed that you received several compliments on your work. Even a close friend of your boss expressed appreciation for your work.

Ms. S: It was a light week at work. I really don't believe they meant what they said.

Nurse: I can see how you can believe that one or two comments are not genuine, but how do you account for four and five good reports on your work?

Ms. S: Well, I don't know.

Nurse: It looks like your beliefs are not supported by your journal entries. Now, what makes you think that your boss wants to fire you after 20 years of service?

BOX **25.7**

BOX 25.7
Thought Distortions and Corrective Statements

THOUGHT DISTORTION	CORRECTIVE STATEMENT
Catastrophizing "This is the most awful thing that has ever happened to me." "If I fail this course, my life is over."	"This is a sad thing, but not the most awful." "If you fail the course, you can take the course again. You can change your major."
Dichotomizing "No one ever listens to me." "I never get what I want." "I can't understand why everyone is so kind at first, then always dumps me when I need them the most."	"Your husband listened to you last night when you told him…" "You didn't get the promotion this year, but you did get a merit raise." "It is hard to remember those kind things and times when your friends have stayed with you when you needed them."
Self-Attribution Errors "If I had just found the right thing to say, she wouldn't have left me." "If I had not made him mad, he wouldn't have hit me."	"There is not a single right thing to say; and she left you because she chose to." "He has a lot of choices in how to respond, and he chose hitting. You are responsible for your feelings and actions."

Management of Transient Psychotic Episodes

During psychotic episodes with auditory hallucinations, the client should be protected from harming self or others. In an inpatient setting, the client should be monitored closely and a determination made as to whether the voices are telling the person to engage in self-harm (command hallucinations). The client may be observed more closely and begin taking antipsychotic medications. In the community setting, the nurse should help the client develop a plan for managing the voices. For example, if the voices return, the individual contacts the clinic and returns for evaluation. There may be a friend or relative who should be contacted or a case manager who can help the person get the necessary protection if it is needed. In some instances, hearing the voices is a prelude to self-injury. Another person can help the individual resist the voices. Once other aspects of the disorder are managed, the episodes of psychosis decrease or disappear.

Teaching and practicing distress tolerance skills help the individual have power over the voices and control intense emotions. When not experiencing hallucinations, the client can practice deep abdominal breathing, which calms the autonomic nervous system. Using brainstorming techniques, the individual identifies early internal cues of rising distress while the nurse writes them on an index card for the client to refer to later. Next, the nurse teaches some skills for tolerating painful feelings or events. To help the client remember, suggest the mnemonic "Wise Mind ACCEPTS" with the following actions:

- **A**ctivities to distract from stress
- **C**ontributing to others, such as volunteering or visiting a sick neighbour

- **C**omparing yourself to people less fortunate than you
- **E**motions that are opposite to what you are experiencing
- **P**ushing away from the situation for awhile
- **T**houghts other than those you are currently experiencing
- **S**ensations that are intense, such as holding ice in your hand (Linehan, 1993b, pp. 165–166)

Client Education

Client education within the context of a therapeutic relationship is one of the most important, empowering interventions for the generalist PMH nurse to use. Teaching individuals skills to resist parasuicidal urges, improve emotional regulation, enhance interpersonal relationships, tolerate stress, and enhance overall quality of life provides the foundation for long-term behavioural changes. These skills can be taught in any treatment setting as a part of the overall facility program (see Box 25-8). If nurses are practicing in a facility where DBT is the treatment model, they can be trained in DBT and can serve as group skills leaders.

Social Domain

Social Assessment

Some individuals with BPD can function very well except during periods when symptoms erupt. They hold jobs, are active in communities, and can perform well. During periods of stress, symptoms often appear.

BOX 25.8

Psychoeducation Checklist: Borderline Personality Disorder

When caring for the client with BPD, be sure to include the following topic areas in the teaching plan:

- Management of medication, if used, including drug action, dosage, frequency, and possible adverse effects
- Regular sleep routines
- Nutrition
- Safety measures
- Functional versus dysfunctional behaviours
- Cognitive strategies (distraction, communication skills, thought stopping)
- Structure and limit setting
- Social relationships
- Community resources

On the other hand, some individuals with severe BPD function poorly; they are always in a crisis, which they have often created.

Social Support Systems

The identification of social supports, such as family, friends, and religious organizations, is the purpose in assessing resources. Knowing how the person obtains social support is important in understanding the quality of interpersonal relationships. For example, some individuals consider their "best friends" to be their nurses, physicians, and other health care personnel. Because this is a false friendship (i.e., not reciprocal), it inevitably leads to frustration and disappointment. Helping the individual find ways to meet other people and encouraging the client's efforts are more realistic.

Interpersonal Skills

An assessment of the person's ability to relate to others is important because interpersonal problems are linked to dissociation and self-injurious behaviour. Information about friendships, frequency of contact, and intimate relationships will provide data about the person's ability to relate to others. Clients with BPD often are sexually active and may have numerous sexual partners. Their need for closeness clouds their judgment about sexual partners, and it is not unusual to find these individuals in abusive, destructive relationships with people with APD. During assessment, nurses should use their own self-awareness skills to examine their personal response to the client. How the nurse responds to the individual can often be a clue to how others perceive and respond to this person. For example, if the nurse feels irritated or impatient during the interview, that is a sign that others respond to this person in the same way; on the other hand, if the nurse feels empathy or closeness, chances are this individual can evoke these same feelings in others.

Self-Esteem and Coping Skills

Coping with stressful situations is one of the major problems for people with BPD. An assessment of their coping skills and their ability to deal with stressful situations is important. Because the individual's self-esteem is usually very low, an assessment of self-esteem can be done with a self-esteem assessment or by interviewing the client and analyzing the assessment data for evidence of personal self-worth and confidence. Self-esteem is highly related to identifying with health care workers. Clients with BPD perceive their families and friends as being weary of their numerous crises and their seeming unwillingness to break the vicious self-destructive cycle. Feeling rejected by their natural support system, these individuals create one within the health system. During periods of crisis or affective instability, especially during the late evening, early morning, or on weekends, they call or visit various psychiatric units, asking to speak to specific personnel who formerly cared for them. They even know different nurses' scheduled days off and make the rounds to several hospitals and clinics. Sometimes they bring gifts to nurses or call them at home. Because their newly created social support system cannot provide the support that is needed, the person continues to feel rejected. One of the goals of the treatment is to help the individual establish a natural support network.

Family Assessment

Family members may or may not be involved with the client. Individuals with BPD are often estranged from their families. In other instances, they are dependent on them, which is also a source of stress. Childhood abuse is common in these families, and the perpetrator may be a family member. Ideally, family members are interviewed for their perspectives on the client's problem. An assessment of any mental disorder in the client's family and of the current level of functioning is useful in understanding the client and identifying potential resources for support.

Nursing Diagnoses for the Social Domain

Defensive coping, chronic low self-esteem, and impaired social interaction are nursing diagnoses that address the social problems faced by clients with BPD.

Interventions for the Social Domain: Modifying Coping Behaviours

Environmental management becomes critical in caring for a person with BPD. Because the unit can be structured to represent a microcosm of the individual's community, clients have an opportunity to identify relationship problems, boundary violations, and stressful situations. When these situations occur, the nurse can help the individual cope by finding alternative explanations for the situation and practicing new skills. Individual sessions help the client try out some skills, such as putting feelings into words without actions. Role playing may help individuals experience different degrees of effectively relating feelings without the burden of hurting someone they care about. Day treatment and group settings are excellent places for clients to learn more effective feeling management and to practice these techniques with each other. The group helps members develop empathy and diffuses attachment to any one person or therapist.

Building Social Skills and Self-Esteem

In the hospital, the nurse can use groups to discuss feelings and ways to cope with them. Women with BPD often benefit from assertiveness classes and women's health issues classes. Many of the women are involved in abusive relationships and lack the ability to resolve these relationships because of their extreme anxiety regarding separating from those they love and their extreme need to feel connected. These women verbalize desires to leave, but they do not have the strength and self-confidence needed to leave. Exposing them to a different style of interaction as well as validation from other people increases their self-esteem and ability to separate from negative influences.

Exploring Social Supports

Dependency on family members is a problem for many people with BPD. In some families, a client's positive progress may be met with negative responses, and individuals in these situations need help in maintaining a separate identity while staying connected to family members for social support. Family support groups sometimes help. Usually, the nurse helps the person explore new relationships that can provide additional social contacts.

Teaching Effective Ways to Communicate

An important area of client education is teaching communication skills. Clients lack interpersonal skills in relating because they often had inadequate modelling and few opportunities to practice. The goals of relationship skill development are to identify problematic behaviour that interferes with relationships and to use appropriate behaviours in improving relationships. The starting point is with communication. The nurse teaches the individual basic communication approaches, such as making "I" statements, paraphrasing what the other party says before responding, checking the accuracy of perceptions with others, compromising and seeking common ground, listening actively, and offering and accepting reactions. Besides modelling the behaviours, the nurse guides clients in practicing a variety of communication approaches for common situations. When role playing, the nurse needs to discuss not only what the skills are and how to perform them but also the feelings clients have before, during, and after the role play.

In day treatment and outpatient settings, the nurse can give the client homework, such as keeping a journal, applying role-playing skills to actual situations, and observing behaviours in others. In the hospital, the individual can experience the same process, and the nurse is available to offer immediate feedback. Whatever the setting, or even the specific problems addressed, the nurse must keep in mind and remind the client that change occurs slowly. Thus, working on the problems occurs gradually, with severity of symptoms as the guide to deciding how fast and how much change to expect.

Spiritual Domain

In addressing the spiritual domain, the qualities of the nurse that have been identified as important include receptivity (e.g., being genuinely available to the client as a person), humanity (e.g., taking time for the "little things" when giving care), competency (e.g., demonstrating safe practice), and positivity (e.g., having a hopeful attitude and fostering a positive spirit; Carr, 2008; see Chapter 13). In nursing clients with BPD, enacting these qualities may be challenging, as characteristics of BPD involving self-dysregulation and interpersonal dysregulation can sometimes promote a negative response to the person in the nurse. If the nurse does not grasp that the client's personality patterns do comprise a mental disorder, she or he may become frustrated with the lack of client behaviour change and progress. As well, trying to understand the worldview of the client with BPD can be difficult. Yet, spiritual care is particularly important for such clients as they often are struggling with issues of self and connection, purpose and meaning. Nurses can play an important role in helping clients with these issues through respectful, knowledgeable, and supportive connection within a therapeutic relationship.

◼◼ EVALUATION AND OUTCOMES

Evaluation and outcomes vary depending on the severity of the disorder, the presence of comorbid disorders, and the availability of resources. For a client with severe symptoms or continual self-injury, keeping the individual safe and alive may be a realistic outcome. Helping the person resist parasuicidal urges may take years. In contrast, individuals who rarely need hospitalization and have adequate resources can expect to recover from the self-destructive impulses and learn positive interaction skills that promote a qualitative lifestyle. Most clients fall somewhere in between, with periods of symptom exacerbation and remission. In these individuals, increasing the symptom-free time may be the best indicator of outcomes.

◼◼ CONTINUUM OF CARE

Treatment of BPD involves long-term therapies. Hospitalization is sometimes necessary during acute episodes involving parasuicidal behaviour, but once this behaviour is controlled, clients are discharged. It is important for these individuals to continue with treatment in the outpatient or day treatment setting. They often appear more competent and in control than they are, and nurses must not be deceived by these outward appearances. They need continued follow-up and long-term therapies, including individual therapy, psychoeducation, and positive role models (see Nursing Care Plan 25-1; Box 25-9).

Nursing Care Plan 25.1

Client With BPD

YJ, a 28-year-old single woman, was brought to the emergency department of a hospital by police officers after finding her in a Burger Chef with superficial self-inflicted lacerations on both forearms. She pleaded with the police not to take her to the hospital. The police report noted that she fluctuated between intense crying and pleading to fighting physically and using foul language. By the time she arrived in the emergency department, however, she was calm, cooperative, pleasant, and charming. When asked why she cut herself, YJ reported that she was not sure but added that her therapist was leaving today for a 4-week trip to Europe. YJ specifically asked the staff not to call her therapist because "she will be angry with me."

After the emergency physician examined YJ, the advanced practice mental health nurse assessed her developmental and psychiatric histories and a summary of recent events, before she reached a provisional diagnosis of BPD with a primary nursing diagnosis of risk for self-mutilation related to abandonment anticipation. YJ had several previous self-destructive episodes with minor injuries, only one requiring sutures, and two hospitalizations. She lives with her boyfriend, who is

currently on a business trip, and she works part time at a bookstore. Her invalid mother lives with her younger sister. There are no other relatives. YJ's father died traumatically in an automobile accident when she was 3 years old. YJ was in the car when it crashed; she received minor injuries.

Because YJ refused to agree not to harm herself, the nurse admitted YJ to the psychiatric unit with suicide precautions. Once on the unit, YJ was assessed by a staff nurse as having a basically normal mental status examination except that her mood was very tearful at times but charming and joking at other times. She said, "Don't mind me, I cry at the drop of a hat sometimes." Toward the middle of the interview she said, "I feel safer here than I ever felt before. It must be you. Are you sure you're just a staff nurse?" YJ agreed to contract for safety just for today, but added, "Are you going to be my nurse tomorrow? I feel safest with you." When the nurse had completed her assessment, she showed YJ around the unit. As the nurse left her in the day room, YJ said, "My therapist doesn't understand me very well. I don't care if she is going out of town. After 4 years, she hasn't helped. If I had you as a therapist, I wouldn't be here now."

Setting: Inpatient Psychiatric Unit in a General Hospital

Baseline Assessment: YJ, a 28-year-old woman, came into the emergency department with superficial self-inflicted wounds on both forearms. There was a marked discrepancy in her behaviour at the scene of the incident reported by emergency medical technicians from her presentation in the emergency department and now on the inpatient unit. She was admitted this time because she refused to agree not to harm herself further if released. She is angry and sad that her therapist is leaving for 4 weeks for a vacation and does not know how she will cope while the therapist is gone. She fears that the therapist will not return.

Psychiatric Diagnosis	Medications
Axis I: Adjustment disorder with depressed mood	Sertraline (Zoloft) 150 mg qd for anxiety and depression
Axis II: BPD	
Axis III: Superficial wounds on both forearms	
Axis IV: Social support (inadequate social support)	
Axis V: Global Assessment of Functioning (GAF) current = 60; GAF past year = 75	

Continued

Nursing Care Plan 25.1 *(Continued)*

Nursing Diagnosis 1: Self-Mutilation

Defining Characteristics	Related Factors
Cuts and scratches on body Self-inflicted wounds	Fears of abandonment secondary to therapist's vacation Inability to handle stress

Outcomes

Initial	Discharge
1. Remain safe and not harm herself. 2. Identify feelings before and after cutting herself. 3. Agree not to harm herself over the next 24 hours.	4. Identify ways of dealing with self-harming impulses if they return. 5. Verbalize alternate thinking with more realistic base. 6. Identify community resources to provide structure and support while her therapist is gone.

Interventions

Interventions	Rationale	Ongoing Assessment
Monitor the client for changes in mood or behaviour that might lead to self-injurious behaviour. Discuss with the client the need for close observation and rationale to keep her safe.	Close observation establishes safety and protection of the client from self-harm and impulsive behaviours. Explanation to the client for the purpose of nursing interventions helps her cooperate with the nursing activity.	Document according to the facility policy. Continue to observe for mood and behaviour changes. Assess her response to the increasing level of observation.
Administer medications as prescribed and evaluate medication effectiveness in reducing depression, anxiety, and cognitive disorganization. After 6–8 hours, present written agreement to not harm herself.	Allows for adjustment of medication dosage based on target behaviours and outcomes. Permits the client time to return to more thoughtful ways of responding rather than her previous reactive response. Also permits her to save face and avoid embarrassment of a losing power struggle if presented much earlier.	Observe for side effects. Observe for her willingness to agree to not harm herself.
Communicate information about the client's risk to other nursing staff.	The close observation should be continued throughout all shifts until the client agrees to resist self-harm urges.	Review the documentation of close observation for all shifts.

Evaluation

Outcomes	Revised Outcomes	Interventions
Remained safe without further harming self. Identified fears of abandonment before cutting herself and relief of anxiety afterward. She identified friends to call when fears return and hotlines to use if necessary.	Use hotlines or call friends if fears to harm self return.	Give the client hotline number and ask her to record her friends' numbers in an accessible place.
Agreed to not harm herself over the next 3 days.	Does not harm self for 3 days.	Remind her to call someone if urges return.
Enrolled in a day hospital program for 4 weeks.	Attend the day hospital program.	Follow-up on enrolment.

Continued

Nursing Care Plan 25.1 (Continued)

Nursing Diagnosis 2: Risk for Loneliness

Defining Characteristics	Related Factors
Social isolation	Fear of abandonment secondary to the therapist's impending vacation

Outcomes

Initial	Discharge
1. Discuss being lonely. 2. Identify previous ways of coping with loneliness.	3. Identify strategies to deal with loneliness while the therapist is away.

Interventions

Interventions	Rationale	Ongoing Assessment
Develop a therapeutic relationship.	People with BPD are able to examine loneliness within the structure of a therapeutic relationship.	Assess her ability to relate and the nurse's response to the relationship.
Discuss her past experience with the therapist being gone with an emphasis on how she was able to survive it.	She has survived the therapist's absences before. By identifying the strategies she used, she can build on those strengths.	Assess her ability to assume any responsibility for "living through it." This will become a strength.
Acknowledge that it is normal to feel angry when the therapist is gone, but there are other strategies that may help the person deal with the loneliness besides cutting.	Acknowledging feelings is important. Helping the client focus on the possibility of other strategies for dealing with the anger helps her regain a sense of control over her behaviour.	Assess whether she is willing to acknowledge that there are other behavioural strategies of handling anger.
Begin immediate disposition planning with a focus on day hospitalization or day treatment for skills training and management of loneliness.	While the client is in hospital, she is out of stressful environment in which she can learn more effective behaviours and use the therapy. Moving out of the hospital and back into the outpatient therapy decreases the possibility of regression and lost learning (Linehan, 1993a, 1993b).	Assess her willingness to learn new skills within a day treatment setting.
Teach her about stress management techniques. Assign her to an anger management group while she is in the hospital.	Learning about ways of dealing with feelings and stressful situations helps the client with BPD choose positive strategies rather than self-destructive ones.	Monitor whether she actually attends the groups. She should be encouraged to attend.

Evaluation

Outcomes	Revised Outcomes	Interventions
YJ was able to verbalize her anger about her therapist leaving and fears of abandonment. The last two times her therapist went on vacation, the client became self-injurious and was hospitalized for 2 weeks.	None.	
YJ was willing to be discharged the next day if she could attend day treatment while her therapist was gone.	Identify other strategies of dealing with the therapist vacations besides cutting.	Attend stress management, communication, and self-comforting classes.

Bulechek, G., Butcher, H., & McCloskey Dochterman, J. (Eds.). (2008). *Nursing interventions classification (NIC)* (5th ed.). St. Louis, MO: Mosby.

BOX 25.9

Research for Best Practice: The Experiences of Suicidal Men

Strike, C., Rhodes, A. E., Bergmans, Y., & Links, P. (2006). Fragmented pathways to care: The experiences of suicidal men. Crisis, 27(1), 31–38.

QUESTION: What is it like for suicidal men with BPD or ASD when they access and use mental health services?

METHOD: In qualitative interviews, 15 men described their experiences with the range of treatment services in Toronto over the previous year. All had a recent history of suicidal behaviour with concurrent substance use, antisocial behaviour, or borderline behaviour.

FINDINGS: The analysis identified patterns of practices by the men and service providers described as "fragmented pathways to care." Participants were slow to identify their needs for mental health services, unable to express their emotions, and challenged to navigate the system. Participants felt mislabelled due, in part, to the failure of care providers to inquire about contextual factors and to do a complete assessment. They felt that they were treated disrespectfully and that providers overrelied on medications.

Participants felt compelled to lie or to attempt suicide to have their needs met, and they were frustrated by involuntary admissions and a lack of dignity.

IMPLICATIONS FOR PRACTICE: The results illuminate the perceived disconnection between what services are desired by suicidal and aggressive men and the various treatment access points and the care that is available. Nurses can ensure that more accessible programs are developed and address stigma and negative behaviours from care providers. These men perceived the disinterest and hostility of staff members toward them, for instance, when nurses were visible in the nursing station yet did not initiate an interaction. They desired greater access to providers and to be kept better informed about treatment and discharge plans. Inquiry about past history, including abuse as children, is meaningful to these men. They desire connections with nurses who show that they are listening and have a willingness to safely encourage suicidal men to express their emotions.

ANTISOCIAL PERSONALITY DISORDER: AGGRANDIZING PATTERN

Clinical Course of Disorder

In the *DSM-IV-TR*, APD is defined as "a pervasive pattern of disregard for, and violation of, the rights of others that begins in childhood or early adolescence and continues into adulthood" (APA, 2000, p. 701).

The term **psychopathy**, which originated in Germany in the late 19th century, initially referred to a number of personality disorders but has gradually become equated with only APD (Lykken, 2006). People with this disorder are behaviourally impulsive and interpersonally irresponsible. They fail to adapt to the ethical and social standards of the community. They act hastily and spontaneously, are shortsighted, and fail to plan ahead or consider alternatives. They lack a sense of personal obligation to fulfill social and financial responsibilities, including those involved with being a spouse, a parent, an employee, a friend, or a member of the community. Disdainful of traditional values, they fail to conform to social norms and values. They enjoy a sense of freedom and relish being unencumbered and unconfined by people, places, or responsibilities. They can be interpersonally engaging, which is often mistaken for a genuine sense of concern for other people. In reality, they lack empathy; are unable to express human compassion; and tend to be insensitive, callous, and contemptuous of others. Easily irritated, they often become aggressive,

disregarding the safety of themselves or others. They lack remorse for transgressions. No matter what the consequences, they are rarely able to delay gratification (APA, 2000).

These individuals have faith only in themselves and are secure only when they are independent from those whom they fear will harm or humiliate them. Their need for independence is based on their mistrust of others, rather than an inherent belief in their own self-worth. They are driven by a need to prove their superiority and see themselves as the centre of the universe. Some of these individuals openly and flagrantly violate laws, ending up in jail. But most people with APD never come in conflict with the law and, instead, find a niche in society, such as in business, the military, or politics, that rewards their competitive, tough behaviour (Millon et al., 2004). The most common social problems statistically associated with APD include substance abuse (Bucholz, Heath, & Madden, 2000; Lejoyeux et al., 2000), sexual assault and other criminal behaviours (Gotz, Johnstone, & Ratcliffe, 1999; Hare, 1999; Smallbone & Dadds, 2000), and family violence (Hanson, Cadsky, Harris, & Lalond, 1997; see Table 25-4). This disorder has a chronic course, but the antisocial behaviours tend to diminish later in life, particularly after the age of 40 years (APA, 2000).

Epidemiology and Risk Factors

The prevalence in nonclinical studies ranges from 2% to 3% of the population, with a median value of

Table 25.4	A Summary of Diagnostic Characteristics of Antisocial Personality Disorder 301.7	DSM IV

Diagnostic Criteria and Target Symptoms	Associated Findings
• Pervasive pattern of disregard for and violation of the rights of others • Failure to conform to social norms with respect to lawful behaviours (repeatedly performing acts that are grounds for arrest) • Deceitfulness (repeated lying, use of aliases, or conning others for personal profit or pleasure) • Impulsivity or failure to plan ahead • Irritability and aggressiveness (repeated physical fights or assaults) • Reckless disregard for the safety of self or others • Consistent irresponsibility (repeated failure to sustain consistent work behaviour or honour financial obligations) • Lack of remorse (being indifferent to or rationalizing having hurt, mistreated, or stolen from another) • Occurring since 15 years of age • At least 18 years of age • Evidence of conduct disorder with the onset before 15 years of age • Not exclusive during the course of schizophrenia or manic episode	*Associated Behavioural Findings* • Lacking empathy • Callous, cynical, and contemptuous of the feelings, rights, and suffering of others • Inflated and arrogant self-appraisal • Excessively opinionated, self-assured, or cocky • Glib, superficial charm; impressive verbal ability • Irresponsible and exploitative in sexual relationships; a history of multiple sexual partners and lack of a sustained monogamous relationship • Possible dysphoria, including complaints of tension, inability to tolerate boredom, and depressed mood

approximately 2% (Moran, 1999). In prison populations, the prevalence of APD rises to 60%.

Age of Onset

To be diagnosed with APD, the individual must have exhibited one or more childhood behavioural characteristics of conduct disorder and ADHD, such as aggression to people or animals, destruction of property, deceitfulness or theft, or serious violation of rules. This requirement of exhibiting antisocial behaviour before 15 years of age is based on older studies of adults with APD (Barry et al., 2000; Faraone, Biederman, Mennin, & Russell, 1998; Myers, Stewart, & Brown, 1998).

Gender

Men receive diagnoses of APD more frequently than do women (Eley, Lichtenstein, & Stevenson, 1999; Marcus, 1999). The best estimate for lifetime prevalence of APD from the Epidemiological Catchment Area (ECA) data is 7.3% for men and 1% for women (Robins, Tipp, & Przybeck, 1991). The cause of this discrepancy between men and women has received considerable speculation. It is generally believed that APD is underdiagnosed in women or manifested differently in men than in women, who usually receive diagnoses of somatization (see Chapter 22) or histrionic disorders (discussed later in this chapter). Some think that males have early onset and adolescent-onset disorder, whereas females primarily have an adolescent-onset disorder (Silverthorn & Frick, 1999), contributing to less

severe symptoms and deficits. Similarly, APD development in females entails more affect dysregulation, resulting in a competing diagnosis of BPD, even though they meet the overall criteria for APD (Zlotnick, 1999; see Box 25-10).

Cultural and Ethnic Differences

People with APD or psychopathic personalities are found in many cultures, including industrialized and nonindustrialized societies. In an analysis of the Inuit of Northwest Alaska, individuals who break the rules when they are known are called *kunlangeta*, meaning "his mind knows what to do but he does not do it" (Murphy, 1976, p. 1026). This term is used for someone who repeatedly lies, cheats, and steals. He is described as someone who does not go hunting and, when the other men are out of the village, takes sexual advantage of the women. In another culture in rural southwest Nigeria, the Yorubas use the word *arankan* to mean a "person who always goes his own way regardless of others, who is uncooperative, full of malice and bullheaded" (Murphy, p. 1026). In both cultures, the healers and shamans do not consider these people treatable.

The number of people within a culture who actually have APD appears to depend on whether the society is individualistic, where competitiveness and independence are encouraged and temporary relationships the norm, or collectivistic, such as in China, where group loyalties and responsibilities are more important than self-expression (Cooke, 1996). Cultural distribution variation may have more to do with

BOX 25.10

Clinical Vignette: Antisocial Personality Disorder: Male Versus Female

Jackson (male) and Stasia (female) are fraternal twins, 22 years old, who received diagnoses of APD. The following are their clinical profiles.

JACKSON

Jackson's juvenile probation officer explained that Jackson came from a very violent family and neighbourhood and described the situation by saying, "If gangs hadn't gotten him, his father would have." His lawyer described him as "a likeable guy, but I wouldn't turn my back on him."

Jackson is currently in prison for the third time. Although his juvenile records begin at age 9 and include minor assault and property damage charges, his burglary conviction is his first adult crime. His school teachers thought that Jackson was very bright but that he had significant difficulty with peers and authority figures. He fought regularly, was described as a bully, and seemed always to be scamming. At age 16, Jackson dropped out of school and joined a gang.

STASIA

Stasia was recently hospitalized for the sixth time when one of her male friends beat her. She has been working as a prostitute for 5 years. Her physical examination noted not only multiple bruises but also tattoos that cover 50% of her body. In addition, she has piercings of her tongue, ears, brow, lips, and nipples. She is emotionally volatile, manipulative, and angry. Stasia has many acquaintances and sexual partners, but none are truly intimate. She has periods when she uses drugs regularly.

Stasia and Jackson's mother was jailed when the twins were 18 months old and did not return until they were 6 years old. They were raised mostly by their paternal grandmother, who hated their mother and reminded Stasia frequently of how much she looked like her mother. Their father, when present, was violent toward Jackson and sexually abused Stasia.

WHAT DO YOU THINK?

- How might gender influence the development of symptoms?
- How might culture influence early recognition of problems and provision of early intervention to prevent future serious mental disorders?
- What are some possible outcomes in this situation?
- How does this case demonstrate the interaction between socialization, biology, and culture?

economic conditions, legal structures, social tolerance, and co-occurring conditions than specific diagnostic factors. Poverty and academic failure were significantly related to delinquency in boys (Pagani, Boulerice, Vitaro, & Tremblay, 1999), and gang entry was seen as a developmental step in boys with conduct disorder (Lahey, Gordon, Loeber, Stouthamer-Loeber, & Farrington, 1999).

Comorbidity

APD is strongly associated with alcohol and drug abuse. Substance-related disorders are common (Lejoyeux et al., 2000; Waldman & Slutske, 2000). The association between substance abuse and APD is stronger in women than in men. It is rare for APD to be the only disorder present. In the ECA study, fewer than 10% of clients with APD had no other diagnoses. In the ECA data, men with active APD were three times more likely to abuse alcohol and five times more likely to abuse drugs than were those without APD. Women with APD were 13 times more likely to use alcohol and 12 times more likely to use drugs (Robins et al., 1991). Other disorders that typically occur with APD include ADHD (Schubiner et al., 2000), depression, and schizophrenia (Nolan, Volavka, Mohr, & Czobor, 1999).

Etiology

Biologic Theories

There appears to be a genetic component in APD, which is five times more common in first-degree biologic relatives of men with the disorder than among the general population. There is a nearly 10 times greater risk to women who are first-degree biologic relatives. Pooled data of 229 pairs of identical twins from seven twin studies conducted in North America, Japan, Norway, Germany, and Denmark showed a concordance rate of 51.5% for APD, whereas data from 316 fraternal twins yielded a corresponding rate of 23.1% (Gottesman & Goldsmith, 1994).

The biochemical basis of antisocial disorder is not clearly understood. However, some curious biologic markers have been identified. Gotz et al. (1999) found a significantly higher antisocial behaviour in adolescent and adult men with XYY sex chromosome abnormality than in control subjects. Another study found a higher concentration of serum testosterone and sex hormone–binding globulin in incarcerated men who met the criteria for APD (Stalenheim, von Knorring, & Wide, 1998). Serotonin deficiency (Dolan, 1994) and low dopamine levels have also been implicated in APD. In a study of 21 hospitalized boys aged 8 to 16 years who had diagnoses of conduct disorder, oppositional deviant disorder, and ADHD, low levels of dopamine activity were found in those who had been abused or neglected before the age of 3 years (Galvin et al., 1991). These researchers suggested that low levels of dopamine may reflect an attachment disruption that occurs at critical times in the lives of abused and neglected boys. This disruption causes the child to be biologically vulnerable, resulting in low levels of dopamine and less effective regulation of the noradrenergic system when activated by stressors. In addition, researchers consistently find dysregulation in catecholamines with changed activity of the dopaminergic pathways in the frontal cortex (Soderstrom, Blennow, Sjodin, & Forsman, 2003). The limbic-prefrontal cortex (Veit et al., 2002) and the dorsolateral prefrontal cortex (Dolan & Park, 2002) are specifically implicated, accounting for poor judgment, emotional distance, aggression, and impulsivity (Kiehl et al., 2001).

Psychological Theories

Learning, social behaviour, empathy, emotional awareness, and regulation are all directly influenced by the nature of the relationship between the caregiver and the child. One of the leading explanations of APD is that these individuals had unsatisfactory attachments in early relationships that led to antisocial behaviours in later life. Normal relationships begin with **attachment**, which can be defined as:

> Behaviour that results in a person's attaining or retaining proximity to some other differentiated and preferred individual. During the course of healthy development, attachment behaviour leads to the development of affectional bonds or attachments, initially between child and parent and later between adult and adult. The forms of behaviour and the bonds to which they lead are present and active throughout the life cycle (Bowlby, 1980, p. 39).

An attachment relationship between the child and the caregiver depends on the response of both parties. The sense of security in any relationship depends on the quality of the responsiveness experienced with the attachment figure (Smallbone & Dadds, 2000). If the parental figures are overanxious or avoidant, the child does not develop a sense of security with others and instead experiences self as an island (Reti et al., 2002). Secure attachments facilitate a balance between the connection to another and the ability to go out into the world autonomously. In a secure attachment, a child feels safe, loved, and valued but also develops the self-confidence to interact with the rest of the world. Experiences in successive relationships interact with prior experiences to determine an individual's trust in others.

Insecure attachments are formed as a result of faulty interactions between the caregiver and the child and are expressed in relationships as ambivalence, avoidance, or disorganization (Ainsworth, 1989). In APD, a failure to make or sustain stable attachments in early childhood can lead to avoidance of future attachments. Studies have found several childhood situations to be risk factors for developing dysfunctional attachments, such as parental abandonment or neglect, loss of parent or primary caregiver, and physical or sexual abuse. However, evidence supports the theory that the ability to foster secure emotional attachments may be a learned parenting skill and that parents who lacked secure attachment relationships in their own childhood may lack the ability to form secure attachment relationships with their own children (Wade, Pevalin, & Brannigan, 1999).

Children are born with a particular **temperament**, a recognizable and distinctive pattern of behaviour that is evident during the first few months of life. Some infants are more relaxed or calm and sleep a lot, whereas others are extremely alert, startled by the slightest noise, cry more, and sleep less. Scientists believe that temperament is neurobiologically determined, and many believe that it is central to understanding personality disorders. Children seem to be born with certain temperaments that remain fairly stable throughout their development.

Temperament consists of the interaction of two behavioural dimensions—activity and adaptability. Activity patterns in individuals vary along a spectrum, from active or intense children, whose actions display decisiveness and vigour as they continuously relate to their environment, to passive children, who are more cautious and slow to relate to their environment (a wait-and-see pattern of behaviour). Adaptability includes a spectrum, with the extreme at one end being the child who is regular in biologic functions such as eating or sleeping, has a positive approach to new stimuli, and maintains a high degree of flexibility in response to changing conditions. At the other end of the adaptability dimension are children who display irregularity in biologic functions, withdrawal reactions to new stimuli, and minimal flexibility in response to change.

Some studies indicate that extreme temperaments make one vulnerable to antisocial behaviour patterns. A difficult temperament is characterized by withdrawal from novel stimuli, low adaptability, and intense emotional reactions. Four key behaviours are present in a difficult temperament: aggression, inattention, hyperactivity, and impulsivity. There is a strong relationship between difficult temperament and problem behaviours such as those of ADHD, oppositional behaviour, and conduct disorder (Dowson, Sussams, Grounds, & Taylor, 2001; Herpertz et al., 2001; Hill, 2002, 2003; Langbehn & Cadoret, 2001).

Hyperactivity alone is not related to the development of antisocial personality in adults; however, hyperactivity occurring with aggression and the other behaviours listed is related to APD (Barry et al., 2000; Giancola, 2000; Schubiner et al., 2000). Temperament and problem behaviours are generally consistent throughout a lifetime. There is a strong relationship between conduct disorder in childhood and antisocial behaviour in adulthood with substance abuse (Myers et al., 1998). In a longitudinal study of 961 children whose temperament related to the development of psychiatric problems in childhood, the children with a difficult temperament were more likely to receive diagnoses of APD in adulthood, be a recidivistic offender, and be convicted of a violent offence (Grann, Lanstrom, Tengstrom, & Kullgren, 1999).

Social Theories

In many cases, individuals with APD come from chaotic families in which alcoholism and violence are the norm. Individuals who have been victims of abuse or neglect, live in a foster home, or had several primary caregivers are more likely to experience antisocial behaviours, especially aggression (Andrews, Foster, Capaldi, & Hop, 2000; Kim, Hetherington, & Reiss, 1999; Pagani et al., 1999). However, it is difficult to separate the influence of social factors on the development of the disorder because the symptoms of APD are social manifestations—unemployment, divorces and separations, and violence.

Interdisciplinary Treatment of Disorder

People with APD rarely seek mental health care because of the disorder itself, but rather for the treatment of depression, substance abuse, or uncontrolled anger, or for forensic evaluation (Black, Baumgard, & Bell, 1995). Clients who are admitted through the courts often have a comorbid diagnosis of APD. Treatment is difficult and involves helping the individual alter his or her cognitive schema. The overall treatment goals are to develop empathy for other people and situations and to live within the norms of society.

Priority Care Issues

Although they can be interpersonally charming, these individuals can become verbally and physically abusive if their expectations are not met. Protection of other clients and staff from manipulative and sometimes abusive behaviour is a priority.

Family Response to Disorder

If there are family members, they have probably been abused, mistreated, or intimidated by these individuals. For example, one client sold his mother's possessions while she was at work. Another would abuse his wife after drinking. However, family members may be fiercely loyal to the person and blame themselves for his or her shortcomings.

■ NURSING MANAGEMENT: HUMAN RESPONSE TO ANTISOCIAL PERSONALITY DISORDER

Biologic Domain

Biologic Assessment

APD does not significantly impair the biologic dimension unless there are coexisting substance abuse or other Axis I disorders. Because substance abuse is a major problem with this population, the physical effects of chronic use of addictive substances must be considered.

Nursing Diagnoses for the Biologic Domain

Common nursing diagnoses in APD include dysfunctional family processes and alcoholism.

Interventions for Biologic Domain

In instances in which there are coexisting disorders, the personality disorder may actually interfere with interventions aimed at improving physical functioning. For example, a client with schizophrenia and APD may not develop enough trust within a relationship to examine his or her delusional thoughts or other aspects of dysfunction, such as alcohol or drug abuse.

Psychological Domain

Psychological Assessment

Many individuals with APD are committed to health care agencies by the court system. An assessment generally involves using basic psychological assessment tools to evaluate aberrant behaviours.

Nursing Diagnoses for the Psychological Domain

Because so many individuals with APD have dysfunctional thinking patterns, common nursing diagnoses include disturbed thought processes and a risk for other directed violence.

Interventions for the Psychological Domain

Therapeutic relationships are difficult to establish because these individuals do not attach to others and are often unable to use the relationship to change behaviour. After the first few meetings with these clients, the nurse may feel that the relationship has a good start, but in reality, a superficial alliance is usually formed. Additional sessions reveal the lack of client commitment to the relationship. These individuals begin to revisit topics discussed in sessions or lose interest in trying to work on problems. By using self-awareness skills and assessing supervision regularly, the nurse can identify blocks in the development of a therapeutic relationship (or lack of) and his or her response to the relationship. The goal of the therapeutic relationship is to identify dysfunctional thinking patterns and develop new problem-solving behaviours.

Self-responsibility facilitation (encouraging a person to assume more responsibility for personal behaviour) is useful with clients with APD (Bulechek et al., 2008). The nursing activities that are particularly helpful include holding the client responsible for his or her behaviour, monitoring the extent that self-responsibility is assumed, and discussing the consequences of not dealing with responsibilities. The nurse needs to refrain from arguing or bargaining about the unit rules, such as time for meals, use of the television room, and smoking. Instead, positive feedback is given to the individual for accepting additional responsibility or changing behaviour.

Self-awareness enhancement (exploring and understanding personal thoughts, feelings, motivation, and behaviours) is another nursing intervention that is important in helping these individuals develop a sense of understanding about relating peacefully to the rest of the world (Bulechek et al., 2008). Encouraging clients to recognize and discuss thoughts and feelings helps the nurse understand how the person views the world. The nurse can then use many of the same communication techniques discussed in the section on BPD.

Teaching Points

Client education efforts have to be creative and thought provoking. In teaching a person with APD, a direct approach is best, but the nurse must avoid lecturing, which the individual will resent. In teaching the client about positive health care practices, impulse control, and anger management, the best approach is to engage the individual in a discussion about the issue and then direct the topic to the major teaching points. These clients often take great delight in arguing or showing how the rules of life do not apply to them. A sense of humour is important, as are clear teaching goals and avoiding being sidetracked (Box 25-11).

BOX 25.11

Psychoeducation Checklist: Borderline Personality Disorder

When caring for the client with APD, be sure to include the following topic areas in the teaching plan:

- Positive health care practices, including substance abuse control
- Effective communication and interaction skills
- Impulse control
- Anger management
- Group experience to help develop self-awareness and impact of behaviour on others
- Analyzing an issue from the other person's viewpoint
- Maintenance of employment
- Interpersonal relationships and social interactions

Social Domain

Social Assessment

The nursing assessment usually focuses on other problems in addition to the response to the personality disorder. In fact, eliciting data may be difficult because of the basic mistrust individuals with APD have toward authority figures. Clients may not give an accurate history or may embellish aspects to project themselves in a more positive light. Often, they deny any criminal activity, even if they are admitted in police custody. Key areas of assessment are determining the quality of relationships, impulsivity, and the extent of aggression. These individuals do not assume responsibility for their own actions and often blame others for their misfortune. Their disregard for others is manifested in their interactions. For example, one individual with human immunodeficiency virus was engaging in unprotected sex with several different women because he wanted to "have fun as long as I can." He was completely unconcerned about the possibility of transmitting the virus. These individuals often make good first impressions. Self-awareness is especially important for the nurse because of the initial charming quality of many of these individuals. Once these clients realize that the nurse cannot be used or manipulated, they lose interest in the nurse and revert to their normal, egocentric behaviours.

Nursing Diagnoses for the Social Domain

Nursing diagnoses for clients with APD are related to their interpersonal detachment, lack of awareness of others, avoidance of feelings, impulsiveness, and discrepancy between their perception of themselves and others' perception of them. Typical diagnoses are ineffective role performance (unemployment), ineffective individual coping, impaired communication, impaired social interactions, low self-esteem, and risk for violence. Outcomes should be short term and relevant to a specific problem. For example, if a person has been chronically unemployed, a reasonable short-term outcome would be to set up job interviews, rather than obtain a job.

Interventions for the Social Domain

These clients have a long-standing history of difficulty in interpersonal relationships. In an inpatient unit, interventions can be more intense and focus on helping the individual develop positive interaction skills and experience a consistent environment. For example, the focus of nursing interventions may be the client's continual disregard of the rights of others. On one unit, a client continually placed orders for pizzas in the name of another person on the unit. This individual had limited intelligence and was genuinely afraid of the person with APD. The victimized person always paid for the pizza and gave it to the other client. When the nursing staff realized what was happening, they confronted the client with APD about the behaviour and revoked his unit privileges.

Group interventions typically are more effective than individual modalities because other individuals on the unit and staff can validate or challenge the client's view of a situation (Messina, Wish, & Nemes, 1999). Problem-solving groups that focus on identifying a problem and developing a variety of alternative solutions are particularly helpful because client self-responsibility is reinforced when fellow clients remind each other of the better alternatives. Clients are likely to confront each other with dysfunctional schemas or thinking patterns. Teaching individuals with APD the same communication techniques as those with BPD will also encourage self-responsibility. These clients often attend groups that focus on the development of empathy.

Milieu interventions, such as providing a structured environment with rules that are consistently applied to clients who are responsible for their own behaviour, are important. While living in close proximity to others, the individual with APD will demonstrate dysfunctional social patterns that can be identified and targeted for correction. For example, these clients often violate ward rules, such as no smoking or limitations on the number of visitors, and may bring contraband, such as illegal drugs, to the unit.

Aggressive behaviour is often a problem for these individuals and their family members. Like clients with BPD, people with APD tend to be impulsive. Instead of self-injury, these individuals are more likely to strike out at those who are perceived to be interfering with their immediate gratification. Anger control assistance (helping to express anger in an adaptive, nonviolent manner) becomes a priority intervention. Because the expression of anger and aggression develops during a lifetime, these individuals can benefit from anger management techniques.

Social support for these individuals is often minimal, just as it is for individuals with BPD, but the reasons are different. These individuals have often taken advantage of friends and relatives who, in turn, no longer trust them. Helping the client build a new support system once new skills are learned is usually the only option. For these individuals to develop friends and reengage family members, they must learn to interact in new ways, develop empathy, and risk an attachment. For many, this never truly becomes a reality.

Family Patterns

Family members of clients with APD usually need help in establishing boundaries. Because there is a long-term pattern of interaction in which family members are responsible for the client's antisocial behaviour, these patterns need to be interrupted. Families need help in recognizing the client's responsibility for his or her actions.

Spiritual Domain

The nature of APD places great limitations on nurses' ability to address the spiritual domain of these clients. Given that spirituality is relational in nature, the APD characteristics of being unable to feel empathy or compassion for others may diminish the person's spiritual capacity. The nurse's ability to provide spiritual care will be limited if meaningful connection with the client cannot be achieved. It may be possible to gain a better understanding of the client's worldview, however, if the client is inclined to share it honestly. Requests for a meeting with a religious leader/guide or for a religious ritual should be taken seriously as with every client. Unfortunately, it is also important to consider that the motivation for such requests may be other than spiritual need. It should not be forgotten that everyone has the potential for spiritual growth, including individuals living with APD.

■ EVALUATION AND OUTCOMES

The outcomes of interventions for individuals with APD need to be evaluated in terms of management of specific problems, such as maintaining employment or developing a meaningful interpersonal relationship. The nurse will most likely see these clients for other health care problems, so adherence to treatment recommendations and the development of health care practices (e.g., reduce smoking and alcohol consumption) can also be factored into the evaluation of outcomes.

■ CONTINUUM OF CARE

People with APD rarely seek mental health care. In one study, only 14.5% of those with a diagnosis of APD had ever discussed any of its symptoms with a physician. Only 4% had visited a mental health provider during the previous 6 months (Robins et al., 1991). Nurses will most likely see these individuals in medical-surgical settings for comorbid conditions. Consistency in interventions is necessary in treating the client throughout the continuum of care.

HISTRIONIC PERSONALITY DISORDER: GREGARIOUS PATTERN

"Attention seeking" and "emotional" describe people with histrionic personality disorders. These individuals are lively and dramatic and draw attention to themselves by their enthusiasm, dress, and apparent openness. They are the "life of the party" and, on the surface, seem interested in others. Their insatiable need for attention and approval quickly becomes obvious. These needs are inflexible and persistent, even after others attempt to meet them. They are moody and often experience a sense of helplessness when others are disinterested in them. They are sexually seductive in their attempts to gain attention and often are uncomfortable within a single relationship. They are highly suggestible and have a tendency to change opinions often. Their appearance is provocative and their speech dramatic. They express strong opinions without supporting facts. Loyalty and fidelity are lacking (APA, 2000; see Table 25-5).

Gender influences the manifestations of this disorder. Women dress seductively, may express dependency on selected men, and may play a submissive role. Men may dress in a very masculine manner and seek attention by bragging about athletic skills or successes in the job. Individuals with this disorder have difficulty achieving any true intimacy in interpersonal relationships. They seem to possess an innate sensitivity to the moods and thoughts of those they wish to please. This hyperalertness enables them to maneuver quickly to gain their attention. Then, they attempt to control relationships by their seductiveness at one level but become extremely dependent on their friends at another level. Their demand for constant attention quickly alienates their friends. They become depressed when they are not the centre of attention.

Epidemiology

The prevalence of histrionic personality disorder is estimated at 2% to 3% of the general population. In mental health settings, the prevalence rate is reported to be

Table 25.5 — A Summary of Diagnostic Characteristics of Histrionic 301.50 and Narcissistic 301.81 Personality Disorders (DSM IV)	
Diagnostic Criteria and Target Symptoms for Histrionic Disorders	**Associated Findings**
• Pervasive and excessive emotionality and attention-seeking behaviour • Feelings of being uncomfortable and unappreciated when not the centre of attention (lively and dramatic in drawing attention to self) • Inappropriately sexually seductive or provocative • Shallow and rapidly shifting emotional expression • Use of physical appearance to draw attention to self • Impressionistic and vague style of speech • Exaggerated expression of emotion, theatricality, and self-dramatization • Highly suggestible • Viewing of relationships as more intimate than they really are	*Associated Behavioural Findings* • Difficulty achieving emotional intimacy in romantic and sexual relationships • Use of emotional manipulation and seductiveness coupled with marked dependency • Impaired relationships with same-sex friends • Constant demanding of attention, leading to alienation of friends • Craving novelty, excitement, and stimulation; easily bored with routines • Difficulty in situations involving delayed gratification • Increased risk for suicidal gestures and threats for attention
Diagnostic Criteria and Target Symptoms for Narcissistic Disorders	**Associated Findings**
• Pervasive pattern of grandiosity; need for admiration; lack of empathy • Grandiose sense of self-importance • Preoccupation with fantasies of unlimited success, power of vigilance, beauty, or ideal love • Belief of own superiority, specialness, and uniqueness; association with individuals of higher or special status • Need for excessive admiration and constant attention • Sense of entitlement (unreasonable expectation of highly favourable treatment) • Exploitation and taking advantage of others • Lack of empathy; difficulty recognizing desires, experiences, and feelings of others • Envious of others; feeling that others are envious of him or her Arrogant, haughty behaviour or attitudes	*Associated Behavioural Findings* • Sensitive to injury from criticism or deficit • Criticism causes inward feelings of humiliation, degradation, hollowness, and emptiness • Social withdrawal • Impaired interpersonal relationships • Impaired performance because of intolerance to criticism • Unwilling to take risk in competitive situation when defeat is possible

10% to 15% (APA, 2000). A higher rate of this disorder has been found among separated and divorced subjects than among married subjects (Nestadt et al., 1990). This disorder co-occurs with borderline, dependent, and antisocial personality disorders. It also exists with anxiety disorders, substance abuse, and mood disorders (Millon et al., 2004). Men with histrionic disorders are more likely to also have substance abuse problems, and women are more likely to experience depressive episodes, suicide attempts, and two or more unexplained medical symptoms (Nestadt et al.).

Etiology

There is a need for research in determining the etiologic factors of histrionic personality disorder. There is speculation that this disorder has a biologic component and that heredity may play a role, but that the biologic influence is less than in some of the previously discussed personality disorders. In infancy and early childhood, these individuals are extremely alert and emotionally responsive. The tendencies for sensory alertness may be traced to responses of the limbic and reticular systems. They demonstrate a high degree of dependence on others and a type of dissociation in which they have a reduced awareness of their behaviour in relation to others (Bornstein, 1998). It is believed that these highly alert and responsive infants seek more gratification from external stimulations during their first few months of life. Depending on the responsiveness of caregivers to them, they develop behaviour patterns in response to their caregivers. It is believed that these children experience brief, highly charged, and irregular reinforcement from multiple caregivers (e.g., parents, siblings, grandparents, foster parents) who are unable to provide consistent experiences.

Parental behaviour and role modelling are also believed to contribute to the development of histrionic personality disorder. Many of the women with this disorder reported that they are just like their mother, who is emotionally labile, bored with the routines of home life, flirtatious with men, and clever in dealing with people. It is believed that through role modelling, these children learn and mimic the behaviours observed in caregivers or adults (Sigmund, Barnett, & Mundt, 1998).

Nursing Management

The ultimate treatment goal for individuals with histrionic personality disorder is to correct the tendency to fulfill all their needs by focusing on others to the exclusion of themselves. When these individuals seek mental health care, they have usually experienced a period of social disapproval or deprivation. Their hope is that the mental health providers will help fulfill their needs. Specific goals are needed to protect the person from becoming dependent on a mental health system. In the nursing assessment, the nurse focuses on the quality of the individual's interpersonal relationships. It is common that the person is dissatisfied with his or her partner, and sexual relations may be nonexistent.

During the assessment, the client will make statements that indicate low self-esteem. Because these individuals believe that they are incapable of handling life's demands and have been waiting for a truly competent person to take care of them, they have not developed a positive self-concept or adequate problem-solving abilities.

Nursing diagnoses that are usually generated include chronic low self-esteem, ineffective individual coping, and ineffective sexual patterns. Outcomes focus on helping the individual develop autonomy, a positive self-concept, and mature problem-solving skills.

A variety of interventions support the outcomes. A nurse–client relationship that allows the client to explore positive personality characteristics and develop independent decision-making skills forms the basis of the interventions. Reinforcing personal strengths, conveying confidence in the person's ability to handle situations, and examining negative perceptions of self can be done within the therapeutic relationship. Encouraging the client to act autonomously can also improve the individual's sense of self-worth (Bulechek et al., 2008). Attending assertiveness groups can help increase the individual's self-confidence and improve self-esteem.

■ NARCISSISTIC PERSONALITY DISORDER: EGOTISTIC PATTERN

People with a narcissistic personality disorder are grandiose, have an inexhaustible need for admiration, and lack empathy. Beginning in childhood, these individuals believe that they are superior, special, or unique and that others should recognize them in this way (APA, 2000). They are often preoccupied with fantasies of unlimited success, power, beauty, or ideal love. They overvalue their personal worth, direct their affections toward themselves, and expect others to hold them in high esteem. They define the world through their own self-centred view. People with narcissistic personality disorder are benignly arrogant and feel themselves above the conventions of their cultural group. They believe that they are entitled to be served and that it is their inalienable right to receive special considerations. These individuals are often successful in their jobs but may alienate their significant others, who grow tired of their narcissism (see Table 25-5). Clinically, those with narcissistic personality disorder show overlapping characteristics of BPD.

Epidemiology

The prevalence of narcissistic personality disorder in the general population is estimated to be less than 1%. In the mental health clinical population, the prevalence ranges from 2% to 16% (APA, 2000). Narcissistic personality disorder is found more frequently in men than in women (Millon et al., 2004). It also commonly occurs in only children and among first-born boys in cultural groups in which males have special privileges. This disorder can coexist with other Axis II disorders, such as antisocial, histrionic, and paranoid disorders, and Axis I disorders of mood, anxiety, and substance abuse.

Etiology

There is little evidence of any biologic factors that contribute to the development of this disorder. One notion about its development is that it is the result of parents' overvaluation and overindulgence of a child. These children are overly pampered and indulged, with every whim catered to. They learn to view themselves as special beings and to expect special treatment and subservience from others. They do not learn how to cooperate, share, or consider others' desires and interests. An alternate explanation is that the child never truly separated emotionally from his or her primary caregiver and therefore cannot envision functioning independently. The underlying basis of the outward aggrandizement may be one of profound self-hatred and inferiority (Bushman & Baumeister, 1998). To avoid feeling this self-hatred, the person develops a defensive need for power over others (Joubert, 1998; Paulhus, 1998).

Nursing Management

The nurse usually encounters persons with narcissistic personality disorder in medical settings and in psychiatric settings with a coexisting psychiatric disorder. They may be difficult clients who present as being snobbish, condescending, and patronizing in their attitudes. It is unlikely that these individuals are motivated to develop sensitivity to others and socially cooperative attitudes and behaviours. Nurses need to use their self-awareness skills in interacting with these clients. The nursing process focuses on the coexisting responses to other health care problems.

■ CONTINUUM OF CARE

Clients with histrionic and narcissistic personality disorders do not seek mental health care unless they have a coexisting medical or mental disorder. They are likely to be treated within the community for most of their lives, with the exception of short hospitalizations for nonpsychiatric problems.

Cluster C Disorders: Anxious-Fearful

■ AVOIDANT PERSONALITY DISORDER: WITHDRAWN PATTERN

Avoidant personality disorder is characterized by avoiding social situations in which there is interpersonal contact with others. This avoidance is purposeful and deliberate because of fears of criticism and feelings of inadequacy. These individuals are extremely sensitive to negative comments and disapproval. They engage in interpersonal relationships only when they receive unconditional approval. The behaviour becomes problematic when they restrict their social activities and work opportunities because of their extreme fear of rejection. They appear timid, shy, and hesitant. In childhood, they are shy, but instead of growing out of the shyness, it becomes worse in adulthood. They distance themselves from activities that involve personal contact with others. They perceive themselves as socially inept, inadequate, and inferior, which in turn justifies their isolation and rejection by others. They rely on fantasy for the gratification of needs, confidence, and conflict resolution. These individuals withdraw into their fantasies as a means of dealing with frustration and anger. They also have underlying feelings of tension, sadness, and anger that vacillate between desire for affection, fear of rebuff, embarrassment, and numbness of feeling (APA, 2000; Millon et al., 2004; see Table 25-6).

Epidemiology

The lifetime prevalence of avoidant personality disorder was estimated at 3.6% (Faravelli et al., 2000). Avoidant personality disorder has been reported in about 10% of outpatients in mental health clinics. The problem with examining the epidemiology of avoidant personality disorder is its potential overlap with the Axis I disorder, generalized social phobia (social anxiety disorder). Several studies found that a significant portion of the clients with diagnoses of social phobia also met the criteria for avoidant personality disorder. Social phobia was found to be more pervasive and characterized by a higher level of interpersonal sensitivity (Perugi et al., 1999). However, avoidant personality disorder involves greater overall psychopathology (Boone et al., 1999). Not surprisingly, social phobia frequently co-occurs with avoidant personality disorder (Moutier & Stein, 1999). Clients with avoidant personality disorder differ from those with generalized social phobia only in the severity of the anxiety symptoms (less than those with social phobia) and in the depressive symptomatology.

Table 25.6   Summary of Diagnostic Characteristics of Cluster C Disorders

Diagnostic Criteria and Target Symptoms

Avoidant Personality Disorder 301.82
- Pervasive pattern of social inhibition with feelings of inadequacy and hypersensitivity to negative evaluation
- Avoidance of activities involving significant personal contact because of fear of criticism, disapproval, or rejection
- Lack of willingness for involvement unless certainty of being liked
- Restraint within intimate relationships for fear of shame or ridicule
- Preoccupation with criticism or rejection in social situations
- Inhibition in new interpersonal situations
- Viewing self as socially inept, personally unappealing, or inferior
- Unusual reluctance to take personal risks or engage in new activities

Dependent Personality Disorder 301.6
- Pervasive and excessive need for being taken care of, resulting in submission and clinging with fears of separation
- Advice and reassurance needed from others for decision making
- Responsibility for major areas of life assumed by others
- Difficulty expressing disagreement with others for fear of loss of support or approval
- Difficulty initiating things by self
- Excessive methods used to obtain support and nurturance from others
- Uncomfortable and helpless when alone
- Urgent seeking of another relationship if the previous one ends
- Unrealistic preoccupation with fears of having to take care of self

Obsessive-Compulsive Personality Disorder 301.4
- Pervasive pattern of preoccupation with orderliness, perfectionism, and mental and interpersonal control at the expense of flexibility, openness, and efficiency
- Major point of activity lost because of preoccupation
- Task completion interfered with because of perfectionism
- Excessive devotion to work and productivity, excluding friends and leisure
- Overly conscientious, scrupulous, and inflexible about morality, ethics, or values
- Difficulty discarding worn-out or worthless objects
- Reluctance to delegate tasks or work with others
- Miserly spending attitude
- Rigidity and stubbornness

Etiology

Experts speculate that individuals with avoidant personality disorder experience aversive stimuli more intensely and more frequently than do others because they may possess an overabundance of neurons in the aversive centre of the limbic system (Millon et al., 2004). A general biologic vulnerability may be inherited and interact with environmental factors. The evidence for this biologic influence is the impact of pharmacotherapies on these individuals. When taking medications (e.g., benzodiazepines, β-blockers, monoamine oxidase inhibitors), symptoms are reduced, but they resume once medication is stopped (Mattick & Newman, 1991).

Research indicates that those with avoidant personality disorder demonstrate significantly less curiosity and novelty seeking than do healthy control subjects. The research postulated that those with avoidant personality disorder had a more tenuous early attachment (Johnston, 1999). In adulthood, they maintain an ambivalent connection with others, wishing deeply for close, enduring relationships but fearing rejection and loss.

Nursing Management

An assessment of these individuals reveals a lack of social contacts, a fear of being criticized, and evidence of chronic low self-esteem. The nursing diagnoses of chronic low self-esteem, social isolation, and ineffective coping can be used. The establishment of a therapeutic relationship is necessary to be able to help these individuals meet their treatment outcomes. The development of the nurse–client relationship is a slow process and requires an extreme amount of patience on the part of the nurse. These individuals have not had positive interpersonal relationships and need time to be able to trust that the nurse will not criticize and demean them. Interventions should focus on refraining from any negative criticism, assisting the client to identify positive responses from others, exploring previous achievements of success, and exploring reasons for self-criticism. The person's social dimension should be examined for activities that increase self-esteem and interventions focused on increasing these self-esteem–enhancing activities. Social skills training may help reduce symptoms.

■▬ DEPENDENT PERSONALITY DISORDER: SUBMISSIVE PATTERN

People with dependent personality disorder cling to others in a desperate attempt to keep them close. Their need to be taken care of is so great that it leads to doing anything to maintain the closeness, including total submission and disregard for self.

Decision making is difficult. They adapt their behaviour to please those to whom they are attached. They lean on others to guide their lives. They ingratiate themselves to others and denigrate themselves and their accomplishments. Their self-esteem is determined by others. Behaviourally, they withdraw from adult responsibilities by acting helpless and seeking nurturance from others. In interpersonal relationships, they need excessive advice and reassurance. They are compliant, conciliatory, and placating. They rarely disagree with others and are easily persuaded. Friends describe them as gullible. They are warm, tender, and noncompetitive. They timidly avoid social tension and interpersonal conflicts (APA, 2000; see Table 25-6). Dependent personality disorder bears a great deal of resemblance to histrionic personality disorder. People with dependent personality disorder demonstrate high levels of self-attributed dependency needs, whereas those with histrionic personality disorder have a greater implicit dependency and will even argue against needing others (Bornstein, 1998).

Epidemiology

Dependent personality disorder is one of the most frequently reported disorders in mental health clinics (APA, 2000). In clinical samples, the prevalence of this disorder ranges from 2% to 55%, with a median of 20% (Widiger, 1991). The diagnosis is made more frequently in women than in men. This gender difference may represent a sex bias by clinicians because when standardized instruments are used, men and women receive diagnoses at equal rates.

Etiology

It is likely that there is a biologic predisposition to develop the dependency attachments of this disorder. However, no research studies support a biologic hypothesis. Dependent personality disorder most often is explained as a result of parents' genuine affection, extreme attachment, and overprotection. Children then learn to rely on others to meet basic needs and do not learn the necessary skills for autonomous behaviour.

Nursing Management

Nurses can determine the extent of dependency by an assessment of self-worth, interpersonal relationships, and social behaviours. They should determine whether there is currently someone on whom the person relies (e.g., parent, spouse) or if there has been a separation from a significant relationship by death or divorce.

Nursing diagnoses that are usually generated from the assessment data are ineffective individual coping, low self-esteem, impaired social interaction, and impaired home maintenance management. Home management skills may be a problem if the client does not have the useful skills and now has to make decisions related to finances, shopping, cooking, and cleaning. The challenge of caring for these individuals is to help them recognize their dependent patterns, motivate them to want to change, and teach them adult skills that have not been developed, such as balancing a check book, planning a weekly menu, and paying bills. Occasionally, if a client is extremely fatigued, lethargic, or anxious and the disorder interferes with efforts at developing more independence, antidepressants or antianxiety agents may be used.

These individuals readily engage in a nurse–client relationship and initially will look to the nurse to make all decisions. The nurse can support these individuals to make their own decisions by resisting the urge to tell them what to do. Ideally, these clients are in individual psychotherapy and working toward long-term personality changes. The nurse can encourage clients to stay in therapy and to practice the new skills that are being learned. Assertiveness training is helpful.

■▬ OBSESSIVE-COMPULSIVE PERSONALITY DISORDER: CONFORMING PATTERN

OCD stands out in Axis II because it bears close resemblance to obsessive-compulsive anxiety disorder (Axis I). A distinguishing difference is that those with the anxiety disorder tend to use obsessive thoughts and compulsions when anxious but less so when anxiety decreases. With OCD, the person does not demonstrate obsessions and compulsions as much as an overall rigidity, perfectionism, and control. Individuals with this disorder attempt to maintain control by careful attention to rules, trivial details, procedures, and lists (APA, 2000). Individuals with OCD may be completely devoted to work, which typically has a rigid character, such as maintaining financial records or tracking inventories. They are uncomfortable with unstructured leisure time, especially vacations. Leisure activities are likely to be formalized (e.g., season tickets to sports, organized tour groups). Hobbies are approached seriously.

Behaviourally, individuals with OCD are perfectionists, maintaining a regulated, highly structured, strictly organized life. A need to control others and situations is common in personal and in work life. They are prone to repetition and have difficulty making decisions and completing tasks because they become so involved in the details. They can be overly conscientious about morality and ethics and value polite, formal, and correct interpersonal relationships. They also tend to be rigid, stubborn, and indecisive and are unable to accept new ideas and customs. Their mood is tense and joyless. Warm feelings are restrained, and they tightly control the expression of emotions (APA, 2000; see Table 25-6).

Epidemiology

The prevalence of OCD is 1% in the general population and 3% to 10% in individuals receiving treatment in mental health clinics (APA, 2000). This disorder is associated with higher education, employment, and marriage. Subjects with this disorder typically have a higher income than do those without this disorder. This disorder is associated with a greater risk for generalized anxiety disorder and simple phobia and lowered risk for alcohol abuse (Nestadt et al., 1990).

Etiology

As with some of the other personality disorders, there is little evidence for a biologic formulation. The basis of the compulsive patterns that characterize OCD is parental overcontrol and overprotection that is consistently restrictive and sets distinct limits on the child's behaviour. Parents teach these children a deep sense of responsibility to others and to feel guilty when these responsibilities are not met. Play is viewed as shameful, sinful, and irresponsible, leading to dire consequences. They are encouraged to resist the natural inclinations toward play and impulse gratification, and parents try to impose guilt on the child to control behaviour.

Nursing Management

These individuals seek mental health care when they have attacks of anxiety, spells of immobilization, sexual impotence, and excessive fatigue. To change the compulsive pattern, psychotherapy is needed. There may be a short-term pharmacologic intervention with an antidepressant or anxiolytic as an adjunct.

The nursing assessment focuses on the client's physical symptoms (sleep, eating, sexual), interpersonal relationships, and social problems. Typical nursing diagnoses include anxiety, risk for loneliness, decisional conflict, sexual dysfunction, disturbed sleep pattern, and impaired social interactions. People with OCD realize that they can improve their quality of life, but they will find it extremely anxiety provoking to make the necessary changes. A supportive nurse–client relationship based on acceptance of the individual's need for order and rigidity will help the person have enough confidence to try new behaviours. Examining the person's belief that underlies the dysfunctional behaviours can set the stage for challenging the childhood thinking. Because the compulsive pattern was established in childhood, it will take a long time to modify the behaviour.

◼◗ CONTINUUM OF CARE

A long-term therapy is ideal for clients with avoidant personality disorder because it takes time to make the changes. Mental health nurses may see these individuals for other health problems. Encouraging the person to continue with the therapy and contacting the therapist when necessary are important in maintaining continuity of care. These individuals are typically hospitalized only for a coexisting disorder.

People with dependent and obsessive-compulsive personality disorders are treated primarily in the community. If there is a coexisting disorder or the person experiences periods of depression, hospitalization may be useful for a short period of time.

Impulse-Control Disorders

This group of mental disorders has an essential feature: irresistible impulsivity. These disorders are not part of other disorders but often coexist with them. The following impulse-control disorders have been identified:

- Intermittent explosive disorder
- Kleptomania
- Pyromania
- Pathologic gambling
- Trichotillomania

These disorders are characterized by an inability to resist an impulse or temptation to complete an activity that is considered harmful to self or others, an increase in tension before the individual commits the act, and excitement or gratification at the time the act is committed. The release of tension is perceived as pleasurable, but remorse and regret usually follow the act (Gallop, McCay, & Esplen, 1992; see Table 25-7).

Table 25.7	Summary of Diagnostic Characteristics for Impulse-Control Disorders	DSM IV

Diagnostic Criteria and Target Symptoms

Intermittent Explosive Episode 312.34
- Discrete episodes of failing to resist aggressive impulses resulting in serious assaultive acts or property destruction
- Degree of aggressiveness grossly out of proportion to provocation or stressor
- Not better accounted for by another psychiatric disorder; not a direct physiologic effect of a substance or general medical condition

Kleptomania 312.32
- Recurrent failure to resist impulse to steal object that is not needed
- Increased tension before theft
- Pleasure, gratification, or relief at the time of theft
- Theft not related to anger or vengeance; not in response to delusion or hallucination
- Not better accounted for by another psychiatric disorder

Pyromania 312.23
- Multiple episodes of deliberate and purposeful fire setting
- Tension or affective arousal before act
- Fascination with, interest in, curiosity about, or attraction to fires
- Regular fire watchers
- False alarm setters
- Pleasure with institution, equipment, and personnel associated with fires·
- Pleasure gratification or tension relief with fire starting, watching its effects or participating in aftermath
- Not done for monetary gain; expression of ideology, anger, or vengeance; concealing criminal activity; improving living conditions; or as a response to hallucination or delusion
- Not better accounted for by another psychiatric disorder

Pathologic Gambling 312.31
- Persistent and recurrent maladaptive gambling behaviour
- Disruption of personal, family, or vocational pursuits
- Preoccupation with gambling
- Increased amounts of money needed to achieve excitement
- Unsuccessful efforts to stop, cut back, or control
- Restlessness and irritability with attempts to control or cut back
- Means of escape from problems or mood
- Chasing of losses; attempts to get even
- Lying to family and others to conceal involvement
- Commission of illegal acts to finance behaviour
- Significant relationships, jobs, or opportunities jeopardized or lost
- Reliance on others for relief of poor financial situation
- Not better accounted for by manic episode

Trichotillomania 312.39
- Recurrent pulling of one's hair with subsequent hair loss
- Brief episodes throughout the day or sustained periods of hours
- Increased during stress and relaxation periods
- Increased tension immediately before the act and with attempts to resist the urge
- Gratification, pleasure, or relief with the act
- Significant distress and impairment of functioning
- Not better accounted for by another psychiatric disorder; not the effect of a general medical condition

■■■ INTERMITTENT EXPLOSIVE DISORDER

Episodes of aggressiveness that result in an assault or destruction of property characterize people with intermittent explosive disorder. The severity of aggressiveness is out of proportion to the provocation. The episodes can have serious psychosocial consequences, including job loss, interpersonal relationship problems, school expulsion, divorce, automobile crashes, or imprisonment. This diagnosis is given only after all other disorders with aggressive components (e.g., delirium, dementia, head injury, BPD, APD, substance abuse) have been excluded. Little is known about this rare disorder. It is more common in men than in women (APA, 2000).

The treatment of this disorder is multifaceted. Psychopharmacologic agents are sometimes used as an adjunct to psychotherapeutic, behavioural, and social interventions. GABA-ergic mood stabilizers have been used. Anxiolytics are used for obsessive clients who experience tension states and explosive outbursts. Medication alone, however, is insufficient.

KLEPTOMANIA

In **kleptomania**, individuals cannot resist the urge to steal, and they independently steal items that they could easily afford. These items are not particularly useful or wanted. The underlying issue is the act of stealing. The term *kleptomania* was first used in 1838 to describe the behaviour of several kings who stole worthless objects (Goldman, 1992). These individuals experience an increase in tension and then pleasure and relief at the time of the theft. It is a rare condition that occurs in fewer than 5% of shoplifters (APA, 2000). There is little information about this disorder, but it is believed to last for years, despite numerous convictions for shoplifting. It appears to be more common in women. About 81% of reported cases of kleptomania involve women (Goldman, 1991; see Table 25-7).

Some shoplifting appears to be related to anxiety and stress, in that it serves to relieve symptoms, although the etiology is not clear (Grant, Kim, & Grosz, 2003). In a few instances, brain damage has been associated with kleptomania. Depression is the most common symptom identified in a compulsive shoplifter.

Kleptomania is difficult to detect and treat. There are few accounts of treatment, but it appears that behaviour therapy is most frequently used. Antidepressant medication that helps relieve the depression has been successful in some cases. More investigation is needed (Schatzberg, 2000).

PYROMANIA

Irresistible impulses to start fires characterize **pyromania**. These individuals are aroused before setting a fire and are fascinated with fires. They are attracted to fires, often becoming regular "fire watchers" or even firefighters. When they intentionally set fires or make an effort at fire setting, they are not motivated by aggression, anger, suicidal ideation, or political ideology. They may make advanced preparation for the fire. Little is known about this disorder. Most fire setting is not done by people with this disorder. This disorder occurs infrequently, mostly in men (APA, 2000; see Table 25-7).

Low serotonin and norepinephrine levels are associated with arson (Virkkunen, Dejong, Bartko, Goodwin, & Linnoila, 1989). Little is known about its treatment, and as with the other impulse-control disorders, no one approach is uniformly effective. A treatment plan should reflect the special needs of the individual (Soltys, 1992). Education, parenting training, behaviour contracting with token reinforcement, problem-solving skills training, and relaxation exercises may all be used in the management of the individual's responses.

PATHOLOGIC GAMBLING

Social gambling becomes pathologic when it becomes recurrent and disrupts personal, family, or vocational pursuits. These individuals are preoccupied with gambling and experience an aroused, euphoric state during the actual betting. They are drawn to the games and begin making bigger and bigger bets. Characteristically, they relentlessly chase their losses in an attempt to win them back. They are unable to control their gaming and may lie to family, friends, and employers to hide their gambling. These individuals are highly competitive, energetic, restless, and easily bored. The prevalence is estimated at 1% to 3% of the population (APA, 2000); another study found a 3.9% lifetime prevalence (Shaffer, Hall, & Vander Bilt, 1999). Of those individuals in treatment for pathologic gambling, 20% have reported attempting suicide (see Table 25-7).

Over the past two decades, there has been a considerable expansion in legalized gambling in Canada as local and provincial governments have sought to stimulate economic development through tourism and the entertainment sector and to develop new revenue possibilities. The introduction of new technologies, including video lottery terminals (VLTs) and Internet-based gambling, has also been a factor in the expansion (Korn, 2001).

It has been challenging for researchers to establish links between the expansion of legalized gambling and the trends with problematic or pathologic gambling (Hargreave & Csiernik, 2003). Shaffer and Hall (2001) have studied prevalence rates for pathologic gambling in the United States and Canada. Although they found similar rates in both countries, they suggested that segments of the population may develop problem patterns for different reasons and that the psychosocial profile of gamblers may differ between the countries. The uncertainty surrounding the impact of legalized gambling continues to fuel a debate in the media where the balance between risk and benefit is challenged. What is known is that pathologic gambling is associated with depression, suicide attempts, alcohol and drug abuse, family violence, unemployment, and crime (Chacko, Palmer, Gorey, & Butler, 2003; Chiu, Copen, Sadek, Cernovsky, & Husni, 2006; King, 1999). Other comorbid disorders include ADHD; Tourette's syndrome; and personality disorders, especially obsessive-compulsive, avoidant, schizoid, paranoid, and antisocial (Black & Moyer, 1998; Crockford & el-Guebaly, 1998).

This disorder is conceptualized as similar to alcohol and other substances of dependence (Hall et al., 2000; Slutske et al., 2000). When substances are used in conjunction with gambling, they cause a deterioration in play and accelerate the progression of the gambling disorder. The disorder has four phases: winning, losing, desperation, and hopelessness. Pathologic gambling can be treated by psychotherapists experienced in this disorder; for many, Gamblers Anonymous is sufficient (Petry & Armentano, 1999).

Pathologic gamblers feel omnipotent in their ability to win back what was lost. This omnipotence serves as self-deception that leads to denial. Care of these clients involves confronting their omnipotent beliefs. These individuals quickly irritate staff by their self-assurance and overbearing attitude. Staff education about the disorder is important. Family involvement is also crucial. Families often have been dealing with the individual in a dysfunctional manner. Relapse prevention involves learning about specific cues that trigger the gambling behaviour (Selzer, 1992).

With the rise in pathologic gambling and its social consequences, there have been greater efforts to identify supportive pharmacotherapy. Because the underlying mechanisms are anxiety and impulsivity, first-line drugs are SSRIs. These have been moderately effective (Hollander et al., 2000), especially when combined with cognitive-behavioural approaches (Oakley-Browne, Adams, & Mobberly, 2000). Mood stabilizing agents, opioid antagonists, and the atypical dopaminergic agent bupropion have demonstrated some efficacy in treating people with pathologic gambling (Chiu et al., 2006).

TRICHOTILLOMANIA

Trichotillomania is chronic, self-destructive hair pulling that results in noticeable hair loss, usually in the crown, occipital, or parietal areas, although sometimes of the eyebrows and eyelashes. The individual has an increase in tension immediately before pulling out the hair or when attempting to resist the behaviour. After the hair is pulled, the person feels a sense of relief. Some would classify this disorder as one of self-mutilation. It becomes a problem when there is a significant distress or impairment in other areas of function. A hair-pulling session can last several hours, and the individual may ritualistically eat the hairs or discard them. Hair ingestion may result in the development of a hair ball, which can lead to anorexia, stomach pain, anaemia, obstruction, and peritonitis. Other medical complications include infection at the hair-pulling site. Hair pulling is done alone, and usually clients deny it. Instead of pain, these individuals experience pleasure and tension release (APA, 2000; Warmbrodt, Hardy, & Chrisman, 1996; see Table 25-7).

The onset of trichotillomania occurs among children before the age of 5 years and in adolescence. For the young child, distraction or redirection may successfully eliminate the behaviour. The behaviour in adolescents may begin a chronic course that may last well into adulthood. This disorder, although it has been described for over 200 years, is poorly understood. Its prevalence is estimated at 2% to 4% of the population. The cause is unknown (APA, 2000). SSRIs, such as clomipramine and fluoxetine, have shown some success in diminishing the hair-pulling behaviour, as have dopamine antagonists, such as haloperidol (van Ameringen, Mancini, Oakman, & Farvolden, 1999), and opioid antagonists (Kim, 1998). An amino acid N-acetylcysteine has been found to reduce hair-pulling symptoms in adults (Grant, Odlaug, & Kim, 2009).

The assessment includes a review of current problems, developmental history (especially school conflicts, learning difficulties), family history, social history, identification of support systems, previous psychiatric treatment, and health history. Hair-pulling history and pattern are also solicited to determine the duration and severity of the disorders. The typical nursing diagnoses include self-mutilation, low self-esteem, hopelessness, impaired skin integrity, and ineffective denial. Within the therapeutic relationship, a cognitive-behavioural approach can be used to help the client to identify when hair pulling occurs, the precipitating events, and the details of the episode. Teaching about the disorder will help individuals understand that they are not alone and that others have also suffered with this problem. The goal of treatment is to help the client learn to substitute positive behaviours for the hair-pulling behaviour through self-monitoring of events that precipitate the episodes.

CONTINUUM OF CARE

Impulse-control disorders require long-term treatment, usually in an outpatient setting. Hospitalization is rare, except when there are comorbid psychiatric or medical disorders.

SUMMARY OF KEY POINTS

☐ Personality is a complex pattern of characteristics, largely outside of the person's awareness, that compose the individual's distinctive pattern of perceiving, feeling, thinking, coping, and behaving. The personality emerges from a complicated interaction of biologic dispositions, psychological experiences, and environmental situations.

☐ Personality disorder is an enduring pattern of inner experience and behaviour that deviates markedly from the expectations of the individual's culture, is pervasive and inflexible, has an onset in adolescence or early adulthood, is stable over time, and leads to distress or impairment.

☐ The severity of personality disorder can be determined by the characteristics of tenuous stability, adaptive inflexibility, and vicious circles of rigid and inflexible behaviour that result in serious interpersonal problems and social dysfunction.

☐ In the *DSM-IV-TR*, personality disorders are on Axis II and are organized around three clusters or dimensions: cluster A, odd-eccentric disorders; cluster B, dramatic-emotional disorders; and cluster C, anxious-fearful disorders. Any of the personality disorders can coexist with Axis I disorders.

☐ People with cluster A personality disorders whose odd, eccentric behaviours often alienate them from others can benefit from interventions such as social skills training, environmental management, and cognitive skill building. Changing the patterns of thinking and behaving is difficult and takes time; thus, client outcomes must be evaluated in terms of small changes in thinking and behaviour.

☐ In cluster A, paranoid personality disorder is characterized by a suspicious pattern, schizoid personality disorder by an asocial pattern, and schizotypal personality disorder by an eccentric pattern.

☐ People with BPD (cluster B) have difficulties regulating emotion and have extreme fears of abandonment, leading to dysfunctional relationships; they often engage in self-injury.

☐ APD (cluster B), often synonymous with psychopathy, includes people who have no regard for and refuse to conform to social rules.

☐ Individuals with cluster B personality disorders often have difficulties with emotional regulation or being able to recognize and control the expression of their feelings, such as anger, disappointment, and frustration. The nurse can help these clients identify feelings and gain control over their feelings and actions by teaching communication skills and techniques, thought-stopping techniques, distraction, or problem-solving techniques.

☐ Cluster C personality disorders are characterized by anxieties and fears and include avoidant, dependent, and obsessive-compulsive disorders. The obsessive-compulsive personality disorder differs from the obsessive-compulsive anxiety disorder because the individual demonstrates an overall rigidity, perfectionism, and a need for control.

☐ For many people with personality disorders, maintaining a therapeutic nurse–client relationship can be one of the most helpful interventions. Through this therapeutic relationship, the individual experiences a model of healthy interaction, establishing trust, consistency, caring, boundaries, and limitations that help to build the client's self-esteem and respect for self and others. In some personality disorders, nurses will find it more difficult to engage the individual in a true therapeutic relationship because of the person's avoidance of interpersonal and emotional attachment (e.g., APD or paranoid personality disorder).

☐ Individuals with personality disorders are rarely treated in an inpatient facility, except during periods of destructive behaviour or self-injury. Treatment is delivered in the community and over time. Continuity of care is important in helping the individual change lifelong personality patterns.

☐ Although not classified as personality disorders, the impulse-control disorders share one of the primary characteristics of impulsivity, which leads to inappropriate social behaviours that are considered harmful to self or others and that give the individual excitement or gratification at the time the act is committed.

CRITICAL THINKING CHALLENGES

1 Compare and contrast the three common features of personality disorders: tenuous stability, adaptive inflexibility, and vicious circles of behaviour.

2 Define the concepts, *personality* and *personality disorder*. When does a normal personality become a personality disorder?

3 Karen, a 36-year-old woman receiving inpatient care, was admitted for depression; she also has a diagnosis of BPD. After a telephone argument with her husband, she approaches the nurse's station with her wrist dripping with blood from cutting. What nursing diagnosis best fits this behaviour? What interventions should the nurse use with the client once the self-injury is treated?

4 A 22-year-old man with BPD is being discharged from the mental health unit after a severe suicide attempt. As his primary psychiatric nurse, you have been able to establish a therapeutic relationship with him but are now terminating the relationship. He asks you to meet with him "for just a few sessions" after his discharge because his therapist will be on vacation. What are the issues underlying this request? What should you do? Explain and justify.

5 Compare the psychoanalytic explanation of the development of BPD with Linehan's biosocial theory.

6 Compare the characteristics, epidemiology, and etiologic theories of antisocial and borderline personality disorders.

7 Discuss the differences between histrionic and borderline personality disorders.

8 Compare and contrast antisocial and narcissistic personality disorders.

9 Define and summarize the three personality disorders of cluster A. Compare the following among the three disorders:
a. Defining characteristics
b. Epidemiology
c. Biologic, psychological, and social theories

d. Key nursing assessment data
e. Nursing diagnoses and outcomes
f. Specific issues related to a therapeutic relationship
g. Interventions

10 Define and summarize the three personality disorders of cluster C. Compare the following among the three disorders:
a. Defining characteristics
b. Epidemiology
c. Biologic, psychological, and social theories
d. Key nursing assessment data
e. Nursing diagnoses and outcomes
f. Specific issues related to a therapeutic relationship
g. Interventions

11 Define and summarize the impulse-control disorders. Compare the following among the five disorders:
a. Defining characteristics
b. Epidemiology
c. Biologic, psychological, and social theories
d. Key nursing assessment data
e. Nursing diagnoses and outcomes
f. Interventions

WEB LINKS

www.bpdcentral.com This is the site of BPD Central, which provides consumer, family, and professional information and resources.

www.bpdworld.org This is the site of BPDWorld, which provides information, advice, and support for those affected by personality disorders and other related conditions.

www.mentalhealth.com Internet Mental Health is a website for mental health disorders.

www.mhsanctuary.com/borderline This is the site of Borderline Personality Sanctuary, a website for consumers that offers a chat room and books.

www.responsiblegambling.org/index.cfm This is the site of the Responsible Gambling Council (RGC), a nonprofit, Ontario-based organization that helps individuals and communities address gambling in a healthy and responsible way.

MOVIES, NOVELS, AND BIOGRAPHIES

Fatal Attraction: 1987. This award-winning film portrays the relationship between a married attorney, Dan Gallagher (played by Michael Douglas), and Alex Forest, a single woman (played by Glenn Close). Their one-night affair turns into a nightmare for the attorney and his family as Alex becomes increasingly possessive and aggressive, demonstrating behaviours characteristic of BPD: anger, impulsivity, emotional lability, fear of rejection and abandonment, vacillation between adulation and disgust, and self-mutilation.

VIEWING POINTS: Identify Alex's behaviours that are characteristics of BPD. Identify the feelings that are generated by the movie. With which characters do you identify? For which characters do you feel sympathy? If Alex had been admitted to your hospital, what would be your first priority?

The Corporation: 2004. This documentary, winner of many international film awards, asks, "If a corporation is legally considered as a 'person' (as it is in Canada), what kind of person is it?" An assessment is carried out using psychiatric diagnostic criteria, and the average corporation is assessed as having an antisocial personality: fundamentally self-interested, callous and deceitful, without guilt, and breaching societal mores and laws for their own ends.

VIEWING POINTS: Although it is not the film makers' intent, consider if the application of diagnostic criteria in this way enables you to better understand the type of person who merits an antisocial personality disorder diagnosis.

REFERENCES

Ainsworth, M. (1989). Attachments beyond infancy. *American Psychologist, 44*(4), 709–716.
American Psychiatric Association. (2000). *Diagnostic and statistical manual of mental disorders* (4th ed., Text revision). Washington, DC: Author.
Andrews, J. A., Foster, S. L., Capaldi, D., & Hop, H. (2000). Adolescent and family predictors of physical aggression, communication, and satisfaction in young adult couples: A prospective analysis. *Journal of Consulting Clinical Psychology, 68*(2), 195–208.
Barry, C. T., Frick, P. J., DeShazo, T. M., McCoy, M. G., Ellis, M., & Loney, B. R. (2000). The importance of callous-unemotional traits for extending the concept of psychopathy to children. *Journal of Abnormal Psychology, 109*(2), 335–340.
Bartholomew, K., & Horowitz, L. (1991). Attachment styles among young adults: A test of a model. *Journal of Social and Personality Psychology, 61*, 226–244.
Best, M., Williams, J. M., & Coccaro, E. F. (2002). Evidence for a dysfunctional prefrontal circuit in patients with an impulsive aggressive disorder. *Processes of the National Academy of Science, 11*(12), 8448–8853.
Black, D. W., & Moyer, T. (1998). Clinical features and psychiatric comorbidity of subjects with pathological gambling behavior. *Psychiatric Services, 49*(11), 1434–1439.
Black, D., Baumgard, C., & Bell, S. (1995). The long-term outcome of antisocial personality disorder compared with depression, schizophrenia, and surgical conditions. *Bulletin of the American Academy of Psychiatry and Law, 23*(1), 43–52.
Black, D., Blum, N., Pfohl, B., & John, D. (2004). The STEPPS group treatment program for outpatients with borderline personality disorder. *Journal of Contemporary Psychotherapy, 34*, 193–210.
Bland, A., Tudor, G., & Whitehouse, D. M. (2007). Nursing care of inpatients with borderline personality disorder. *Perspectives in Psychiatric Care, 43*(4), 204–212.
Bohus, M., Haaf, B., Stiglmayr, C., Pohl, U., Bohme, R., & Linehan, M. (2000). Evaluation of inpatient dialectical-behavioral therapy for

borderline personality disorder—a prospective study. *Behavior Research and Therapy*, *38*(9), 875–887.

Bohus, M. F., Landwehrmeyer, G. B., Stiglmayr, C. E., Limberger, M. F., Bohme, R., & Schmahl, C. G. (1999). Naltrexone in the treatment of dissociative symptoms in patients with borderline personality disorder: An open-label trial. *Journal of Clinical Psychiatry*, *60*(9), 598–603.

Boone, M. L., McNeil, D. W., Masia, C. L., Turk, C. L., Carter, L. E., Ries, B. J., et al. (1999). Multimodal comparisons of social phobia subtypes and avoidant personality disorder. *Journal of Anxiety Disorders*, *13*(3), 271–292.

Bornstein, R. F. (1998). Implicit and self-attributed dependency needs in dependent and histrionic personality disorders. *Journal of Personality Assessment*, *71*(1), 1–14.

Boughn, S. (2005). Evidence-based nursing care of patients suffering from trichotillomania. *New Jersey Nurse*, *35*(3), 13.

Bowlby, J. (1980). *Loss: Sadness and depression*. New York, NY: Basic Books.

Bucholz, K. K., Heath, A. C., & Madden, P. A. (2000). Transitions in drinking adolescent females: Evidence from the Missouri adolescent female twin study. *Alcohol Clinical Experimental Research*, *24*(6), 914–923.

Bulechek, G., Butcher, H., & McCloskey Dochterman, J. (Eds.). (2008). *Nursing interventions classification (NIC)* (5th ed.). St. Louis, MO: Mosby.

Bushman, B. J., & Baumeister, R. F. (1998). Threatened egotism, narcissism, self-esteem, and direct and displaced aggression: Does self-love or self-hate lead to violence? *Journal of Personality Social Psychology*, *75*(1), 219–229.

Cadenhead, K. S., Perry, W., Shafer, K., & Braff, D. L. (1999). Cognitive functions in schizotypal personality disorder. *Schizophrenia Research*, *37*(2), 123–132.

Campbell, R. J. (2004). *Campbell's psychiatric dictionary* (8th ed.). New York, NY: Oxford University Press.

Cardish, R. J. (2007). Psychopharmacologic management of suicidality in personality disorders. *The Canadian Journal of Psychiatry*, *52*(6 Suppl. 1), 115–127.

Carr, T. (2008). Mapping the processes and qualities of spiritual nursing care. *Qualitative Health Research*, *18*(5), 686–700.

Chacko, J., Palmer, M., Gorey, K., & Butler, N. (2003). Social work with problem gamblers: A key informant survey of service needs. In R. Csiernik & W. Rowe (Eds.), *Responding to the oppression of addiction: Canadian social work perspectives* (pp. 335–343). Toronto, ON: Canadian Scholars' Press.

Chiu, S., Copen, J., Sadek, G., Cernovsky, Z., & Husni, M. (2006, December). Pathological gambling: Co-morbidity and pharmacological treatment. *Canadian Society of Addiction Medicine Bulletin*, *10*(3), 14–19.

Clarkin, J. F., Yeomans, F. E., & Kernberg, O. F. (2006). *Psychotherapy for borderline personality: Focusing on object relations*. Washington, DC: American Psychiatric Press.

Cloninger, C., Bayon, C., & Svrakic, D. (1998). Measurement of temperament and character in mood disorders: A model of fundamental states as personality types. *Journal of Affective Disorders*, *51*(1), 21–32.

Coccaro, E. F. (1998). Clinical outcome of psychopharmacologic treatment of borderline and schizotypal personality disordered subjects. *Journal of Clinical Psychiatry*, *59*(Suppl. 1), 30–35.

Coccaro, E. F., Kavoussi, R. J., Hauger, R. L., Cooper, T. B., & Ferris, C. F. (1998). Cerebrospinal fluid vasopressin levels: Correlates with aggression and serotonin function in personality-disordered subjects. *Archives of General Psychiatry*, *55*(8), 708–714.

Cooke, D. (1996). Psychopathic personality in different culture: What do we know? What do we need to find out? *Journal of Personality Disorders*, *10*(1), 23–40.

Crichton, R. (1959). *The great impostor*. New York, NY: Random House.

Crockford, D. N., & el-Guebaly, M. (1998). Psychiatric comorbidity in pathological gambling: A critical review. *Canadian Journal of Psychiatry*, *43*(1), 43–50.

Dean, M. (2006). *Borderline personality disorder: The latest assessment and treatment strategies* (3rd ed.). Kansas City, MO: Compact Clinicals.

Dolan, M. (1994). Psychopathy: A neurobiological perspective. *British Journal of Psychiatry*, *165*(2), 151–159.

Dolan, M., & Park, I. (2002). The neuropsychology of antisocial personality disorder. *Psychological Medicine*, *32*(3), 417–427.

Dowson, J. H., Sussams, P., Grounds, A. T., & Taylor, J. C. (2001). Associations of past conduct disorder with personality disorders in "nonpsychotic" psychiatric inpatients. *European Psychiatry: The Journal of the Association of European Psychiatrists*, *16*(1), 49–56.

Driessen, M., Herrmann, J., Stahl, K., Zwaan, M., Meier, S., Hill, A., et al. (2000). Magnetic resonance imaging volumes of the hippocampus and the amygdala in women with borderline personality disorder and early traumatization. *Archives of General Psychiatry*, *57*(12), 1115–1122.

Eley, T. C., Lichtenstein, P., & Stevenson, J. (1999). Sex differences in the etiology of aggressive and nonaggressive antisocial behavior: Results from two twin studies. *Child Development*, *70*(1), 155–168.

Erikson, E. (1968). *Identity: Youth and crisis*. New York, NY: Norton.

Farabaugh, A., Fava, M., Mischoulon, D., Sklarsky, K., Petersen, T., & Alpert, J. (2005). Relationships between major depressive disorder and comorbid anxiety and personality disorders. *Comprehensive Psychiatry*, *46*(4), 266–271.

Faravelli, C., Zucchi, T., Viviani, B., Salmoria, R., Perone, A., Paionni, et. al. (2000). Epidemiology of social phobia: A clinical approach. *European Psychiatry*, *15*(1), 17–24.

Faraone, S. V., Biederman, J., Mennin, D., & Russell, R. (1998). Bipolar and antisocial disorders among relatives of ADHD children: Parsing familial subtypes of illness. *American Journal of Medical Genetics*, *81*(1), 108–116.

Farmer, C. M., O'Donnell, B. F., Niznikiewicz, M. A., Voglmaier, M. M., McCarley, R. W., & Shenton, M. E. (2000). Visual perception and working memory in schizotypal personality disorder. *American Journal of Psychiatry*, *157*(5), 781–788.

Feigenbaum, J. (2007). Dialectical behaviour therapy: An increasing evidence base. *Journal of Mental Health*, *16*(1), 51–68.

Gallop, R., McCay, E., & Esplen, J. (1992). The conceptualization of impulsivity for psychiatric nursing practice. *Archives of Psychiatric Nursing*, *6*(6), 366–373.

Galvin, M., Shekhar, A., Simon, J., Stilwell, B., Ten Eyck, R., Laite, G., et al. (1991). Low dopamine-beta-hydroxylase: A biological sequela of abuse and neglect? *Psychiatry Research*, *39*(1), 1–11.

Gerull, F., Meares, R., Stevenson, J., Korner, A., & Newman, L. (2008). The beneficial effect on family life in treating borderline personality. *Psychiatry*, *71*(1), 59–70.

Giancola, P. R. (2000). Temperament and antisocial behavior in preadolescent boys with or without a family history of a substance use disorder. *Psychological Addictive Behaviors*, *14*(1), 56–68.

Goldman, M. (1991). Kleptomania: Making sense of the nonsensical. *American Journal of Psychiatry*, *148*(8), 986–999.

Goldman, M. (1992). Kleptomania: An overview. *Psychiatric Annals*, *22*(2), 68–71.

Gottesman, I., & Goldsmith, H. (1994). Developmental psychopathology of antisocial behavior: Inserting genes into its ontogenesis and epigenesis. In C. Nelson (Ed.), *Threats to optimal development: Integrating biological, social, and psychological risk factors* (Vol. 27, pp. 69–104). Hillsdale, NJ: Erlbaum.

Gotz, M. J., Johnstone, E. C., & Ratcliffe, S. G. (1999). Criminality and antisocial behavior in unselected men with sex chromosome abnormalities. *Psychological Medicine*, *29*(4), 953–962.

Grann, M., Lanstrom, N., Tengstrom, A., & Kullgren, G. (1999). Psychopathy (PCL-R) predicts violent recidivism among criminal offenders with personality disorders in Sweden. *Law & Human Behavior*, *23*(2), 205–217.

Grant, J., Kim, S., & Grosz, R. (2003). Perceived stress in kleptomania. *Psychiatric Quarterly*, *74*(3), 251–258.

Grant, J. E., Odlaug, B. L. & Kim, S. W. (2009). *N*-Acetylcysteine, a glutamate modulator, in the treatment of Trichotillomania: A double-blind, placebo-controlled study. *Archives of General Psychiatry*, *66*(7), 756–763.

Greene, H., & Ugarriza, D. (1995). The "stably unstable" borderline personality disorder: History, theory, and nursing intervention. *Journal of Psychosocial Nursing*, *33*(12), 26–30.

Gregory (2007). Borderline attributions. *American Journal of Psychotherapy*, *61*(2), 131–147.

Grilo, C. (2002). Are there gender differences in DSM-IV personality disorders? *Comprehensive Psychiatry*, *43*(6), 427–430.

Grover, K. E., Carpenter, L. L., Price, L. H., Gagne, G. G., Mello, M., F., & Tyrka, A. R. (2007). The relationship between childhood abuse and adult personality disorder symptoms. *Journal of Personality Disorders*, *21*(4), 442–447.

Gurvits, I. G., Koenigsberg, H. W., & Siever, I. J. (2000). Neurotransmitter dysfunction in patients with borderline personality disorder. *Psychiatric Clinics of North America*, *23*(1), 27–40.

Hall, G. W., Carriero, N. J., Takushi, R. Y., Montoya, I. D., Preston, K. L., & Gorelick, D. A. (2000). Pathological gambling among cocaine-dependent outpatients. *American Journal of Psychiatry*, *157*(7), 1127–1133.

Hanson, R. K., Cadsky, O., Harris, A., & Lalond, C. (1997). Correlates of battering among 997 men: Family history, adjustment, and attitudinal difference. *Violence and Victims, 12*(3), 191–208.

Hare, R. D. (1999). Psychopathy as a risk factor for violence. *Psychiatric Quarterly, 70*(3), 181–197.

Hargreave, C., & Csiernik, R. (2003). An examination of gambling and problem gambling in Canada. In R. Csiernik & W. Rowe (Eds.), *Responding to the oppression of addiction: Canadian social work perspectives* (pp. 313–333). Toronto, ON: Canadian Scholars' Press.

Hayward, B. A. (2007). Cluster A personality disorders: Considering the 'odd-eccentric' in psychiatric nursing. *International Journal of Mental Health Nursing, 16*, 15–21.

Health Canada. (2002). A report on mental illness in Canada: Chapter 5: Personality Disorders. Retrieved August 1, 2008, from http://www.phac-aspc.gc.ca/publicat/miic-mmac/chap_5-eng.php

Herpertz, S. C., Kunnert, H. J., Schwenger, U. B., & Sass, H. (1999). Affective responsiveness in borderline personality disorder: A psychophysiological approach. *American Journal of Psychiatry, 156*(10), 1550–1556.

Herpertz, S. C., Wenning, B., Mueller, B., Qunaibi, M., Sass, H., & Herpertz-Dahlmann, B. (2001). Psychophysiological responses in ADHD boys with and without conduct disorder: Implications for adult antisocial behavior. *Journal of the American Academy of Child & Adolescent Psychiatry, 40*(10), 1222–1230.

Hill, J. (2002). Biological, psychological and social processes in the conduct disorders. *Journal of Child Psychology & Psychiatry & Allied Disciplines, 43*(1), 133–164.

Hill, J. (2003). Early identification of individuals at risk for antisocial personality disorder. *British Journal of Psychiatry-Supplementum, 44*, S11–S14.

Hoffman, P. D., Fruzzetti, A. E., & Buteau, E. (2007). Understanding and engaging families: An education, skills and support program for relatives impacted by borderline personality disorder. *Journal of Mental Health, 16*(1), 69–82.

Hollander, E., DeCaria, C. M., Finkell, J. N., Begaz, R., Wong, C. M., & Carwight, C. (2000). A randomized double-blind fluvoxamine/placebo crossover trial in pathologic gambling. *Biological Psychiatry, 47*(9), 813–817.

Hollander, E., Tracy, K. A., Swann, A. C., Coccaro, E. F., McElroy, S. L., Wozniak, P., et al. (2003). Divalproex in the treatment of impulsive aggression: Efficacy in cluster B personality disorders. *Neuropsychopharmacology, 28*(6), 1186–1197.

Holm, A. L., & Severinsson, E. (2008). The emotional pain and distress of borderline personality disorder: A review of the literature. *International Journal of Mental Health Nursing, 17*(1), 27–35.

Horsfall, J. (1999). Towards understanding some complex borderline behaviours. *Journal of Psychiatric Mental Health Nursing, 6*(6), 425–432.

Hurlemann, R., Hawellek, B., Maier, W., & Dolan, R. (2007). Enhanced emotion-induced amnesia in borderline personality disorder. *Psychological Medicine, 37*(7), 971–981.

Johnson, J. G., Cohen, P., Brown, J., Smailes, E. M., & Bernstein, D. P. (1999). Childhood maltreatment increases risk for personality disorders during early adulthood. *Archives of General Psychiatry, 56*(7), 607–608.

Johnson, D. M., Sheahan, T. C., & Chard, K. M. (2003). Personality disorders, coping strategies, and posttraumatic stress disorder in women with histories of childhood sexual abuse. *Journal of Child Sexual Abuse, 12*(2), 19–39.

Johnston, M. A. (1999). Influences of adult attachment in exploration. *Psychological Reports, 84*(1), 31–34.

Jordan, J. V. (2004). Personality disorder or relational disconnection. In J. J. Magnavita (Ed.), *Handbook of personality disorders* (pp. 120–134). Hoboken, NJ: John Wiley.

Joubert, C. E. (1998). Narcissism, need for power, and social interest. *Psychological Report, 82*(2), 701–702.

Kavoussi, R. J., & Coccaro, E. F. (1998). Divalproex sodium for impulsive aggressive behavior in patients with personality disorder. *Journal of Clinical Psychiatry, 59*(12), 676–680.

Kiehl, K. A., Smith, A. M., Hare, R. D., Mendrek, A., Forster, B. B., Brink, J., et al. (2001). Limbic abnormalities in affective processing by criminal psychopaths as revealed by functional magnetic resonance imaging. *Biological Psychiatry, 50*(9), 677–684.

Kim, S. W. (1998). Opioid antagonists in the treatment of impulse-control disorders. *Journal of Clinical Psychiatry, 59*(4), 159–164.

Kim, J. E., Hetherington, E. M., & Reiss, D. (1999). Associations among family relationships, antisocial peers, and adolescents' externalizing behaviors: Gender and family type differences. *Child Development, 70*(5), 1209–1230.

King, A. (1999). *Diary of a powerful addiction.* Tyndall, MB: Crown.

Korn, D. A. (2001). Research as a foundation for action on gambling. *Canadian Journal of Public Health, 92*(3), 165–166.

Krause, E. D., Mendelson, T., & Lynch, T. R. (2003). Childhood emotional invalidation and adult psychological distress: The mediating role of emotional inhibition. *Child Abuse & Neglect, 27*, 199–213.

Lahey, B. B., Gordon, R. A., Loeber, R., Stouthamer-Loeber, M., & Farrington, D. P. (1999). Boys who join gangs: A prospective study of predictors of first gang entry. *Journal of Abnormal Child Psychology, 27*(4), 261–276.

Langbehn, D. R., & Cadoret, R. J. (2001). The adult antisocial syndrome with and without antecedent conduct disorder: Comparisons from an adoption study. *Comprehensive Psychiatry, 42*(4), 272–282.

LeGris, J., & van Reekum, R. (2006). The neuropsychological correlates of borderline personality disorder and suicidal behaviour. *Canadian Journal of Psychiatry, 51*(3), 131–142.

Lejoyeux, M., Boulenguiez, S., Fichelle, A., McLoughlin, M., Claudon, M., & Ades, J. (2000). Alcohol dependence among patients admitted to psychiatric emergency services. *General Hospital Psychiatry, 22*(3), 206–212.

Lenzenweger, M. F., & Clarkin, J. F. (2005). The personality disorders: History, classification, and research issues. In M. F. Lenzenweger & J. F. Clarkin (Eds.), *Major theories of personality disorders* (pp. 1–42). New York, NY: Guilford.

Linehan, M. (1993a). *Cognitive-behavioral treatment of borderline personality disorder.* New York, NY: Guilford.

Linehan, M. (1993b). *Skills training manual for treating borderline personality disorder.* New York, NY: Guilford.

Links, P. S., Heslegrave, R., & van Reekum R. (1998). Prospective follow-up study of borderline personality disorder: Prognosis, prediction of outcome, and Axis II comorbidity. *Canadian Journal of Psychiatry, 43*(3), 265–270.

Links, P. S., & Stockwell, M. (2004). Couples therapy with a paranoid personality-disordered client. In M. M. MacFarlane (Ed.), *Family treatment of personality disorders: Advances in clinical practice* (pp. 361–380). New York, NY: Haworth.

Lykken, D. T. (2006). Psychopathic personality: The scope of the problem. In C. J. Patrick (Ed.), *Handbook of psychopathy* (pp. 3–13). New York, NY: Guilford.

Lyons, M. (1995). Epidemiology of personality disorders. In M. Tsuang, M. Tohen, & G. Zahner (Eds.), *Textbook in psychiatric epidemiology.* New York, NY: Wiley-Liss.

Magnavita, J. J. (Ed.). (2004). The relevance of theory in treating personality dysfunction. In *Handbook of personality disorders: Theory and practice* (pp. 56–77). Hoboken, NJ: John Wiley & Sons.

Mahler, M., Pine, F., & Bergman, A. (1975). *The psychological birth of human infant: Symbiosis and individuation.* New York, NY: Basic Books.

Marcus, R. F. (1999). A gender-linked exploratory factor analysis of antisocial behavior in young adolescents. *Adolescence, 34*(133), 33–46.

Martin, E. A. (Ed.). (2007). *Concise medical dictionary* (7th ed.). London, UK: Oxford.

Matta, I., Sham, P. C., Gilvarry, C. M., Jones, P. B., Lewis, S. W., & Murray, R. M. (2000). Childhood schizotypy and positive symptoms in schizophrenic patients predict schizotypy in relatives. *Schizophrenia Research, 44*(2), 129–136.

Mattick, R., & Newman, C. (1991). Social phobia and avoidant personality disorder. *International Review of Psychiatry, 3*(2), 163–173.

McDougle, C. J., Kresch, L. E., & Posey, D. J. (2000). Repetitive thoughts and behavior in pervasive developmental disorders: Treatment with serotonin reuptake inhibitors. *Journal of Autism & Development Disorders, 30*(5), 427–435.

Messina, N. P., Wish, E. D., & Nemes, S. (1999). Therapeutic community treatment for substance abusers with antisocial personality disorder. *Journal of Substance Abuse Treatment, 17*(1–2), 121–128.

Meyer, B., & Pilkonis, P. A. (2005). An attachment model of personality disorders. In M. F. Lenzenweger & J. F. Clarkin (Eds.), *Major theories of personality disorders* (pp. 231–281). New York, NY: Guilford.

Miller, S. (1994). Borderline personality disorder from a patient's perspective. *Hospital and Community Psychiatry, 45*(12), 1215–1219.

Millon, T., & Davis, R. (1999). *Personality disorders in modern life.* New York, NY: John Wiley.

Millon, T., Millon, C., Meagher, S., Grossman, S., & Ramnath, R. (2004). *Personality disorders in modern life* (2nd ed.). New York, NY: John Wiley.

Moran, P. (1999). The epidemiology of antisocial personality disorder. *Social Psychiatry & Psychiatric Epidemiology, 34*(5), 231–242.

Moutier, C. Y., & Stein, M. B. (1999). The history, epidemiology, and differential diagnosis of social anxiety disorder. *Journal of Clinical Psychiatry, 60*(Suppl. 9), 4–8.

Murphy, J. (1976). Psychiatric labeling in cross-cultural perspective: Similar kinds of disturbed behavior appear to be labeled abnormal in diverse cultures. *Science, 191*(4231), 1019–1028.

Myers, M. G., Stewart, D. G., & Brown, S. A. (1998). Progression from conduct disorder to antisocial personality disorder following treatment for adolescent substance abuse. *American Journal of Psychiatry, 155*(4), 479–485.

Nehls, N. (1998). Borderline personality disorder: Gender stereotypes, stigma and limited system of care. *Issues in Mental Health Nursing, 19*(2), 97–112.

Nehls, N. (1999). Borderline personality disorder: The voice of patients. *Research in Nursing & Health, 22*(4), 285–293.

Nestadt, G., Romanoski, A., Chahal, R., Merchant, A., Folstein, M., Gruenberg, E., et al. (1990). An epidemiological study of histrionic personality disorder. *Psychological Medicine, 20*(2), 413–422.

Nolan, K. A., Volavka, J., Mohr, P., & Czobor, P. (1999). Psychopathy and violent behavior among patients with schizophrenia or schizoaffective disorder. *Psychiatric Services, 50*(6), 787–792.

Oakley-Browne, M. A., Adams, P., & Mobberly, P. M. (2000). Interventions for pathological gambling. *Cochrane Database System Review, 2*, CD001521.

O'Donohue, W., Fowler, K., & Lilienfeld, S. (Eds.). (2007). *Personality disorders: Toward the DSM-V.* Los Angeles, CA: Sage.

Oquendo, J. A., & Mann, J. J. (2000). The biology of impulsivity and suicidality. *Psychiatric Clinics of North America, 23*(1), 11–25.

Pagani, L., Boulerice, B., Vitaro, F., & Tremblay, R. E. (1999). Effects of poverty on academic failure and delinquency in boys: A change and process model approach. *Journal of Child Psychology & Psychiatry, 40*(8), 119–120.

Paris, J. (2007). *Half in love with death: Managing the chronically suicidal patient.* Mahwah, NJ: Lawrence Erlbaum.

Paulhus, D. L. (1998). Interpersonal and intrapsychic adaptiveness of trait self-enhancement: A mixed blessing? *Journal of Personality and Social Psychology, 74*(5), 1197.

Perugi, G., Nassini, S., Socci, C., Lenzi, M., Toni, C., Simonini, E., et al. (1999). Avoidant personality in social phobia and panic-agoraphobia disorder: A comparison. *Journal of Affective Disorders, 54*(3), 277–282.

Petry, N. M., & Armentano, C. (1999). Prevalence, assessment, and treatment of pathological gambling: A review. *Psychiatric Services, 50*(8), 1021–1027.

Pezze, M. A., & Feldon, J. (2004). Mesolimbic dopaminergic pathways in fear conditioning. *Progress in Neurobiology, 74*(5), 301–320.

Pinto, O. C., & Akiskal, H. S. (1998). Lamotrigine as a promising approach to borderline personality: An open case series without concurrent DSM-IV major mood disorder. *Journal of Affective Disorder, 51*(3), 333–343.

Reti, I. M., Samuels, J. F., Eaton, W. W., Bienvenu, O. J. III, Costa, P. T., Jr., & Nestadt, G. (2002). Adult antisocial personality traits are associated with experiences of low parental care and maternal overprotection. *Acta Psychiatrica Scandinavica, 106*(2), 126–133.

Robins, L., Tipp, J., & Przybeck, T. (1991). Antisocial personality. In L. N. Robins & D. Reiger (Eds.), *Psychiatric disorders in America: The epidemiological catchment area study* (pp. 258–291). New York, NY: Free Press.

Rouff, L. (2000). Schizoid personality traits among the homeless mentally ill: A quantitative and qualitative report. *Journal of Social Distress and Homelessness, 9*(2), 127–141.

Rushton, J., & Irwing, P. (2008). A general factor of personality (GFP) from two meta-analyses of the Big Five: Digman (1997) and Mount, Barrick, Scullen, and Rounds (2005). *Personality and Individual Differences, 45*, 679–683.

Schatzberg, A. F. (2000). New indications of antidepressants. *Journal of Clinical Psychiatry, 61*(Suppl. 11), 9–17.

Schubiner, H., Tzelepis, A., Milberger, S., Lockhart, N., Kruger, M., Kelley, B. J., et al. (2000). Prevalence of attention-deficit/hyperactivity disorder and conduct disorder among substance abusers. *Journal of Clinical Psychiatry, 61*(4), 244–251.

Selzer, J. (1992). Borderline omnipotence in pathological gambling. *Archives of Psychiatric Nursing, 6*(4), 215–218.

Shaffer, H. J., & Hall, M. N. (2001). Updating and refining prevalence estimates of disordered gambling behaviour in the United States and Canada. *Canadian Journal of Public Health, 92*(3), 168–172.

Shaffer, H. J., Hall, M. N., & Vander Bilt, J. (1999). Estimating the prevalence of disordered gambling behavior in the United States and Canada: A research synthesis. *American Journal of Public Health, 89*(9), 1369–1376.

Sigmund, D., Barnett, W., & Mundt, C. (1998). The hysterical personality disorder: A phenomenological approach. *Psychopathology, 31*(6), 318–330.

Silk, K. R. (2000). Borderline personality disorder. Overview of biologic factors. *Psychiatric Clinical North America, 23*(1), 61–75.

Silverthorn, P., & Frick, P. J. (1999). Developmental pathways to antisocial behavior: The delayed-onset pathway in girls. *Developmental Psychopathology, 11*(1), 101–126.

Skodol, A. E., Siever, L. J., Livesley, W. J., Gunderson, J. G., Pfohl, B., & Widiger, T. A. (2002). The borderline diagnosis II: Biology, genetics, and clinical course. *Biological Psychiatry, 51*, 951–963.

Slutske, W., Eisen, S., True, W., Lyons, M., Goldberg, J., & Tsuang, M. (2000). Common genetic vulnerability for pathological gambling and alcohol dependence in men. *Archives of General Psychiatry, 57*(7), 666–673.

Smallbone, S. W., & Dadds, M. R. (2000). Attachment and coercive sexual behavior. *Sex Abuse, 12*(1), 3–15.

Soderstrom, H., Blennow, K., Sjodin, A. K., & Forsman, A. (2003). New evidence for an association between the CSF HVA: 5-HIAA ratio and psychopathic traits. *Journal of Neurology, Neurosurgery & Psychiatry, 74*(7), 918–921.

Soloff, P. H. (2000). Psychopharmacology of borderline personality disorder. *Psychiatric Clinics of North America, 23*(1), 169–192.

Soloff, P., Lis, J., Kelly, T., Cornelius, J., & Ulrich, R. (2004). Risk factors for suicidal behavior in borderline personality disorder. *American Journal of Psychiatry, 151*(9), 1316–1323.

Soltys, S. (1992). Pyromania and firesetting behaviors. *Psychiatric Annals, 22*(2), 79–83.

Stahl, S. M., & Grady, M. M. (2005). *Essential psychopharmacology: The prescriber's guide.* Cambridge, UK: Cambridge University Press.

Stalenheim, E. G., von Knorring, L., & Wide, L. (1998). Serum levels of thyroid hormones as biological markers in a Swedish forensic psychiatric population. *Biological Psychiatry, 43*(10), 755–761.

Stern, A. (1938). A psychoanalytic investigation and therapy in the borderline group of neuroses. *Psychoanalytic Quarterly, 7*, 467–489.

Strike, C., Rhodes, A. E., Bergmans, Y., & Links, P. (2006). Fragmented pathways to care: The experiences of suicidal men. *Crisis, 27*(1), 31–38.

Teplin, D., O'Connell, T., Daiter J., & Varenbut, M. (2004). A psychometric study of the prevalence of DSM-IV personality disorders among office-based methadone maintenance patients. *American Journal of Drug and Alcohol Abuse, 30*(3), 515–524.

Torgersen, S., Kringlen, E., & Cramer, V. (2001). The prevalence of personality disorders in a community sample. *Archives of General Psychiatry, 58*(6), 590–596.

Tuohig, G., Saffle, J., Sullivan, J., Morris, S., & Lento, S. (1995). Self-inflicted patient burns: Suicide versus mutilation. *Journal of Burn Care and Rehabilitation, 16*(4), 429–436.

van Ameringen, M., Mancini, C., Oakman, J. M., & Farvolden, P. (1999). The potential role of haloperidol in the treatment of trichotillomania. *Journal of Affective Disorders, 56*(2–3), 219–226.

van den Bosch, L. M., Verheul, R., Schippers, G. M., & van den Brink, W. (2002). Dialectical behavior therapy of borderline patients with and without substance use problems: Implementation and long-term effects. *Addictive Behaviors, 27*(6), 911–923.

van Reekum, R. (1993). Acquired and developmental brain dysfunction in borderline personality disorder. *Canadian Journal of Psychiatry, 38*(1), 54–58.

Van Wel, B., Kockmann, I., Blum, N., Pfohl, B., Black, D., & Heesterman, W. (2006). STEPPS group treatment for borderline personality disorder in the Netherlands. *Annals of Clinical Psychiatry, 18*(1), 63–67.

Veit, R., Flor, H., Erb, M., Hermann, C., Lotze, M., Grodd, W., et al. (2002). Brain circuits in emotional learning in antisocial behavior and social phobia in humans. *Neuroscience Letters, 328*(3), 233–236.

Virkkunen, M., Dejong, J., Bartko, J., Goodwin, F. K., & Linnoila, M. (1989). Relationship of psychobiological variables to recidivism in violent offenders and impulsive fire setters. *Archives of General Psychiatry, 46*(7), 600–603.

Voglmaier, M. M., Seidman, L. J., Niznikiewicz, M. A., Dickey, C. C., Shenton, M. E., & McCarley, R. W. (2000). Verbal and nonverbal neuropsychological test performance in subjects with schizotypal personality disorder. *American Journal of Psychiatry, 157*(5), 787–793.

Wade, T., Pevalin, D., & Brannigan, A. (1999). The clustering of severe behavioural, health and educational deficits in Canadian children: Preliminary evidence from the National Longitudinal Survey of Children and Youth. *Canadian Journal of Public Health, 90*(4), 253–259.

Waldeck, T. L., & Miller, L. S. (2000). Social skills deficits in schizotypal personality disorder. *Psychiatry Research, 93*(3), 237–246.

Waldman, I. D., & Slutske, W. S. (2000). Antisocial behavior and alcoholism: A behavioral genetic perspective on comorbidity. *Clinical Psychological Review, 20*(2), 255–287.

Ward, R. K. (2004). Assessment and management of personality disorders. *American Family Physician, 70*(8), 1505–1512.

Warmbrodt, L., Hardy, E., & Chrisman, S. (1996). Understanding trichotillomania. *Journal of Psychosocial Nursing, 34*(12), 11–15.

Widiger, T. (1991). *DSM-IV* reviews of the personality disorders: Introduction to special series. *Journal of Personality Disorders, 5*(2), 122–134.

Widiger, T., & Samuel, D. (2005). Diagnostic categories or dimensions? A question for the Diagnostic and Statistical Manual of Mental Health Disorders–Fifth Edition. *Journal of Abnormal Psychology, 114*(4), 494–504.

Widiger, T., & Weissman, M. (1991). Epidemiology of borderline personality disorder. *Hospital & Community Psychiatry, 42*(10), 1015–1021.

Wilkinson-Ryan, T., & Westen, D. (2000). Identity disturbance in borderline personality disorder: An empirical investigation. *American Journal of Psychiatry, 157*(4), 528–541.

Yen, S., Shea, M. T., Battle, C. L., Johnson, D. M., Zlotnick, C., Dolan-Sewell, R., et al. (2002). Traumatic exposure and posttraumatic stress disorder in borderline, schizotypal, avoidant and obsessive-compulsive personality disorders: Findings from the Collaborative Longitudinal Personality Disorders Study. *Journal of Nervous and Mental Disease, 190,* 510–518.

Yeomans, F., Hull, J., & Clarkin, J. (1994). Risk factors for self-damaging acts in a borderline population. *Journal of Personality Disorders, 8*(1), 10–16.

Young, J. E. (1999). *Cognitive therapy for personality disorders: A schema-focused approach* (3rd ed.). Sarasota, FL: Professional Resource Press.

Zanarini, M. C., Frankenburg, F. R., Reich, D. B., Silk, K. R., Hudson, J. I., & McSweeney, L. B. (2007). The subsyndromal phenomenology of borderline personality disorder: A 10-year follow-up study. *American Journal of Psychiatry, 164*(6), 929–935.

Zanarini, M. C., Ruser, T., Frankenburg, F. R., & Hennen, J. (2000). The dissociative experiences of borderline patients. *Comprehensive Psychiatry, 41*(3), 223–227.

Zanarini, M. C., Williams, A. A., Lewis, R. E., Reich, R. B., Vera, S. C., Marino, M. F., et al. (1997). Reported pathological childhood experiences associated with the development of borderline personality disorder. *American Journal of Psychiatry, 154*(8), 1101–1106.

Zlotnick, C. (1999). Antisocial personality disorder, affect dysregulation and childhood abuse among incarcerated women. *Journal of Personality Disorders, 13*(1), 90–95.

Zweig-Frank, F., Paris, J., & Guzder, J. (1994a). Dissociation in female patients with borderline and non-borderline personality disorders. *Journal of Personality Disorders, 8*(3), 203–209.

Zweig-Frank, F., Paris, J., & Guzder, J. (1994b). Psychological risk factors for dissociation and self-mutilation in female patients with borderline personality disorder. *Canadian Journal of Psychiatry, 39*(5), 259–264.

UNIT V

Children and Adolescents

Mental Health Promotion With Children and Adolescents

Wendy Austin

Adapted from the chapter "Mental Health Promotion with Children and Adolescents" by Jean Robinson Hughes, Catherine Gray Deering, Lawrence Scahill, Nazilla Khanlou, and Freida Chavez

LEARNING OBJECTIVES

After reading this chapter, the student will be able to:

*   Describe the protective factors in the mental health promotion of children and adolescents.
*   Identify the risk factors for the development of psychopathology in childhood and adolescence.
*   Analyze the role of the nurse in mental health promotion with children and families.

KEY CONCEPTS

*   grief in childhood
*   invincibility fable

KEY TERMS

• attachment • bibliotherapy • child abuse and neglect • developmental delay • early intervention programs • family preservation • fetal alcohol spectrum disorder • formal operations • normalization • protective factor • psychoeducational programs • resilience • risk factor • social skills training

C hildren and adolescents respond to the stresses of life in different ways according to their developmental levels. This chapter examines the importance of childhood and adolescent mental health, identifies core prevention strategies, discusses the effects of common childhood stressors, identifies stressors that create risk for psychopathology, and provides guidelines for mental health promotion and risk reduction. Nurses are in a key position to identify and intervene with children and adolescents at risk for psychopathology by virtue of their close contact with families in health care settings and their roles as educators. Knowing the difference between normal child development and psychopathology is crucial in helping parents to view their children's behaviour realistically and to respond appropriately.

CHILDHOOD AND ADOLESCENT MENTAL HEALTH

According to the goals of Canada's National Children's Agenda (Federal/Provincial/Territorial Council on Social Policy Renewal, 2000), children's needs include physical and emotional health, safety and security, success at learning, and social engagement and responsibility. Supportive social networks and positive childhood and adolescent experiences maximize the mental health of children and adolescents. Children are more likely to be mentally healthy if they have normal physical and psychosocial development, an easy temperament (e.g., adaptable, low intensity, positive mood), and a secure **attachment** at an early age. These three areas are considered in the mental health assessment of children (see Chapter 27). **Developmental delays** not only slow the child's progress but also can interfere with the development of positive self-esteem. Children with an easy temperament can adapt to change without intense emotional reactions. A secure attachment helps the child test the world without fear of rejection. Parents, in particular, play a critical role in preventing adverse outcomes in their children and, if needed, can be assisted to learn ways of being optimally responsive to their children. Families transmit and interpret values to their children and teach them how to make connections with, and get along in, the larger world—particularly during the early years of life (Schor & the American Academy of Paediatrics Task Force on the Family, 2003).

• CRNENOTE

Attachment and temperament are key concepts in the behaviour of children and adolescents in any health care setting. Consider how you would apply these concepts to the care of any paediatric patient.

■■■ COMMON CHILDHOOD STRESSORS

Stress is an inevitable part of life and may originate in any one area, or several common areas, including the following:

- The community: violence, poverty, lack of safety and supports, inadequate housing.
- The home/family environment: disorganization, conflict, transience, breakup, lack of supplies and resources.
- Parent–child interactions: parent shows insensitivity or responses of rejection, angry or harsh discipline, frightened behaviour, a failure to protect the child; the child may lack eye contact or manipulate the parent.
- Parent: lack of parenting knowledge and skills, lack of education, negative attributions to the child, unresolved loss/trauma, developmental delay, a history of parenting difficulties, high stress, chronic health problems, substance abuse.
- Child: difficult temperament, birth difficulties (e.g., prematurity, developmental delay, failure to thrive), extreme sensitivity to sensory experiences, suspected abuse/neglect, loss of a significant caregiver, withdrawal, extreme activity level, aggressive behaviour and

emotional dysregulation/reactivity, substance abuse (Infant Mental Health Promotion, 2005, p. 2).

Regardless of the origin, stress usually causes conflict and difficulty with family relationships. These responses to stress can disrupt parenting as well as the interactions between the parent and the child and can lead to short-term or lasting poor outcomes. The earlier these events begin and the longer that the disruption lasts, the worse the outcomes for children (Schor et al., 2003).

Loss: Death and Grief

It is important for nurses to recognize that death and grief are universally experienced by children and therefore are the most common stresses encountered. It is of paramount importance for nurses to understand that children do not respond in the same way as adults. The most common losses experienced are death of a grandparent, parental divorce, death of a pet, and loss of friends through moving or changing schools. Learning to mourn losses can lead to a renewed appreciation of the precious value of life and close relationships. Vast research shows that both children and adults who experience major losses are at risk for mental health problems, particularly if the natural grieving process is impeded. The grieving process differs somewhat between children and adults (Table 26-1).

KEY CONCEPT **Grief in childhood** is shaped by both developmental stages and experiences (Pfund, 2006). Similar to the experience of adults, children's grief is experienced in stages. Children's grief usually begins without understanding the full effects of the loss, and they experience some numbness or dulling of emotional pain. This stage progresses to a greater acceptance of the reality of the loss, which leads to more intense psychological pain. Finally, they undergo a reorganization of identity to incorporate the loved person, which may involve engaging in new activities and interests.

Children's responses to loss reflect their developmental level, as well as their previous experience. As early as age 3 years, children can have some concept of death. For example, the death of a goldfish provides an opportunity for the child to grasp the idea that the fish will never swim again. However, not until about age 7 years can most children understand the permanence of death. Before this age, they may verbalize that someone has "died" but in the next sentence ask when the dead person will be "coming back." Even though the finality of death is understood by early adolescence (Brown, 2009), adolescents sometimes flirt with death by driving dangerously or engaging in other risky behaviours, as if they believe that they are

Table 26.1	Grieving in Childhood, Adolescence, and Adulthood	
Children	**Adolescents**	**Adults**
• View death as reversible: do not understand that death is permanent until about age 7 years • Experiment with ideas about death by killing bugs, staging funerals, acting out death in play • Mourn through activities (e.g., mock funerals, playing with things owned by the loved one); may not cry • May not discuss the loss openly, but express grief through regression, somatic complaints, behaviour problems, or withdrawal • Need repeated explanations to fully understand the loss; it may be helpful to read children's books that explain death	• Understand that death is permanent but may flirt with death (e.g., reckless driving, unprotected sex) due to omnipotent feelings • May be fascinated by death, enjoy morbid books and movies, listen to rock music about death and suicide • Mourn by talking about the loss, crying, and reflecting on it, sometimes becoming dramatic (e.g., overidentifying with the lost person, developing poetic or romantic ideas about death) • Often withdraw when mourning or seek comfort through peer groups; may feel parents do not understand their feelings • Need permission to grieve openly because they may believe they should act strong or take care of the adults involved; need acceptance of their sometimes extreme reactions	• Understand that death is permanent: may struggle with spiritual beliefs about death • May try not to think about death, depending on cultural background • Mourn through talking about the loss, crying, reviewing memories, and thinking privately about it • Usually discuss loss openly, depending on level of support available; may feel there is a "time limit" on how long it is socially acceptable to grieve • Need friends, family, and other supportive people to listen and allow them to mourn for however long it takes; need opportunities to review their feelings and memories

immune to death. This phenomenon is known as the *invincibility fable* because adolescents view themselves in an egocentric way, as unique and invulnerable to the consequences experienced by others.

> ⊛ **KEY CONCEPT Invincibility fable** is an aspect of egocentric thinking in adolescence that causes teens to view themselves as immune to dangerous situations, such as unprotected sex, fast driving, and drug abuse.

The concept of death is difficult to grasp, and adults should be sensitive to the child's struggle to understand and cope with it. Most children closely watch their parents' response to grief and loss and use fantasy to fill the gaps in their understanding. In many cases, family members take turns grieving, and some children may sense that their parents are so overwhelmed by their own emotional pain that they cannot bear the children's grief.

It has been recently recognized that children and adolescents may experience complicated grief. *Complicated grief* is a form of bereavement-related distress that can include such symptoms as being preoccupied with thoughts of the deceased, including difficulty accepting the death, and numbness, bitterness, or a sense of futility (Dillen, Fontaine, & Verhofstadt-Denève, 2009; Melhem, Moritz, Walker, Shear, & Brent, 2007). An indication

that bereaved children may need mental health services is related to such things as level of functioning (e.g., grief responses), coping, self-esteem, and aspects of their family environment (e.g., stressors, parenting) (Brown, Sandler, Tein, Liu, & Haine, 2007).

Loss and Preschool-Aged Children

The preschool-aged child may react more to the parents' distress about a death than to the death itself. Young children who depend totally on their parents may be frightened when they see their parents upset. Anything the parent can do to alleviate the child's anxiety, such as reassuring him or her that the parent will be okay and continuing the child's normal routine (e.g., normal bedtimes, snacks, play times), will help the child to feel secure. Because preschool-aged children have limited ability to verbalize their feelings, they may need to express them through fantasy play and activities, such as mock funerals. Books that explain death, such as *Charlotte's Web* by E. B. White, may also be helpful. Parents should take care not to use euphemisms that could fuel misconceptions of death, such as "He went to sleep" or "Jesus took him." Young children may interpret these messages literally and fear going to sleep (because they might die) or focus their natural, grief-related anger on the irrational idea that the person deliberately has not returned. The best approach is to explain honestly that the person has died and is not coming back, elicit the child's understanding

Developmental level

Does the child have a basic understanding of death, an awareness that adults' emotional upset is not catastrophic, and good coping skills?

Child's wishes

Does the child express a desire to go to the funeral and display a basic understanding of what will happen?

Does the ethnic group have an open approach to death? Do children commonly attend funerals?

Is there a familiar adult who is coping adequately with their own grief available to monitor the child's needs?

Ethnic/ cultural background

Support & supervision

FIGURE 26.1 Factors that influence whether a child should attend a funeral.

and questions about what has happened, and then repeat this process continually as the child gradually begins to grasp the reality of the situation. The decision of whether to take a small child to a funeral may be particularly complex. Figure 26-1 enumerates some factors to consider.

Loss and School-Aged Children

School-aged children understand the permanence of death more clearly than do preschoolers, but they may be unable to express their feelings in a grown-up way. Children in this age group may express their grief through somatic complaints; finding comfort in behaviours engaged in during earlier developmental stages, also known as regression; behaviour problems; withdrawal; and even hostility toward parents. They may think that others expect them to cry and react with immediate emotional intensity to the death; when they do not react this way, they may feel guilty.

Loss and Adolescents

Adolescents who are in Piaget's stage of formal operations can better understand death as an abstract concept. **Formal operations** is the period of cognitive development characterized by the ability to use abstract reasoning to conceptualize and solve problems. Because adolescents tend to be idealistic and to think in extremes, they may even have poetic or romantic notions about death. Many teenagers become fascinated with morbid rock music, movies, and books. Although they may be able to express

their thoughts and feelings about death more clearly than younger children, they often are reluctant to do so for the fear of being viewed as childish. Some adolescents assume a parental role in the family after a death, denying their own needs. School settings may be particularly helpful in providing group and individual support for grieving adolescents, particularly as a preventive intervention (Van Epps, Oppie, & Goodwin, 1997).

Separation and Divorce

According to the Institute of Marriage and Family Canada (2009), separation and divorce are realities for a good number of children in Canada—224 per 1,000 in 2003, about half the rate reported for the United States. Trends show that divorce now occurs earlier in a child's life, and although joint custody is becoming more common (13%), mothers retain the sole custody of the children in about 79% of the cases (Child Support Team of the Department of Justice, 2000). In addition, about 40% of the children rarely or never have contact with the other parent after the family breaks up. Although many families adapt to separation and divorce without long-term negative effects for the children, research points out that youth often show at least temporary difficulties dealing with this common stressor in our society (Pruett, Williams, Insabella, & Little, 2003). Parental separation and divorce create changes in the family structure, usually resulting in a substantial reduction in the contact that children have with one of their parents. The child's response to divorce can be similar to the response to death. In some ways, divorce may be harder for the child to understand because the noncustodial parent is gone but still alive, and the parents have made a conscious choice to separate. Research shows that children of divorce are at increased risk for emotional, behavioural, and academic problems. However, the analysis of data from Canada's Longitudinal Survey of Children and Youth shows that children who grow up in a married biologic-parent household do not have better short-term behavioural outcomes than those who do not (Wu, Hou, & Schimmele, 2008). Rather, behavioural outcomes are related to such things as income, family dysfunction, and parental nurturance. The response to the loss that divorce imposes varies depending on the child's predivorce experience (Kelly, 2003); the child's temperament; the parents' interventions; and the level of stress, change, and conflict surrounding the divorce (Hetherington & Kelly, 2002). Major changes in socioeconomic status, that is, moving from a dual-earner status to a single-parent family status, may account for much of the variation in levels of distress among divorcing families (Jeynes, 2002; Sun & Li, 2002). In fact, single mothers (31%) represent the largest group of families living in poverty in Canada (Child Support Team, 2000). In addition, Statistics Canada (2004a) shows that in 1999,

20% of the single-parent mothers who worked full time lived in poverty.

The first 2 or 3 years after the couple's breakup tend to be the most difficult. Typical childhood reactions include confusion, guilt, depression, regression, somatic symptoms, acting-out behaviours (e.g., stealing, disobedience), fantasies that the parents will reunite, fear of losing the custodial parent, and alignment with one parent against the other. After an initial adjustment period, children usually accept the reality of the situation and begin coping adaptively. If the divorced parents remarry new partners, this often imposes another period of coping difficulties for the children. Children with stepparents and stepsiblings are at renewed risk for emotional and behavioural problems as they struggle to cope with the new relationships (Reifman, Villa, Amans, Rethinam, & Telesca, 2001).

Protective factors against emotional and behavioural problems in children of divorce include parental nurturance, parents' mental health, joint custody, and low parental conflict (Kelly, 2003). For children of divorce and remarriage, protective factors also include a structured home and school environment with reasonable and consistent limit setting and a warm, supportive relationship with stepparents (Hetherington & Kelly, 2002). Helpful interventions for children of divorce include education regarding children's reactions; promotion of regular and predictable visitation; reduction of conflict between the parents through counselling, mediation, and clear visitation policies; continuance of usual routines; and family counselling to facilitate adjustment after remarriage (Table 26-2). Some evidence shows that it is not the divorce itself but rather the continuing conflict between the parents that is most damaging to the child. Parents manage divorce better if they can remember that children naturally idealize and identify with both parents and need to view both of them positively. Therefore, it is helpful for parents to reinforce each other's good qualities and focus on evidence of their former partner's love and respect for the child.

Sibling Relationships

Until recently, the role of siblings in a child's development was underemphasized. A growing body of research shows that sibling relationships significantly influence personality development. Moreover, research shows that positive sibling relationships can be protective factors against the development of psychopathology, particularly in troubled families in which the parents are emotionally unavailable (Brody, 1998). A Canadian longitudinal study revealed that sibling affection moderated the effects of stressful life events on "internalized symptomatology" (e.g., being anxious, depressive, overcontrolled) (Gass, Jenkis, & Dunn, 2007). Thus, nurses should emphasize that whatever parents can do to minimize sibling rivalry

and maximize cooperative behaviour among their children will benefit their children's social and emotional development throughout life. Sibling rivalry begins with the birth of the second child. It is a natural experience, and some sibling rivalry is inevitable. Often, the birth of a sibling is traumatic for the first child who, up until then, was the sole focus of the parents' attention. The older sibling usually reacts with anger and may reveal not-so-subtle fantasies of getting rid of the new sibling (e.g., "I dreamed that the new baby died"). Parents should recognize that these reactions are natural and allow the child to express feelings, both positive and negative, about the baby while reassuring the child that he or she has a very special place in the family. Allowing the older child opportunities to care for the baby and reinforcing any nurturing or affectionate behaviour will promote positive bonding.

Though some sibling rivalry is natural, intense rivalry and conflict between siblings correlate with behaviour problems in children (Moser & Jacob, 2002). One factor that can exacerbate this problem is differential treatment of children. Although it is natural and appropriate for parents to use different methods to manage children with different personalities, parents must be sensitive to their children's perceptions of their behaviour and emphasize each child's strengths. Helping each child to develop a separate identity based on unique talents and interests can help address sibling rivalry and perceptions of favouritism.

Children with siblings experiencing mental illness are at increased risk, themselves, for mental health problems and behavioural disorders. Nurses should be alert to behaviour problems and include siblings in family interventions (Sharpe & Rossiter, 2002).

Physical Illness

Many children experience a major physical illness or injury at some point during development. The experience of hospitalization and intrusive medical procedures is at least acutely traumatic for most children. The likelihood of lasting psychological problems resulting from physical illness depends on the child's developmental level and previous coping mechanisms, the family's level of functioning before and after the illness, and the nature and severity of the illness. As with any major stressor, the perception of the event (i.e., meaning of the illness) will influence the family's ability to cope.

Common childhood reactions to physical illness include developmental regression (e.g., in toilet training, social maturity, autonomous behaviour), sleep and feeding difficulties, behaviour problems (e.g., negativism, withdrawal), somatic complaints that mask attempts at emotional expression (e.g., headaches, stomachaches), and depression. Infants and children younger than school age are particularly vulnerable to separation anxiety

Table 26.2 Play Therapy With a 4-Year-Old Child Whose Parents Are Divorcing		
Child Statement	**Nurse Response**	**Analysis and Rationale**
(The child smashes two cars together and makes loud, crashing sound.)	That's a loud crash. They really hit hard.	The child may be experiencing anger and frustration nonverbally through play. The nurse attempts to establish rapport with the child by relating at the child's level, using age-appropriate vocabulary.
Crrrash!	I know a boy who gets so mad sometimes that he feels like smashing something.	The child is engrossed in fantasy play, typical of preschoolers. Children often use toys as symbols of human figures. The nurse uses an indirect method of eliciting the child's feelings because preschoolers often do not express feelings directly. Reference to another child's anger helps to normalize this child's feelings.
Yeah!	Sounds like you feel angry too sometimes… the same way the other boy feels.	The child is beginning to relate to the nurse and sense her empathy. The nurse reflects the child's feelings to facilitate further communication.
Yeah, when my mom and dad fight.	It's tough to listen to parents fighting. Sometimes it's scary. You wonder what's going to happen.	The child is experiencing frustration and helplessness related to family conflict. The nurse expresses empathy and attempts to articulate the child's feelings because preschool children have a limited ability to identify and label feelings.
My mom and dad are getting a divorce.	That's too bad. Children often feel mixed up when their parents get divorced. What's going to happen when they get the divorce?	The child has a basic awareness of the reality of parents' divorce but may not understand this concept. The nurse expresses empathy and attempts to assess the child's level of understanding of the divorce.
Dad's not going to live in our house.	Oh, I guess you'll miss having him there all the time. It would be nice if you all could live together, but I guess that's not going to happen.	The preschool child focuses on the effects the divorce will have on him (egocentrism). The child seems to have a clear understanding of the consequences of the divorce. The nurse articulates the child's perspective and reinforces the reality of the divorce to avoid fuelling the child's possible denial and reconciliation fantasies.
(Silently moves cars across the floor.)	What do you think is the reason your parents decided to get a divorce?	The child expresses sadness nonverbally. The nurse further attempts to assess the child's understanding of the circumstances surrounding the divorce.
Because I did it.	What do you mean—you did it? How?	The child provides a clue that he may be feeling responsible. The nurse uses clarification to fully assess the child's understanding.
I made them mad because I left my bike in the driveway and dad ran over it.	Do you think that's why they're getting the divorce?	The child uses egocentric thinking to draw a conclusion that his actions caused the divorce. The nurse continues to clarify the child's thinking. The goal is to elicit the child's perceptions so that misperceptions can be corrected.
Yeah, they had a big fight.	They may have been upset about the bike, but I don't think that's why they're getting a divorce.	The nurse goes on to explain why parents get divorced and to provide opportunities for the child to ask questions.
Why?	Because parents get divorced when they're upset with *each other*—when they can't get along—not when they're upset with their children.	

during illness and may regress to earlier levels of anxiety about strangers, becoming fearful of health care providers. Young children often have magical thinking about the illness, and their tendency to process information in concrete terms may lead to misperceptions about the illness and treatment procedures (e.g., dye = die; stretcher = stretch her) (Deering & Cody, 2002). Adolescents may be concerned about their body image and maintaining their sense of independence and control.

Nurses must remember that parents are the primary resource to the child and the experts who know the child's needs and reactions. Thus, nurses must maintain a collaborative approach in working with parents of physically ill children. If the child is a sick infant, nurses should take care to allow the normal attachment process between parents and the infant to unfold, despite health care professionals' efforts to assume some parenting functions. Parents who view their children as physically and emotionally fragile will feel disempowered in decision making and limit setting and may develop helpless or overprotective styles of dealing with their children.

Many parents react with guilt to their child's illness or injury, especially if the illness is genetically based or partially the result of their own behaviour (e.g., drug or alcohol abuse during pregnancy). Parents may project their guilt onto each other or health care professionals, lashing out in anger and blame. Nurses should view this behaviour as part of the grieving process and help parents to move forward confidently in caring for their children. Teaching parents how to care for their children's health needs and reinforcing their successes in doing so will help. For example, rather than reacting to what may appear to be an abdication of parenting responsibilities, nurses can, instead, use empathy to acknowledge the parent's feelings and discuss ways to help the parent regain a sense of control with comments, such as,

> It's pretty confusing to know how best to respond to your child's behaviour. Before receiving her diagnosis, you felt comfortable setting reasonable limits on her behaviour, but now that seems to have changed. Sometimes parents feel guilty and are even afraid of setting limits because they know how sick their child is.... It may seem odd, but children actually feel safer and more secure when their parents set some limits.... Let's talk about some of the limits that you might feel most comfortable setting for your daughter to help her feel safe and secure while she is so ill?

Chronic physical illness in childhood presents a unique set of challenges, with survival rates of previously fatal diseases at an all-time high (Martinez & Ercikan, 2009). Although studies show that most children with chronic illnesses and their families are remarkably resilient and adjust to the stressors and regimens involved in their care (LeBlanc, Goldsmith, & Patel, 2003), research shows that children with chronic health conditions are at higher risk for developing anxiety-related disorders, academic problems, and learning disabilities (Martinez & Ercikan, 2009). Children with chronic health conditions are also three to four times more likely to experience psychiatric symptoms than are their healthy peers (Lewis & Vitulano, 2003). Conditions that affect the central nervous system (CNS) (e.g., infections, metabolic diseases, CNS malformations, brain and spinal cord trauma) are particularly likely to result in psychiatric difficulties. Nurses who understand pathophysiologic processes are in a unique position to assess the interaction between biologic and psychological factors that contribute to mental health problems in chronically ill children (e.g., lethargy from high blood sugar levels or respiratory problems; mood swings from steroid use). Inactivity and a lack of sensory stimulation from hospitalization or bed rest may contribute to neurologic deficits and developmental delays. The major challenge for a chronically ill child is to remain active despite the limitations of the illness and to become fully integrated into school and social activities. Children who view themselves as different or defective will experience low self-esteem and be more at risk for depression, anxiety, and behaviour problems. Studies show that parental perceptions of the child's vulnerability predict greater adjustment problems, even after controlling for age and disease severity (Anthony, Gil, & Schanberg, 2003). Educating parents about these facts and helping them to foster maximum independence within the limitations of the child's health problem is the key. For example, nurses might comment,

> Having kidney disease is certainly no fun... and it would be wonderful if wrapping your son in a cocoon would ensure that he came to no harm. Unfortunately, there is no such way of protecting him completely.... But we know that children seem to manage better with their illness when their parents believe that they have possibilities. Even with all the limitations, what are the best things your son has going for him?

Adolescent Risk-Taking Behaviours

Adolescence is a time of growing independence and, consequently, experimentation. Emotional extremes prevail. To adolescents, the world seems great one day and terrible the next; people are either for them or against them. Adolescents are struggling to consolidate their abilities to control their impulses and react to the many "crises" that may seem trivial to adults but are very important to teens. Biologic changes (e.g., the onset of puberty, height and weight changes, hormonal changes), psychological changes (e.g., increased ability for abstract thinking), and social changes (e.g., dating, driving, increased autonomy) are all significant. The primary developmental task of identity formation leads teenagers to test different roles and struggle to find a peer group that fits their unfolding self-image.

Adolescence is a time of pushing and exploring social and personal boundaries. This often involves experimentation, which can increase the risk of poor physical health, mental health problems, substance use including tobacco, risky sexual behaviours, and psychological distress (Canadian Population Health Initiative, 2005). Pregnancy occurs in approximately 4% of Canadian females aged 15 to 19 years annually (Dryburgh, 2000), and sexually transmitted infections (STIs) are most common among younger Canadians (Health Canada, 2000). Of those adolescents aged 15 to 24, 18% report symptoms associated with a major mental disorder, while 8% report substance dependence (Statistics Canada, 2004a). Some adolescents engage in truancy or criminal behaviours and running away from home. Although most youths eventually become more conventional in their behaviour, some develop harmful behaviour patterns and addictions that endanger their mental and physical health. Adolescents whose psychiatric problems have already developed are particularly vulnerable to engaging in risky behaviours because they have limited coping skills, may attempt to self-medicate their symptoms, and may feel an increased pressure to fit in with other teens. Moreover, research shows that risky behaviours tend to be interrelated (Eggert, Thompson, Randell, & Pike, 2002).

Research shows that enhanced life skills and supportive school and family environments can mediate the effect of stressful life events (Burns, Andrews, & Szabo, 2002). Programs that enhance the school environment are associated with improved behaviour and well-being. Interventions that teach cognitive skills are associated with a reduction in one of the most prevalent mental health problems affecting adolescents, depression (Puskar, Sereika, & Tusaie-Mumford, 2003). Current evidence suggests that for an intervention to be sustainable, it must encompass multiple components across several levels, including the classroom, curriculum, whole school, and school–community boundaries. Several approaches to mental health promotion with adolescents are recommended. First, intervening at the peer group level through educational programs, alternative recreational activities, and peer counselling are most successful. Adolescents are sceptical of authority figures and tend to take cues from one another. Nurses working with teenagers find it helpful to use a discussion approach that encourages questioning and argument, as opposed to talking down to or "talking at" teenagers (Deering & Cody, 2002).

Second, research has shown that training in values clarification, decision making, problem solving, social skills, and assertiveness helps give adolescents the skills to cope with situations in which they are pressured by their peers (Botvin, 2000). Social psychological research shows that if just one person can find the strength to express an unpopular viewpoint in a group and decline to participate in a destructive activity, others will quickly follow. It takes enormous courage, as well as concrete knowledge and practice with assertiveness, to speak up in these situations.

A third type of intervention is a program that uses team efforts by teachers, parents, community leaders, and teen role models. These programs help at-risk youth by building self-esteem, setting positive examples, and working to involve the youth in community activities. It is important to note that teaching interpersonal skills, including cognitive and problem-solving skills, should be coupled with the promotion of positive school and family environments to prevent mental health problems in young people, notably depression (Burns, Andrews, & Szabo, 2002). Approaches that have not proved effective include more education and information about dangerous activities without behaviour training, as well as programs that provide inadequate training and support for the professionals implementing them.

███ PROTECTIVE FACTORS AGAINST CHILDHOOD PATHOLOGY

Protective factors include individual, family, and community characteristics that alleviate the impact of risk factors by interacting together to foster resilience in children (Waddell, McEwan, Sheperd, Offord, & Hua, 2005). In the child, these protective factors include learning abilities, social skills, a sense of competence, positive beliefs about one's purpose in the larger world, and long-term support from at least one adult (Werner & Smith, 1992). In the family, low stress, stable employment, adequate resources for child care, and higher socioeconomic status can serve as protective factors. In the community, protective factors include positive and cohesive families, schools, and neighbourhoods (Box 26-1) (Schoor, 1997).

███ RISK FACTORS FOR CHILDHOOD PSYCHOPATHOLOGY

Poverty and Homelessness

An estimated 14.9% of children in Canada live in poverty (UNICEF, 2005), and 9% of these children had lived in poverty for more than 5 years (Campaign, 2000). Forty percent of people of Aboriginal descent, 40% of immigrants, and 34% of visible minority groups also live in poverty in Canada. The effects of poverty on child development and family functioning are numerous and pervasive. Lack of proper nutrition and access to prenatal and mother–infant care place children from poor families at risk for physical and mental health problems. Children from poor rural areas often lack access to educational

Khanlou, N., & Crawford, C. (2006). Post-migratory experiences of newcomer female youth: Self-esteem and identity development. Journal of Immigrant and Minority Health, 81(1), 45–46. The study was supported by a research contract from Status of Women Canada's Policy Research Fund.

BOX 26.1
Research for Best Practice

THE QUESTION: This study explored the postmigratory experiences of newcomer female youth attending secondary school within a multicultural context. The impact of the resettlement process on the self-esteem and identity of newcomer females was considered.

METHODS: Focus groups were held with 10 newcomer female youth in Toronto. Data were also collected through focus groups or in-depth interviews with school educators, parents, and school and community health centre workers. Also, the Current Self-Esteem (CSE) instrument was used to examine the global self-esteem of youth and the influences on their self-esteem.

FINDINGS: Participants' average age was 17 years; average age at the time of immigration to Canada was 13.9 years. The mean for CSE scores was 7.9, indicating that respondents felt, in general, good about themselves. Among the influences on youth's self-esteem were those related to self, school, relationships, achievements, and lifestyle. The emerging subthemes of the self-concept theme, arising from the qualitative data, consisted of dynamic self, silenced self, cultural identity, female role models, and future aspirations.

IMPLICATIONS FOR NURSING PRACTICE: This study is an example of a community-based mental health promotion study. The researchers concluded that, in multicultural and postmigration societies, context-specific strategies in mental health promotion are needed for youth. Their published report (Khanlou et al., 2002) provides policy recommendations for health, social services, and educational systems and for resettlement services.

and other resources. Urban children living in poor, often inner-city neighbourhood areas are vulnerable to violent crimes, crowded living conditions, and an increased access to drugs (Leventhal & Brooks-Gunn, 2000). Although crime, drug abuse, gang activity, and teenage pregnancy are seen in adolescents from all socioeconomic backgrounds, children living in poverty are more vulnerable to these problems because they may have limited opportunities for change (Kelly & Caputo, 2007). The obstacles inherent in overcoming the effects of poverty can seem insurmountable to young people.

A major focus of preventive nursing interventions for disadvantaged families involves simply forming an alliance that conveys respect and willingness to work as an advocate to help patients gain access to resources. In terms of Maslow's need hierarchy, families living in poverty may be more focused on survival needs (e.g., food, shelter) than on self-actualization needs (e.g., insight-oriented psychotherapy for themselves or their children). Unless the nurse can work as a partner with the family and address the issues most pressing for the family with an active, problem-solving approach, other types of intervention may be fruitless. At the same time, it is inappropriate to assume that poor families will be resistant to or unable to benefit from psychotherapies or other mental health interventions.

Contrary to a popular opinion, homelessness is a very complex phenomenon, and the homeless are not a homogenous population. Canada has a growing number of homeless women, children, youth, families, new immigrants, people with mental illness, ethnic minorities, and Aboriginal people (Begin, Casavant, Chenier, & Dupuis, 1999). Homelessness among children and teens may result from a variety of events, including a loss of

shelter for the entire family, running away, being thrown out of one's home (Kelly & Caputo, 2007), or, in the case of youth, being abandoned by the social service system. Risk factors for becoming homeless or street involved include problems at home, failure of the social welfare and educational systems, substance abuse, participation in criminal activities, lack of employability or affordable housing, and personal issues. There is no accurate understanding of the numbers of homeless people in Canada, much less the number of homeless youth. However, emergency shelters alone accounted for, on average, 6,500 homeless people in Toronto per night in 1997 (Begin et al., 1999).

Research reveals an increased risk for physical health problems (e.g., nutritional deficiencies, infections, chronic illnesses, injuries as a result of violence, STIs), mental health problems (particularly developmental delays in language, fine or gross motor coordination, and social development; depression, anxiety, posttraumatic stress disorder, and psychotic symptoms; disruptive behaviour disorders; substance abuse), and educational underachievement in homeless youth. Many homeless youth have been physically or sexually abused, leading to elevated rates of externalizing disorders for boys and internalizing disorders for girls (Cance et al., 2000). Evidence suggests that at least 50% of homeless youth suffer from serious mental health and drug addiction problems (Adlaf & Zdanowicz, 1999) and are now more likely to be homeless than adults (Ringwalt, Greene, Robertson, & McPheeters, 1998). For adolescents, running away from abusive conditions at home often thrusts them onto the street and into environments where staying alive and developing self-reliance are a daily struggle (Kelly & Caputo 2007; Rew, 2003). The living conditions of many shelters place children at risk for lead poisoning and communicable diseases and make the regular sleep, feeding, play, and bathing patterns important for normal development nearly impossible. Nurses working with homeless families need to be aware of the effects of this lifestyle on children because they have a limited ability to speak for themselves and because their needs are often overlooked. Studies show that the demands of parenting often overwhelm parents in homeless shelters. The unstable nature of their living conditions limits the ability of these parents to nurture their children (Gorzka, 1999).

Though a heterogeneous population, typically street youth have experienced extreme stress in the course of their lives even before they run away, with most fleeing temporary living arrangements (e.g., foster homes, friends, relatives) (Kelly & Caputo, 2007; Warren, Gary, & Moorhead, 1997). Thus, their runaway experience serves only to compound an already chronic history of trauma and disruption. The key is to prevent the conditions that preceded the runaway behaviour. Unfortunately, much of the response to homelessness has resulted in greater social control measures (e.g., rendering panhandling illegal, excluding the homeless from the community) rather than strategies to address the underlying causes (Begin et al., 1999). Street nurses are often one of the few resources available to marginalized populations who face a variety of barriers to accessing traditional health care services, such as mental health problems, criminal involvement, lack of transportation, lack of ability to pay for prescriptions, lack of specialized or knowledgeable providers, and provider discrimination (Self & Peters, 2005). Street services are effective because they are delivered wherever the person feels comfortable: a school, a drop-in centre, a mall, a youth centre, or simply the street.

Child Abuse and Neglect

Each year, thousands of Canadian children suffer intentional physical or emotional abuse, neglect, or sexual exploitation as the result of their parents' action or inaction (Wolfe, 1998). A recent study (Trocme et al., 2001) confirmed close to half (45%) of the 135,573 child maltreatment investigations in 1998. Child abuse may affect every aspect of a child's life and may have varying consequences depending on its form, duration, severity, and child's gender (Maguire, Mann, Sibert, & Kemp, 2005; Trocme et al., 2001). The effects may appear immediately or surface only in adolescence or adulthood and may differ according to the nature of the response to the abuse and whether the abuse was disclosed or reported. In some cases, the consequences are fatal (Canadian Centre for Justice Statistics, 2001). Maltreated children often have difficulty managing emotions (Campbell, 1995), communicating effectively (Browne & Sagi, 1988), developing satisfying relationships with others (Crittenden, 1996), and learning in productive ways (Doherty, 1997). Early recognition and a reduction of risk factors are the keys to preventing **child abuse and neglect** (Box 26-2).

Risk factors for child abuse and neglect include high levels of family stress, drug or alcohol abuse, a stepparent or parental boyfriend or girlfriend who is unstable or unloving toward the child, and lack of social support for the parents. In addition, young children (particularly those younger than 3 years) and children with a history of prematurity, medical problems, and severe emotional problems are at high risk because they place great demands on the parents. Abuse has a well-known intergenerational pattern, such that children who are abused and neglected are more likely to repeat this behaviour when they become parents (Helfer, Kemper, & Kongman, 1997). However,

---

BOX 26.2

Research for Best Practice: The Impact of a Proven Parenting Program on a High-Risk Population

Hughes, J. R., & Gottlieb, L. N. (2004). The effects of the Webster-Stratton parenting program on maltreating families: Fostering strengths. Child Abuse and Neglect, 28, 1081–1097.

THE QUESTION: This study examined the effects of the nurse-developed, research tested, Webster-Stratton parenting program on the parenting skills of maltreating mothers and on the autonomy of their children (3–8 years of age).

METHODS: Twenty-six maltreating families were randomly assigned to one of two conditions: the 16-hour weekly intervention group or the 4-month wait list control group. Preintervention and postintervention independent assessments included a 2-hour home visit involving videotaped mother–child interactions during two prescribed (structured and unstructured), 10-minute play activities.

FINDINGS: Compared with the control group, treatment group mothers demonstrated significant improvement in involvement and marginally significant improvement in autonomy support. Treatment group children showed no significant improvement in autonomy when compared with control group children.

CONCLUSIONS AND IMPLICATIONS FOR NURSING PRACTICE: This parenting program proved effective with maltreating parents. The lack of demonstrated effect on children may reflect the need for a larger and more sustained treatment dose and/or the need to include parent–child interaction opportunities in the program. This study shows that conventional promotion programs may need additional supports to be effective with high-risk populations.

intergenerational abuse is not a foregone conclusion. Evidence shows that among abused and nonabused children, having a strong commitment to school, having parents and peers who disapprove of antisocial behaviour, and being involved in a religious community lowered the rates of lifetime violence, delinquency, and status offences (Herrenkohl, Tajima, Whitney, & Huang, 2005).

Table 26-3 lists types of abuse in children. Research clearly documents that child abuse is a risk factor for later psychopathology, especially depression and substance abuse (Putnam, 2003). Nurses should be aware that they are legally mandated to report any reasonable suspicion of abuse and neglect to the appropriate provincial and child protection systems. Mandated reporting laws are designed to allow the provinces and child protection systems to investigate the possibility of abuse, provide protection to children, and link families with the support and services that they need to reduce the risk for further abuse. Nurses are ethically and legally responsible for reporting abuse. The decision to report abuse sometimes poses an ethical dilemma for nurses as they try to balance the need to maintain the family's trust against the need to protect the child. This decision is further complicated by the knowledge that, if temporary out-of-home placement is necessary, the quality of the placement may not be optimum, and the child and the family may suffer in the process of the separation.

Experts recommend that, when possible, nurses report abuse in the presence of the parents, preferably with the parent initiating the telephone call, and that the professional should explain the reporting as necessary to provide safety for the child and to obtain services for the family. If the parents cannot be present when the report is made, the nurse should, at minimum, notify the family that the report was made and explain the reasons. A major protective factor against psychopathology stemming from abuse and neglect is the establishment of a supportive relationship with at least one adult, who can provide empathy, consistency, and, possibly, a corrective experience (e.g., a foster parent or other family member) for the child (Taussig, 2002).

The prevention of child abuse and neglect can occur with interventions that support the parents with physical, financial, mental health, and medical resources that will

Table 26.3	Types and Rates of Abuse in Canada	
Type	**Description**	**Rate**
Neglect	Is often chronic and usually involves repeated incidents of failing to provide what a child needs for his or her physical, psychological, or emotional development and well-being.	3.66 confirmed cases per 1,000 children
Physical abuse	May consist of just one incident or happen repeatedly. It involves deliberately using force against a child in such a way that the child is either injured or is at risk for being injured. Injuries may include bruises, lacerations, burns, and fractures caused by another person or object (e.g., belt, cords, cigarette). *Note:* Many injuries do not represent child abuse; therefore, when abuse is suspected, bruising must be assessed in the context of medical, social, and developmental histories; the explanation given; and the patterns of nonabusive bruising (Maguire, Mann, Sibert, & Kemp, 2005).	2.25 confirmed cases per 1,000 children
Emotional abuse	Involves harming a child's sense of self. It includes acts (or omissions) that result in, or place a child at risk for, serious behavioural, cognitive, emotional, or mental health problems.	2.20 confirmed cases per 1,000 children
Sexual abuse and exploitation	Involves using a child for sexual purposes, resulting in physical wounds such as bruises or bleeding of the genitals or rectum, STIs, sore throat, enuresis/encopresis, pregnancy, and foreign objects in the vagina or rectum. The child may also display sophisticated knowledge/behaviour/preoccupation with sexual activities, withdrawal, hypervigilance, or sleep difficulties.	0.86 confirmed cases per 1,000 children

From Trocme, N., MacLaurin, B., Fallon, B., et al. (2001). *Canadian incidence study of reported child abuse and neglect.* Ottawa, ON: Minister of Public Works and Government Services Canada.

reduce stress within the family system. Early intervention and family support programs are considered the cornerstones of preventive efforts. Nurses working with abused children should resist the temptation to view the child as the only victim. Remembering that most abusive parents were abused themselves as children and, therefore, may have limited coping mechanisms or little access to positive parental role models will help the nurse maintain empathy toward the parents. Once agencies intervene to establish the child's safety, a family systems approach that is supportive of the whole family unit is most effective.

Child and Family Services

The tendency to blame parents and view out-of-home placement as a refuge for children has sharply declined in recent years. This change in attitude results from public awareness of the deficiencies in the foster care system, greater support for parents' rights, and increased knowledge of the biologic basis for many of the disorders of parents and children that lead to out-of-home placement. **Family preservation** involves efforts made by professionals to preserve the family unit by preventing the removal of children from their homes by providing support and education to secure the attachment between children and parents. Today, children are removed from their homes only as a last resort. Family support services are designed to assist families with access to resources and education regarding childrearing, to monitor and facilitate the development of the bond between the child and the caregiver, and to increase the caregiver's confidence in his or her abilities (MacLeod & Nelson, 2000).

IN A LIFE

Charleen Touchette (1954–)

Public Persona

Charleen Touchette is a celebrated artist, writer, and activist. Her book, *It Stops With Me: Memoirs of a Canuck Girl*, is her own rich story of hope and self-discovery that is grounded in her French Canadian and Aboriginal heritage. The artwork and text of the book tell of her healing from childhood abuse and her determination that abuse would no longer be a family legacy: "[C]'est fini. No more. It stops with me" (Touchette, 2004, p. 245).

Personal Realities

As a child, Charleen's family life was shaped by anger, alcohol abuse, and physical violence. She writes, "At eight, I wrote a letter to my future grown-up self. Never forget how it feels to be a little kid with a crazy mean daddy" (p. 19). She left her birthplace, a French Canadian community in Rhode Island, United States, at 17 and began a journey that took her to the world of art, Aboriginal culture, marriage, and motherhood. Today, she shares what she learned about healing in her books and painting.

However, despite recent trends toward family preservation, an increasing number of children are placed in foster homes, group homes, or residential treatment centres—in many cases, for months to years. Factors leading to the increased number of children in out-of-home placement include increased willingness of the public and professionals to report child abuse and neglect, the epidemic proportions of substance abuse and cases of AIDS, and the increasing number of families living in poverty, which may lead to abuse, neglect, and homelessness. In 2003, 76,183 children and youth in Canada were under the protection of Child and Family Services across the country. Infants who are abandoned by drug-abusing parents and children with HIV whose parents are sick or deceased need permanent out-of-home placements, which are often difficult to find.

The adjustment to an out-of-home placement can be viewed through the conceptual framework of Bowlby's stages of coping with parental separation. According to Bowlby (1960), the child initially responds to separation from parents with protest (crying, kicking, screaming, pleading, and attempting to elicit the parent's return). The child then moves to a state of despair (listlessness, apathy, and withdrawal, which lead to some acceptance of caregiving by others, but a reluctance to reattach fully). Finally, the child experiences detachment if the child and the new parent cannot manage to form an emotional bond. Because children often experience multiple placements, the potential for a disrupted attachment may be great by the time the child faces the prospect of a permanent family. After repeatedly undergoing separation and mourning, the child learns that rejection is inevitable and may automatically maintain a distance from a new caregiver.

Typical coping styles seen in children exposed to multiple placements include detachment, diffuse rage, chronic depression, antisocial behaviour, low self-esteem, and chronic dependency or exaggerated demands for nurturing and support. Sometimes these symptoms develop into attachment disorders that can be difficult to treat (O'Connor, Bredenkamp, & Rutter, 1999). It takes a very committed and resilient parent to continue caring for a child who does not reinforce attempts at caregiving and who exhibits these kinds of significant emotional and behavioural problems.

Parent With Mental Illness

Children who grow up with a depressed parent, the most common form of mental illness among adults (approximately 8% of the adult population) (Health Canada, 2002), are themselves at increased risk for mental illness—both in childhood and in later life (Health Canada & Canadian Mental Health Association, 1999). These children are also more likely to be at sociodemographic disadvantage—they are more likely to be living with a single mother and living on low income (Federal/Provincial/Territorial Advisory Committee on Population Health, 1999). Infants whose mothers experience post-partum depression (approximately 10%) or are otherwise troubled are at most risk for losing the opportunity to establish a secure attachment (Federal/Provincial/Territorial Advisory Committee on Population Health). Many children know that something is wrong when a parent has a mental illness but may not be able to identify the problem specifically (Health Canada & Canadian Mental Health Association, 1999). They feel alone, left out, distanced, and powerless to participate in decisions. They report feeling angry, sad, and guilty that somehow they are to blame for their parent's illness. They also worry that they will, in turn, become ill and fear the stigma that surrounds mental illness. Fortunately, the likelihood or severity of these problems can be reduced or eliminated when families have the knowledge and support they need. Children need information, their questions answered, an opportunity to talk about how they feel, and routine childhood experiences. As with other family stressors, it is important to keep children informed, in manageable ways and doses, and at times that the children determine (Health Canada & Canadian Mental Health Association). Nurses can help parents get started by modelling.

> Mommy isn't feeling well. She feels sad, it's because of an illness and it's not her fault. It is a sad time for all of us but I'm here to talk with you about it when you need to.

Children need hope that depression is treatable and that their mother will get better. They also need to be reassured that their parents love them—no matter what the challenge involves… or how long it takes (Health Canada & Canadian Mental Health Association, 1999). Children also need supportive relationships outside the home with someone (e.g., a teacher, coach, neighbour) who can provide a listening ear, extra support, and a measure of respite for the family. Children need to know that their routine in life will continue, including the fun times, and that their relationship with both parents is valued by the parents. Evidence shows that when children and their families are given information about the affected parent's mental illness, they show improved knowledge and long-standing positive effects in how they problem solve (a resilient-related quality) around parental illness (Beardslee, Gladstone, Wright, & Cooper, 2003).

Parent With a Substance Abuse Problem

A number of Canadian children live in homes (in urban or rural communities) with a parent who is dependent on alcohol (2.6% of adults: men 3.8%, women 1.3%) or illicit drugs (0.7% of adults: men 1.0%, women 0.4%)

(Statistics Canada, 2004a). Many of the parents with an alcohol or illicit substance dependence are also suffering or have suffered from depression, which acts as both a precursor and an outcome of heavy substance use, and are more likely to be living on a low income and have a relatively low education level (Statistics Canada, 2004b). Children whose parents are dependent on alcohol live in an unpredictable family environment, coping with stress that may disrupt their ability to perform in school and lead to other emotional problems (Casa-Gil & Navarro-Guzman, 2002). Many individuals with alcoholism become polysubstance abusers, addicted to other drugs as well. The codependency movement, which emphasizes the effects of addiction on family members, and groups such as Adult Children of Alcoholics (ACOA) and Al-Anon have brought increasing attention to the effects of parental substance abuse on child development. Any review of this topic must examine the role of biologic-genetic mechanisms and environmental mechanisms in creating an increased risk for psychological problems among children of those who abuse substances (see Chapter 24).

Biologic factors affecting children of those who abuse substances include **fetal alcohol spectrum disorder,** nutritional deficits stemming from neglect, and neuropsychiatric dysfunction related to overstimulation or understimulation (Kaemingk & Paquette, 1999). Genetic factors are at least partly responsible for the well-documented increased risk for substance abuse. Studies are beginning to link a family history of mental disorders and alcoholism with genetically transmitted mental disorders, which may be a precursor to alcohol abuse. The precise mechanism of family transmission of alcoholism remains unknown. Recent studies suggest that children of those who abuse substances may inherit a predisposition to a nonspecific form of biologic dysregulation that may be expressed phenotypically, either as alcoholism or as some other psychiatric disorder (e.g., hyperactivity, conduct disorder, depression), depending on the individual's developmental history.

Children of persons who abuse substances are at high risk for both substance abuse and behaviour disorders (Mylant, Ide, Cuevas, & Meehan, 2002). Moreover, some evidence shows that other factors related to addiction, such as family stress, violence, divorce, dysfunction, and other concurrent parental psychiatric disorders (e.g., depression, anxiety), are as important as the alcoholism itself in increasing this risk (Ritter, Stewart, Bernet, Coe, & Brown, 2002). The experience of growing up in a substance-abusing family is marked by unpredictability, fear, and helplessness because of the cyclic nature of addictive patterns.

The literature on children of parents who are alcoholic has described several typical roles that children assume, including the "hero" (overly responsible children who may ignore their own needs to take care of parents and other children), "scapegoat" (problem children who divert the attention away from the parent with alcoholism), "mascot" (family clowns who relieve tension and mask feelings through joking), and "lost child" (children who suffer in silence but may exhibit difficulties at school or in later life) (Veronie & Freuhstorfer, 2001). These roles, combined with the enabling behaviours of other family members who attempt to cover up and minimize the effects of the addiction, may become so rigid and effective in masking the problem that children of substance abusers may not come to the attention of mental health professionals until after the parent stops drinking and family roles are disrupted.

Even for children who do not experience significant psychopathology, the experience of growing up in a substance-abusing family can lead to a poor self-concept when children feel responsible for their parents' behaviour, the child becoming isolated and learning to mistrust his or her own perceptions because the family denies the reality of the addiction. Despite the well-documented risk for children in substance-abusing families, there is no uniform pattern of outcomes, and many children demonstrate resilience (Harter, 2000). **Resilience** is the phenomenon by which some children at risk for psychopathology—because of genetic or experiential circumstances—attain good mental health, maintain hope, and achieve healthy outcomes (Masten, 2001). Again, individual protective factors and preventive interventions are paramount.

▪■◖ MENTAL ILLNESS AMONG CHILDREN AND ADOLESCENTS

Fourteen percent of children aged 4 to 17 years experience mental health disorders (more than 50% have at least two concurrent disorders) that cause significant distress and impairment at home, at school, and in the community (Federal/Provincial/Territorial Advisory Committee on Population Health, 1999; Waddell et al., 2005). Suicide is the second leading cause of death among youth (24%) (Health Canada, 2002), and the rates are two to seven times higher among Aboriginal populations (Federal/Provincial/Territorial Advisory Committee on Population Health, 2000). Sadly, fewer than 25% of the children with a mental disorder receive treatment, and youth rate professionals as the last resource, behind peers and parents, for seeking assistance regarding depression, drugs, and alcohol (Federal/Provincial/Territorial Advisory Committee on Population Health). Fortunately, there is growing recognition of these service challenges (Geist & Simon, 1999) and a growing interest in understanding better which approaches are most effective in preventing mental illness during the early years (Goldner, 2002).

▪■◖ INTERVENTION APPROACHES

Mental health promotion with children, adolescents, and their families encompasses the full range of preventive efforts discussed in Chapter 2. Current thinking argues that a mix of psychological and social determinants affects health overall and mental health in particular (Health Canada, 2002, p. 23).

> At the individual level, such factors as secure attachment, good parenting, friendship and social support, meaningful employment and social roles, adequate income, physical activity, and internal locus of control will strengthen mental health and, indirectly, reduce the impact or incidence of some mental health problems.

At a system level, strategies that create supportive environments, strengthen community actions, develop personal skills, and orient health services can help to ensure that the population has some control over the psychological and social determinants of mental health.

Professional nursing emphasizes an interdisciplinary approach in which the nurse acts as the collaborator, coordinator, case manager, and advocate to establish linkages with physicians and nurse practitioners, teachers, speech and language specialists, social workers, and other professionals to develop and implement comprehensive preventative interventions (Box 26-3). A view of parents as partners should be foremost. In the past, parents have been viewed as the culprits in creating children's mental health problems and were treated as patients themselves. Recent insights into the biologic and genetic origins of psychiatric disorders have contributed to a shift from blaming parents to seeking their collaboration in treatment. Promotion and prevention programs incorporate a range of techniques to provide reassurance and education, skills training, or direct intervention. The programs may use face-to-face techniques (e.g., home visits, educational groups), literature (e.g., pamphlets, books), phone (e.g., crisis lines), or electronic mechanisms (e.g., Internet, telehealth).

Psychoeducational programs are a particularly effective form of mental health intervention. These programs are designed to teach parents and children basic coping skills for dealing with various stressors. Among other techniques, they use the process of **normalization** (i.e., teaching families what are normal behaviours and expected responses) and provide families with information about normal child development and expected reactions to various stressors so that the families will feel less isolated, know what to expect, and put their reactions into perspective. For example, if families learn that anger is a natural part of grieving, they will be less likely to view it as abnormal and more likely to accept and cope with it constructively. Parallel curricula can be established with concurrent psychoeducational groups for adults

---

BOX 26.3

Clinical Vignette: Preventive Interventions With an Adolescent in Crisis

- Ben and Rita were just transferred to a second foster home after being removed from their mother's care when she relapsed on cocaine and left them unattended. The plan is for the two children to return to their mother's home after she completes a 30-day drug treatment program. Ben, a high school freshman, is in the school nurse's office asking for aspirin for another headache.

- The nurse notices that Ben's nose looks inflamed, he is sniffling, and he seems more "hyper" than usual. In a concerned tone of voice, she asks him if he has been using cocaine and he snaps back, "Just because my mother's a coke head doesn't give you the right to suspect me!" When the nurse gently says, "Tell me about what's been happening with your mother; I had no idea," Ben responds less defensively and explains the situation about the foster home and his mother's drug problem. He says that if it were not for Rita, his younger sister, he would have run away by now. His foster parents are "making him" go to school, but he is going to drop out as soon as he returns to live with his mother. The only thing that he likes about school is playing basketball, and the basketball coach, who is his gym teacher, wants him on the team.

- After a lengthy talk with Ben, the nurse finishes the assessment interview and concludes that he is at risk for drug abuse, running away, and dropping out of school. He is also showing symptoms of depression, which he may be attempting to medicate with cocaine. Protective factors for Ben include his strong attachment to his sister, his ability and willingness to express his thoughts and feelings, his interest in basketball, and a positive relationship with the basketball coach.

- The nurse develops a plan with Ben to attend the weekly drug and alcohol discussion group at the school, so that he can talk with other teens from substance-abusing families and learn coping skills to prevent addiction. The nurse contacts the basketball coach, who agrees to find a student mentor who can shoot hoops with Ben and help him come up with a plan to stay in school, maybe find a part-time job, and join the basketball team. Ben agrees to check in regularly with the nurse to report how the plan is working and revise it if needed. The nurse feels optimistic that with support from his peers, coach, mentor, and herself, Ben can overcome what is probably a genetically based risk for depression and addiction. Ben shows signs of resilience. He is motivated to "keep his act together for Rita," capable of forming positive attachments, and willing to seek help when he knows where to find it.

---

and children. Most foster care agencies now provide a program of education and training for prospective foster parents to help them know what to expect and how to help the child adjust to placement.

Social skills training is one psychoeducational approach that has been useful with youth who have low self-esteem, aggressive behaviour, or a high risk for substance abuse (Cavell, Ennett, & Meehan, 2001). Social skills training involves instruction, feedback, support, and practice with learning behaviours that help children to interact more effectively with peers and adults. When combined with assertiveness training, social skills training can be particularly helpful in providing children with coping skills to resist engaging in addictive or antisocial behaviours and to prevent social withdrawal under stress. Social skills training may be particularly helpful for children who are bullies or who are rejected by their peers (Fopma-Loy, 2000).

Bibliotherapy is the therapeutic use of books, stories, and other reading materials. It can be used to help children, adolescents, and families to gain information and understanding about life stressors, illness, and recovery. It is a particularly potent form of intervention because it empowers families to learn and develop coping mechanisms on their own. A wide variety of books are available to help children understand issues such as death, divorce, chronic illness, stepfamilies, adoption, and the birth of a sibling. For instance, Baker (2007) describes the way stories about being in foster care can help foster children, parents, and caseworkers in discussing their own situation.

By using eight stories to reveal the themes found in accounts of foster care (e.g., the fear of foster children in developing attachments; the way siblings can play a powerfully supportive role; the importance of recognizing the humanity of the biologic parents), she highlights the benefits of this therapeutic approach. Children and adolescents can find comfort and increased understanding through stories that reflect their own experience. Parents can use stories as a way to learn about their children's concerns: the adventures and/or tribulations of a story's characters can be a means to discover their child's thoughts and feelings about an experience. Some health centres and hospitals have patient library services available (Anglin, 2008). Many mental health organizations such as the Canadian Mental Health Association, public health agencies, and Health Canada have pamphlets or website information designed for parents or children and youth about various physical and psychological problems. In addition to providing concrete information and advice, these reading materials help to reduce anxiety by pointing out common reactions to the various stressors so that families do not feel alone.

Support groups are available for just about every kind of stressor that a family can experience, including substance abuse, death, divorce, and coping with a chronic illness. Both parents and children in groups can experience Yalom's (1985) healing effects of group therapy, including group cohesiveness, universality (awareness of the normalcy and commonality of one's reactions), catharsis, hope, and altruism (being able to help others).

Early intervention programs, possibly the most important form of primary prevention available to children and families, offer regular home visits, support, education, and concrete services to those in need. Research supports the effectiveness of these programs, which may be the key to preventing the placement of children outside the home (Gimpel & Holland, 2003; Tomlin & Viehweg, 2003). The assumption underlying these programs is that parents are the most consistent and important figures in children's lives, and they should be afforded the opportunity to define their own needs and priorities. With support and education, parents will be empowered to respond more effectively to their children.

Canada invests in early intervention to promote healthy child development by enhancing such programs as paid parental leave (now 1 year), child care, family resource centres, and early learning (Waddell et al., 2005). A number of jurisdictions have introduced promotion and prevention programs aimed at high-risk families (low-income, lone parents) around the birth of a newborn (e.g., Better Beginnings Better Futures in Ontario; Healthy Beginnings: Enhanced Home Visiting in Nova Scotia). Many of these programs involve nurse home visitation. There is growing evidence that intensive postpartum support (more than antenatal support) provided by a health care professional prevents postpartum depression (Dennis, 2005) and that early interventions are effective in preventing child maltreatment among disadvantaged first-time mothers (MacMillan & Canadian Task Force on Preventive Health Care, 2000). Other population-based early intervention initiatives are aimed at older children in socioeconomically disadvantaged communities. These universal programs are directed toward the child (e.g., classroom enrichment, quality child care), parent (e.g., home visiting, parent help/information/crisis phone lines, parent–child play groups), and neighbourhood (information that engages families and connects them to community supports), with an emphasis on providing intensive services to children directly. They have demonstrated improvements in children's emotional problems, behavioural problems, social skills, and a decreased need for special education during the early years (ages 4 to 8 years) (Peters, Petrunka, & Arnold, 2003).

Current thinking around prevention and promotion programs designed for adolescent mental health argues that offerings should support and educate youth (e.g., through peer mentoring in community organizations and schools); enhance self-help and self-responsibility, coping skills, self-esteem, and skill development in ways that foster mental health; and teach youth when and how to seek assistance for problems (Federal/Provincial/Territorial Advisory Committee on Population Health, 2000). Particular emphasis has been given to ways of creating healthy images related to gender, body image, and empowerment.

Historically, nurses have been underused in school-based mental health efforts, although schools are good locations for other early intervention programs because they are physically near the families they serve and are less intimidating than mental health centres. Programs can be targeted for very young children before symptoms have time to develop. Studies show that by fourth grade, a large number of young children already use some kind of substance (e.g., inhalants, which are toxic); therefore, prevention efforts may be crucial in the early grades (Finke et al., 2002). In numerous schools throughout Canada, Youth Health Centres have become familiar resources.

The number of promotion and early intervention mental health services provided through electronic media (e.g., Internet, telehealth) is growing. Targeted support groups are increasingly available through the Internet. Dedicated websites providing both universal mental health information and confidential intervention services by e-mail are also available through some school systems. Similar services around specific mental health issues are also being tested with high-risk populations. Telehealth, which involves telephone and video support to rural and remote Canada, is increasingly offered both to practitioners and to children or their parents (Urness, Hailey, Delday, Callanan, & Orlik, 2004). The full capacity of these approaches is largely unknown, and contrary to professional fears, the users are generally more than satisfied with the services (Williams, May, & Esmail, 2001). Some users even prefer the anonymity of electronic media. Nurses are playing instrumental roles in many of these initiatives, both as direct service providers and as on-site support services (Elford, 1998).

Although a number of children's mental health promotion and prevention programs have proven effective on their own, less understood are the effects of programs that include an array of comprehensive health care services, parent education, and support on the mental health of children and youth (Breton, 1999; Peters et al., 2003). Best thinking to date suggests that the most effective strategies for reducing the burden of suffering from child psychiatric disorders are those that consist of a number of concurrent steps (Offord, Kraemer, Kazdin, Jensen & Harrington, 1998). First, effective universal programs should be in place. Targeted programs should follow for those not helped sufficiently by the universal programs. Finally, for those unaffected by the targeted programs, clinical services should be available. To be effective, prevention programs need to start early, continue long term, and involve multiple domains in a child's life (Offord & Bennett, 2002).

In conclusion, undertaking interventions to promote the mental health of children and adolescents is time and effort well spent. Many adult mental health problems can be prevented, coped with more effectively, or at least reduced in their scope and severity through focused intervention with children, youth, and families. Children and youth lack the power and voice to fight for their own needs, making them one of the most vulnerable groups in society. By virtue of their close interaction with families, nurses are in a key position to identify the mental health needs of children and youth and to intervene, particularly in times of crisis.

■ NEW DIRECTIONS IN COMMUNITY-BASED MENTAL HEALTH PROMOTION

Mental health promotion with children and youth can occur at individual, familial, community, and global levels. There is growing recognition that multiple factors affect mental well-being, that mental health does not equate to a lack of mental illness, that mental health is also affected by the social determinants of mental well-being, and that health promotion efforts need to span across systems (Khanlou, 2003; Khanlou, Beiser, Cole, Friere, Hyman, & Kilbride, 2002). Mental health promotion initiatives need to be individualized to the circumstances of the children and youth with whom we work (including their familial and social resources), must be sensitive to context (e.g., rural setting or urban multicultural setting), and must incorporate the latest empirical and theoretical developments (see Box 26-1). Among children and youth, in addition to the health and social services systems, the education system can be among the sites where mental health promotion initiatives take place.

SUMMARY OF KEY POINTS

☐ Nurses working with children and adolescents are in a key position to identify risk and protective factors for psychopathology and to intervene to reduce risk.

☐ Nurses who are aware of normal developmental processes can educate parents about their children's behaviours, help them better understand their children's reactions to stress, and decide when intervention may be warranted.

☐ If the process of normal biologic maturation in childhood is disrupted through trauma or neglect, developmental delays and disorders can occur, some of which may have irreversible effects.

☐ From early infancy, children exhibit different kinds of temperaments that are at least partially biologically determined.

☐ Studies of attachment show that the quality of the emotional bond between the child and the parental figure is an important determinant of the success of later relationships.

☐ Research shows that children who experience major losses, such as death or divorce, are at risk for developing mental health problems.

☐ Sibling relationships have significant effects on personality development. Positive sibling relationships can be protective factors against the development of mental health problems.

☐ Medical problems in childhood and adolescence may cause psychological problems when illness leads to behaviours common to an earlier developmental stage (regression) or lack of full participation in family, school, and social activities.

☐ Striving for identity and independence may lead adolescents to participate in high-risk activities (e.g., substance use, including tobacco; unprotected sex; delinquent behaviours) that may lead to mental health problems.

☐ Poverty, homelessness, abuse, neglect, and parental alcoholism all create conditions that undermine a child's ability to make normal developmental gains and contribute to the child's vulnerability for various emotional and behavioural problems.

☐ Children who experience disrupted attachments because of out-of-home placements may have difficulty forming close relationships with their new parents and trusting others.

☐ Family support services and early intervention programs are designed to prevent the removal of the child from the family as a result of abuse or neglect and to maintain a strong, nurturing family system.

CRITICAL THINKING CHALLENGES

1　Analyze a case of a family that is grieving a loss and compare the parents' and children's reactions. Include an evaluation of how each child's reactions differ, depending on his or her developmental level.

2　Watch a movie or read a book that provides a child's view of death, divorce, or some other loss and consider how adults may be insensitive to the child's reactions.

3　Examine your own developmental history and pinpoint periods when stressful life events might have increased the risk for emotional problems for you or other family members. What protective factors in your own personality and coping skills, as well as in the environment around you, helped you to maintain your good mental health?

4　What aspects of life are more stressful for children than for adults (i.e., how is it different to experience life as a child)?

5　Examine how your own social and cultural background may either facilitate or create barriers to your ability to interact with families from other ethnic backgrounds or those who are poor or homeless.

6 Allow yourself to reflect on how your own attitudes might interfere with your ability to communicate effectively with families who have abused or neglected their children.

7 Why is the process of normalization of feelings such a powerful intervention with children and families? What kinds of mental health issues, developmental processes, or both would benefit from teaching related to normal reactions? How can nurses incorporate this kind of intervention into their practice roles?

8 How can nurses expand their roles to have maximal effects on primary, secondary, and tertiary mental health interventions with children, youth, and families?

WEB LINKS

www.phac-aspc.gc.ca This is the website of the Public Health Agency of Canada. At this site, various information and resources on child health can be found, including the National Clearinghouse on Family Violence, Canada's resource centre for information on violence within relationships, can be found here. The Public Health Agency of Canada also serves as the Centres of Excellence for Children's Well-Being website (**www.phac-aspc.gc.ca/dca-dea/ allchildren_touslesenfants/centres_main-eng. php**), which provides the latest information on issues concerning the National Children's Agenda in Canada. It also hosts the Health Canada Mental Health Promotion website (**www.phac-aspc.gc.ca/mh-sm/ mhp-psm/**), which provides extensive publications, including information on capacity building in youth mental health promotion as well as youth projects.

www.ccf-fcsge.ca/docs/cccf/rs050_en.htm The website of the Child and Family Canada represents about 50 not-for-profit organizations and provides public education on children and families.

www.canadiancrc.com This website of the Canadian Children's Right's Council includes the 2005 article, "Homeless Children and Youths in Canada."

MOVIES, NOVELS, AND BIOGRAPHIES

My Girl: 1991. This story lovingly portrays a young girl coping with her mother's death. It provides a thoughtful general analysis of death because the family runs a funeral parlour.

VIEWING PIONTS: How is the depiction of the child's grieving process in this film typical of childhood mourning? What aspects of it appear to be uniquely influenced by her family and the circumstances? How could the adults in the film have been more sensitive to the child's fears and anxieties about death?

To Kill a Mockingbird: 1962. The narrator of this beautiful film is a young girl growing up in the southern United States. The story illustrates several important factors that can influence a child's development, including single-parent families, cultural factors, the effects of abuse and alcoholism, and the child's attempt to reconcile good and evil forces in the world.

VIEWING PIONTS: How effective is this single-parent family in coping with life stresses and developmental changes? What aspects of the family's functioning appear particularly strong? Compare Scout and Jem's upbringing to that of the young woman from the family with alcoholism. In what ways does this young girl appear to be at risk for developing mental health problems?

The Breakfast Club: 1985. This funny, poignant portrayal of adolescence is told through the eyes of several teens from different backgrounds brought together when they are assigned to all-day Saturday detention. It illustrates the heightened sense of drama that typifies adolescence, identity concerns, and peer relationship struggles.

VIEWING PIONTS: Which of these adolescents do you consider to be most at risk for having mental health problems? State the reasons for your choice. What are some factors that appear to be contributing to the risk-taking and acting-out behaviours among these adolescents?

What's Eating Gilbert Grape?: 1997. Johnny Depp plays Gilbert, a frustrated young man who struggles to be free from emotional stagnation, his sleepy Iowa town, and his 500-pound reclusive mother. This story highlights complex family dynamics and revolves around Gilbert's relationship with his mentally handicapped brother, played by Leonardo Di Caprio.

Significance: Family interaction centres on food and the impact of the mother's obesity on the rest of the family.

VIEWING PIONTS: Observe the interaction of the family during meal times. How has the mother's disability affected the family? How would you provide nursing care to this very complex family?

REFERENCES

Adlaf, E. M., & Zdanowicz, Y. M. (1999). A cluster-analytic study of substance problems and mental health among street youths. *American Journal of Drug and Alcohol Abuse, 25*(4), 639–660.

Anglin, C. (2008). Providing pediatric psychosocial support through patient library services in an outpatient hematology/oncology clinic. *Primary Psychiatry, 15*(7), 78–83.

Anthony, K. K., Gil, K. M., & Schanberg, L. E. (2003). Parental perceptions of child vulnerability in children with chronic illness. *Journal of Pediatric Psychology, 28*(3), 185–190.

Baker, A. (2007). Fostering stories: Why caseworkers, foster parents, and foster children should read stories about being in foster care. *The American Journal of Family Therapy, 35*, 151–165.

Beardslee, W. R., Gladstone T. R., Wright, E. J., & Cooper, A. B. (2003) A family-based approach to the prevention of depressive symptoms in children at risk: Evidence of parental and child change. *Paediatrics, 112*(2), e119–e131.

Begin, P., Casavant, L., Chenier, N. M., & Dupuis, J. (1999). *Homelessness*. Ottawa, ON: Library of Parliament, Parliamentary Research Branch.

Botvin, G. J. (2000). Preventing drug abuse in schools: Social and competence enhancement approaches targeting individual-level etiologic factors. *Addictive Behaviors, 25*(6), 887–897.

Bowlby, J. (1960). Grief and mourning in infancy and early childhood. *Psychoanalytic Study of the Child, 15*, 9–52.

Breton, J. J. (1999). Complementary development of prevention and mental health promotion programs for Canadian children based on contemporary scientific paradigms. *Canadian Journal of Psychiatry, 44*(3), 227–234.

Brody, G. H. (1998). Sibling relationship quality: Its causes and consequences. *Annual Review of Psychology, 49*, 1–24.

Brown, E. (2009). Helping bereaved children and young people. *British Journal of School Nursing, 4*(2), 69–73.

Brown, A., Sandler, I., Tein, J., Liu, X., & Haine, R. (2007). Implications of parental suicide and violent death for promotion of resilience of parentally-bereaved children. *Death Studies, 31*, 301–335.

Browne, K., & Saqi, S. (1988). Approaches to screening for child abuse and neglect. In K. Browne, C. Davies, & P. Stratton (Eds.), *Early prediction and prevention of child abuse* (pp. 57–85). Toronto, ON: John Wiley & Sons.

Burns, J. M., Andrews, G., & Szabo, M. (2002). Depression in young people: What causes it and can we prevent it? *Medical Journal of Australia, 177*(Suppl.), S93–S96.

Campaign 2000. *One million too many: Implementing solutions to child poverty in Canada*. 2004 Report Card on Child Poverty. Available at: http://www.campaign2000.ca.

Campbell, S. (1995). Behaviour problems in preschool children: A review of recent research. *Journal of Child Psychiatry, 36*, 113–149.

Canadian Centre for Justice Statistics. (2001). Family violence in Canada: A statistical profile. Cat. No. 85–224-XPE. Ottawa, ON: Statistics Canada.

Canadian Population Health Initiative. (2005). *Improving the health of young canadians*. Ottawa, ON: Canadian Institutes for Health Information.

Cance, A. M., Paradise, M., Ginzler, J. A., Embry, L., Morgan, C. J., Lohr, Y., et al. (2000). The characteristics and mental health of homeless adolescents: Age and gender differences. *Journal of Emotional & Behavior Disorders, 8*(4), 230–239.

Casa-Gil, M. J., & Navarro-Guzman, J. I. (2002). School characteristics among children of alcoholic parents. *Psychological Reports, 90*(1), 341–348.

Cavell, T., Ennett, S. T., & Meehan, B. T. (2001). Preventing alcohol and substance abuse. In J. N. Hughes, A. M. LaGreca, & J. C. Conoley (Eds.), *Handbook of psychological services for children and adolescents* (pp. 133–160). Oxford, UK: Oxford University Press.

Child Support Team. (2000). *Selected statistics on Canadian families and family law* (2nd ed.). Ottawa, ON: Department of Justice Canada.

Crittenden, P. M. (1996). Research on maltreating families: Implications for intervention. In J. Briere, L. Berliner, A. Bulkey, C. Jenny, & T. Reid (Eds.), *The APSAC handbook on child maltreatment* (pp. 158–174). Thousand Oaks, CA: Sage.

Deering, C. G., & Cody, D. J. (2002). Communicating effectively with children and adolescents. *American Journal of Nursing, 102*(3), 34–42.

Dennis, C. L. (2005). Psychosocial and psychological interventions for prevention of postnatal depression: Systematic review. *British Medical Journal, 331*(7507), 15–24.

Dillen, L., Fontaine, J., & Verhofstadt-Denève, L. (2009). Confirming the distinctiveness of complicated grief from depression and anxiety among adolescents. *Death Studies, 33*, 437–461.

Doherty, G. (1997). *Zero to six: The basis for school readiness*. Hull, Quebec: Applied Research Branch, Human Resources Development Canada.

Dryburgh, H. (2000). Teenage pregnancy. *Health Reports, 12*, 9–19.

Eggert, L. L., Thompson, E. A., Randell, B. P., & Pike, K. (2002). Preliminary effects of brief school-based prevention approaches for reducing youth suicide: Risk behaviors, depression, and drug involvement. *Journal of Child and Adolescent Psychiatric Nursing, 15*(2), 48–64.

Elford, R. (1998). Telemedicine activities at memorial University of Newfoundland: A historical review, 1975–1997. *Telemedicine Journal, 4*(3), 207–224.

Federal/Provincial/Territorial Advisory Committee on Population Health (1999). *Toward a healthy future: Second report on healthy Canadians*. Cat. N(o): H39–468/1999E. Ottawa, ON: Author.

Federal/Provincial/Territorial Advisory Committee on Population Health. (2000). *The opportunity of adolescence: The health sector contribution*. Cat. N(o): H39–548/200E. Ottawa, ON: Author.

Federal/Provincial/Territorial Council on Social Policy Renewal. (2000). *Public report: Dialogue on the national children's agenda—Developing a shared vision*. Ottawa, ON: Author.

Finke, L., Williams, J., Ritter, M., Kemper, D., Kersey, S., Nightenhauser, J., et al. (2002). Survival against drugs: Education for school-age children. *Journal of Child and Adolescent Psychiatric Nursing, 15*(4), 163–169.

Fopma-Loy, J. (2000). Peer rejection and neglect of latency age children: Pathways and group psychotherapy model. *Journal of Child and Adolescent Psychiatric Nursing, 13*, 29–38.

Gass, K., Jenkins, J., & Dunn, J. (2007). Are sibling relationships protective? A longitudinal study. *Journal of Child Psychology and Psychiatry, 48*(2), 167–175.

Geist, R., & Simon, L. (1999). Innovative continuing medical education program for paediatricians: A model for the delivery of mental health services. *Paediatrics & Child Health, 4*(2), 119–123.

Gimpel, G., & Holland, M. (2003). *Emotional and behavioral problems of young children: Effective interventions in the preschool and kindergarten years*. New York, NY: The Guilford Press.

Goldner, E. (2002). Sharing the learning: The health transition fund-synthesis series. *Mental Health*. Cat. N(o): H13–6/2002–8. Ottawa, ON: Health Canada.

Gorzka, P. (1999). Homeless parents' perceptions of parenting stress. *Journal of Child and Adolescent Psychiatric Nursing, 12*, 7–16.

Harter, S. (2000). Psychosocial adjustment of adult children of alcoholics: A review of recent empirical literature. *Clinical Psychology Review, 20*(3), 311–337.

Health Canada. (2000). *1998/1999 Canadian sexually transmitted disease surveillance report. Centre for Infectious Disease Prevention*. Canada Communicable Disease Report (CCDR), 26S6, 1–46. Available at: http://www.phac-aspc.gc.ca

Health Canada. (2002). *A report on mental illness in Canada*. Cat. N(o): 0–662–32817–5. Ottawa, ON: Author.

Health Canada & Canadian Mental Health Association. (1999). *All together now: How families are affected by depression and manic depression*. Cat. N(o): H39–461/1999E. Ottawa, ON: Author.

Helfer, M. E., Kemper, S., & Kongman, R. D. (1997). *The battered child*. Chicago, IL: University of Chicago Press.

Herrenkohl, T. I., Tajima, E. A., Whitney, S. D., & Huang, B. (2005). Protection against antisocial behavior in children exposed to physically abusive discipline. *Journal of Adolescent Health, 36*(6), 457–465.

Hetherington, E. M., & Kelly, J. (2002). *For better or for worse: Divorce reconsidered*. New York, NY: WW Norton.

Hughes, J. R., & Gottlieb, L. N. (2004). The effects of the Webster-Stratton parenting program on maltreating families: Fostering strengths. *Child Abuse and Neglect, 28*, 1081–1097.

Infant Mental Health Promotion. (2005). *Core prevention and intervention for the early years*. Toronto, ON: The Hospital for Sick Children.

Institute of Marriage and Family Canada. (2009). *Canadian divorce statistics. Quick Stats: Social Policy Statistics at a Glance*. Ottawa, ON: Author.

Jeynes, W. (2002). *Divorce, family structure, and the academic success of children*. New York, NY: Haworth Press.

Kaemingk, K., & Paquette, A. (1999). Effects of prenatal alcohol exposure on neuropsychological functioning. *Developmental Neuropsychology, 15*, 111–140.

Kelly, J. (2003). Changing perspectives on children's adjustment following divorce: A view from the United States. *Childhood, 10*(3), 237–254.

Kelly, K., & Caputo, T. (2007). Health and street/homeless youth. *Journal of Health Psychology, 12*(5), 726–736.

Khanlou, N. (2003). Mental health promotion education in multicultural settings. *Nursing Education Today, 23*, 96–103.

Khanlou, N., & Crawford, C. (2006). Post-migratory experiences of newcomer female youth: Self-esteem and identity development. *Journal of Immigrant and Minority Health, 81*(1), 45–56.

Khanlou, N., Beiser, M., Cole, E., Freire, M., Hyman, I., & Kilbride, K. M. (2002). Mental health promotion among newcomer female youth: Post-migration experiences and self-esteem. Ottawa, ON: Status of Women Canada (English and French versions). Available at: http://dsp-psd.communication.gc.ca

LeBlanc, L. A., Goldsmith, T., & Patel, D. R. (2003). Behavioral aspects of chronic illness in children and adolescents. *Pediatric Clinics of North America, 50*(4), 859–878.

Leventhal, T., & Brooks-Gunn, J. (2000). The neighborhoods they live in: The effects of neighborhood residence on child and adolescent outcomes. *Psychological Bulletin, 126*, 309–337.

Lewis, M., & Vitulano, L. A. (2003). Biopsychosocial issues and risk factors in the family when the child has a chronic illness. *Child & Adolescent Psychiatric Clinics of North America, 12*(3), 389–399.

MacLeod, J., & Nelson, G. (2000). Programs for the promotion of family wellness and the prevention of child maltreatment: A meta-analytic review. *Child Abuse & Neglect, 24*(9), 1127–1149.

MacMillan, H. L., & Canadian Task Force on Preventive Health Care. (2000). Preventive health care, 2000 update: Prevention of child maltreatment. *Canadian Medical Association Journal, 163*(11), 1451–1458.

Maguire, S., Mann, M. K., Sibert, J., & Kemp, A. (2005). Are there patterns of bruising in childhood which are diagnostic or suggestive of abuse? A systematic review. *Archives of Diseases in Childhood, 90*(2), 182–186.

Martinez, Y., & Ercikan, K. (2009). Chronic illnesses in Canadian children: What is the effect of illness on academic achievement, and anxiety and emotional disorders? *Child: Care, Health And Development, 35*(3), 391–401.

Masten, A. S. (2001). Ordinary magic: Resilience processes in development. *American Psychologist, 56*(3), 227–238.

Melhem, N., Moritz, G., Walker, M., Shear, M. K., & Brent, D. (2007). Phenomenology and correlates of complicated grief in dhildren and adolescents. *Journal of Academic Child Adolescent Psychiatry, 46*(4), 493–499.

Moser, R. P., & Jacob, T. (2002). Parental and sibling effects in adolescent outcomes. *Psychological Reports, 91*(2), 463–479.

Mylant, M. L., Ide, B., Cuevas, E., & Meehan, M. (2002). Adolescent children of alcoholics: Vulnerable or resilient? *Journal of the American Psychiatric Nurses Association, 8*(2), 57–64.

O'Connor, T. G., Bredenkamp, D., & Rutter, M. (1999). Attachment disturbances and disorders in children exposed to early severe deprivation. *Infant Mental Health Journal, 20*(1), 10–29.

Offord, D. R., & Bennett, K. J. (2002). Prevention. In M. Rutter & E. Taylor (Eds.), *Child and adolescent psychiatry* (4th ed.). Oxford, UK: Blackwell Science.

Offord, D. R., Kraemer, H. C., Kazdin, A. E., Jensen, P. S., & Harrington, R. (1998). Lowering the burden of suffering from child psychiatric disorder: Trade-offs among clinical, targeted, and universal interventions. *Journal of the American Academy of Child and Adolescent Psychiatry, 37*(7), 686–694.

Peters, R., Petrunka, K., & Arnold, R. (2003). The better Beginnings, Brighter Futures Project: A universal, comprehensive, community-based prevention approach for primary school children and their families. *Journal of Clinical Child and Adolescent Psychology, 32*, 215–227.

Pfund, R. (2006). *Palliative care nursing for children and young people.* Oxford: Radcliffe.

Pruett, M. K., Williams, T. Y., Insabella, G., & Little, T. D. (2003). Family and legal indicators of child adjustment to divorce among families with young children. *Journal of Family Psychology, 17*(2), 169–180.

Puskar, K. R., Sereika, S., & Tusaie-Mumford, K. (2003). Effect of the Teaching Kids to Cope (TKC) Program on outcomes of depression and coping among rural adolescents. *Journal of Child and Adolescent Psychiatric Nursing, 16*(2), 71–80.

Putnam, F. W. (2003). Ten-year research update review: Child sexual abuse. *Journal of the American Academy of Child & Adolescent Psychiatry, 42*(3), 269–278.

Reifman, A., Villa, L. C., Amans, J. A., Rethinam, V., & Telesca, T. Y. (2001). Children of divorce in the 1990's: A meta-analysis. *Journal of Divorce and Remarriage, 35*(1–2), 27–36.

Rew, L. (2003). A theory of taking care of oneself grounded in experiences of homeless youth. *Nursing Research, 52*(4), 234–241.

Ringwalt, C. L., Greene, J. M., Robertson, M., & McPheeters, M. (1998). The prevalence of homelessness among adolescents in the United States. *American Journal of Public Health, 88*(9), 1325–1329.

Ritter, J., Stewart, M., Bernet, C., Coe, M., & Brown, S. A. (2002). Effects of childhood exposure to familial alcoholism and family violence on adolescent substance use, conduct problems, and self-esteem. *Journal of Traumatic Stress, 15*(2), 113–122.

Schoor, L. B. (1997). *Common purpose: Strengthening families and neighborhoods to rebuild America.* New York, NY: Doubleday.

Schor, E. L., & the American Academy of Pediatrics Task Force on the Family. (2003). Family pediatrics: Report of the task force on the Family. *Pediatrics, 111*(6 Pt 2), 1541–1571.

Self, B., & Peters, H. (2005). Street outreach with no streets. *Canadian Nurse, 101*(1), 20–24.

Sharpe, D., & Rossiter, L. (2002). Siblings of children with a chronic illness: A meta-analysis. *Journal of Pediatric Psychology, 27*(8), 699–710.

Statistics Canada. (2004a). *Canadian community health survey: Mental health and well-being.* Ottawa, ON: Author.

Statistics Canada. (2004b). *Health reports: How healthy are Canadians? 2004 Annual Report.* Supplement to Vol. 15. Cat. N(o): 82–003-S1E. Ottawa, ON: Author.

Sun, U., & Li, Y. (2002). Children's well-being during parents' marital disruption process: A pooled time-series analysis. *Journal of Marriage and the Family, 64*(2), 472–488.

Taussig, H. N. (2002). Risk behaviors in maltreated youth placed in foster care: A longitudinal study of protective and vulnerability factors. *Child Abuse & Neglect, 26*(11), 1179–1199.

Tomlin, A. M., & Viehweg, S. A. (2003). Infant mental health: Making a difference. *Professional Psychology: Research and Practice, 34*(6), 617–625.

Trocme, N., MacLaurin, B., Fallon, B., Daciuk, J., Billingsley, D., Tourigny, M., et al. (2001). *Canadian incidence study of reported child abuse and neglect.* Ottawa, ON: Minister of Public Works and Government Services Canada.

UNICEF. (2005). *Child poverty in rich countries, 2005.* Innocenti Report Card No.6. Florence, Italy: UNICEF Innocenti Research Centre. Available at: http://www.unicef.org/irc

Urness, D., Hailey, D., Delday, L., Callanan, T., & Orlik, H. (2004). The status of telepsychiatry services in Canada: A national survey. *Journal of Telemedicine and Telecare, 10*(3), 160–164.

Van Epps, J., Opie, N. D., & Goodwin, T. (1997). Themes in the bereavement experience of inner city adolescents. *Journal of Child and Adolescent Psychiatric Nursing, 10*, 25–36.

Veronie, L., & Freuhstorfer, D. B. (2001). Gender, birth order and family role identification among children of alcoholics. *Current Psychology: Developmental, Learning, Personality, Social, 20*(1), 53–67.

Waddell, C., McEwan, K., Shepherd, C. A., Offord, D. R., & Hua, J. M. (2005). A public health strategy to improve the mental health of Canadian children. *Canadian Journal of Psychiatry, 50*(4), 226–233.

Warren, J. K., Gary, F. A., & Moorhead, M. S. (1997). Runaway youths in a Southern community: Four critical areas of inquiry. *Journal of Child and Adolescent Psychiatric Nursing, 10*(2), 26–35.

Werner, E. E., & Smith, R. S. (1992). *Overcoming the odds: High risk children from birth to adulthood.* Ithaca, NY: Cornell University Press.

Williams, T. L., May, C. R., & Esmail, A. (2001). Limitations of patient satisfaction studies in telehealthcare: A systematic review of the literature. *Telemedicine Journal and E-Health, 7*(4), 293–316.

Wolfe, D. A. (1998). *Prevention of child abuse and neglect.* Ottawa, ON: Health Canada.

Wu, Z., Hou, F., & Schimmele, C. (2008). Family structure and children's psychosocial outcomes. *Journal of Family Issues, 29*(12), 1600–1624.

Yalom, I. D. (1985). *The theory and practice of group psychotherapy* (2nd ed.). New York, NY: Basic Books.

Mental Health Assessment of Children and Adolescents

Wendy Austin

Adapted from the chapter "Mental Health Assessment of Children and Adolescents" by Jean Robinson Hughes, Vanya Hamrin, Catherine Gray Deering, and Lawrence Scahill

KEY CONCEPT

- maturation

LEARNING OBJECTIVES

After studying this chapter, you will be able to:

- Define the assessment process for children and adolescents.
- Discuss the techniques of data collection used with children and adolescents.
- Discuss the synthesis of bio/psycho/social/spiritual assessment data for children and adolescents.
- Delineate the important bio/psycho/social/spiritual areas of assessment for children and adolescents.

KEY TERMS

- assortative mating • attachment • attachment disorganization • developmental delays • egocentrism • maturation • temperament

*T*he mental health assessment of children and adolescents is challenging. At any given time, 14% of children aged 4 to 17 years (more than 800,000 in Canada) experience mental disorders that cause significant distress and impairment at home, at school, and in the community (Waddell, McEwan, Shepherd, Offord, & Hua, 2005). Yet, fewer than 25% of these children receive specialized treatment services. There are a number of reasons for this situation. First, mental health services are woefully inadequate in many regions of Canada and often are limited to urban areas (e.g., Breton, Plante, & St-Georges, 2005). Second, evidence from large studies using national survey data shows that differences in government policies and healthcare system characteristics cause variances in service use (Sturm, Ringel, & Andreyeva, 2003). Third, some children do not

get help when those who serve as gatekeepers to treatment (parents, teachers, and physicians) either fear the stigma that children will carry with mental illness (Jellnick, Patel, & Froehle, 2003) or fail to recognize mental illness as a childhood problem or the impact of early emotional experience on a child's capacity to develop relationships and to learn (Carter, Briggs-Gowan, & Davis, 2004). Given the evidence that the largest determinants of service provision to youth are provider assessment of mental health problems and provider knowledge of service resources (Stiffman et al., 2000), it is crucial that health professionals be knowledgeable and proficient in these areas.

The assessment of children and adolescents is a specialized process that considers their unique problems and responses within the context of their development.

The *Standards of Psychiatric-Mental Health Nursing Practice* (3rd ed.) (Canadian Federation of Mental Health Nurses [CFMHN], 2005) serves as a guide for this process. These standards argue that effective diagnosis and monitoring are dependent on a client-centred approach, one that incorporates both theory and an understanding of the meaning of the health or illness experience from the perspective of the client. The nurse acknowledges clients as valued and respected partners throughout the decision-making process and supports them in drawing on their own assets and resources for self-care and mental health promotion. The nurse also incorporates knowledge of family dynamics as well as knowledge of cultural values and beliefs about families in the assessment. The assessment of children and adolescents generally follows the same format as that for adults (see Chapter 11), but there are significant differences. Children think in more concrete terms; thus, the nurse needs to ask more specific and fewer open-ended questions than would typically be asked of adults. The nurse should use simple phrasing because children have a narrower vocabulary than do adults. Examples include saying "sad" instead of "depressed" or "nervous" instead of "anxious." The nurse needs to corroborate information that children offer with more sources (e.g., parents, teachers) than they would for adults. The nurse may want to use artistic and play media (e.g., puppets, family drawings) to engage children and evaluate their perceptions, inner worlds, fine motor skills, and intellectual functions. Children have a less specific sense of time and a less developed memory than do adults. When children are asked about a sequence of events or specific times when events occurred, they may not be able to provide accurate information.

Mental health assessment involves much more than completing assessment tools and considers far more than the individual. A conceptual framework used as a guide can assist in planning the goals of the assessment, as well as identify the factors, types of information and sources, and the elements within the environment to be considered. A framework that is bio-ecological (Bronfenbrenner, 1986), transactional (Sameroff & Chandler, 1975), and developmental in nature reinforces the importance of placing information about the child's social-emotional functioning and psychopathologic symptoms within the context of the child's cognitive and developmental functioning, family relationships, cultural values and beliefs, and broader family and community risk factors (Carter et al., 2004).

The Canadian Mental Health Association's Framework for Support (Trainor, Pomeroy, & Pape, 2004) clusters such knowledge in three resource bases: the Person Resource Base, the Knowledge Resource Base, and the Community Resource Base. By focusing on the *Person Resource Base*, the nurse acknowledges that the child is far more than a repository of illness and symptoms and that positive change builds on existing strengths. Hence, when approaching assessment, the nurse considers children's understanding of their mental health problem/illness as well as their self-esteem, sense of belonging (within their family and community), and sense of purpose and meaning in the world. The nurse also assesses children's skills and capacities (sense of personal control, confidence, resilience, hope) to confront illness. By focusing on the *Knowledge Resource Base*, the nurse takes into consideration not only medical-clinical and social science knowledge but also experiential (first-hand experience) and traditional knowledge (cultural ways). The nurse's assessment considers how children experience mental illness and how the family and community (public attitudes and conventional wisdom) accept it. A critical analysis of such information assists the nurse in building a rich understanding of children and guards against drawing inaccurate assumptions. It can also identify inaccuracies and misconceptions that may be held within the family or community about mental illness. By focusing on the *Community Resource Base*, the nurse gains an understanding of the many factors and social determinants (housing, education, income, meaningful work) that affect the everyday life of children (Trainor et al., 2004, pp. 8–10). The Community Resource Base also acknowledges the importance of both formal services (mental health services, generic community services) and the network of natural supports (family and friends, self-help and consumer organizations) available to promote mental health and recovery. Equally important, it recognizes the person (child or youth) as having the power (age-appropriate) to make choices about resources to use, if any, and to participate fully in decision making.

The Framework for Support helps the nurse focus assessment on outcomes and, in particular, on those outcomes that play a critical role in recovery from mental illness. Specifically, it assesses whether a child has access to the social determinants of good mental health (housing, school, family, friends, a sense of purpose), feels good and has a sense of personal control, and has various personal resources in place and ways to connect with the formal service system if needed. Finally, the framework assesses how the individual's age (child or youth) and life circumstances (e.g., breakup or death in family, being dropped from sport team) have challenged the child.

A comprehensive evaluation includes a bio/psycho/social/spiritual history, mental status examination, additional testing (e.g., cognitive or neuropsychological)—if necessary, records of the child's school performance and medical-physical history, and information from other agencies that may be providing services (e.g., department of child and family services, juvenile court). The nurse may use various assessment tools, including the Child Attention Profile (CAP) and the Devereux Early Childhood Assessment (DECA), the Behaviour Assessment System for Children (BASC), the Child Behaviour Checklist (CBCL), or the Children's Depression Inventory (CDI).

DATA COLLECTION IN THE CLINICAL INTERVIEW

The clinical interview is the primary assessment tool used in child and adolescent psychiatry. A unique set of skills is necessary for interviewing children and adolescents. How the nurse obtains mental health information depends on the developmental level of each child, specifically considering the child's language and cognitive, social, and emotional skills. For example, the nurse should simplify questions for young children or children with developmental delays (e.g., mental retardation, Asperger's syndrome, pervasive developmental disorder) so that these children can understand and respond appropriately.

The assessment interview may be the initial contact between the child and parent or guardian and the nurse. The first step is to establish a helping relationship, and the second is to assess the interactions between the child and the parent. It is important to understand that children cannot be considered apart from their caregivers and the context in which they live. However, defining the caregiving context is sometimes a challenge (Carter et al., 2004). The nurse needs to identify the child's primary *caregivers*, the patterns of current caregiving relationships (e.g., how often the child goes to other caregivers), and the history of these relationships (e.g., multiple transitions, abrupt losses) (p. 114). The nurse should also explore the family's definition of *family* and identify those included in the family constellation—both biologic and psychological relationships (e.g., friends, neighbours) (pp. 114–115).

Treatment Alliance: The Helping Relationship

The nurse can establish rapport by greeting the child or adolescent in a friendly, polite, open manner, and putting him or her at ease. Speaking clearly and at a normal volume and using friendly, reassuring tones are essential measures. The nurse can establish a helping relationship by recognizing the child's individuality and showing respect and concern for that child. The nurse should demonstrate sensitivity, objectivity, and confidentiality. The child will be more forthcoming if he or she believes that the nurse is listening carefully and is interested in what he or she has to say.

Child and Parent Observation

Because the child's primary environment is most often with the parent, child–parent interactions provide important data about the child–parent attachment and parenting practices. The nurse's observations focus on both the child alone and the child within the family. The nurse can actually make some of these observations while the family is in the waiting area, noting behaviours identified in Barnard's parent–child interaction model (1994):

- Sensitivity/clarity/responsiveness to cues
  - How the child and parent get each other's attention
  - How parent and child interact with and talk to each other (clarity of cues)
  - How frequently each initiates conversation and how promptly each responds
  - How the child and parent separate
  - Whether the parent and child play together
  - How responsive the parent is to the child's attention-seeking initiatives
  - How the parent and child show affection to each other
  - How attached the parent and the child appear
- Response to distress
  - Whether the parent starts/stops/notes the distress/changes in activity
  - How the parent consoles the child
  - How the parent disciplines the child (clear directive voice, yells, hits)
- Social-emotional growth fostering
  - Use of talking/smiling/laughing/singing/touching (praising or criticising)
- Cognitive growth fostering
  - Parent talks about/describes objects/ideas using developmentally appropriate and stimulating language
  - Parent provides child with/points out objects of interest
  - Parent encourages and/or allows the child to explore.

Interview Techniques

To get an accurate picture of the child, the nurse should interview the child and parent individually for some part of the session because each can provide unique, meaningful information. Research has shown that during times when parent and child are interviewed separately in a structured interview about the child's psychopathology, they rarely agree on the presence of diagnostic criteria, regardless of the diagnostic type (Jensen et al., 1999). Generally, children provide better information about internalizing symptoms (e.g., mood, sleep, suicide ideation), and parents provide better information about externalizing symptoms (e.g., behaviour disturbances, oppositionality, relationship with parents).

Discussion With the Child

After talking with the parent and child together, the nurse should ask to speak with the child alone for a while. Young children may fear separating from their parents. The nurse can reassure children by showing them where the waiting area is and telling them, "Mommy and Daddy are going to be waiting right here for you. You and I are going to be in a room close by. But if you get scared, we can come back out here to check on them." Introducing a toy or game or giving the child a transitional object to hold may help. For example, young children often like holding the family car or house keys, knowing that their parents cannot go anywhere without them. Remember that observing how the child separates from the parent is part of the data needed to complete the assessment.

Adolescents may act indifferent or even hostile when the nurse asks to speak with them alone. Teens tend to be sceptical that adults can really understand their experience, suspicious that they will be blamed for their problems, and fearful that their thoughts and feelings are abnormal. The nurse should be patient with adolescents and show empathy for their concerns through comments such as, "I can see that you're pretty angry about being here. There might be a way that I can help.... But in order to help, I need to know from *you* what is going on that is making you so angry. I want to assure you that I am not here to judge or blame. I can also promise you that if you tell me anything that I think needs to be shared with your parents, then I will tell you first." If the child is particularly silent, the nurse might comment, "You've been pretty quiet during the last few minutes.... I'm not sure if that means you're having trouble expressing yourself.... That can be really frustrating. If that is the case, then, maybe if you just start talking, we can try to find some words together to express your ideas.... On the other hand, you may be wondering if it is safe to tell me what you're thinking. It can be really frightening to trust a stranger with your most private thoughts.... You may be wondering whether I really meant what I said about confidentiality/keeping things private.... or about not judging you.... I guess the dilemma/problem is whether it is safer to keep holding on to those tormenting thoughts and feelings or taking a chance that someone might be able to help."

To begin the initial assessment of a child, the nurse introduces himself or herself and explains briefly what they will be doing together. For children younger than 11 years of age, the nurse should explain that he or she helps worried or upset children by talking, playing, and together with his or her parents, thinking of ways to make things better. The nurse should then ask about the child's understanding of why he or she is there. This question often helps to identify children's misconceptions (e.g., believing the nurse is going to give them an injection, thinking that they have done something bad) that could create barriers to working with them. When conducting the child interview, the nurse will need to get several releases of information from the child's guardian to obtain corroborating reports, such as the child's physical assessment from the paediatrician or paediatric nurse practitioner; the school's report about the child's academic (report card) and behavioural performance (interactions with peers and adults); and records of diagnosis and treatment from any previous psychiatric provider. Youth are often very sensitive when reports are requested from school. They worry about repercussions if they have had prior difficulties (e.g., disciplinary problems). It is important that the nurse explain how these reports will be used, whether the school will be involved in the development of treatment plans, and how the youth and family will participate.

The nurse must adapt communication to the child's age level (Box 27-1). The challenge is to avoid using overly complex vocabulary or talking down to children.

BOX 27.1

Strategies for Interviewing Children

- Use a simple vocabulary and short sentences tailored to the child's developmental and cognitive levels.
- Be sure that the child understands the questions and that you do not lead the child to give a particular response. Presenting polar opposite choices (never... or all the time), or scaled questions (1–10), is helpful. For example, "Some people feel angry all the time, some only feel angry at certain times, and others don't seem to feel angry at all. On a scale of 1–10, where 1 means never and 10 means all the time, how often do you feel angry?" If the child chooses a number greater than 1, she can be asked to describe times when she is angry.
- Select the questions for your interview on an individual basis, using judgment and discretion and considering the child's age and developmental level.
- Be sure that the manner and tone of your voice do not reveal any personal biases.
- Speak slowly and quietly, and try to allow the interview to unfold, using the child's verbalizations and behaviour as guides.
- Use simple terms (e.g., "sad" for "depressed") in exploring affective reactions, and ask the child to give examples of how he or she behaves or how other people behave when emotionally aroused.
- Assume an accepting and neutral attitude toward the child's communications.
- Learn about children's current interests by looking at Saturday morning television programs, talking with parents, visiting toy stores, looking at children's books, and visiting day care centres and schools to observe children in their natural habitat (Sattler, 1998).

Young children often express themselves more easily in the context of play than through adult-like conversation. For example, a child may re-enact a conversation that he had with a sibling or parent using puppets. Children respond well to third-person conversation prompts, such as "Some kids don't like being compared to their brothers and sisters," or "I know a kid who was so sad when he lost his dog that he thought he would never be happy again."

Early in the interview, the goal is to explain the nurse's purpose, elicit any concerns the child may have about what is happening, and establish rapport with the child by engaging in unthreatening discussion. Many adults rarely ask children about things that truly interest them, but expect children to respond readily to adult conversation. The nurse can establish a high degree of credibility simply by taking note of and asking about things that are obviously important to children (e.g., a sport that they participate in, a rock group displayed on a shirt, a toy they have brought with them). However, children have an uncanny natural "radar" for dishonest adult behaviour. Attempts to establish rapport work only when the nurse is genuinely interested in the child's life.

Discussion With the Parents

After meeting alone with the child, the nurse should discuss with the child that she or he would now like to talk with the parents alone, just as she or he did with the child. The nurse should be careful to reiterate that she or he wants to help and will not judge anyone in the family. The nurse should ensure that the child has a safe place to wait and age-appropriate activities. When the nurse meets with the parents, she or he should review the expectations and provide similar reassurances around confidentiality, building trust, and being nonjudgmental as those given to the child. The nurse would then proceed to ask parents to describe their view of the problem. When alone, parents often feel more comfortable discussing their children in depth and sharing their frustrations. Parents need this opportunity to speak freely, without being constrained by concern for the child's feelings. Although children often have a pretty good sense about their parents' reactions, it may not be constructive for them to hear the full force of the parents' complaints and feelings, such as their sense of helplessness, anger, or disappointment. Parents sometimes feel guilty and need permission to express their negative feelings without feeling judged. This session is the nurse's opportunity to enlist the help of parents as partners in understanding and addressing the child's problem. This time is also good for filling in any gaps in the history and clarifying the data obtained from the interview with the child.

Parents need the chance to describe the presenting problem in their own words. The nurse can encourage them by asking general questions, such as, "It is not easy for parents to recognize that childhood is sometimes unhappy and that their child needs help. A child's emotions and behaviour can be pretty confusing, even frightening, and most parents hope that, with time, the problems will disappear on their own. Sadly, that is sometimes not the case, and if left unattended over time, the problems can worsen. It takes great courage to seek help, and you took a big step in coming here today. I hope that by working together with your child, we will find some ways of assisting. I am interested in *your* story. Tell me what brings *you* here *today*." The nurse should then reflect his or her understanding of the problem, showing empathy and respect for both parent and child. Asking any other family members about their view of the problem is always a good idea to clarify discrepancies, obtain additional data, and communicate awareness that different family members experience the same problem in different ways.

Building Rapport

To reduce anxiety about the evaluation, the nurse must develop rapport with the family members. Establishing rapport can be facilitated by maintaining appropriate eye contact; speaking slowly, clearly, and calmly with friendliness and acceptance; using a warm and expressive tone; reacting to communications objectively; showing interest in what families are saying; and making the interview a joint undertaking (Sattler, 1998). Suggestions for building rapport with children and adolescents are also addressed in each of the developmental sections that follow. Building rapport, which is often challenging, is fundamental to any mental health assessment of children and youth. The developmental transitions throughout childhood and adolescence are rapid, and there are few guidelines about how information from many sectors should be integrated, how impairment levels should be determined, or how assessing function that may be specific to context (relational or cultural) or caregiver (e.g., parents, relatives, day care staff, school teacher) can be achieved practically (Carter et al., 2004). The information in Box 27-2 can serve as a guide to asking specific questions during a comprehensive assessment of the child. The Community Resource Base of the Framework for Support (Trainor et al., 2004) provides a useful guide for identifying a range of stakeholders from the child's daily living activities (e.g., parent, school, day care, recreation, arts) as well as services (formal or informal) that might be consulted (with family permission) for related information about the various contexts in which the child interacts. These stakeholders can provide complementary information (formal or informal) about how the child is functioning in critical developmental domains (language and literacy, physical, cognitive, social, and emotional). They also provide an understanding of how the child is treated within, and copes with, various peer environments involving diverse cultures

BOX 27.2

Semi-Structured Interview With School-Aged Children

This guide identifies a range of areas and sample questions that can be addressed during an interview with a school-aged or adolescent child. The nurse should note that children generally prefer to be engaged in a conversation rather than peppered with questions. The interview should be tailored in a way that is comfortable and relevant for the child. Although some direct questions are inevitable, open-ended questions are preferable (Hill & O'Brien, 1999). Similarly, phrasing questions to get at what a child is thinking (e.g., "I can see you are trying to tell me something" or "tell me more") is preferable to asking "why" questions that tend to put people on the defensive (Plutchik, 2000). Finally, trying to match the child's emotional state (unless hostile) helps people feel understood (Forgatch & Patterson, 1989). The interview can begin with a simple greeting, such as the following: "Hi, I am (your name and title). You must be Tom Brown. Come in."

FOR ALL SCHOOL-AGED CHILDREN

PRESENTING CONCERN

Thank you for coming to talk with me today. To begin, it would help me if I knew what, if anything, you have been told about why you are here or what will go on today.... Can you tell me *your* story of how you came to be here today (if necessary, probe with specific questions below)? Let the child take the lead and explore issues as he or she raises them. If the child raises a problem, explore it in detail.

DEMOGRAPHIC INFORMATION

I'd like to know you better. Could you tell me about yourself?

Probes

1. How old are you?
2. When is your birthday?
3. Where do you live? (address)
4. And your telephone number is…?

SCHOOL

Tell me about your school.

Probes

5. Which school do you go to? Is it close to your home? How do you get there each day?
6. Where do you go after school (home, sitter, etc.)… and who is there (parent/relative, sitter, no one)?
7. What do most kids think about your school?… What is it like for you?
8. What grade are you in? What do most kids think about it?… What is it like for you?
9. What subjects do you like the best?… Like least?
10. What subjects give you the least trouble?… Most trouble?
11. How well do you do in school—about the same as, better than, or not as well as other kids in your class?
12. On the whole, would you say that you are doing better or worse than last year?
13. What activities do you participate in at school?
14. How well do you get along with your classmates?
15. How well do you get along with your teachers?
16. Tell me how you spend a usual day at school.

HOME AND FAMILY

To help me understand your family, can you name each of the people who live with you… and then other important family members who live somewhere else… and I'll put them into a picture… Now using the picture, tell me a little about your family.

(A **genogram** [pronounced: *jen-uh-gram*] [Wright & Leahey, 2005] provides a useful diagram of family relationships. It resembles a family tree but includes additional relationships among individuals. It permits the nurse and the child to quickly see patterns in family history. It maps relationships and traits that may otherwise be missed and includes basic information about number of families, number of children in each family, birth order, and deaths. Some genograms include information on disorders running in the family such as alcoholism, depression, diseases, alliances, and living situations. Older children can provide additional information [e.g., about separation/divorce, death] for understanding family dynamics.)

Probes

17. Tell me a little about each of them.
    * Who makes you happy and who makes you sad/angry/worried? Explain.
    * Do you have a favourite photo of you and your family? Tell me about it… and why you like it.
18. What does your father do during the day—does he work? (other activities at home/with friends)?
19. What does your mother do during the day—does she work? (other activities at home/with friends)?
20. Tell me what your home is like.
21. Tell me about your room at home.
22. What chores do you do at home?
23. How do you get along with your father?
24. What does he do that you like?… Don't like?
25. How do you get along with your mother?
26. What does she do that you like?… Don't like?
27. (Where relevant) Some brothers and sisters get along well, whereas others don't get along at all… How do you get along with your brothers and sisters?
28. What do (does) they (he/she) do that you like?… That you don't like?
29. Who handles the discipline at home?
30. Tell me about how they (he/she) handle (handles) it.
    * When you do something good, what happens and who is involved?
    * When you get in trouble, what happens and who is involved?
    * If you want to do something different from the rest of your family, would that be okay? Explain… Who would support you?
    * If you need help, what would you do? Would someone support you? Explain.
    * Are there other relatives who are important to you? Tell me about who they are and how they connect with you (if not already discussed with the genogram).

Continued

- Would you say that your family is like most other families in your school/neighbourhood or different? Explain. Does that make it easy or difficult for you/your family… and in what ways and in what types of situations? This question gets at culture (ethnicity, socio-economic status, language, beliefs/values, etc.) in a broad way.

INTERESTS

Now let's talk about the things you like to do?

Probes

31. What hobbies and interests do you have?
32. What do you do in the afternoons/evenings after school?
33. Tell me what you usually do on Saturdays and Sundays.
    - What do you do on special holidays? Tell me about the best holiday you ever had.
    - When you are having fun, what are you doing, who are you with? Tell me about a time when you were really having a good time.

Friends

Tell me about your friends.

Probes

34. What do you like to do with your friends?
    - Any best friends?
    - If you needed help, could you count on them to support you? Give an example.
    - If you wanted to do something different from them, would that be okay?

MOODS AND FEELINGS

Probes

35. Everybody feels happy at times. What things make you feel happiest?
36. What are you most likely to get sad about?
37. What do you do when you are sad?
38. Everybody gets angry at times. What things make you angriest?
39. What do you do when you are angry?

FEARS AND WORRIES

Probes

40. All children get scared sometimes about some things. What things make you feel scared?
41. What do you do when you are scared?… What takes away the fear?
    - How well does that work?
42. Tell me what you worry about… What takes away the worry?
    - How well does that work?
43. Any other things?

SELF-CONCERNS

Probes

44. What do you like best about yourself?… Anything else?
45. What do you like least about yourself?… Anything else?
46. Tell me about the best thing that ever happened to you.
47. Tell me about the worst thing that ever happened to you.
    - What did you do about this situation?
    - How well does that work?
    - Overall, how much would you say you believe in yourself?

SOMATIC CONCERNS

Probes

48. Do you ever get headaches?
49. (If yes) Tell me about them. (How often? What do you usually do?)
50. Do you get stomachaches?
51. (If yes) Tell me about them. (How often? What do you usually do?)
52. Do you get any other kinds of body pains?
53. (If yes) Tell me about them.
    - What do you do to ease these problems?
    - How well does that work?

THOUGHT DISORDER

Probes

54. Do you ever hear things that seem funny or unusual?
55. (If yes) Tell me about them. (How often? How do you feel about them? What do you usually do?)
56. Do you ever see things that seem funny or unreal?
57. (If yes) Tell me about them. (How often? How do you feel about them? What do you usually do?)

HELP-SEEKING

Probes

58. Tell me about a time when you have needed help. What did you do? Who did you ask for help? What kind of help did you get? How did things work out?
59. Have you ever gone to see a counsellor before? Explain. Did it help?

MEMORIES AND FANTASY

Probes

60. What is the first thing you can remember from the time when you were a very little baby?
61. Tell me about your dreams.
62. Which dreams come back again?
63. Who are your favourite television characters?
64. Tell me about them.
65. What animals do you like best?
66. Tell me about these animals.
67. What animals do you like least?
68. Tell me about these animals.
69. What is your happiest memory?
70. What is your saddest memory?
71. If you could change places with anyone in the whole world, who would it be?
72. Tell me about that.
73. If you could go anywhere you wanted to right now, where would you go?
74. Tell me about that.
75. If you could have three wishes, what would they be?
76. What things do you think you might need to take with you if you were to go to the moon and stay there for 6 months?

ASPIRATIONS

77. What do you plan on doing when you become an adult?
78. What things will help you be successful? Is there anything standing in the way of you being successful?
    - How hopeful are you that you might be successful? (suggestion–using a visual analogue with a series of faces on a line [sad face-to-very happy face] ask child to choose the face that best describes their hopefulness)

Continued

BOX 27.2

Semi-Structured Interview With School-Aged Children (Continued)

79. If you could do anything you wanted when you become an adult, what would it be?

CONCLUDING QUESTIONS

80. Do you have anything else that you would like to tell me about yourself?
81. Do you have any questions that you would like to ask me?
   • What are you hoping will happen as a result of our talking today?

FOR ADOLESCENTS

These questions can be inserted after number 57 (the help-seeking section).

SEXUAL RELATIONS

Adolescence is a very confusing time emotionally. Our bodies change as we begin to look more like adults. Our relationships also change. While our sexual relationships are new and exciting, they can also be puzzling, frustrating, or even frightening.

1. Do you have any romantic feelings or relationship(s) with guys or girls? Do you feel comfortable talking about them? With girls/guys/or both?
2. What makes you feel good about it/them?
3. What makes you feel not so good about them?
4. Do you have any special girlfriend (boyfriend)?
5. (If yes) Tell me about her (him). Most people have lots of questions about their sexual relationships and yet are not sure whom to trust to talk openly…
6. What kind of sexual concerns do you have?
7. (If present) Tell me about them.

8. (If applicable) What do you think might be helpful to do about your concerns? (getting information, talking to someone, getting a check-up/some medication)
9. Are you interested in getting help? Would you like me to help you make the right connections?

DRUG AND ALCOHOL USE

10. Do your parents/sister/brothers drink?
11. (If yes) Tell me about their drinking. (How much, how frequently, and where?)
12. Do your friends drink alcohol?
13. (If yes) Tell me about their drinking.
14. Do you drink alcohol?
15. (If yes) Tell me about your drinking.
16. Do your parents use drugs?
17. (If yes) Tell me about the drugs they use. (How much, how frequently, and for what reasons?)
18. Do your friends use drugs?
19. (If yes) Tell me about the drugs they use.
20. Do you use drugs?
21. (If yes) Tell me about the drugs you use. (Sattler, 1998)
22. Are you worried about the way your parents/siblings/friends use alcohol or drugs?
23. Are you worried about the way you use alcohol/drugs?
24. (If yes) Are you interested in getting help?
25. (If applicable) What do you think might be helpful to do regarding your concerns?

(e.g., ethnic, socioeconomic, language) and activities (e.g., scholastic, recreational, artistic). This information can assist the nurse in formulating a well-balanced and integrated mental health assessment (strengths and limitations from multiple contexts) of the child.

Children's Rating Scales

There are a number of instruments available for conducting bio/psycho/social/spiritual assessments. They vary according to age and target areas of interest as well as purpose. Observational assessment and parent-report questionnaires are generally used for screening, whereas in-depth surveys and interviews help formulate diagnoses of psychopathology. Evidence shows that *screening* for early problems is both feasible and effective in improving rates of referral for mental health services (Murphy et al., 1996). Screening can be administered in stages starting with short screens of groups of children (e.g., in clinics, day care, school) followed by more in-depth screens involving parents and observations of those identified to be at elevated risk. Most effective screening methods involve brief standardized measures that are easy to administer, score, and interpret

(Carter et al., 2004). The Ages and Stages Questionnaire–Social-Emotional Version (Squires, Bricker, & Twombly, 2002) is a promising parent-report screen for measuring social-emotional and behavioural problems and competencies from birth to 5 years. It is important to remember, however, that screening measures have proved most effective in evaluating the level of risk for children with socioemotional problems within a population (e.g., a community, school) and are less effective in identifying with certainty an individual at risk (Costello, Egger, & Angold, 2005). This means that the nurse should not rely on one source of evidence but, instead, use multiple sources of data to understand a child's emotional well-being.

The BASC, developed by Reynolds and Kamphouse (1998), is a tool to measure behaviours and emotions in children aged 2 to 18 years. The scales include a teacher rating scale, parent rating scale, and 180-item self-report of personality. The scale evaluates several dimensions, including attitude toward school, attitude toward teachers, sensation seeking, atypicality, locus of control, somatization, social stress, anxiety, depression, sense of inadequacy, relations with parents, interpersonal relations, self-esteem, and self-reliance. The CBCL developed by Achenbach and Edelbrock (1983) is a 113-item, self-report tool to identify forms of psychopathology and competencies that occur in children ages 4 to 16 years. This instrument provides scores on internalizing and externalizing behaviours.

Several scales are useful for diagnosing specific problems in children and adolescents. The CDI developed by Kovacs (1982) is a 27-item self-rated symptom orientation scale for children aged 7 to 17 years that is useful for diagnosing physical symptoms, harm avoidance, social anxiety, and separation or panic disorder. The Multidimensional Anxiety Scale for Children (MASC) developed by March (1997) is a 39-item self-rating scale that assesses severity of anxiety in children and adolescents. The paediatric anxiety rating scale (PARS) developed by the RUPP Anxiety Study Group (2002) is a clinician-administered, 50-item semi-structured interview to assess the severity of anxiety in children aged 6 to 17 years.

The SNAP-IV developed by Swanson (1983) is a 90-item teacher and parent rating scale containing items from the Conners' questionnaire for measuring inattention and overactivity; it is useful for diagnosing attention deficit hyperactivity disorder (ADHD—inattentive and impulsive types) and oppositional defiant disorder. The Children's Yale-Brown Obsessive Compulsive Scale developed by Goodman et al. (1989) is a 19-item scale that can help diagnose childhood obsessive-compulsive disorder in children aged 6 to 17 years.

Assessments performed for *diagnostic* purposes often require trained administrators and interpreters and are more time consuming and rigorous to administer than screens. However, evidence shows that they are very useful because they highlight both positive and negative aspects of the child and identify delays, evaluate the relative degree of impairment associated with extant problem behaviours, and facilitate the design of interventions that capitalize on children's strengths (Carter et al., 2004).

Preschool-Aged Children

When interviewing preschool-aged children, the nurse should understand that these children may have difficulty putting feelings into words and provide assistance (e.g., "When I see your face all wrinkled up, it tells me that you are mixed up—confused"). The nurse should also understand that young children think in very concrete terms. For example, when talking to a young boy (3 to 6 years) about the death of his father, the nurse needs to recognize that, although children can acknowledge physical death, they consider it as temporary or gradual and not fully separate from life. The young boy may believe that his father continues to live (in the ground where he was buried) and ask questions about his activities (e.g., how is Dad eating, going to the toilet, breathing, playing?) (National Cancer Institute, 2005). The child may also believe that something

the child thought or did actually caused the father's illness and subsequent death. In response to death, children younger than 5 years will often exhibit disturbances in eating, sleeping, and bladder or bowel control that may result in a parent's seeking help (Grollman, 1990). The nurse should keep language simple and tailored to the child's developmental level. Any discussion about death should include proper words (e.g., cancer, died, death) and avoid euphemisms (e.g., "he passed away," "he is sleeping," "we lost him") because they can confuse children and lead to misinterpretations (Wass & Corr, 1984).

The nurse can achieve rapport with preschool-aged children by joining their world of play. Play is an activity by which the child transforms an experience from real life into a symbolic, nonliteral representation. Play encourages verbalizations, promotes manual strength, teaches rules and problem solving, and helps children master control over their environment (Moore-Taylor, Menarchek-Fetkovich, & Day, 2000). With children younger than 5 years of age, the nurse may conduct the assessment in a playroom. Useful materials are paper, pencils, crayons, paints, paint brushes, easels, clay, blocks, balls, dolls, doll houses, puppets, animals, dress-up clothes, and a water supply. The nurse must inform preschool-aged children about any rules for the play. For example, the nurse must tell the child that the nurse must ensure safety so that there will be no hitting in the playroom.

When observing the child in a free play setting, the nurse should pay attention to initiation of play, energy level, manipulative actions, tempo, body movements, tone, integration, creativity, products, age appropriateness, and attitudes toward adults. In addition, themes of play, expression of emotions, and temperament are important to observe. The nurse must allow children to direct and initiate these themes. When evaluating the young child's peer relationships through play therapy in a play group or school setting, observe play settings and themes, initiation of play, response to peer initiations of play, integration of affect and action during play, resolution of conflicts, responses to suggestions of others during play, and the ability to engage in role taking and role reversals (Howes & Matheson, 1992).

The nurse's roles are to be a good listener; to use appropriate vocabulary; to tolerate a child's anxious, angry, or sad behaviour; and to use reflective comments about the child's play. Through play, the nurse can assess the child's sensory-motor skills, cognitive style, adaptability, language functioning, emotional and behavioural responsiveness, social level, moral development, coping styles, problem-solving techniques, and approaches to perceiving and interpreting the surrounding world. For example, when assessing a child's problem-solving skills, the nurse might say to a preschooler, "I can see that you've noticed the tent in the corner and would like to check it out. Yes, the tent does look interesting... but I can also see that you have a problem... the tent looks a little scary to you... and you do not want to check it out alone. Hmmm... can you think of someone whom you would like to take with you?" Then, in response to the child's answer, the nurse says, "Mr. Bear... because he protects you.... Oh, then Mr. Bear is a great choice. You chose a friend who would be sure to keep you safe.... You made a good decision."

In any assessment, the nurse should be careful to assess both strengths and limitations and then build on the strengths to address the child's problem areas. For example, the nurse might engage a preschooler with the comment, "Sara, you are a great storyteller; I wonder if you could tell me a story about this doll, Jane, who is afraid at day care just like you."

Lidz (2003) developed a tool that the clinician can use to assess preschoolers' play (Box 27-3). Analyzing children's perceptions of fairy tales can provide the clinician with clues to culture, problems, solutions, and elements of mental functioning (LeBuffe & Naglieri, 1999; Trad, 1989).

Drawings are also used in child assessment to illuminate the child's intellect, creative talents, neuropsychological deficits, body image difficulties, and perceptions of family life (Fig. 27-1). Types of drawings used in child assessments are free drawings; self-portraits; the kinetic family drawing; tree, person, house drawing; and a picture of someone of the opposite sex (Cepeda, 2000). The DECA (LeBuffe & Naglieri, 2003) screening instrument measures protective factors of attachment, self-control, and initiative in children 2 to 5 years of age. The DECA tool is used in the preschool classroom setting with the goal of promoting positive resilience in children.

FIGURE 27.1 Me and my mom going for ice cream. Drawing and writing by a 5-year-old girl.

School-Aged Children

Unlike preschool-aged children, school-aged (5 to 11 years) children can use more constructs, provide longer descriptions and make better inferences of others, and acquire more complete conceptions of various social roles. Children in middle school are more capable of verbal exchange and can tolerate limited periods of direct questioning (Box 27-4). The nurse can establish rapport with school-aged children by using competitive board games, such as checkers and playing cards. A therapeutic game helpful in assessing the child's perceptions, cognition, and emotions and in establishing rapport between clinician and child is the thinking–feeling–doing game. In this game, the clinician and the child take turns drawing cards that pose hypothetical situations and ask what a person might think, feel, or do in such scenarios. For example, one card might say, "A boy has something on his mind that he is afraid to tell his father. What is he scared to talk about?" Another might read, "A girl heard her parents fighting. What were they fighting about? What was the girl thinking while she listened to her parents?"

Adolescents

Adolescents have an increased command of language concepts and have developed the capacity for abstract and formal operations thinking. Their social world is also more complex. Some early adolescents tend to assume that their subjective experiences are real and congruent with objective reality, which can lead to egocentrism (Shave & Shave, 1989). **Egocentrism** is a pre-occupation with one's own appearance, behaviour, thoughts, and feelings. For

---

BOX 27.3

Lidz Assessment Tool

Child's Name: _____ Birth Date: _____ Age: _____

Assessor: _____ Date of Assessment: _____

Describe typical play style/sequence.

Describe range of levels of play from lowest to highest level with age estimates and within contexts of independent/ facilitated, familiar/unfamiliar, single/multiple toys.

Describe language and evidence of self-talk and internalized speech.

Describe interpersonal interactions with assessor and facilitator (if not assessor).

Describe content of any play themes.

What held the child's attention the longest? (For how long?) And what were the child's toy/play preferences?

Describe the child's affective state during play.

Implications of above for intervention:

From Lidz, C. S. (2003). *Early childhood assessment.* Hoboken, NJ: Wiley & Sons, Inc. Copyright 2003, John Wiley & Sons. Used with permission.

BOX 27.4

Bio/psycho/social/spiritual Psychiatric Nursing Assessment of Children and Adolescents

1. **Identifying information**
   Name
   Sex
   Date of birth
   Age
   Birth order
   Grade
   Ethnic background
   Religious preference
   List of others living in household

2. **Major reason for seeking help**
   Description of presenting problems or symptoms
   When did the problems (symptoms) start?
   Describe both the child's and the parent's perspectives.

3. **Psychiatric history**
   Previous mental health contacts (inpatient and outpatient)
   Other mental health problems or psychiatric diagnosis (besides those described currently)
   Previous medications and compliance
   Family history of depression, substance abuse, psychosis, etc., and treatment

4. **Current and past health status**
   Medical problems
   Current medications
   Surgery and hospitalizations
   Allergies
   Diet and eating habits
   Sleeping habits
   Height and weight
   Hearing and vision
   Menstrual history
   Immunizations
   If sexually active, birth control method used
   Date of last physical examination
   Paediatrician or nurse practitioner's name and telephone number

5. **Medications**
   Prescription (dosage, side effects)
   OTC drugs

6. **Neurologic history**
   Right handed, left handed, or ambidextrous
   Headaches, dizziness, fainting
   Seizures
   Unusual movement (tics, tremors)
   Hyperactivity
   Episodes of weakness or paralysis
   Slurred speech, pronunciation problems
   Fine motor skills (eating with utensils, using crayon or pencil, fastening buttons and zippers, tying shoes)
   Gross motor skills and coordination (walking, running, hopping)

7. **Responses to mental health problems**
   What makes problems (symptoms) worse or better?
   Feelings about those experiences (what helped and did not help)

What interventions have been tried so far?
Major losses or changes in past year
Fears, including punishment

8. **Mental status examination**
   Appearance, gait, posture, dress, nutrition, gestures
   Motor/motility
   Interaction with nurse, eye contact
   Psychosis, hallucinations, delusions
   Mood, affect, anxiety
   Speech (clarity, speed, volume), language (articulation, tone, modulation, coherence).
   Writing/reading (comprehension), content
   Thought patterns (organization, thought content)
   Intellectual ability, judgment, insight, general knowledge, orientation to date, time, person
   Activity level, stereotypes, mannerisms, obsessions or compulsions, attention, phobia

9. **Developmental assessment**
   Mother's pregnancy, delivery
   Child's Apgar score, whether preterm or fullterm, weight at birth
   Physical maturation
   Psychosocial
   Language
   Developmental milestones: walking, talking, toileting

10. **Attachment, temperament/significant behaviour patterns**
    Attachment
    Concentration, distractability
    Eating and sleeping patterns
    Ability to adjust to new situations and changes in routine
    Usual mood and fluctuations
    Excitability
    Ability to wait, tendency to interrupt
    Responses to discipline
    Lying, stealing, fighting, cruelty to animals, fire-setting

11. **Self-concept**
    Beliefs about self
    Body image
    Self-esteem
    Personal identity

12. **Risk assessment**
    History of suicidal thoughts, previous attempts
    Suicide ideation, plan, lethality of plan, accessibility of plan
    History of violent, aggressive behaviour
    Homicidal ideation

13. **Family relationships**
    Relationship with parents
    Deaths/losses
    Family strengths and conflicts (nature and content)
    Nurturing and disciplinary methods
    Quality of sibling relationship
    Sleeping arrangements
    Who does the child relate to or trust in the family?
    Relationships with extended family

Continued

BOX 27.4

Bio/psycho/social/spiritual Psychiatric Nursing Assessment of Children and Adolescents (Continued)

14. **School and peer adjustment**
    Learning difficulties and strengths
    Behaviour problems and strengths at school
    School attendance
    Relationship with teachers
    Special classes
    Best friend
    Relationships with peers
    Dating
    Drug and alcohol use
    Participation in sports, clubs, other activities
    After-school routine

15. **Community resources**
    Professionals or agencies working with child or family
    Day care resources

16. **Functional status**
    GAF scale

17. **Stresses and coping behaviours**
    Psychosocial stresses
    Coping behaviours (strengths)

18. **Summary of significant data**

example, a preteen may think that he caused his parents to divorce because he fought with his father the day before the parents announced their decision to separate. Because teenagers have a heightened sense of self-consciousness, they may be preoccupied during the interview with applying makeup or other self-grooming tasks.

During early adolescence, cognitive changes include increased self-consciousness, fear of being shamed, and demands for privacy and secrecy. An adolescent's willingness to talk to a nurse will depend partly on his or her perception of the degree of rapport between them. The nurse's ability to communicate respect, cooperation, honesty, and genuineness is important. Rejection by the adolescent, even outright hostility, during the first few interactions is not uncommon, especially if the teen is having behaviour problems at home, at school, or in the community. The nurse should be patient and avoid jumping to conclusions. Hostility or defiance may be a test of how much the teen can trust the nurse, a defence against anxiety, or a transference phenomenon (see Chapter 8).

Adolescents are likely to be defensive in front of their parents and concerned with confidentiality. At the start of the interview, the nurse should clearly convey to the adolescent what information will and will not be shared with parents. Adolescents generally prefer a straightforward, candid approach to the interview because they often distrust those in authority. Making a commitment to adolescents that they do not have to discuss anything that they are not ready to reveal is important so that they will feel in control while they gradually build trust.

■ BIO/PSYCHO/SOCIAL/SPIRITUAL PSYCHIATRIC NURSING ASSESSMENT OF CHILDREN AND ADOLESCENTS

As discussed, the comprehensive assessment of the child or adolescent includes interviews with the child and parents, child alone, and parents alone. After completing these components, the nurse should bring the child and parents back together to summarize his or her view of their concerns and to ask for feedback regarding whether these perceptions agree with theirs. The nurse must give the family a chance to share additional information and ask questions. The nurse should then thank them for their willingness to talk and give them some idea of the next steps. The use of an assessment tool is helpful in organizing data for mental health planning and intervention. The nurse should also ask for feedback on the suggested next steps of both child and parents and discuss any areas of disagreement to find a plan with which all can live.

When interviewing both child and parents, the nurse's directly asking the child as many questions as possible is generally the best way to get accurate, first-hand information and to reinforce interest in the child's viewpoint. Asking the child questions about the history of the current problem, previous psychiatric experiences (both good and bad), family psychiatric history, medical problems, developmental history (to get an idea of what the child has been told), school adjustment, peer relationships, and family functioning is particularly important. If necessary, the nurse can ask some or all of these same questions of the parents to get consensus or another opinion about the matter, attain supplemental information, or both. Keep in mind that developmental research shows moderate to low correlation between parent and child reports of family behaviour. It is helpful to discuss openly with the family the fact that different perspectives exist and to note that the nurse's role is not to judge or side with one view, but rather to understand the different perspectives and how they might be affecting the family.

Biologic Domain

Nurses should include a thorough history of psychiatric and medical problems in any comprehensive assessment. A physical assessment is necessary to rule out any medical problems that could be mistaken for psychiatric symptoms (e.g., weight loss resulting from diabetes, not depression; drug-induced psychosis). Pharmacologic assessment should include prescription and over-the-counter (OTC) medications. Nurses should ask about any allergies to food, medications, or environmental triggers.

Genetic Vulnerability

The line between nature and nurture is not always clear. Characteristics that appear to be inborn may influence parents and teachers to respond differently toward different children, thus creating problems in the family environment. A phenomenon called **assortative mating**, the tendency for individuals to select mates who are similar in genetically linked traits such as intelligence and personality style, may contribute to the genetic transmission of psychiatric disorders. Research increasingly shows that major psychiatric disorders (e.g., depression, anxiety disorder, schizophrenia, bipolar disorder, substance abuse) run in families. Thus, having a parent or sibling with a psychiatric disorder usually indicates an increased risk for the same or another closely related disorder in a child or adolescent. In addition, many childhood psychiatric disorders, such as autism, developmental learning disorders, some language disorders (e.g., dyslexia), ADHD, Tourette's syndrome, enuresis (bed wetting) and other trisomy disorders (e.g., Down syndrome) appear to be genetically transmitted (American Psychiatric Association, 2000; Health Canada, 2002; Rutter, Silberg, O'Connor, & Simonoff, 1999; State, Lombroso, Pauls, & Leckman, 2000). Certain disorders (e.g., ADHD, enuresis, stuttering) are more common in boys than in girls.

Neurologic Examination

A full neurologic evaluation is beyond the scope of practice for a baccalaureate-level or master's-level nurse without specific neuropsychiatric training. However, a screening of neurologic soft signs can help establish a database that will clarify the need for further neurologic consultation. The nurse should ask the child directly the brief neurologic screening questions suggested in Box 27-4 and also should note any soft signs of neurologic dysfunction, such as slurred speech, unusual movements (e.g., tics, tremors), hyperactivity, and coordination problems. The nurse can ask young children to hop on one foot, skip, or walk from toe to heel to assess their gross motor coordination and to draw with a crayon or pencil or to play pick-up sticks or jacks to assess their fine motor coordination.

Psychological Domain

Children can usually identify and discuss what improves or worsens their problems. The assessment may be the first time that someone has asked the child to explain his or her view of the problem. It is also a perfect opportunity to discuss any life changes or losses (e.g., death of grandparents or pets, parental divorce) and fears, especially of punishment.

Mental Status Examination

The mental status examination of children combines observation and direct questioning. The nurse should note the child's general appearance, including size, cleanliness, dress, masculinity or femininity, and level of attractiveness. Although it perhaps should not be so, social-psychological research shows that the appearance and attractiveness of both children and adults strongly influence their social relationships (Eagly, Ashmore, Makhijani, & Kennedy, 1991). The nurse also should note the child's nonverbal behaviour, including posture, tone of voice, eye contact, and mannerisms. How active is the child? Does he or she seem to have difficulty focusing on the interview, sitting still, refraining from impulsive behaviour, and listening without interrupting (possible signs of ADHD)? Does the child seem underactive, lethargic, distant, or hopeless (possible signs of depression)?

The nurse should observe the child's sentence structure and vocabulary for a general sense of his or her intellectual functioning. Does the child seem to be able to form a relationship with the nurse, or does the child seem distant, uninterested, or in his or her own world? Speech patterns, such as rate (overly fast or slow), clarity, and volume, and any speech dysfluencies (e.g., stuttering, halting), are important in screening for mood disorders (e.g., depression, mania), language disorders, psychotic processes, and anxiety disorders (see Chapter 21).

Asking children general questions about their everyday lives and observing the content and process of their play (e.g., ability to focus on an activity, play themes, boundaries between themselves and others) helps to reveal the level of organization and content of their thinking. The nurse should also note the level of speech organization. Young children normally shift subjects rather abruptly, but adolescents should continue with one train of thought before moving to another. The nurse should note any morbid or eccentric thoughts, violent fantasies, and self-deprecating statements that could reflect a poor self-concept. Assessment of preteens and adolescents should address substance use and sexual activity because responses may provide useful information about high-risk behaviour or harmful substance use. In addition, the nurse should inquire about any obsessions or compulsions (e.g., worries about germs, severe hand washing).

Developmental Assessment

Children respond to life's stresses in different ways and in accordance with their developmental level. Knowing the difference between normal child development and psychopathology is crucial in helping parents view their children's behaviour realistically and respond appropriately. The key areas for assessment include maturation, psychosocial development, and language.

Maturation

Healthy development of the brain and nervous system during childhood and adolescence provides the foundation for successful functioning throughout life. Such development, called **maturation**, unfolds through sequential and orderly growth processes. These processes are biologically and genetically based but depend on constant interactions with a stimulating and nurturing environment.

> **KEY CONCEPT** **Maturation** is the process of completing a state of development; a ripening.

If trauma or neglect impairs the process of normal biologic maturation, **developmental delays** and disorders that may not be fully reversible can result. For example, babies born with fetal alcohol syndrome experience permanent brain damage, often resulting in mental retardation (Roebuck, Mattson, & Riley, 1999). A pregnant woman's use of crack cocaine deprives the fetus of nutrients and oxygen, leading to developmental delays, deformities, and behaviour disorders (e.g., impulsivity, withdrawal, hyperactivity). The nurse can assess for developmental delays by asking questions from specific sections of the mental status examination:

- *Intellectual functioning*: Evaluate the child's creativity, spontaneity, ability to count money and tell time, academic performance, memory, attention, frustration tolerance, and organization.
- *Gross motor functioning*: Ask child to hop on one foot, throw a ball, walk up and down hall, and run.
- *Fine motor functioning*: Ask the child to draw a picture or pick up sticks.
- *Cognition*: The nurse can evaluate the child's general level of cognition by assessing the child's vocabulary, level of comprehension, drawing ability, and responsiveness to questions. Testing, such as the Wechsler Intelligence Scale for Children (WISC-III), provides measures of intelligence quotient. A psychologist usually performs such tests. The nurse can request cognitive testing if he or she has concerns about developmental delays or learning disabilities.
- *Thinking and perception*: Evaluate level of consciousness; orientation to date, time, and person; thought content; thought process; and judgment.
- *Social interactions and play*: Assess the child's organization, creativity, drawing capacity, and ability to follow rules. Children experiencing developmental delays

may remain engaged solely in parallel play, instead of moving to reciprocal play. They may consistently play with toys designed for younger children, draw crude body pictures, or display receptive (understanding) or expressive (communicative) language problems.

Psychosocial Development

Assessment of psychosocial development is very important for children with mental health problems. Various theoretical models are available from which to choose; the most commonly used model is Erikson's stages of development. When considering this model, the nurse should examine the child's gender and cultural background for appropriateness. The nurse also may use the Baker Miller model for girls (see Chapter 8).

Language

At birth, infants can emit sounds of all languages. Maturation of language skills begins with babbling, or the utterance of simple, spontaneous sounds. By the end of the 1st year, children can make one-word statements, usually naming objects or people in the environment. By age 2 years, they should speak in short, telegraphic sentences consisting of a verb and noun (e.g., "want cookie"). Between ages 2 and 4 years, vocabulary and sentence structure develop rapidly. In fact, the preschooler's ability to produce language often surpasses motor development, sometimes causing temporary stuttering when the child's mind literally works faster than the mouth.

Language development depends on the complex interaction of physical maturation of the nerves, development of head and neck musculature, hearing abilities, cognitive abilities, exposure to language, educational stimulation, and emotional well-being. Social needs create a natural inclination toward communication, but the child needs reinforcement to develop correct pronunciation, vocabulary, and grammar.

Before a diagnosis of a communication disorder (i.e., impairment in language expression, comprehension, or both) can be made, the child must be tested to rule out hearing, visual, or other neurologic problems. Brain damage, especially to the left hemisphere (dominant for language in most individuals), can seriously impair the development of communication abilities in children. Any child who has experienced brain damage from anoxia at birth, congenital trauma, head injury, infection, tumour, or drug exposure should be closely monitored for signs of a communication disorder. Before the age of 5 years, the brain has amazing plasticity, and sometimes other intact areas of the brain can take over functions of damaged areas, especially with immediate speech therapy. Genetically based disorders, such as autism, cause language delays that are sometimes permanent and severe. Children with language delays need particular encouragement to communicate properly because they tend to compensate by using nonverbal signals (Tanguay, 2000).

The nurse must recognize normal variations in child development and assess lags in the development of vocabulary and sentence structure during the critical preschool years. Delays in this area can seriously affect other areas, such as cognitive, educational, and social development. Many children who receive psychiatric treatment have speech and language disorders that are sometimes undetected, either leading to or compounding their emotional problems. Cantwell and Baker (1991) studied 600 consecutive child referrals to an urban community clinic for speech and language disorders and found that the psychiatric prevalence was 50% for any diagnosis, 26% for behaviour disorders, and 20% for emotional disorders. The most common individual psychiatric diagnoses were ADHD (19%), oppositional defiant disorder (7%), and anxiety disorders (10%). Beitchman, Cohen, Konstantareas, and Tannock (1996) found that children with receptive language disorders also had a high prevalence of ADHD (59%).

Attachment: The Caregiving Context

Current thinking among researchers and clinicians who assess early emerging social-emotional and behavioural problems holds that children must be evaluated in relation to their primary caregivers (Carter et al., 2004). Although parents usually serve as the primary caregivers, in today's world, other family members (biologically or psychologically related), babysitters, day care, and club activity staff, to name a few, often play a significant role in the development of child attachment and should be assessed. In addition, recognizing that children respond differently in different situations, the routine environments in which the child interacts need to be evaluated. Finally, the contexts of culture (values, beliefs, and practices), race, and ethnicity need to be considered (Garcia-Coll & Magnuson, 2000). For meaningful assessments, nurses need to be culturally competent, as suggested in the *Standards of Psychiatric-Mental Health Nursing Practice* (CFMHN, 2005). Studies of **attachment** show that the quality of the emotional bond between the infant and parental or caregiver figures provides the groundwork for future relationships. The need to touch and be close to a parental figure appears biologically driven and has been demonstrated in classic studies of monkeys who bonded with a terrycloth surrogate mother (Harlow, Harlow, & Suomi, 1971). A secure attachment is based on the caretaker's consistent, appropriate response to the infant's attachment behaviours (e.g., crying, clinging, calling, following, protesting). Children who have developed a secure attachment protest when their parents leave them (beginning at about age 6 to 8 months), seek comfort from their parents in unfamiliar situations, and playfully explore the environment in the parent's presence. When

parents are unresponsive to a child's attachment behaviours, the child may develop an insecure attachment, evidenced by clinging and lack of exploratory play when the parent is present, intense protest when the parent leaves, and indifference or even hostility (Thompson, 2002) when the parent returns (Ainsworth, 1989).

Secure attachments in early childhood produce cooperative, harmonious parent–child relationships in which the child is responsive to the parents' socialization efforts and likely to adopt the parents' viewpoints, values, and goals. Securely attached young children also socialize competently, are popular with well-acquainted peers during the preschool years, and have warm relationships with important adults in their lives. Securely attached children see themselves and others constructively and have relatively sophisticated emotional and moral understanding (Thompson, 2002).

Although the importance of the parent's responsiveness is unquestionable in determining the development of a secure attachment, the process works both ways. Some babies seem to encourage attachment naturally with their parents by responding positively to holding, cuddling, and comforting behaviours. Others, such as those with developmental delays or autistic disorders, may respond less readily and even reject parental attempts at connecting. The interrelatedness of child behaviour and the parenting context is not only reciprocal but also extends over time (Sameroff, 2000). The goodness of fit of the caregiving relationship is, at least in part, dependent on infant temperament, parental perceptions, and the parenting style used, which either lessens or heightens the risk for later psychopathology (Seifer, 2000).

Attachment Theories

Bowlby's early studies (1969) of maternal deprivation formed the initial framework for attachment theory, based on the notion that the infant tends to bond to one primary parental figure, usually the mother. Although this pattern is common, recent studies show that although children make multiple attachments to parents and other caregivers, the high-quality, intense bonds remain essential for healthy development. Contemporary nursing theories, such as Barnard's parent–child interaction model (1994), have stressed the importance of the interaction between the child's spontaneous behaviour and biologic rhythms and the mother's ability to respond to cues that signal distress (Baker et al., 1994). The model provides the foundation for the development of several scales measuring dimensions of attachment. These standardized, observational assessment scales use routine parent–child interaction activities involving feeding (NCAFS scale—76 items, birth to 1 year) and teaching (NCATS scale—73 items, birth to 3 years) to assess a dyad's strengths and limitations during the early years. Areas assessed include contingency (reciprocal communication patterns between caregiver and child), positioning (caregiver's sensitivity to child developmental stage and needs), verbalness (ability to stimulate language development), sensitivity (psychological availability and responsivity to the child), affect (positive or negative quality of communication patterns), and attention regulation (engaging and disengaging behaviours). Such measures can provide informed assessments to nurses in a variety of settings, such as postpartum hospital care, the home (e.g., public health newborn visits), or primary care settings (e.g., mental health nurse in community health centre). Doyle, Markiewicz, Brendgen, Lieberman, and Voss (2000) studied 216 parents' attachment style and marital adjustment and found that mothers having an anxious attachment style uniquely predicted that children's attachment to both mother and father would be insecure. Child–mother attachment was associated uniquely with perceived global self-worth and physical appearance for both younger and older children, whereas child–father attachment was associated uniquely with child-perceived school competence and, only for older children, with global self-worth. Although most attachment research has been done with mothers, the father's role in child development has become better understood through research done during the past two decades. Economic support of the family constitutes a major role in which fathers contribute to the rearing and emotional health of their children (Lamb, 1997). Fathers' emotional support tends to enhance the quality of mother–child relationships and facilitates positive adjustment by children, whereas when fathers are unsupportive and marital conflict is high, children suffer (Cummings & O'Reilly, 1997).

Fathers play an important role in children's play, which affects the quality of the child's attachment. Playful interactions involving emotional arousal provide an especially good opportunity to learn how to get along with peers, with fathers' modelling and reinforcing turn taking, affect regulation, and acceptable ways of competing, as well as the sports skills that facilitate acceptance into peer groups. Fathers are also important as role models who assist in their sons' identity formation and serve as models of gender-appropriate behaviour, particularly around aggressive behaviour (DeKlyen, Speltz, & Greenberg, 1998). Biller and Lopez-Kimpton's (1997) review of the literature found that children who have active, committed, and involved fathers generally perform better cognitively, academically, athletically, and socially than do children who do not benefit from such involvement. All these data support the importance of including the father in the mental health assessment of his child, whereas traditionally, the clinician has had contact only with the mother.

Disrupted Attachments

Disrupted attachments resulting from deficits in infant attachment behaviours, lack of responsiveness by caregivers to the child's cues, or both may lead to reactive attachment disorder, feeding disorder, failure to thrive, or anxiety disorder. A reactive attachment disorder is a state in which a child younger than 5 years of age fails to initiate or respond appropriately to social interaction and the caregiver subsequently disregards the child's physical and emotional needs. O'Connor and Rutter (2000) studied 163 adopted children with early severe deprivation at 4 years of age and again at 6 years of age. Longitudinal findings showed that attachment disorder behaviours were correlated with attention and conduct problems. Solomon and George (1999) reviewed the research on a new classification of attachment disorder titled attachment disorganization. **Attachment disorganization** is a consequence of extreme insecurity that results from feared or actual separation from the attached figure. Disorganized infants appear to be unable to maintain the strategic adjustments in attachment behaviour, represented by organized avoidant or ambivalent attachment strategies, with the result that an alteration in both behavioural and physiologic behaviour occurs. Frightening and frightened caregivers can contribute to disorganized attachment in infants. Preschoolers with disorganized attachment manifest behaviours of fear, contradictory behaviour, or disorientation or disassociation in the caregivers' presence.

Temperament and Behaviour

Temperament is a person's characteristic intensity, activity level, threshold of responsiveness, rhythmicity, adaptability, energy expenditure, and mood. According to research findings, temperamental differences can be observed early in life, suggesting that they are at least partly biologically determined, and patterns of temperament can be correlated with emotional and behavioural problems (Kagan, 1999). One basic aspect of temperament, the tendency to approach or avoid unfamiliar events, appears moderately stable over time and has been associated with distinct, apparently genetically based, physiologic profiles in 2-year-old children (Caspi & Silva, 1995; Schwartz, Snidman, & Kagan, 1999; Snidman, Kagan, Riordan, & Shannon, 1995). When looking at the cerebral asymmetry of the brain in children with inhibited compared with uninhibited temperaments, Davidson (1994) found that inhibited children in the third year of life showed greater electroencephalographic activation on the right frontal area under resting conditions.

The classic New York Longitudinal Study (Thomas, Chess, & Birch, 1968) identified three main patterns of temperament seen in infancy that often extend into childhood and later life:

- **Easy temperament**, characterized by a positive mood, regular patterns of eating and sleeping, positive approach to new situations, and low emotional intensity
- **Difficult temperament**, characterized by irregular sleep and eating patterns, negative response to new stimuli, slow adaptation, negative mood, and high emotional intensity
- **Slow-to-warm-up temperament**, characterized by a negative, mildly emotional response to new situations that is expressed with intensity and initially slow adaptation but evolves into a positive response

On the positive side, an easy temperament can serve as a protective factor against the development of psychopathology. Children with easy temperaments can adapt to change without intense emotional reactions. Difficult temperament places children at high risk for adjustment problems, such as with adjustment to school or bonding with parents.

Temperament has a major influence on the chances that a child may experience psychological problems; however, temperament is not unchangeable, and environmental influences can change or modify a child's emotional style. Kerr and Mcgehee (1964) found that temperament remained stable from childhood to adulthood only in those children who were extremely inhibited or uninhibited.

The concept of temperament provides an excellent example of the interaction between biologic–genetic factors and environmental factors in producing child psychopathology. Although a child may be born with a particular temperament, longitudinal studies show that the temperament itself is less influential than the "goodness of fit" (Chess & Thomas, 2002) between the child's temperament and the reactions of parents and significant others. Difficult children in particular may evoke negative reactions in parents and teachers, thereby creating environments that exacerbate their biologically based behaviour problems, initiating a vicious cycle. Vanden Boom and Hoeksma (1994) found that infants with difficult temperaments received less sensitive caring than did other children, and parents of 2-year-old children with difficult temperaments often resorted to angry, punitive discipline.

Most research in temperament has focused on the child with a difficult temperament. Studies show that the difficult temperament is correlated with the development of child psychopathology, but only if such temperament persists beyond 3 years of age. Furthermore, the effects of a difficult temperament are more significant in psychiatric populations than in nonpsychiatric populations (Tubman, Lerner, Lerner, & Von Eye, 1992). Extremely difficult temperament shows an association with the development of oppositional and conduct disorders as well as ADHD (Dulcan & Martini, 1999; McClowry, 1995). McClowry developed a school-age temperament inventory for parental report of children 8 to 11 years old. Four empirically derived dimensions were proposed: task persistence, negative reactivity, approach/withdrawal, and energy.

The nurses working with parents of young children need to understand temperament so that they can educate families about this concept, particularly because many parents of children with difficult temperaments blame themselves for their children's behaviour. Parents may compare the child with a difficult temperament to children with easier temperaments and wonder what they have done wrong or attribute negative motives to the child. The nurse can help parents accept biologically based differences in their children and learn to adapt their behaviour to each child's needs to improve "fit." Linder (1993) developed a worksheet to assist the clinician in evaluating the child's temperament during play that is divided into measures of activity level, adaptability, and reactivity (Box 27-5).

Self-Concept

For young children, eliciting their view of themselves and the world through projective techniques is helpful. For example, the nurse should ask them what they would wish for if they had three wishes. Answers can be revealing. An inability to wish for anything beyond a nice meal or place to live may reflect hopelessness, whereas wishes to conquer the world or put one's teacher in jail may indicate feelings of grandiosity. Another technique is to tell a story and ask the child to make up an ending for it. For example, a baby bird fell out of a nest—what happened to it?… or, a little girl went to the mall with her mother but got lost—what happened to her? The nurse may design stories to elicit particular fears or concerns that he or she suspects may be relevant for the individual child.

Drawings also provide an excellent window into the child's internal world (Fig. 27-2). Asking the child to draw a picture of a person can provide data about the child's self-concept, sexual identity, body image, and developmental level. By age 3 years, children should be able to draw some facial features and limbs, but their drawings may have an "x-ray" quality, in which clothing is transparent and the body can be seen underneath. Older children should produce more sophisticated drawings, unless they are resistant to the task. After the child has finished the drawing, the nurse can ask what the person in the drawing is thinking and feeling, using this device to assess the child's mental processes.

BOX 27.5

Social-Emotional Observation Worksheet

Name of child: _____ Date of birth: _____ Age: _____

Name of observer: _____ Discipline or job title: _____ Date of assessment: _____

On the following pages, note specific behaviours that document the child's abilities in the social-emotional categories. Qualitative comments should also be made. The format provided here follows that of the Observation Guidelines for Social-Emotional Development in Transdisciplinary Play-Based Assessment. It may be helpful to refer to the guidelines while completing this form.

1. Temperament
   A. Activity level
      1. Motor activity:
      2. Specific times that are particularly active
         a. Beginning, middle, or end:
         b. During specific activities:
   B. Adaptability
      1. Initial response to stimuli
         a. Persons:
         b. Situations:
         c. Toys:
      2. Demonstration of interest or withdrawal (*circle one*):
         a. Smiling, verbalizing, touching
         b. Crying, ignoring or moving away, seeking security

3. Adjustment time:
4. Adjustment time after initially shy or fearful response (*circle one*):
   a. Self-initiation
   b. Adult as base of security
   c. Resists; stays uninvolved
C. Reactivity
   1. Intensity of stimuli for discernible response:
   2. Type of stimulation needed to interest child (circle those that apply):
      a. Visual, vocal, tactile, combination
      b. Object, social
   3. Level of affect and energy:
   4. Common response mode:
   5. Response to frustration:

From Linder, T. W. (1993). *Transdisciplinary play-based assessment: A functional approach to working with young children* (Revised ed.). Baltimore, MD: Paul H. Brookes Publishing Co., Inc. Copyright © 1993 by Paul H. Brookes Publishing Co., Inc. Used with permission.

FIGURE 27.2 Self-portrait of a girl, age 5.

For example, one adolescent with school phobia drew a person fully dressed, in great detail, but with no feet. When asked about the drawing, he said that the boy could not go anywhere because his mother was afraid to let him leave home.

Other ways to assess children's self-concepts include asking them what they want to do when they grow up, what their best subjects are in school, what things they are really good at, and how well-liked they are at school. Before concluding the individual interview with a child, the nurse should always ask whether the child has any other information to share and whether he or she has any questions.

Risk Assessment

The nurse must ask the child about any suicidal or violent thoughts. The best way to assess these areas is to ask straightforward questions, such as, "Have you ever thought about hurting yourself? Have you ever thought about hurting someone else? Have you ever acted on these thoughts? Have you thought about how you would do it? What did you think would happen if you hurt yourself? Have you ever done anything to hurt yourself before?" Contrary to popular belief, talking about suicide with someone who can help can provide great relief to a child or youth. Further, no age should be exempt from assessment because even young children attempt suicide, and they are capable of violent acts toward other children, adults, and animals. When a child shares the intent to commit a suicidal or violent act, the nurse must remind him or her that the nurse will have to discuss this concern with the parent to keep the child and others safe. It is helpful to ask the child if he or she wants anything in particular to be said to the parent and if he or she wants to be present when the nurse talks with the parents. Although painful, such conversations can serve as an abrupt halt to the charade of happiness that the child may feel forced to portray to the outside world, and often opens honest dialogue within a family in which none has occurred for some time. Alternatively, the conversation can sometimes give words to what the family has long been fearing but lacks the skills or courage to break the silence. The nurse provides a safe environment for the family to begin to face the issues.

Substance use disorders across the life span account for more deaths, illness, and disabilities than any other preventable health condition. Screening for potential use and abuse of substances is becoming a priority in mental health assessment of adolescents. An interview guide has been adapted from questions on substance use developed by Adlaf (Adlaf & Zdanowicz, 1999) to serve as a useful screen for identifying substance use problems in youth. Given that many younger children engage in substance use (see Chapter 24), the nurse should consider assessing younger children as well (Box 27-6).

Social Domain

Family Relationship

Children depend on adults to create a safe, nurturing, and appropriate environment to support their development. The nurse should assess the quality of the home in terms of its ability to provide appropriate physical space (living space, sleeping arrangements, safety, cleanliness), child care arrangements (age-appropriate supervision), and stimulation (activities or resources), either through a home visit or by discussing these issues with the family. The Home Observation for Measurement of the Environment (HOME) scale (Caldwell & Bradley, 1984) is a widely used, standardized measure to assess the quality of the home environment for fostering child development at any age according to cognitive, social, and emotional growth. It is a 45-item binary (yes/no) scale and best administered in the home through parent interview and observation. The scale addresses six areas: emotional and verbal responsivity of caregiver, avoidance of restriction and punishment, organization of the environment, provision of appropriate play material, caretaker

involvement with child, and opportunities for variety in daily stimulation.

When gathering a family history, a genogram and timeline are also useful tools to map family members according to birth order and medical and psychiatric histories; family roles, norms, boundaries, strengths, and subgroups; birth dates, deaths, and relationships; stage in the family cycle; and critical events. To understand fully the family's values, goals, and beliefs, the nurse must consider the family's ethnic, cultural, and economic background throughout the assessment (Carter & McGoldrick, 1999). A comprehensive family assessment should be considered (see Chapter 17).

School and Peer Adjustment

The child's adjustment to school is also significant. Often, children are referred for a mental health assessment as a result of changes in behaviour at school. Falling grades, loss of interest in normal activities, decreased concentration, or withdrawal from or aggression toward peers may indicate that the child is experiencing emotional problems. It is very important that the nurse obtain signed permission from the parents to talk to the child's teacher for his or her observations of the child. The nurse may want to observe the child in school, if feasible, to see how the child functions there. The parent can request a treatment planning conference in which the teacher, parent, and nurse discuss the child's school performance and plan ways to promote the child's emotional, cognitive, and social functioning in school. For older children, and in particular youth, the nurse should include the child, if even for only a portion of the meeting. It is critically important that children feel that they are consulted and have an opportunity to participate in the planning processes. Although such involvement is not always comfortable or even desired by all parties, it provides formal recognition of each participant involved in the change process. Suggestions emanating from such planning sessions may range from having the child tested (e.g., for learning disabilities) to designing strategies for addressing predictable situations that routinely dissolve into chaos, in which rewards result for each party (e.g., extra computer time for the child, quiet time for the parent) for improved functioning.

Community

Assessing the child's economic status, access (psychologically, geographically, economically) to health and other services, housing and home environment, exposure to environmental toxins (e.g., lead), neighbourhood safety, and exposure to violence is important in understanding the social context of children and families.

BOX 27.6

Practice Note 0.1: An Interview Protocol for Reviewing Chemical Use in Youths

As with other topics, questions about substance use are interactive—the answers given determine, to some extent, the subsequent questions. The questions can be used for investigating the use of tobacco, alcohol, and drugs.

TOBACCO
- Many youth smoke, do you?
- Do you ever feel you should smoke less?
- Do you wish you could smoke less than you do now?
- Have others bothered you by complaining about your smoking?
- Have you felt bad or guilty because of your smoking?
- Have you thought you had a problem because of your smoking?
- Have you ever had a medical problem as a result of your smoking?
- Have you been in hospital because of your smoking?
- Have you gone to anyone for help for a smoking problem?
- How many of your friends smoke occasionally/regularly?
- How many of your family smoke occasionally/regularly?

ALCOHOL
- Many youth drink, do you?
- Are you always able to stop drinking when you want?
- Have you felt you should drink less?
- Have others bothered you by complaining about your drinking?
- Have you felt bad or guilty because of your drinking?
- Have you been arrested or warned by police because of your drinking?
- Have you ever had "blackouts" or "flashbacks" due to your drinking?
- Have you drunk in the early morning or drunk to get rid of a hangover?
- Have you ever had any medical problem as a result of your drinking?
- Have you been in hospital because of your drinking?
- Have you gone to anyone for help for a drinking problem?
- How many of your friends drink occasionally/regularly?
- How many of your family drink occasionally/regularly?

DRUGS
- Many youth use drugs, do you?
- Do you ever feel concerned about your drug use?
- Are you always able to stop using drugs when you want?
- Have you been arrested or warned by police because of your drug use?
- Have you ever had "blackouts" or "flashbacks" due to your drug use?
- Do you wish you could use fewer drugs than you do now?
- Have you ever had any medical problems as a result of your drug use?
- Have you gone to anyone for help for a drug problem?
- Have you ever seen a doctor or been in the hospital because of your drug use?
- How many of your friends use drugs occasionally/regularly?
- How many of your family use drugs occasionally/regularly?

Adapted from Adlaf, E. M., & Zdanowicz, Y. M. (1999). A cluster-analytic study of substance problems and mental health among street youths. *American Journal of Drug and Alcohol Abuse, 25*(4), 639–660.

Such assessment is also important given the evidence from large, longitudinal population-based studies that have demonstrated the links between social disadvantage (socioeconomic, residential stability, community efficacy, and willingness to help neighbours) and mental illness in children (Xue, Levanthal, Brooks-Gunn, & Earls, 2005) and adults (Fryers, Melzer, Jenkins, & Brugha, 2005).

Children and adolescents function better if they are linked to community supports, such as churches, recreational programs, park district programming, and after-school programming. A number of voluntary organizations such as the YWCA or Big Brothers and Big Sisters offer mentoring relationship programs for children in communities. Before making a commitment, a family should visit the organization and talk with staff to ensure that the programs are well organized and monitored by trained staff. The mentor may perform a wide range of services, from taking a child to community events, helping with homework, or talking about how the child can achieve his or her dreams and goals. Some towns offer community-based juvenile justice programs to rehabilitate children who have had an altercation with the legal system. Juvenile justice programs provide support, such as individual and family counselling and prosocial recreational activities; teach children how to make positive choices about spending free time; and closely monitor their behaviours.

Functional Status

Functional status can be evaluated in children and adolescents using such scales as the Global Assessment of Functioning (GAF) scale (American Psychological Association, 2000), which tallies behaviours related to school, peers, activity level, mood, speech, family relationships, behavioural problems, self-care skills, and self-concept. The GAF scale ranges from 0 to 100; the lower the score, the higher the level of impairment, indicated by psychiatric symptoms and level of general functioning. For example, a score of 30 may indicate that the child is severely homicidal or suicidal and has made previous attempts; that hallucinations or delusions influence the child's behaviour; or that the child has serious impairment in communication or judgment. Moderate impairment scores usually fall in the range of 51 to 69. Indications of moderate impairment include difficulty in one area, such as school phobia that hinders school attendance or performance, while the child is functioning well within other areas, such as with family and peers. Children in this category are not homicidal or suicidal and usually respond well to outpatient interventions. A score of 70 to 100 usually indicates that the child is functioning well in relation to school, peers, family, and community. The GAF is always measured at the initial assessment so that treatment can be evaluated over time in terms of symptom improvement.

Stresses and Coping Behaviours

Biologic, behavioural, and personality predispositions, family, and community environment may affect a child's ability to cope with stressful life events. Stressful experiences for children include the death of a loved person or pet, parental divorce, violence, physical illness (especially chronic illness), mental illness, social isolation, racial discrimination, neglect, and physical and sexual abuse. The Difficult Life Circumstances (DLC) scale (Barnard, 1989) is a 28-item self-report measure, administered in interview format to a parent, to identify the existence of chronic family problems in a variety of activities of daily life (e.g., partner in jail, financial problems, partner or child abuse).

Spiritual Domain

Nurses and other health professionals are increasingly aware that spiritual assessment is an important aspect of the assessment of children and adolescents. Although adult spiritual assessment tools exist, to date no validated instrument exists for use with children and adolescents. Rubin and colleagues (2009) assessed the applicability of two adult scales (The Spiritual Involvement and Beliefs Scale; The Spirituality Well-Being Scale) with chronically ill and healthy adolescents and their parents. The conclusion made was that there is a need to develop a specific spirituality scale for adolescents, as less than half the adolescents in the study considered either scale as an effective measure of their spiritual well-being. Parents, too, did not feel find the scales to be adequate measures of their own spirituality. Measuring spirituality, even with adults, continues to have its challenges and limits.

Spiritual beliefs (the way spirituality is understood by an individual) are shaped by experience, family, friends, community, culture, and religious affiliation. With children and adolescents, in particular, developmental level is a significant factor. This can be seen in children's response to loss, for instance (see Chapter 26). In addressing the spiritual domain with children and adolescents, openness and receptivity to their questions and concerns, as well as sensitivity to their level of understanding are important. Nurses can use stories to open discussion about the way a child or an adolescent understands and gives meaning to their experiences. There is a wide range of classic and contemporary literature (across levels of development) that address spiritual concerns such as loneliness, illness, injury, disability, and death. For instance, *Charlotte's Web* by E.B. White (1952) and *The Ten Good Things about Barney* by Viorst (1972) are stories about the death of beloved animals that can help young children to express themselves about death and dying. Adolescents may be particularly hesitant to raise their spiritual concerns unless "an open, acceptable attitude and atmosphere" is available, and they feel safe and comfortable in revealing their feelings and beliefs (Callaghan, 2005, p. 115). Importantly, pediatric nurses describe approaching the spiritual domain primarily at the family level (Whitehead, 2008). There is recognition that establishing a relationship with the family, as well as the child, is foundational to understanding spiritual beliefs, values, and needs (see Chapter 6).

Spiritual assessment, including the expressed values and beliefs of children, youth, and families should be appropriately documented so that other health professionals can be involved in spiritual care (Callaghan, 2005). Pastoral care services are a resource in many health services, and representatives of the family's religious or cultural community may be utilized as a resource under the family's direction. For example, Aboriginal elders and/or cultural workers have been described by pediatric nurses as being very helpful in the provision of spiritual care to Aboriginal families (Whitehead, 2008).

Evaluation of Child Abuse

Thousands of Canadian children suffer maltreatment (intentional physical or emotional abuse, neglect, or sexual exploitation) each year as the result of their parents' action or inaction (Trocmé, McPhee, & Tam, 1995; Wolfe, 1998). The 2003 Canadian Incidence Study of Reported Child Abuse and Neglect (Trocmé et al., 2005) revealed an incidence rate of 21.71 substantiated investigations per 1,000 children in 2003. The three most common categories of substantiated maltreatment comprised neglect (30%), exposure to domestic violence (28%), and physical abuse (24%). Emotional maltreatment accounted for another 15% of cases, whereas sexual abuse cases represented only 3% of all substantiated investigations. Most cases (52%) involved children living in two-parent families, and most referrals (75%) came from professionals (police and school).

The effects of family-engendered maltreatment can result in a lifetime of debilitating bio/psycho/social/spiritual problems. A maltreated child may have difficulty managing emotions (Campbell, 1995), communicating effectively (Browne & Sagi, 1988), developing satisfying relationships with others (Crittenden, 1996), and learning in productive ways (Aber, Allen, Carlson, & Cicchetti, 1989; Doherty, 1997). Consequently, there is increasing awareness among Canadian policy makers (Canadian Council on Social Development, 1997; Edwards, 1999; King & Coles, 1992; Steinhauer, 1998; Wolfe, 1998) of the need for child maltreatment policy to concentrate more on ways of building child competence, resilience, and health potential (i.e., autonomous self-regulation) (Wolfe, 1998) than simply on issues of protection and deviance.

Although the cause of child abuse is not absolutely clear, best thinking suggests that an ecological model better captures the influencing factors of child abuse and neglect because it understands the child within the context of the family and the larger community (Wachtel, 1999). Such a model uses a broad multifactorial approach for assessment. Such assessment takes into consideration the child's current developmental level and understands that compromises to his or her early development may continue in various ways through all the developmental stages that follow. It is child centred (child welfare is critical), family focused (most child abuse occurs within the family), has a community context (forms a key part of the child's environment), and is culturally sensitive (the nurse must be culturally competent). It also involves gathering information from a number of stakeholders and ensures that information is gathered in a coordinated way to maximize the integrity of the data collection.

Although a number of assessment tools exist, three general areas should be addressed in any assessment (English, 1996):

1. Are the child's immediate circumstances unsafe? Does the child have to be taken into care or removed to a safe place?
2. For current cases, what is the assessed risk of repeat abuse? What are the issues that merit intervention on a priority basis?
3. For ongoing cases, to what extent are interventions working? What is the current situation of the child, the family, and any substitute care arrangement?

There are several special considerations in interviewing an abused child. First, the nurse must establish a safe and supportive environment in which to conduct the evaluation. Second, the nurse needs to understand the forensic implications of assessment so that the interview format will be acceptable for disclosure in a court hearing. The Canadian Psychiatric Association (1992) offers practice guidelines for evaluating children who may have been abused. The *Standards of Psychiatric-Mental Health Nursing Practice* (CFMHN, 2005) also identifies a nurse's role in assessing clients for the risk of victim violence and abuse. The American Academy of Child and Adolescent Psychiatry (1997) offers practice guidelines for evaluating children who may have been abused. If the child reports abuse, the nurse has a legal responsibility to report the abuse to the child protection agencies. The nurse must use the same language and vocabulary that the child uses to describe the abuse, or anatomical terms, and ask nonleading questions. Nursing professionals who regularly interview children who have been abused may have special training in the use of anatomically correct dolls to obtain information about the abuse.

In the case of family-perpetrated child abuse, the nurse should consider very carefully whether the report will be made *with* or *without* the knowledge of the child's family. The nurse should consider factors such as whether she or he has developed a relationship with the family, the degree of imminent risk to the child, and whether she or he is likely to continue working with the family. The reality is that maltreatment is a complex phenomenon, and families tend to stay connected with services for long periods. Finding ways to build a positive working relationship with families becomes a crucial, yet challenging, goal for nurses. When nurses are open, honest, and direct, families know what to expect. If nurses have an established working relationship with families, they can often share their specific observations about parenting practices and the need to involve child protection services. Nurses might also invite the family to make the call themselves with the nurse's support. For example, the nurse might say, "I know that you love your child but your actions are causing harm... I don't think your child is safe.... He needs help.... I need to call child protection services to get some help for your family. I know this is scary for you... but you could take an important step in the right direction by making the first call and asking for help for your child and you. I would be happy to support you while you make that call right now... before I make my call." See Chapter 37 for further understanding of caring for abused persons.

Evaluation of Childhood Sexual Abuse

The use of anatomically correct dolls is beneficial because it does not overstimulate or distress the child; assists in identifying and naming specific body parts; increases verbal productivity during the examination; helps to prompt memory; and is useful with immature, language-impaired, or cognitively delayed children (Cepeda, 2000). White (2000) provides a detailed chapter on the use of these dolls in interviewing preschoolers. Some questions that may be asked in forensic evaluation of a child for sexual abuse are presented in Box 27-7.

Risk and Protective Factors

The number of stressful events that a child experiences, the supports that the child has in place, and the child's developmental stage may also influence his or her ability to cope with stressors. Werner (1989) performed a longitudinal study of 500 Hawaiian youths considered to be at high risk for mental health problems because they were born into poverty, homelessness, single-parent families, or families whose parents had little education or were alcoholic or mentally ill. Other risk factors included low birth weight, difficult temperament, mental retardation, childhood trauma, exposure to racism, poor schools, and community and domestic violence. One third of the children born at risk did not experience mental health problems by the age of 18 years. Protective factors that were identified in these children were the following:

- Individual attributes, such as resilience, problem-solving skills, sense of self-efficacy, accurate processing

---

BOX 27.7

Assessing Possible Sexual Abuse of a Child

1. Have you ever been touched on any part of your body?
2. Have you ever touched a part on anybody else's body?
3. Have you ever been hurt on any part of your body?
4. Have you ever hurt a part on anybody else's body?
5. Has anyone done something you didn't like to your body?
6. Have you ever been asked to do something you didn't like to someone else's body?
7. Has anyone put anything on or in any part of your body?
8. Have you ever been without your clothes?
9. Has anyone else asked you to take off your clothes?
10. Have you seen anyone else without clothes?
11. Has anyone asked you not to tell something about your body?
12. Has anyone said that something bad might happen to you or to someone else if you told some secret about your body?
13. Has anyone ever kissed you?
14. Has anyone ever kissed you when you didn't want them to?
15. Has anyone ever taken your picture?
16. Has anyone ever taken your picture without your clothes on?

From White, S. (2000). Using anatomically detailed dolls in interviewing preschoolers. In K. Gitlin-Weiner, A. Sandgrund, & C. Schaefer (Eds.), *Play diagnosis and assessment* (2nd ed., pp. 210–227). New York, NY: Wiley & Sons, Inc. Used with permission.

---

of interpersonal cues, positive social orientation, and activity level
- A supportive family environment, including attachment with adults in the family, low family conflict, and supportive relationships
- Environmental supports, including those that reinforce and support coping efforts and recognize and reward competence.

Doll's and Lyon's (1998) review of the literature about resilience found that children who show resilience in the face of adversity typically have good intellectual functioning, positive and easygoing temperament, positive social orientation, strong self-efficacy, achievement orientation with high expectations, positive self-concept, faith, high rate of involvement in productive activities, close affective relationship with at least one caregiver, effective parenting, access to positive extrafamilial models, and strong connections with prosocial institutions. Similarly, Steinhausen's (2006) longitudinal study of the determinants and processes of mental disorders in adolescence identified that self-esteem, active coping, parental warmth, and peer acceptance, in different combinations, acted as protective factors against internalizing and externalizing mental disorders.

SUMMARY OF KEY POINTS

☐ Mental health assessment of children and adolescents includes evaluating the child's biologic, psychological, social, and spiritual factors.

☐ Assessment of children and adolescents differs from assessment of adults in that the nurse must consider the child's developmental level, specifically addressing the child's language, cognitive, social, and emotional skills. Establishing a treatment alliance and building rapport are essential to obtaining a good mental health history.

☐ The mental status examination includes observations and questions about the child's appearance, speech, language, vocabulary, orientation, knowledge base (including reading, writing, and math skills), attention level, activity level, memory, social skills, peer relationships, relationship to interviewer, mood, affect, suicidal or homicidal tendencies, thinking (presence or absence of hallucinations or delusions), substance use, and behaviours.

☐ Assessment of the child and caregiver together provides important information regarding child–parent attachment and parenting practices.

☐ The three main types of temperament include the easy temperament, difficult temperament, and slow-to-warm-up temperament. Temperament can be evaluated by assessing the child's sleep and eating habits, mood, emotional intensity, and responses to new stimuli.

☐ A child's self-concept can be evaluated using tools such as play, stories, asking three wishes, and asking the child to draw a picture of himself or herself.

☐ If a child reveals suicidal ideation in the interview, the nurse must determine whether the child has a plan, let the parent know the child is suicidal, and make a plan to keep the child safe, including consideration of inpatient hospitalization.

☐ If a child reports to the nurse neglect or physical or sexual abuse, the nurse must by law report the child's disclosure to Child Protection Services.

☐ Protective factors that promote resiliency in children are active coping and the ability to solve problems, a sense of self-efficacy, self-esteem, accurate processing of social cues, supportive family environment, peer acceptance, and environmental supports that promote coping efforts and recognize and reward competence.

CRITICAL THINKING CHALLENGES

1   An adolescent is hostile and refuses to talk in an interview. How would you respond?

2   What are some strategies for building rapport with children?

3   A child reports that he or she is suicidal. What would be your next question? What measures would you take next?

4   What are some techniques and media for obtaining information about a child's inner world, such as self-concept, sexual identity, body image, and developmental level?

5   Explain why it may be detrimental to interview a child in front of his or her parent. Why may it be detrimental to interview a parent in front of his or her child? Why is it useful, in most cases, to ensure that both parent and child are also interviewed together?

6   Why is obtaining the mental health histories of parents relevant to the child's mental health assessment?

7   What are useful tools in obtaining a family history from the child and parent?

8   Anatomically correct dolls are used in what specific type of child assessment?

9   Describe five characteristics of the resilient child.

WEB LINKS

www.cccf-fcsge.ca   This website of the Canadian Child Care Federation is a unique public education resource representing 50 Canadian nonprofit organizations. This easy-to-navigate website provides quality, credible resources on children and families.

www.cich.ca   The Canadian Institute of Child Health (CICH) is the only national charitable organization dedicated solely to improving the health of children and youth in Canada. It has three main functions: monitoring children's health; educating professionals, caregivers, and policy makers; and advocating for legislation and policies that improve child health.

www.nncc.org   The website of the National Network for Child Care gives detailed accounts of expected developmental milestones from birth through adulthood and links to numerous articles on child development and parenting.

www.aacap.org   The website of the American Academy of Child and Adolescent Psychiatry provides an exhaustive list of links to short articles on many mental health issues and is geared toward families and consumers.

www.phac-aspc.gc.ca/ncfv-cnivf/index-eng.php   National Clearinghouse on Family Violence, operated by the Public Health Agency of Canada. The NCFV is

Canada's resource centre for information on violence within relationships of kinship, intimacy, dependency, or trust.

REFERENCES

Aber, J. L., Allen, J. P., Carlson, V., & Cicchetti, D. (1989). The effects of maltreatment on development during early childhood: Recent studies and their theoretical, clinical, and policy implications. In D. Cicchetti & V. Carlson (Eds.), *Child maltreatment: Theory and research on the causes and consequences of child abuse and neglect* (pp. 570–619). New York, NY: Cambridge University Press.

Achenbach, T. M., & Edelbrock, C. (1983). *The Child Behavior Checklist: Manual for the child behavior checklist and revised child behavior profile.* Burlington, VT: Queen City Printers.

Adlaf, E. M., & Zdanowicz, Y. M. (1999). A cluster-analytic study of substance problems and mental health among street youths. *American Journal of Drug and Alcohol Abuse, 25*(4), 639–660.

Ainsworth, M. D. S. (1989). Attachments beyond infancy. *American Psychologist, 44,* 709–716.

American Academy of Child and Adolescent Psychiatry. (1997). Practice parameters for the forensic evaluation of children and adolescents who may have been physically or sexually abused. *Journal of the American Academy of Child and Adolescent Psychiatry, 36*(10 Suppl), 37S–56S.

American Psychiatric Association. (2000). *Diagnostic and statistical manual of mental health disorders* (4th ed., Text revision). Washington, DC: Author.

Baker J. K., Borchers, D. A., Cochran, D. T., et al. (1994). Parent–child interaction model (of Kathryn Barnard). In A. Marriner-Tomey (Ed.), *Nursing theorists and their work.* St. Louis, MO: Mosby.

Barnard, K. E. (1989). *Difficult life circumstances manual.* Seattle, WA: NCAST Publications, University of Washington, School of Nursing.

Barnard, K. E. (1994). The Barnard model. In G. Sumner, & A. Spitz, *NCAST caregiver/parent–child interaction feeding manual* (pp. 6–14). Seattle, WA: NCAST Publications, University of Washington, School of Nursing.

Beitchman, J. H., Cohen, N. J., Konstantareas, M. M., & Tannock, R. (Eds.). (1996). *Language, learning, and behavior disorders: Developmental, biological, and clinical perspectives.* New York, NY: Cambridge University Press.

Biller, H., & Lopez-Kimpton, J. (1997). The father and the school-aged child. In M. Lamb (Ed.), *The role of the father in child development* (3rd ed., pp. 143–161). New York, NY: Wiley & Sons.

Bowlby, J. (1969). *Attachment* (Vol. 1 of *Attachment and loss*). New York, NY: Basic Books.

Breton, J. J., Plante, M. A., & St-Georges, M. (2005). Challenges facing child psychiatry in Quebec at the dawn of the 21st century. *Canadian Journal of Psychiatry, 50*(4), 203–212.

Bronfenbrenner, U. (1986). Ecology of the family as a context for human development: Research perspectives. *Developmental Psychology, 22,* 723–742.

Browne, K., & Saqi, S. (1988). Approaches to screening for child abuse and neglect. In K. Browne, C. Davies, & P. Stratton (Eds.), *Early prediction and prevention of child abuse* (pp. 57–85). Toronto, ON: John Wiley & Sons.

Caldwell, B., & Bradley, R. (1984). *Home observation for measurement of the environment.* Little Rock, AK: University of Little Rock at Arkansas.

Callaghan, D. M. (2005). The influence of spiritual growth on adolescents' initiative and responsibility for self-care. *Pediatric Nursing, 31*(2), 91–115.

Campbell, S. (1995). Behaviour problems in pre-school children: A review of recent research. *Journal of Child Psychiatry, 36,* 113–149.

Canadian Council on Social Development. (1997). Safer communities: A social strategy for crime prevention in Canada. *Canadian Journal of Criminology, 31,* 359–401.

Canadian Federation of Mental Health Nurses. (2005). *The standards of psychiatric-mental health nursing practice* (3rd ed.). Available at: http://www.cfmhn.ca/standards.html

Canadian Psychiatric Association. (1992). *Guidelines for the evaluation and management of family violence.* Available at: http://www.epa-apc.org/publications/position-papers/violence.asp

Cantwell, D. P., & Baker, L. (1991). *Psychiatric and developmental disorders in children with communication disorders.* Washington, DC: American Psychiatric Press.

Carter, B., & McGoldrick, M. (1999). *The expanded family life cycle: Individual, family, and social perspectives* (3rd ed.). Needham Heights, MA: Allyn & Bacon.

Carter, A. S., Briggs-Gowan, M. J., & Davis, N. O. (2004). Assessment of young children's social-emotional development and psychopathology: Recent advances and recommendations for practice. *Journal of Child Psychology and Psychiatry, 45*(1), 109–134.

Caspi, A., & Silva, P. A. (1995). Temperamental qualities at age 3 predict personality traits in young adulthood: Longitudinal evidence from a birth cohort. *Child Development, 66,* 486–498.

Cepeda, C. (2000). *The concise guide to the psychiatric interview of children and adolescents.* Washington, DC: American Psychiatric Press.

Chess, S., & Thomas, A. (2002). Temperament and its clinical applications. In M. Lewis (Ed.), *Child and adolescent psychiatry: A comprehensive textbook* (3rd ed.). Philadelphia, PA: Lippincott, Williams & Wilkins.

Costello, E. J., Egger, H., & Angold, A. (2005). Ten-year research update review: The epidemiology of child and adolescent psychiatric disorders. I. Methods and public health burden. *Journal of American Academy of Child and Adolescent Psychiatry, 44*(10), 972–986.

Crittenden, P. M. (1996). Research on maltreating families: Implications for intervention. In J. Briere, L. Berliner, A. Bulkey, C. Jenny, & T. Reid (Eds.), *The APSAC handbook on child maltreatment* (pp. 158–174). Thousand Oaks, CA: Sage.

Cummings, E. M., & O'Reilly, A. (1997). Fathers in family context: Effects of marital quality on child adjustment. In M. Lamb (Ed.), *The role of the father in child development* (3rd ed.). New York, NY: Wiley.

Davidson, R. J. (1994). Asymmetric brain function, affective style, and psychopathology. *Developmental Psychopathology, 6,* 741–758.

DeKlyen, M., Speltz, M., & Greenberg, M. (1998). Fathering and early onset conduct problems: Positive and negative parenting, father–son attachment, and the marital context. *Child and Family Psychology Review, 1,* 3–21.

Doherty, G. (1997). *Zero to six: The basis for school readiness.* Ottawa, ON: Human Resources Development Canada, Applied Research Branch, Strategic Policy.

Doll, B., & Lyon, M. A. (1998). Risk and resilience: Implications for delivery of educational and mental health services in the schools. *School Psychology Review, 27*(3), 348–363.

Doyle, A., Markiewicz, D., Brendgen, M., Lieberman, M., & Voss, K. (2000). Child attachment security and self-concept: Associations with mother and father attachment style and marital quality. *Merrill-Palmer Quarterly, 46*(3), 514–539.

Dulcan, M., & Martini, D. R. (1999). *Child and adolescent psychiatry.* Washington, DC: American Psychiatric Press.

Eagly, A. H., Ashmore, R. D., Makhijani, M. G., & Kennedy, L. (1991). What is beautiful is good, but...: A meta-analytic review of research on physical attractiveness stereotype. *Psychological Bulletin, 110,* 109–128.

Edwards, P. (1999). *Fostering knowledge development on the health and well-being of children in Canada: A division paper.* Prepared for Health Canada and the Interim National Expert Advisory Committee for the Centres of Excellence for Children's Well-being.

English, D. T. (1996). *The promise and reality of risk assessment: Protecting children.* Ottawa, ON: Public Health Agency of Canada. Retrieved November 21, 2005, from http://www.phac-aspc.gc.ca/ncfv-cnivf/familyviolence/html/nfntsptprevention_e.html

Forgatch, M., & Patterson, G. (1989). *Parents and adolescents: Living together (Part 2: Family problem-solving).* Eugene, OR: Castalia Publishing Company.

Fryers, T., Melzer, D., Jenkins, R., & Brugha T. (2005, September 5). The distribution of the common mental disorders: Social inequalities in Europe. *Clinical Practice in Epidemiology and Mental Health, 1,* 14.

Garcia-Coll, C., & Magnuson, K. (2000). Cultural differences as sources of developmental vulnerabilities and resources. In J. P. Shonkoff & S. J. Meisels (Eds.), *Handbook of early education intervention* (2nd ed., pp. 94–114). New York, NY: Cambridge University Press.

Goodman, W. K., Price, L. H., Rasmussen, S. A., Mazure, J. C., Fleischmann, R. L., Hill, C. L., et al. (1989). The Children's Yale-Brown Obsessive Compulsive Scale (CYBOCS). I. Development, use, and reliability. *Archives of General Psychiatry, 46,* 1006–1011.

Grollman, E. A. (1990). *Talking about death: A dialogue between parent and child* (3rd ed.). Boston, MA: Beacon Press.

Harlow, H. F., Harlow, M. K., & Suomi, S. J. (1971). From thought to therapy: Lessons from a private laboratory. *American Scientist, 59*(5), 538–549.

Health Canada. (2002). *A report on mental illness in Canada*. Cat. 0–662–32817–5. Ottawa, ON: Author.

Hill, C. E., & O'Brien, K. M. (1999). *Helping skills: Facilitating exploration, insight and action*. Washington, DC: American Psychological Association.

Howes, C., & Matheson, C. (1992). Sequences in the development of competent play with peers: Social and social pretend play. *Developmental Psychology, 28*(5), 961–974.

Jellnick, M., Patel, B. P., & Froehle, M. C. (2003). Bright futures in practice: Mental health (Vol. 1, practice guide and Vol. 2, tool kit). *Journal of the American Academy of Child and Adolescent Psychiatry, 1–2*, 507–508.

Jensen, P., Rubio-Stipac, M., Carnio, G., et al. (1999). Parents and child contributions to diagnosis of mental disorder: Are both informants always necessary? *Journal of the American Academy of Child and Adolescent Psychiatry, 38*(12), 1569–1579.

Kagan, J. (1999). The concept of behavioral inhibition. In L. Schmidt & J. Schulkin (Eds.), *Extreme fear, shyness, and social phobia: Origins, biological mechanisms, and clinical outcomes. Series in affective science.* New York, NY: Oxford University Press.

Kerr WA, Mcgehee EM. (1964). Creative temperament as related to aspects of strategy and intelligence. *Journal of Social Psychology, 62*, 211–216.

King, A., & Coles, B. (1992). *The health of Canada's youth*. Ottawa, ON: Health and Welfare Canada.

Kovacs, M. (1982). *Children's depression inventory*. North Tonawanda, NY: Multi-Health Systems.

Lamb, M. E. (Ed.). (1997). *The role of the father in child development* (3rd ed.). New York, NY: Wiley & Sons.

LeBuffe, P. A., & Naglieri, J. A. (1999). *Devereux early childhood assessment*. The Devereux Foundation. Lewisville, NC: Kaplan Press.

LeBuffe, P. A., & Naglieri, J. A. (2003). *The Devereux early childhood assessment clinical form (DECA)*. Lewisville, NC: Kaplan Press.

Lidz, C. S. (2003). *Early childhood assessment*. Hoboken, NJ: Wiley & Sons.

Linder, T. W. (1993). *Transdisciplinary play-based assessment: A functional approach to working with young children* (Rev ed.). Baltimore, MD: Paul H. Brookes Publishing.

March, J. (1997). *Multidimensional anxiety scale for children*. North Tonawanda, NY: Multi-Health Systems.

McClowry, S. G. (1995). The development of the School-Age Temperament Inventory. *Merrill-Palmer Quarterly, 41*(3), 271–285.

Moore-Taylor, K. M., Menarchek-Fetkovich, M., & Day, C. (2000). In K. Gitlin-Weiner, A. Sandgrund, & C. Scafer (Eds.), *The play history, interview play diagnosis and assessment* (2nd ed.). New York, NY: Wiley.

Murphy, J. M., Ichinose, C., Hicks, R. C., Kingdon, D., Crist-Whitzel, J., Jordan, P., et al. (1996). Utility of the pediatric symptom checklist as a psychosocial screen to meet the federal Early and Periodic Screening, Diagnosis, and Treatment (EPSDT) standards: A pilot study. *Journal of Pediatrics, 129*, 864–869.

National Cancer Institute, US National Institutes of Health. (2005). *Supportive care around bereavement*. Retrieved November 7, 2005, from http://www.cancer.gov/cancertopics/pdq/supportivecare/bereavement/Health-Professional/page8#Section_83

O'Connor, T., & Rutter, M. (2000). Attachment disorder behavior following early severe deprivation: Extension and longitudinal follow-up. *Journal of the American Academy of Child and Adolescent Psychiatry, 39*(6), 709–712.

Plutchik, R. (2000). *Emotions in the practice of psychotherapy*. Washington, DC: American Psychological Association.

Research Unit on Pediatric Psychopharmacology (RUPP) Anxiety Study Group (2002). The pediatric anxiety rating scale (PARS): Development and psychometric properties. *Journal of the American Academy of Child and Adolescent Psychiatry, 41*, 1061–1069.

Reynolds, C. R., & Kamphouse, R. W. (1998). *Behavior assessment system for children (BASC)*. Circle Pines, MN: American Guidance Service.

Roebuck, T. M., Mattson, S. N., & Riley, E. P. (1999). Behavioural and psychosocial profiles of alcohol-exposed children. *Alcoholism: Clinical and Experimental Research, 23*(6), 1070–1076.

Rubin, D., Dodd, M., Desai, N., Pollock, B., & Graham-Pole, J. (2009). Spirituality in well and ill adolescents and their parents: The use of two assessment scales. *Pediatric Nursing, 35*(1), 37–42.

Rutter, M., Silberg, J., O'Connor, T., & Simonoff, E. (1999). Genetics and child psychiatry. I. Advances in qualitative and molecular genetics. *Journal of Psychological Psychiatry, 40*, 3–18.

Sameroff, A. J. (2000). Dialectical processes in developmental psychopathology. In A. J. Sameroff, M. L. Lewis, & S. M. Miller (Eds.), *Handbook of developmental psychopathology* (2nd ed., pp. 23–40). New York, NY: Kluwer Academic.

Sameroff, A., & Chandler, M. (1975). Transactional models in early social relations. *Human Development, 18*, 65–79.

Sattler, J. (1998). *Clinical and forensic interviewing of children and families*. San Diego, CA: Jerome Sattler Publisher.

Schwartz, C., Snidman, N., & Kagan, J. (1999). Adolescent social anxiety as an outcome of inhibited temperament in childhood. *Journal of the American Academy of Child and Adolescent Psychiatry, 38*(8), 1008–1015.

Seifer, R. (2000). Temperament and goodness of fit: Implications for developmental psychopathology. In A. J. Sameroff, M. L. Lewis, & S. M. Miller (Eds.), *Handbook of developmental psychopathology* (pp. 257–276). New York, NY: Kluwer Academic.

Shave, D., & Shave, B. (1989). *Early adolescence and search for self: A developmental perspective*. New York, NY: Praeger Publishers.

Snidman, N., Kagan, J., Riordan, L., & Shannon, D. C. (1995). Cardiac function and behavioural reactivity. *Psychopathology, 32*, 199–207.

Solomon, J., & George, C. (1999). *Attachment disorganization*. New York, NY: Guilford Press.

Squires, J., Bricker, D., & Twombly, E. (2002). *The ASQ: SE user's guide*. Baltimore, MD: Paul H. Brookes Publishing.

State, M., Lombroso, P., Pauls, D., & Leckman, J. (2000). The genetics of childhood psychiatric disorders: A decade of progress. *Journal of the American Academy of Child and Adolescent Psychiatry, 39*(8), 946–962.

Steinhauer, P. D. (1998). *Developing resiliency in children from disadvantaged populations*. Ottawa, ON: Health Canada.

Steinhausen, H. C. (2006). Developmental psychopathology in adolescence: Findings from a Swiss study–the NAPE Lecture 2005. *Acta Psychiatr Scand, 113*(1), 6–12.

Stiffman, A. R., Hadley-Ives, E., Dore, P., Polgar, M., Horvath, V. E., Striley, C., et al. (2000). Youths' access to mental health services: The role of providers' training, resource connectivity, and assessment of need. *Mental Health Services Research, 2*(3), 141–154.

Sturm, R., Ringel, J. S., & Andreyeva, T. (2003). Geographic disparities in children's mental health care. *Pediatrics, 112*(4), e308.

Swanson, J. M. (1983). *The SNAP-IV*. Irvine, CA: University of California, Irvine.

Tanguay, P. (2000). Pervasive developmental disorders: A 10-year review. *Journal of the American Academy of Child and Adolescent Psychiatry, 39*, 1079–1095.

Thomas, A., Chess, S., & Birch, H. G. (1968). *Temperament and behavior disorders in childhood*. New York, NY: New York University Press.

Thompson, R. (2002). Attachment theory and research. In M. Lewis (Ed.), *Child and adolescent psychiatry: A comprehensive textbook* (3rd ed.). Philadelphia, PA: Lippincott, Williams & Wilkins.

Trad, P. (1989). *The pre-school child assessment, diagnosis and treatment*. New York, NY: Wiley.

Trainor, J., Pomeroy, E., & Pape, B. (2004). *A framework for support*. (3rd ed.). Toronto, ON: Canadian Mental Health Association.

Trocmé, N., Fallon, B., MacLaurin B., Daciuk, J., Felstiner, C. Black, T., et al. (2005). *Canadian incidence study of reported child abuse and neglect 2003: Major findings*. Ottawa, ON: Minister of Public Works and Government Services Canada.

Trocmé, N., McPhee, D., & Tam, K. K. (1995). Child abuse and neglect in Ontario: Incidence and characteristics. *Child Welfare, 74*, 563–586.

Tubman, J. G., Lerner, R. M., Lerner, J. V., & Von Eye, A. (1992). Temperament and adjustment in young adulthood: A 15-year longitudinal analysis. *American Journal of Orthopsychiatry, 62*, 564–574.

Vanden Boom, D. C., & Hoeksma, J. B. (1994). The effect of infant irritability on mother–infant interaction: A growth curve analysis. *Developmental Psychology, 30*, 581–590.

Viorst, J. (1972). *The Ten Good Things about Barney*. New York, NY: Simon & Schuster.

Wachtel, A. (1999). *"State of the art" in child abuse prevention*. Prepared for the Family Violence Prevention Unit, Health Canada. Cat. H72–21/151–1997E. Ottawa, ON: Minister of Public Works and Government Services Canada, National Clearing House on Family Violence.

Waddell, C., McEwan, K., Shepherd, C. A., Offord, D. R., & Hua, J. M. (2005). A public health strategy to improve the mental health of Canadian children. *Canadian Journal of Psychiatry, 50*(4), 226–233.

Wass, H., & Corr, C. A. (1984). *Childhood and death*. Washington, DC: Hemisphere Publishing.

Werner, E. E. (1989). High-risk children in young adulthood: A longitudinal study from birth to 32 years. *American Journal of Orthopsychiatry, 59,* 72–81.

White, E.B. (1952*). Charlotte's Web*. New York, NY: HarperCollins.

White, S. (2000). Using anatomically detailed dolls in interviewing preschoolers. In K. Gitlin-Weiner, A. Sandgrund, & C. Schaefer (Eds.), *Play diagnosis and assessment* (2nd ed., pp. 210–227). New York, NY: Wiley & Sons.

Whitehead, M. (2008). *Pediatric nurses' perspectives of spirituality and spiritual care within nurse-patient relationships: An interpretive description*. Unpublished Master Thesis, University of Alberta, Canada.

Wolfe, D. A. (1998). *Prevention of child abuse and neglect*. Ottawa, ON: Health Canada.

Wright, L. M., & Leahey, M. (2005). The three most common errors in family nursing: How to avoid or sidestep. *Journal of Family Nursing, 11*(2), 90–101.

Xue, Y., Leventhal, T., Brooks-Gunn, J., & Earls, F. J. (2005). Neighborhood residence and mental health problems of 5- to 11-year-olds. *Archives of General Psychiatry, 62*(5), 554–563.

Psychiatric Disorders Diagnosed in Children and Adolescents

Julia Gajewski-Noel

Adapted from the chapter "Psychiatric Disorders Diagnosed in Children and Adolescents" by Lawrence Scahill, Vanya Hamrin, and Catherine Gray Deering

LEARNING OBJECTIVES

After studying this chapter, you will be able to:
- Identify the disorders usually first diagnosed in infancy, childhood, or adolescence, according to the *Diagnostic and Statistical Manual of Mental Disorders*, 4th ed., Text revision (*DSM-IV-TR*).
- Identify the bio/psycho/social/spiritual dimensions of the developmental disorders of childhood.
- Discuss the nursing care of children with pervasive developmental disorders.
- Compare the disruptive behaviour disorders: attention deficit hyperactivity disorder, oppositional defiant disorder, and conduct disorder.
- Relate the assessment data of children with attention deficit hyperactivity disorder to the development of nursing diagnoses, interventions, and evaluation of outcomes.
- Discuss the epidemiology, etiology, psychopharmacologic interventions, and nursing care of children with disorders of mood and anxiety, including posttraumatic stress disorder.
- Discuss the epidemiology, etiology, psychopharmacologic interventions, and nursing care of children with tic disorders.
- Discuss the behavioural intervention strategies for the treatment of encopresis.

KEY TERMS

• ascertainment bias • autism • communication disorders • concordant • dyslexia • encopresis • enuresis • externalizing disorders • internalizing disorders • learning disorders • school phobia • stereotypic behaviour

For much of the 20th century, the predominant theoretical perspectives in the mental health fields were that child and adolescent mental disturbances were directly linked to faulty parenting. With such professional blame firmly established, the shame of admitting a child or adolescent's mental disorder also served to limit help-seeking. Thus, stigmatization of child and adolescent disorders and the blame of parenting practices as causally responsible for them are important considerations for child and adolescent mental health (Hinshaw, 2005).

The understanding of child psychiatric disorders has benefited from advances in several related fields, including developmental biology, neuroanatomy, psychopharmacology, genetics, and epidemiology. Before the introduction of the third edition of the American Psychiatric Association's (APA's) *Diagnostic and Statistical Manual of Mental Disorders (DSM-III)* in 1980, clinicians based their diagnostic decisions on subjective impressions, rather than on clearly defined diagnostic criteria. Because the clinician's theoretic orientation directly influenced these subjective impressions, psychiatric diagnoses were notoriously unreliable. The *DSM-III* provided a reliable method for making psychiatric diagnoses, a necessary factor for strengthening research efforts concerning the etiology and outcome of childhood and adolescent disorders. In addition, the clear diagnostic criteria and the multiaxial system introduced by the *DSM-III* facilitated communication among clinicians.

This chapter uses criteria from the current *Diagnostic and Statistical Manual of Mental Disorders*, 4th ed. Text revision (*DSM-IV-TR*; APA, 2000) in defining childhood disorders. The *DSM-IV-TR* contains 10 categories of disorders, as listed in Table 28-1. Childhood and adolescent disorders are generally coded under Axis 1, except for mental retardation, which is categorized under Axis 11.

Child psychopathology can be classified according to several broad categories: developmental disorders, disruptive behaviour disorders, mood and anxiety disorders, tic disorders, and psychotic disorders. The prevalence of child psychiatric disorders varies across these categories. For example, child schizophrenia is rare, whereas attention deficit hyperactivity disorder (ADHD) is relatively common. In cited estimates of prevalence for psychiatric disorders of childhood, the numbers usually include adolescents; however, it should be noted that some of these disorders vary with age. For example, depression is more common in adolescents than in younger children. Gender ratio may also vary with some disorders according to age. For example, depression is probably more common in boys in children younger than 12 years of age but is more common in girls during adolescence.

The Canadian Pediatric Society (2006) contends that mental health problems among children and youth have increased in recent years and are predicted to increase by 50% by the year 2020. In Canada, at any given time, approximately 14% of children aged 4 to 17 years (more than 800,000) experience mental disorders that cause significant distress and impairment at home, at school, and in the community—fewer than 25% of these children receive specialized treatment (Waddell, McEwan, Shepherd, Offord, & Hua, 2005). This discrepancy appears to be the result of limited access to treatment facilities, either because of financial constraints or because appropriate mental health services for children are simply unavailable. Psychiatric problems are less easily diagnosed in children than they are in adults. One factor contributing to this difference is that sometimes the symptoms of disorders are difficult to distinguish from the turbulence of normal growth and development. For example, a 4-year-old child who has an invisible imaginary friend is normal; however, an adolescent with an invisible friend might be experiencing a hallucination. The certainty of current estimates for the frequency of the various psychiatric disorders is also inconsistent, partly because of changing definitions of these disorders.

This chapter presents an overview of the childhood disorders that the psychiatric–mental health nurse may encounter and discusses the nursing care of children with these challenges. Because it is beyond the scope of this text to present all child and adolescent psychiatric disorders, this chapter focuses on developmental disorders (excluding mental retardation/intellectual disability), disruptive behaviour disorders, mood, anxiety, and tic disorders. Attention deficit hyperactivity disorder is reviewed in detail. Childhood schizophrenia and elimination disorders are also briefly described.

> **▪ CRNENOTE**
>
> **CRNENOTE** All of the psychiatric disorders of childhood and adolescence should be viewed within the context of growth and development models. Safety and self-esteem are priority considerations.

Developmental Disorders of Childhood

Under the primary influences of genes and environment, development may be said to proceed along several pathways, such as attention, cognition, language, affect, and social and moral behaviours. The developmental disorders of childhood include several conditions that are etiologically unrelated; however, their common feature is a significant delay in one or more lines of development. Some of these developmental pathways and developmental delays are closely interwoven. For example, a language delay can interfere with a child's social development and contribute to behaviour problems (Russell & Grizzle, 2008). The *DSM-IV-TR* classifies developmental disorders in several categories, including mental retardation/intellectual disability, pervasive developmental disorders, and specific developmental disorders.

Table 28.1 Disorders Usually First Diagnosed in Infancy, Childhood, or Adolescence	
Disorder	**Characteristics**
Mental Retardation/Intellectual Disability	
Mild	Significantly below-average intellectual functioning (IQ about 70 or below) with onset before the age of 18 years and concurrent impairments in adaptive functioning
Moderate	
Severe	
Profound	
Severity unspecified	
Learning Disorders	
Reading disorder	Academic functioning substantially below that expected given the person's chronologic age, measured intelligence, and age appropriate education
Mathematics disorder	
Disorder of written expression	
Learning disorders not otherwise specified	
Motor Skills Disorders	
Developmental coordination disorder	Motor coordination substantially below that expected given the person's chronologic age and measured intelligence
Communication Disorders	
Expressive language disorder	Significant delay or deviance in speech or language
Mixed receptive–expressive language disorder	
Phonologic disorder	
Stuttering	
Communication disorder not otherwise specified	
Pervasive Developmental Disorders	
Autistic disorder	Severe deficits in multiple areas of development; these include impairment in reciprocal social interaction, impairment in communication, and the presence of stereotyped behaviour, restricted interests, and activities
Asperger's disorder	
Pervasive developmental disorder not otherwise specified	
Rett's disorder	
Childhood disintegrative disorder	
Attention Deficit and Disruptive Behaviour Disorders	
Predominantly inattentive type	Prominent symptoms of inattention and/or hyperactivity–impulsivity
Predominantly hyperactive–impulsive type	
Combined type	
Conduct disorder	A pattern of behaviour that violates the basic rights of others or major age-appropriate societal norms or rules
Oppositional defiant disorder	A pattern of negativistic hostile, and defiant behaviour
Feeding and Eating Disorders of Infancy or Early Childhood	
Pica	Persistent disturbances in feeding and eating
Rumination disorder	
Feeding disorder of infancy or early childhood	
Tic Disorders	
Tourette disorder	Vocal or motor tics
Chronic motor or vocal tic disorder	
Transient tic disorder	
Tic disorder not otherwise specified	
Elimination Disorders	
Encopresis	Repeated passage of feces into inappropriate places
Enuresis	Repeated voiding of urine into inappropriate places
Other Disorders of Infancy, Childhood, or Adolescence	
Separation anxiety disorder	Developmentally inappropriate and excessive anxiety concerning separation from home or those to whom the child is attached
Selective mutism	A consistent failure to speak in specific social situations despite speaking in other situations
Reactive attachment disorder of infancy or early childhood	Markedly disturbed and developmentally inappropriate social relatedness that occurs in most contexts and is associated with physical and/or emotional neglect
Stereotypic movement disorder	Repetitive, seemingly driven, and nonfunctional motor behaviour that markedly interferes with normal activities and at times may result in bodily injury

Data from American Psychiatric Association. (2000). *Diagnostic and statistical manual of mental disorders* (4th ed., Text revision, pp. 39–41). Washington, DC: Author.

PERVASIVE DEVELOPMENTAL DISORDERS

Children with pervasive developmental disorders (PDDs) may or may not have an intellectual disability, but they commonly show an uneven pattern of intellectual strengths and weaknesses. Children with PDDs may show a lifelong pattern of being rigid in style, intolerant of change, and prone to behavioural outbursts in response to environmental demands or changes in routine (Box 28-1).

KEY CONCEPT **Developmental delay** means that the child's development is outside the norm, including delayed socialization, communication, peculiar mannerisms, and idiosyncratic interests.

KEY CONCEPT **Pervasive developmental disorders** are a group of syndromes marked by severe developmental delays in several areas that cannot be attributed to an intellectual disability.

Types

The *DSM-IV-TR* includes five categories of PDDs: autistic disorder, Asperger's disorder, Rett's disorder, childhood disintegrative disorder, and pervasive developmental disorder not otherwise specified (Perry & Condillac, 2003). This section focuses on autistic and Asperger's disorders.

Autistic Disorder

Autistic disorder, or **autism**, has been a subject of considerable interest and research effort since its original description more than 50 years ago, when Leo Kanner

BOX 28.1

History and Hallmarks of Childhood and Adolescent Disorders

- Maternal age and health status during pregnancy
- Exposure to medication, alcohol, or other substances during pregnancy
- Course of pregnancy, labour, and delivery
- Infant's health at birth
- Eating, sleeping, and growth in first year
- Health status in first year
- Interest in others in first 2 years
- Motor development
- Mastery of bowel and bladder control
- Speech and language development
- Activity level
- Response to separation (e.g., school entry)
- Regulation of mood and anxiety
- Medical history in early childhood
- Social development
- Interests

(1943) described the profound isolation of these children and their extreme desire for sameness. Two features distinguish autism from other PDDs: early age of onset (before the age of 30 months) and severe disturbance in social relatedness. These children appear aloof and indifferent to others and often seem to prefer inanimate objects.

The impairment in communication is severe and affects both verbal and nonverbal communication (APA, 2000). Children with autism manifest delayed and deviant language development, as evidenced by *echolalia* (repetition of words or phrases spoken by others), and a tendency to be extremely concrete in the interpretation of language. Pronoun reversals and abnormal intonation are also common. Other common features of autism categorized as **stereotypic behaviour** include repetitive rocking, hand flapping, and an extraordinary insistence on sameness. The child may also engage in self-injurious behaviour, such as hitting, head banging, or biting. For some children, their unusual interests may evolve into fascination with specific objects, such as fans or air conditioners, or a particular topic, such as Prime Ministers of Canada.

KEY CONCEPT **Autistic disorder** is a marked impairment of development in social interaction and communication with a restrictive repertoire of activity and interest.

Epidemiology and Etiology

There has been a dramatic rise in the incidence of autistic disorder, from 2–5 to 15–60 per 10,000 children during the past two decades. The use of broader diagnostic criteria, more systematic assessment practices, and increased awareness and attention by health care professionals are factors that may be contributing to this apparent increase (Persico & Bourgeron, 2006).

Autism occurs in boys more often than in girls, with the ratio ranging from 2:1 to 5:1. However, when girls are affected, they tend to be more severely impaired and have poorer outcomes (Volkmar, Klin, & Paul, 2004). About half of children with autism are intellectually disabled, and about 25% have seizure disorders.

The etiology of autism disorder remains elusive, though research continues in the areas of genetics, neurology, and metabolic disorders. Numerous theories suggest various causes for autism, including genetics, perinatal insult, and impaired parent–child interactions (Volkmar et al., 2004). It was fashionable in the 1950s and 1960s to believe that the "indifference" of professional parents was a contributing cause of autism. This explanation is no longer seriously considered and almost certainly reflected an **ascertainment bias** (a bias that occurs when the method of identifying cases creates a sample that differs from the population it purports to represent) because professional families were more likely to use the services of major medical centres. It also represents a failure to recognize that the child's disability may have contributed to disturbed parent–child interactions, rather than being an effect of these interactions.

Low IQ and autism recur at a higher than expected rate in the siblings of children with autism, and monozygotic twins are more likely to be **concordant** (mutually affected) than are dizygotic twins, suggesting that genetic factors play a role in the disorder. Other proposed causes include perinatal complications, such as exposure to infectious agents or medications during gestation; prematurity; and gestational bleeding. The role of environment in autistic disorder has been conclusively demonstrated only for prenatal or perinatal exposure to viral agents, such as rubella and cytomegalovirus, and prenatal exposure to thalidomide and valproic acid. Vaccinations have also recently drawn attention as possible causative factors due to their high content of thimerosal, a preservative containing mercury, and due to the proposed causal link between autism and the measles–mumps–rubella vaccine. However, recent epidemiological studies have excluded a widespread causal role for vaccines in autism (Persico & Bourgeron, 2006). The specific cause remains unknown and may result from multiple factors. Studies of genetic, epigenetic, and environmental factors are finally beginning to provide some insights into solving the complexities of autistic disorder. Structural and functional imaging studies also provide intriguing leads for future inquiry (Fig. 28-1).

The literature quite clearly supports the need for early screening and referral programs to promote early diagnosis and treatment (Pinto-Martin, Souders, Giarelli, & Levy, 2005). Some early developmental indicators which suggest that a child should be referred for a full assessment include lack of babbling or gestures at 12 months,

FIGURE 28.1 The client with autism (*right*) may have decreased metabolic rates in the cingulate gyrus and other associated areas; however, wide heterogeneity in brain metabolic patterns is seen in clients with autism. (Courtesy of Monte S. Buchsbaum, MD, Mount Sinai Medical Centre and School of Medicine, New York, NY.)

lack of single words by 16 months, lack of two-word combinations by 18 months, and any regression or loss of words or skills. Other developmental indicators include lack of joint attention (pointing to show), lack of response to name, and unusual or absent eye contact and the use of facial expression (Perry & Condillac, 2003). Parents who report concerns about their chid's development should be taken seriously. Early identification through screening followed by psychosocial support and education about the disorder and treatment options can help families to adjust and cope (Pinto-Martin et al.). Nursing has a pivotal role to play in all these areas.

Psychopharmacologic Interventions

No medication has proved effective at changing the core social and language deficits of autism. However, numerous psychiatric medications have been used to treat the associated behavioural difficulties in PDDs (Palermo & Curatolo, 2004; Witwer & Lecavalier, 2005). Medications can reduce the frequency and intensity of behavioural disturbances, including hyperactivity, agitation, mood instability, aggression, self-injury, and stereotypic behaviour. Haloperidol, a typical antipsychotic medication, has demonstrated efficacy in reducing hyperactivity, stereotypic behaviour, emotional lability, temper outbursts, and social withdrawal (McDougle & Posey, 2003). In combination with behavioural language training, it was found to be more effective than either haloperidol or language training alone in facilitating the imitation of new words. Despite these reported benefits, haloperidol is associated with a range of side effects, including sedation and dystonic reactions. In addition, long-term use can be followed by the development of treatment-related involuntary movements including tardive dyskinesia, both during administration and following withdrawal from medication (Palermo & Curatolo). Given these findings, drug holidays every 6 to 12 months are often recommended to observe the child's continued need for medication. The less potent antipsychotics, such as chlorpromazine, tend to cause excessive sedation without clinical improvement.

A large number of studies have documented the efficacy of several atypical antipsychotics in a variety of clinical domains of autism, including risperidone, olanzapine, quetiapine, and clozapine. Risperidone, however, appears to be the most effective in treating core social-cognitive symptoms and other domains (stereotyped and repetitive behaviours) that are compromised in autism. Furthermore, its efficacy in improving working memory, executive function, and attention in schizophrenia, in addition to the clinical improvements in conditions that share certain clinical features with autism, such as obsessive-compulsive spectrum disorder, further strengthens evidence for its use. Due to the possible side effects of hyperprolactinemia and severe weight gain, children and adolescents on risperidone should be monitored closely, as the long-term consequences of elevated serum prolactin are not clear (Shea et al., 2004). Although considerable research has been conducted on the use of risperidone in treating autism, the long-term risks of use in children needs further study (Anderson et al., 2007).

The serotonin reuptake inhibitors, both selective (fluoxetine, sertraline, and paroxetine) and nonselective (clomipramine), also have a role in the treatment of interfering behaviours of autism, specifically repetitive and aggressive ones, and have been found to improve social relatedness in autistic children, more so in the presence of a positive family history for affective disorders (Palermo & Curatolo, 2004), while continued research is needed in children with PDD (McDougle & Posey, 2003).

Continuum of Care

Autism is a chronic disorder usually requiring long-term care at various levels of intensity. Children and adolescents with autism are a heterogeneous group and as such they have diverse needs. It is essential that intervention treatment plans be based on individual patterns of strengths and limitations (Perry & Condillac, 2003). Intervention treatment consists of designing academic, interpersonal, and social experiences that support the child's development. Children with autism, even those who are severely affected, may be able to live at home and attend a special school for children with autism that uses behavioural modification. Other outpatient services may include family counselling, home care, and medication. As the child moves toward adulthood, living at home may become more difficult, given the appropriate need for greater independence. The level of structure required depends primarily on IQ and adaptive functioning. Ongoing support and respite for the family are critical and an essential part of the intervention treatment plan in which nursing plays an integral role.

Asperger's Disorder

Although Asperger's disorder was also described about 50 years ago, it was not included in the *DSM-III* or *DSM-III-R*. It has been incorporated into the *DSM-IV-TR* and is defined as severe and sustained impairment in social interaction and restricted, repetitive patterns of behaviour, interests, and activities (APA, 2000). Children with Asperger's disorder have profound social deficits marked by an inappropriate initiation of social interactions, an inability to respond to usual social cues, and a tendency to be concrete in their interpretation of language. They also display stereotypic behaviours, such as rocking and hand flapping, and highly restricted areas of interest, such as train schedules, fans, air conditioners, dogs, or British royalty. Signs of developmental delay may not be apparent until preschool or school age, when social deficits become evident (Box 28-2). Such deficits and behaviour patterns are not associated with intellectual disability in Asperger's disorder, and the communication deficits are less severe than in autism. The differences in intelligence, language development, and age of clear onset suggest that Asperger's disorder is distinguishable from autism. However, it may not be differentiated from autism in the literature (Volkmar et al., 2004).

BOX 28.2

*Clinical Vignette: **Frank (Asperger's Disorder)***

A paediatrician refers Frank, age 5 years 6 months, for an evaluation because of Frank's unusual preoccupation with ceiling fans and lawn sprinklers. According to his mother, Frank became interested in ceiling fans at the age of 3 years when he began drawing them, tearing pictures of them out of magazines, and engaging others in discussions about them. In the months before the evaluation, Frank also became fascinated by lawn sprinklers. These preoccupations so dominated Frank's interactions with others that he was practically incapable of discussing any other topics. He remained on the periphery of his kindergarten class and had few friends. Although he tried to make friends, his approaches were inept, and he had trouble reading others.

Frank was the product of a full-term uncomplicated pregnancy, labour, and delivery to his then 25-year-old mother. It was her first pregnancy, and both parents eagerly anticipated Frank's birth. As an infant, Frank was healthy but seemed to cry a lot and was difficult to comfort, causing his mother to feel inadequate and depleted. His motor development was also delayed, and at the age of 3 years, nonfamily members had difficulty understanding his speech. His articulation, however, was within normal limits at the time of consultation. Frank received regular paediatric care and had no history of serious illness or injury. There was no family history of intellectual disability or psychiatric illness; results of genetic testing for chromosomal abnormality were negative.

In addition to his unusual preoccupations and social deficits, Frank resisted any change in his routine, was easily frustrated, and was prone to temper tantrums. His parents sharply disagreed about the nature of and appropriate response to his problems.

WHAT DO YOU THINK?
- What effect do you think Frank's preoccupation may have on his family and their relationships?
- What kind of teaching program would you develop if you were the nurse assigned to this family?

Epidemiology and Etiology

The etiology of Asperger's disorder is not completely understood but is believed to have genetic causes combined with environmental factors (Schnur, 2005). The prevalence of this disorder is difficult to determine because of shifts in its definition and lack of population data on the newly established diagnostic criteria. The current estimate is in the range of 1 to 3 per 10,000. Asperger's disorder appears to be more common in boys. Although no genetic marker has been identified, the disorder often runs in families, with high recurrence in fathers (Schnur; Volkmar et al., 2004).

Psychopharmacologic Interventions

Pharmacologic interventions in children with Asperger's disorder have recently been gaining attention. Medications, including selective serotonin reuptake inhibitors (SSRIs), antidepressants, and atypical antipsychotics and anticonvulsants, may alleviate troublesome symptoms and behaviours or cormorbid conditions such as depression, but they do not cure the underlying Asperger's disorder (Schnur, 2005). Although no medication studies have been conducted on children with carefully diagnosed Asperger's disorder, approaches to the treatment of depression and anxiety disorders would be the same as those used in typically developing young children.

Continuing Care

Asperger's disorder is a social and communication disability, knowledge of which is still evolving through research. As with autism, the family needs education and help in supporting the child's development and managing symptoms.

▪ NURSING MANAGEMENT: HUMAN RESPONSE TO PERVASIVE DEVELOPMENTAL DISORDER

Biologic Domain

Assessment

The assessment of children with PDD is a complex endeavour (Pinto-Martin et al., 2005; Sherer & Schreibman, 2005). Biologic assessment should include a review of physical health and neurologic status, giving particular attention to coordination, childhood illnesses, injuries, and hospitalizations. The nurse should assess sleep, appetite, and activity patterns because they may be disturbed in these children. Lack of adequate sleep can increase irritability. Sleep problems are common in children with PDD, but research findings suggest that children with Asperger's disorder have sleep problems that are more resistant to behavioural treatment, have more disoriented wakening, and have generally more symptoms of sleep disturbance (Polimeni, Richdale, & Francis, 2005). Comorbid seizure disorders are common in autism, and depression is often seen concurrently with Asperger's disorder. Thus, the nurse should also consider these conditions in his or her assessment of the child.

Youngsters with additional psychiatric disorders or seizures may be receiving multiple medications and require the care of several clinicians. Therefore, the assessment should include a careful review of current medications and treating clinicians.

Nursing Diagnoses for the Biologic Domain

Assessment data generate a variety of potential nursing diagnoses, including self-care deficits, impaired verbal communication, disturbed sensory perceptions, delayed growth and development, and disturbed sleep patterns. Treatment outcomes need to be individualized to the child, family, and social environment.

Interventions for the Biologic Domain

In teaching self-care skills, the nurse needs to consider the child's current adaptive skills and language limitations. Developing a list of activities for the child to post in his or her bedroom may be effective for some children. Drawings or symbols may be useful for nonverbal children. Physical safety is an important concern for children who are cognitively delayed and may have impaired judgment.

As noted earlier, children with PDD may be treated with multiple medications in novel combinations (Martin, Van Hoof, Stubbe, Sherwin, & Scahill, 2003). In some cases, these unusual combinations are the result of careful management; in other cases, the combinations are the result of clinical mismanagement, perhaps because of poor coordination among treating prescribers. Consequently, the nurse should carefully review the target symptoms for each drug treatment with the parents. This review includes possible drug interactions that are especially important for this clinical population.

Psychological Domain

Assessment

Critical elements to be evaluated include intellectual ability, communication skills, and adaptive functioning. Direct behavioural observation is critical to evaluate the child's ability to relate to others, to verify the selection of age-appropriate activities, and to watch for stereotypic behaviours. Children with PDD often need specific behavioural interventions to reduce the frequency of inappropriate or aggressive behaviour. These interventions follow from a careful evaluation of the circumstances that precede or accompany the behaviour and the usual consequences of the behaviour (Volkmar et al., 2004). For example, a child may exhibit angry outbursts in response to routine transitions. If the tantrum is dramatic, the consequence may be that the transition does not take place. By structuring the environment and using visual cues to signal the end of one activity and the start of another, it may be possible to reduce the number and intensity of responses to transitions.

Nursing Diagnoses for the Psychological Domain

Assessment data generate a variety of potential nursing diagnoses, including anxiety and disturbed thought processes. Because of the long-term nature of these disorders, outcomes may change with time.

Interventions for the Psychological Domain

Managing the repetitive behaviours of these children will depend on the specific behaviour and its effects on others or the environment. If the behaviour, such as rocking, has no negative effects, ignoring it may be the best approach. If the behaviour, such as head banging, is unacceptable, redirecting the child and using positive reinforcement are recommended. In some cases, especially in severely delayed children, these strategies may not work, and environmental alterations and perhaps protective headgear are needed.

Social Domain

Assessment

The nursing assessment is an ongoing process in which attention is given to establishing a positive relationship with the child and the family. The assessment should include a review of the child's capacity for self-care and maladaptive behaviours (Pinto-Martin et al., 2005; Sherer & Schreibman, 2005). Self-injury and aggression are sometimes present, and children may need to be protected from hurting themselves and others. Inquiry should also include the presence of perseverative behaviours and preoccupation with restricted interests. These odd behaviours may not necessarily cause a problem, but they often interfere with the child's relationships.

Another important domain to consider in the nursing assessment is the effect of the child's developmental delays on the family. Having a child with PDD is bound to influence family interaction, and responding to the child's needs may adversely affect family functioning. For example, sleep disruption in family members who care for these children may increase family stress.

Nursing Diagnoses for the Social Domain

Assessment data generate a variety of potential nursing diagnoses, including social isolation. The family may be grieving the loss of the normal child it had expected and is trying to cope with the multitude of problems inherent in raising a child with a disability. Because of the long-term nature of these disorders, the aims of treatment may change with time. However, throughout childhood, the focus should be on the development of age-appropriate adaptive and social skills.

Interventions for the Social Domain

Planning interventions for youngsters with severe developmental problems considers the child, family, and community supports, such as schools, rehabilitation centres, mental health centres, or group homes and available respite services. First and foremost, the various clinicians involved in the child's treatment should collaborate with the family toward the same general goals. As the number of clinicians and educators involved increases, the chance of fragmentation in treatment planning also increases. The nurse can serve as a case coordinator to ensure that the plan of care is both comprehensive and appropriate in meeting the needs of both the child and the family.

Promoting Interaction

Many of the core deficits in PDD fall within the domain of social development, regardless of the level of cognitive functioning of the particular child or adolescent. The goal of intervention in the social domain is to increase meaningful relationships by teaching skills that support the development of social interest, social initiation, social responsiveness, empathy, and understanding of the other's perspective. It is critical that intervention treatment plans include strategies to enhance social understanding, social relating, and play skills and that these strategies take into account the individual's cognitive, learning, linguistic, and developmental abilities (Perry & Condillac, 2003). Interventions fostering nonverbal social interactions may sometimes be more useful than those based on speech. For higher functioning children, activities such as getting the mail, passing out snacks, or taking turns in the context of simple games can engage them in social activities without requiring the use of their limited language skills. Structuring social interactions so that the child has to share a task with another, such as carrying a load of books, may help to boost confidence in relating to others.

Ensuring Predictability and Safety

When children with PDD are hospitalized, milieu management—a consistent, structured environment with predictable routines for activities, mealtimes, and bedtimes—is necessary for successful treatment. Changes in routine may provoke disorganization in the child with PDD, leading to emotional disequilibrium and explosive behaviour. The safety of the inpatient unit offers an opportunity to try behavioural strategies, such as rewards for managing transitions. Health care professionals can explore with family strategies that have been successful for managing behaviours in the past and can also share new successful strategies with parents or primary caretakers.

Managing Behaviour

Because children with PDD have difficulty relating to others, they should spend most of their time within the therapeutic environment of the unit. These children can learn social and communication skills, such as taking turns in conversation and warning the listener before changing the subject in the context of milieu. If a child requires isolation for control of aggressive or assaultive behaviour, a brief "time out" followed by prompt re-entry into unit activities is optimum.

Autism and related disorders are chronic conditions that call for extraordinary patience and determination. Unfortunately, lack of integration of medical, psychiatric, social, and educational services can add to the family's burden. Family stress research has repeatedly demonstrated that parents (especially mothers) of children with PDDs experience greater stress, depression, and mental health difficulties than parents of children with other types of disability (Perry & Condillac, 2003). Parents may manifest feelings of denial, grief, guilt, anger, and sorrow at various points as they adjust to their child's disability. The nurse can offer parents the opportunity to express their frustrations and disappointments and can be alert for indications that parents are in need of additional assistance, such as parent support groups or respite care.

Residential care may be necessary in some cases. After making the decision to place a child into a residential facility, family members may experience guilt, loss, and a sense of failure concerning their inability to care for the child at home.

Supporting Family

Family interventions include support, education, counselling, and referral to self-help groups. Whenever possible, the nurse provides education to help parents determine appropriate expectations for their child with PDD and to meet the child's special needs.

The following are examples of potentially useful nursing interventions focusing on the family:

- Interpreting the treatment plan for parents and the child
- Modelling appropriate behaviour modification techniques
- Including the parents as cotherapists for the implementation of the care plan
- Assisting the family members in identifying and resolving their sense of loss related to the diagnosis
- Coordinating support systems for parents, siblings, and family members
- Maintaining interdisciplinary collaboration
- Facilitating access to and encouraging families to use formal support services such as respite care
- Assisting parents to advocate/lobby on behalf of their child and children with disabilities.

Spiritual Domain

As spirituality is about who we are and our connections with one another and the sacred, it shapes our lives (see Chapter 6). Children with PDD may face particular challenges in terms of evolving and sustaining their spirituality. Children understand themselves and the world around them based on their level of development and experience (Smith & McSherry, 2004). Children with PDD will need spiritual support (e.g., help to express their spiritual needs) based on their individual capacity for understanding and interacting with others. A major challenge, however, is that the spiritual lives of children with special needs or disabilities can be devalued or ignored. A study of parents/caregivers of such children revealed that they were disillusioned or alienated from potential spiritual support when, for instance, they found their children to be unwelcome at their church or synagogue (Speraw, 2006). No participant in this study perceived nurses as being aware of or interested in their family's spiritual needs. Yet this is where spiritual care must begin: with an explicit regard for the importance of this domain to one's clients (see Chapter 27 for ways to address children's spiritual domain).

■ EVALUATION AND TREATMENT OUTCOMES

Evaluation of client and family outcomes is an ongoing process. Short-term outcomes might consist of discrete behavioural improvements, such as reducing self-injurious behaviour by 50%. The long-term goal is for the client to achieve the highest level of functioning. The prognosis depends on the severity of the impairments, the interventions available, and the cognitive ability of the child. The use of standardized rating scales before and after the treatment can improve the precision of outcome measurement (Perry & Condillac, 2003).

SPECIFIC DEVELOPMENTAL DISORDERS

In contrast to intellectual disability and PDD, specific developmental disorders are characterized by a narrower range of deficits. These more discrete delays can occur in various developmental domains. However, some children have more than one specific developmental disorder, and some of these disorders may have a common etiology (Shaywitz, 2003). Current data also suggest that psychiatric disorders occur two to three times more often in children with developmental disorders than in children without (Fox, Keller, Grede, & Bartosz, 2007).

Types

Specific developmental disorders are generally classified as learning, communication, and motor skills disorders. This section focuses primarily on learning disorders, with a focus on dyslexia and communication disorders.

Learning Disorders

Learning disorders (also called learning disabilities) are one of the most common neurobehavioural disorders in children and are typically defined as difficulties in an academic area. They constitute an invisible handicap and are viewed as important causes of poor school performance. Learning disorders refer to a heterogeneous group of disorders manifested by unexpected, specific, and persistent difficulties in the acquisition and use of efficient reading (dyslexia), writing (dysgraphia), or mathematical (dyscalculia) abilities despite conventional instructions, intact senses, normal intelligence, proper motivation, and adequate sociocultural opportunities. The child's ability to achieve in the specific academic area is below what is expected for the child's age, educational level, and intelligence. The difficulty experienced by the child is severe enough to interfere with academic achievements and/or age-appropriate activities of daily living (Karande, Sawant, Sandeep, Kanchan, & Sholapurwala, 2005).

For children with learning disabilities, the negative effects of low achievement or failure may be manifested in low self-esteem and reduced academic effort. Some children and adolescents may also exhibit difficulties in age-appropriate social interactions. Postsecondary students with learning disabilities have been observed to exhibit poor self-concepts, have problems with interpersonal skills, and have deficits in processing and study skills (Ransby & Swanson, 2003). Research also suggests that children and adolescents with learning disorders experience more feelings of loneliness, depression, stress, and suicidal ideations than their peers without learning disabilities (Buysse, Goldman, & Skinner, 2003).

Dyslexia, a reading disability, is the most common and most carefully researched of the learning disabilities, affecting 80% of all identified as learning disabled. The incidence of dyslexia in Canadian school children is about 5%. In clinical samples, dyslexia affects boys more often than girls; however, a large community-based sample of children with reading disorders found no gender difference. This discrepancy suggests that the observed difference in clinical samples may be related to biases in seeking treatment, rather than a true gender difference (Shaywitz, 2003).

Substantial evidence has established that children with dyslexia have deficits in phonologic awareness. According to this phonologic-deficit hypothesis, dyslexic children have difficulty developing an awareness that words both written and spoken can be broken down into smaller units of sound and that the letters constituting the written word represent the sound heard in the spoken word (Karande et al., 2005).

Communication Disorders

Communication disorders involve speech or language impairments. Speech refers to the motor aspects of speaking; language consists of higher order aspects of formulating and comprehending verbal communication. Language delay in young children is a common problem. Using the widely accepted criterion of a parent-reported expressive vocabulary of less than 50 words and/or no combination of words, the prevalence of developmental language delay is estimated to be 15% at age 24 to 29 months. Children with isolated expressive language delay generally have a good prognosis. However, early language delay can be an indicator for several neurological developmental problems. First, language delay can reflect specific language impairment (SLI). Children with SLI can have either expressive language lags or they show deficits in both expressive and receptive language abilities. Second, language delay can be caused by neurological disorder or be associated with general cognitive impairment. Third, language delay can be the first presenting symptom of an autism spectrum disorder. Finally, persistent hearing loss in children can affect speech, language, social, emotional, and cognitive development. The most common cause of hearing loss in children is persistent otitis media with effusion. Its prevalence is between 15% and 40% in children from infancy to 5 years of age (Buschmann et al., 2008).

A delay in speech or language development can adversely affect the child's socialization and education. For example, peers may rebuff or tease a child with an articulation defect or stutter, contributing to withdrawal and a negative self-image. The resulting isolation could limit opportunities to negotiate rules, take turns, and learn cooperation. These same tasks could also be difficult for children with language delay. Moreover, language appears to play a role in the regulation of behaviours and impulses. Parents and teachers tend to perceive children with delayed language as temperamentally difficult and hard to manage compared with children who are developing language normally (Law & Garrett, 2004). Currently, there is a lack of clarity in the relationship between early language, learning, and emotional and behavioural difficulties (Law & Garrett).

Nursing Management

The nursing assessment of children with a known specific developmental disorder includes (1) evidence of interference in daily life, (2) determination of the youngster's ability (and limitations) to communicate during the interview, (3) assessment of the child's perception about his or her disability, (4) observation for impaired learning and communication, and (5) past and current interventions for the learning or communication deficit, with data gathered through a direct interview of the child and significant others such as parents. Several nursing diagnoses can be generated from these data, such as impaired verbal communication, social isolation, and chronic or situational low self-esteem. For the child with learning disabilities, nurses can focus on building self-confidence and helping the family connect with guidance and educational resources that support the child's development into adulthood. For the child with communication disorders, the interventions focus on fostering social and communication skills and making referrals for specific speech or language therapy. Modelling appropriate communication in spontaneous situations with the child can be a useful intervention for some children. The following is an overview of nursing interventions for the child with specific developmental difficulties:

- Educate parents about the disorder.
- Introduce strategies for increasing communication skills (e.g., initiating conversation, taking turns in conversation, facing the listener).
- Identify and develop specific intervention strategies for problems secondary to learning communication disorders, such as low self-esteem.
- Provide parental support for coping with the disorder.
- Maintain interdisciplinary medical, psychiatric, dental, speech therapy, and educational collaboration.
- Refer to a learning or speech specialist for evaluation and assistance.

■■◖ CONTINUUM OF CARE

Children with learning disabilities obviously require careful psychoeducational and cognitive testing to identify their strengths and deficits. School or clinical psychologists usually perform this type of specialized testing. When a learning disability has been identified, families may need help in advocating for the required services.

The same is true for children with communication disorders, although the services requested may be different. Speech pathologists conduct the diagnostic assessment of speech and language disorders. Services such as speech therapy (directed at the motor aspects of speaking) or social skills groups (directed at the social and interpersonal aspects of language) may be available in some school districts and can be obtained if a speech or language disorder has been identified. For some children with communication disorders, the services offered by the school may be insufficient. In such cases, the nurse can help the family locate resources that can provide these needed services.

Disruptive Behaviour Disorders

The disruptive behaviour disorders, which include ADHD, oppositional defiant disorder, and conduct disorder, are a group of syndromes marked by significant problems of conduct. Because these disorders are characterized by "acting out" behaviours, they are sometimes referred to as **externalizing disorders**. By contrast, disorders of mood (e.g., anxiety, depression) are classified as **internalizing disorders** because the symptoms tend to be within the child.

The disruptive behaviour disorders are more common in boys and are associated with lower socioeconomic status, urban living, learning disabilities, and language delay (Biederman & Faraone, 2005). These disorders are relatively common in school-aged children and are frequently presenting complaints in child psychiatric treatment settings.

■■◖ ATTENTION DEFICIT HYPERACTIVITY DISORDER

All children have occasional experiences with inattention and high energy levels. For most children, these occurrences do not interfere with daily life. Attention deficit hyperactivity disorder is a neuropsychiatric developmental disorder affecting 8% to 12% of children worldwide. It is associated with functional impairments such as school dysfunction, peer problems, and family conflicts. The relatively high frequency of ADHD and associated behaviour problems virtually guarantees that nurses will meet these children in all paediatric treatment settings (Biederman & Faraone, 2005).

Clinical Course and Diagnostic Criteria

Attention deficit hyperactivity disorder is a persistent pattern of inattention, hyperactivity, and impulsiveness that is pervasive and inappropriate for developmental level (APA, 2000).

Parents and teachers describe children with ADHD as restless, always on the go, highly distractible, unable to wait their turn, heedless, and frequently disruptive. Indeed, it is often disruptive behaviour that brings these children into treatment. The historical debate concerning the nature of ADHD is reflected in the labels used to describe it: organic brain syndrome, hyperkinetic impulse disorder, minimal brain dysfunction, hyperkinetic reaction of childhood, hyperkinesis, attention deficit disorder, and most recently, in *DSM-IV-TR*, ADHD. This long list of terms also implies the various theories

regarding the cause and the presumed site of the primary defect. The *DSM-IV-TR* represents yet another formulation by defining ADHD as predominantly hyperactive type, predominantly inattentive type, or combined type (Table 28-2). Despite the historical shifts in terminology and the various proposals regarding the etiology of ADHD, the accumulated consensus during the past several decades is that three core symptoms define the disorder: inattention, impulsiveness, and hyperactivity.

Attention is a complex mental process that involves the ability to concentrate on one activity to the exclusion of others, as well as the ability to sustain focus. Children with ADHD are easily distracted and lack persistence in the performance of age-appropriate tasks, reflecting an inability to filter stimuli, sustain attention, or both. The inability to screen stimuli leaves the child unable to identify salient stimuli. The child may then treat all incoming stimuli with

Table 28.2	**Key Diagnostic Characteristics of Attention Deficit Hyperactivity Disorder** **DSM IV** **314.10:** Attention deficit hyperactivity disorder, combined type **314.00:** Attention deficit hyperactivity disorder, predominantly inattentive type **314.01:** Attention deficit hyperactivity disorder, predominantly hyperactive–impulsive type **314.9:** Attention deficit hyperactivity disorder, not otherwise specified

Diagnostic Criteria and Target Symptoms	Associated Features

• Symptoms of inattention (at least six)
  Lacks close attention to details; makes careless mistakes in activities
  Has difficulty sustaining attention
  Appears to not listen when spoken to directly
  Has difficulty following through on instructions; fails to finish work or activities
  Has difficulty organizing tasks and activities
  Has difficulty with tasks requiring sustained mental effort; commonly avoids, dislikes, or is reluctant to engage in them
  Loses items necessary for tasks
  Is easily distracted by outside stimuli
  Is often forgetful in daily activities
 • Symptoms of hyperactivity–impulsivity (at least six)
  Hyperactivity
  Fidgets or squirms
  Gets up when expectation is to remain seated
  Excessively runs about or climbs inappropriately
  Has difficulty with quiet leisure activities
  Often appears "on the go" or "driven by a motor"
  Talks excessively
  Impulsivity
  Blurts out answers before question completion
  Has difficulty awaiting turn
  Is interruptive or intrusive or others
 • Symptoms are maladaptive and inconsistent with developmental level, persisting for at least 6 months
 • Some symptoms present before the age of 7 years
 • Evidence of significant impairment in social, academic, or occupational functioning
 • Not exclusive during other psychiatric disorder; not better accounted for by another mental disorder
	• Low frustration tolerance
	 • Temper outbursts
	 • Bossiness, stubbornness
	 • Excessive and frequent insistence for requests to be met
	 • Mood lability
	 • Demoralization
	 • Dysphoria
	 • Rejection by peers
	 • Low self-regard
	 • Resentment and antagonism within family
	 • Reduced vocational achievement

equal regard and respond to multiple incoming stimuli. Alternatively, it has been argued that the distractibility seen in ADHD is the result of stimulus-seeking behaviour. Given the heterogeneity of ADHD, either of these models may be true for subgroups of affected children.

Both clinical observations and laboratory studies support the conclusion that children with ADHD are prone to impulsive, risk-taking behaviour (Biederman & Faraone, 2005).

 KEY CONCEPT Attention is a complex process that involves the ability to concentrate on one activity to the exclusion of others and the ability to sustain that focus.

A fundamental question that some have raised is whether impulsiveness is truly separate from distractibility or hyperactivity. Alternatively, some have argued that children with ADHD have an impaired capacity to learn through reinforcement, which predisposes them to impulsive behaviour. In behavioural terms, children with ADHD often fail to consider the consequences of their actions, exercise poor judgment, and tend to have more than the usual lumps, bumps, and bruises because of their risk-taking behaviour. They often require a high degree of structure and supervision.

KEY CONCEPT Impulsiveness is the tendency to act on urges, notions, or desires without adequately considering the consequences.

Although hyperactivity is a characteristic often associated with ADHD, controversy is long-standing about whether attention deficit can occur without overactivity. The decision by *DSM-IV-TR* to define ADHD as predominately hyperactive, predominately inattentive, or combined offers a compromise in the debate regarding attention deficit disorder with or without hyperactivity. Even those who argue in favour of attention deficit disorder without hyperactivity acknowledge that it is probably much less common than attention deficit disorder with hyperactivity.

In many cases, it is the hyperactivity that prompts the search for treatment. Parents typically report that the child's hyperactivity was manifest early in life and evident in most situations. These behaviours, although challenging, were not deemed problematic until the child entered a more structured environment like daycare, kindergarten, or school.

KEY CONCEPT Hyperactivity is an excessive motor activity, as evidenced by restlessness, inability to remain seated, and high levels of physical motion and verbal output.

IN A LIFE

Temple Grandin (1949–)
Scientist and a Person With Autism

Public Persona

Dr. Temple Grandin is a gifted scientist and world-renowned expert on cattle. Her book, *Thinking in Pictures and Other Reports of My Life With Autism* (1996), is an astonishing revelation of the profoundly different way in which a person with autism conceives and experiences the world. Her story shows the extraordinary way in which she uses her visual thinking ability to develop her field of animal science. It gives us a view of her world and helps us understand the reason she identifies with Data, the android in *Star Trek*.

Personal Realities

As a child, Temple experienced life as chaotic, full of engulfing sensations of sound, smell, and touch. She would scream, rock, or spin continually and shut the world out by fixing for hours on one object. At first thought to be deaf when she did not learn to speak, she was taken to a neurologist and labelled "brain-damaged." Although she gained a sense of language and speech, connecting with others was affected by her inability to understand them or them, her. She dreamed of a magic machine that could give her safe "hugging." Her mother's dedication to her and the guidance of a gifted science teacher enabled her to create a life as a scientist.

Epidemiology and Risk Factors

Attention deficit hyperactivity disorder is the most common psychiatric disorder of childhood (Klassen, Miller, & Fine, 2004).

Boys are three times more likely to have ADHD than girls and six to nine times more likely than girls to be seen with ADHD among clinic-referred children. Longitudinal studies that followed up groups of children with ADHD into adulthood have shown that symptoms did persist into adulthood (Biederman & Faraone, 2005). There is clearly an age-dependent decline in symptoms, but even when symptoms are not prominent, they are frequently associated with clinically significant impairments. Older adolescents and young adults with a history of ADHD were more likely to have a history of poor occupational performance, engage in antisocial behaviour, and have more traffic violations and accidents than individuals without the diagnosis of ADHD (Biederman & Faraone).

Etiologic Factors

In the 20th century, ADHD emerged as the first psychiatric disorder to be diagnosed and treated in children, with studies of stimulant treatment since 1937 and regulatory approval of stimulant treatment for children beginning in the 1960s (Doyle, 2004). Attention deficit hyperactivity disorder has emerged from the 20th century with a large amount of scientific work investigating its validity and clarifying clinical controversies. Hypotheses about the cause of ADHD have evolved from simple one-cause theories to the view that it is a complex, multifactoral disorder caused by the coming together of many different types of risk factors (i.e., genetic, biologic, environmental, psychosocial), with every type having a small effect on the increasing vulnerability to the disorder through their additive and interactive effects. According to the multifactoral theory of ADHD, no one causal factor is necessary or sufficient to trigger the disorder, and all these risk factors are interchangeable. What is critical is the total number of risk factors (Biederman & Faraone, 2005).

Biologic Factors

There have been various theories on the neurobiological site of presumed dysfunction in ADHD.

One such theory is that the pattern of neuropsychological deficit in individuals with ADHD is caused by the dysregulation of the frontal-subcortical circuits. That finding has now been confirmed by structural and functional neuroimaging studies showing those individuals to have small volume reductions in these regions (Faraone & Biederman, 2004). Other findings suggest that aberrant frontal-subcortical circuitry is not sufficient to explain the pathophysiology of the disorder. One study has shown widespread but small volume reductions throughout the brain and another has shown widespread cortical abnormalities (Sowell, et al., 2003). A later study has implicated structures such as the cerebellum and the corpus callosum which are outside the frontal-subcortical circuits (Seidman, Valera, & Bush, 2004). Molecular imaging studies suggest that abnormalities of the dopamine transporter lead to impaired neurotransmission (Durston et al., 2003). A study using MRI scans of the putamen in 44 males (25 recruited from a residential treatment centre and having comorbid ADHD and psychopathic traits and 19 healthy community controls) found no differences in the total left or right volume of the putamen. The study did, however, find a reversal of symmetry in the ADHD group compared to the control group. The ADHD children's group generally had a larger right putamen than left, whereas control children's group had a larger left putamen than right (McMahon-Wellington, Semrud-Clikeman, Gregory, Murphy, & Lancaster, 2006).

For many decades, studies have shown that ADHD is transmitted in families (Faraone, 2004). According to twin and adoption studies carried out in Australia, Sweden, the United Kingdom, and the United States, genes have a substantial role in familial transmission. The data from this study also suggest that estimates of heritability have not changed from 1973 to 2004. Adoptive studies also implicate genetic causes. Adoptive relatives of children with ADHD are less likely than biologic relatives to have the disorder or associated syndrome (Biederman & Faraone, 2005).

Molecular genetic studies are beginning to unravel the complex genetics of ADHD. Genome scans of individuals with ADHD have used the method of linkage analysis to screen the genome for regions that might include disease-related susceptibility genes (Bakker et al., 2003). Candidate gene studies of ADHD have produced substantial evidence implicating several genes in the etiology of the disorder (Faraone et al., 2005).

Numerous environmental exposures, including food sensitivity, food additives, and lead poisoning, have been examined as potential causes of ADHD and generally have been found to be false (Biederman & Faraone, 2005). There is increasing evidence, however, that a relative lack of Omega-3 fatty acids may contribute to many psychiatric and neurodevelopmental disorders including ADHD (Richardson, 2006). A positive correlation has been found between obstetrical complications and ADHD and learning disorders. A Quebec study of 64 children aged 6 to 12 diagnosed with ADHD was conducted to assess for a history of obstetrical complications using the Kinney Medical and Gynecological Questionnaire. Children with ADHD and a learning disability in mathematics or reading had a higher rate of neonatal complications than children with ADHD and no disability (Bhat, Grizenko, Ben-Amor, & Joober, 2005). These results further support what has already been shown for ADHD and learning disorders individually: that the events in the early life of a child are critical to brain development.

Psychological and Social Factors

Although genetic endowment clearly plays a fundamental role in the etiology of ADHD, psychosocial factors are also important. Children with ADHD live in families with a host of problems that both affect and are affected by the child. Parents of children with ADHD report more frequent and severe interparental discord and child-rearing disagreements, more negative parenting practices, greater caregiver strain, and more psychopathology themselves. Children with ADHD are generally bossy, intrusive, immature, boisterous, aggressive, and less aware of social cues. Such behaviours can contribute to parental unwillingness to take their ADHD child on social outings or vacations. These children are also often rejected from sports teams and other recreational and social groups (Pelham, Fabiano, & Massetti, 2005).

▪ NURSING MANAGEMENT: HUMAN RESPONSE TO ATTENTION DEFICIT HYPERACTIVITY DISORDER

Biologic Domain

The nursing assessment for the biologic domain may be initiated either before or after the diagnosis of ADHD is made. In the school setting, the teacher may suspect ADHD and consult the school nurse. The nurse in collaboration with the teacher will collect assessment data similar to that collected by the nurse in a psychiatric facility.

Assessment

In the school setting, the primary focus of the assessment is the impact of ADHD on classroom behaviour and school performance. In the hospital, the nurse tries to determine the contribution of ADHD to the acute psychiatric problem. In both cases, the nurse collects assessment data through direct interview, observation of the child and parent, and teacher ratings. Because children with ADHD may have difficulty sitting through long sessions, interviews are typically brief. Parents and teachers are extremely important sources for assessment data. To this end, the nurse can make use of several standardized instruments (Box 28-3).

As with other psychiatric disorders with onset in childhood, the nursing assessment of children with ADHD begins with the identification and exploration of the presenting problem. This typically entails a review of the child's developmental course, the onset and pattern of the current symptoms, factors that have worsened or improved the child's problems, and prior treatment or self-initiated efforts to remedy the situation. The association of ADHD and communication disorders suggests a need for careful consideration of language

BOX 28.3

Standardized Tools for ADHD Diagnosis

The Conners Parent Questionnaire is a 48-item scale that a parent completes about his or her child. Each item is a statement that the parent rates on a four-point scale from 0 (not at all) to 3 (very much). The Conners Teacher Questionnaire is a 28-item questionnaire that the child's teacher completes according to the same four-point scale as the Parent Questionnaire. Both questionnaires have been standardized by age and gender for a mean of 50 and a standard deviation of 10 (Conners, 1989; Goyette, Conners, & Ulrich, 1978).

The ADHD Rating Scale is a recently developed measure that asks parents or teachers to respond directly to 18 items in the *DSM-IV-TR* criteria (see Barkley, 1998, for a description of this scale). A similar scale called the SNAP-IV is available online for free at www.adhd.net. The SNAP-IV was used as the primary outcome measure in the MTA Cooperative Group Study (1999).

The Child Behaviour Checklist (CBCL) is a 118-item questionnaire that a parent completes. In addition to the 118 questions about specific behaviours and psychiatric symptoms, the CBCL also includes questions concerning the child's competence in social and academic spheres as well as age-appropriate activities. Normative data are available allowing the conversion of raw scores to standard scores for age and gender. There is also a teacher version of this scale.

Note that the diagnosis of ADHD is not made on the basis of questionnaires alone. Data from these rating scales augment the information gathered through interview and observation. These questionnaires can be especially useful before and after initiating a treatment plan to measure the change.

development and current language functioning. Medical history is also essential, consisting of perinatal course, childhood illnesses, hospital admissions, injuries, seizures, tics, physical growth, general health status, and timing of the child's last physical examination. Family history is also an important part of assessment data.

Behaviour of these children is characteristically very active and can often be observed in the office. They cannot sit still. They fidget. Even in sleep, they may be more active than normal children. Thus, a careful assessment of eating, sleeping, and activity patterns is essential. Assessing daily food intake, typical diet, and frequency of eating will help identify any nutrition problems. Caffeinated products can contribute to hyperactivity. Sleep is often disturbed for children with ADHD and, consequently, the family. A detailed sleep assessment can provide points for interventions and help the interpretation of drug effects.

Nursing Diagnoses for the Biologic Domain

Depending on the severity of the responses, family situation, and school environment, several nursing diagnoses could be generated from the assessment data, including self-care deficit, risk for imbalanced nutrition, risk for injury, and disturbed sleep pattern. The outcomes should be individualized to the child.

Interventions for the Biologic Domain

The planning of nursing interventions must be done within the context of the family, treatment setting, and school environment. With the parents, clinical team members, and school personnel, the nurse participates in designing a plan of care that fits the child's and family's needs. Medication can help the hyperactivity, impulsiveness, and inattention; therefore, teaching the parent, child, and school personnel about the importance of the medication in ADHD and the potential side effects is a place to begin. Explaining to the child that the medication improves concentration and the ability to sit still can help strengthen the client's motivation and compliance.

For 40 years, the main treatment for ADHD has been the stimulant drugs methylphenidate, D-amphetamine, and L-amphetamine (Table 28-3). Although each of these medications has demonstrated efficacy in controlled studies, methylphenidate has received considerably more research effort and has emerged as the first-line effective therapy to treat ADHD (Flapper & Schoemaker, 2008). The stimulant pemoline is less frequently used because of concerns about liver toxicity. It should be noted that stimulants are not effective in all cases; thus, alternatives to the stimulants, such as trycyclic antidepressants, have been prescribed for children

Table 28.3	Stimulant Medications Used in Treating ADHD	
Medication	**Total Daily Dosage***	**Common Side Effects**
Methylphenidate	10–60 mg in two or three divided doses	Loss of appetite, insomnia, rebound activation, increase in tics or compulsive behaviour, psychotic reaction
Metadate CD	Once daily capsule children 6 and over. 18 mg daily	
Concerta	Maximum dose 54 mg daily Once daily capsule 18 mg daily Maximum 72 mg daily Dosage not to exceed 2 mg/kg daily	
D-Amphetamine	5–40 mg in two divided doses	Similar to methylphenidate
D, L-Amphetamine	5–40 mg in two divided doses	Similar to methylphenidate

*Dosage ranges are similar for long-acting products Concerta, Metadate, and Adderall.

BOX 28.4

Drug Profile: Methylphenidate (Ritalin)

DRUG CLASS: CNS stimulant

RECEPTOR AFFINITY: The mechanisms of effect are not completely clear. At low doses, it provides mild cortical stimulation similar to that of amphetamines. This stimulation results from methylphenidate's ability to promote release and interfere with the reuptake of dopamine in the synaptic cleft. Main sites appear to be the cerebral cortex, striatum, and pons.

INDICATIONS: Treatment of narcolepsy, attention deficit disorders, and hyperkinetic syndrome; unlabelled uses for the treatment of depression in older adults and persons with cancer or stroke.

ROUTES AND DOSAGE: Available in 5- to 10-mg immediate-release tablets and 20-mg sustained-release tablets (Ritalin-SR). Newer long-acting preparations such as Concerta and Metadate, in various dose strengths, are also available.

Adult Dosage: Must be individualized; range from 10 to 60 mg/day orally in divided doses bid to tid, preferably 15–30 minutes before meals. If insomnia is a problem, drug should be administered before 6 PM.

Child Dosage: The immediate-release formulation can be started at 5 mg twice or three times daily on a 4-hour schedule with weekly increases depending on response. Starting doses of the long-acting preparations are equivalent to the total tid dose (e.g., 5 tid of short-acting preparations would translate into 18 mg of Concerta). Usually given on a tid schedule, with the last dose being roughly half that of the first and second dose. Daily dosage of >60 mg not recommended. Discontinue after 1 month if no improvement.

PEAK EFFECT: 1 hour; *half-life:* 3–4 hours for the immediate-release preparations.

SELECT ADVERSE REACTIONS: Nervousness, insomnia, dizziness, headache, dyskinesias (including tics), toxic psychosis, anorexia, nausea, abdominal pain, increased pulse and blood pressure, palpitations, tolerance, and psychological dependence.

WARNING: The drug is discontinued periodically to assess the client's condition. Contraindications include marked anxiety, tension and agitation, glaucoma, severe depression, and obsessive-compulsive symptoms. Use cautiously in clients with a personal or family history of tic disorders, seizure disorders, hypertension, drug dependence, alcoholism, or emotional instability.

SPECIFIC CLIENT/FAMILY EDUCATION

- Do not chew or crush sustained-release tablets—they must be swallowed whole.
- Take the drug exactly as prescribed; if insomnia is a problem, time and dose may need adjustment. The drug is rarely taken after 5 pm.
- Avoid alcohol and OTC products, including decongestants, cold remedies, and cough syrups—these could accentuate side effects of the stimulant.
- Keep appointments for follow-up, including evaluations for monitoring the child's growth and the use of parent and teacher ratings to monitor benefit.
- Note that the prescriber may discontinue the drug periodically to confirm the effectiveness of the therapy.

---

who do not respond to the stimulants or who develop tics when taking them. However, for many years, reduced efficacy and anticholinergic side effects have restricted their use (Biederman & Faraone, 2005).

Two clinically important developments in the treatment of ADHD have been the use of long-acting formulations and the nonstimulant drug amoxetine.

Immediate-release stimulants like methylphenidate are short-acting medications that peak in about 90 minutes to 2 hours and have a total duration of action of about 4 hours (Box 28-4). Thus, parents or teachers often describe a return of overactivity and distractibility as the first dose of medication wears off, and multiple doses are required to maintain effectiveness through the day.

The change in behaviour and the need for additional doses of medication created embarrassment and stigma for school-aged children, who typically had to go to the nurse or principal's office for the medication. The long-acting stimulants have shown effectiveness and side effects similar to those seen with short-acting stimulants (Biederman & Faraone, 2005). In addition, they may be seen as contributing to improving the quality of school life for children with ADHD by eliminating the need for additional doses during the day.

Psychological Domain

Assessment

Hyperactivity, impulsivity, and inattention are typically pervasive problems that are evident both at school and at home. Discipline is frequently an issue because parents may have difficulty controlling their child's behaviour, which is disruptive and occasionally destructive.

Nursing Diagnoses for the Psychological Domain

Assessment of the psychological domain may generate several diagnoses, including anxiety and defensive coping. The outcomes should be individualized to the child.

Interventions for the Psychological Domain

As a complement to medication, behavioural programs based on rewards for positive behaviour, such as waiting turns and following directions, can foster new social skills. Interventions may also include specific cognitive behavioural techniques in which the child learns to "stop, look, and listen" before doing. A combined behavioural-psychosocial and medication approach allows for significantly lower doses of medication than a medication-only approach in achieving treatment outcomes and decreasing the risk of side effects (Chronis, Jones, & Raggi, 2006).

Social Domain

Assessment

Dysfunctional interactions can develop within the family. Reviewing the problematic behaviours and the situations in which they occur is a way to identify negative interaction patterns. These children are often behind in their work at school because of poor organization, off-task behaviour, and impulsive responses. They can exhaust their parents, aggravate teachers, and annoy siblings with their intrusive and disruptive behaviours. Because ADHD often occurs in the context of psychosocial adversity, it is important to review the family situation, including parenting style, stability of household membership, consistency of rules and routines, and life events, such as divorce, moves, deaths, and job loss. Identification of these factors can be useful in shaping a care plan that builds on potential strengths and mitigates the effects of environmental factors that may perpetuate the child's disruptive behaviour. Data regarding school performance, behaviour at home, and comorbid psychiatric disorders are essential for developing school interventions and behaviour plans and establishing the baseline severity for medication.

Nursing Diagnoses for the Social Domain

Depending on the severity of the child's responses, family situation, and school environment, several nursing diagnoses could be generated from the assessment data, including impaired social interaction, ineffective role performance, and compromised family coping. Short-term outcomes, such as decreasing the number of classroom ejections within a 2-week period, may be useful for one child, whereas reducing the frequency and amplitude of angry outbursts at home may be relevant to another child.

Interventions for the Social Domain

Family treatment is nearly always a component of cognitive behavioural treatment approaches with the child. This may involve parent training that focuses on the principles of behaviour management, such as appropriate limit setting and the use of reward systems, as well as revising expectations about the child's behaviour. School programming often involves increasing structure in the child's school day to offset the child's tendency to act without forethought and to be easily distracted by extraneous stimuli. Specific remediation is required for the child with comorbid deficits in learning or language. Some children may require small, self-contained classrooms.

Spiritual Domain

There needs to be concerted effort on the part of nurses and other health care professionals to address the spiritual domain of children with ADHD. Their environment must be, in addition to being calm and predictable, one in which they have the opportunity to express their questions, fears, and hopes about life, death, and the sacred. The expression of their spiritual needs should not be dismissed, but encouraged appropriately and understood in terms of stage of development and life experience. There needs to be openness to families' spiritual needs as well. ADHD symptoms in a child can overwhelm a family and disconnect them from sources of spiritual support when such symptoms are not tolerated by others.

EVALUATION AND TREATMENT OUTCOMES

As with most mental health disorders in children, the aim of treatment for ADHD is to decrease symptoms, enhance functionality, and improve well-being for the child and his or her close contacts (Fig. 28-2). Children may not notice any effects after taking medications, but people in their environment do. Often, within 1 to 2 weeks of initiating therapy, children with ADHD become more attentive, less impulsive, and less active. However, measurement of treatment response is often limited to measuring a reduction in symptoms using behavioural rating scales completed by parents and teachers. Because so much focus has been on measuring symptom reduction, little research has been done to study the effects of ADHD on other aspects of the child's health. The current development of an increasing number of multidimensional health-related quality of life questionnaires now affords the opportunity to measure the health of children with ADHD more comprehensively (Klassen, Miller, & Fine, 2004).

CONTINUUM OF CARE

Treatment of ADHD typically is conducted in community clinic settings. Optimal treatment is multimodal (includes several types of interventions), encompassing four main areas: individual treatment for the child, family treatment, school accommodations, and medication. Well-managed medication is the most important intervention for the core symptoms of ADHD (Biederman & Faraone, 2005). Parent training and social skills training also help

FIGURE 28.2 Long-term outcomes of optimal treatment for clients with attention deficit hyperactivity disorder.

diminish disruptive and defiant behaviours (see Nursing Care Plan 28-1). Treatment plans need regular upgrading to address important social, cognitive, psychological, and physical changes that occur as the child ages (Child's Health Policy Centre, Simon Fraser University, 2007).

OPPOSITIONAL DEFIANT DISORDER AND CONDUCT DISORDER

Oppositional defiant disorder is characterized by a persistent pattern of disobedience, argumentativeness, angry outbursts, low tolerance for frustration, and a tendency to blame others for misfortunes, large and small. Conduct disorder is characterized by serious violations of social norms, including aggressive behaviour, destruction of property, and cruelty to animals. Children with oppositional defiant

---

Nursing Care Plan 28.1

Attention Deficit Hyperactivity Disorder

Jamie, age 6 years, comes to the mental health clinic with his mother Lillian because of motor restlessness, distractibility, and disruptive behaviour in the classroom. According to Lillian, Jamie had a reasonably good year in kindergarten, but early in the first grade, the teacher began to report disruptive behaviour. On reflection, Lillian recalls that kindergarten was a half-day program with more activity. By contrast, Jamie is expected to sit in his seat and pay attention for longer periods in first grade.

Jamie's medical history is unremarkable. Lillian's pregnancy with Jamie was her first and unplanned. Although there were no complications during the pregnancy, the period was marked by significant marital discord, culminating in divorce before Jamie's first birthday. Jamie was born by cesarean section after a long, unproductive labour. He was healthy at birth and grew normally, with no developmental

delays. Despite genuine interest in other children, his intrusive style and inability to wait his turn resulted in frequent conflicts with them. The family history is positive for substance abuse in his father. In addition, Lillian reports that her ex-husband was disruptive in school, had trouble concentrating, and was highly impulsive. These problems have continued into adulthood.

During the two evaluation sessions, Jamie is active but cooperative. His speech is fluent and normal in tone and tempo, but somewhat loud. His discourse is coherent, but at times, he makes rather abrupt changes in conversation without warning his listeners. Psychological testing done at the school revealed average to above-average intelligence. Parent and teacher questionnaires concurred that Jamie was overactive, impulsive, inattentive, and quarrelsome, but not defiant.

Continued

Nursing Care Plan 28.1 (Continued)

Setting: Mental Health Centre—Child and Adolescent Services

Baseline Assessment: Jamie is a 6-year-old boy with prominent hyperactivity and disruptive behaviour. He lives with Lillian, his single mother. These problems interfere with his interpersonal relationships and academic progress. Lillian is discouraged and feels unable to manage Jamie's behaviour.

Associated Psychiatric Diagnosis	Medications

Axis I: Attention deficit hyperactivity disorder
Axis II: None
Axis III: None
Axis IV: Problems with primary support (mother is exhausted)
    Educational problems (failing in school)
    Economic problems (mother in entry-level job with no health insurance)
Axis V: GAF = 52
	Methylphenidate 5 mg at breakfast and lunch (i.e., at 8 AM and 12 noon), then adding 5 mg at 4 PM. The likely dose would be 7.5 mg at 8 am and 12 noon and 5 mg at 7 PM.

Nursing Diagnosis 1: Impaired Social Interaction

Defining Characteristics	Related Factors
Cannot establish and maintain developmentally Appropriate social relationships Has interpersonal difficulties at school Is not well accepted by peers Is easily distracted Interrupts others Cannot wait his turn in games Speaks out of turn in the classroom	Impulsive behaviour Overactive Inattentive Risk-taking behaviour (tried to climb out the window to get away from Lillian) Failure to recognize the effects of his behaviour on others

Outcomes

Initial	Discharge
1. Decrease hyperactivity and disruptive behaviour. 2. Improve attention and decrease distractibility. 3. Decrease the frequency of acting without forethought.	4. Improve capacity to identify alternative responses in conflicts with peers. 5. Improve capacity to interpret behaviour of age-mates.

Interventions

Interventions	Rationale	Ongoing Assessment
Educate the mother and teach her about ADHD and the use of stimulant medication.	Better understanding helps to ensure adherence; also parents and teachers often miscast children with ADHD as "troublemakers."	Determine the extent to which the parent or teacher "blames" Jamie for his problems.
Monitor adherence to medication schedule.	Uneven compliance may contribute to a failed trial of medication.	Administer parent and teacher questionnaires; inquire about behaviour across entire day.
Ensure that the medication is both effective and well tolerated.	Stimulants can affect appetite and sleep and can cause "behavioural rebound" (Biederman & Faraone, 2005).	Administer parent and teacher questionnaires; check height and weight; ask about sleep and appetite.

Evaluation

Outcomes	Revised Outcomes	Interventions
Jamie shows decreased hyperactivity and less disruption in the classroom. Jamie shows improved attention and decreased distractibility.	Improve the ability to identify disruptive classroom behaviour. Improve school performance.	Initiate a point system to reward appropriate behaviour. Move to the front of the classroom as an aid to attention.

Continued

Nursing Care Plan 28.1 (Continued)

Evaluation

Outcomes	Revised Outcomes	Interventions
Mother and teacher attest to Jamie's decreased impulsive behaviour. Jamie identifies alternative responses such as walking away until it is his turn. Jamie improves interpretation of motives and behaviours of others.	Increase Jamie's capacity to recognize the effects of his behaviour on others. Increase the frequency of acting on these alternative approaches. Improve acceptance by peers.	Encourage participation in structured activities. Inquire about social skills group at school, if available. Encourage participation in community activities.

Nursing Diagnosis 2: Ineffective Coping (Lillian)

Defining Characteristics	Related Factors
Verbalizes discouragement and inability to handle the situation with Jamie	Chronicity of ADHD More than average child-rearing problems

Outcomes

Initial	Discharge
1. Verbalize frustration at trying to raise a child with ADHD alone. 2. Identify positive methods of interacting with and disciplining Jamie that will support the parent–child relationship as well as meet Jamie's developmental needs.	3. Identify coping patterns that decrease the sense of frustration and increase parental competence. 4. Initiate a collaborative relationship with the teacher. 5. Identify sources of support in the community and begin to access these resources.

Interventions

Interventions	Rationale	Ongoing Assessment
Assess the mother's discouragement and feelings about parenting, identifying specific problem areas.	Helping the mother verbalize her feelings and identify problem areas helps in formulating problem-solving strategies.	Assess the severity of the problems with which she is living.
Refer the mother to a community health centre for free parenting class.	Parent training based on clear directives and rewards can be effective for decreasing impulsive and disruptive behaviours.	Monitor the mother's level of confidence and perceived change in Jamie's behaviour.
Refer the mother to a self-help organization.	Parent groups such as Children and Adults with Attention Deficit Disorder (CHAAD) can be sources of support and information.	Determine whether contact was made and whether it was helpful.
Make contact with school to enhance collaboration with the mother.	Assess the effectiveness of medication and other interventions, need feedback from teachers.	Determine whether the mother has been able to contact the teacher.

Evaluation

Outcomes	Revised Outcomes	Interventions
After four sessions, Lillian expresses her frustrations, but she has begun to identify different ways of relating to Jamie and his developmental needs. Through attending the parenting class and joining a support group, Lillian begins to change her coping patterns, decrease her frustrations, and increase parental competence. Lillian initiates a collaborative relationship with Jamie's teacher.	None

Complete the parenting class; attend at least two support group meetings each month.

Lillian and Jamie's teacher mutually develop and implement behaviour plans for home and school. | None

If necessary, refer for additional parent counselling.

Have the mother observe in the classroom; have the mother visit highly structured classroom. |

Clinical Vignette: Leon (Conduct Disorder)

Leon, a 14-year-old boy, was admitted to the child psychiatric inpatient service from the emergency department after a fight with his mother. His mother reported that she and Leon had argued earlier in the evening and that he stormed out of the house screaming and vowing that he would never return. Several hours later, Leon came back, yelling and demanding entry into the apartment. Leon's father was working. While his mother was getting up to open the door, Leon continued to yell and scream, waking the neighbours. This led to further arguing between Leon and his mother. Before long, the police were called, and Leon was taken to the emergency department.

The admission interview revealed that Leon had run away on several occasions and had even stayed away overnight. Although he strongly denied drug use, he had gotten drunk on several occasions. He had also been in several fights, the latest of which resulted in an expulsion from school. Three months before admission, he was caught trying to steal a CD from a music store. More recently, he boasted that he and his

friends had snatched a purse at an outdoor concert and had broken into a car to steal its contents. Leon's school performance has been declining; he was truant on several occasions and will probably have to repeat ninth grade.

Leon was born in Cape Breton, N.S., and is the oldest of three children. His family moved to Toronto shortly after his birth. His father is employed as a janitor and is illiterate. His mother works as a secretary and has recently completed a BA in English. There is much marital discord at home. Leon has received no treatment except for consultation with the school social worker.

WHAT DO YOU THINK?

- When conducting a nursing assessment, what would you want to learn about Leon's school performance?
- What information could you provide Leon's parents about pharmacotherapy? About behaviour management?
- How would you present the material so it meets the learning needs of both parents?

disorder have trouble making friends and often find themselves in conflict with adults. This disorder is distinguishable from conduct disorder, which is characterized by more serious violations of social norms. Youngsters with conduct disorder often lie to achieve short-term ends, may be truant from school, may run away from home, and may engage in petty larceny or even mugging (Box 28-5).

The prevalence of conduct disorder is greater in boys and ranges from 6% to 16%, compared with a range of 2% to 9% in girls. Conduct disorder is one of the most frequently diagnosed disorders in children in mental health facilities. Individuals with conduct disorder are at greater risk for experiencing mood or anxiety disorders and substance-related disorders (APA, 2000). Other common comorbid conditions that may precede conduct disorder include specific developmental delays, such as learning disabilities and language delay, ADHD, oppositional defiant disorder, and depressive and anxiety disorders (Maughan, Rowe, Messer, Goodman, & Meltzer, 2004).

Children with ADHD, a learning disability, or a language deficit may frequently encounter failure and acquire a bitter and hostile attitude. Appropriate treatment focussed on the ADHD or the specific developmental delay may foster more positive interactions and promote success at school. Success in these areas may lead to more positive behaviour in some cases.

The etiology of oppositional defiant disorder and conduct disorder is complex. More attention has been paid to conduct disorder, probably because it is the more serious of the two. Models used to understand antisocial personality disorder (see Chapter 25) and aggressiveness (see Chapter 36) are useful in examining these childhood disorders, which appear to have both genetic

and environmental components. For example, the risk for conduct disorder is increased in the offspring of individuals with conduct disorder. However, harsh parenting, family disruption, parental psychopathology, poverty, single parenthood, and being physically harmed also increase the risk for conduct disorder in biologic or adopted children (Kim-Cohen, et al., 2005).

■ NURSING MANAGEMENT: HUMAN RESPONSE TO OPPOSITIONAL DEFIANT DISORDER

Biologic Domain

Assessment

The nurse gathers data from multiple sources and domains, including biologic, psychological (e.g., mood, behavioural, cognitions), and social domains. These adolescents are at high risk for physical injury as a result of fighting and impulsive behaviour. Sexual promiscuity is common, resulting in an increased frequency of pregnancy and sexually transmitted diseases.

Another important aspect of assessment of adolescents presenting with defiance or aggressive behaviour is to rule out comorbid conditions that may partially explain or complicate their lack of behavioural control. These conditions include ADHD, learning disabilities, chemical dependency, depression, bipolar illness, or generalized anxiety. Young people who are chronically depressed may be irritable and easily frustrated. Given the tendency of adolescents to act out their frustration, chronic depression may exacerbate their behaviour.

Conduct problems can also elevate the risk for depression, because young people who regularly elicit negative attention from parents and teachers and are constantly at odds with their environment may become despondent.

Nursing Diagnoses for the Biologic Domain

Typical nursing diagnoses in the biologic domain are risk for other-directed violence, risk for self-directed violence, and impaired verbal communication. Although the outcomes are individualized for each client, some outcomes for these clients are as follows:

- Maintenance of physical safety in the milieu (or other treatment setting)
- Decreased frequency of verbal and physical aggressive episodes

Interventions for the Biologic Domain

Children with oppositional defiant disorder or conduct disorder who also have specific developmental disorders should be referred to appropriate programs for remediation. If a diagnosis of ADHD or depression emerges from the evaluation, appropriate pharmacotherapy should be considered (see previous discussion of ADHD and after the discussion regarding depression).

Limited evidence is available on the efficacy of medications in treating conduct disorder. In the past, several medications have been used to treat extremely aggressive behaviour, including typical antipsychotics, such as haloperidol and thioridazine; the anticonvulsant carbamazepine; the α-blocking agent propranolol; the antimanic medication lithium carbonate; the stimulant methylphenidate; and tricyclic antidepressants. More recently, several placebo-controlled studies have shown that low doses of two atypical antipsychotic medications, risperidone and olanzapine, have been found effective for the treatment of aggression in children with conduct disorder. Olanzapine has also been found effective in treating children with severe, treatment-resistant conduct disorder (Masi et al. 2006). Weight gain is a side effect of both these medications, which may affect willingness to comply with therapy in children and adolescents. Medication should always be a part of a multipronged approach to therapy for children and adolescents with conduct disorders. Other approaches include individual, group, and family therapies, as well as family education programs (Masi et al.).

Psychological Domain

Assessment

Adolescents with conduct problems are usually brought or coerced into the mental health system by family, school, or the court system because of fighting, truancy, speeding tickets, car accidents, petty crimes, substance abuse, or suicide attempts. These young people may be hostile, sarcastic, defensive, and provocative. At the same time, they may appear calm, outgoing, and engaging. Inconsistencies, distortions, and misrepresentations of the truth are common when interviewing these children, so obtaining a clear history may be difficult. Therefore, instead of asking if an event or behaviour occurred, it may be better to ask when it occurred and the circumstances surrounding the event. A structured interview such as the revised Child Psychopathy Scale focuses on affective and interpersonal traits and contains a proneness-to-boredom scale (Lynam & Gudonis, 2005). These adolescents have difficulty with trust and are adept at changing the subject and diverting discussion from sensitive issues. They often use denial, projection, and externalization of anger as defence mechanisms when asked for self-disclosure. The assessment, which may take several sessions, should be conducted in an open and nonjudgmental manner.

Nursing Diagnoses for the Psychological Domain

In the psychological domain, a typical nursing diagnosis is ineffective coping. Outcomes are individualized for each client but can include the following:

- Increased personal responsibility for behaviour
- Increased use of problem-solving skills as evidenced by decreased interpersonal conflicts
- Decreased rule violations and conflicts with authority figures
- Improved peer relationships
- Realistic assessment of own strengths and limitations

Interventions for the Psychological Domain

In planning interventions for clients with oppositional defiant disorder or conduct disorder, the focus is on problem behaviours. There has been some empirical support for child-focused cognitive-behavioural approaches also targeting anger, control, and coping (Beauchaine, Webster-Stratton, & Reid, 2005). Therapeutic progress may be slow, at least partly because these clients often lack trust in authority figures.

Social Skills Training

The nurse should communicate behavioural xpectations clearly and enforce them consistently. Consequences of appropriate and inappropriate actions also should be clear. Specific approaches for improving social and problem-solving skills are fundamental features for school-aged children and adolescents. Insofar as children and adolescents with conduct problems fail to recognize the adverse effects of their verbal and nonverbal behaviours, their deficit can be formulated as an interpersonal problem. Social skills training teaches adolescents with these behaviour disorders to recognize the ways in which their actions affect others. Training involves techniques such as role playing, modelling by the therapist, and giving positive reinforcement to improve interpersonal relationships and enhance social outcomes.

Problem-Solving Therapy

In contrast to social skills training, which proposes that problems of conduct are the result of poor interpersonal skills, problem-solving therapy conceptualizes conduct problems as the result of deficiencies in cognitive processes. These processes include assessment of situations, interpretation of events, and expectations of others that are congruent with behaviour. These children often misinterpret the intentions of others and may perceive hostility with little or no cause (Webster-Stratton, Reid, & Hammond, 2004). Problem-solving skills training teaches these children to generate alternative solutions to social situations, to sharpen thinking concerning the consequences of those choices, and to evaluate responses after interpersonal conflicts.

Social Domain

Assessment

Adolescents with conduct disorder display behaviours that violate social norms and the basic rights of others. Some of the behaviours evident in conduct disorder consist of aggression toward people and animals, bullying, threatening behaviours, and sexual aggression (Redston-Iselin, 2005). High levels of marital conflict, family violence, parental substance abuse, and parental antisocial behaviour often mark the family history.

Nursing Diagnoses for the Social Domain

In the social domain, nursing diagnoses include compromised family coping and impaired social interaction. Some outcomes for these clients are as follows:

- Increased use of problem-solving skills as evidenced by decreased interpersonal conflicts
- Decreased rule violations and conflicts with authority figures
- Demonstrating socially acceptable behaviour in the community
- Increased attendance and active participation in school.

Interventions for the Social Domain

Parent education for preschool- and school-aged children with disruptive behaviour problems appears to be the most effective psychosocial intervention (Beauchaine et al., 2005). Also proven effective have been teacher-focused educational approaches aimed at improving classroom management of problem behaviours (Webster-Stratton et al., 2004).

Management Training

Parent training begins with educating parents about disruptive behaviour disorders, focusing particularly on impulsiveness, impaired judgment, and self-control. Children with long-standing problems in these areas often elicit punitive responses and negative attributions about their behaviour from their parents. Ironically, because these parental responses focus on the child's failure, they may contribute to the child's behaviour problems. An important second step is to clarify parental expectations and interpretation of the child's behaviour. Parent management training may be offered to a group of parents or to individuals (Kazdin & Weisz, 2003).

Educating Parents

The aims of education are to provide parents with new ways of understanding their child's behaviour and to promote improved interactions between parents and the child. The most commonly presented techniques include the importance of positive reinforcement (praise and tangible rewards) for adaptive behaviour, clear limits for unacceptable behaviour, and the use of mild punishment, such as time out (Box 28-6). Improving parental competence, strengthening social skills in children, and creating a positive classroom environment are strategies that have proved effective in preventing and reducing conduct disorder (Webster-Stratton et al., 2004).

Spiritual Domain

As spirituality is essentially relational and about the way one lives one's life, children with oppositional defiant disorder or conduct disorder may have particular difficulty understanding and expressing their spiritual needs. They may not be able to sustain relationships that offer spiritual support; they may reject what any institutionalized religion has to offer. At the same time, such children can be experiencing existential angst, involving fear of death, a deep sense of isolation, hopelessness about the future, and a belief that life has no meaning. Their families tend to be under duress and unable to offer the spiritual guidance a child needs. Nurses need to look beyond the defiant social behaviours of these children and be responsive whenever a chance to explore and address their spiritual distress arises.

■ EVALUATION AND TREATMENT OUTCOMES

The nurse can review treatment goals and objectives to assess the child's progress with respect to verbal and physical aggression, socially appropriate resolution of

BOX 28.6

Time Out

TIME-OUT PROCEDURE

- *Labelling behaviour:* Identify the behaviour that the child is expected to perform or cease. The aim of this statement is to make clear what is required of the child. It typically takes the form of a simple declarative sentence: "Threatening is not acceptable."
- *Warning:* In this step, the child is informed that if he or she does not perform the expected behaviour or stop the unacceptable behaviour, he or she will be given a "time out." "This is a warning: if you continue threatening to hit people, you'll have a time out."
- *Time out:* If the child does not heed the warning, he or she is told to take a time out in simple straightforward terms: "Take a time out."
- *Duration:* The usual duration for a time out is 5 minutes for children 5 years of age or older.
- *Location:* The child sits in a designated time-out chair without toys and without talking. The chair should be located away from general activity but within view. A kitchen timer can be used to mark the time, but the clock does not start until the child is sitting quietly in the designated spot.
- *Follow-up:* The child is asked to recount why he or she was given the time out. The explanation need not be detailed, and no further discussion of the matter is required. Indeed, long discourse about the child's behaviour is not helpful and should be avoided.

conflicts, compliance with rules and expectations, and better management of frustration. As is true for the initial assessment, evaluation of treatment outcomes relies on input from parents, teachers, and other team members.

CONTINUUM OF CARE

Children and adolescents with disorders of conduct may be involved in many different agencies in the community, such as child and family services, school authorities, and the legal system. Mental health services are requested when a child or adolescent's behaviour is out of control or a comorbid disorder is suspected. Helping the youngster and the family negotiate their way through this maze of services may be an essential part of the treatment plan.

Disorders of Mood and Anxiety

ANXIETY DISORDERS

Anxiety disorders are the most prevalent mental illness in Canadian children between 4 and 17 years of age.

Approximately 6 in 100 children have severe problems with worries and fears warranting a clinical diagnosis (Children's Health Policy Centre, SFU, 2007; Waddell, Godderis, Hua, McEwan, & Wong, 2004). Many childhood fears are developmentally normal: it is common for toddlers to fear the dark, for school-aged children to fear animals, and for teenagers to worry about relationship with peers. These typical anxiety experiences do not usually interfere with the child's development and functioning (Children's Health Policy Centre, SFU). Children with anxiety disorders, however, experience excessive, prolonged, or recurrent fears or symptoms of anxiety, with accompanying impairment in age-appropriate functioning at home, at school, and with peers (Manassis, 2004). To screen quickly for one or more anxiety disorders in children, the following questions may be useful: (1) Does the child worry or ask for parental reassurance everyday? (2) Does the child consistently avoid age-appropriate situations or activities or avoid doing them without a parent? (3) Does the child have frequent episodes of stomach aches, headaches, or hyperventilation? (4) Does the child have daily repetitive rituals? These four questions address the main thoughts, behaviours, and feelings related to anxiety seen in children (Manassis). This section focuses on separation anxiety, a disorder diagnosed in childhood, and obsessive-compulsive disorder (OCD), a disorder that occurs in both adults and children (see Chapter 21).

SEPARATION ANXIETY DISORDER

Some have suggested that separation anxiety disorder is the childhood equivalent of panic disorder in adults. Although many children experience some discomfort on separation from their mothers or major attachment figures, children with separation anxiety disorder suffer great distress when faced with ordinary separations, such as going to school. In most cases, the mother is the focus of the child's concern, but this may not be so, especially if the mother is not the primary caregiver. The child may exhibit extraordinary reluctance or even refusal to separate from the primary caregiver. When asked, most children with separation anxiety disorder will express worry about harm or permanent loss of their major attachment figure. Other children may express worry about their own safety (Table 28-4).

A common manifestation of anxiety is **school phobia**, in which the child refuses to attend school, preferring to stay at home with the primary attachment figure. However, it should be noted that school phobia is a common presenting complaint in child psychiatric clinics and may be part of separation anxiety disorder, general anxiety disorder, social phobia, OCD, depression, or conduct disorder. In rare cases, school phobia can be a side effect of antipsychotic medication (Scahill, Leckman, Schultz, Katsovich, & Peterson, 2003). The term "school phobia"

Table 28.4 ⬙ Key Diagnostic Characteristics of Separation Anxiety Disorder 309.21		DSM IV
Diagnostic Criteria and Target Symptoms	**Associated Findings**	

• Inappropriate and excessive anxiety about being away from home or the primary attachment figure
  Excessive distress when separation occurs or is anticipated
  Persistent, excessive worry about losing or having harm come to attachment figures
  Persistent and excessive worry about an event that might cause separation from attachment figure
  Persistent reluctance or refusal to go to school or somewhere else because of separation anxiety
  Reluctance to be alone without attachment figures at home or without significant adults in other settings
  Persistent reluctance or refusal to go to sleep without being near the attachment figure or sleep away from home
  Repeated nightmares about being separated
  Repeated complaints of physical symptoms when separated or when separation from attachment figures is anticipated
• Duration of at least 4 weeks
• Onset before the age of 18 years (for early onset type, onset before the age of 6 years)
• Not exclusively occurring during the course of other psychotic disorders; not better accounted for by panic disorder with agoraphobia
	• Social withdrawal, apathy
	• Difficulty concentrating
	• Fears of other situations, such as animals, monsters, accidents, and plane travel
	• Concerns about death and dying
	• School refusal and subsequent academic difficulties
	• Anger or lashing out with the prospect of separation
	• Unusual perceptual experiences when alone
	• Demanding and needing constant attention and reassurance
	• Somatic complaints
	• Depressed mood
	• Other recurring worries that do not involve attachment figures	

was coined to distinguish it from truancy—whether it is a phobia in the usual sense is a matter of some debate. When another disorder such as depression is identified, it becomes the focus of treatment. In some cases, the school phobia may resolve when the primary disorder is successfully treated.

Separation anxiety disorder is excessive anxiety on separation from home or major attachment figure before the age of 18 years. It is manifested by acute distress, frequent nightmares about separation, and reluctance or refusal to separate. It lasts for at least 1 month and causes clinically significant impairment in social or academic functioning.

Epidemiology and Etiology

The prevalence of separation anxiety disorder is estimated at 4% of school-aged children; thus, it is relatively common. Anxiety disorders run in families, and it appears that both environmental and genetic factors affect the risk for separation anxiety disorder. For example, it may emerge after a move, change to a new school, or death of a family member or pet. By contrast, recent evidence suggests that traits such as shyness and behavioural inhibition (reluctance in new situations) are inherited (Rapee & Spence, 2004). Furthermore, not only are children with an enduring "inhibited" temperament at greater risk for anxiety disorders themselves, but their immediate family members are also at greater risk for anxiety disorders compared

with a psychiatric control group. Others have argued in favour of environmental determinants of separation anxiety, contending that anxious parents communicate to the child that the world is inhospitable and menacing to keep the child near. Available data suggest that the long-term outcome of childhood disorders is favourable in many cases but may evolve and take other forms in adulthood. For example, separation anxiety in childhood may re-emerge as panic disorder in adults (Koda, Charney, & Pine, 2003).

Psychopharmacologic Interventions

Selective serotonin reuptake inhibitors (SSRIs) are currently considered first-line medications for treating children with anxiety disorders. All SSRIs have been used for children, and no clear evidence suggests that one is superior to another. Recent findings suggesting increased suicidal ideations in children taking paroxetine have resulted in a Health Canada warning to avoid this medication in children. All SSRIs can result in nausea or changes in sleep patterns early in treatment, but these usually resolve within a week. In the past, tricyclic antidepressants were used for treating anxiety disorders in children but are currently considered second-line medications due to the risk of cardiac conduction disturbances (Manassis, 2004). If tricyclic antidepressants are used, baseline and follow-up electrocardiograms are recommended (King, Scahill, Lombroso, & Leckman, 2003).

Nursing Management

School phobia is often what prompts the family to seek consultation for the child. The onset of school refusal may be gradual or acute. Because school phobia can be a behavioural manifestation of several different child psychiatric disorders, it requires careful assessment. Issues to consider are whether the parents have been aware that the child is avoiding school (separation versus truancy); what efforts the family has made to return the child to school; the presence of significant subjective distress in the child with anticipation of going to school; and whether the school refusal occurs in the context of other behavioural, social, or emotional problems. The nurse should also review the purpose and dose of current medications.

The child's developmental history and response to new situations and prior separations provide essential background information for understanding the child's current separation anxiety. The assessment should also include a review of recent life events and the methods the family has used to promote the child's return to school. Finally, the family history with respect to anxiety, panic attacks, or phobias is also informative.

Most clinicians agree that the child should return to school as soon as possible because resistance to attending school invariably mounts the longer the child remains absent. Several therapeutic approaches are used in treating separation anxiety disorder, including individual psychotherapy, behavioural treatment, and pharmacotherapy. Although individual psychotherapy is a common treatment, data to support this approach are sparse. By contrast, evidence suggests that behavioural techniques can be effective in reducing separation anxiety. These techniques include flooding (rapid and forcible return to school) and desensitization in which the child is gradually returned to school (Labellarte & Ginsberg, 2003). To be successful, these techniques require close collaboration with the family and the school and may also include medication (Labellarte & Ginsberg).

■■◖ OBSESSIVE-COMPULSIVE DISORDER

OCD is characterized by intrusive thoughts that are difficult to dislodge (obsessions) or ritualized behaviours that the child feels driven to perform (compulsions) to prevent or reduce anxiety. The most common obsessions in children are fears of contamination. Worries about personal and family safety are also frequent. The most common compulsions are excessive washing, cleaning, and checking actions. Historically, OCD was regarded as a neurosis, and the primary symptoms were viewed as the expression of unresolved sexual and aggressive impulses. Recent evidence from family genetic studies, pharmacologic trials,

and neuroimaging studies has dramatically shifted the conceptualization of OCD (see Chapter 21). The notion that OCD is the manifestation of internal conflicts concerning sexual and aggressive impulses has given way to a more biologic model (Stewart et al., 2007).

Epidemiology and Etiology

Until recently, OCD was considered uncommon in adults and even rarer in children, but research over the last two decades has identified OCD as one of the most common psychiatric illnesses in both children and adults. Prevalence in the pediatric population has been reported to be in the range of 1% to 3% (Stewart et al., 2004). OCD can affect the child's or adolescent's physical, psychological, social, and emotional well-being.

Family studies and twin studies indicate that genetic determinants play a significant role in the etiology of anxiety disorders, including OCD, and recur with a greater-than-expected frequency in the families of clients with OCD or Tourette disorder (Van Grootheest, Cath, Beekman, & Boomsma, 2005). Many biologic theories of OCD hypothesize that abnormalities in serotonin metabolism and frontal-striatal circuitry operation are responsible for the creation of OCD symptomatology. The serotonin hypothesis is based on the observation that, in most cases, individuals with OCD respond to SSRIs as opposed to nonserotonergic medications or placebos (Cameron, 2007). Neuroimaging studies and neurosurgical evidence suggest that OCD is associated with hyperactive operation in the frontal-striatal circuitry of the brain, which includes the orbital frontal cortex, anterior cingulated cortex, caudate nucleus, and the thalamus (Leonard, Ale, & Freeman, 2005). Despite advances in the genetics, diagnosis, and treatment of OCD in children and adolescents, little is known about the disorder's long-term outcome (Stewart et al., 2004).

 KEY CONCEPT Obsessions are unwanted persistent, intrusive thoughts, impulses, or images related to anxiety

KEY CONCEPT Compulsions are unwanted behavioural acts or patterns.

Psychopharmacologic Interventions

Current and past studies suggest that psychotropic medications can be introduced to supplement psychosocial interventions in the treatment of OCD but should never be used as the sole form of intervention (Cameron, 2007). The tricyclic antidepressant clomipramine was the first drug reported to be effective for treating OCD (Clomipramine Collaborative Study Group, 1991).

In recent years, SSRIs have become the pharmacological intervention of choice for OCD. Effective SSRIs include fluoxetine, sertraline, and fluvoxamine. These SSRIs have demonstrated effectiveness in older children and adolescents, although little is known about their efficacy with preschool or younger school-aged children (Leonard et al., 2005). Parental education regarding SSRI treatment should include a discussion of the medication's action and potential side effects and a realistic assessment of potential outcomes (Cameron).

Nursing Management

Recurrent worries and ritualistic behaviour can occur normally in children at particular stages of development. The first step in the assessment of OCD in children is to distinguish between normal childhood rituals and worries and pathologic rituals and obsessional thoughts (Cameron, 2007). Obsessional thoughts are recurrent, nagging, and bothersome. Although children may describe obsessions as occurring "out of the blue," external events may trigger obsessions. For example, a child may fear contamination whenever he or she is in contact with a certain person or object. Likewise, compulsions waste time, cause distress, and interfere with daily living (Box 28-7).

The severity of the child's and family's response to OCD will determine the appropriate nursing diagnoses. When the obsessions and compulsions emerge, these children or adolescents are in distress because of the disturbing and relentless nature of the symptoms. What distinguishes OCD families from families of children with other mental disorders is the inextricable way that they are brought into the illness. Parents may be pulled into the child's rituals. The term *family accommodation* is often used to refer to family responses that are direct (e.g., participation in or assistance with the ritual) or indirect (e.g., modification in the family's lifestyle around the OCD symptomatology) (Cameron, 2007). Ineffective coping, compromised family coping, and ineffective role performance are likely nursing diagnoses for these families.

Treatment goals focus on reducing the obsessions and compulsions and their effects on the child's development. Cognitive behavioural therapy, particularly exposure and response prevention (ERP), was found to be an effective intervention in children with OCD (Bolton & Perrin, 2008). Exposure consists of gradual confrontation with events or situations that trigger obsessions and cause the urge to ritualize. According to the theory behind ERP therapy, repeated exposure works because the client learns that the immediate anxiety will subside even if he or she does not complete the ritual. Response prevention complements exposure and consists of instructing the client to delay the execution of the ritual. When exposure and response prevention are combined, the client is confronted with a triggering stimulus such as dirt (exposure) but agrees not to do the hand washing for a brief period (response prevention) and tracks the anxiety level during the exercise. Successful cognitive behavioural treatment of children with OCD includes parents, both to include them in the treatment plan and to reduce parental involvement in the ritualized behaviour. For example, the child may demand that the parent participate in a

---

BOX 28.7

Clinical Vignette: Kimberly and OCD

Kimberly, an 11-year-old fifth grader, comes for evaluation because her mother and teacher have become increasingly concerned about her repetitive behaviours. In retrospect, Kim's mother recalls first noticing repetitive rituals about 2 years ago, but she did not become alarmed about these behaviours until recently when they began to interfere with daily living. At the time of referral, Kim exhibits complicated jumping rituals that involve a specific number of jumps and a particular manner of jumping. She also turns light switches off and on and performs complex movements, such as blinking in patterns and thrusting her arms back and forth a certain number of times. Her mother also reports Kim's near-constant request for reassurance about her own safety. In recent months, her incessant demands for reassurance have been more frequent and elaborate. For example, Kim's mother has to answer three times that everything is all right and then say, "I swear to it."

At the evaluation, Kim expresses fears that some ill fate, such as catastrophic illness or injury, will befall her. This fear is triggered by contact with any individual who seems sick,

chance exposures to foul smells or dirt, or minor scrapes or bumps. Once the fear is triggered, she becomes increasingly anxious and consumed with the fear that she will develop an illness and die. Sometimes her fears are specific, such as cancer or AIDS; other times, her fears are more ambiguous, as evidenced by statements that "something bad will happen" if she doesn't complete the ritual. Kim acknowledges that the ritual is probably not related to the feared event, but she is reluctant to take a chance. If the ritual does not reduce her anxiety, she seeks reassurance from her mother.

Kim's medical history was negative for serious illness or injury; she was born after an uncomplicated pregnancy, labour, and delivery and achieved developmental milestones at appropriate times. Indeed, her mother could recall no unusual problems in the first few years of life except that Kim was typically anxious in new situations. Kim's mother reports a prior history of panic attacks, but the family history is otherwise negative for anxiety disorders, including OCD.

washing and checking ritual (Bolton & Perrin). Because of the dynamic impact OCD in children and adolescents has on families, they should be involved in psychosocial interventions whenever possible (Cameron, 2007).

POSTTRAUMATIC STRESS DISORDER

Stressful or traumatic events in early childhood may have long-lasting effects on brain development, affecting the neural and endocrine systems that mediate the response to stress and exhibiting persistent alterations after trauma (Mulvihill, 2005). Posttraumatic stress disorder (PTSD) can occur in children as a response to personal experience of an event where there is actual or threatened serious injury or death, as in war or natural disaster; in response to childhood abuse or neglect; or threat of serious injury or death to a family member or close friend (see Chapter 26). Symptoms of PTSD last at least a month and include re-experiencing; reenactment of traumatic events in plays, drawings, or verbalizations; avoidance or numbing where the child tries to block out reminders of events; detachment from others; and loss of interest in normal activities. The last symptom present is hyperarousal, which includes difficulty sleeping and concentrating, irritability, angry outbursts, hypervigilance, and an exaggerated startle response (Garner-Evans & Oehler-Stinnet, 2006; McDermott, Lee, Judd, & Gibbon, 2005).

MOOD DISORDERS: MAJOR DEPRESSIVE DISORDER

The *DSM-IV-TR* includes several mood disorders, such as major depressive disorder, dysthymic disorder, bipolar I and bipolar II disorders, and cyclothymic disorder. Although these disorders occur in children and adolescents, they are less common in prepubertal children. These disorders are reviewed in detail in Chapter 20. Thus, this section is confined to a brief discussion of major depressive disorder in children and adolescents.

Depression in childhood and adolescence is a challenging problem for those affected, including parents, siblings, peers, and teachers. Depression is characterized by profound sadness, loss of interest in usual activities, loss of appetite with weight loss, sleep disturbance, loss of energy, feeling worthless or guilty, and recurrent thoughts of death or suicide, and it prompts significant use of mental health services. To meet *DSM-IV-TR* criteria, the symptoms must be present on a daily basis and persist for at least 2 weeks (see Chapter 20). Childhood bipolar disorder is among the most severe disabling psychiatric conditions affecting children. It is associated with great severity of the illness and impairment. Because pediatric bipolar disorder has been assumed to be extremely rare or nonexistent, very little is known thus far about the treatment (Biederman et al., 2005).

Epidemiology

Before reaching the age of 18, about one in five children and adolescents will experience an episode of major depressive disorder that is characterized by a high recurrence rate, persistent psychosocial impairment, and increased risk of suicide (Garland, 2004). Boys appear to be at higher risk for depression until adolescence, when depression becomes more common in girls. The influence of hereditary factors on susceptibility to major depression has been documented based on twin and adoption studies (Strauss et al., 2005).

Nursing Management

The clinical picture of a child with depression may be similar to that of an adult, but children may not spontaneously express feelings of sadness and worthlessness. Some children and adolescents with depression do not have actual "depressed mood" and instead experience increased irritability, which may occur with or without depressed mood (Cheung, Emslie, & Mayes, 2006). Thus, clinical experience is helpful when trying to elicit symptoms of depression from young children. Reports from parents are important sources of information about changes in sleep patterns, appetite, activity level and interests, and emotional stability. A common presentation is a teenager who has a sudden drop in grades; experiences frequent irritability; has a change in friends; participates in fewer social or recreational activities; has recently changed eating or sleeping patterns; has frequent fatigue; and frequently experiences feelings of worthlessness, hopelessness, or suicidal thinking. In addition, many adolescents with depression may be at risk for substance abuse and attempted or completed suicide (Cheung et al.).

Nursing diagnoses for children or adolescents who are depressed are similar to those for adults, including ineffective coping, chronic low self-esteem, disturbed thought processes, self-care deficit, imbalanced nutrition, disturbed sleep pattern, impaired social interaction, and risk for self-injury.

Treatment goals include improving the depressed mood and restoring sleep, appetite, and self-care. Interventions for responses to major depressive disorder in children and adolescents are also similar to those for adults. The psychiatric nurse develops a therapeutic relationship with the child and provides parent education and support. These children may act out their feelings rather than discuss them. Thus, behaviour problems may accompany

BOX **28.8**

Questions, Choices, and Outcomes

Mrs. S has just returned with her son Jared to the child psychiatric inpatient services following an overnight pass. She reports that the visit did not go well due to Jared's anger and defiance. She remarked that this behaviour was distressingly similar to his behaviour before the hospitalization. She expressed additional concern because of the upcoming discharge from the hospital. After saying goodbye to Jared, she pulled the nurse aside and stated that she had decided to file for divorce.

Mrs. S indicated that she had not told her husband or the family therapist. When asked whether Jared knew about her decision, Mrs. S suddenly realized that he may have overheard her discussing the matter with her sister on the telephone during this home visit.

How should the nurse approach this situation?

CHOICE	POSSIBLE OUTCOMES
Discuss her hypothesis about Jared's behaviour and his uncertainty	Mother can see the relationship between Jared's behaviour and her plan for divorce
	Mother ignores the nurse
	Mother is interested but does not see the connection
Ignore the statement	Child and family did not learn about the connection between Jared's behaviour and the events at home
Encourage mother to sort out her problems	The focus is then on mother's problems

ANALYSIS

The best response is focusing on the possible relationship between Jared's recent behavioural deterioration and his uncertainty of his family's future. If the nurse ignores the statement or focuses on the mother's interpretation of Jared's behaviour, the mother is less likely to appreciate the connection between pending divorce and Jared's behaviour. The nurse should also emphasize the importance of discussing the matter in family therapy.

---

depression. Younger children may respond to the use of art or play therapy as a safe way to encourage the expression of painful feelings. Older children and adolescents may also respond positively to board games that have been specifically designed to encourage the expression of emotions. Developing sensitivity to the influence of environmental events on the child is important for the nurse, parents, and teachers (Box 28-8).

These children are likely to be treated with an antidepressant medication and may also undergo psychotherapy with a mental health professional. Antidepressants prescribed to adults are used to treat children and adolescents. Because of the lack of beneficial effects with tricyclic antidepressants in pediatric cases, SSRIs and serotonin-norepinephrine reuptake inhibitors have been increasingly used. The increased research conducted on treatment with SSRIs with this population triggered the recent controversy about the safety and efficacy of SSRI use. Following months of reviewing safety data, regulatory agents in Canada, the United States, and the United Kingdom have issued warnings about the increased risk of suicidal behaviour in children and adolescents using these medications (Cheung et al., 2006). It is critical that the nurse educate the family about the risk for suicide. Parents will also need information on how to assess for risk and what steps to take if the risk is apparent (see Chapter 37). Ongoing research is needed to confirm

the best methods for treating children with major depression and bipolar disorder.

Tic Disorders and Tourette Disorder

Motor tics are usually quick, jerky movements of the eyes, face, neck, and shoulders, although they may involve other muscle groups as well. Occasionally, tics involve slower, more purposeful, or dystonic movements. Phonic tics typically include repetitive throat clearing, grunting, or other noises but may also include more complex sounds, such as words, parts of words, and, in a minority of clients, obscenities. Transient tics, by definition, do not endure over time and appear to be fairly common in school-aged children. Tics are most prevalent in children aged 9 to 11 years, have a higher incidence in males than females, and are more common in children with ADHD (Singer, 2005).

KEY CONCEPT **Tics** are sudden, rapid, repetitive, stereotyped motor movements or vocalizations.

Tic disorder is a general term encompassing several syndromes that are chiefly characterized by motor tics,

Table 28.5	Key Diagnostic Characteristics of Tourette Syndrome 307.23	DSM IV

Diagnostic Criteria and Target Symptoms	Associated Findings

• Multiple motor tics and one or more vocal tics
   Sudden, rapid, recurrent, nonrhythmic, stereotyped motor movements or vocalizations
   Motor tics typically involving the head and other parts of body
   Vocal tics typically involving throat clearing, grunting, and occasionally words or parts of words
• Tics occurring many times a day, present for at least 1 year
   Appear simultaneously or at different periods during the illness
   No tic-free period of more than 3 consecutive months
• Onset before the age of 18 years
• Not a direct physiologic effect of a substance or general medical condition
	• Obsessions and compulsions
	• Hyperactivity, distractibility, and impulsivity
	• Social discomfort, shame, self-consciousness, and depressed mood
	• Impaired social, academic, and occupational functioning
	• Possible interference with daily activities if tics are severe

phonic tics, or both. The *DSM-IV-TR* includes four tic disorders: Tourette syndrome or disorder, chronic motor or vocal tic disorder, transient tic disorder, and tic disorder not otherwise specified. This section focuses on the most severe tic disorder, Tourette disorder (Table 28-5). No diagnostic laboratory tests exist to test for tic disorder. In addition to clinical assessment, the diagnosis is made from the person's family, birth, developmental, school, and medical histories (Singer, 2005). The Yale Global Tic Severity Scale was found to be a reliable and valid instrument for the assessment of pediatric Tourette syndrome (Storch et al., 2005). A major focus of the assessment is the careful exploration of how the tics are affecting the child's physical, psychological, social, and academic well-being. Tourette disorder is undetectable in CAT, PET, and MRI scans (Murray, 2008).

The typical age of onset for tics is about 7 years, and motor tics generally precede phonic tics. Parents often describe the seeming replacement of one tic with another. In addition to this changing repertoire of motor and phonic tics, Tourette disorder exhibits a waxing and waning course. The child can suppress the tics for brief periods. Thus, it is not uncommon to hear from parents that their child has more frequent tics at home than at school. Older children and adults may describe an urge or a physical sensation before having a tic. Tics commonly increase during periods of anticipation, emotional upset, and fatigue and generally tend to subside when the child is absorbed in activities, concentrating, pleased, or asleep. Tics have different degrees of severity, and no two children have the same pattern (Singer, 2005). Tourette disorder is defined by multiple motor and phonic tics for at least 1 year.

Epidemiology and Etiology

The prevalence of Tourette disorder is estimated to be between 1 and 10 per 1,000 in school-aged children,

with boys being affected three to six times more often than girls. Tourette disorder is common in children with autism, Asperger's disorder, and other autistic-spectrum disorders (Singer, 2005). The specific causes of Tourette disorder remain unclear. The disturbance is not due to direct physiological effects of a medical condition. Direct and indirect evidence has found that cortico-striatal-thalamocortical pathways are involved in its expression. There is a general concensus that there is a circuit abnormality in the area but the pathophysiology is speculative (Singer, Mink, Hallett, & Lombroso, 2004). The possibility of dopaminergic abnormality also continues to receive much attention because of the therapeutic response to neuroleptics in vocal and motor tics (Singer).

In the 1980s, data from family genetic studies suggested that Tourette disorder is inherited as a single autosomal dominant gene. Later studies have found that the disorder results from a combination of major genes, modifying genes, and environmental factors that can increase or decrease the severity of symptoms (McMahon, Carter, Fredine, & Pauls, 2003). Currently, many approaches are being used to search for a genetic site, including cytogenetics, candidate gene studies, and molecular genetic studies. Linkage analyses have suggested several chromosomal locations, without a clear reproducible locus or convergence of findings (Singer, 2005). Genetic studies may provide the most promising answers to the question of causation.

Psychopharmacologic Interventions

There is no cure for tics, and all pharmacotherapies must be regarded as symptomatic therapy. The goal of treatment with medication is not to completely stop all motor and phonic tics, but to reduce them so that they no longer cause substantial psychosocial disturbance (Singer, 2005). Historically, the most commonly used antipsychotics include haloperidol and pimozide. These potent dopamine blockers are often effective at low doses. Attempts to eradicate all tics by increasing the dosages of these antipsychotics almost certainly result in diminishing therapeutic returns and additional side effects. The most frequently encountered side effects include drowsiness, dulled thinking, muscle stiffness, akathisia, increased appetite and weight gain, and acute dystonic reactions. Long-term use carries a small risk for tardive dyskinesia. Currently, the atypical antipsychotics ziprasidone, risperidone, quetiapine, and olanzapine are being used to suppress tics in children and adolescents (Singer). In this group, risperidone has been studied most extensively. When compared with drugs previously used in the suppression of tics, risperidone was equally effective as clonidine and superior to pimozide. Reported side effects include weight gain, social phobia, depression, and sedation (Kim, Lee, Hwang, Shin, & Cho, 2005). Olanzapine has been found to significantly reduce both aggressive behaviour and tic frequency and severity. However, weight gain has also been found to be a significant side effect (Stephens, Bassel, & Sandor, 2004). Monitoring weight gain at regular intervals and educating parents about the need to monitor their child's diet and level of exercise are critical nursing interventions when working with families whose child has been prescribed either olanzapine or risperidone.

Nursing Management

The nursing assessment of a child with tics includes a review of the onset, course, and current level of the symptoms. The goals of the assessment are to identify the frequency, intensity, complexity, and interference of the tics and their effects on functioning; determine the child's level of adaptive functioning; identify the child's areas of strength and weakness in general and in school; and identify social supports for the child and family (Singer, 2005). Another important aspect of the assessment is to determine the effects of the tic symptoms on the child and family. Some children and families adjust well; however, others are embarrassed or devastated and tend to withdraw socially. About half of school-aged children with Tourette disorder have ADHD, and a substantial percentage have symptoms of OCD (Roessner, Becker, Banaschewski, & Rothenberger, 2007). Therefore, in addition to inquiring about tics, the nurse should assess the child's overall development, activity level, and capacity to concentrate and persist with a single task, as well as explore repetitive habits and recurring worries. The completion of a family history of tic disorder may also provide some critical assessment data.

Nursing diagnoses could include ineffective coping, chronic low self-esteem, impaired social interaction, anxiety, and compromised family coping. Children with Tourette disorder typically have normal intelligence, although clinical samples may show a higher frequency of learning problems. These learning problems may include subtle problems of organization and planning or more severe problems with reading (Burd, Freeman, Klug, & Kerbeshian, 2005). Handwriting, including both speed and legibility, is another common problem for these youngsters. The use of a computer can obviate difficulties with handwriting in some cases.

The approach to planning nursing interventions depends on the primary source of impairment: tics themselves, OCD symptoms, or the triad of hyperactivity, inattention, and poor impulse control. The nurse can provide counselling and education for the client, education for the parents, and consultation for the school. Most children and their families need some education about Tourette disorder. Individual psychotherapy with a mental health specialist (such as a psychologist or an advanced practice nurse) may be indicated for some children and adolescents with Tourette disorder to deal with maladaptive responses to the chronic condition.

Before the evaluation and diagnosis of Tourette disorder, most families struggle with various explanations for the child's tics. Because tics fluctuate in severity with time and may be more prominent in some settings than in others, family members may have difficulty understanding their involuntary nature. Some parents may be convinced that the tics are deliberate and done to secure attention; others may judge that the tics are "nervous habits" indicative of underlying trouble. Such views require reconciliation with the currently accepted view that tics are involuntary. Some parents may conclude that the child is incapable of controlling any behaviour because of Tourette disorder. They may subsequently feel uncertain about setting limits. In these families, delineating the boundaries of Tourette disorder can be helpful (Singer, 2005).

On learning that this disorder is probably genetic, some parents may harbour guilt for having passed it on to their child. The nurse can assist such families by listening to these concerns and providing information about the natural history of Tourette disorder—it is not a progressive condition, tics often diminish in adulthood, and it need not restrict what the child can achieve in life.

Teaching

Students who have Tourette disorder have unique academic, social, emotional, and physical needs in the classroom. Teachers, guidance counsellors, and school nurses may need current information about Tourette disorder and related problems. Discussions with school personnel often include issues such as how to deal with tic behaviours that are disruptive in the classroom, how to manage teasing from other children, and how to handle medication side effects. A careful discussion of the boundaries

Therapeutic Dialogue: *Tics and Disruptive Behaviours*

INEFFECTIVE APPROACH

Teacher: I see the tics. He jerks his head, makes faces, and flicks his hands.

Nurse: What do you do about them?

Teacher: What can I do? If he isn't disrupting the class, I leave him alone. Even when he is throwing spitballs.

Nurse: Spitballs! He shouldn't be allowed to throw spitballs.

Teacher: Oh, I thought that was a part of his problem.

Nurse: Well, throwing spitballs has nothing to do with tics.

EFFECTIVE APPROACH

Teacher: I see the tics. He jerks his head, makes faces, and flicks his hands.

Nurse: He cannot help the tics that you are seeing. Tic disorders can exhibit a wide range of severity, from mild to severe and from simple to complex. Some complex tics may be difficult to distinguish from habits or rituals.

Teacher: What about things like throwing spitballs? When he does things like that, I try to ignore that behaviour.

Nurse: Sounds like you give him the benefit of the doubt. (Validation) However, throwing a spitball is not a tic behaviour.

Teacher: What should I do?

Nurse: How do you usually handle that type of behaviour? (A modification of reflection)

Teacher: I'd ask him to stop and sometimes go into the hall.

Nurse: Disruptive behaviour that is voluntary in a student with a tic disorder should be handled as you would handle any other child.

CRITICAL THINKING CHALLENGE

- Compare the responses of the nurse in these scenarios. What made the difference in the teacher's responsiveness to the nurse?

of Tourette disorder and tic symptomatology usually can resolve these matters. Teachers who understand the involuntary nature of tics can often generate creative solutions, such as excusing the child for errands. This maneuver allows the child to step out of the classroom briefly to release a bout of tics, thereby reducing stress. In some situations, a brief presentation about Tourette disorder to the class will reduce teasing and help both teachers and classmates tolerate the tic symptoms (Prestia, 2003) (see Box 28-9). Such presentations foster openness and understanding and help students with Tourette disorder feel included and academically adept.

Before initiating these interventions, it is essential to identify the child's needs and to pursue these strategies in collaboration with the family and other clinical team members. If evidence shows that Tourette disorder is hindering academic progress, the nurse can help families negotiate with the school to obtain appropriate services.

Childhood Schizophrenia

Childhood schizophrenia, defined as an onset of psychosis before the age of 13, is diagnosed by the same criteria as those used in adults (Greenstein et al., 2006) (see Chapter 18). The difficulty in diagnosing a psychiatric disorder in children has led to years of debate and controversy regarding whether childhood schizophrenia differs from the adult type or is merely an early manifestation of the same disorder. For many years, it was believed that autism represented the childhood form of schizophrenia. However, in recent years, autism and childhood schizophrenia have

been differentiated (Volkmar et al., 2004). As currently defined, childhood schizophrenia (occurring before the age of 13 years) is rare, with an estimated 2 cases per 100,000 in the population. Other forms of psychosis, falling short of diagnostic criteria for schizophrenia, can occur in children.

Childhood schizophrenia is usually characterized by poorer premorbid functioning than later-onset schizophrenia. Common premorbid difficulties include social, cognitive, linguistic, attentional, motor, and perceptual delays (Volkmar et al., 2004). Taken together, these findings suggest that early onset schizophrenia is a more severe form of the disorder.

Nursing care for these children follows an approach similar to that used in the treatment of PDDs. Antipsychotic medication is prescribed for symptoms (Sikich, Hamer, Bashford, Sheitman, & Lieberman, 2004). Risperidone and olanzapine are widely used as the first-line treatment to ameliorate psychotic symptoms in youth, but their abilities to specifically treat children and adolescents presenting with psychotic symptoms have not been rigorously studied in the past (Sikich et al.). In a current first-randomized, double-blind trial of olanzapine and risperidone in youth presenting for the treatment of psychotic symptoms, it was found that these medications are effective in reducing both the positive and the negative effects of schizophrenia. However, the study also provided evidence that both these medications are associated with more prevalent and severe side effects than those found in adults with psychosis. The majority of participants experienced mild to moderate extra-pyramidal effects. Although no cases of tardive dyskinesia were identified in the study, the acute extra-pyramidal effects observed in some of the participants suggest the need to monitor for tardive dyskinesia in children and adolescents taking atypical antipsychotics (Sikich et al.). See Chapters 10 and 14 for more detailed description of the atypical antipsychotics.

Development of an individualized care plan for children with schizophrenia begins with nursing assessment to identify functional problems specific to the child. Similarly, the recognition that childhood schizophrenia is a chronic and severe condition should guide the identification of outcomes. Goals should be realistic, and the nurse should pay special attention to the child's support systems. Parent education about the disorder, medications (including side effects), and long-term management (including the use of community resources) is an essential part of the treatment plan. Long-term management also requires monitoring of chronic antipsychotic therapy. Weight gain is a side effect of the newer atypical antipsychotics. Children treated with these medications may be at risk for chronic health problems associated with obesity, such as diabetes, hypertension, cardiovascular disease, and osteoarthritis (Sikich et al., 2004). Parental education about diet and exercise is an important part of the treatment plan.

Elimination Disorders

■◗ ENURESIS

Enuresis usually means involuntary bedwetting, although repeated urination on clothing during waking hours can occur (diurnal enuresis). For nocturnal enuresis, the *DSM-IV-TR* specifies that bedwetting occurs at least twice per week for a duration of 3 months and that the child is at least 5 years of age. Even without treatment, 50% of these children can achieve dryness by the age of 10 years.

Enuresis is the involuntary excretion of urine after the age at which the child should have attained bladder control.

Epidemiology and Etiology

The prevalence of nocturnal enuresis varies with age and gender, being most common in young boys—an estimated 15% of 5-year-old boys, 7% of boys aged 7 to 9 years, and 1% of 14-year-old boys have nocturnal enuresis. The frequency in girls is about half that of boys in each age group. The etiology of enuresis is unknown, with probably no single cause. Most children with nocturnal enuresis are urologically normal. The prevalence of nocturnal enuresis decreases from early childhood to adolescence, and time is the cure for bedwetting in the majority of cases (Nield & Kamat, 2004).

Nursing Management

The nursing assessment should include the child's developmental history, the onset and course of enuresis, prior treatment, presence of emotional problems, medical history, and family history of enuresis, diabetes, or kidney disease. Psychosocial issues such as a change in living arrangements, a new child in the family, or a death should also be documented because stresss can be a contributing factor to the problem (Nield & Kamat, 2004). The nurse should also explore the family's home environment and family attitudes about the child's enuresis. Routine laboratory tests such as urinalysis and a urine culture are used to determine the presence of infection. The nurse should obtain baseline data regarding toileting habits, including daytime incontinence, urinary frequency, and constipation. He or she should refer children with persistent daytime enuresis for consultation with a urologist (Reiner, 2003).

The nurse can explore and dispel myths that parents may have about bedwetting, such as the child is misbehaving and needs to be punished for wetting the bed. In addition, education about bedwetting and its causes may help to alleviate parents' feelings of frustration and the child's feelings of humiliation and shame. The nurse can also encourage parents to limit fluid intake in the evening and treat constipation (if present).

Pharmacologic Interventions

If conservative methods fail, both drug and behavioural treatments have been beneficial for nocturnal enuresis. Imipramine (Tofranil), a tricyclic antidepressant, has shown efficacy in the treatment of enuresis. The nasal spray preparation or tablet form of desmopressin (DDAVP) has also shown promise, but beneficial effects may not endure. DDAVP is a synthetic antidiuretic hormone that actually inhibits the production of urine. Although both these medications are fairly safe, DDAVP can lead to water intoxication and electrolyte abnormalities and the tricyclic antidepressants can have the multiple systemic side effects of anticholinergics (see Chapter 13). Both tricyclic antidepressants and DDAVP are effective when actively administered to the child, but the majority of children will relapse once the medication is stopped (Nield & Kamat, 2004). This can cause recurrence of parental frustration, and shame and humiliation in addition to feelings of failure in the child.

Behavioural Interventions

The most effective nonpharmacologic treatment is the bedwetting alarm. In this form of behavioural treatment, the bed is equipped with a pad that sets off a buzzer if the child wets. The buzzer then wakes up the child, thereby reminding the child to void. Six to sixteen weeks of alarm treatment may be necessary for the majority of children to experience two consecutive weeks of dry nights. Many families, especially those of adolescents, may want a quicker result than the alarm can provide. It is critical that the nurse spend time explaining the benefits of this intervention which provides the best chance for long-term successful treatment (Nield & Kamat, 2004).

■ ENCOPRESIS

Encopresis involves soiling clothing with feces or depositing feces in inappropriate places. Additional diagnostic criteria include that the child is older than 4 years, that the soiling occurs at least once per month, and that the soiling is not the result of a medical disorder, such as aganglionic megacolon (Hirschsprung's disease). The most common form of encopresis is fecal impaction accompanied by leakage around the hardened mass of stool. Because of the loss of muscle tone in the lower bowel, the child loses the usual urge to defecate and may not feel the leakage. Surprisingly, the child may not detect the smell of the stool because the olfactory apparatus becomes accustomed to the odor. If left untreated, this problem generally resolves independently by middle adolescence (North American Society for Pediatric Gastroenterology, Hepatology and Nutrition, 2006). Encopresis can affect the lives of children in the following areas: physical, psychological, educational, social, emotional, and in the area of self-esteem.

Epidemiology and Etiology

The problem of encopresis has received less attention in pediatric literature compared with enuresis. As with enuresis, encopresis is more common in boys, and the frequency of the condition declines with age. Recorded prevalence of encopresis varied between studies from 1% to 4% in children older than 4 years of age, 1% to 2% in children 7 years of age, and 1.6% in those 10 to 11 years of age, with boys three to four times more likely to have encopresis than girls (Bongers, Tabbers, & Benninga, 2007). Fecal incontinence is reported to be responsible for 3% of referrals to health care professionals.

The diagnosis of encopresis includes both retentive fecal incontinence and nonretentive fecal incontinence which presents as a single symptom without any organic cause or signs of constipation (Bongers et al., 2007). The reasons for withholding stool and starting the cycle of fecal impaction are unclear but are usually not the result of physical causes. However, as noted, once the fecal impaction occurs, there is a loss of tone in the bowel and leakage.

Nursing Management

The assessment includes a detailed interview with the child and parent regarding the pattern of the encopresis.

A calm, matter-of-fact approach can help to reduce the child's embarrassment. A physical examination is also necessary; thus, collaboration with the child's family physician or consulting paediatrician is essential. The presence of encopresis does not necessarily signal severe emotional or behavioural disturbances, but the nurse should inquire about other psychiatric disorders. The diagnosis of encopresis is presumed given a history of intermittent constipation and soiling. Collaboration with the family physician and paediatrician often is helpful to rule out rare medical conditions, such as Hirschsprung's disease.

Teaching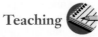

Effective intervention begins with educating the parents and the child about normal bowel function and the self-perpetuating cycle of fecal impaction and leakage of stool around the hardened mass of feces. The short-term goal of this educational effort is to decrease the anger and recrimination that often complicate the picture in these families. It is important for parents to understand that soiling from overflow incontinence is not a willful and defiant maneuver. Parents are encouraged to maintain a consistent, positive, and supportive attitude in all aspects of treatment (North American Society for Pediatric Gastroenterology, Hepatology and Nutrition, 2006). Because encopresis often results in a loss of bowel tone, it may help to motivate children by emphasizing the need to strengthen their muscles. In many cases, cleaning out the bowel is necessary before initiating behavioural treatment. The bowel catharsis is usually followed by the administration of mineral oil, which is often continued during the bowel retraining program. A high-fiber diet is often recommended.

The behavioural treatment program involves daily sitting on the toilet after each meal for a predetermined period (e.g., 10 minutes). The child and parents can measure the time with an ordinary kitchen timer, and the parents can encourage the child to read or look at picture books while sitting. They can give the child rewards in the form of stars, stickers, or points for complying with the retraining program and add bonuses for successful defecation. The family can tally stickers or points on a calendar, and the child can "cash in" collected points for small prizes (Reiner, 2003). Children with nonretentive fecal incontinence should not be treated with laxatives. After the exclusion of underlying organic diseases, the treatment is based on the following aspects: education, toilet training, a daily bowel diary with a reward system, and medication. Loperamide has been found effective in the short-term treatment of nonretentive fecal incontinence (Bongers et al., 2007).

All the disorders discussed in this chapter are summarized in Table 28-6 (Box 28-10).

Table 28.6	Summary of Diagnostic Characteristics
Disorder	**Diagnostic Characteristics**

Pervasive Developmental Disorder Not Otherwise Specified	• Impairment of reciprocal social interaction
	  Marked impairment in use of nonverbal behaviours
	  Failure to develop appropriate peer relationships
	  Absence of spontaneously seeking to share enjoyment, interest, or achievements (e.g., pointing out things of interest)
	  Lack of social or emotional reciprocity (oblivious to others, not noticing another's distress)
	• Repetitive and stereotypic behaviour patterns and activities
	  Preoccupation with a pattern that is abnormal in intensity or focus
	  Inflexible adherence to nonfunctional routines or rituals
	  Stereotypic, repetitive motor mannerisms
	  Persistent preoccupation with idiosyncratic interests (e.g., train schedules, air conditioners)

Autism	• As listed above for pervasive developmental disorders
	• Severe impairment in communication
	  Delay or total lack of spoken language
	  Impaired ability to initiate or sustain a conversation
	  Use of stereotypic, repetitive, or idiosyncratic language
	  Lack of varied, spontaneous make-believe or social imitative play
	• Abnormal social interaction, use of language for social communication, or symbolic or imaginative play before the age of 3 years
	• Not better accounted for by another psychiatric disorder

Asperger's disorder	• As listed above for pervasive developmental disorders • Clinically significant impairment in social, occupational, or other areas of functioning • No general delay in language • Less likely to have delay in cognitive development or daily living skills • Overfocus on an area of restricted interest is a prominent feature • Not better accounted for by another pervasive developmental disorder or schizophrenia
Learning Disorders Reading disorders Mathematics disorders Disorders of written expression	• Discrepancy between academic achievement and intellectual ability • Reading achievement substantially below that expected for age, intelligence, and education • Mathematic ability substantially below that expected for age, intelligence, and education • Writing skills substantially below that expected for age, intelligence, and education

Communication Disorders
Expressive language disorder
	• Interference with academic or occupational achievement or social communication
	• Deficits not explained by retardation or deprivation
	• Impairment of expressive language development
	  Limited amount of speech
	  Limited range of vocabulary
	  Vocabulary errors
	  Sentence structure problems
	  Unusual word order
	  Slow rate of language development
	  Difficulty in communication, both verbally and with sign language
	• As listed above for communication disorders
	• Deficits cannot be explained by pervasive developmental disorder

Mixed receptive– expressive language disorder	• Impairment of receptive and expressive language development
	  Markedly limited vocabulary
	  Errors in tense
	  Difficulty recalling words or appropriate-length sentences
	  General difficulty expressing ideas
	  Difficulty understanding words, sentences, or types of words or statements
	  Multiple disabilities such as inability to understand basic vocabulary or simple sentences; deficits in sound discrimination, storage, recall, and sequencing
	• As listed above for communication disorders
	• Deficits not explained by pervasive developmental disorder

Phonologic disorder	• Failure to use appropriate developmentally expected speech sounds
	  Errors in sound production
	  Substitution of one sound for another
	  Omission of sounds
	• As listed above for communication disorders

Continued

Table 28.6	Summary of Diagnostic Characteristics *(Continued)*
Disorder	**Diagnostic Characteristics**

Stuttering	• Disturbed fluency and timing patterns of speech
	    Repetition of sounds and syllables
	    Prolongation of sound
	    Interjections
	    Broken words
	    Filled or unfilled pauses in speech
	    Substitutions of words to avoid problematic sounds
	    Production of words with an excess of physical tension
	    Repetitions of monosyllabic whole word
	• As listed above for communication disorders

Disruptive Behaviour Disorders
Conduct disorder
	• Significant impairment in social, academic, or occupational functioning
	• Not accounted for by antisocial personality disorder if older than 18 years
	• Repetitive and persistent behaviour that violates the rights of others or major age-appropriate societal norms
	    Aggression to people and animals
	    Destruction of property
	    Deceitfulness or theft
	    Serious violations of rules
	• As listed above for disruptive behaviour disorders

Oppositional defiant disorder	• Negativistic, hostile behaviour pattern
	    Loss of temper
	    Frequently argumentative
	    Active defiance or refusal to comply with adult requests or rules
	    Deliberate annoyance of others
	    Blaming of others for own mistakes or misbehaviour
	    Anger and resentment
	    Spitefulness and vindictiveness
	• As listed above for disruptive behaviour disorders
	• Not exclusive during the course of psychotic or mood disorder

Anxiety Disorders Obsessive-compulsive disorders	See Chapter 21
Mood Disorders Major depressive disorder	See Chapter 20
Tic Disorders	• Single or multiple tics • Onset before the age of 18 years • Not due to a substance (e.g., amphetamine) or general medical condition
Chronic motor or vocal tic disorder, 307.22	• Motor or vocal tics occurring many times per day nearly every day or intermittently throughout more than 1 year, no tic-free period greater than 3 months • As listed above for tic disorders
Transient tic disorder, 307.21	• Motor or vocal tics occurring many times during the day for at least 4 weeks; not longer than 12 consecutive months
Tourette disorder	• Motor and phonic tics lasting more than 12 months
Childhood Schizophrenia	See Chapter 18
Elimination Disorders Enuresis, 307.6	• Repeated voiding into bed or clothes (involuntary or intentional) • Occurring twice a week for at least 3 consecutive months or significant impairment in social, academic, or other area of functioning • At least 5 years of age or developmental equivalent • Not a physiologic effect of a substance or general medical condition

Encopresis
  307.7 without constipation and overflow incontinence
  787.6 with constipation and overflow incontinence
	• Repeated passage of feces into inappropriate places, such as clothing or floor
	• Occurring at least once a month for at least 3 months
	• At least 4 years of age or developmental equivalent
	• Not the physiologic effect of a substance or general medical condition except involving constipation

BOX 28.10

Research for Best Practice

From Luther, E. H., Canham, D. L., Young-Cureton, V. (2005). Coping and social supports for parents of children with autism. Journal of School Nursing, 21(1), 40–47.

QUESTIONS: What are the perceived levels of informal and formal social supports among families of autistic children? What are the coping strategies used by parents of children with autism?

METHODS: The conceptual framework for this study was the Resiliency Model of Family Stress, Adjustment, and Adaptation. The study used a descriptive survey design and a convenience sample. Participants were parents of children with autism (ages 5–13) who were enrolled in selected special education classes. A convenience sample of 72 was identified; however, only 18 families completed and returned the questionnaires. Participants completed a demographic questionnaire, which included questions about concurrent stressors in the family, and two Likert-type scales that examined coping strategies and formal and informal types of social support.

FINDINGS: Significant stressors in addition to a child's autism were reported by 50% of the families. Identified stressors were finances, unemployment, absentee fathers, transportation problems, recent divorce, and concurrent chronic health problems such as diabetes and asthma. Reframing scored highest as a coping strategy for participants. Reframing enabled families to define problems in more positive ways to avoid becoming depressed. Social support ranked second as a coping method for families. There were individual differences in accessing social supports because of difficulties such as inability to speak English, low income, and lack of

transportation. Approximately 50% of the parents indicated that they attended or were interested in attending a support group. Eighty-three percent of participants strongly agreed with the statement that having faith in God was a way of coping; however, fewer than half coped by attending church services or sought the advice of a minister, priest, or rabbi. Participants scored high on the Passive Appraisal subscale. This subscale focussed on inactive or passive behaviour that the families might use, such as avoidance of responses based on a lack of confidence in their ability to change the situation. Passive behaviours may also be used as a means of coping with stress. Responses regarding formal and informal social support were consistently high for close friends and family members; few, however, relied on neighbours for help or support. Responses for obtaining help when needed and feeling comfortable within the community were variable. The variation may have resulted from differing cultural and socioeconomic levels, as well as differing lengths of time families may have resided in the neighbourhood.

IMPLICATIONS FOR NURSING PRACTICE: This study found that half of the children with autism had coexisting medical conditions. School nurses are the link between educational and medical institutions and are valuable members of the educational intervention team. The school nurse can assist parents or caregivers to examine information and make informed decisions about the child's needs. Understanding parents' preferred coping strategies and their access to informal and formal support systems will assist nurses as they strive to help them meet their own and their families' needs.

SUMMARY OF KEY POINTS

☐ Improved methods of assessing and defining psychiatric disorders have enhanced appreciation for the frequency of psychiatric disorders in children and adolescents.

☐ An estimated 14% of children 4–17 years of age (more than 800,000) in Canada experience mental disorders that cause significant distress and impairment at home, at school, and in the community.

☐ The developmental disorders include intellectual disability, pervasive developmental disorders (PDDs), and specific developmental disorders. Assessment findings should guide nursing management. Specific developmental disorders include communication disorders and learning disorders. These disorders are fairly common in the general population, but they are more common in children with other primary psychiatric disorders.

☐ Child psychiatric disorders can be divided into externalizing and internalizing disorders. Externalizing disorders include the disruptive behaviour disorders: attention deficit hyperactivity disorder (ADHD), oppositional defiant disorder, and conduct disorder. Internalizing disorders include depression and anxiety disorders.

☐ ADHD is defined by the presence of inattention, impulsiveness, and, in most cases, hyperactivity. As currently defined, ADHD is the most common disorder of childhood. This heterogeneous disorder affects boys more often than girls.

☐ Effective treatment of ADHD often involves multiple approaches, including medication and parent training.

☐ Primary features of oppositional defiant disorder include persistent disobedience, argumentativeness, and tantrums.

☐ Conduct disorder is characterized by lying, truancy, stealing, and fighting.

☐ Assessment of children with disruptive behaviour problems involves securing data from multiple sources, including the child, parents, and school personnel.

☐ Standardized rating instruments can assist data collection from multiple informants.

☐ Separation anxiety and OCD are relatively common anxiety disorders in school-aged children. (OCD becomes more common in adolescents.)

☐ Treatment of separation anxiety and OCD may include medication, behavioural therapy, or a combination of these treatments.

◻ Major depression in children is believed to be similar to major depression in adults.

◻ The efficacy of antidepressant medications is less well established in children and adolescents than in adults.

◻ Tourette disorder is a tic disorder characterized by motor and phonic tics. Common comorbid conditions include ADHD and OCD.

◻ Childhood schizophrenia is a rare disorder.

◻ Elimination disorders include encopresis and enuresis. Behavioural therapy approaches are the most effective treatment for these disorders. Medication may also be used.

CRITICAL THINKING CHALLENGES

1 Analyze how genetic and environmental factors may interact in the etiology of child psychiatric disorders.

2 Learning disabilities and communication disorders are more common in children with psychiatric disorders than in the general population. How might a learning disability or a communication disorder complicate a psychiatric illness in a school-aged child?

3 Compare and contrast nursing approaches for a child with ADHD with those used for a child with autistic disorder. How are they different? How are they similar?

4 Many children have imaginary playmates. What are the benefits to the child? At what age level is this appropriate? When does it become inappropriate?

5 Discuss what effect you think extensive television coverage of the wars in Afghanistan and Iraq has on newly arrived refugee children to Canada? What factors might serve as protective factors to these previously traumatized children?

6 How would you help parents differentiate between normal adolescent mood and behaviour and depression?

WEB LINKS

www.chadd.org This site of the Children and Adults With Attention-Deficit/Hyperactivity Disorder (CHADD) organization provides information and resources on ADHD.

www.tourette.ca This web site contains information and resources about Tourette disorder.

kidshealth.org/parent/medical/brain/asperger.html This web site describes Asperger's disorder.

www.autism.org The web site of the Centre for Study of Autism contains information and resources about autism and related disorders.

www.bpkids.org This is the site of the Child & Adolescent Bipolar Foundation.

REFERENCES

American Psychiatric Association. (2000). *Diagnostic and statistical manual of mental disorders* (4th ed., Text revision). Washington, DC: Author.

Anderson, G., Scahill, L., McCracken, J., McDougle, C., Aman, M., Tierney, E., et al. (2007). Effects of short- and long-term risperidone treatment on prolactin levels in children with autism. *Biological Psychiatry, 61*(4), 545–550.

Bakker, S. C., van der Meulen, E. M., Buitelaar, J. K., Sandkuijl, L. A., Pauls, D. L., Monsuur, A. J., et al. (2003). A whole-genome scan in 164 Dutch sib pairs with attention-deficit/hyperactivity disorder: Suggestive evidence for linkage on chromosones 7p and 15q. *American Journal of Human Genetics, 72*(5), 1251–1260.

Beauchaine, C., Webster-Stratton, C., & Reid, J. (2005). Mediators, moderators, and predictors of 1-year outcomes among children treated for early-onset conduct problems: A latent growth curve analysis. *Journal of Consulting and Clinical Psychology, 73*(3), 371–388.

Bhat, M., Grizenko, N., Ben-Amor, L., & Joober, R. (2005). Obstetric complications in children with attention deficit/hyperactivity disorder and learning disability. *McGill Journal of Medicine, 8*(2), 109–113.

Biederman, J., & Faraone, S. (2005). Attention-deficit hyperactivity disorder. *Lancet, 366*(7), 237–248.

Biederman, J., Mick, M., Wozniak, J., Aleardi, M., Spencer, T., & Faraone, S. (2005). An open-label trial of risperidone in children and adolescents with bipolar disorder. *Journal of Child and Adolescent Psychopharmacology, 15*(2), 311–317.

Bolton, D., & Perrin, S. (2008). Evaluation of exposure with response-prevention for obsessive compulsive disorder in children and adolescents. *Journal of Behaviour Therapy and Experimental Psychiatry, 39*(1), 11–22.

Bongers, M., Tabbers, M., & Benninga, M. (2007). Functional nonretentive fecal incontinence in children. *Journal of Pediatric Gastroenterology and Nutrition, 44*(1), 5–13.

Burd, L., Freeman, R., Klug, M., & Kerbeshian, J. (2005). Tourette syndrome and learning disabilities. *BMC Pediatrics, 5*(34). Retrieved May 15, 2007, from http://www.biomedcentral.com/1471-2431/5/34

Buschmann, A., Jooss, B., Rupp, A., Dockter, S., Blaschtikowitz, H., Heggen, I., et al. (2008). Children with developmental language delay at 24 months of age: Results of a diagnostic work-up. *Developmental Medicine & Child Neurology, 50*(3), 223–229.

Buysse, V., Goldman, B. D., & Skinner, M. L. (2003). Seeing effects on friendship formation among young children with and without disabilities. *Exceptional Children, 68*(4), 503–517.

Cameron, C. L. (2007). Obsessive-compulsive disorder in children and adolescents. *Journal of Psychiatric and Mental Health Nursing, 14*(7), 696–704.

Canadian Pediatric Society. (2006). Mental health of children and adolescents. Retrieved November 24, 2009, from http://www.cps.ca/english/Advocacy/MentalHealth.htm

Cheung, A., Emslie, G., & Mayes, T. (2006). The use of antidepressants to treat depression in children and adolescents. *Canadian Medical Association Journal, 174*(2), 193–200.

Children's Health Policy Centre, Simon Fraser University. (2007). Addressing attention problems in children. *Children's Mental Health Research Quarterly*, Fall. Retrieved November 24, 2009, from http://www.childhealthpolicy.sfu.ca/research_quarterly_08/rq-pdf/RQ-4-07-Fall.pdf

Chronis, A. M., Jones, H., & Raggi, V. (2006). Evidence-based psychosocial treatments for children and adolescents with attention deficit/hyperactivity disorder. *Clinical Psychology Review, 26*(4), 486–502.

Clomipramine Collaborative Study Group. (1991). Clomipramine in the treatment of patients with obsessive compulsive disorder. *Archives of General Psychiatry, 48*(8), 730–738.

Doyle, R. (2004). The history of attention deficit/hyperactivity disorder. *Psychiatric Clinics of North America, 27*(2), 203–214.

Durston, S., Tottenham, N. T., Thomas, K. M., Davidson, M. C., Eigsti, I., Yang, Y., et al. (2003). Differential patterns of striatalactivation in young children with and without ADHD. *Biological Psychiatry, 53*, 871–878.

Faraone, S. V. (2004). Genetics of adult attention deficit hyperactivity disorder. In T. Spencer (Ed.), *Psychiatric Clinics of North America* (pp. 303–321). Philadelphia, PA: Saunders Press.

Faraone, S. V., & Bierderman, J. (2004). The neurobiology of attention deficit hyperactivity disorder. In D. S. Charney, E. J. Nestler, & Bunney, B. S. (Eds.), *Neurobiology of Mental Illness* (2nd ed., pp. 979–999). New York, NY: Oxford University Press.

Faraone, S. V., Perlis, R. H., Doyle, A. E., Smoller, J. W., Goralnick, J. J., Holmgren, M. A., et al. (2005). Molecular genetics of attention-deficit/hyperactivity disorder. *Biological Psychiatry, 57*(11), 1313–1323.

Flapper, B., & Schoemaker, M. (2008). Effects of methylphenidate on quality of life in children with both developmental coordination disorder and ADHD. *Developmental Medicine and Child Neurology, 50*(4), 294–299.

Fox, R., Keller, K., Grede, P., & Bartoz, A. (2007). A mental health clinic for toddlers with developmental delays and behaviour problems. *Research in Developmental Disabilities, 28*(2), 119–129.

Garland, E. J. (2004). Facing the evidence: antidepressant treatment in children and adolescents. *Canadian Medical Association Journal, 170*(4), 489–491.

Garner-Evans, L., & Oehler-Stinnett, J. (2006). Structure and prevalence of PTSD symptomology in children who have experienced a severe tornado. *Psychology in the Schools, 43*(3), 283–295.

Goyette, G. H., Conners, C. K., & Ulrich, R. F. (1978). Normative data on the revised Connors parent and teacher rating scales. *Journal of Abnormal Child Psychology, 6*, 221–236.

Greenstein, D., Lerch, J., Shaw, P., Clasen, L., Giedd, J., Gochman, P., et al. (2006). Childhood onset of schizophrenia: Cortical brain abnormalities as young adults. *Journal of Child Psychology and Psychiatry, 47*(10), 1003–1012.

Hinshaw, S. (2005). The stigmatization of mental illness in children and parents: developmental issues, family concerns, and research needs. *Journal of Child Psychology and Psychiatry, 46*(7), 714–734.

Kanner, L. (1943). Autistic disturbances of affective contact. *Nervous Child, 2*, 217–250.

Karande, S., Sawant, S., Kulkarni, M., Kanchan, S., & Sholapurwala, R. (2005). Cognition in specific learning disability. *Indian Journal of Pediatrics, 72*, 1029–1043.

Kazdin, A. E., & Weisz, J. K. (2003). *Evidence-based psychotherapies for children and adolescents.* New York, NY: Guilford.

Kim, B. N., Lee, C., Hwang, J., Shin, M., & Cho, S. (2005). Effectiveness and safety of risperidone for children and adolescents with chronic tic or tourette disorders in Korea. *Journal of Child and Adolescent Psychopharmacology, 15*(2), 318–324.

Kim-Cohen, J., Arsenault, L., Caspi, A., Tomás, M. P., Taylor, A., & Moffitt, T. (2005). Validity of DSM-IV conduct disorder in 4½-5-year-old children: A longitudinal epidemiological study. *American Journal of Psychiatry, 162*(6), 1108–1117.

King, R. A., Scahill, L., Lombroso, P. J., & Leckman, J. F. (2003). Tourette's syndrome and other tic disorders. In A. Martin, L. Scahill, D. S. Charney, & J. F. Leckman (Eds.), *Pediatric psychopharmacology: Principles and practice* (1st ed., pp. 526–542). New York, NY: Oxford University Press.

Klassen, A., Miller, A., & Fine, S. (2004). Health-related quality of life in children and adolescents who have a diagnosis of attention-deficit/hyperactivity disorder. *Pediatrics, 114*(5). Retrieved April 21, 2008, from http://www.pediatrics.org/cgi/content/full/114/5/e541

Koda, V. H., Charney, D. S., & Pine, D. S. (2003). In A. Martin, L. Scahill, D. S. Charney, J. F. Leckman (Eds.), *Pediatric psychopharmacology: Principles and practice* (1st ed., pp. 138–149). New York, NY: Oxford University Press.

Labellarte, M. J., & Ginsberg, G. S. (2003). Anxiety disorders. In A. Martin, L. Scahill, D. S. Charney, J. F. Leckman (Eds.), *Pediatric psychopharmacology: Principles and practice* (1st ed., pp. 497–510). New York, NY: Oxford University Press.

Law, J., & Garrett, Z. (2004). Speech and language therapy: Its potential role in CAMHS. *Child and Adolescent Mental Health, 9*(2), 50–55.

Leonard, H. L., Ale, C. M., & Freeman, J. B. (2005). Obsessive-compulsive disorder. *Child and Adolescent Clinics of North America, 14*, 727–743.

Lynam, D., & Gudonis, L. (2005). The development of psychopathology. *Annual Review of Clinical Psychology, 1*, 381–407.

Manassis, K. (2004). Childhood anxiety disorders: Approach to interventions. *Canadian Family Physician, 50*, 379–384.

Martin, A., Van Hoof, T., Stubbe, D., Sherwin, T., & Scahill, L. (2003). Multiple psychotropic pharmacotherapy in children and adolescents: A study of Connecticut Medicaid managed care recipients. *Psychiatric Services, 54*, 72–77.

Masi, G., Milone, A., Canepa, G., Millepiedi, S., Mucci, M., & Muratori, F. (2006). Olanzapine treatment in adolescents with severe conduct disorder. *European Psychiatry, 21*, 51–57. Retrieved April 23, 2008, from www.sciencedirect.com

Maughan, B., Rowe, R., Messer, J., Goodman, R., & Meltzer, H. (2004). Conduct disorder and oppositional defiant disorder in a national sample: Developmental epidemiology. *Journal of Child Psychology and Psychiatry, 45*(3), 606–621.

McDermott, B., Lee, E., Judd, M., & Gibbon, P. (2005). Posttraumatic stress disorder and general psychopathology in children and adolescents following a wildfire disaster. *Canadian Journal of Psychiatry, 50*(3), 137–143.

McDougle, C. J., & Posey, D. J. (2003). Autistic and other pervasive developmental disorders. In A. Martin, L. Scahill, D. S. Charney, & J. F. Leckman (Eds.), *Pediatric psychopharmacology: Principles and practice* (1st ed., pp. 563–579). New York: Oxford.

McMahon, W., Carter, A., Fredine, N., & Pauls, D. (2003). Children at familial risk for Tourette's disorder: Child and parent diagnoses. *American Journal of Medical Genetics Part B: Neuropsychiatric genetics, 121B*(1), 105–111. Retrieved May 12, 2008, from http://www3interscience.wiley.com/cgi-bin/fulltext/104537823/main.html,ftx abs

McMahon-Wellington, T., Semrud-Clikeman, M., Gregory, A. L., Murphy, J. M., & Lancaster, J. L. (2006). Magnetic resonance imaging volumetric analysis of the putamen in children with ADHD: Combined type versus control. *Journal of Attention Disorders, 10*(2), 171–180. Retrieved May 8, 2008, from http://jad.sagepub.com/cgi/content/abstract/10/2/171

Mulvihill, D. (2005). The health impact of childhood trauma: An interdisciplinary review, 1997–2003. *Issues in Comprehensive Pediatric Nursing, 28*(2), 115–136.

Murray, B. (2008). Disorders diagnosed in infancy, childhood or adolescence. In P. O'Brien, W. Kennedy, & K. Ballard (Eds.), *Psychiatric mental health nursing: An introduction to theory and practice* (pp. 207–234). Boston, MA: Jones and Bartlett Publishers.

Nield, L., & Kamat, D. (2004). Enuresis: How to evaluate and treat. *Clinical Pediatrics, 43*(5), 409–415.

North American Society for Pediatric Gastroenterology, Hepatology and Nutrition (2006). Evaluation and treatment of constipation in infants: Clinical practice guidelines. *Journal of Pediatric Gastroenterology and Nutrition, 43*(3), 1–13.

Palermo, M., & Curatolo, P. (2004). Pharmacologic treatment of autism. *Journal of Child Neurology, 19*(3), 155–164.

Pelham, W., Fabiano, G., & Massetti, G. (2005). Evidence-based assessment of attention deficit hyperactivity disorder in children and adolescents. *Journal of Clinical Child and Adolescent Psychology, 34*(3), 449–476.

Perry, A., & Condillac, R. (2003). Evidence-based practices for children and adolescents with autism spectrum disorders: Review of the literature and practice guide. Toronto, Ontario: Children's Mental Health.

Persico, A., & Bourgeron, T. (2006). Searching for ways out of the autism maze: Genetic, epigenetic and environmental clues. *Trends in Neuroscience, 29*(7), 349–358.

Pinto-Martin, J., Souders, M., Giarelli, E., & Levy, S. (2005). The role of the nurse in screening for autistic spectrum disorder in pediatric primary care. *Journal of Pediatric Nursing, 20*(3), 163–169.

Polimeni, M. A., Richdale, A. L., & Francis, J. P. (2005). A survey of sleep problems in autism, Asperger's disorder and typically developing children. *Journal of Intellectual Disability Research, 49*(4), 260–268.

Prestia, K. (2003). Tourette's syndrome: Characteristics and interventions. *Intervention in School and Clinic, 39*(2), 67–71.

Ransby, M., & Swanson, H. L. (2003). Reading comprehension skills of young adults with childhood diagnosis of dyslexia. *Journal of Learning Disabilities, 36*(6), 538–555.

Rapee, R., & Spence, S. (2004). The etiology of social phobia: Empirical evidence and an initial model. *Clinical Psychology Review, 24*, 737–767.

Redston-Iselin, A. (2005). Adolescent psychiatric nursing. In G. Wiscarz-Stuart & M. Laraia (Eds.), *Principles and practice of psychiatric nursing* (pp. 753–776). St. Louis, MO: Elsevier Mosby.

Reiner, W. G. (2003). Elimination disorders: Enuresis and encopresis. In A. Martin, L. Scahill, D. S. Charney, & J. F. Leckman (Eds.), *Pediatric psychopharmacology: Principles and practice* (1st ed., pp. 686–698). New York, NY: Oxford University Press.

Richardson, A. (2006). Omega-3 fatty acids in ADHD and related neurodevelopmental disorders. *International Review of Psychiatry, 18*(2). Retrieved May 10, 2008, from http://www.ingentaconnect.com/apl/cirp/2006/00000018/00000002/art00009

Roessner, V., Becker, A., Banaschewski, T., & Rothenberger, A. (2007). Psychopathological profile in children with chronic tic disorder and co-existing ADHD: Additive effects. *Journal of Abnormal Child Psychology, 35*, 79–85.

Russell, R., & Grizzle, K. (2008). Assessing child and adolescent pragmatic language competencies: Toward evidence-based assessments. *Clinical Child and Family Psychology Review, 11*(1), 59–73.

Scahill, L., Leckman, J. F., Schultz, R. T., Katsovich, L., & Peterson, B. S. (2003). A placebo-controlled trial of risperidone in Tourette syndrome. *Neurology, 60*, 1130–1135.

Schnur, J. (2005). Asperger syndrome in children. *Journal of the American Academy of Nurse Practitioners, 17*(8), 302–308.

Seidman, L. J., Valera, E. M., & Bush, G. (2004). Brain function and structure in adults with attention-deficit/hyperactivity disorder. *Psychiatric Clinics of North America, 27*(2), 323–347.

Shaywitz, S. E. (2003). *Overcoming dyslexia* (1st ed.). New York, NY: Knopf.

Shea, S., Turgay, A., Carroll, A., Schulz, M., Orlik, H., Smith, et al. (2004). Risperidone in the treatment of disruptive behavioral symptoms in children with autistic and other pervasive developmental disorders. *Pediatrics, 114*(5), e634–e641.

Sherer, M. R., & Schreibman, L. (2005). Individual behavioral profiles and predictors of treatment effectiveness for children with autism. *Journal of Consulting and Clinical Psychology, 75*, 525–538.

Sikich, L., Hamer, R. M., Bashford, R. A., Sheitman, B. B., & Lieberman, J. A. (2004). A pilot study of risperidone, olanzapine, and haloperidol in psychotic youth: A double-blind, randomized, 8-week trial. *Neuropsychopharmacology, 29*, 133–145.

Singer, H. S. (2005). Tourette's syndrome: From behaviour to biology. *Lancet Neurology, 4*(3), 149–159.

Singer H. S., Mink, J. W., Hallett, J. J., & Lombroso, P. J. (2004). Is the microinfusion of antineuronal antibodies into rodent striatum a valid method to evaluate autoimmunity in pediatric movement disorders? *Annals of Neurology, 56*(Suppl. 8), S89.

Smith, J., & McSherry, W. (2004). Spirituality and child development: A concept analysis. *Journal of Advanced Nursing, 45*(3), 307–315.

Sowell, E. R., Thompson, P. M., Welcome, S. E., Henkenius, A. L., Toga, A. W., & Peterson, B. S. (2003). Cortical abnormalities in children and adolescents with attention-deficit hyperactivity disorder. *Lancet, 362*(9397), 1699–1707.

Speraw, S. (2006). Spiritual experiences of parents and caregivers who have children with disabilities or special needs. *Issues in Mental Health Nursing, 27*, 213–230.

Stephens, R. J., Bassel, C., & Sandor, P. (2004). Olanzapine in the treatment of aggression and tics in children with Tourette's syndrome: A pilot study. *Journal of Child and Adolescent Psychopharmacology, 14*(2), 255–266.

Stewart, S. E., Geller, D. A., Jenike, M., Pauls, D., Shaw, D., Mullin, B., et al. (2004). Long-term outcome of pediatric obsessive-compulsive disorder: A meta-analysis and qualitative review of the literature. *Acta Psychiatrica Scandinavica, 110*(1), 4–13.

Stewart, S. E., Rosario, M. C., Brown, T. A., Carter, A. S., Leckman, J. F., Sukhodolsky, D., et al. (2007). Principal components analysis of obsessive-compulsive disorder symptoms in children and adolescents. *Biological Psychiatry, 61*, 285–291.

Storch, E. A., Murphy, T. K., Geffken, G. R., Sajid, M., Allen, P., Roberti, J. W., et al. (2005). Reliability and validity of the Yale Global Tic Severity Scale. *Psychological Assessment, 17*(4), 486–491.

Strauss, J., Barr, C. L., George, C. J., Devlin, B., Veto, A., Baji, I., et al.; The International Consortium for Childhood Onset Mood Disorders. (2005). Brain-derived neurotropic factor variants are associated with childhood-onset mood disorder: Confirmation in a Hungarian sample. *Molecular Psychiatry, 10*, 861–867.

Van Grootheest, D., Cath, D., Beekman, A., & Boomsma, D. (2005). Twin studies on obsessive compulsive disorder: a review. *Twin Research and Human Genetics, 8*(5), 450–458.

Volkmar, F. R., Klin, A., & Paul, R. (2004). *Handbook of autism and pervasive developmental disorders* (3rd ed.). New York, NY: Wiley.

Waddell, C., Godderis, R., Hua, J., McEwan, K., & Wong, W. (2004). Preventing and treating anxiety disorders in children and youth. *Children's Mental Health Policy Research Program*. Vancouver: British Columbia Ministry of Children and Family Development.

Waddell, C., McEwan, K., Shepherd, C., Offord, D., & Hua, J. M. (2005). A public health strategy to improve the mental health of Canadian children. *Canadian Journal of Psychiatry, 50*(4), 226–233.

Webster-Stratton, C., Reid, J., & Hammond, M. (2004). Treating children with early-onset conduct problems: Interventions outcomes for parent, child, and teacher training. *Journal of Clinical Child and Adolescent Psychology, 33*(1), 105–124.

Witwer, A., & Lecavalier, L. (2005). Treatment incidence and patterns in children and adolescents with autism spectrum disorder. *Journal of Child and Adolescent Psychopharmacology, 15*(4), 671–681.

Acknowledgments

The original work was supported in part by the following: United States Public Health Service grants: Children's Clinical Research Center Grant RR06022; Program Project Grant MH49351 from the National Institute of Mental Health; Program Project Grant HD-03008 from the National Institute of Child Health and Human Development; Research Units on Pediatric Psychopharmacology; contract MH-70009 from the National Institute of Mental Health.

UNIT *VI*
Older Adults

CHAPTER 29

Mental Health Promotion With the Older Adult

Sharon L. Moore

Adapted from the chapter "Mental Health Promotion With the Older Adult" by Mary Ann Boyd

LEARNING OBJECTIVES

After studying this chapter, you will be able to:

- Identify the important bio/psycho/social/spiritual factors occurring in late adulthood.
- Identify the risk factors related to geriatric psychopathology.
- Analyze the nurse's role in mental health promotion with older adults and their families.
- Discuss mental health prevention and promotion interventions that are especially effective with older adults.

KEY CONCEPT

- late adulthood

KEY TERMS

- gerotranscendence • middle-old • old-old • young-old

C anada, like many other countries, is experiencing a boom in population growth of seniors. At the beginning of the 21st century, nearly 4 million of the 30 million Canadians were older adults. Statistics Canada estimates this number will grow to 5.7 million by the year 2016 and will double to more than 9 million by the year 2031 (National Advisory Council on Aging [NACA], 2003, 2005; Turcotte & Schellenberg, 2007). In 2007, individuals older than 65 years comprised 13.4% of the population, up from 12.7% in 2002 (Statistics Canada, 2007). It is predicted that by the year 2031, they will account for 25% of the population. NACA reports that seniors are the fastest growing age group in the country. Because women tend to live longer than men, they dominate the fastest growing segment of the senior population, those older than 80 years (Edwards & Mawani, 2006).

Mental health concerns among older adults are a significant problem in Canada. With the increase in aging population, there is a concomitant increase in the number of older adults with psychiatric disorders. The Southern Alberta Geriatric Mental Health Working Group (2003) reported 15% to 30% prevalence rates in the community, while the Canadian Coalition for Seniors' Mental Health (2003) reported a 50% to 80% prevalence rate for mental disorders within nursing homes and long-term care settings in Canada.

These disorders can substantially impair functioning and can result in unnecessary hospitalizations and nursing home placement, poorer health outcomes, and increased rates of mortality. For example, older persons who suffer from depression have worse outcomes after medical events such as hip fractures, heart attacks, or cancer, and individuals who are age 75 and older have the highest suicide rate of any age group (National Alliance on Mental Illness, 2001, p. 1). It is also well documented that, for older adults, it takes less alcohol to exacerbate medical and mental problems, and, in turn, medical and emotional problems may contribute to further alcohol use (Public Health Agency of Canada, 2002; Sattar, Petty, & Burke, 2003).

Older adults' mental health needs are not easily addressed within generic treatment programs as older adults have "unique attributes that distinguish their mental health needs from those of other groups" (Standing Senate Committee on Social Affairs, Science and Technology, 2006, p. 158). Mental health promotion and mental illness prevention efforts that are targeted at meeting the needs of older adults are needed to help them maintain optimum health and quality of life. It is important for nurses to understand and respond well to the unique needs of this special population.

This chapter explains the effect of aging on mental health and identifies risk factors related to geriatric psychopathology.

MENTAL HEALTH OF THE OLDER ADULT

KEY CONCEPT Late adulthood can be divided into three chronologic groups: *young-old* (ages 65 to 74 years), **middle-old** (ages 75 to 84 years), and *old-old* (age 85 years and older).

Adults 85 years and older are the most rapidly growing segment of the Canadian population. From 1921 until 1998, the population of **old-old** adults has increased 20 times (Lindsay & Almay, 1999). The transition from **young-old** to old-old is more than a series of birthdays; it is a gradual bio/psycho/social/spiritual process that may be viewed as both positive and negative. From a positive perspective, the later years provide time for personal growth and development, providing an opportunity to do all the things that were impossible when work and family responsibilities took precedence. Travelling, visiting friends, and engaging in neglected hobbies enhance quality of life and improve well-being.

In late adulthood, changes in health status can lead to negative outcomes. A loss in physical functioning can lead to a loss in independence, which can result in an unplanned change in residence. Family relationships change, as once-dependent children grow into adulthood and become parents themselves. Friendships change, and losses occur. Many older adults retire from meaningful lifelong work and are faced with establishing new meaning in life. To have a sense of meaning and purpose is a critical factor in older adults' mental health and is one of the factors that serves as a protection against suicide and despair in later life (Moore, 1997; Moore, Metcalf, & Schow, 2000).

In all health care settings, communication is an integral factor in nursing care. Communication with older adults requires special attention to verbal interactions and environmental influences. Box 29-1 highlights some necessary considerations.

BOX 29.1

Communicating With Older Adults

- Focus the person's attention on the exchange of communication; the older adult may need extra time to begin to process information.
- Face the person when speaking to him or her.
- Minimize distractions in the room, including other people, objects in your hands, noise, and other activities.
- Reduce glare from room lighting by dimming too-bright lights. Conversely, avoid sitting in shadows.
- Speak slowly and clearly. Older adults may depend on lip reading, so ensure that the individual can see you. Speak loudly, but do not shout. It is not necessary to over enunciate with exaggerated lip movements.
- Use short, simple sentences and be prepared to repeat or revise what you have said.
- Limit the number of topics discussed at one time to prevent information overload.
- Ask one question at a time to minimize confusion. Allow plenty of time for the person to answer and express ideas.
- Frequently summarize the important points of the conversation to improve understanding and comprehension.
- Avoid the urge to finish sentences.
- If the communication exchange is going poorly, postpone it for another time.

Biologic Domain

During the later years of adulthood, changes in vital biologic structure and processes can occur in a particular organ or tissue or in the whole body. Changes may occur from disuse after the function of the organ has been fulfilled (e.g., the uterus or thymus gland) or from disuse associated with insufficient exercise or movement (e.g., in neuromusculoskeletal systems). Body fat increases (18% to 36% in men, 33% to 48% in women), total body water decreases (10% to 15%), and muscle mass decreases. Distinguishing whether changes occur because of decreased physical activity, level of motivation, influence of societal expectations, or cumulative effects of disease is difficult.

When changes occur in the organ systems, functional capacity is often decreased. However, many older adults can integrate profound decrements in physical capacity without affecting the ability to function under normal conditions. It is only when functional reserves are needed, such as during an infection, that the absence of these reserves is observed. The following sections highlight significant biologic changes that occur in later adulthood.

Renal Changes

Even without disease, a predictable decline in glomerular filtration and tubular secretion occurs with aging. Renal blood flow decreases by as much as 10% every decade after age 40. Renal clearance is estimated to decrease by as much as 35% between the ages of 20 and 90 years. These changes result in decreased renal excretion, which is of particular concern because the kidneys excrete most drugs (Tiao, Semmens, Masarei, & Lawrence-Brown, 2002).

Gastrointestinal Changes

Blood flow in the liver tends to decline with advancing age, decreasing as much as 40% to 50% by the age of 65. Reduced cardiac output is the major factor slowing blood flow through the liver. Reduced blood flow decreases the liver's opportunity to metabolize medications; consequently, medications may remain in the blood longer, increasing the risk for toxicity. As a result, fat-soluble drugs become sequestered in fatty tissue, rather than remaining in the circulating plasma. These factors increase the risk for accumulation and drug toxicity (Anantharaju, Feller, & Chedid, 2002).

Neurologic Changes

Nervous system changes that occur with aging include central and peripheral neuronal cell loss; slowed transmission of nerve impulses; slowed reaction time; diminished proprioception, balance, and postural control; poor thermoregulation; and altered sleep patterns. The effects of changes in the nervous system are confounded by changes in other systems, such as the cardiovascular system (e.g., decreased arterial elasticity) and the respiratory system (e.g., diminished response to hypoxia and hypercapnia). Physiologic changes occurring with physical illness may precipitate altered mental status (e.g., delirium) or exacerbate symptoms of existing psychiatric illness (e.g., depression).

The brain, like most other body organs, undergoes changes with aging. Although brain weight begins to decline after the age of 30, visible atrophy is not apparent until about 60 years of age. Brain weight decreases by about 10% from early life to the 9th decade; this change is reflected in enlarged ventricles and widened sulci. Brain atrophy may result from a net loss of neurons (Scahill et al., 2003).

Sensory Changes

All five senses decline with age. This factor is important to remember when assessing older adult patients with psychiatric illnesses because diminished senses may affect attention and perception, potentially affecting interpretation of standard mental status examinations. Structural changes in the eye include rigidity of the iris, accumulation of yellow substance in the lens, and diminished lens elasticity. These changes result in decreased pupil size, alteration in colour perception, presbyopia, impaired adaptation to darkness, and significant vision impairment in the presence of glare (Bakker, 2003). Auditory changes are noticeable as early as 40 years of age; however, age of onset varies according to lifestyle (e.g., previous exposure to occupational noise). Cochlear neurons are lost, resulting in hearing loss that may affect performance on intelligence tests. Several other factors beyond loss of hearing can influence age-related differences in performance on intelligence tests. Research on taste, touch, and smell is sparse, but a uniform dulling of these senses occurs with aging. The rate of decline is highly variable among individuals.

Sexuality

Misinformation and attitudinal barriers continue to plague the study of sexuality in the aging individual. Several generalizations, however, have emerged: older adults retain interest in sex, frequency of sexual activity is less than desired, and increasing problems with sexual performance are associated with increasing age in both men and women. Although several physical changes with aging affect sexual functioning, interest in and enjoyment of sexual activities can continue until one's death. Health, the desire to remain sexually active, access to a partner, and a conducive environment contribute to positive sexual functioning.

Physiologic changes in women include decreasing estrogen levels, alterations in the structural integrity of the vagina (e.g., decreased blood flow, decreased flexibility, diminished lubrication, and diminished response during orgasm), and decreased breast engorgement during arousal (Wright, 2001). The sexual response continues as in younger women but with less intensity. Even with chronic illness, many older women remain interested in and satisfied with a variety of sexual activities. Although being older is often associated with a decrease in sexual interest in women, sexual attitudes and knowledge are also important predictors of interest, participation, and satisfaction with sexual activity. In reality, sexual activity in aging women often depends on availability of a partner.

Physiologic changes in men include a decline in testosterone production, increased time to achieve erection, less firm erections, decreased urgency for ejaculation, decreased sperm production, and a longer refractory period (i.e., the amount of time before the man can achieve another erection; Wright, 2001). Problems with sexual performance in aging men are usually associated with erectile dysfunction.

In men, frequency and desired frequency for sexual activity decline as age increases. Men are more likely to be sexually active but are less satisfied with their level of sexual activity than are women. As with women, partner availability and willingness influence the frequency of sexual activity.

Access to a conducive environment may be hindered if the parent resides with an adult child or in a nursing home. Although nursing home residents may remain interested in maintaining sexual relationships, the attitudes of the staff and physicians constitute an additional barrier for this population beyond those noted previously (Bauer, 1999; Gott & Hinchliff, 2003).

Psychological Domain

Cognitive Function

Changes in cognition are most likely accounted for by structural and functional changes in the brain (Rosenzweig & Barnes, 2003). These alterations are probably highly specific because aspects of cognitive decline are very specific (e.g., secondary memory), and many abilities are preserved. Moreover, external factors, including activity levels, socioeconomic status, education, and personality, may modify the development or the expression of age-related changes in cognition (see Chapter 30). Normal aging does not impair consciousness. Alertness is required for attention, but the alert patient may not necessarily be able to attend. Attention has two aspects: sustained attention (vigilance) and selective attention (ability to extract relevant from irrelevant information). Numerous studies indicate that older adults perform well on tests of sustained and selective attention (Ebersole, Touhy, Hess, & Jett, 2007; Yevchak, Loeb, & Fick, 2008). Earlier findings of poor performance on tests of selective attention have been attributed to lack of control for perceptual difficulties (e.g., vision and hearing deficits).

Slower reaction time may affect how quickly an older adult responds to questions. Hurrying older adults to answer questions may interfere with their ability to provide the correct answer. This has been labelled the *speed-accuracy shift*, by which the older adult focuses more on accuracy than on speed in responding. Caution tends to increase, whereas risk-taking behaviour tends to decrease; older adults are more likely to make errors of omission (leaving the answer out) than errors of commission (making a guess; Zimprich, 2002).

Learning

Intelligence and personality are stable across the life span in the absence of disease; however, the learning abilities of older adults may be more selective, requiring motivation ("How important is this information?"), meaningful content ("Why do I need to know this?"), and familiarity with the idea or content. Although age causes no differences in the ability to process knowledge to learn a skill, younger people are more likely to employ strategies to learn tasks. Level of education needs to be considered in evaluating responses on mental status examinations because it may represent socioeconomic status and occupation.

Memory

Other than overall intelligence, age-related memory alterations have been more widely studied than any other aspect of cognition. Contrary to popular belief, memory loss is not a normal part of aging. To remember events, individuals must first attend to information and process it. Older adults may well dismiss information that is not important to them. Memory problems in later life are believed to result from encoding problems or "getting" the information in the first place. This problem may be related to sensory problems, not paying attention, or a general failure to link the "to be remembered" information to existing knowledge through association or to strengthen the memory through repetition. However, it is important not to confuse decline with deficit. Although a decline in memory ability may be frustrating for the older individual, it does not necessarily hamper his or her ability to function daily. Threats to memory include medications, depression (impairs concentration and attention), poor nutrition, infection, heart and lung disease (lack of oxygen), thyroid problems (can cause symptoms of depression or confusion that mimic memory loss), alcohol use, and sensory loss (interferes with perception).

Development

Late-life adult developmental phenomena have not been well-defined (see Chapter 8). Although Erik Erikson identified "integrity versus despair" as a developmental task specific to late adulthood, his wife recently published an extension of his theory that included old age as a ninth stage, **gerotranscendence** (Erikson & Erikson, 1997). Gerotranscendence is a psychosocial theory of aging that regards aging as the final stage in a "possible natural progression towards maturation and wisdom" (Tornstam, 2005, p. 1) that generally results in increased satisfaction and meaning in life. Rather than emphasizing decrements in physical capacity for function, gerotranscendence theory provides for continued growth in dimensions such as spirituality and inner strength (Wadensten, 2007; Wadensten & Carlsson, 2007a, 2007b; see Box 29-2).

The concept of gerotranscendence may be used in establishing health promotion interventions. Research suggests that the following guidelines may help the staff support older adults in their process toward gerotranscendence:

- Accept the possibility that behaviours resembling the signs of gerotranscendence are normal signs of aging.
- Reduce preoccupation with the body.
- Allow alternative definitions of time.
- Allow thoughts and conversations about death.
- Choose topics of conversation that facilitate and further older people's personal growth.

BOX 29.2

Research for Best Practice

Marziali, E., McDonald, L., & Donahue, P. (2008). The role of coping humor in the physical and mental health of older adults. Aging & Mental Health, 12(6), 713–718.

QUESTION: Is the use of humour as a coping strategy related to the older adult's maintenance of a supportive social network, spiritual belief system, self-efficacious belief system, and self-perception of mental and physical health status?

METHOD: An exploratory survey of personal/social factors and health status of 73 community dwelling older adults in a Canadian city was implemented. A home interview was conducted and several questionnaires completed, including the Health Status Questionnaire and two mental health status self-report scales (depression and anxiety) as dependent variable measures. Independent variable measures included the Coping Humor Scale, the Multidimensional Scale of Perceived Social Support, the Spiritual Involvement and

Beliefs Scale, and a self-efficacy scale, based on Bandura's model (see Chapter 8).

FINDINGS: Significant positive correlations were found among social support, self-efficacy, and coping humour. Unlike previous research, associations between social support and physical health and between spirituality and both physical and mental health statuses were not found. The researchers note the small sample size as a limitation and query the type of scale they used to measure spirituality.

IMPLICATIONS FOR PRACTICE: Being able to use one's sense of humour to cope with stress may converge with possessing a sense of self-efficacy. Humour may be a self-efficacious strategy for coping with adversity. Coping humour, self-efficacy, and social support may be factors that balance self-attributes with social connectedness.

- Accept, create, and introduce new types of activities.
- Encourage and facilitate quiet and peaceful places and times (Wadensten & Carlsson, 2003).

Relationship Strains

As family relationships change, interpersonal relationship strains can develop. Disappointments with lifestyles of adult children and changes in caregiving responsibilities may affect the quality of a longtime family relationship. In some instances, young-old adults assume caregiving responsibilities for their old-old relatives. It is also common for grandparents to assume some caregiving responsibilities for their grandchildren. A change in work status of grandparents (the fact that many of them work today) has drastically changed the "face" of grandparenting in Canada.

With Canadians living longer and healthier lives, grandparents are playing a larger part in the lives of their families. A century ago, grandparents could expect to have only 10 years with their grandchildren; that statistic has doubled to 20 years today. As most Canadian women can expect to live to be at least 82 years of age, many will spend nearly half of their lives as grandmothers. As well, many more Canadians can expect to become great-grandparents than those in the past (NACA, 2005). While there are positive benefits to grandparents being able to spend more time with their grandchildren, clinical experience suggests that this can also be problematic in cities where there have been large immigrant populations where grandparents who immigrate to provide child care can become extremely isolated, contributing to mental health problems.

Social Domain

Functional Status

Functional status, the extent to which a person can independently carry out personal care, home management, and social functions in everyday life in a way that has meaning and purpose, often changes during the later years (see Chapter 30). Estimates of the prevalence of functional dependency vary, but, in general, studies show that difficulty in performing activities of daily living (ADLs) increases with advancing age and that rates of dependency are significantly higher for women than for men, particularly for women who live alone (von Strauss, Aguero-Torres, Kareholt, Winblad, & Fratiglioni, 2003).

Although older women and men have similar paths to life satisfaction, a Canadian study conducted by Bourque, Pushkar, Bonneville, and Beland (2005) reported that there are important differences. Men's greater independence allows them to be less dependent on environmental and social factors for life satisfaction; women's greater social embeddedness enables them to be as satisfied as men with life in general, even though their life circumstances may be poorer.

Retirement

A trend toward early retirement is becoming more common in Canada (mostly in the public sector). Between 1987 and 2000, 29% of adults retired before the age of 60. From 1997 until 2005, 42% of adults retired before the age of 60 (Charron, 2007).

The transition from a paid work role to a potentially less structured and purposeful pattern of living can lead to alterations in self-concept. While retirement is often chosen, it is frequently characterized as a stressful life event that may bring psychological, social, and economic uncertainty. It affects social roles, income, use of health services, and participation in leisure activities. Although these changes are often associated with negative myths and stereotypes, most people do very well in retirement. Adequate pensions, savings/investments, and social assistance contribute to its success.

Cultural Impact

As the population ages in Canadian society, it is also becoming more culturally diverse. Our North American communities are increasingly a reflection of multiple ethnic histories and values (Hayes-Bautista, Hsu, Perez, & Gamboa, 2002). Before the 1960s, immigrants to Canada were mostly from Europe; since the late 1980s, immigrants are increasingly from Asia, Central and South America, and Africa (Tam, Fletcher, & Chi, 2004). Wide cultural variations exist in family expectations of and responsibilities for the older adult. Some groups, such as Aboriginal and Asian cultures, tend to highly value the experience and wisdom of their older family members, and younger family members feel a responsibility for their care. This cultural belief can create additional pressures for younger family members who may not have the resources to fulfill these expectations.

Immigrants and refugees who come to Canada constitute a heterogeneous group who frequently experience loneliness, uprootedness, "brokenness" and "woundedness." Older adults, in addition to facing such problems, often do not speak the language, become further isolated, and have difficulty expressing mental health needs (Standing Senate Committee on Social Affairs, Science and Technology, 2006).

Further research is needed to understand and address the relationships between cultural issues related to aging, health, and health care delivery. We do know that treatment and intervention are most effective when patients, families, and the health care team can work together to integrate patients' beliefs and cultural values into the plan of care.

Social Activities

While the majority of older adults acknowledge that their health is good, there are health conditions that may prevent participation in home maintenance and leisure activities, especially walking, gardening, and active sports. Among serious health conditions in the years after retirement, lung disease and diabetes most seriously affect leisure activities. As age increases, participation decreases. Higher education levels are associated with increased participation in both formal and informal activities (Holmes & Dorfman, 2000). Interestingly, in a study of older adults volunteering for Habitat for Humanity, it was found that these volunteers were not physically healthier than community counterparts, but were mentally healthier (Brown, Mefford, Chen, & Brown,

2009). Positive attitudes around notions of "everyone contributes" and "adjusting to limitations" were displayed.

Impacts of Aging on Housing and Communities

The aging of the Canadian population is requiring a reshaping of the pattern of housing needs, the demand for services, and the ways in which communities are being structured to make them more responsive to individuals with disabilities (Canada Mortgage and Housing Corporation [CMHC], 2008). CMHC further reports that while life expectancy for men is increasing, women in their 80s outnumber men by almost 50% and by more than 50% among older adults in their 90s. These trends are placing additional demands for a variety of services responsive to the needs of this population.

Most older adults prefer to age in surroundings that are familiar to them until their health prohibits them from doing so. CMHC (2008) reported that 85% of individuals surveyed older than 55 years said they planned to remain in their own homes as long as possible, even if health challenges required additional support for home maintenance or personal care from government and private service providers. Implications for health promotion are such that nurses need to be vigilant in their assessment skills, providing ongoing support and facilitating early intervention when needed.

The types of facilities and supports to assist older adults to age in place vary across the country and seem to depend in large part on provincial funding. All provinces will need to address the changing demographics that require a variety of community and residential housing options.

> The rapid growth in numbers of older seniors who live alone, are frail, or have disabilities will necessitate considerable expansion of supportive housing choices that enable them to stay in the community rather than in long-term health facilities, such as nursing homes. (CMHC, 2008, p. 5)

Residential Care

Various residential care models are in part a response to the medical model emphasized in most long-term care facilities and the need to develop alternatives to nursing home care. Residential care models include a spectrum of residential living environments, such as foster care homes, family homes, personal care homes, residential care facilities, and assisted living arrangements.

According to Statistics Canada, approximately 7% of seniors live in nursing homes and health care facilities, and "the proportion of seniors that enter those facilities rises steadily with age, to 13% of those 75 and older" (CMHC, 2008, p. 5). Residential facilities are seeing increased numbers of older adults with mental and physical health challenges, presenting both opportunities and challenges to supporting these individuals.

Assisted Living

The assisted living concept has emerged as an important long-term care alternative for older adults who are mentally and physically frail. Assisted living provides community-based residential services for older adults and adults with physical disabilities who need help with ADLs. Assisted living services combine housing, personal services, and light medical or nursing care. Perhaps the most important feature of these assisted living facilities is the orientation toward the older resident that empowers the frail older adult by sharing responsibilities for care and ADLs, enhancing their choices, and managing risks.

Spiritual Domain

Humanists suggest that the main purpose of life is to find meaning and that this can be accomplished through creations (or accomplishments), experiences in the world, and attitude toward suffering (Frankl, 1963). In nursing, spirituality is recognized as a basic quality, inherent in all humans. The spiritual perspective includes three critical attributes:

- Connectedness (with other humans, nature, universal forces, or God)
- Beliefs in powers or forces beyond the self and a faith that affirms life
- A creative energy

The spiritual perspective also can provide a path for the quest for the meaning of life and can organize and guide human values and motivations.

Spirituality can be extremely important to the older adult and can positively affect attitude, particularly as health declines (Lowry & Conco, 2002).

▨ RISK FACTORS FOR GERIATRIC PSYCHOPATHOLOGY

Chronic Illnesses

Although the frequency of acute conditions declines with advancing age, about 90% of older adults have chronic medical conditions that can adversely affect function. Poor physical health is a well-established risk factor for mental disorders. The major chronic conditions experienced by older adults are ischemic heart disease, hypertension, vision impairment, hearing impairment, musculoskeletal impairment, and diabetes (U.S. Department of Health and Human Services, 2001). Chronic illnesses can reduce physiologic capacity and consequently increase functional dependency. In addition, during acute episodes of illness, many older adults lose functional ability because they have limited reserves or cannot mobilize reserves to regain their premorbid performance levels.

Polypharmacy

Polypharmacy, the use of several medications, is often associated with chronic illness and long-term drug therapy (see Chapter 30). The Canadian Broadcasting Corporation (CBC; 2007) reports that seniors in Canada take more prescription drugs than the general population and account for almost 40% of all prescription medications. In 2005, through an analysis of Health Canada data, CBC estimated that "3,330 seniors die every year due to adverse drug reactions," a number which probably underestimates the actual number of deaths. In addition, many more older adults are impacted by adverse drug reactions. The Canadian Institute for Health Information (CIHI) notes that "seniors are at greater risk for adverse effects due to complex drug therapies and age related changes to the body" (2007, p. 19). Adverse drug reactions create a significant economic burden on the health care system.

Beer's criteria is an internationally recognized list of drugs, developed by Dr. Mark Beers, that identifies "potentially inappropriate" drugs to prescribe to seniors due to a heightened risk of adverse effects. CBC reported that in 2004, almost one and a half million—or more than 1/3 of Canadian seniors—were prescribed such drugs, even though safer alternatives were available (CBC, 2005). According to a study carried out by CIHI (2007), the percentage of Canada's older adults taking potentially harmful drugs dropped from 34% in 2000–2001 to 17% in 2005–2006 based on an analysis of drug claims in four Canadian provinces. While this is encouraging, the study also noted an increase in the use of other drugs, such as the antidepressant amitriptyline.

Serious problems result when coordination of the care delivery and treatment regimen specific to prescribed medications is lacking. These problems are compounded when the patient uses over-the-counter drugs, herbal remedies, and home or folk remedies without considering their potential interaction with prescribed drugs. Nurses can follow the principles delineated in Box 29-3 to improve drug therapy with older adults.

Bereavement and Loss

Older adults experience many losses—friends and family members die, physical health compromises, and social status diminishes. Loss of one's spouse, particularly when the relationship has been long and satisfying, constitutes a major life event. Women are more likely to lose their spouses and tend to be widowed at a younger age than are men. Consequently, women have more time to adjust and develop substitute social relationships to replace the spouse. Conversely, men tend to lose their wives at an older age, have fewer social networks to replace the spouse, and express feelings of loneliness and abandonment. Because of differences in longevity,

BOX 29.3

Drug Therapy Interventions

- Administer priority/life essential medications first.
- Minimize the number of drugs that the person uses, keeping only those drugs that are essential.
- Always consider alternatives among different drug classifications or dosage forms that are more suitable for older adults. Monitor the claim trends for Beers drugs.
- Implement preventive measures to reduce the need for certain medications. Such prevention includes health promotion through proper nutrition, exercise, and stress reduction.
- Most age-dependent pharmacokinetic changes lead to potential accumulation of the drug; therefore, medication dosage should start low and go slow.
- Exercise caution when administering medication with a long half-life or in an older adult with impaired renal or liver function. Under these conditions, the time may be extended between doses.
- Be knowledgeable of each drug's properties, including such factors as half-life, excretion, and adverse effects. For example, venlafaxine HCl (Effexor), a structurally novel

antidepressant that inhibits the reuptake of serotonin and norepinephrine, requires regular monitoring of the older person's blood pressure.
- Assess the individual's clinical history for physical problems that may affect excretion of medications to assess for orthostatic hypotension and the potential for falls.
- Monitor laboratory values (e.g., creatinine clearance) and urinary output in patients receiving medications eliminated by the kidneys.
- Monitor plasma albumin levels in patients receiving drugs that have high binding affinity to protein
- Regularly monitor the older person's reaction to all medications to ensure a therapeutic response.
- Look for potential drug interactions that may complicate therapy. Antacids lower gastric acidity and may decrease the rate at which other medications are dissolved and absorbed.
- Remind older adults to consult with their health care provider before taking any over-the-counter medications.

---

men and women usually experience life events at different ages.

Gender differences in reactions to loss through death have been reported. One study (Benedict & Zhang, 1999) asked 391 individuals who had lost a spouse, parent, child, other relative, or friend to recall their experiences at the time of the loss. Significantly, more women than men recalled being highly emotional at the time of the loss; the recovery period after the loss was longer for women. However, more men than women wished that they could have changed past relationships with their families. One possible explanation for the findings in this study is that a significantly higher percentage of women (38.5%) than men (15.1%) had lost a spouse; whereas, men more often reported the loss of a parent (52.4% for men versus 39.8% for women).

Regardless of gender differences, survivors are at higher risk for depression and face financial issues after the death of a loved one. Health care professionals should work closely with grieving survivors to help them understand that their lives will be displaced for some time. Support sessions on the grief process and financial and employment planning could become a standard part of care.

Poverty

Because retirement and losing a spouse are common events in later life, older adults (particularly women) can be at higher risk for poverty than other age groups. Two groups of poor older adults include those who have lived in poverty all their lives and those who become impoverished in late life. Poverty may result from inadequate

retirement income, illness, discrimination against women in pension plans, and financial exploitation of older individuals. Poverty has significant effects on this population, including higher mortality rates, poorer health, lower health-related quality of life, lower likelihood of participating in health screening programs, and higher likelihood of using the emergency department for acute illness (Fleming, Evans, & Chutka, 2003).

Suicide and the Lack of Social Support

Suicide is a leading cause of preventable death in Canada and worldwide. The Canadian Association for Suicide Prevention (CASP) reports that more than 400,000 Canadians engage in some type of self-harm behaviour every year and that in the past 30 years, many of the 100,000 people who have died by suicide in Canada have been older adults (CASP, 2004). Older adults tend to use more lethal methods than younger people in their suicide attempts. Firearms are the most common method of suicide for men, while women tend to use self-poisoning or suffocation (Moore, Grek, Heisl, & Jackson, 2006). The general population engages in suicidal behaviour approximately 20 times for every death to suicide; older adults, in contrast, may do so fewer than four times (Conwell et al., 1998; McIntosh, Santos, Hubbard, & Overholser, 1994). "The lethality of suicidal behaviour and related likelihood of death among older adults are especially disturbing in light of large estimated increases in the older Canadian population in coming years" (Statistics Canada, 2005, p. 1).

A lack of social support has been linked to the rate of suicide in older adults (Heisl, 2004; Heisl & Duberstein,

2005), the highest rates being for divorced or widowed men. Risk factors for suicide in older adults include being white, male, widowed or divorced, retired or unemployed, living alone in an urban area, in poor health (including poor mental health) or lonely, and having a history of poor interpersonal relationships (Waern, Rubenowitz, & Wilhelmson, 2003).

MENTAL ILLNESS PREVENTION AND MENTAL HEALTH PROMOTION

There is growing evidence of the cumulative benefits of regular physical activity when sustained over time (Health Canada, 2002; Mental Health Commission of Canada [MHCC], 2009; Shields & Martel, 2006). An improvement in mental health and psychological well-being has been noted, and there is some early, promising evidence that links participation in regular physical activity with a decreased likelihood of developing dementia (Larson et al., 2006; Wang, Larson, Bowen, & van Belle, 2006). While these benefits are widely known, Health Canada (2002) notes that a large number of older Canadians do not participate in enough activity to maintain or promote their health and well-being.

Mental health promotion efforts of nurses should include facilitating appropriate levels and types of increased physical activity for older adults. There is substantial evidence to show the positive benefits and improvements not only in physical well-being but also in mental and emotional well-being (Health Canada, 2002; Ministry of Healthy Living and Support, 2008; Shields & Martel, 2006). Health Canada notes that "increasing daily energy expenditure by all Canadians of every age is a well-known health promotion and disease prevention resource that is as important as smoking cessation for public health" (p. 4).

Mental Illness

Preventing Depression and Suicide

Mental illness prevention is aimed at addressing the risk factors associated with mental illness and "enhancing the protective factors that inhibit its onset or shorten its duration" (Standing Senate Committee on Social Affairs, Science and Technology, 2006, p. 515). Depression is one of the most common mental disorders in older adults (see Chapter 20). Recognition and early intervention are the keys to preventing ongoing depressive episodes. Early indications of symptomatology can be identified in primary care settings. Several preventive interventions, such as grief counselling for widows and widowers, self-help groups, and social activities, are helpful. Community-based projects have been effective in significantly reducing

suicide rates in older adults (Heisl & Duberstein, 2005). By assessing and addressing cognitive and social-cognitive vulnerability factors and by focusing on the promotion of life satisfaction, nurses can help not only to prevent suicide but also to assist the older adult in achieving a healthier and more meaningful life (Grek, 2007; Heisl, 2004, 2006). Increasingly, studies are exploring concepts such as meaning and hope and the role that these play in helping older adults live well (Heisl & Duberstein; Moore, 1997).

Reducing the Stigma of Mental Health Treatment

The stigma of mental illness continues to interfere with the willingness of older adults to seek treatment. Today's older Canadians grew up during a time when institutionalization in asylums, electroconvulsive treatments, and other treatment approaches were regarded with fear. This fear can lead to denial of problems. The work of the MHCC has recognized the critical importance of combating stigma and discrimination. The commission has launched a 10-year antistigma campaign, recognizing that combating stigma requires a multi-pronged effort sustained over a long period of time and includes: ongoing community based education and action, media campaigns, and forums of exchange between affected individuals and other Canadians to enhance public awareness, and professional awareness campaigns to reduce structural discrimination in the health care system and in the mental health system itself. (Standing Senate Committee on Social Affairs, Science and Technology, 2006, p. 25)

Nurses are in a primary position to participate in these initiatives at local and national levels. They can also assist older adults in understanding mental health concerns when they arise and encourage them to access appropriate services.

> **· CRNENOTE**
>
> Safety concerns are a priority. Carefully explore any suicidal ideation and develop a plan for intervention and prevention.

Use of Medications

With the approval of new medications, older adults will be able to treat health problems with pharmacologic agents that were not previously available. Side effects and drug interactions should be carefully monitored to detect untoward symptoms and delirium (see Chapter 31).

Education of older adults and their families regarding a medication regimen is crucial to ensure adherence and to minimize untoward effects. Basic principles regarding neurobiologic changes in normal aging (as previously discussed) should be applied when designing teaching strategies. The nurse must consider the older adult's pace of learning as well as any visual and hearing deficits. Education should include the reason for administering the drug and important side effects of the drug. The nurse should provide instructional aids, large-print labelling, and devices such as medication calendars that encourage adherence to the treatment plan. Patients should be aware that they can reject childproof containers for their medications if they have trouble opening them.

Avoiding Premature Institutionalization

In Canada, as in many countries around the world, health care reform has drastically affected how health care is delivered. Such reform has focused on a move from institutional care to home care. Research has demonstrated that there is significant potential for home care to support the mental health and well-being of seniors in the community (Parent, Anderson, & Huestis, 2002). Supportive community-based services can help to avoid premature institutionalization in seniors. There is evidence that governments are increasingly recognizing the impacts of population aging and looking to make necessary changes. These include appropriate adaptations to "facilitate mobility, improve safety and security, and to permit ADL without strain or injury"; improved access to transportation and to location of services; proper housing management practices; and newer housing and infrastructures that include a wider range of housing choices, accessible community facilities, and opportunities for active living and volunteer involvement (CMHC, 2008, p. 14). There are housing initiatives across Canada with alternate levels of care to facilitate increased access to health services for seniors. There are innovative trends in housing design that combine assisted living with programs such as active living and creative arts. Other programs across Canada (e.g., the Alberta Centre for Active Living in Edmonton, Meanderthals hiking groups, and elder hostels) are also directed at promoting active lifestyles and the physical and mental well-being of seniors.

Mental Health

Social Support Transitions

Older adults may compensate for loss of family by expanding friendship networks, and employment may become an important method of establishing a network in later life. The older adult can be prepared for the transition by receiving information about internal developmental processes, sources of social support, and opportunities for personal growth and role supplementation.

Lifestyle Support

Lifestyle interventions, such as exercise promotion and nutrition counselling, are particularly important in later life because a tendency to slow down and to become more sedentary usually accompanies aging. For many, retirement provides an opportunity to restructure the time that was previously spent working. Developing regular exercise habits can help maintain physical and psychological well-being. Self-help programs generally include components of exercise, nutrition, health screening, and health habits.

Spiritual Support

Supporting contact with spiritual leaders important to the patient is an ongoing mental health promotion intervention. The nurse can also support a patient's spiritual growth by exploring the meanings that a particular life change has for the elder. In later life, existential issues such as experiencing losses, redefining meanings in existence,

IN A LIFE

Verna Splane (1914–) and Dr. Helen Mussallem (1915–)
Outstanding Canadian Nurses Acknowledged at Dr. Mussallem's Birthday Party, 2005

Dr. Helen Mussallem
(*right*) celebrated her 90th birthday in 2005. Currently living in Ottawa, she is a former chairperson of the Board of the Victorian Order of Nurses, a Companion of the Order of Canada, and Canada's most decorated nurse. She holds seven Honourary Doctorates and is a recipient of the Florence Nightingale Medal of the International Red Cross. Beginning her career in 1937, she has dedicated her life to nursing.

Verna Splane
(*left*) celebrated her 90th birthday in 2004. She was Chief Nursing Officer in National Health and Welfare and worked with the World Health Organization in International Nursing and Public Health. She was also Vice President of the International Council of Nurses (ICN). She continues to meet with nursing students at the University of British Columbia who have an interest in international nursing.

and living in the present become the standard, replacing the performance and future orientation that characterize earlier adulthood.

Community Services

More emphasis should be placed on community care options, services that provide both sustenance and growth. Examples of supportive services that foster independent community living include information and referral services; transportation and nutrition services; legal and protective services; comprehensive senior centres; home-maker and handyman services; matching of older with younger individuals to share housing; and use of the supports available through churches, community groups, or mental health and other community agencies (e.g., area agencies on aging) to maintain elderly individuals in the community for as long as possible. The availability and accessibility of these services vary greatly, and eligibility requirements may exist. A Canadian Mental Health Association project, funded by Population Health in Canada, examined seniors' mental health and home care using mental health promotion principles. A variety of methods grounded in the principle of participation explored the perspectives of seniors, family caregivers, and home care providers. A policy guide was developed as an outcome of the project to provide direction for a holistic model of care, incorporating both medical and psychosocial supports to meet the needs of seniors (McCourt, 2004).

Summary

Home care can contribute to a holistic approach to the health and well-being of older adults (Canadian Mental Health Association, 2002). While recognizing that effective mental health promotion requires a comprehensive, interdisciplinary, and cross-sectoral approach, nurses in particular are well situated in institutions, in home care, and in community settings to provide important interventions, guidance, and support for seniors in Canada.

SUMMARY OF KEY POINTS

□ Major changes in social roles with aging include retirement, loss of partner, and residence.
□ The brain changes with aging; these changes include a decline in weight and reduction in synapses.
□ The nervous system has a considerable degree of plasticity and can sustain some structural losses without losing function.
□ All five senses (sight, hearing, touch, taste, and smell) decline with age.
□ Intelligence and personality are stable throughout the life span; however, reaction time slows with age.

□ The concept of gerotranscendence emphasizes continued spiritual growth and development of inner strength rather than decrements in physical capacity in the last stage of life.
□ Threats to memory in the older adult include medications, depression, poor nutrition, infection, heart and lung disease, thyroid problems, alcohol use, and sensory loss.
□ Polypharmacy is prevalent in older adults, particularly in nursing homes. Ongoing assessment of medication is needed to prevent inappropriate medication administration.
□ Older adults are at higher risk for poverty and suicide.
□ Although older adults experience many physical changes, they can desire and have the urge to remain sexually active.
□ Aging affects pharmacokinetics, including drug absorption, distribution, metabolism, and excretion; aging also affects the strength and number of protein-binding sites.
□ Residential care environments ideally emphasize family-oriented care that optimizes existing functional capacities.
□ Assisted living is a supportive housing environment that provides routine nursing services within a philosophy of patient empowerment.

CRITICAL THINKING CHALLENGES

1 Compare the three late adulthood chronologic groups in terms of age. Using the recommendations in Box 29-1, interview people representing each of the three chronologic groups about their views of mental health.
2 Describe strategies that might facilitate older adults finding or renewing a sense of purpose and meaning in their lives.
3 Hypothesize why IQ tests and personality do not change with time.
4 Use the concept of *gerotranscendence* to explain differences between the young-old and the old-old.
5 Identify positive and negative perspectives of retirement.
6 Explain why chronic illnesses, polypharmacy, and poverty are all risk factors for mental health problems in later life.
7 Describe mental health promotion interventions that relate to social support transitions, lifestyle support, and self-care.

WEB LINKS

www.ccsmh.ca This is the site of the Canadian Coalition for Seniors' Mental Health, established in 2002, which has as its goal to support collaborative initiatives that will facilitate positive mental health for seniors through innovation and dissemination of best practices.

www.cgna.net This is the site of the Canadian Gerontological Nursing Association, which represents nurses who work with and for older adults in a wide variety of settings. Its interests include education, research, and clinical practice. It encourages and supports members through research grants, scholarships, conference funding, and certification study sessions.

www.dcri.duke.edu/ccge/curtis/beers.html This is the site for Potentially Inappropriate Medications for the Elderly According to the Revised Beers Criteria.

www.nami.org This is the site for the National Alliance on Mental Illness, which includes a guide book written for older adults with mental health concerns and their family members and caregivers.

www.nia.nih.gov/AboutNIA/NACA This is the site of the NACA, which was created on May 1, 1980 to assist and advise the Minister of Health on all matters related to the aging of the Canadian population and the quality of life of seniors.

www.nicenet.ca/home.aspx This is the site of the National Initiative for the Care of the Elderly (NICE), which is an international network of researchers, practitioners, and students dedicated to improving the care of older adults, both in Canada and abroad.

www.phac-aspc.gc.ca/mh-sm/index-eng.php Mental health promotion website for the Public Health Agency of Canada.

www.seniorsmentalhealth.ca/PolicyLensENG_17_06. pdf Seniors Mental Health Policy Lens (SMHPL) was developed as part of a national project "Psychosocial Approaches to the Mental Health Challenges of Late Life" awarded to the BC Psychogeriatric Association by Health Canada, Population Health Fund.

▓▓▓ ▪▪▪▪▪▪▪▪▪▪▪▪▪▪▪▪▪▪▪▪▪▪▪▪▪▪▪▪▪
MOVIES, NOVELS, AND BIOGRAPHIES
▪▪▪▪▪▪▪▪▪▪▪▪▪▪▪▪▪▪▪▪▪▪▪▪▪▪▪▪▪

The Bucket List: 2007. This movie, starring Jack Nicholson and Morgan Freeman, tells the story of two terminally ill men who are fulfilling a list of things they want to do before they die, or as they put it, "kick the vbucket." Carter Chambers is a mechanic and Edward Cole is a billionaire hospital magnate who meet in the hospital, both having a diagnosis of cancer. Their "bucket list" ranges from "laugh till I cry" to "get a tattoo" to "ride the Great Wall of China."

VIEWING POINTS: Consider what this movie suggests about the developmental tasks of later life. How realistic

is the movie regarding the physical capacity of Carter and Edward? What do you think of the items on the list? How would your list be different if you were Carter or Edward? Are any items on their bucket list spiritual in nature? If so, which ones?

Emile: 2004. Emile returns to western Canada to receive an honorary degree for his life achievements. Ironically, in this reconnection with his past, he must face things left undone. This movie, part of a trilogy on self-transition, is about searching for one's identity in the latter part of life.

VIEWING POINTS: What were the turning points in Emile's life? Do you believe he would truly choose differently if he could live his life over? Is Emile's experience an example of gerotranscendence or not?

Driving Miss Daisy: 1989. This film, starring Jessica Tandy as Daisy Werthan, a cantankerous old woman, and Morgan Freeman as Hoke Colburn, Daisy's chauffeur, examines a relationship between two people who have more in common than just growing old. The film also challenges some of the myths about aging.

VIEWING POINTS: Identify the normal behaviours in the growth and development of the older adult. Observe the verbal and nonverbal communication of Daisy and Hoke. How do they support each other?

REFERENCES

Anantharaju, A., Feller, A., & Chedid, A. (2002). Aging liver: A review. *Gerontology, 48*(6), 343–353.

Bakker, R. (2003). Sensory loss, dementia, and environments. *Generations, 27*(1), 46–51.

Bauer, M. (1999). Their only privacy is between their sheets: Privacy and the sexuality of elderly nursing home residents. *Journal of Gerontological Nursing, 25*(8), 37–41.

Benedict, A., & Zhang, X. (1999). Reactions to loss among men and women: A comparison. *Activities, Adaptation & Aging, 24*(1), 29–38.

Bourque, P., Pushkar, D., Bonneville, L., & Beland, F. (2005). Contextual effects on life satisfaction of older men and women. *Canadian Journal on Aging, 24*(1), 31–44.

Brown, J., Mefford, L., Chen, S., & Brown, A. (2009). Health and function of older persons volunteering for Habitat for Humanity. *Southern Online Journal of Nursing Research, 9*(3).

Canada Mortgage and Housing Corporation. (2008). *Impacts of the aging of the Canadian population on housing and communities: Research highlights.* Retrieved November 20, 2009, from http://www.cmhc-schl.gc.ca/odpub/pdf/65913.pdf

Canadian Association for Suicide Prevention. (2004). *CASP: Blueprint for a Canadian National Suicide Prevention Strategy.* Edmonton, AB: Author.

Canadian Broadcasting Corporation. (2005). *CBC news in depth: Seniors and drugs: Prescribed to death.* Retrieved November 20, 2009, from http://www.cbc.ca/news/background/seniorsdrugs/prescribed-to-death.html

Canadian Broadcasting Corporation. (2007). *Drugs seniors should avoid—the Beer's criteria.* Retrieved November 20, 2009, from http://www.cbc.ca/news/background/seniorsdrugs/beers_table_more.html

Canadian Coalition for Seniors' Mental Health. (2003). Depression fought in seniors. *Canadian Coalition for Seniors' Mental Health, 1*(4), 2.

Canadian Institute for Health Information. (2007). *Drug claims by seniors: An analysis focusing on potentially inappropriate medication use, 2000 to 2006.* Retrieved June 27, 2008, from http://secure.cihi.ca/cihiweb/en/downloads/Potentially_Inappropriate_Medications_EN.pdf

Canadian Mental Health Association. (2002). *Supporting seniors' mental health through home care: A policy guide.* Toronto, ON: Author. Retrieved

November 20, 2009, from http://www.cmha.ca/data/1/rec_docs/158_smhhc_polguide.pdf

Charron, L. (2007). *Canada's pension predicament: The widening gap between public and private sector retirement trends and pension plans.* Retrieved November 20, 2009, from http://ebnc.benefitnews.com/attachment-cache/pdfs/ebnc/partners/CFIBreport.pdf

Conwell, Y., Lyness, J. M., Duberstein, P. R., Cox, C., Seidlitz, L., & Caine, E. D. (1998). *Physical illness & suicide among elderly patients in primary care practices.* Abstract. Toronto, ON: American Psychiatric Association.

Ebersole, P., Touhy, T. A., Hess, P., & Jett, K. (2007). *Toward healthy aging: Human needs and nursing response.* Philadelphia, PA: Mosby.

Edwards, P., & Mawani, A. (2006). *Healthy aging in Canada: A new vision, a vital investment from evidence to action. A background paper prepared for the Federal, Provincial and Territorial Committee of Officials.* Ottawa, ON: Author. Retrieved March 10, 2009 from http://www.phac-aspc.gc.ca/seniors-aines/pubs/haging_newvision/pdf/vision-rpt_e.pdf

Erikson, E. H., & Erikson, J. M. (1997). *The lifecycle completed, extended version.* New York, NY: WW Norton.

Fleming, K. C., Evans, J. M., & Chutka, D. S. (2003). A cultural and economic history of old age in America. *Mayo Clinic Proceedings, 78*(7), 914–921.

Frankl, V. (1963). *Man's search for meaning: An introduction to logotherapy.* New York, NY: Pocket Books.

Gott, M., & Hinchliff, S. (2003). How important is sex in later life? The views of older people. *Social Science Medicine, 56*(8), 1617–1628.

Grek, A. (2007). Clinical management of suicidality in the elderly: An opportunity for involvement in the lives of older patients. *The Canadian Journal of Psychiatry, 56*(Suppl. 1), 47S–57S.

Hayes-Bautista, D. E., Hsu, P., Perez, A., & Gamboa, C. (2002). The "browning" of the graying of America: Diversity in the elderly population and policy implications. *Generations, 26*(3), 15–24.

Health Canada. (2002). *Physical activity and older adults.* Division of aging and seniors. Ottawa, ON: Minister of Public Works and Government Services Canada. Retrieved November 20, 2009, from http://www.phac-aspc.gc.ca/seniors-aines/pubs/workshop_healthyaging/pdf/physical_activity_e.pdf

Heisl, M. J. (2004). Suicide ideation in the elderly. *Psychiatric Times, XXI*(3)., 1–2. Retrieved November 20 from http://www.psychiatrictimes.com/display/article/10168/48656?pageNumber=2

Heisl, M. J. (2006). Suicide and its prevention among older adults. *Canadian Journal of Psychiatry, 51*(3), 143–154.

Heisl, M. J., & Duberstein, P. R. (2005). Suicide prevention in older adults. *Clinical Psychology: Science and Practice, 12*(3), 242–259.

Holmes, J. S., & Dorfman, L. T. (2000). The effects of specific health conditions on activities in retirement. *Activities, Adaptation & Aging, 25*(1), 47.

Larson, E. B., Wang, L., Bowen, J. D., McCormick, W. C., Teri, L., Crane, P., et al. (2006). Exercise is associated with reduced risk for incident dementia among persons 65 years of age and older. *Annals of Internal Medicine, 144*, 73–81.

Lindsay, C., & Almay, M. (1999). *A portrait of seniors in Canada.* Ottawa, ON: Statistics Canada.

Lowry, L. W., & Conco, D. (2002). Exploring the meaning of spirituality with aging adults in Appalachia. *Journal of Holistic Nursing, 20*(4), 388–402.

Marziali, E., McDonald, L., & Donahue, P. (2008). The role of coping humor in the physical and mental health of older adults. *Aging & Mental Health, 12*(6), 713–718.

Mental Health Commission of Canada. (2009). *Toward recovery and well-being. A framework for a mental health strategy for Canada (draft).* Ottawa, ON: Author. Available at: http://www.mentalhealthcommission.ca/SiteCollectionDocuments/Key_Documents/en/2009/Mental_Health_ENG.pdf

McCourt, P. A. (2004). *Seniors' mental health policy lens.* British Columbia: BC Psychogeriatric Association, Retrieved November 20, 2009, from http://www.seniorsmentalhealth.ca/PolicyLensENG_17_06.pdf

McIntosh, J. L., Santos, J. F., Hubbard, R. W., & Overholser, J. C. (1994). *Elder suicide research, theory & treatment.* Washington, DC: American Psychological Association.

Ministry of Healthy Living and Support. (2008). *Seniors in British Columbia: A healthy living framework.* British Columbia: Author. Retrieved November 20, 2009, from http://www.hls.gov.bc.ca/seniors/PDFs/seniors_framework_web.pdf

Moore, S. L. (1997). A phenomenological study of meaning in life in suicidal older adults. *Archives in Psychiatric Nursing, XI*(1), 29–36.

Moore, S. L., Grek, A., Heisl, M., & Jackson, F. (2006). *Canadian Coalition for Seniors Mental Health: National guidelines initiative. Suicide assessment and prevention.* Toronto, ON: Canadian Coalition for Seniors Mental Health.

Moore, S. L., Metcalf, B., & Schow, E. (2000). Meaning in life: Examining the concept. *Geriatric Nursing, 21*(1), 27–29.

National Advisory Council on Aging. (2003). *Interim report card: Seniors in Canada.* Ottawa, ON: Government of Canada.

National Advisory Council on Aging. (2005). *Grandparenting today.* Ottawa, ON: Government of Canada.

National Alliance on Mental Illness. (2001). *Mental illness, healthy aging: A NH guide for older adults and caregivers.* Retrieved November 20, 2009, from, http://www.nami.org/Content/ContentGroups/Home4/Home_Page_Spotlights/Spotlight_1/Guidebook.pdf

Parent, K., Anderson, M., & Huestis, L. (2002). *Supporting seniors' mental health through home care: A policy guide.* Toronto, ON: Canadian Mental Health Association.

Public Health Agency of Canada. (2002). *A report on mental illnesses in Canada.* Ottawa, ON: Author. Retrieved November 20, 2009, from http://www.phac-aspc.gc.ca/publicat/miic-mmac/

Rosenzweig, E. S., & Barnes, C. A. (2003). Impact of aging on hippocampal function: Plasticity, network dynamics and cognition. *Progress in Neurobiology, 69*(3), 143–179.

Sattar, S. P., Petty, F., & Burke, W. J. (2003). Diagnosis and treatment of alcohol dependence in older alcoholics. *Clinics in Geriatric Medicine, 19*, 743–764.

Scahill, R. I., Frost, C., Jenkins, R., Whitwell, J. L., Rossor, M. N., & Fox, N. C. (2003). A longitudinal study of brain volume changes in normal aging using serial registered magnetic resonance imaging. *Archives of Neurology, 60*(7), 989–994.

Shields, M., & Martel, L. (2006). Healthy living among seniors. *Supplement to Health Reports, 16*, 7–20. Retrieved March 10, 2009 from http://www.statcan.ca/english/freepub/82–003-SIE/2005000/pdf/82–003-SIE20050007445.pdf

Southern Alberta Geriatric Mental Health Working Group (SAGMHS). (2003, September). *Summary report of the Southern Alberta Geriatric Mental Health Working Group* (pp. 1–12). Calgary, AB: Author.

Standing Senate Committee on Social Affairs, Science and Technology. (2006). *Out of the shadows at last: Transforming mental health, mental illness and addictions in Canada.* Ottawa, ON: Government of Canada.

Statistics Canada. (2005). *Population projections, 2005 to 2031.* Retrieved March 10, 2009 from, http://www.statcan.ca/Daily/English/051215/d051215b.htm

Statistics Canada. (2007). *Canada's population by age and sex.* Retrieved November 20, 2009, from http://www.statcan.ca/Daily/English/071129/d071129c.htm

Tam, E. Y., Fletcher, P. C., & Chi, I. (2004). Cultural and gender diversity in health. *STRIDE, 1.* Retrieved December 18, 2005, from http://www.stridemagazine.com

Tiao, J. Y., Semmens, J. B., Masarei, J. R., & Lawrence-Brown, M. M. (2002). The effect of age on serum creatinine levels in an aging population: Relevance to vascular surgery. *Cardiovascular Surgery, 10*(5), 445–451.

Tornstam, L. (2005). *Gerotranscendence: A developmental theory of positive aging.* New York, NY: Springer.

Turcotte, M., & Schellenberg, G. (2007). *A portrait of seniors in Canada 2006.* Ottawa, ON: Statistics Canada.

U.S. Department of Health and Human Services. (2001). *Older adults and mental health: Issues and opportunities.* Washington, DC: Administration on Aging.

von Strauss, E., Aguero-Torres, H., Kareholt, I., Winblad, B., & Fratiglioni, L. (2003). Women are more disabled in basic activities of daily living than men only in very advanced ages: A study on disability, morbidity, and mortality from the Kungsholmen Project. *Journal of Clinical Epidemiology, 56*(7), 669–677.

Wadensten, B. (2007). The theory of gerotranscendence as applied to gerontological nursing-Part I. *International Journal of Older People Nursing, 2*, 289–294.

Wadensten, B., & Carlsson, M. (2003). Theory-driven guidelines for practical care of older people, based on the theory of gerotranscendence. *Journal of Advanced Nursing, 41*(5), 462–470.

Wadensten, B., & Carlsson, M. (2007a). Adoption of an innovation based on the theory of gerotranscendence by staff in a nursing home–Part III. *International Journal of Older People Nursing, 2*, 302–314.

Wadensten, B., & Carlsson, M. (2007b). The theory of gerotranscendence in practice: Guidelines for nursing–Part II. *International Journal of Older People Nursing, 2,* 295–301.

Waern, M., Rubenowitz, E., & Wilhelmson, K. (2003). Predictors of suicide in the old elderly. *Gerontology, 49*(5), 328–334.

Wang, L., Larson, E. B., Bowen, J. D., & van Belle, G. (2006). Performance-based physical function and future dementia in older people. *Archives of Internal Medicine, 166,* 1115–1120.

Wright, L. (2001). Sexuality-reproductive pattern: Normal changes with aging. In M. L. Maas, K. C. Buckwalter, M. D. Hardy, et al. (Eds.), *Nursing care of older adults: Diagnoses, outcomes, and interventions* (pp. 729–732). St. Louis, MO: Mosby.

Yevchak, A. M., Loeb, S. J., & Fick, D. M. (2008). Promoting cognitive health and vitality: A review of clinical implications. *Geriatric Nursing, 29*(5), 302–310.

Zimprich, D. (2002). Cross-sectionally and longitudinally balanced effects of processing speed on intellectual abilities. *Experimental Aging Research, 28,* 231–251.

Mental Health Assessment of the Older Adult

Annette M. Lane

Adapted from the chapter "Mental Health Assessment of the Older Adult" Mary Ann Boyd and Mickey Stanley

LEARNING OBJECTIVES

After studying this chapter, you will be able to:

- Compare changes in normal aging with those associated with mental health problems in older adults.
- Select various techniques in assessing older adults who have mental health problems.
- Delineate the important areas of assessment for the biologic domain in completing the geriatric mental health nursing assessment.
- Delineate the important areas of assessment for the psychological domain in completing the geriatric mental health nursing assessment.
- Delineate the important areas of assessment for the social domain in completing the geriatric mental health nursing assessment.

KEY CONCEPTS

- bio/psycho/social/spiritual geriatric mental health nursing assessment
- normal aging

KEY TERMS

- dysphagia • functional activities • insomnia • polypharmacy
- xerostomia

*I*n 1920, the average life span in Canada was 60 years (Statistics Canada, 2005). By 2004, this life span increased to 77.8 years for men and 82.6 years for women (Statistics Canada, 2006). Health care providers will face new and increased challenges as the baby boomers move into the ranks of older adults. By the year 2021, projections are that there will be almost 7 million older adults (65 years of age and older), composing 19% of the Canadian population. The fastest growing segment of the older population is the group 85 years of age and older (Public Health Agency of Canada, 2005a).

Normal aging is associated with some physical decline, such as decreased sensory abilities and decreased pulmonary and immune functions, but many important functions do not change. Intellectual function, capacity for change, and productive engagement with life remain stable. Many myths exist about normal aging. Some people believe that "senility" is normal or that depression or hopelessness is natural for older individuals. If older adults and family members believe these myths, they will be less likely to seek treatment for themselves or their elders with real problems. Even if they seek help for themselves or their older adults, health care providers may fail to identify depression or simply attribute symptoms to normal aging (Rabheru, 2004). Approximately 15% to 30% of older adults experience symptoms of mental illness (SAGMHS, 2003). Older adults with mental health problems comprise different population groups. One group consists of those with long-term mental illnesses who have reached the ranks of the older adult population. These individuals usually understand their disorders and treatments. Unfortunately, the changes associated with aging can affect a client's control of his or her chronic mental illness. Symptoms may reappear, and medications may need to be adjusted. Another group includes individuals who are relatively free of mental health problems until their later years. These individuals, who may already have other health problems, develop late-onset mental disorders, such as depression, psychotic symptoms, or dementia. For these individuals and their family members, the development of a mental disorder can be very traumatic.

Mental health problems in older adults can be especially complex because of coexisting medical problems and treatments. Many symptoms of somatic disorders mimic or mask psychiatric disorders. For example, fatigue may be related to anaemia, but it also may be symptomatic of depression. In addition, older individuals are more likely to report somatic symptoms, rather than psychological ones, making identification of a mental disorder even more difficult.

The purpose of this chapter is to present a comprehensive geriatric mental health nursing assessment process that serves as the basis of care for older individuals (discussed in Chapters 29 and 31). A mental health assessment is necessary when psychiatric or mental health issues are identified or when clients with mental illnesses reach their later years (usually about age 65 years). The assessment generally follows the same format as described in Chapter 11. However, the overall health care issues for older adults can be very complex, so it follows that certain components of the geriatric mental health nursing assessment are unique. Thus, the geriatric assessment emphasizes some areas that are less critical to the standard adult assessment.

> **KEY CONCEPT** **Normal aging** is associated with some physical decline, such as decreased sensory abilities and decreased pulmonary and immune functions, but many important functions do not change.

■ TECHNIQUES OF DATA COLLECTION

The nurse assesses the older client using an interview format that may take a few sessions to complete. She or he also may rely on self-report standardized tests, such as depression and cognitive functioning tools. A wide variety of physiologic disorders may cause changes in mental status for older adults; thus, results of laboratory tests often are significant. For example, urinalysis can detect a urinary tract infection that has affected a client's cognitive status. Box 30-1 contains a representative listing of common physiologic causes of changes in mental status. In addition, medical records from other health care providers are useful in developing a complete picture of the client's health status.

BOX 30.1

Changes That Affect Mental Status

- Acid–base imbalance
- Dehydration
- Drugs (prescribed and over-the-counter)
- Electrolyte changes
- Hypothyroidism
- Hypothermia and hyperthermia
- Hypoxia
- Infection and sepsis

An important source of client data is family members, who often notice changes that the older individual overlooks or fails to recognize. A client with memory impairment may be unable to give an accurate history. By interviewing family members, the nurse expands the scope of the client assessment. Moreover, the nurse has an opportunity to evaluate the caregivers themselves to determine whether they can care for the older individual adequately and how they are coping with the situation. For example, a husband may be unable to care for his wife but is unwilling to admit it. If the nurse can establish rapport with the husband, the nurse may use the assessment interview as an opportunity to help the husband to examine his wife's care requirements realistically. The nurse may be able to explain to the husband the impact of caregiving on his health. For instance, it is not uncommon for the caregiving spouse to experience significant physical and mental health decline because of the extreme and prolonged stresses.

■ BIO/PSYCHO/SOCIAL/SPIRITUAL GERIATRIC MENTAL HEALTH NURSING ASSESSMENT

> **KEY CONCEPT** A **bio/psycho/social/spiritual geriatric mental health nursing assessment** is the comprehensive, deliberate, and systematic collection and interpretation of bio/psycho/social/spiritual data that are based on the special needs and problems of older adults to determine current and past health, functional status, and human responses to mental health problems, both actual and potential (Box 30-2).

At the beginning of the assessment, the nurse should determine the client's ability to participate. For example, if a client is using a wheelchair, he or she may have physical limitations that prevent full participation in the assessment. The older client must be able to hear the nurse. For a client with compromised hearing, the nurse must attend to voice projection and volume. Shouting

BOX 30.2

Bio/Psycho/Social/Spiritual Geriatric Mental Health Nursing Assessment

I. Major reason for seeking help _____

II. Initial information

   Name _____

   Age _____ Current marital status _____

   Gender _____ Caregiver's name _____

   Living arrangements _____

III. Level of independence:

   High (needs no help) _____

   Moderate (lives independently, but needs some help with instrumental activities) _____

   Low (relies on others for help in meeting functional and instrumental activities) _____

   Physical limitations _____

   Level of education completed _____

	Normal	Treated	Untreated
Physical functions: system review	☐	☐	☐
Activity/exercise	☐	☐	☐
Sleep patterns	☐	☐	☐
Appetite and nutrition	☐	☐	☐
Hydration	☐	☐	☐
Elimination	☐	☐	☐
Existing physical illnesses	☐	☐	☐

   List any chronic illnesses _____

   Presence of pain (Use standardized instrument if pain is present.) No _____ Yes _____

   Score _____ Treatment of pain _____

Medication (prescription and over-the-counter)	Dosage	Side Effects	Frequency of Side Effects

Significant Laboratory Tests	Values	Normal Range

IV. Responses to mental health problems

   Major concerns regarding mental health problem _____

   Major loss/change in past year: No _____ Yes _____

   Fear of violence: No _____ Yes _____

   If yes, type of violence _____

   Strategies for managing problems/disorder _____

Continued

BOX 30.2

Bio/Psycho/Social/Spiritual Geriatric Mental Health Nursing Assessment (Continued)

V.   Mental status examination

Ｇeneral observation (appearance, psychomotor activity, attitude) _____

Orientation (time, place, person)

Mood, affect, emotions (Geriatric Depression Scale should be used if evidence of depression)

Speech (verbal ability, speed, use of words correctly) _____

Thought processes (hallucinations, delusions, tangential, logic, repetition, rhyming of words, loose connections, disorganized) (*Describe the content of hallucinations, delusions.*)

Cognition and intellectual performance (*Use standardized test scores as well as observations.*)

Attention and concentration _____

Abstract reasoning and concentration _____

Memory (recall, short-term, long-term) _____

Judgment and insight _____

(MMSE, CASI scores) _____

VI.   Significant behaviours (psychomotor, agitation, aggression, withdrawn) (*Use standardized test if behaviours are problematic.*) _____

When did problem behaviour begin? Has it gotten worse?

VII.   Self-concept (beliefs about self—body image, self-esteem, personal identity)

VIII.   Risk assessment

Suicide: High _____ Moderate _____ Low _____ Assault/homicide: High _____ Low _____

Suicide thoughts or ideation: No _____ Yes _____

Current thoughts of harming self _____ Plan _____

Means _____

Means available

Assault/homicide thoughts: No _____ Yes _____

What do you do when angry with a stranger? _____

What do you do when angry with family or partner? _____

Have you ever hit or pushed anyone? No _____ Yes _____

Have you ever been arrested for assault? No _____ Yes _____

Current thoughts of harming others _____

IX.   Functional status (*Use standardized test such as FAQ.*) _____

X.   Cultural assessment

Cultural group _____

Cultural group's view of health and mental illness _____

By what cultural rules do you try to live? _____

Special, cultural foods that are important to you _____

XI.   Stresses and coping behaviours

Social support _____

Family members _____

Which members are important to you? _____

On whom can you rely? _____

Community resources _____

XII.   Spiritual assessment _____

XIII.   Economic status _____

XIV.   Legal status _____

XV.   Quality of life _____

Summary of significant data that can be used in formulating a nursing diagnosis:

SIGNATURE/TITLE _____ Date _____

at the older individual is unnecessary. The nurse should remember to lower the pitch of her or his voice because higher-pitched sounds are often lost with presbycusis (loss of hearing sensitivity associated with aging). The nurse should eliminate distracting noises, such as from a television or radio, and ensure that the client's hearing aid is in place and turned on. Facing the client and using distinct enunciation will help lip-reading clients understand what is being said. Sometimes, deafness is mistaken for cognitive dysfunction. If a client's hearing is questionable, the nurse should examine the client for build-up of cerumen. If this is not believed to be contributing to hearing loss, the nurse can enlist the help of a speech and language specialist. Generally, the pace of the interview should mirror the older adult's ability to move through the assessment. Usually, the pace will be slower than the nurse uses with younger populations.

Biologic Domain

Collecting and analyzing data for the assessment of the biologic domain include areas similar to those discussed in Chapter 11. The assessment components include present and past health status, physical examination results, physical functioning, and a pharmacology review. When focusing on the biologic domain, the nurse pays special attention to the client's general physical appearance as well as any observable manifestations of illness. The nurse should assess how all physical problems affect the client's mental well-being. For example, pain and immobility are physical problems that can negatively affect mental health. Low energy level may be immediately apparent. Women with obvious osteoporosis are experiencing pain most of the time. Men undergoing radiation for prostate cancer worry about sexual functioning and urinary incontinence.

Present and Past Health Status

A review of the older adult's current health status includes examining health records and collecting information from the client and family members. The nurse must identify chronic health problems that could affect mental health care. For example, the client's management of diabetes mellitus could provide clues to the likelihood of complications such as retinopathy or neuropathy, which in turn will affect the individual's ability to follow a mental health treatment regimen. The nurse must document a history of psychiatric treatment.

Physical Examination

The psychiatric and mental health (PMH) nurse reviews the physical examination findings, paying special attention to recent laboratory values, such as urinalysis, white and red blood cell counts, and fasting blood glucose data (see

Chapter 11). Results of neurologic tests could indicate compromise of the neuromuscular systems. Many psychiatric medications lower the seizure threshold, making a history of seizures, which can cause behavioural changes, an important assessment component. The nurse should note any evidence of movement disorders, such as tremors, abnormal movements, or shuffling. If a client has been taking conventional antipsychotics, the nurse should consider assessment for symptoms of tardive dyskinesia, using one of the appropriate assessment tools (see Chapter 18 for additional discussion of tardive dyskinesia).

The nurse should take routine vital signs during the assessment. She or he should note any abnormalities in blood pressure (i.e., hypertension or hypotension) because many psychiatric medications affect blood pressure. Generally, these medications may cause orthostatic hypotension, which can lead to dizziness, unsteady gait, and falls. A baseline blood pressure is needed for future monitoring of medication side effects. Lying, sitting, and standing blood pressures are especially useful in assessing for orthostatic hypotension.

Physical Functions

The nurse must consider the older client's physical functioning within the context of the normal changes that accompany aging and the presence of any chronic disorders. The nurse should note the client's use of any personal devices, such as canes, walkers, wheelchairs, or oxygen, or environmental devices, such as grab bars, shower benches, or hospital beds. Specific areas to consider are nutrition and eating, elimination, and sleep patterns.

Nutrition and Eating

An assessment of the type, amount, and frequency of food eaten is standard in any assessment of the older adult. The nurse should note any unintentional weight loss of more than 4.5 kg. She or he must consider such nutrition changes in light of mental health problems. For example, is a client's weight loss related to an underlying physical problem or to the client's belief that she is being poisoned, which makes her afraid to eat? Or, is the older adult not eating because of an active wish to die?

Eating is often difficult for older adults, who may experience a lack of appetite. The nurse must assess eating and appetite patterns because many psychiatric medications can affect digestion and may impair an already compromised gastrointestinal tract. A common problem of older individuals who live in long-term care facilities is **dysphagia**, or difficulty swallowing. Dysphagia can lead to dehydration, malnutrition, pneumonia, or asphyxiation. People who have been exposed to conventional antipsychotics (e.g., haloperidol, chlorpromazine) may have symptoms of tardive dyskinesia, which can make swallowing difficult. Thus, the nurse should evaluate any client who has been exposed to the older psychiatric medications for symptoms of tardive dyskinesia.

Xerostomia, or dry mouth, which is common in older adults, also may impair eating. The nurse should pay particular attention to those who are currently receiving treatment for mental illnesses, particularly with medications that have anticholinergic properties. Dry mouth is also a side effect of many other anticholinergic medications, such as cimetidine, digoxin, and furosemide. Frequent rinsing with a non–alcohol-based mouthwash will help to correct the dry condition. Decreased taste or smell is common among older adults and may reduce the pleasure of eating so that the client may eat less. Making meal times social and relaxing experiences can help the older individual compensate for some of the loss of pleasure associated with decreased taste or smell. Preparing favourite foods will also enhance the quality of meals and meal times.

The nurse also must determine the client's use of alcohol. Alcoholism is a growing problem in the older adult population. According to the Canadian Addiction Survey (Adlaf, Begin, & Sawka, 2005), just over 20% of older adults aged 65 to 74 years and 24% of individuals over 75 years of age admit to consuming alcohol four or more times per week. The incidence of drinking frequency is approximately double that of younger adults. There is a substantially increased mortality risk for heavy drinkers and a slightly reduced risk for lighter drinkers. Limited data suggest a more favourable mortality experience for drinkers of wine than for drinkers of liquor or beer (Klatsky, Friedman, Armstrong, & Kipp, 2003). The use of the CAGE questionnaire (see Appendix G) or the SMAST-G (Short Michigan Alcoholism Screening Test—Geriatric Version) (University of Michigan Alcohol Research Centre, 1991) may be helpful in this area. If an older adult screens negatively for problem drinking using one of these scales, yet the nurse believes that he or she may have an alcohol problem, the nurse might choose to retest the older adult using the other instrument. According to one study (Moore, Seeman, Morgenstern, Beck, & Reuben, 2002) that compared the CAGE instrument with the SMAST-G, less than half of the older individuals who tested positive on one screening tool did so on the other. They concluded that each instrument may target different facets of problem drinking.

Elimination

The nurse must assess the client's urinary and bowel functions. Older individuals are more likely to experience constipation because the peristaltic movement of the bowel slows. Medications with anticholinergic properties can cause constipation, leading to fecal impaction. Abuse of laxatives is common among older adults and requires evaluation. Although the addition of fiber is recommended for constipation, such measures may cause bloating and excessive gas production. Older clients are also more likely to experience urinary frequency because the strength of the sphincter muscle decreases. Because many older adults drink fewer fluids to manage urinary incontinence, fluid intake also becomes an important factor in assessing urinary functioning and constipation. The nurse should remember that urinary incontinence is a symptom of a disorder that requires follow-up and treatment.

Sleep

During the normal aging process, sleep patterns change, and clients often sleep less than they did when younger. The nurse must assess any recent changes in sleep patterns and evaluate whether they are related to normal aging or are symptomatic of an underlying disorder. **Insomnia,** the inability to fall or remain asleep throughout the night, can be related to depression (Box 30-3) and

---

BOX 30.3

Research for Best Practice: Sleep Difficulties and Depression in Community Residing Older Adults

Almeida, O. P., & Pfaff, J. J. (2005). Sleep complaints among older general practice patients: Association with depression. British Journal of General Practice, 55, 864–866.

THE QUESTION: This research study examined the incidence of insomnia and depression among 1,029 Australian adults, 60 years of age and older.

METHODS: A cross-sectional study, using self-report questionnaires [The Centre for Epidemiologic Studies Depression Scale (CES-D)] and three questions from the Cambridge Examination for Mental Health Disorders of the Elderly, Revised (CAMDEX-R), was conducted. Researchers contacted offices of family physicians (54 out of 500 agreed to participate), who then each recruited 15–30 older adults to complete the questionnaires.

FINDINGS: In this study, 63% of the 1,029 older adults reported insomnia. Older adults who admitted to experiencing sleep difficulties were 3.7 times more likely to be depressed than those who did not experience sleep problems. The researchers conclude that family physicians should assess older adults for depression when they indicate concerns about insomnia.

IMPLICATIONS FOR NURSING: Nurses should ask older clients who report insomnia about symptoms of depression, and if present, they should encourage their clients to see their family physicians. They should also assess for the use of alcohol, over-the-counter drugs, and prescription drugs that may impact sleep or be used as sleep aids.

lead to the regular use of sleep medications. Clients with insomnia report that they cannot sleep at night and do not feel rested in the morning. They often sleep during the day. In a large 3-year study of 10,430 women, 70 to 75 years of age, more than 60% reported difficulty sleeping and 15% reported using sleep medications (Byles, Mishra, Harris, & Nair, 2003). Sleep problems are also often linked to the use of alcohol. If an older individual reports sleep problems, the nurse should ask about his or her use of alcohol, over-the-counter medications, and prescription drugs.

Pain

Older adults are more likely to experience pain than younger adults because they are at increased risk for chronic illness and may be suffering from the consequences of a lifetime of injuries. For a number of older individuals, pain is a constant companion; for instance, in 1999, 27% of home-dwelling older adults admitted to living with chronic pain (Public Health Agency of Canada, 2005b). The experience of chronic pain often contributes to unexplained behaviour and personality changes. To assess pain, the nurse can use many pain instruments. One of the most popular instruments is the Wong-Baker FACES Pain Rating Scale, initially developed for children but now used for all age groups (Fig. 30.1). This scale is especially useful in communicating with people from different cultures and languages than the nurse's. See Chapter 33 for further discussion of pain.

The assessment of pain is especially critical for those older adults who are cognitively impaired and living in long-term care institutions. In one study, researchers utilized interviews and focus groups to examine attitudes and beliefs of physicians and nurses about administering pain medications to cognitively impaired residents in four long-term care facilities in Ontario (Kaasalainen et al., 2007). They found that physicians and nurses expressed uncertainty about assessing pain in cognitively impaired individuals, admitted reluctance to administer opioids, and voiced concerns about overmedicating these residents. These results suggest that pain may be underrecognized and undertreated in older adults with cognitive impairment.

Pharmacologic Assessment

One of the most important areas of the biologic domain is the pharmacologic assessment. **Polypharmacy**, the concurrent use of several different medications, is common in older individuals. The nurse must ask the client and family to list all medications and times that the client takes them. Asking family members to bring in all the medications that the client is taking, including over-the-counter medications, vitamins, and herbal supplements, is a good idea. Because older adults are more sensitive than younger people to medications, the possibility of drug–drug interactions is greater. Adverse drug interactions may cause delirium in older adults and constitute a medical emergency which may result in death (see Chapter 14). Also, when considering potential drug interactions, the nurse should ask the older individual about his or her consumption of grapefruit juice, which contains narginin, a compound that inhibits the CYP3A4 enzyme involved in the metabolism of many medications (e.g., antidepressants, antiarrhythmics, erythromycin, several statins).

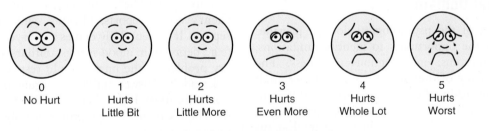

Wong-Baker FACES Pain Rating Scale

Each face represents a person who is happy or sad depending on how much or how little pain he/she has:

0 "a person who is very happy because he/she doesn't hurt at all"
1 "it hurts just a little bit"
2 "it hurts a little more"
3 "it hurts even more"
4 "it hurts a whole lot"
5 "it hurts as much as you can imagine, but you don't have to be crying to feel this bad"

Subject ID #:_____ Date:____/____/____ Visit #_____

Pt. name:_____

RA:_____

FIGURE 30.1 Wong-Baker FACES Pain Rating Scale.

BOX 30.4

Therapeutic Dialogue: Assessment Interview

Tom, 79 years old, is being seen for the first time in a geriatric mental health clinic because of recent changes in his behaviour and his accusations that family members are trying to steal his house and car. He locked his wife out of the house, accusing her of being unfaithful. When Susan, the PMH nurse assigned to his case, is conducting the assessment interview, Tom cooperates and is very pleasant until the nurse begins to assess the psychological domain.

INEFFECTIVE APPROACH

Nurse: Have there been times when you have had problems with any members of your family?

Client: No. (Silence)

Nurse: Have you noticed that lately you have been getting more upset than usual?

Client: No. Who has been talking to you?

Nurse: Your wife seems to think that you may be getting a little more upset than usual.

Client: You are just like her. She keeps telling me something is wrong with me. (Getting very agitated)

Nurse: Please, I'm trying to help you. I understand that you locked your wife out of the house last week.

Client: Leave me alone. (Gets up and leaves)

EFFECTIVE APPROACH

Nurse: How have things been going at home?

Client: All right.

Nurse: (Silence)

Client: Well, my wife and I sometimes argue.

Nurse: Oh. Most husbands and wives argue. Any special arguments?

Client: No. Just the usual. I don't pick up after myself enough. I don't dress right to suit her. But, lately, she's gone a lot.

Nurse: She is gone a lot?

Client: Yeah! A lot.

Nurse: The way you say that, it sounds like you have some feelings about her being gone.

Client: You're damned right I do—and you would, too.

Nurse: I'm missing something.

Client: Well, if you must know, I think she's having an affair with the man next door.

Nurse: Really? That must upset you to think your wife is having an affair.

Client: I am devastated. I feel so bad.

Nurse: Would you say that you are depressed?

Client: Well, wouldn't you be? Yes, I'm feeling pretty low.

CRITICAL THINKING CHALLENGE

- How do the very first questions differ in the two interviews?
- What therapeutic techniques did the nurse use in the second interview to avoid the pitfalls the nurse encountered in the first scenario?
- How did the nurse in the second scenario elicit the client's delusion about his wife's affair?
- From the data that the second nurse gathered, how many of the client's problems can be identified?

Psychological Domain

The assessment of the psychological domain provides the nurse with the opportunity to identify limitations, behavioural symptoms, and reactions to illness. The nurse assesses many of the same areas as in other adult assessments, but again, the emphasis may be different. The following discussion focuses on the responses of older adults to mental health problems, mental status examinations, behavioural changes, stress and coping patterns, and risk assessments.

Responses to Mental Health Problems

Many older clients are reluctant to admit that they have psychiatric symptoms, particularly if their culture stigmatizes mental illness, and may deny having mental or emotional problems. They may also fear that if they admit to any symptoms, they may be placed outside their home. If clients do not recognize or admit to having psychiatric symptoms, their vulnerability to being taken advantage of or injured increases.

Throughout the assessment, the nurse evaluates the client's verbal reports, obvious symptoms, and family reports. If a client flatly denies any psychiatric symptoms (e.g., depression, mood swings, outbursts of anger, memory problems), the nurse should respectfully accept the older adult's answer and avoid arguments or confrontation (Box 30-4). If the client's family members contradict the client's report or symptoms are obvious during the interview, the nurse can approach the issue while planning care. Nurses may need to use conflict resolution strategies in helping families and clients obtain appropriate care despite disagreement about symptoms experienced by the older adults.

Mental Status Examination

The areas of special interest in the mental status examination are mood and affect, thought processes, and cognitive functioning. The nurse should interpret the results in light of any accompanying physical problems, such as chronic pain, or life changes, such as loss of a spouse.

BOX 30.5

Research for Best Practice: Geriatric Depression Scale (Short Form)

	Yes	No
1. Are you basically satisfied with your life?	Yes	No
2. Have you dropped many of your activities and interests?	Yes	No
3. Do you feel that your life is empty?	Yes	No
4. Do you often get bored?	Yes	No
5. Are you in good spirits most of the time?	Yes	No
6. Are you afraid that something bad is going to happen to you?	Yes	No
7. Do you feel happy most of the time?	Yes	No
8. Do you often feel helpless?	Yes	No
9. Do you prefer to stay at home rather than go out and do new things?	Yes	No
10. Do you feel you have more problems with memory than most?	Yes	No
11. Do you think it is wonderful to be alive now?	Yes	No
12. Do you feel pretty worthless the way you are now?	Yes	No
13. Do you feel full of energy?	Yes	No
14. Do you feel that your situation is hopeless?	Yes	No
15. Do you think that most people are better off than you are?	Yes	No

Score: _____ /15 One point for "No" to questions 1, 5, 7, 11, 13

One point for "Yes" to other questions

Normal	3 ± 2
Mildly depressed	7 ± 3
Very depressed	12 ± 2

Adapted from Sheikh, J. I., & Yesavage, J. A. (1986). Geriatric Depression Scale (GDS): Recent evidence and development of a shorter version. In T. L. Brink (Ed.), *Clinical gerontology: A guide to assessment and intervention* (pp. 165–173). Binghamton, NY: Haworth Press. © By the Haworth Press, Inc. All rights reserved. Reprinted with permission.

Mood and Affect

Depression in older adults is common and associated with the following risk factors: loss of spouse, physical illness, education below high school, impaired functional status, and heavy alcohol consumption. In older people, other disorders may mask depression. When symptoms are present, they may be attributed to normal aging or atherosclerosis or other age-related problems. Older clients are less likely to report feeling sad or worthless than are younger clients. As a result, family members and primary care providers often overlook depression in older adults.

Depressive symptoms are much more common than a full-fledged depressive disorder, as characterized by the *Diagnostic and Statistical Manual of Mental Disorders* (APA, 2000). Between 10% and 15% of older adults living in the community experience depressive symptoms (Conn, 2002). Approximately 50% of older adults living in long-term care facilities show signs of depression (Canadian Coalition for Seniors Mental Health, 2003). Research suggests that untreated depression in older adults may result in the overuse of health care services, longer hospital stays, decreased treatment compliance, and increased morbidity and mortality (Conn, 2002). The Geriatric Depression Scale (GDS) is a useful screening tool with demonstrated validity and reliability (Hyer & Blount, 1984). The GDS was designed as a self-administered test, although it also has been used in observer-administered formats. One advantage of the test is its "yes/no" format, which may be easier for older adults than the Hamilton Rating Scale for Depression (HAM-D), which uses a scale from 0 to 4 (see Chapter 20). This tool is easy to administer and provides valuable information about the possibility of depression (Box 30-5). If results are positive, the nurse should refer the client to a psychiatrist or advanced practice nurse for further evaluation.

Among residents in long-term care facilities, the usefulness of the GDS depends on the degree of cognitive impairment. Residents who are mildly impaired may be able to answer yes/no questions; however, moderately to severely impaired older adults will be unable to do the same. The best validated scale for individuals with dementia is the Cornell Scale for Depression in Dementia (CSDD) (Alexopoulos, Abrams, Young, & Shamoian, 1998). The CSDD is an interview-administered scale that uses information both from the client and an outside informant.

Anxiety is another important mood for nurses to assess in older adults because it can interfere with normal functioning. In dementia, anxiety is common (Lopez et al., 2003). The Rating Anxiety in Dementia (RAID) scale was developed as a global scale to assess anxiety in clients with dementia (Shankar, Walker, Frost, & Orrell, 1999). The domains that the RAID scale assesses include worry, apprehension and vigilance, motor tension, autonomic hyperactivity, and phobias and panic attacks.

Thought Processes

Thought processes and content are critical in the assessment of older adults. Can the client express ideas and thoughts logically? Can the client understand questions and follow the conversation of others? If the older adult shows any indication of hallucinations or delusions, the nurse should explore the content of the hallucination or delusion. If the client has a history of mental illness, such as schizophrenia, these symptoms may be familiar to family members, who can validate whether they are old or new problems. If this is the first time the client has experienced these abnormal thought processes, the nurse should further evaluate the content. Suspicious and delusional thoughts that characterize dementia often include some of the following beliefs:

- People are stealing my things.
- My spouse is having an affair.
- My relative is an impostor.

If a client shares any such thoughts, the nurse can complete further assessment by using the Behavioural Pathology in Alzheimer's Disease rating scale (BEHAVE-AD). This 25-item scale is based on caregivers' reports within the previous 2 weeks (Reisberg & Ferris, 1985). The BEHAVE-AD measures thought and behavioural disturbances in seven major categories, with each item scored on a four-point scale of severity (0 to 3), including delusions, hallucinations, activity disturbances, aggressiveness, diurnal rhythm disturbances, mood disturbances, and anxieties and phobias. The BEHAVE-AD also contains a four-point global assessment of the overall magnitude of the behaviour symptoms in terms of disturbance to the caregiver, dangerousness to the client, or both. The reliability of the BEHAVE-AD (0.95 and 0.96; $p < 0.01$) is comparable to that of the Mini-Mental State Examination (MMSE) (Reisberg, Auer, & Monteiro, 1996).

Cognition and Intellectual Performance

Cognitive functioning includes such parameters as orientation, attention, short- and long-term memories, consciousness, and executive functioning. Intellectual functioning, also considered a cognitive measure, is rarely formally assessed with a standardized intelligence test in older adults. Considerable variability among individuals depends on lifestyle and psychosocial factors. Some changes in cognitive capacity accompany aging, but important functions are spared. Normal cognitive changes during aging include a slowing of information processing and memory retrieval. Abnormalities of consciousness, orientation, judgment, speech, or language are not related to age but to underlying neuropathologic changes. Cognitive changes in older adults are associated with delirium or dementia (see Chapter 31) or with schizophrenia (see Chapter 18).

The assessment includes the number of years of education. An inverse relationship between Alzheimer's disease and the number of years of education exists. When assessing cognitive functioning, the nurse should use standardized instruments and not rely on observations or chart documentations, as health care professionals tend to underrecognize cognitive impairment in older adults residing in hospitals and long-term care facilities (Barton, Miller, & Yaffe, 2006) (Box 30-6). Of such instruments, the MMSE, discussed in Chapter 11, is recommended for use in screening for cognitive functioning related to dementia (Leifer, 2009). Various studies suggest that an MMSE score below 24 of 30 has a reasonable sensitivity (80% to 90%) and specificity (80%) for discriminating between those

---

BOX 30.6

Improved Evaluation and Management of Cognitive Impairment: Results of a Comprehensive Intervention in Long-term Care

THE QUESTION: How can recognition, diagnosis, and treatment of cognitive impairment be improved within long-term care facilities? Will an intervention program make a difference in the diagnosis and treatment of cognitive impairment in residents within one long-term care facility?

METHODS: This study was a preevaluation and postevaluation of residents' charts following an intervention program. Prior to the initiation of an educational program for nursing staff, charts of 60 residents admitted to a home care unit were examined to assess how many residents were cognitively impaired (as determined by an MMSE score or by a diagnosis of dementia), had received a diagnosis of a specific type of dementia, and had a physician management plan as well as a multidisciplinary plan. Following the administration of an educational program for unit nurses (including focus groups, training sessions, strategies to improve the documentation of cognitive status, and consultation with dementia professionals), 60 other charts were examined for the same measures as the preintervention charts.

FINDINGS: The researchers determined that the educational intervention enhanced the documentation of residents' cognitive status and greater consultation with dementia professionals, resulting in greater specification of the types of dementias experienced by residents. The educational intervention program also resulted in better management plans for individuals on this unit.

IMPLICATIONS FOR NURSING: This study suggests that educating nurses in long-term care units may enhance their abilities to document cognitive impairment, increase their efforts to seek consultation with dementia professionals, and motivate them to develop management plans to assist residents suffering from dementias.

Barton, C., Miller, B., & Yaffe, K. (2006). Improved evaluation and management of cognitive impairment: Results of a comprehensive intervention in long-term care. *Journal of American Medical Directors Association, 7*(2), 84–89.

with dementia and those without. However, some data suggest that the MMSE may have a built-in bias against those with fewer than 8 years of education or among those who belong to ethnic minority groups (Mulgrew et al., 1999).

Evidence suggests that severe cognitive deterioration may occur in older individuals with schizophrenia. In assessing the cognitive status of this population, the Cognitive Abilities Screening Instrument (CASI) demonstrates greater specificity than does the MMSE (Sherrell, Buckwalter, Bode, & Strozdas, 1999). The CASI is a 25-item instrument test developed as a research instrument and piloted in Japan and the United States (Teng et al., 1994). The total score ranges from 0 (poor) to 100 (good), with a suggested cutoff of 74 for classifying dementia. The CASI provides quantitative assessment of nine domains: attention, concentration, orientation, long-term memory, short-term memory, language, visual construction (copying pentagons), fluency (naming four-legged animals), and abstraction and judgment. Because it determines the level of cognitive impairment, the CASI could be used in establishing individualized care plans.

Behaviour Changes

Behaviour changes in older adults can indicate neuropathologic processes and thus require nursing assessment. If such changes occur, it is most likely that family members will notice them before the client does. Apraxia (the inability to execute a voluntary movement despite normal muscle function) is not attributed to age but indicates an underlying disease process, such as Alzheimer's disease, Parkinson's disease, or other disorders. Various other behaviour problems are associated with psychiatric disorders in older individuals, including irritability, agitation, apathy, and euphoria. Other behaviours in older adults who are experiencing psychiatric problems include wandering and aggressive behaviours. The BEHAVE-AD identifies these behaviours.

The Neuropsychiatric Inventory (NPI) was developed in 1994 to assess behaviour problems associated with dementia. The scale assesses 10 behaviour problems: delusions, hallucinations, dysphoria, anxiety, agitation/aggression, euphoria, disinhibition, irritability/lability, apathy, and aberrant motor behaviour (Cummings et al., 1994). The NPI was subsequently refined to include two more behavioural problems: night-time behavioural disturbances such as difficulties with sleep and changes in eating patterns. The NPI also added a component to assess for caregiver distress (Cummings, 1997). This very popular tool is used in many medication clinical trials. There are two versions. The standard version is used when the client is still at home, whereas a different version is used when the client is in a long-term care facility.

Stress and Coping Patterns

Identifying stresses and coping patterns is just as important for older individuals as it is for younger adults. Unique stresses for older clients include living on a fixed income, handling declining health, losing partners and friends, and ultimately confronting death. Coping ability varies, depending on clients' unique circumstances. For example, some older adults respond to stressful events with amazing adaptability, whereas others become depressed and suicidal.

Loss of a spouse is common in late life, especially for women in older age groups. For instance, women constitute 52% of the population aged 65 to 69 years of age, but by the age of 80 to 84 years, this percentage jumps to 61% (Schellenberg & Turcotte, 2006). Bereavement, a natural response to the death of a loved one, includes crying and sorrow, anxiety and agitation, insomnia, and loss of appetite. These symptoms, while overlapping with those of major depression, do not constitute a mental disorder. Only when these symptoms persist for 2 months or longer can a diagnosis of either adjustment disorder or major depressive disorder be made (APA, 2000). Although bereavement is a normal response, the nurse must identify it and develop interventions to help the individual successfully resolve the loss. Bereavement is an important and well-established risk factor for depression. Factors such as previous mental or physical health conditions in the surviving spouse, high levels of caregiver strain before the death of the spouse, and a lack of social support increase the likelihood of depression post bereavement (Schum, Lyness, & King, 2005).

Risk Assessment

Suicide is a major mental health risk for older adults. Men 85 years of age and older have the highest suicide rate of all age groupings in Canada (Government of Canada, 2006). Most older individuals who commit suicide have visited their family physician within the month of their death (Juurlink, Herrmann, Szalai, Kopp, & Redelmeier, 2004).

When caring for the older client with mental health problems, the nurse always should consider the individual's potential to commit suicide. Depression is the greatest risk factor for suicide. In assessing an older client, the nurse should consider the following characteristics as indications of high risk for committing suicide:

- Depression
- Attempted suicide in the past
- Family history of suicide
- Firearms in the home
- Abuse of alcohol or other substances
- Unusual stress
- Chronic medical condition (e.g., cancer, neuromuscular disorders)
- Social isolation

Social Domain

An assessment of the social domain includes determining the client's interactions with others in his or her family and community. The nurse targets social support because it is so important to the well-being of older adults, functional status because of the potential physical changes that can affect this area, and social systems, which encompass all community resources.

Social Support

Remaining active throughout one's life is one of the best predictors of mental health and wellness in an older individual. People obtain their sense of self-worth through their interactions with others in their environment. A sense of "who one is" is closely tied to the roles that a person plays in life. When older adults relinquish such roles because of physical disabilities, become isolated from friends and family, or begin to sense that they are a burden to those around them, rather than contributing members of society, a sense of hopelessness and helplessness may follow.

The role of social support is critical to assess in this age group. Social support is a reciprocal concept, meaning that simply receiving assistance increases the person's sense of being a burden. Those older individuals who also believe that they contribute to the welfare of others are most likely to remain mentally healthy. For this reason, pets are often "life savers" for older adults who live alone. Nothing can be more understanding and accepting of an older adult's behaviour or disabilities than a beloved pet.

The nurse should assess the client's number of formal and informal social contacts. The nurse should ask about the frequency of contacts with others (in person and through telephone calls, letters, and cards) that the older adult has. The amount of social support currently experienced should be compared with the amount and kinds of support the client received in the past. Determining whether these contacts are actually satisfying and supporting to the client is essential. If family members are important to the client's well-being, the nurse should complete a more in-depth family assessment (see Chapter 17).

The nurse can use the following questions to focus on social support (Kane, 1995):

- In the past 2 weeks, how often would you say that others let you know that they care about you?
- In the past 2 weeks, how often has someone provided you with help, such as giving you a ride somewhere or helping around the house?

- Do you have any one special person you could call or contact if you needed help? Who?
- In general, other than your children, how many relatives do you feel close to and have contact with at least once a month?

For older clients who are isolated with few social contacts, the nurse can develop interventions to improve social support.

Functional Status

As part of a complete assessment, the nurse will need to assess the older adult's functional status. **Functional activities** or activities of daily living (ADLs) are the activities necessary for self-care (i.e., bathing, toileting, dressing, transferring). Instrumental ADLs (IADLs) include those that facilitate or enhance the performance of ADLs (i.e., shopping, using the telephone, using transportation). These aspects are critical to consider for any older adult living alone. When possible, the older adult should be observed for his or her ability to complete ADLs, rather than relying on self-report or report of the family. Common tools used to assess functional status include the Index of Independence in Activities of Daily Living and the Instrumental Activities of Daily Living Scale (Katz & Akpom, 1976). The Functional Activities Questionnaire (FAQ) measures an adult's functional abilities based on the information from family members and caregivers. The older person is rated on 10 complex, higher-order activities, such as writing checks, assembling tax records, and driving (Pfeffer, Kursaki, Harrah, Chance, & Filos, 1982). The Functional Autonomy Measuring System (Hebert, Guilbeault, & Pinsonnault, 2002; McKye, Naglie, Tierney, & Jaglal, 2009) is designed for use in a community setting and measures's a person's actual performance on a task (e.g., performs task alone; with cueing or help; total help needed). Client and family reports can be used in completing it.

Social Systems

Community resources are essential to an older adult's ability to maintain mental health and wellness, as well as to his or her ability to remain at home throughout the later years. Senior centres are federally or provincially funded community resources that provide a wide array of services to Canada's older population. They may provide daily balanced meals at a nominal cost. In addition, they provide opportunities for socialization, which is key to combating loneliness and social isolation. Many senior centres provide annual influenza and pneumonia vaccination clinics and education on such topics as fall prevention and the recognition and prevention of elder abuse. Additional community resources that are specific to older individuals include geriatric assessment clinics and adult day programs.

During the assessment, the nurse must determine which community resources are available and if the older client uses them. Lack of transportation to and from these community resources may be a barrier to use. Most communities have buses available for older or handicapped individuals. The nurse may need to assist the older adult in accessing this important resource.

One in five older adults in Canada is classified as living in a low-income situation (Public Health Agency of Canada, 2005c). Low income is particularly prevalent among older women living on their own (Government of Canada, 2008). A number of older adults rely on Canada Pension Plan (CPP) (or for older adults living in Quebec, the Quebec Pension Plan), Old Age Security (OAS), and Guaranteed Income Supplement (GIS) for their monthly income. For these older individuals, this financial support, although less than adequate in most instances, is their only source of income. The nurse should assess a client's sources of financial support. Sometimes, nurses are uncomfortable asking for financial information, fearing that they are invading the client's privacy. However, such data are important for the nurse to determine whether an older individual's resources adequately meet his or her needs. The source of financial support is also important. For example, a client whose income is adequate and comes from personal resources is more likely to be independent than is a client who depends on family members for income.

The nurse should ask the client about accessible health care facilities; available transportation to and from health care facilities; formal supports such as physicians, nurses, and other health care professionals; and the client's ability to pay for medications and health aids. Information about available health care resources beyond standard provincial health care (e.g., plans to pay for additional services such as medications or foot care) will alert the nurse to what services the client currently can and cannot access. In urban areas that are likely to have adequate health care resources, cultural and language barriers may prohibit access. People who live in rural areas where health care resources are limited are less likely to enjoy the full range of health care resources than are those in urban areas. For instance, older adults in Canadian rural settings have greater difficulty accessing geriatric mental health services than those in urban sites (Conn, 2003). Even in centres with geriatric mental health services, however, many older adults are reluctant to access services because of a lack of awareness of available help, stigma, or cultural issues (Sadavoy, Meier, & Ong, 2004).

Legal Status

A growing trend in Canada and the United States is to view older adults as a special population whose rights deserve increased attention. Instances of elder abuse are far too common. Every nurse must consider herself or himself a client advocate and be vigilant in recognizing the signs of neglect or abuse, such as unexplained injuries. At times, abuse can take the form of another individual (sometimes an adult child) usurping the rights of the older person.

Unless the older person is medically and legally determined to be incompetent, he or she has the same rights to personal decision making as any other adult, including the right to refuse treatment.

Spiritual Domain

Spiritual needs are basic for all age groups and are requirements for establishing meaning and purpose, love and relatedness, and forgiveness. Spirituality is sometimes expressed through commitment to organized religion and, other times, is expressed differently. Aging is a process that can bring individuals closer to understanding the finite nature of existence and evokes an awareness of their spiritual needs. With advanced age, many people begin to reflect on their successes and failures. During such reflection, many seek out God or a higher being to make sense of the past and establish hope for the future.

The process of spiritual assessment involves active listening, thoughtful observing, and sensitive questioning. The nurse may simply ask if the older adult would find comfort from a visit from a minister or a spiritual leader. Many forms of religion use various rituals that are important to the older individual's daily routine. The nurse should explore and honour these aspects to the extent possible (see Chapters 6 and 13).

A sense of quality of life is closely tied to values and beliefs about life's meaning. For many older individuals, quality of life is not reflected in material possessions or physical health but more by contentment over how the person has lived life and the extent to which his or her life has had meaning and purpose. Keeping close personal contacts with friends and family and having the opportunity to share stories of lifetime experiences are important to mental health and spiritual well-being. For older individuals, physical illnesses may affect the quality of life more than psychiatric disorders. The assessment of quality of life becomes especially important when assessing a client living in a continuing care facility or isolated in his or her own home. The assessment of quality of life of older adults is similar to that for younger adults (see Chapter 11).

SUMMARY OF KEY POINTS

☐ Normal aging is associated with some physical decline, but most functions do not change. Intellectual functioning, capacity for change, and productive engagement with life remain stable.

☐ Mental health assessments are necessary when older clients face psychiatric or mental health issues. The bio/psycho/social/spiritual geriatric mental health nursing assessment examines many sources of data, including self-reports, laboratory test results, and reports from family members.

□ The bio/psycho/social/spiritual geriatric mental health nursing assessment is based on the special needs and problems of older individuals. This assessment examines current and past health, functional status, and human responses to mental health problems.

□ The assessment of the biologic domain involves collecting data about the past and present health status, physical examination findings, physical functions (i.e., nutrition and eating, elimination patterns, sleep), pain, and pharmacologic information.

□ The assessment of the psychological domain includes the client's responses to mental health problems, mental status examination, behavioural changes, stress and coping patterns, and risk assessment.

□ When conducting an assessment, the nurse may find several tools useful. For clients with possible depression, the GDS may be helpful. For clients with anxiety, nurses can use the RAID scale. In addition to a careful interview, the nurse can use the BEHAVE-AD scale to determine delusions, hallucinations, activity disturbances, aggressiveness, diurnal rhythm disturbances, mood disturbances, anxieties, or phobias.

□ The nurse can conduct cognitive assessments using the MMSE or the CASI.

□ Coping with the stresses of aging varies among clients. Determining stresses and coping skills for dealing with stresses is important.

□ Social support is critical to clients in this age group and requires assessment.

□ Determination of the client's ability to perform functional and instrumental ADLs is critical in the assessment of older adults. The FAQ measures the functional abilities based on information from others.

□ Social systems, spiritual assessment, legal information, and the quality of life are components within the social domain that the nurse should consider.

CRITICAL THINKING CHALLENGES

1 The director of your church's senior centre has asked you to be the guest speaker at the monthly meeting of the Retired Active Citizens group. The subject is to be "Maintaining Your Mental Health After Retirement." What key points will you touch on in your presentation? What activities or handouts will you use to highlight your talk?

2 When asking about current illnesses, a client begins telling you her whole life story. What approach would you take to elicit the most important information needed to develop an individualized plan of care for your older client?

3 A caregiver tells you that her mother has become suspicious of the neighbours and other family members.

How would you assess this perceptual experience? What other data should you gather from this client?

4 A caregiver brings a bag of medications to the client's assessment interview. What information should you obtain from the caregiver regarding the older individual's use of these medications?

5 A woman brings her father, who has a long history of frequent psychiatric hospitalizations for depression, to the clinic. The client's wife recently died, and the daughter fears that her father is becoming depressed again. What approach would you use in assessing for changes in mood?

6 Obtain a listing of the social services available in your community. Examine the list for areas of duplication and omission of services needed by an older adult living alone in his or her own home.

WEB LINKS

www.alzheimer.ca The Alzheimer Society of Canada website includes information about the society, Alzheimer's disease (AD), how to care for someone with AD, and research updates.

www.canada.gc.ca The Government of Canada website provides information on government financial plans for older adults (e.g., CPP).

www.ccsmh.ca The Canadian Coalition for Seniors Mental Health (CCSMH) website explains the mission of this organization and offers resources for education, assessment, and treatment for older adults living with mental illness.

www.cgna.net The Canadian Gerontological Nursing Association (CGNA) website provides information about the CGNA, access to CGNA newsletters, links to other useful websites pertaining to the care of older adults, and information about upcoming events for gerontological nurses.

www.cmhc-schl.gc.ca The Canada Mortgage and Housing Corporation (CMHC) website provides information about how older adults can adapt their homes for increasing disabilities and financial assistance programs for housing for older adults.

MOVIES, NOVELS, AND BIOGRAPHIES

On Golden Pond: 1981. In this classic film, Henry Fonda portrays a crotchety, retired professor named Norman Thayer. Norman is angry that he is 80 years old and scared that he may lose his cognitive abilities. His wife, played by Katherine Hepburn, provides support and encouragement in maintaining his independence.

The story revolves around Norman's relationship with his estranged daughter (played by Jane Fonda) as they try finally to understand each other during Norman's later years.

VIEWING POINTS: Identify the physical impairments that are obvious throughout the movie. Identify specific memory problems that Norman experiences. Are these problems part of normal aging? If you were Norman Thayer's nurse, what key assessment areas would you explore?

REFERENCES

Adlaf, E. M., Begin, P., & Sawka, E. (Eds.). (2005). *Canadian Addiction Survey (CAS): A national survey of Canadians' use of alcohol and other drugs: Prevalence of use and related harms: Detailed report.* Ottawa, ON: Canadian Centre on Substance Abuse.

Alexopoulos, G. S., Abrams, R. C., Young, R. C., & Shamoian, C. (1998). Cornell scale for depression in dementia. *Biological Psychiatry, 23,* 271–284.

Almeida, O. P., & Pfaff, J. J. (2005). Sleep complaints among older general practice patients: Association with depression. *British Journal of General Practice, 55,* 864–866.

American Psychiatric Association. (2000). *Diagnostic and statistical manual of mental disorders* (4th ed., Text revision). Washington, DC: Author.

Barton, C., Miller, B., & Yaffe, K. (2006). Improved evaluation and management of cognitive impairment: Results of a comprehensive intervention in long-term care. *Journal of the American Directors Association, 7*(2), 84–89.

Byles, J. E., Mishra, G. D., Harris, M. A., & Nair, K. (2003). The problems of sleep for older women: Changes in health outcomes. *Age and Ageing, 32*(2), 123–124.

Canadian Coalition for Seniors Mental Health. (2003). Depression fought in seniors. *Canadian Coalition for Seniors Mental Health, 1*(4), 2.

Conn, D. K. (2002). An overview of common mental disorders among seniors. *National Advisory Council on Aging, Writing in Gerontology, Mental Health and Aging.* Minister of Public Works and Government Services Canada.

Conn, D. K. (2003). Oral presentation to the Standing Senate Committee on Social Affairs, Science and Technology. *Bulletin of the Canadian Academy of Geriatric Psychiatry, 10*(3), 5–8.

Cummings, J. L. (1997). The Neuropsychiatric Inventory: Assessing psychopathology in dementia patients. *Neurology, 48*(5) (Suppl. 6), S10–S16.

Cummings, J. L., Mega, M., Gray, K., Rosenberg-Thompson, S., Carusi, D. A., & Gornbein, J. (1994). The Neuropsychiatric Inventory: Comprehensive assessment of psychopathology in dementia. *Neurology, 44*(12), 2308–2314.

Government of Canada. (2006). *The human face of mental health and mental illness in Canada – 2006* (Cat. No. HP5–19/2006E). Minister of Public Works and Government Services Canada.

Government of Canada. (2008). *Reducing poverty among older women: The potential of retirement income policies.* Retrieved April 17, 2008, from www.swc-cfc.gc.ca/pubs/pubspr/0662659271/200008_0662659271_9_e.html

Hebert, R., Guilbeault, J. & Pinsonnault, E. (2002). *Functional Autonomy Measuring System User Guide.* Sherbrooke, Quebec: Centre d'expertise de l'Institut universitaire de geriatrie de Sherbrooke.

Hyer, L., & Blount, J. (1984). Concurrent and discriminant validities of the geriatric depression scale with older psychiatric inpatients. *Psychological Reports, 54,* 611–616.

Juurlink, D. N., Herrmann, N., Szalai, J. P., Kopp, A., & Redelmeier, D. A. (2004). Medical illness and the risk of suicide in the elderly. *Archives of Internal Medicine, 164*(11), 1179–1184.

Kaasalainen, S., Coker, E., Dolovich, L., Papaioannou, A., Hadjstavropoulous, T., Emili, A. & Ploeg, J. (2007). Pain management decision making among long-term care physicians and nurses. *Western Journal of Nursing Research, 29*(5), 561–580.

Kane, R. A. (1995). Assessment of social functioning: Recommendations for comprehensive geriatric assessment. In Z. Rubenstein, D. Wieland, & R. Bernabei (Eds.), *Geriatric assessment technology: The state of the art* (pp. 91–110). New York, NY: Springer.

Katz, S., & Akpom, A. (1976). A measure of primary sociobiological functions. *International Journal of Health Science, 6,* 493.

Klatsky, A. L., Friedman, G. D., Armstrong, M. A., & Kipp, H. (2003). Wine, liquor, beer, and mortality. *American Journal of Epidemiology, 158*(6), 585–595.

Leifer, B. (2009). Alzheimer's disease: seeing the signs early. *Journal of the Academy of Nurse Practitioners, 21,* 588–595.

Lopez, O. L., Becker, J. T., Sweet, R. A., Klunk, W., Kaufer, D. I., Saxton, J., Habeych, M. & DeKosky, S. (2003). Psychiatric symptoms vary with the severity of dementia in probable Alzheimer's disease. *Journal of Neuropsychiatry and Clinical Neuroscience, 15*(3), 346–353.

McKye, K.A., Naglie, G., Tierney, M. & Jaglal, S. (2009). Comparison of older adults' and occupational therapists' awareness of functional abilities at discharge from rehabilitation with actual performance in the home. *Physical & Occupational Therapy in Geriatrics, 27*(3), 229–244.

Moore, A. A., Seeman, T., Morgenstern, H., Beck, J. C., & Reuben, D. B. (2002). Are there differences between older persons who screen positive on the CAGE questionnaire and the Short Michigan Alcoholism Screening Test – Geriatric Version? *Journal of the American Geriatrics Society, 50*(5), 858–862.

Mulgrew, C., Morgenstern, N., Shetterly, S., Baxter, J. Barón, A. & Hamman, R. (1999). Cognitive functioning and impairment among rural elderly Hispanics and non-Hispanic whites as assessed by the Mini-Mental State Examination. *Journals of Gerontology, 54B*(4), 223–230.

Pfeffer, R., Kurosaki, T., Harrah, C., Chance, J. & Filos, S. (1982). Measurement of functional activities in older adults in the community. *Journal of Gerontology, 37*(3), 323–329.

Public Health Agency of Canada. (2005a). *A growing population: Statistical snapshot #1.* Statistics Canada. Retrieved July 25, 2005, from http://www.phac.aspc.gc.ca/seniors-aines

Public Health Agency of Canada. (2005b). *Seniors experiencing chronic pain: Statistical snapshot # 34.* Statistics Canada. Retrieved July 25, 2005, from http://www.phac.aspc.gc.ca/seniors-aines

Public Health Agency of Canada. (2005c). *Low income across the country: Statistical snapshot #18.* Statistics Canada. Retrieved July 25, 2005, from http://www.phac.aspc.gc.ca/seniors-aines

Rabheru, K. (2004). Special issues in the management of depression in older patients. *Canadian Journal of Psychiatry, 49*(Suppl. 1), 41S–50S.

Reisberg, B., & Ferris, S. (1985). A clinical rating scale for symptoms of psychosis in Alzheimer's disease. *Psychopharmacology Bulletin, 21,* 101–104.

Reisberg, B., Auer, S., & Monteiro, I. (1996). Behavioural Pathology in Alzheimer's Disease (BEHAVE-AD) rating scale. *International Psychogeriatrics, 8*(3), 301–308.

Sadavoy, J., Meier, R., & Ong, A. Y. M. (2004). Barriers to access to mental health services for ethnic seniors: The Toronto study. *Canadian Journal of Psychiatry, 49*(3), 192–199.

SAGMHS (Southern Alberta Geriatric Mental Health Working Group). (2003, September). *Summary Report of the Southern Alberta Geriatric Mental Health Working Group,* 1–12.

Schellenberg, G., & Turcotte, M. (2006). *A portrait of Seniors in Canada* (Cat. No. 89–519-XWE). Statistics Canada.

Schum, J. L., Lyness, J. M., & King, D. A. (2005). Bereavement in late life: Risk factors for complicated bereavement. *Geriatrics, 60*(4), 18–20, 24.

Shankar, K. K., Walker, M., Frost, D., & Orrell, M. W. (1999). The development of a valid and reliable scale for rating anxiety in dementia (RAID). *Aging & Mental Health, 3*(1), 39–49.

Sheikh, J. I., & Yesavage, J. A. (1986). Geriatric Depression Scale (GDS): Recent evidence and development of a shorter version. In T. L. Brink (Ed.), *Clinical gerontology: A guide to assessment and interventions* (pp. 165–177). Binghamton, NY: Haworth Press.

Sherrell, K., Buckwalter, K., Bode, R., & Strozdas, L. (1999). Use of the cognitive abilities screen instrument to assess elderly persons with schizophrenia in long-term care settings. *Issues in Mental Health Nursing, 20,* 541–558.

Statistics Canada. (2005). Life expectancy at birth, by sex, by provinces. Retrieved June 06, 2005, from http://www.40.statcan. ca/l01/cst01/health26.htm

Statistics Canada. (2006). The Daily: Deaths 2004. Retrieved May 01, 2008, from http://www.statcan.ca/Daily/English/061220/d061220b.htm

Teng, E., Kazuo Hasegawa, K., Homma, A., Imai, Y., Larson, E., Graves, A., et al. (1994). The cognitive abilities screen instrument (CASI): A practical test for cross-cultural epidemiological studies of dementia. *International Psychogeriatrics, 6*(1), 45–58.

University of Michigan Alcohol Research Centre. (1991). Short Michigan Alcoholism Screening Test – Geriatric Version (SMAST-G). Retrieved April 23, 2008, from http://www.hartfordign.org/publications/trythis/issue17.pdf

CHAPTER 31

Delirium, Dementias, and Other Related Disorders

Mary Haase

Adapted from the chapter "Delirum, Dementials, and Related Disorders" by Mary Ann Boyd, Linda Garand, Linda A. Gerdner, Bonnie J. Wakefield, and Kathleen Buckwalter

C ognition and memory are important in many psychiatric disorders, but in this chapter, they are the key concepts. Cognition is the ability to think and know. The definition is further refined to be understood as a relatively high level of intellectual processing in which perceptions and information are acquired, used, or manipulated.

KEY CONCEPT Cognition is based on a system of interrelated abilities, such as perception, reasoning, judgment, intuition, and memory, that allow one to be aware of oneself and one's surroundings. Impairments in these abilities can result in a failure of the afflicted person to recognize that he or she is not well and is in need of treatment.

Cognition involves both how reality is perceived and how those perceptions are understood in relation to internal representations of reality previously acquired. In the broadest sense, cognition denotes how the brain processes information. Cognition includes a number of specific functions, such as the acquisition and use of language, the ability to be oriented in time and space, and the ability to learn and solve problems. It includes judgment, reasoning, attention, comprehension, concept formation, planning, and the use of symbols, such as numbers and letters used in mathematics and writing.

Memory, a facet of cognition, refers to the ability to recall or reproduce what has been learned or experienced. It is more than simple storage and retrieval; it is a complex cognitive mental function that includes most areas of the brain, especially the hippocampus, which is believed to be essential to the transfer of some memories from short-term to long-term storage. Defects of memory are an essential feature of many cognitive disorders, particularly dementia.

> **KEY CONCEPT Memory** is a facet of cognition concerned with retaining and recalling past experiences, whether they occurred in the physical environment or internally as cognitive events.

The disorders discussed in this chapter—delirium, dementia, and related cognitive disorders—are characterized by deficits in cognition or memory that represent a clear-cut deterioration from a previous level of functioning. Delirium is a disorder of acute cognitive impairment and can be caused by a medical condition (e.g., infection) or substance abuse, or it may have multiple etiologies. Dementia is characterized by chronic cognitive impairments and is differentiated by the underlying cause, not by symptom patterns, which are often similar. Some dementias are irreversible and progressive. Some organic compounds and chemicals, such as lead, manganese, and toluene (one of the toxins in glue and paint), may produce the symptoms of dementia (Table 31-1). Once a person with chemically induced symptoms is evaluated and treated, the symptoms of dementia may resolve.

> **KEY CONCEPT Delirium** is a disorder of physical origin that develops over a short period of time, and is characterized by fluctuating consciousness and attention.

> **KEY CONCEPT Dementia** is characterized by chronic cognitive impairment and is differentiated by underlying cause, not by symptom patterns, which are often similar. Dementia can be further classified as cortical or subcortical to denote the location of the underlying pathology.

Table 31.1	Selected Compounds and Chemicals That May Produce Dementia
Substance	**Related Symptoms**
Arsenic	Headache
	Drowsiness
	Confusion
Mercury	Tremors
	Extrapyramidal signs
	Upper and lower extremity ataxia
	Depression
	Confusion
Lead	Abdominal cramps
	Anemia
	Peripheral neuropathy
	Encephalopathy (rare)
Manganese	Extrapyramidal symptoms
	Delirium
Toluene (methyl benzene)	Profound cognitive impairment
	Tremor
	Ataxia
	Loss of vision and hearing

Cortical dementia results from a disease process that globally afflicts the cortex. **Subcortical dementia** is caused by dysfunction or deterioration of deep grey- or white-matter structures inside the brain and brain stem. Symptoms of subcortical dementia may be more localized and tend to disrupt arousal, attention, and motivation, but they can produce a variety of clinical behavioural manifestations. In this chapter, a type of cortical dementia, Alzheimer's disease (AD), is highlighted because it is the most prevalent form of dementia in Canada.

Delirium

CLINICAL COURSE OF DISORDER

Delirium is a disorder of physical origin that develops over a short period of time, and it is characterized by fluctuating consciousness and attention. Delirium is usually reversible if treated promptly. It is a serious disorder that is associated with high morbidity and mortality.

Emergency!

"Delirium is an acute, complex disorder that requires immediate interventions to prevent permanent brain damage and death" (RNAO, 2004, p. 30). It is associated with mortality rates of 25%–33% (Inouye, 2000).

Table 31.2 Key Diagnostic Characteristics of Delirium Caused by a General Medical Condition 293.0	
Diagnostic Criteria	**Associated Findings**

• Disturbance of consciousness
  Reduced clarity of awareness
  Decreased ability to focus, sustain, or shift attention
• Developing over a short period of time—usually hours to days; fluctuating during the course of the day
• Cognitive changes
  Memory deficit, disorientation, language disturbance
    Development of perceptual disturbance not better accounted for by a preexisting, established, or evolving dementia
• History, physical examination, or laboratory tests indicating change as a direct cause of physiologic effects of medical condition
 	
Etiologies
• Substance intoxication delirium
• Substance withdrawal delirium
• Multiple etiologies (due to more than one medical condition, substance effect, or medication side effect)
• Not otherwise specified
	Associated Behavioural Findings
	• Attention wandering
	• Perseveration
	• Easily distracted
	• Recent memory changes
	• Dysnomia, dysgraphia
	• Speech is rambling, irrelevant, incoherent
	• Misinterpretations, illusions, and hallucinations
	
	Associated Physical Findings
	• Daytime sleepiness
	• Nighttime agitation
	• Difficulty falling asleep
	• Restlessness, hyperactivity, or sluggishness and lethargy
	• Anxiety, fear, irritability, anger, euphoria, and apathy
	• Rapid unpredictable shifts from one emotional state to another
	
	Associated Laboratory Findings
	• Abnormal electroencephalogram

DIAGNOSTIC CRITERIA

There are no specific tests available to diagnose delirium; the diagnosis is made on the basis of clinical presentation (White & Bayer, 2007). Impaired consciousness is the key diagnostic criterion. The patient becomes less aware of his or her environment and loses the ability to focus, sustain, and shift attention. Associated cognitive changes include problems in memory, orientation, and language. The patient may not know where he or she is, may not recognize familiar objects, or may be unable to carry on a conversation. An important diagnostic indicator is that delirium develops rapidly, usually over hours or days. Table 31-2 presents the diagnostic criteria of delirium caused by a general medical condition. Delirium is different from dementia, but the presenting symptoms are often similar, and it is possible to have a delirium superimposed on a dementia. Figure 31-1 shows the kaleidoscope of care strategies of delirium, dementia, and depression.

• CRNENOTE
Delirium can be life threatening; identifying potential underlying causes of symptoms is a priority.

DELIRIUM IN SPECIAL POPULATIONS

Children

Delirium can occur in children and may be related to medications (anticholinergic agents) or fever. Children seem to be especially susceptible to this disorder, probably because of their immature brain. However, delirium may be hard to diagnose and may be mistaken for uncooperative behaviour.

Older Adults

Although delirium may occur in any age group, it is most common among the older adults. Nurses must recognize that delirium, dementia, and depression present with overlapping clinical features and may coexist in the older adult (Registered Nurses Association of Ontario [RNAO], 2003).

EPIDEMIOLOGY AND RISK FACTORS

Statistics concerning the prevalence of delirium are based primarily on older individuals in acute care settings. Estimated prevalence rates range from 10% to 30% of patients. In nursing homes, the prevalence is much higher, approaching 60% of those older than the age of 75 years. Delirium occurs in as many as 30% of patients hospitalized for cancer and in 30% to 40% of those hospitalized with acquired immunodeficiency syndrome (AIDS). Near death, 80% of patients experience delirium (American Psychiatric Association [APA], 2000).

The most powerful risks for developing delirium are present before admission, for example, old age, severe illness, dementia, visual/hearing impairments, polypharmacy, alcohol abuse, fracture, infection, pain, and renal impairment (British Geriatrics Society, 2006; Vollmer, Rich, & Robinson, 2007). One study concluded

FIGURE 31.1 Kaleidoscope of care strategies for delirium, dementia, and depression (RNAO, 2004, p. 19).

that patients with or without dementia had persistent symptoms of delirium up to 12 months after diagnosis. The same study found that a quicker in-hospital recovery is associated with better outcomes (McCusker, Cole, Dendukuri, Han, & Belzile, 2003). Patients experiencing mental confusion are also more likely to be victims of falls and fractures. Box 31-1 lists the proposed risk factors for delirium, and Box 31-2 presents a vignette of a patient who experienced delirium after using an over-the-counter (OTC) sleeping medication.

ETIOLOGY

The etiology of delirium is complex and usually multifaceted. A lack of generally accepted theories of causation has resulted in considerable variability in the research.

BOX **31.1**

Risk Factors for Delirium

- Advanced age
- Preexisting dementia
- Functional dependence
- Preexisting illness
- Bone fracture
- Infection
- Medications (both number and type)
- Changes in vital signs (including hypotension and hyper- or hypothermia)
- Electrolyte or metabolic imbalance
- Admission to a long-term care institution
- Postcardiotomy
- AIDS
- Pain

BOX 31.2

*Clinical Vignette: **Delirium***

Mrs. Campbell, a widowed 72-year-old woman living in her own home, has been having trouble sleeping. Her daughter visits her and suggests that Mrs. Campbell try an OTC sleeping medication. Mrs. Campbell has also been taking antihistamines for allergies and the antidepressant amitriptyline. Three nights later, a neighbour calls the daughter, concerned because she encountered Mrs. Campbell wandering the streets, unable to find her home. When the neighbour approached Mrs. Cambell to help her home, Mrs. Campbell began to scream and strike out at the neighbour.

The daughter visits immediately and discovers that her mother does not know who she is, does not know what time it is, appears disheveled, and is suspicious that people have been in her home stealing the things she cannot find. Mrs. Campbell does not recall taking any medication, but when her daughter investigates she finds that 10 pills of the new sleeping aid have already been used. Mrs. Campbell is irritable and refuses to go to the hospital, but over the course of a few hours, she appears to calm down, and her daughter is able to take her to see her physician the following morning. After hearing the history, the physician hospitalizes Mrs. Campbell, withholds all medication, and provides intravenous hydration. Within 3 days, Mrs. Campbell is again able to recognize her daughter, and her mental status appears to be greatly improved.

WHAT DO YOU THINK?

- Identify risk factors that may have contributed to Mrs. Campbell experiencing delirium.
- How could the addition of an OTC sleeping medication interact with the antihistamine and antidepressant to be responsible for Mrs. Campbell's delirium?

Thus, integrating the research and applying it to practice have been difficult. To date, studies focus almost exclusively on biologic causes of delirium, with psychosocial factors viewed as contributing or facilitating. Because environmental and psychosocial factors have been explored only in small, uncontrolled studies, conclusions cannot be drawn about these factors. For this reason, the following discussion of etiology covers biologic theories of cause.

The most commonly identified causes of delirium, in order of frequency, follow:

- Medications
- Infections (particularly urinary tract and upper respiratory)
- Fluid and electrolyte imbalance; metabolic disturbances
- The probability of the syndrome developing increases if certain predisposing factors, such as advanced age, brain damage, or dementia, are present. Sensory overload or underload, immobilization, sleep deprivation, and psychosocial stress also contribute to delirium

Because delirium has multiple causes, a wide variety of brain alterations may also be responsible for its development. Major theories of causation follow:

- A general reduction in brain functioning, which can result from a decrease in the supply, uptake, or use of substances for metabolic activity
- Damage of enzyme systems, the blood–brain barrier, or cell membranes
- Reduced brain metabolism resulting in decreased acetylcholine synthesis
- Imbalance of neurotransmitters, such as acetylcholine, norepinephrine, and dopamine

- Increased plasma cortisol level in response to acute stress, which affects attention and information processing
- Involvement of the white matter, especially in the thalamocortical projections (Tune, 2000)

■ INTERDISCIPLINARY TREATMENT AND PRIORITY CARE ISSUES

Delirium may be recognized and diagnosed in any health care setting and the interdisciplinary team needs to act promptly to reverse the symptoms (Heidrich, 2007). The management of delirium includes four key steps: (1) elimination or correction of the underlying cause(s), (2) management of behavioural disturbances, (3) anticipation and prevention of complications of delirium, and (4) support and restoration of functional needs (White & Bayer, 2007).

When developing a treatment plan for a patient in whom delirium is suspected, close attention must be paid to correcting any organic or disease-related factors. Initially, life-threatening illnesses, such as cerebral hypoxia, hypertensive encephalopathy, intracranial hemorrhage, meningitis, severe electrolyte and metabolic imbalances, hypoglycemia, and intoxication, must be ruled out or corrected. If possible, the use of all suspected medications should be stopped and vital signs monitored at least every 2 hours. Many patients with delirium are seriously ill and excellent nursing care is vital. The plan of care requires close observation for changes in vital signs, behaviour, and mental status. Patients are monitored until the delirium subsides. If the delirium still exists at discharge, it is critical that referrals for postdischarge follow-up assessment and care be implemented.

NURSING MANAGEMENT: HUMAN RESPONSE TO DELIRIUM

By definition, a biologic insult must be present for delirium to occur, but psychological and environmental factors are often involved. Because delirium develops quickly during a matter of hours or days and has been associated with increased mortality, nurses should be particularly vigilant in assessing patients who are at increased risk for this syndrome. (If the patient is a child, the assessment process presented in Chapter 27 should be used.) If the patient is an older person, the assessment that follows will serve as a guide. Special efforts should be made to include family members in the nursing process.

• CRNENOTE

Nurses need to be able to differentiate between the characteristics of dementia and those of delirium. Remember it is possible to have DSD; therefore, if agitation and a sudden change in mental status occur, assess the person for delirium.

Biologic Domain

Biologic Assessment

The onset of symptoms is typically signalled by a rapid or acute change in behaviour. To assess the symptoms, the nurse needs to know what is normal for the individual. Caregivers, family members, or significant others may be the only resource for accurate information and should be interviewed.

Current and Past Health Status

History should include a description of the onset, duration, range, and intensity of associated symptoms. Chronic physical illness, dementia, depression, or other psychiatric illnesses should be identified. Sorting out historical information may be particularly problematic when delirium accompanies acute illness, recent surgery, or infection.

Physical Examination and Review of Systems

In an attempt to discover the underlying cause of suspected delirium, monitoring of vital signs is crucial. An examination of body systems is conducted. Laboratory data, including complete blood count, glucose, blood urea nitrogen, creatinine, electrolyte analyses, liver function, and oxygen saturation, are gathered. Fluid balance, signs of constipation, or a recent history of diarrhea should be assessed.

Physical Functions

A functional assessment includes physical functional status (activities of daily living), the use of sensory aids (eyeglasses and hearing aids), usual activity level and any recent changes, and pain assessment. Sleep disturbances are a symptom of delirium and may precipitate confusion. Often, the sleep-wake cycle of the patient becomes reversed, with the individual attempting to sleep during the day and be awake at night. Restoration of a normal sleep cycle is extremely important.

Pharmacologic Assessment

A substance use history (including alcohol intake and smoking history) should be obtained (see Chapters 24 and 32). Information regarding medication use must be obtained, with particular attention given to new medications or changes in the dose of current medications. Table 31-3 lists some of the drugs that can cause an acute change in mental status. Special attention should be given to combinations of these medications because drug interactions can cause delirium.

Information regarding OTC medications should be included in this assessment. OTC medications are often thought of as harmless, but several medications, such as cold medications, taken in sufficient quantities may produce confusion, especially in older individuals.

Findings from the medication and physical assessments are integrated. Chronic pain may lead an individual to use more medication than has been intended. The increase in medication then results in delirium. Careful monitoring of the effectiveness of pain medications may lead to the order of a more effective medication that results in less potential misuse. Because many classes of medications have been associated with delirium, the focus is on changes in the type and number of medications and how medications relate to other findings in the history and physical assessment.

Nursing Diagnoses for the Biologic Domain

The nursing diagnoses typically generated from assessment data are acute confusion, disturbed thought processes, or disturbed sensory perception (visual or auditory; North American Nursing Diagnosis Association [NANDA], 2006). However, an astute nurse will also use nursing diagnoses based on other indicators, such as hyperthermia, acute pain, risk for infection, and disturbed sleep pattern.

Interventions for the Biologic Domain

Important interventions for a patient experiencing acute confusional state include providing a safe and therapeutic environment, maintaining fluid and electrolyte balance,

Table 31.3	Categories of Drugs That Can Cause "Acute Change in Mental Status"*
Mnemonic: Drug Category	**Examples of Drugs**
Antiparkinsonian drugs	Trihexyphenidyl, benzatropine, bromocriptine, levadopa, selegiline (deprenyl)
Corticosteroids	Prednisolone
Urinary incontinence drugs	Oxybutinin (Ditropan), flavoxate (Urispas)
Theophylline	Theophylline
Emptying drugs (motility drugs)	Metoclopramide (Reglan), cisapride (Prepulsid)
Cardiovascular drugs (including antihypertensives)	Digoxin, quinidine, methaldopa, reserpine, beta blockers (propanolol—to a less amount), diuretics, ACE inhibitors (captopril, Enalapril), calcium channel antagonists (nifedipine, verapamil, diltiazem)
H$_2$ blockers	Cimetidine (uncommon on its own but increased risk with renal impairment)
Antimicrobials	Cephalosporins, penicillin, quinolones, others
NSAIDs	Indomethacin, ibuprofen, naproxen, salicylate compounds
Geropsychiatry drugs	1. Tricylic antidepressants (e.g., amitriptyline, desipramine—to a lesser extent, imipramine, nortriptyline) 2. SSRIs—safer but watch if hyponatremia present 3. Benzodiazepines (e.g., diazepam) 4. Antipsychotics (e.g., haloperidol [Haldol], chlorpromazine, risperidone)
ENT drugs	Antihistamines, decongestants, cough syrups in OTC preparations
Insomnia	Nitrazepam, flurazepam, diazepam, temazepam
Narcotics	Meperdine, pentazocine (risky)
Muscle relaxants	Cyclobenzaprine (Flexeril), methocarbamol (Robaxin)
Seizure drugs	Phenytoin, primidone

*This table notes some examples of possible medications that can contribute to delirium. It is the physiologic status of the older adult and the combination of medications, among other factors, that increase risk. Therefore: "Watch and Beware."

Reprinted from Flaherty, J. H. (1998). Commonly prescribed and over-the-counter medications: Causes of confusion. *Clinics in Geriatric Medicine, 14*(1), 101–125, copyright (1998), with permission from Elsevier.

ensuring adequate nutrition, and preventing aspiration and decubitus ulcers. Other interventions, related to a particular nursing diagnosis, focus on individual symptoms and underlying causes, for example, for patients with disturbed sleep patterns, the Sleep Enhancement intervention is appropriate (McCloskey & Bulechek, 2000). Interventions to prevent delirium can reduce the length of hospital stay (White & Bayer, 2007).

Safety Interventions

Behaviours exhibited by the delirious patient, such as hallucinations, delusions, **illusions**, aggression, or agitation (restlessness or excitability), may pose safety problems. The patient must be protected from physical harm by using low beds, guardrails (use caution when putting up both bedrails as a confused person may try to climb over the rail), bed alarms, and careful supervision. The intervention "Surveillance: Safety or Fall Prevention" may be implemented (McCloskey & Bulechek, 2000) for any patient at risk for falls.

Pharmacologic Interventions

There is a lack of research to support the use of drugs in the management of delirium; in fact, they may worsen symptoms (White & Bayer, 2007). However, the goal of psychopharmacologic management is treatment of the behaviours associated with delirium, such as agitation, inattention, sleep disorder, and psychosis, with the goal of making the patient comfortable. The decision to use medications should be based on the specific symptoms. Dosages are usually kept very low. Medications should be chosen in light of the potential side effects (particularly anticholinergic effects, hypotension, and respiratory suppression). The use of antipsychotic agents in older individuals is discussed in greater detail later in the chapter. Benzodiazepines should be used only when the delirium is related to alcohol withdrawal. In some patients, the sedation effect may further impair cognition or a paradoxic agitation may develop (Gleason, 2003).

Administering and Monitoring Medications

Patients experiencing delirium may resist taking medications because of their confusion. If a medication is given, ideally it should be oral. Medications should never be hidden in food.

Monitoring and Managing Side Effects. Monitoring drug action and side effects is especially important because the cause of the delirium may not be known, and the patient may inadvertently be affected by the medication. Patients should be monitored for sedation, hypotension, or extrapyramidal symptoms. Although mental status often fluctuates during delirium, it may also be influenced by these medications, and any changes or worsening of mental status after the administration of the medication should be reported immediately to the prescriber. Some side effects may also be confused with the symptoms of delirium. For example, akathisia (see Chapter 14) may appear to be agitation or restlessness. The patient's physical condition and concurrent medication regimen may also influence the bioavailability, metabolism, and elimination of these medications. Adequate hydration and nutrition must be maintained. When using antipsychotic medications, closely monitor the patient for symptoms of neuroleptic malignant syndrome (see Chapter 14). The appearance of these symptoms may be confused with those related to delirium and therefore missed.

The use of medications for treating symptoms related to delirium should be discontinued as soon as possible. These medications should be withdrawn gradually during a period of several days or weeks.

Identifying Drug Interactions. The etiology of delirium is often a drug–drug interaction. OTC sleeping, cold, or allergy medication may be the cause. If medication is the underlying cause, it is important to identify accurately which medications are involved before administering any other drugs. A consultation with a clinical pharmacist may also be helpful.

Teaching Points

To prevent future occurrences, the nurse needs to educate the patient, family, and caregivers about the underlying cause of delirium. If the delirium is not resolved before discharge, caregivers need to know how to care for the patient at home.

Psychological Domain

Assessment

The psychological assessment of the individual with delirium focuses on cognitive changes revealed through the mental status examination as well as the resulting behavioural manifestations. Changes in mental status must be monitored frequently for an early detection of delirium, especially in older individuals. In addition, other factors, such as stressors and environmental changes, may contribute to the symptoms.

Mental Status

Rapid onset of global cognitive impairment that affects multiple aspects of intellectual functioning is the hallmark of delirium. Mental status evaluation reveals several changes:

- Fluctuations in the level of consciousness with a reduced awareness of the environment
- Difficulty focusing and sustaining or shifting attention
- Severely impaired memory, especially immediate and recent memory

Patients may be disorientated to time and place but rarely to person. Environmental perceptions are often disturbed. The patient may believe that shadows in the room are really people. Thought content is often illogical, and speech may be incoherent or inappropriate to the context. Each variation in mental status tends to fluctuate over the course of the day. During the same day, an individual with delirium may appear confused and uncooperative, whereas later, the individual may be lucid and able to follow instructions. Nurses must continually assess the cognitive status of the individual throughout the day so that interventions can be modified accordingly.

Calculations, orientation (especially to time), and recall are most affected in delirium, whereas naming and registration are relatively preserved. Several rating scales are available for use in assessing the cognitive and behavioural fluctuations of delirium (Box 31-3).

Behaviour

Delirious patients exhibit a wide range of behaviours, complicating the process of making a diagnosis and planning interventions. At times, the individual may be restless or agitated, and at other times, lethargic and slow to respond. Delirium can be categorized into three types:

- **Hyperactive delirium** involves behaviours such as being overly alert, exhibiting psychomotor hyperactivity, and marked excitability (may hallucinate).
- **Hypoactive delirium** is marked by lethargy, sleepiness, apathy, and psychomotor slowing; this is the "quiet" patient for whom the diagnosis of delirium often is missed.
- **Mixed delirium** involves behaviour that fluctuates between the hyperactive and the hypoactive states over brief or long periods.

Nursing Diagnoses for the Psychological Domain

The nursing diagnosis of acute confusion is also associated with impaired cognitive functioning. Although the

BOX 31.3

Therapeutic Dialogue: Rating Scales for Use With Delirium

THE CONFUSION ASSESSMENT METHOD (CAM)
Inouye, S. K., van Dyck, C. H., Alessi, C. A., Balkin, S., Siegal, A. P., & Horwitz, R. I. (1990). Clarifying confusion: The confusion assessment method. *Annals of Internal Medicine, 113*, 941–948.

CONFUSION RATING SCALE (CRS)
Williams, M. A., Ward, S. E., & Campbell, E. B. (1988). Confusion: Testing versus observation. *Journal of Gerontological Nursing, 14*(1), 25–30.

DELIRIUM SYMPTOM INTERVIEW
Levkoff, S., Liptzin, B., Cleary, P., Reilly, C. H., & Evans, D. (1991). Review of research instruments and techniques used to detect delirium. *International Psychogeriatrics, 3*, 253–271.

DELIRIUM RATING SCALE (DRS)
Trzepacz, P. T., Baker, R. W., & Greenhouse, J. (1988). A symptom rating scale for delirium. *Psychiatry Research, 23*, 89–97.

VISUAL ANALOG SCALE FOR ACUTE CONFUSION (VASAC)
Cacchione, P. Z. (2002). Assessment. Four acute confusion assessment instruments: Reliability and validity for use in long-term care facilities. *Journal of Gerontological Nursing, 28*(1), 12–19.

underlying cause of confusion is physiologic, nursing care should focus on the psychological domain, as well as the physical. Other typical nursing diagnoses related to the psychological domain include disturbed thought process, ineffective coping, and disturbed personal identity.

Interventions for the Psychological Domain

Staff members should have frequent interactions with patients and support them if they are confused, experiencing illusions, or hallucinating. Patients should be encouraged to express their fears and discomforts that result from frightening or disconcerting psychotic experiences. Adequate lighting, easy-to-read calendars and clocks, a quiet noise level, and frequent verbal orientation may reduce this frightening experience. If the patient wears eyeglasses or uses a hearing aid, these devices should be used. Including familiar personal possessions in the environment may also help. Interventions that may be useful for these individuals are discussed in detail later in the chapter (see the section on dementia).

Social Domain

Assessment

Discussions should be initiated with the family to determine whether the patient's behaviours are new.

An assessment of living arrangements may provide information about sensory stimulation or social isolation. Cultural and educational background must be considered when the patient's mental capacity is evaluated. Individuals from certain ethnic backgrounds may not be familiar with the information used in tests of general knowledge (e.g., names of prime ministers, geographic knowledge), memory (e.g., date of birth in cultures that do not routinely celebrate birthdays), and orientation (e.g., sense of placement and location may be conceptualized differently in some cultures; APA, 2000). Some cultural practices may involve using substances such as elixirs that contain chemicals that may exacerbate delirium. The assessment should address these practices.

Family Roles

Family support for the individual and understanding of the disorder must be assessed. The behaviours exhibited by the person experiencing delirium may be frightening or at least confusing for family members. Some family members may actually contribute to the patient's increased agitation. Assessing family interactions and family members' ability to understand delirium is important. If feasible, family presence may help to calm and reassure the patient.

Nursing Diagnoses for the Social Domain

Several nursing diagnoses associated with the social domain can be generated. Interrupted family processes, ineffective protection, ineffective role performance, and risk for injury are the most typical. Risk for injury is a high-priority diagnosis because individuals with delirium are more likely to fall or injure themselves during a confused state (Carpenito-Moyet, 2004).

Interventions for the Social Domain

The environment needs to be safe to protect the patient from injuries. A predictable, orienting environment will help to reestablish order to the patient's life. That is, a calendar, clocks, and other items may be provided to help orient the patient to time, place, and person. If the patient is agitated, de-escalation techniques should be used (see Chapter 13). Physical restraint should be avoided.

Support from Families

Families can be encouraged to work with staff members to reorient the patient and provide a supportive environment. Families need to understand that important decisions requiring the patient's input should be delayed if at all possible until the patient has recovered. Although patients may be able to participate in decision making, they may not remember the decision later; therefore, it is important to have several witnesses present.

Spiritual Domain

Because delirium involves global cognitive impairment, including fluctuations in the level of consciousness and severely impaired memory, and may include agitation or lethargy, persons with delirium are very dependent on others for their comfort, dignity, and spiritual well-being. Communication and connection with others is often seriously affected and the nurse will need to enact well the critical qualities of spiritual care: receptivity, humanity, competency, and positivity (see Chapter 13). Patients experiencing hallucinations, delusions, and/or illusions in delirium may understand them as having a spiritual cause or purpose. This can make them more or less frightening at the time, depending on the meaning attributed to them. Once the delirium passes, the person may want to discuss such experiences (if remembered). The confusion of delirium necessitates, for the most part, that spiritual care of the patient is intensively "in the moment," as the nurse strives to sustain the person through the episode.

▨ EVALUATION AND TREATMENT OUTCOMES

The primary treatment goal is the prevention or resolution of the delirious episode with return to previous cognitive status. Outcome measures include

- Correction of the underlying physiologic alteration
- Resolution of confusion
- Family member verbalization of understanding of confusion
- Prevention of injury

Resolution of confusion is the primary goal; however, the nurse makes important contributions to all four of these outcomes. The end result of delirium is full recovery, incomplete recovery, incomplete recovery with some residual cognitive impairment, or a downward course leading to death.

▨ CONTINUUM OF CARE

The nurse may encounter patients with delirium in a number of treatment settings (e.g., home, nursing home, ambulatory care, day treatment, outpatient setting, hospital). Patients usually are admitted to an acute care setting for rapid evaluation and treatment of the underlying etiology. An abrupt change in cognitive status can also occur while the patient is hospitalized for another reason. Delirium often persists beyond discharge from the hospital. Discharge planning should routinely include family education and referrals to community health care providers. If the patient will return to a residential

BOX 31.4

Psychoeducation Checklist: Delirium

When caring for the patient with delirium, be sure to include the caregivers, as appropriate, and address the following topic areas in the teaching plan:

- Psychopharmacologic agents, if used, including drug action, dosage, frequency, and possible adverse effects
- Underlying cause of delirium
- Mental status changes
- Safety measures
- Hydration and nutrition
- Avoidance of restraints
- Decision-making guidelines

long-term care setting, communication with facility staff about the patient's hospital stay and treatment regimen is crucial. For more information on caring for patients with delirium, see Box 31-4.

Delirium superimposed on dementia (DSD) occurs when a patient with dementia develops a delirium (Fick, Hodo, Lawrence, & Inouye, 2007). DSD is often poorly identified or misdiagnosed. Fick and colleagues used case vignettes to assess experienced nurses' recognition of DSD. The researchers found that nurses were more able to recognize dementia and hyperactive delirium than dementia and hypoactive delirium (or hypoactive delirium alone). These case vignettes can be used as a learning tool for nurses. This remains an area for further research.

Dementia

Dementia is an irreversible syndrome that is characterized by ongoing decline in intellectual functioning sufficient to disrupt social and/or occupational functioning. There are four primary types of dementia: AD, vascular dementia, dementia with Lewy Bodies (DLB), and frontotemporal dementia (FTD).

Alzheimer's Disease

▨ CLINICAL COURSE OF DISORDER

AD is a degenerative, progressive neuropsychiatric disorder that results in cognitive impairment, emotional and behavioural changes, physical and functional decline, and ultimately death. Gradually, the patient's ability to carry out activities of daily living declines, although physical status often remains intact until late in the disease. Primarily a disorder of older individuals, AD has been diagnosed in patients as young as age 35 years.

Early Stage (2–4 years)	Middle Stage (2–10 years)	Late Stage (1–3 years)
Mild forgetfulness Difficulty processing new information Reduced concentration Communication difficulties Problems with orientation Mood shifts Passive Restless	Deterioration in mental abilities, mood and behaviour Disorientation Personality changes Wandering, pacing Disinhibited Assistance needed for ADL	Mental capacities severely compromised Restricted emotions Increased sleep Incontinent Unable to perform ADL Increasingly nonverbal

FIGURE 31.2 Signs and symptoms of the stages of Alzheimer's disease (National Advisory Council on Aging, 2004).

Two subtypes have been identified: the less common, early-onset AD (age 65 years and younger) and the more rapidly progressing, late-onset AD (age older than 65 years). AD is also routinely conceptualized in terms of three stages: early, middle, and late. Signs and symptoms of AD change as the patient passes from one stage of the illness to another (Fig. 31-2).

It is unclear whether all patients with AD pass through a specific sequence of deterioration and whether the staging of a patient at initial assessment has any prognostic implications in terms of speed of decline. Nevertheless, staging is a useful technique for determining the patient's current cognitive status and provides a sound basis for decisions in clinical management.

DIAGNOSTIC CRITERIA

The diagnosis of AD is made on clinical grounds, and verification is confirmed at autopsy by abnormal degenerative structures, neuritic plaques, and neurofibrillary tangles. The essential feature of AD is multiple cognitive deficits, especially memory impairment, and at least one of the following cognitive disturbances: **aphasia** (alterations in language ability), **apraxia** (impaired ability to execute motor activities despite intact motor functioning), **agnosia** (failure to recognize or identify objects despite intact sensory function), or a **disturbance of executive functioning** (ability to think abstractly, plan, initiate, sequence, monitor, and stop complex behaviour).

The cognitive deficits must be sufficiently severe to impair occupational or social functioning and must represent a decline from a previously higher level of functioning (APA, 2000). These symptoms are common to all presentations of dementia, regardless of the underlying pathology. Table 31-4 lists essential symptoms of dementia, along with other possible behavioural and psychological changes that may or may not be present. To make a diagnosis of AD, all other known causes of dementia must be excluded (e.g., vascular, AIDS, Parkinson's disease, others). Box 31-5 lists 10 warning signs of AD.

BOX 31.5
Ten Warnings Signs of AD

To help the public know the warning signs of AD, the Alzheimer Society of Canada lists the following:

1. Memory loss that affects day-to-day function
2. Difficulty performing familiar tasks
3. Problems with language
4. Disorientation of time and place
5. Poor or decreased judgment
6. Problems with abstract thinking
7. Misplacing things
8. Changes in mood and behaviour
9. Changes in personality
10. Loss of initiative

See http://www.alzheimer.ca for more information.

Mild Cognitive Impairment

When people experience memory problems but do not meet the diagnostic criteria for dementia, they are thought to have mild cognitive impairment (MCI). In some studies, about 40% of these individuals develop AD within 3 years. Others never develop AD (United States Department of Health and Human Services [U.S. DHHS], 2003).

EPIDEMIOLOGY AND RISK FACTORS

The 2006 Canadian census indicates that those aged 55 to 64 years are the country's fastest-growing population group with an increase in percentage of 28.1% since 2001. This number is expected to reach 30% by 2017. This group is followed by those over the age of 80 years. Canadian's over 65 has surpassed the 4-million mark for the first time in history. The number of seniors has increased from 13% in 2001 to 13.7% in 2006 (Statistics Canada, 2007). The people born between 1947 and 1966

Table 31.4	Key Diagnostic Characteristics for Dementia of the Alzheimer's Type 290	DSM IV

With early onset:
With delirium 290.11
With delusions 290.12
With depressed mood 290.13
Uncomplicated 290.10

With late onset:
With delirium 290.3
With delusions 290.20
With depressed mood 290.21
Uncomplicated 290.0

Diagnostic Criteria	Target Symptoms and Associated Findings
• Development of multiple cognitive deficits • Involvement of both memory impairment and one or more of the following cognitive disturbances: aphasia, apraxia, agnosia, or disturbance in executive functioning • Significant impairment in social or occupational functioning resulting from cognitive deficits; significant decline from previous level of functioning • Cognitive deficits not due to other CNS conditions causing progressive deficits in memory or cognition; systemic conditions known to cause dementia; substance-induced conditions • Not occurring exclusively during course of a delirium • Not better accounted for by another Axis I disorder Early onset: age 65 years or less Late onset: over age 65 years	• Memory impairment • Cognitive disturbances *Associated Behavioural Findings* • Spatial disorientation and difficulty with spatial tasks • Poor judgment and poor insight • Little or no awareness of memory loss or other cognitive abnormalities • Unrealistic assessment of abilities; underestimation of risks involved in activities • Possible suicidal behaviours (usually in early stages when individual is more capable of carrying out a plan of action) • Possible gait disturbances and falls • Disinhibited behaviour, such as inappropriate jokes, neglect of personal hygiene, undue familiarity with strangers, or disregard for conventional rules of social conduct • Delusions, especially ones involving persecution • Superimposed delirium *Associated Physical Examination Findings* • Few motor or sensory signs (in the first year of illness) • Myoclonus and gait disorder (later) • Seizure possible *Associated Laboratory Findings* • Brain atrophy (with computed tomography or magnetic resonance imaging) • Senile plaques, neurofibrillary tangles, granulovascular degeneration, neuronal loss, astrocytic gliosis, and amyloid angiopathy on microscopic examination

are beginning to enter their 60s and thereby the age of greatest risk for dementia (Forbes & Neufeld, 2008). In 1991, 8% of the Canadian population 65 years and older suffered from dementia. It is estimated that the number of Canadians with dementia will have tripled between 1991 and 2031 (Canadian Study of Health and Aging Working Group, 1994).

To date, only age, a family history and genetics (ApoE gene), diabetes, Down's syndrome, MCI, female gender, head trauma, and low level of formal education are identified as risk factors for AD (Alzheimer Society of Canada, 2009). Studies evaluating other factors, including race,

impaired immunity, lifestyle, and environmental toxins, are ongoing. Forbes, Morgan, and Janzen (2006) found that there are more young-old (50 to 64 years of age) females with dementia living in rural areas compared to those living in urban areas. Forbes raises the question, "Are young-old females with dementia more likely to live in rural areas or does living in rural areas increase the risk of developing dementia?"

AD can run in families. Compared with the general population, first-degree biologic relatives of individuals with early-onset AD are more likely to experience the disorder. A systematic meta-analysis of studies aimed at uncovering AD risk genes suggests that more than 20 loci have modest but significant risk effects (Tanzi & Bertram, 2008). Studies point toward genetically related risk factors only in familial AD, which accounts for only a small proportion of cases of AD (less than 5%; Cummings, 2003). Genetically, AD displays no single or simple mode of inheritance.

The hypothesis that low educational level may increase the risk for AD remains a matter of controversy. It is currently thought that keeping mentally active throughout one's life lessens the risk of developing dementia. Prior head injury leading to unconsciousness may represent a significant risk factor for the later development of AD for Canadians (Rapoport, Verhoeff, & van Reekum, 2004).

▪◀ ETIOLOGY

Researchers have yet to identify a definitive cause of AD. In general, the brain appears normal in the early stages of AD, but it undergoes widespread atrophy as the disease advances. Although causation remains in question, new research using a brain scan–based computer program that measures brain metabolism in the hippocampus supports the possibility of screening for early AD (Mosconi et al., 2005).

Beta-Amyloid Plaques

One piece of the puzzle is partially explained by a leading theory that, in AD, beta-amyloid deposits destroy cholinergic neurons, in a manner similar to cholesterol causing atherosclerosis. It is hypothesized that **beta-amyloid plaques**, dense, mostly insoluble deposits of protein and cellular material outside and around neurons, gradually

---

IN A LIFE

Dame Iris Murdoch (1919–1999)

Public Persona

Born in Dublin, Ireland, Dame Iris Murdoch became a much loved philosopher and writer, the author of 36 novels, several plays, essays and philosophical works, and a critical study of Jean-Paul Sartre. Over her life, she filled 95 diaries with her aspirations and self-analysis of her own shortcomings. Her book, *The Sea, The Sea* won the Booker Prize in 1978. Iris Murdoch was elected as a fellow to St. Anne's College, Oxford in 1948 and remained a tutor there until 1963.

Personal Realities

Iris Murdoch married John Bayley in 1956. In the mid-1990s, she began to show signs of AD. Her extensive vocabulary became diminished; she had difficulty in answering questions, and there was a noticeable decline in the quality of her last book, *Jackson's Dilemma*. She died of AD in 1999. Her husband's book about her life, an *Elegy for Iris* (1999), was made into a movie, *Iris*, in 2001.

---

increase in number and are abnormally distributed throughout the cholinergic system. Plaques are partly made of a protein, beta-amyloid protein, which is a fragment snipped from a larger protein called amyloid precursor protein (APP) and apolipoprotein A (apoA) cores. Neuritic plaque densities are highest in the temporal and occipital lobes, intermediate in the parietal lobes, and lowest in the frontal and limbic cortex. Symptoms such as aphasia and visuospatial abnormalities are attributable to plaque formation (Cummings, 2003). Study continues as investigators examine the process by which APP releases beta-amyloid protein, how the fragments accumulate in the brain, and whether the plaques cause AD or are a by-product.

Neurofibrillary Tangles

Neurofibrillary tangles are made of paired helical filaments of a chemically altered protein, or tau proteins, that disrupt normal intracellular transport and result in cell death. They are initially found in the limbic area and then progress to the cortex. Neurofibrillary tangles contribute to memory disturbance and psychiatric symptoms (Cummings, 2003). It is thought that the formation of these neurofibrillary tangles is related to the apolipoprotein E$_4$ (apoE$_4$). Apolipoprotein (apoE) is a normal cholesterol-carrying protein produced by a gene on chromosome 19, which has three forms: apoE$_2$, apoE$_3$, and apoE$_4$. It appears that apoE$_3$ protects against abnormal changes in proteins that lead to neurofibrillary tangles, associated with late-onset dementia, but apoE$_4$ appears to leave these proteins unprotected and increases the patient's risk for AD (Stahl, 2000) (Fig. 31-3).

Cell Death and Neurotransmitters

In patients with AD, neurotransmission is reduced, neurons are lost, and the hippocampal neurons degenerate. Several major neurotransmitters are affected. **Acetylcholine** (ACh) is associated with cognitive functioning, and the disruption of cholinergic mechanisms damages memory in animals and humans (see Chapter 10). Cell loss in the nucleus basalis leads to deficits in the synthesis of cortical acetylcholine, but the number of ACh receptors is relatively unchanged. The reduced ACh is related to a decrease in *choline acetyltransferase* (a critical enzyme in the synthesis of ACh), especially in the forebrain. That is, there are fewer enzymes available to synthesize ACh, which leads to a reduction in cholinergic activity. Positron emission tomography (PET) scans, such as those in Figure 31-4, show changes in brain function.

Other neurotransmitters that are affected include norepinephrine and serotonin. Deficiencies in norepinephrine are associated with the loss of cells in the locus ceruleus, and neuronal loss in the raphe nuclei leads to a loss of serotoninergic activity (Cummings, 2003).

FIGURE 31.3 Series comparison of older adult control subjects (*top row*) and patients with Alzheimer's disease (*bottom row*). Although there are some decreases in metabolism associated with age, in most patients with AD, there are marked decreases in the temporal lobe, an area important in memory functions. (Courtesy of Monte S. Buchsbaum, MD, The Mount Sinai Medical Centre and School of Medicine, New York, NY.)

FIGURE 31.4 Metabolic activity in a subject with AD (*left*) and in a control subject (*right*). (Courtesy of Monte S. Buchsbaum, MD, The Mount Sinai Medical Center and School of Medicine, New York, NY.)

Genetic Factors

Approximately half of the cases of early-onset AD appear to be transmitted as a pure genetic, autosomal dominant trait caused by mutations in genes on chromosomes 1 and 14 (Rogaeva, 2002; Suh & Checler, 2002). Mutations on chromosome 14 account for most cases of early-onset familial AD (Taddei et al., 2002). Chromosome 21 is also associated with AD because amyloid plaques and neurofibrillary tangles accumulate consistently in older people with Down's syndrome (trisomy 21) who have AD. The role of chromosome 19 in the production of apoE was previously discussed.

Oxidative Stress and Free Radicals

One theory of aging and neurodegeneration is that damage from oxygen free radicals (highly reactive molecules) can build up in neurons over time. This *oxidative stress* can modify or damage cellular molecules, such as proteins, lipids, and nucleic acids. This type of damage has been observed in AD, especially in the late stages when the beta-amyloid plaques and neurofibrillary tangles are present. However, it is not known whether the oxidative stress causes or results from the process of plaque formation (U.S. DHHS, 2003).

Inflammation

Inflammation in the brain is one of the early hallmarks of AD, but it is unknown whether it is a cause or effect. The use of certain medications, such as nonsteroidal anti-inflammatory drugs and estrogen, may delay the onset of the disorder (Tarkowski, Andreasen, Tarkowski, & Blennow, 2003).

▬ INTERDISCIPLINARY TREATMENT

In designing services and interventions, the interdisciplinary team must keep in mind that AD has a progressively deteriorating clinical course and that the anatomic and neurochemical changes that occur in the brain are accompanied by impairments in cognition, sensorium, affect (facial expression representing mood), behaviour, and psychosocial functioning. The nature and range of services needed by patients and families throughout the illness can vary dramatically at different stages.

Initial assessment of the patient suspected of having dementia has three main objectives: (1) confirmation of the diagnosis, (2) establishment of baseline levels in a number of functional spheres, and (3) establishment of a therapeutic relationship with the patient and family that will continue through subsequent phases of the disease. Treatment efforts currently focus on managing the cognitive symptoms, delaying the cognitive decline

(e.g., memory loss, confusion, and problems with learning, speech, and reasoning), treating the noncognitive symptoms (e.g., psychosis, mood symptoms, agitation), and supporting the caregivers as a means of improving the quality of life for both patients and their caregivers. Nurses have an important role in initiating and supporting patient referrals to specialized services (Edwards, Davies, Ploeg, Virani, & Skelly, 2007).

▬ PRIORITY CARE ISSUES

The priority of care will change throughout the course of AD. Initially, the priority is delaying cognitive decline and supporting family members. Later, the priority changes to protecting the patient from injury. Near the end, the physical needs of the patient are the focus of care.

▬ FAMILY RESPONSE TO DISORDER

Families are often the first to be aware of the cognitive problems of a loved one. The patient may be unaware of the extent of memory impairment. When finally confirmed, the actual diagnosis can be devastating to the family and patient (Werezak & Stewart, 2002). Although, Carpenter et al. (2008) concluded that most patients and their families do not have a catastrophic emotional reactions to diagnosis. A diagnosis of AD means long-term care responsibilities, while the essence of a family member diminishes day by day. Most families keep their relative at home as long as possible to maintain contact and to avoid costly nursing home placement. The two symptoms that often result in nursing home placement are incontinence that cannot be managed and behavioural problems, such as wandering and aggression.

The needs of family members should also be considered. Caring for a family member with dementia takes its toll. Caregivers' health is often compromised, and normal family functioning is threatened. Caregiver distress is a major health risk for the family, and "caregiver burnout" is a common cause of the institutionalization of patients with dementia.

▬ NURSING MANAGEMENT: HUMAN RESPONSE TO ALZHEIMER'S DISEASE

The development and implementation of appropriate, effective, and safe nursing services for the care and support of patients with dementia and their families are a particular challenge because of the complex nature of the illness. Although AD is caused by biologic changes, the psychological and social domains are seriously

BOX 31.6

Research for Best Practice: Losing One's Memory in Early AD

From Parsons-Suhl, K., Johnson, M. E., McCann, J. L., & Solberg, S. (2008). Losing one's memory in early Alzheimer's disease. Qualitative Health Research, 18*(1), 31–42.*

THE QUESTION: Most research has focused on obtaining greater knowledge of the impact of dementia on the person with AD and their caregivers. A few studies have looked at the lived experience of AD in later stages of the illness. This study addresses the lived experience of a person in the early stage of AD or with MCI.

METHODS: A Heideggerian hermeneutical phenomenological research method was used to investigate the experience of memory loss in 12 individuals with early stage AD or MCI. The understanding of the participants' lived world was uncovered in the textual analysis and interpretation of taped face-to-face interviews.

FINDINGS: From the analysis of interview data, three constitutive patterns with relational themes were identified. The first pattern, experiencing breakdown, consisted of two themes: awakening to breakdown and living with forgetting. The second pattern, temporality, consisted of three themes: being-in-the-nothing, forgetting the past, and looking ahead. The third pattern, managing forgetting, consisted of four themes: remembering with cues, writings things down, recognizing what made remembering better or worse, and laughter.

IMPLICATIONS FOR NURSING: It is hoped that this study will provide nurses with a better understanding of the lived experience of AD and MCI. All interactions are meaningful, and it is important for nurses to truly listen.

affected by this disorder (see Box 31-6). The assessment of the patient with AD should follow the geriatric mental health nursing assessment in Chapter 30.

Biologic Domain

Assessment

The nursing assessment should include a medical history; current medication profile (prescription and OTC medications or home remedies); substance use history (including alcohol intake and smoking history); chronic physical or psychiatric illness; and a description of the onset, duration, range, and intensity of symptoms associated with dementia. The onset of symptoms in dementia is typically gradual, with insidious changes in behaviour. To conduct a thorough assessment of the patient with dementia, the nurse needs to know what is typical for the individual; therefore, caregivers, family members, or significant others can be sources of valuable information.

Physical Examination and a Review of Body Systems

A review of body systems must be conducted on each patient suspected of having dementia. Specific biologic assessment parameters include vital signs, neurologic status, nutritional status, bladder and bowel function, hygiene, skin integrity, rest and activity level, sleep patterns, and fluid and electrolyte balance. The neurologic function is usually preserved through the early and middle stages of AD, although seizures, gait disturbances, and tremors may occur at any time. Morgan et al. (2007) reviewed the literature about the relationship between gait and dementia. They concluded that careful assessment of gait, balance, and movement during the early stages of dementia has the potential to contribute

to differential diagnosis of the type of dementia. In the later stages of the disease, neurologic signs, such as flexion contractures and primitive reflexes, are prominent features.

Physical Functions

At first, limitations may primarily involve instrumental activities, such as shopping, preparing meals, and performing other household chores. Later in the disease process, basic physical dysfunctions occur, such as incontinence, ataxia, dysphagia, and contractures. Incontinence can be a major source of stress and a considerable burden to family caregivers.

Assessment of physical functions includes activities of daily living, recent changes in functional abilities (dressing, toileting, and feeding), use of sensory aids (glasses and hearing aids), activity level, and assessment of pain. Eyeglasses and hearing aids may need to be in place before other assessments can be made.

Self-Care

Alterations in the central nervous system (CNS) associated with dementia impair the patient's ability to collect information from the environment, retrieve memories, retain new information, and give meaning to current situations. Therefore, patients with dementia often neglect self-care activities. Periodically, biologic assessment parameters need to be reevaluated because patients with dementia may neglect activities such as bathing, eating, or skin care.

Sleep-Wake Disturbances

The sleep-wake disturbances that commonly occur in dementia are hypersomnia, insomnia, and reversal of the sleep-wake cycle. These disturbances may be attributable partly to physiologic changes, neurotransmitters, or metabolic changes resulting from a dementia-causing disease or injury, but they are often of environmental or iatrogenic origin. Patients with dementia have frequent daytime napping and nighttime periods of wakefulness, with little rapid eye movement (REM) sleep. Lowered levels of REM sleep are associated with restlessness, irritability, and general sleep impairment (Wolkove, Elkholy, Baltzan, & Palayew, 2007).

Activity and Exercise

One of the earliest symptoms of AD is withdrawal from normal activities. The patient may just sit staring at a blank wall.

Nutrition

Eating can become a problem for a patient with dementia. As the disease progresses, patients may lose the ability to feed themselves or recognize what is offered as food. The hyperactive patient requires frequent feedings of a high-protein, high-carbohydrate diet in the form of finger foods (which they can carry while on the go). Most patients with dementia prefer to feed themselves with their fingers rather than have someone feed them.

Some patients with dementia are bulimic or hyper-oral (eating or chewing almost everything possible, including inedible objects, and sometimes with an insatiable appetite). Other patients with dementia experience anorexia and have no appetite. It is important to monitor patients with altered appetites for hydration and electrolyte imbalances. Maintaining weight and proper hydration status are signs of effective nursing interventions.

Pain

Assessment and documentation of any physical discomfort or pain the patient may be experiencing are a part of any geropsychiatric nursing assessment (see Chapter 11). Although AD is not usually thought of as a physically painful disorder, patients often have other comorbid physical diseases. In the early stages of AD, the patient can usually respond to verbal questions regarding pain. Later, it may be difficult to assess the comfort level objectively, especially if the patient cannot communicate. Some patients in the end stage of dementia become hypersensitive to touch.

Pain can be assessed through physical examination and use of a pain assessment scale (see Chapter 11; see http://www.hartfordign.org/ for resources for pain assessment). The Pittsburgh Agitation Scale may allow the nurse to assess both agitation and uncommunicated pain. The authors suggest trialing pain medication and then reassessing agitation (Zieber, Hagen,

Armstrong-Esther, & Aho, 2005). Laboratory tests may identify the source of discomfort. Subtle behavioural changes, such as lethargy, anxiety, or restlessness, or more obvious physical signs, such as pyrexia, tachypnea, or tachycardia, may be the only indications of actual or impending illness. Observing for changes in patterns of nonverbal communication, such as facial expressions, may help the nurse identify indicators of pain. Hypervocalizations, restlessness, and agitation are other possible signs of pain.

Nursing Diagnoses for the Biologic Domain

The unique and changing needs of these patients present a challenge for nurses in all settings. A sample of common nursing diagnoses include imbalanced nutrition: less (or more) than body requirements; feeding self-care deficit; impaired swallowing; bathing/hygiene self-care deficit; dressing/grooming self-care deficit; toileting self-care deficit; constipation (or perceived constipation); bowel incontinence; impaired urinary elimination; functional incontinence; total incontinence; deficient fluid volume; risk for impaired skin integrity; impaired physical mobility; activity intolerance; fatigue; disturbed sleep pattern; pain; chronic pain; ineffective health maintenance; and impaired home maintenance.

Interventions for the Biologic Domain

The numerous interventions for the biologic domain vary throughout the course of the disorder. Initially, the patient requires simple directions for self-care activities and initiation of psychopharmacologic treatment. At the end of the disorder, total patient care is required.

Self-Care Interventions

Promotion of self-care supports cognitive functioning and a sense of independence. In the early stages, the nurse should maximize normal perceptual experiences by making sure that the patient and family have appropriate eyeglasses and working hearing aids. If eyeglasses and hearing aids are needed, but not used, patients are more likely to have false perceptual experiences. Ongoing monitoring of self-care is necessary throughout the course of AD. Oral hygiene can be a problem and although this may be difficult, requires excellent basic nursing care (see http://www.marep.uwaterloo.ca/ for resource materials). Aging and many medications reduce salivary flow, leading to a painfully dry and cracking oral mucosa. Drugs that have xerostomia (dry mouth) as a side effect and are commonly prescribed for patients with progressive dementia include antidepressant, antispasmodic, antihypertensive, bronchodilator, and some antipsychotic agents. For patients with xerostomia, hard candy or chewing gum may stimulate salivary flow, or modification of the drug regimen may be necessary. Glycerol mouthwash can provide as much relief from xerostomia as artificial saliva.

Nutritional Interventions

Maintenance of nutrition and maintenance of hydration are essential nursing interventions. The patient's weight, oral intake, and hydration status should be monitored carefully. Patients with dementia should eat well-balanced meals that are appropriate to their activity level and eating abilities, with special attention given to electrolyte balance and fluid intake.

When swallowing is a problem for the patient, thick liquids or semisoft foods are more effective than traditionally prepared foods. If a patient is likely to choke or aspirate food, semisolid foods should be offered because liquids flow into the pharyngeal cavity more quickly and cause choking.

The dining environment should be calm and food presentation appealing. If the patient eats only a small portion of food at one meal, reduce the presentation of food in terms of the amount and number of choices. One-dish meals (e.g., a casserole) are ideal. If the patient is distressed delay feeding because eating, chewing, and swallowing difficulties are accentuated and choking becomes a risk.

As dementia progresses, intensive feeding efforts are needed to ensure adequate food and fluid intake. If food intake is low, vitamin and mineral supplements may be indicated. If weight loss cannot be stopped by skillful feeding or dietary adjustments, then enteral or parenteral feedings may be considered. The patient's quality of life is an important issue to consider when the family or other health care proxy must decide whether to use artificial feeding mechanisms. By inserting a feeding tube, the goal of sustaining weight can be met, but patient comfort may be jeopardized, especially if restraints are used to keep the tube in place.

The patient with dementia should be presented food that is appropriate for their individual needs (see http://www.hartfordign.org/ for publication on nutrition). In the later stages of progressive dementia, some patients hoard food in their mouths; others swallow too rapidly or fail to chew their food sufficiently before attempting to swallow. The nurse needs to watch for swallowing difficulties that place the patient at risk for aspiration and asphyxiation. Swallowing difficulties may result from changes in esophageal motility and decreased secretion of saliva.

Supporting Bowel and Bladder Function

Urinary or bowel incontinence affects many patients with dementia. During middle stage of the disease, incontinence may be caused by the patient's apathy or inability to communicate the need to use the toilet or locate a toilet quickly, undress appropriately to use the toilet, or recognize the sensation of fullness signalling the need to urinate or defecate.

For the patient who is incontinent because of an inability to locate the toilet, reorientation may be helpful. Displaying pictures or signs on bathroom doors provides visual cues while verbal promts promote reorientation to the environment.

If the patient cannot recognize the need to void because of an impaired sensory perception of fullness, increasing fluid intake can help to fill the bladder sufficiently to give a clear message of the need to urinate. Getting to know the patient's habits and moods can help the nurse identify signals that indicate a need to void. The patient can then be assisted to reach the bathroom in time. Positioning the patient near the toilet or placing a portable commode nearby may help if the patient cannot reach a toilet quickly. If the patient demonstrates dressing apraxia (cannot undress appropriately), clothing can be modified with easy-to-open fasteners in place of zippers or buttons. For nocturnal incontinence limiting the amount of fluid consumed after the evening meal and taking the patient to the toilet just before going to bed or upon awakening during the night should reduce or eliminate nocturia.

Indwelling urinary catheters are contraindicated in patients with dementia because they are generally not well tolerated and because hand restraints are often used to prevent them from removing the catheter. Indwelling urinary catheters foster the development of urinary tract infections and may compromise the patient's dignity and comfort. Urinary incontinence can be managed with the use of disposable incontinent products.

Patients with dementia often experience constipation, although they may not be able to tell the nurse about this change. Therefore, subtle signs such as lethargy, reduced appetite, and abdominal distention need to be assessed frequently. Medications, decreased food and liquid intake, lack of motor activity, and decreased intestinal motility contribute to developing constipation. The patient's diet should be rich in fiber, including bran or whole grains, vegetables, and fruit. Adequate oral intake (minimum of 1,500 to 2,000 mL per day) helps to prevent constipation. A gentle laxative such as milk of magnesia (1 to 2 tablespoons every other evening) is commonly used to promote bowel elimination. Enemas and harsher chemical cathartics should be avoided because they may increase pain or discomfort. Care must be taken to ensure that the patient does not become dehydrated in the process of treating constipation.

Sleep Interventions

Disturbed sleep cycles are particularly stressful to both family caregivers and nursing staff. Disturbed sleep is difficult to manage from a behavioural perspective, and the patient's overall level of health may suffer because sleep serves a restorative function. Sedative–hypnotic agents may be prescribed for a short time for restlessness or insomnia, but they may also cause a paradoxic reaction of agitation and insomnia (especially in older adults).

Sleep hygiene interventions are appropriate for patients with dementia, although morning and afternoon naps (or rest periods for patients who do not nap) may be the most effective intervention for a patient with altered diurnal rhythms. Morning naps are likely to produce REM sleep patterns and may help patients who are restless from a loss of REM sleep, whereas afternoon naps produce deep sleep and are suitable for restlessness associated with fatigue. Rest periods (in reclining chairs) in the morning and afternoon may help to eliminate late-day confusion (sundowning) and nighttime awakenings.

Activity and Exercise Interventions

Activity and exercise are important nursing interventions for patients with dementia. To promote a feeling of success, any activity or exercise plan must be culturally sensitive and adapted to the patient's functional ability and interests. The activity or exercise must be designed to prevent excess stress (both physical and psychological). If the program of rest, activity, and exercise is truly individualized, the resultant feelings of value and competency will enhance the patient's physical comfort, morale, and sleep pattern.

Pain and Comfort Management

Nursing care of noncommunicative patients who have dementia and pain can be challenging. Common behaviours associated with pain may be difficult to interpret or absent. Symptoms such as aggressive behaviour may be attributed to the dementia, but indeed may be an indication of pain. Because of the difficulty in identifying and monitoring pain, patients are often undertreated. This undertreatment may result in further cognitive and behavioural problems. Astute nurses may spot the signs of pain by a patient's facial expression, movement, or breathing.

Relaxation

Approaching patients in a calm, confident, unhurried manner; maintaining a soothing, quiet environment; avoiding unnecessary noise or chatter around patients and lowering vocal tone and rate when addressing them; maintaining eye contact; and using touch judiciously are likely to promote a sense of security conducive to patient relaxation and comfort. Simple relaxation exercises can be used to reduce stress and should be performed by the patient.

Administering and Monitoring Medications

Because no medication can cure AD, psychopharmacologic interventions have two goals: restoration or maintenance of cognitive function and treatment of related psychiatric and behavioural disturbances that cause discomfort for the individual, interfere with treatment, or worsen the individual's cognitive status. However, medications for AD must be used with caution. Doses must be kept extremely low, and individuals should be monitored closely for any side effects or worsening of cognitive status. "Start low and go slow" is the principle guiding the administration of psychopharmacologic agents to older adults.

Often, convincing the patient to take the medication is one of the biggest nursing challenges. Patients may be unwilling, even though they previously agreed to take the drugs. The nurse will need to investigate and hypothesize the reason for their reluctance to take medication. It may be because of difficulty swallowing pills, paranoid ideas, or lack of understanding. The underlying reason for medication refusal will determine the strategy. If the patient has difficulty swallowing, most medications come in concentrate liquid form and can be easily swallowed. Medications should never be mixed in food without the patient being made aware. If suspicion or paranoia is the reason, the nurse will need to try to identify the conditions under which the patient feels safe to take the medication, such as in the presence of favourite nurse or relative.

Cholinesterase Inhibitors. Acetylcholinesterase (AChE) is the key enzyme that inactivates the neurotransmitter acetylcholine. AChE is found in high concentrations in the brain and is one of the two cholinesterase enzymes capable of breaking down ACh. **Butyrylcholinesterase** (BuChE), a nonspecific cholinesterase, is also found in the brain, but especially in the glial cells. Both AChE and BuChE work in the gastrointestinal tract. If these enzymes are inhibited, the destruction of ACh will be delayed, resulting in an increase in ACh activity. The increase in ACh activity helps maintain cognitive functioning and delay its decline. **Acetylcholinesterase inhibitors** (AChEIs) are the mainstay of pharmacologic treatment of dementia because they inhibit AChE, resulting in an enhancement of cholinergic activity. Because these medications have been shown to delay the decline in cognitive functioning, but generally do not improve cognitive function once it has declined, it is important that this medication be started as soon as the diagnosis is made. The primary side effect of these medications is gastrointestinal distress—nausea, vomiting, and diarrhea. Three AChEI drugs have been approved for use in Canada: donepezil (Aricept), rivastigmine

(Exelon), and galantamine (Reminyl). Tacrine (Cognex) has not been approved for use in Canada. In 2004, Memantine (Ebixa), a neuropeptide-modifying agent, was approved for use in the treatment of moderate to severe dementia. Clinical trials have demonstrated that people with mild to severe AD treated with these medications experience modest improvements in cognition, function, behaviour, or global clinical state (Keren, 2006). The earlier in the disease process these medications are initiated, the more likely they will delay cognitive decline. Doses at the higher end of the recommended ranges are associated with greater benefits, but more side effects. The main side effects are nausea, vomiting, and diarrhoea. These three drugs are only effective in the treatment of mild to moderate AD. The lack of Canadian clinical guidelines for the discontinuation of these drugs means a decision to discontinue use is based on clinical judgment (Keren, 2006).

NMDA Antagonists. Overstimulation of the *N*-methyl-D-aspartate (NMDA) receptor by glutamate (excitatory neurotransmitter) is considered to have a role in AD. Approximately 70% of all excitatory synapses in the CNS are stimulated by this neurotransmitter. Dysfunction of glutamatergic neurotransmission is involved in the pathology of dementia. In dementia, it is hypothesized that there is a chronic release of glutamate that causes a permanent increased intracellular calcium concentration that leads to neuronal degeneration. Memantine is an NMDA-receptor antagonist that has been shown to improve cognition and global function in patients with mild to severe symptoms of dementia (Raina et al., 2008).

Antipsychotic Agents. Antipsychotic agents are often effective in reducing psychosis, agitation, or aggressive behaviours that are common in the moderate to severe stages of AD. Hagen et al. (2005) found that up to 40% of long-term care older adult patients were prescribed tranquilizers. This compares with approximately 8.63% to 10.3% of older adult patients in general hospitals (Kwasny, Hagen, & Armstong-Esther, 2006). These researchers warn that the risk with tranquilizers with older adults warrants ongoing prudence by health care professionals.

Health Canada (2005) issued an advisory that studies have shown that demented older adult patients who were prescribed atypical antipsychotics had a 1.6 times greater death rate than those taking a placebo. Risperidone (Risperdal), quetiapine (Seroquel), olanzepine (Zyprexa), and clozapine (Clozaril) are not approved for treating behavioural disorders in older patients with dementia (Health Canada). Gill et al. (2007) found the risk of death may be greater with conventional antipsychotics than atypical antipsychotics.

Antidepressant Agents and Mood Stabilizers. A depressed mood is common in patients with dementia, and they often experience response to psychotherapeutic intervention alone (individual or group therapy) or in combination with pharmacotherapy. Low doses of the selective serotonin reuptake inhibitors and other newer antidepressive agents should be considered.

Antianxiety Medications (Sedative–Hypnotics). Antianxiety medications, also known as benzodiazepines, should be used with caution in older patients and, if used, should be administered on a short-term basis. An antianxiety medication may be considered in an emergency, but ideally, the patient should try a nonbenzodiazepine before being prescribed a benzodiazepine. In older people, the benzodiazepines can cause a paradoxic reaction.

Other Medications. Clinical observations indicate that older patients with defects in the cholinergic system are more vulnerable to the effects of anticholinergic drugs that can cause confusion and amnesia. Anticholinergic medications should be avoided in patients with AD if at all possible. See Box 31-7 for examples of medications that are commonly prescribed to older adults, all of which have anticholinergic receptor activity.

Psychological Domain

Psychological Assessment

As the disease progresses, personality changes can take the form of either an accentuation or a marked alteration of a patient's previous lifelong character traits. The neural substrates underlying personality change in AD are not understood, but researchers have identified two contrasting patterns. One is marked by apathy, lack of spontaneity, and passivity. The other involves growing

---

BOX 31.7

*Medications With Anticholinergic Effects**

Captopril (Capoten)
Codeine
Cimetidine (Tagamet)
Digoxin (Lanoxin)
Dipyridamole (Trental)
Furosemide (Lasix)
Isosorbide (Ismotic)
Nifedipine (Procardia)
Prednisolone
Ranitidine (Zantac)
Theophylline (Bronkodyl)
Triamterene (Dyrenium) and hydrochlorothiazide (HCTZ)
Warfarin (Coumadin)

*These medications are commonly prescribed for older adults.

irritability, sarcasm, self-preoccupation, and intolerance of and lack of concern for others.

Cognitive Status

Cognitive disturbance is the clinical hallmark of dementia. The intellectual status of the patient is usually assessed by the traditional, neurologically oriented mental status assessment including use of the minimental state examination (MMSE). If cognitive deterioration occurs rapidly, delirium should be suspected. The patient should be quickly evaluated by a physician because delirium calls for immediate attention to diagnose and treat the underlying cause (Box 31-8).

Memory. The most dramatic and consistent cognitive impairment is in memory. Patients with early stage dementia appear mildly forgetful and repetitive in conversation. They misplace objects, miss appointments, and forget what they were just doing. They may lose track of a conversation or television story. Initially, they may complain of memory problems, but rapidly in the course of the illness, insight is lost and they become unaware of what is lost. Sometimes, they may confabulate, making what appears to be an appropriate explanation of why the information or object is missing. Eventually, all aspects of memory are impaired. Short-term memory loss is usually readily evident by the patient's inability to recall three or four words given to him or her at the beginning of an assessment. Often, the earliest symptom of AD is the inability to retain new information.

Language. Language is progressively impaired. Individuals with AD may initially have agnosia, difficulty finding a word in a sentence or in naming an object. They may be able to talk around it, but the loss is noticeable. Later, fluent aphasia develops, comprehension diminishes, and, finally, they become mute and unresponsive to directions or information.

Visuospatial Impairment. Deficits in visuospatial tasks that require sensory and motor coordination develop early, drawing is abnormal, and the ability to write may change. Inaccurate drawings on the MMSE or clock drawings (see Chapter 11) are diagnostic of impairment. Sequencing tasks, such as cooking or other self-care skills, become impaired. The individual becomes unable to complete complex tasks that require calculations, such as balancing a cheque book.

Executive Functioning. Judgment, reasoning, and the ability to problem solve or make decisions are also impaired in the late stage of AD It is hypothesized that as the disease progresses, the degeneration of neurons is spread diffusely throughout the neocortex.

BOX 31.8

Rating Scales for Use With Dementia

MENTAL STATUS QUESTIONNAIRES
Mini-Mental State Examination (MMSE)
Folstein, M. F., Folstein, S. E., & McHugh, P. R. (1975). "Mini mental state": A practical method for grading the cognitive state of patients for the clinician. *Journal of Psychiatric Research, 12*, 189–198. See Chapter 11.

Cognitive Abilities Screening Instrument (CASI)
Teng, E. L., Hasegawa, K., Homma, A., et al. (1994). The Cognitive Abilities Screening Instrument (CASI): A practical test for cross-cultural epidemiological studies of dementia. *International Psychogeriatrics, 6*, 45–58.

Montreal Cognitive Assessment (MoCA)
Nasreddine, Z. S., Phillips, N. A., Bedirian, V., Charbonneau, S., Whitehead, V., Collin, I., et al. (2005). The Montreal Cognitive Assessment, MoCA: A Brief Screening Tool for Mild Cognitive Impairment. *Journal of the American Geriatrics Society, 53*(4), 695–699. See www.mocatest.org for more details.

COMBINATION OF COGNITIVE AND FUNCTIONAL ASSESSMENT
Brief Cognitive Rating Scale
Reisberg, B., Schneck, M. K., & Ferris, S. H. (1983). The Brief Cognitive Rating Scale (BCRS): Findings in primary degenerative dementia. *Psychopharmacology Bulletin, 19*, 47–50.

Includes five scales: concentration, recent memory, remote memory, orientation, and functioning and self-care.
Agitation Scale
Rosen, J., Burgio, L., Killar, M., Cain, M., Allison, M., Fogleman, M., et al. (1994). The Pittsburg agitation scale: User-friendly instrument for rating agitation in dementia patients. *The American Journal of Geriatric Psychiatry, 2*(1), 52–59.

RATING SCALES OF ACTIVITIES OF DAILY LIVING
Progressive Deterioration Scale (PDS)
DeJong, R., Osterlund, O. W., & Roy, G. W. (1989). Measurement of quality-of-life changes in patients with Alzheimer's disease. *Clinical Therapeutics, 11*, 545–554.

Dependence Scale
Stern, Y., Albert, S. M., Sano, M., et al. (1994). Assessing patient dependence in Alzheimer's disease. *Journal of Gerontology, 49*, M216–M222.

RATINGS SCALES FOR RELATIVES
Geriatric Evaluation by Relatives Rating Scale Instrument (GERRI)
Schwartz, G. E. (1983). Development and validation of the Geriatric Evaluation by Relatives Rating Instrument (GERRI). *Psychological Reports, 53*, 478–488.

Psychotic Symptoms

Suspiciousness, Delusion, and Illusions. During the early and middle stages of dementia, many patients are aware of their cognitive losses and compensate with hyperalertness. In a hyperalert state, one becomes aware of many environmental stimuli one does not readily understand. Illusions (mistaken perceptions) and visual or tactile hallucinations are common in people with dementia. These experiences can be very frightening for the patient and family. A kind, caring approach by the nurse is needed.

As the disease progresses, delusions develop in 34% to 50% of the people with dementia. These characteristic delusions are different from those discussed in the psychotic disorders. Common delusional beliefs include the following:

- Belief that his or her partner is engaging in marital infidelity
- Belief that other patients or staff are trying to hurt him or her
- Belief that staff or family members are impersonators
- Belief that people are stealing his or her belongings
- Belief that strangers are living in his or her home
- Belief that people on television are real.

Hallucinations. Hallucinations occur frequently in dementia and are usually visual or tactile (they can also be auditory, gustatory, or olfactory). A frequent concern is that children, adults, or strange creatures are entering the house or the patient's room. These hallucinations may not seem unusual to the patient. If possible, the content and form of hallucination should be ascertained because this information may suggest a treatable disorder. For example, an auditory hallucination commanding the patient to commit suicide may be caused by a treatable depression, not dementia.

Mood Changes

Recognition of coexisting (and often treatable) psychiatric disorders in patients with dementia is often missed. One of the challenges of caring for a patient with dementia is when there is the coexistence of depression (Metzger, 2008). Depression is characterized by alterations in sleep, anhedonia, lack of eye contact, feelings of sadness, expression of somatic concerns, and decrease in self-care (RNAO, 2004). A depressed mood is common and is reported in 40% to 50% of AD cases. A diagnosis of major depression is less common, occurring in 10% to 20% of patients with AD. A number of people with AD experience one or more depressive episodes with symptoms such as psychomotor retardation, anxiety, feelings of guilt and worthlessness, sadness, frequent crying, insomnia, loss of appetite, weight loss, and suicidal rumination. Depressive symptoms are most prevalent in the early stages of dementia, which may be attributed to the patient's awareness of cognitive changes, memory loss, and functional decline. However, dysphoric symptoms can occur at any stage, even in the most disoriented older patients. In more advanced stages of dementia, an assessment of depression depends more on changes in behaviour than on the verbal expression of concerns.

Anxiety. It is common to observe symptoms of anxiety with depression; therefore, it is important to assess for depression when signs of anxiety appear. Moderate anxiety is a natural reaction to the fear engendered by gradual deterioration of intellectual function and the realization of impending loss of control over one's life. Failure to complete a task once regarded as simple creates a source of anxiety in the patient with AD. As patients with AD become unsure of their surroundings and the expectations of others, they frequently react with fear and distress. It is thought that anxious behaviour occurs when the patient is pressed to perform beyond his or her ability.

Catastrophic Reactions. Catastrophic reactions are overreactions or extreme anxiety reactions to everyday situations. Catastrophic responses occur when environmental stressors are allowed to continue or increase beyond the patient's threshold of stress tolerance. Behaviours indicative of catastrophic reactions typically include verbal or physical aggression, violence, agitated or anxious behaviour, emotional outbursts, noisy behaviour, compulsive or repetitive behaviour, agitated night awakening, and other behaviours in which the patient is cognitively or socially inaccessible. Factors that contribute to catastrophic responses in patients with progressive cognitive decline include fatigue; change in routine (pace or caregiver); demands beyond the patient's ability; overwhelming sensory stimuli; and physical stressors, such as pain or hunger.

Behavioural Responses

Apathy and Withdrawal. Apathy, the inability or unwillingness to become involved with one's environment, is common in AD, especially in moderate to late stages. Apathy leads to withdrawal from the environment and a gradual loss of empathy for others. The lack of empathy is very difficult for families and friends to understand. Staal and colleagues (2007) found that the use of a multi-sensory room (Snoezelen therapy) may reduce apathy in dementia patients.

Restlessness, Agitation, and Aggression. Restlessness, agitation, and aggression become more prominent in the middle to late stages of dementia. Restlessness should be further evaluated to determine its underlying cause. If the restlessness occurs during medication change or adjustment, side effects should be suspected.

Agitation and aggressive physical contacts are among the most dangerous behaviour management problems encountered in any setting. They often result in the placement of a family member in a nursing home. Careful evaluation of the antecedents of the behaviour enables the nurse to plan nursing care that prevents future occurrences.

Aberrant Motor Behaviour. Symptoms such as fidgeting, picking at clothing, wringing hands, loud vocalizations, and wandering may all be signs of underlying conditions such as dehydration, medication reaction, pain, or infection (suggesting delirium). One of the most difficult behaviours for which to determine an underlying cause is hypervocalization; the screams, curses, moans, groans, and verbal repetitiveness that are common in the later stages of dementia. In the assessment of these hypervocalizations, it is important to identify when the behaviour is occurring and any antecedents to the behaviour. Gotell, Brown, and Ekman (2009) concluded that caregiver singing and background music can enable the hypervocal patient to express positive emotions and moods.

Disinhibition. One of the most frustrating symptoms of AD is disinhibition, acting on thoughts and feelings without exercising appropriate social judgment. The patient may decide that he or she is more comfortable naked than with clothes. Or the patient may not be able to find his or her clothes and may walk into a room of people without any clothes on. This behaviour is extremely disconcerting to family.

Hypersexuality. A closely related symptom is hypersexuality, inappropriate and socially unacceptable sexual behaviour. The patient may begin talking and behaving in ways that are uncharacteristic of premorbid behaviour.

Stress and Coping Skills. Patients with dementia seem extremely sensitive to stressful situations and often do not have the coping abilities to deal with the situation. A careful assessment of the triggers that precede stressful situations will help in understanding a provoking event.

Nursing Diagnoses for the Psychological Domain

A multitude of potential nursing diagnoses can be identified for the psychological domain of this population.

A sample of common nursing diagnoses includes impaired memory, disturbed thought processes, chronic confusion, disturbed sensory perception, impaired environmental interpretation syndrome, risk for violence: self-directed or directed at others, risk for loneliness, risk for caregiver role strain, ineffective sexuality patterns, ineffective individual coping, hopelessness, and powerlessness (Carpenito-Moyet, 2004).

Interventions for the Psychological Domain

The therapeutic relationship is the basis for interventions for the patient and family with dementia. Care of the patient entails a long-term relationship, needing much support and expert nursing care.

Cognitive Impairment

Validation Therapy. Validation therapy emerged in the 1970s as a method for communicating with patients with AD. It was developed as a contrast to reality therapy, which attempted to provide a here-and-now, factual focus to the interaction. *Validation therapy* focuses on the emotions and subjective reality of the patients. In validation therapy, individuals with cognitive impairment are viewed on one of four stages of a continuum: malorientation, time confusion, repetitive motion, and vegetation. The benefits of validation therapy for patients are reported as restoration of self-worth, less withdrawal from the outside world, communication and interaction with other people, reduction of stress and anxiety, help in resolving unfinished life tasks, and facilitation of independent living for as long as possible. These outcomes are highly desirable, but no substantive research supports its effectiveness (Neal & Briggs, 2003). Validation therapy is a useful model for nursing care of the patient with dementia. The nurse does not try to reorient the patient, but rather respects the individual's sense of reality.

Memory Enhancement. Interventions for progressive memory impairment should always be a part of the treatment plan. The sooner patients begin taking AChE inhibitors, the slower the cognitive decline. However, pharmacologic agents are only a small part of the intervention picture. The nursing goal is to maintain memory functioning as long as possible. The nurse should make a concerted effort to reinforce short- and long-term memory. For example, reminding patients what they had for breakfast, which activity was just completed, or who their visitors were a few hours ago will reinforce short-term memory. Encouraging patients to tell the stories of their earlier years will help bring long-term memories into focus. In the earlier stages of AD, there is considerable frustration when the patient realizes that he or she has short-term memory loss.

In a matter-of-fact manner, the nurse should "fill in the blanks" and then redirect to another activity. Pictures of familiar people, places, and activities are also important tools in memory retrieval. Using scents (perfume, shaving lotions, spices, different foods) to stimulate memory retrieval and asking patients to relate memories are also useful. Formalized reminiscence groups also help patients relive their earlier experiences and support long-term memories.

Orientation Interventions. To enhance cognitive functioning, attempts should be made to remind patients of the day, time, and location. However, if the patient begins to argue that he or she is really at home or that it is really 1992, the patient need not be confronted by facts. Any confrontation could easily escalate into an argument. Instead, the nurse should either redirect the patient or focus on the topic at hand (see Box 31-9).

Maintaining Language. Losing the ability to name an object (agnosia) is frustrating. For example, the patient may describe a flower in terms of colour, size, and fragrance but never be able to name it a flower. When this happens, the nurse should immediately say the name of the item. This reinforces cognitive functioning and prevents disruption in the interaction. Referral to speech therapists may also be useful if the language impairment impedes communication.

Supporting Visuospatial Functioning. The patient with visuospatial impairments loses the ability to sequence automatic behaviours, such as getting dressed or eating with silverware. For example, patients often put their clothes on backward, inside out, or with undergarments over outer garments. Once dressed, they become confused as to how they arrived at their current state. If this happens, the nurse should begin

---

BOX 31.9

Therapeutic Dialogue: The Patient With Dementia of the Alzheimer Type

Lois's daughter has told the home care nurse that on several occasions, Lois has been found cowering and fearful under the kitchen table, saying she was hiding from voices. The nurse also knows that Lois denies having any difficulty with her memory or her ability to care for herself.

INEFFECTIVE APPROACH

Nurse: I'm here to see you about your health problems.

Patient: I have no problems. Why are you here?

Nurse: I'm here to help you.

Patient: I do not need any help. I think there is a mistake.

Nurse: Oh, there is no mistake. Your name is Ms. W, isn't it?

Patient: Yes, but I don't know who you are or why you are here. I'm very tired, please excuse me.

Nurse: OK. I will return another day.

EFFECTIVE APPROACH

Nurse: Hello, my name is Susan Miller. I'm the home health nurse and I will be spending some time with you.

Patient: Oh, alright. Come in. Sit here.

Nurse: Thank you.

Patient: There is nothing wrong with me, you know.

Nurse: Are you wondering why I am here? Tell me what is on your mind (open-ended statement).

Patient: I know why you are here. My children think that I cannot take care of myself.

Nurse: You're feeling concerned and perhaps a little worried your family seems to think you need more help at home?

Patient: Of course I can care for myself. When people get older they slow down. I'm just a little slower now and that upsets my children.

Nurse: You are a little slower and that's what you think is concerning your children.

Patient: I sometimes forget things.

Nurse: Such as... (open-ended statement)

Patient: Sometimes, I cannot remember a telephone number or a name of a food.

Nurse: ....and that causes problems.

Patient: According to my children, it does!

Nurse: What about you? What causes problems for you?

Patient: Sometimes the radio says terrible things to me.

Nurse: That must be frightening to experience while listening to the radio.

Patient: It's terrifying. Then, my daughter looks at me as if I am crazy. Am I?

Nurse: Some people, when they become older, experience challenges with their memory. Also for some people, the daily living tasks which used to be carried out easily become more challenging. For you it seems doubly scary because you doubt yourself and you're afraid your daughter doesn't understand.

Patient: Oh, OK. Will you tell my daughter that I am not crazy?

Nurse: Sure, I would be happy to meet with both you and your daughter if you would like (acceptance).

CRITICAL THINKING CHALLENGE

• How did the nurse's underlying assumption that the patient would welcome the nurse in the first scenario lead to the nurse's rejection by the patient?

• What communication techniques did the nurse use in the second scenario to open communication and set the stage for the development of a sense of trust?

to place clothes for dressing in a sequence so that the patient can move from one article to the next in the correct sequence. This same technique can be used in other situations, such as eating, bathing, and toileting.

Managing Suspicions, Illusions, and Delusions. Patients' suspiciousness and delusional thinking must be addressed to be certain that patients do not endanger themselves or others. Often, delusions are verbalized when patients are placed in a situation they cannot master cognitively. The principle of nonconfrontation is most important in dealing with suspiciousness and delusion formation. No efforts should be made to ease the patient's suspicions directly or to correct delusions. Efforts should be directed at determining the circumstances that trigger suspicion or delusion formation and creating a means of avoiding these situations.

Frequent causes of suspicion are changes in daily routine and strangers. The common accusations that "Someone has entered my room," or "Someone has changed my room," can be managed by asking, "Do you want to see if anything is missing?" Such accusations usually arise when a patient cannot remember what the room looked like or when the room was rearranged or cleaned.

Patients with dementia often hide or misplace their belongings and later complain that the item is missing. It is helpful if the nurse and other caregivers pay attention to the patient's favourite hiding places and communicate this so that objects can be more easily retrieved. An outburst of delusional accusations after a social outing or other activity may indicate that the activity was too long, the setting was too stimulating, there was too much activity, or the pace was too fast for the patient. All these elements can be modified, or it may be necessary to engage the patient in quieter activities.

Patients with dementia may have delusions that a spouse, child, or other significant person is an impostor. If this situation occurs, it is important to assert in a matter-of-fact manner, "This is your wife Barbara" or "I am your daughter Jenny." More vigorous assertions, such as offering various types of proof, tend to increase puzzlement as to why a person would go so far to impersonate the spouse or child.

When patients experience illusions, the nurse needs to find the source of the illusion and remove it from the environment if possible. For example, if a patient is watching a television program featuring animals and then verbalizes that the animal is in the room, switch the channel and redirect the conversation. Some patients with dementia may no longer recognize the reflection in the mirror as self and become agitated, thinking that a stranger is staring at them. Potentially misleading or disturbing stimuli, such as mirrors or art work, can be easily covered or removed from the environment.

Managing Hallucinations. Reassurance and distraction may be helpful for the hallucinating patient. For example, an 89-year-old patient with AD in a residential care facility would get up each night, walk to the nursing station, and whisper to the nurses, "There's a man in my bed who won't let me sleep. You should patrol this place better!" If the hallucination is not too disturbing for the patient, it can often be dismissed calmly with diversion or distraction. Because this patient did not seem too concerned by the man in her bed, the nurse may gently respond by saying, "I'm sorry you have to put up with so much. Just wait here (or come with me) and I'll make sure your room is ready for you." The nurse should then take the patient back to her room and help her into bed.

Frightening hallucinations and delusions usually require antipsychotic medications to dampen the patient's emotional reactions, but they can also be dealt with by optimizing perceptual cues (cover mirrors or turn off the television) and by encouraging patients to stay physically close to their caregivers. For example, one patient complained to her visiting nurse that she was being poisoned by deadly bugs that crawled up and down her arms and legs while she tried to sleep at night. Antipsychotic medication may help this patient sleep at night, and she would also likely benefit from reassurance and protection. Patients benefit more if nurses give them a specific distracting intervention to alleviate anxiety and to help diminish the hallucination, such as applying moisturizing lotion to her legs and arms to repel the bugs at night. The nurse does not agree with the patient's hallucination or delusion but lets the patient know that the feelings are justified based on the patient's perception of the threat.

Interventions for Mood Changes

Managing Depression. Psychotherapeutic nursing interventions for depression that accompanies dementia are similar to interventions for any depression. It is important to spend time alone with patients and to personalize their care as a way of communicating the patient's value. Encouraging the expression of negative emotions is helpful because patients can talk honestly to a nonjudgmental person about their feelings. Although depressed patients with dementia are likely to be too disorganized to commit suicide, it is wise to remove potentially harmful objects from the environment (Box 31-10).

Do not force depressed patients to interact with others or participate in activities, but encourage activity and exercise. One of the psychogenic aspects of depression is a sense of lowered worth related to the patient's actual decreased competence to work and to deal with the problems of daily living. Therefore, it may be helpful to

BOX 31.10

Clinical Vignette: A Nurse's Dilemma

It is 8 o'clock and you are working as a nurse on an inpatient general medical unit of a large urban hospital. A 72-year-old man is admitted to your unit with symptoms of disorientation to time and place, and he is intermittently exhibiting signs of agitation. He thinks you are his child, and he falls asleep while you ask him questions about his symptoms. When you ask him to sign a consent form and hand him a pen, he looks at you as if he didn't understand your request.

The patient's wife tells you that he has had trouble with his memory for the past 3 or 4 years but that her husband has been "acting strange for the past 4 days." The patient's wife denies any history of substance abuse or head injury, but states that her husband has been recently diagnosed as having dementia of the Alzheimer's type.

The patient's physician gives a verbal order to restrain the patient "as needed" while writing orders for lab work.

WHAT DO YOU THINK?

- What assessment techniques would you use to determine whether this patient has dementia, delirium, or both?
- What nursing diagnosis would be included in the patient's plan of care?
- What nursing interventions would promote comfort and safety for this patient?
- Is this patient able to give consent?
- What would be the possible outcomes of physically restraining this patient (e.g., would restraints be helpful or harmful for the patient)?

involve the person in a simple repetitive task or project (such as folding linens or setting the table), especially one that involves helping someone else. Assist the patient to meet self-care needs while encouraging independence when possible.

Managing Anxiety. Cognitively impaired patients are particularly vulnerable to anxiety. As patients with dementia become increasingly unsure of their surroundings or of what is expected of them, they tend to react with fear and distress. They may feel lost, insecure, and left out. Failure to complete a task once regarded as simple creates anxiety and agitation. Often, they cannot explain the source of their anxiety. The difficulty in developing interventions for the anxious patient with dementia is that the symptoms may also be a sign of underlying illnesses, such as depression, pain, infection, or other physical illnesses.

In many cases, lowering the demands, or perceived demands, on the patient will be conducive to promoting comfort. Although maintaining autonomy in any remaining function is a high priority in nursing care of the patient with dementia, it may decrease the patient's anxiety or stress level to have things done for him or her at certain points along the illness continuum. Frequently, as the day progresses and the patient becomes more fatigued, their ability to cope with stressors is increasingly challenged. Many patients with dementia experience "sundowning" where they have an increased restlessness and agitation as the day draws to a close. In addition, being sensitive to the pronounced startle reflexes and potential hypersensitivity to touch also helps reduce stress.

The threshold for stress is progressively lowered in AD and other progressive dementias. A healthy person frequently uses cognitive coping strategies when under stress, whereas the person with dementia can no longer use many of these strategies. Effective nursing interventions include simplifying routines, making routines as consistent and predictable as possible, reducing the number of choices the patient must make, identifying areas in which control can be maintained, and creating an environment in which the patient feels safe. With any of the therapeutic interventions discussed, the nurse is reminded that each patient has relative strengths and weaknesses and that sound nursing judgment must be used in each situation.

Commonly used therapeutic approaches may exacerbate anxiety in a patient with dementia. For example, reality orientation is usually an effective intervention for acutely confused patients in the early stages of their illness. Reality orientation is contraindicated in the later stages of dementia because it is possible that the patient's disoriented behaviour or language has inherent meaning. If the disoriented behaviour or language is continuously neglected or corrected by the nurse, the patient's sense of isolation and anxiety may increase.

Another therapeutic intervention that may (or may not) be contraindicated in patients with dementia is providing the patient with information before a difficult or painful procedure. Anticipatory preparation for non-routine events may produce anxiety because the patient is unable to retain information, use reasoning skills, or make sound judgments. Telling the patient that he or she is scheduled for an upcoming diagnostic test only communicates, on an emotional level, that something distressing is about to happen. A simple explanation immediately before the event may be more helpful.

Managing Catastrophic Reactions. If a patient reacts catastrophically, the nurse needs to remain calm, minimize environmental distractions (quiet the environment), get the patient's attention, and softly assure the patient that he or she is safe. Give information slowly, clearly, and simply, one step at a time. Let the patient know that you understand the fear or other emotional response, such as anger or anxiety.

As the nurse becomes skilled at identifying antecedents to the patient's catastrophic reactions, it becomes possible to avoid situations that provoke such reactions. Patients with AD respond poorly to change and respond well to structure. Attempts to argue or reason with them only escalate their dysfunctional responses.

Interventions for Behaviour Problems

Managing Apathy and Withdrawal. As the patient withdraws and becomes more apathetic, the nurse is challenged to engage the patient in meaningful activities and interactions. To provide this level of care, the nurse must know the premorbid functioning of the patient. Close contact with family helps give the nurse ideas about meaningful activities.

Managing Restlessness and Wandering. Restlessness and wandering are major concerns for caregivers, especially in the community (home) or long-term care setting. The principal means of dealing with restless patients who wander into other patient's rooms or out the door is to have an adequate number of staff (or caregivers, in the home setting) to provide supervision, as well as electronically controlled exits. Wandering behaviour may be interrupted in more cognitively intact patients by distracting them verbally or visually. Colour and structure of the care setting can serve as cues to enable patients to locate their own rooms (Gibson, MacLean, Barrie, & Geiger, 2004). Patients who are beyond verbal distraction can be distracted by physically joining them on their walk and then interrupting their course of action and gently redirecting them back to the house or facility. Many times, wandering is a result of a patient's inability to find his own room; window boxes that contain photographs of family, personal mementoes, or pieces of art may cue a patient to identify their room.

Managing Aberrant Behaviour. When patients are picking in the air or wringing hands, simple distraction may work. Hypervocalizations have meaning to the patient. The nurse should develop strategies to try to reduce the frequency of vocalizations such as offering comfort measures (change of position, a snack or drink, or warm face cloth to refresh the patient's hands and face).

Managing Agitated Behaviour. Omelan (2006) suggests the following strategies when dealing with an agitated patient with dementia:

- Examine patient for any physical causes (pain or infection)

- Review medications (check for any anticholinergic drugs)
- Observe the environment for contributing factors (noise or activity)
- Assess for depression and/or anxiety
- Focus on one behaviour at a time (reduce confusion for the patient)
- Constantly be aware of safety issues for the patient.

Reducing Disinhibition. Anticipation of disinhibiting behaviour is the key to nursing interventions for this problem. Disinhibition can take many forms, from undressing in a public setting to touching someone inappropriately to making cruel statements. This behaviour can usually be viewed as normal by itself, but abnormal within its social context. With keen behavioural assessment of the patient, the nurse should be able to anticipate the likely socially inappropriate behaviour and redirect the patient or change the context of the situation. If the patient starts undressing in the dining room, offering a robe and gently escorting him or her to another part of the room might be all that is needed. If a patient is trying to fondle a staff member or another patient, having the person leave the immediate area or redirecting the patient may alleviate the situation.

Social Domain

Social Assessment

Dementia interferes with a person's ability to interact socially as much as it disrupts intellectual functioning. The social domain assessment should include those areas explained in Chapter 30, including functional status, social systems, legal status, and quality of life (see Chapter 11). The Global Assessment of Functioning scale presented in Chapter 11 also can be used.

The patient's whole social network is affected by dementia, and the the primary caregiver of a person with dementia is often considered a copatient. It is important to assess the family caregiver's ability to use supportive mechanisms to maintain his or her own integrity throughout the disease process.

The extent of the primary caregiver's personal, informal, and formal support systems must also be assessed, as well as personal resources, skills, and stressors. The assessment of the social domain provides objective data on the patient's social circumstances and impressions of the patient's family structure, sociocultural beliefs, attitudes toward health and disease, myths about dementia, patterns of communication, and degree of psychopathology (such as potential for abuse). If the patient still resides in the community, a home visit will prove useful because it gives the nurse information about the patient in his/her own environment.

From this assessment, the nurse can identify the situational and psychosocial stressors that affect the family and patient and can begin to develop interventions to strengthen coping strategies.

Nursing Diagnoses for the Social Domain

Typical nursing diagnosis for the social domain are deficient diversional activity, impaired social interaction, social isolation, risk for loneliness, caregiver role strain, ineffective coping, hopelessness, and powerlessness (Carpenito-Moyet, 2004). Outcomes are determined according to nursing diagnoses.

Interventions for the Social Domain

Safety Interventions

One of the primary concerns of the nurse should be patient safety. In the early stages of the illness, safety may not seem to be a prime. However, early behaviours suggesting dementia are often related to safety, such as the patient getting lost while driving or going the wrong way on a highway. Determining the ability of a dementia patient to drive is recognized as a challenge for health care providers (Byszewski et al., 2003). Safety continues to be an issue in the home when patients engage in unsupervised cooking, cleaning, or household tasks. Day care centres provide a safe and structured environment for these individuals. Family members should be encouraged to continually assess the abilities of the patient to live at home safely.

During hospitalizations or nursing home care, the safety issues are different. By the time dementia patients are admitted to a facility, they are in the middle to late stage of their illness. Cognitive impairments are more pronounced and safety is of greater concern. Most geropsychiatric units are locked, and in a dementia unit, there often is an electronic alarm system to alert the staff of patients attempting to leave the secured floor. Staff and visitors need to be vigilant for perilous situations.

Environmental Interventions

The need for stimulation can also be an antecedent to catastrophic reactions. The need for stimulation varies from individual to individual and can change, depending on many factors, including cognitive intactness, alertness, emotional state, and physical state. The amount of stimulation received also influences each patient's behaviour. Lack of stimulation or intense stimulation may cause emotional distress and aggression. Generally speaking, the more severe the dementia, the less stimulation can be integrated. The nurse should attempt to determine each patient's optimal level of stimulation at various times of the day. Hicks-Moore and Robinson (2008), from the University of New Brunswick, have found that music and hand massage are effective in reducing agitation in patients with dementia.

Socialization Activities

Overlearned social skills are rarely lost in patients with AD. It is not unusual for the patient with dementia to respond appropriately to a handshake or smile well into the disease process. Even patients who are no longer able to communicate coherently will carry on long discussions with people who are willing to listen and respond. There is a strong risk for social isolation in patients with dementia because of communication difficulties. Reinforcing social remarks and gestures, such as eye contact, smiling, greetings, and farewells, can promote a sense of competency and self-esteem (Box 31-11). Pet therapy may enhance social interaction in cognitively impaired individuals. It is important to remember that patients with dementia do not lose their ability to laugh and play, and the psychosocial benefits of humor are well known.

The nurse who engages a patient with dementia in an activity is encouraged to (1) avoid confrontation; (2) allow the level of autonomy best tolerated by the patient; (3) simplify activities and directions to the point that they can be mastered; (4) provide adequate structure; and (5) recognize that instructions may not be carried out correctly. It is important to monitor the length of time, crowding, and noise level when the patient participates in a group activity because all these factors may increase the patient's stress level.

Activities that elicit pleasant memories from an earlier time in the patient's life (reminiscence) may produce a soothing effect. Eliciting pleasant memories may be enhanced by gentle stimulation of the patient's senses, for example, viewing and discussing photo albums, looking at personal memorabilia, providing a favourite food item, playing a musical instrument, or listening to music the person preferred in younger years.

It may be useful to incorporate movement or dance along with a singing exercise. If the patient with dementia resists structured exercise, it may be because of a fear of falling or injury, or of demonstrating to others that his or her health is failing. Patients with dementia often forget how to move or how to coordinate their movements in relation to objects. Therefore, exercise should be light and enjoyable. Encourage the patient to take rest periods at intervals throughout the activity in an effort to minimize stress.

Home Visits

Changes in the delivery of health care in Canada have resulted in a shift from the hospital to the community.

BOX 31.11

Research for Best Practice: Nurse–Patient Communication in Dementia

From Perry, J., Galloway, S., Bottorff, J. I., & Nixon, S. (2005). Nurse-patient communication in dementia: Improving the odds. Journal of Gerontological Nursing, 31(4), 43–52.

THE QUESTIONS: What are the communication strategies used by expert nurses in communication with people diagnosed with advanced dementia? How effective are these strategies in supporting participation in social conversations?

METHOD: This is a descriptive study of interactions in a weekly socialization group composed of eight women with advanced dementia (MMSE 0–19) in a residential facility and led by two researchers. Ten sessions, 30–50 minutes in length, were audiotaped and then transcribed. There were no specific agendas for the groups, but the leaders addressed topics such as holidays, the weather, unit activities, and members' well-being. A line-by-line analysis of the first group session by the researchers resulted in two taxonomies that were used to code the other nine transcripts.

FINDINGS: With effective support and prompting, people with advanced dementia were able to engage in social conversations beyond what would be expected given their diagnosis and MMSE scores.

IMPLICATIONS FOR NURSES: Communication strategies should be adapted to the nursing situation at hand. Useful strategies included clarifying (attempting to ensure that the nurse understood the resident), exploring (searching for information about the resident and helping the resident to articulate experience or thoughts), moderating (initiating and maintaining the conversation), validating (recognizing expressed or inferred feelings), and rescuing (suggesting relevance for specific, isolated, or unconnected sentences). The use of socialization groups to enrich conversation with institutionalized individuals with dementia may be a cost-effective way of enhancing quality of life.

The goal of in-home– and community-based long-term care services is to maintain patients in a self-determining environment that provides the most home-like atmosphere possible, allows maximum personal choice for care recipients and caregiver, and encourages optimal family caregiving involvement without overwhelming the resources of the family network. All services for patients with dementia and their families must be provided within a context of continuity of care, a concept that mandates access to a variety of health and supportive services over an unpredictable and changing clinical course.

Community Actions

Nurses working with patients with dementia are especially knowledgeable about all aspect of the illness and care. These nurses are often involved in local organizations, such as the Alzheimer Society of Canada. Issues of care and safety and access to services often require professional expertise and influence.

Family Interventions

Caregivers are faced with extreme pressures. Caregivers are either spouses of the person with AD or children, usually a daughter, who also have other responsibilities, such as children and a job. The caregiver often feels isolated, frustrated, and trapped. The potential for patient abuse is significant, especially if agitated and aggressive behaviours are present in the relative. The use of home care nurses has been investigated relative to their impact on the burden and depression of older caregivers. Caregivers welcome visits from a nurse and

thankful for support offered by other members of the multidisciplinary team.

It is important the nurse recognize the need of the caregivers for support and relief from the 24-hour responsibility. Determining the availability of family members or friends to assist with personal care of the patient should be included in the assessment (see Box 31-12). Caregivers should be encouraged to attend support groups and carve out personal time. Educational and training programs may help in understanding the complex nature of the disorder. Community resources, such as day care centres, home care agencies, and other community services, can be an important aspect of nursing care for the patient with dementia (see Box 31-13).

BOX 31.12

Psychoeducation Checklist: Tips for Caregivers

When caring for the patient with dementia, be sure to include the caregivers, as appropriate, and address the following topic areas in the teaching plan:

- Psychopharmacologic agents, if used, including drug action, dosage, frequency, and possible adverse effects
- Rest and activity
- Consistency in routines
- Nutrition and hydration
- Sleep and comfort measures
- Protective environment
- Communication and social interaction
- Diversional measures
- Community resources

BOX 31.13

Research for Best Practice: Services for Seniors in Small-Town Canada: The Paradox of Community

From Skinner, M. W., Rosenberg, M. W., Lovell, S. A., Dunn, J. R., Everitt, J. C., Hanlon, N., et al. (2008). Services for seniors in small-town Canada: The paradox of community. Canadian Journal of Nursing Research, 40*(1), 80–101.*

THE QUESTION: There is a prevailing argument that what small towns lack in formal services is made up for in close ties among rural people and a shared understanding of the notion of community. The objective of this study was to determine whether this perspective reflects the reality of in-home and community care in rural communites.

METHODS: The researchers used a grounded theory approach to analyze the results of in-depth interviews with key informants. In total, 110 interviews were conducted (and 55 analyzed) with a variety of informants from government, health and social care institutions, voluntary sector organizations, and community groups.

FINDINGS: Belief in community, small-town milieu, and services for seniors emerged as themes. The descriptive findings show that belief in community, rurality (the small-town milieu), and service provisioning are important yet complex themes for understanding the health and social care of seniors living in small towns. The results of this study suggest that assumptions about community, rurality, and services for seniors are predicted on positive perceptions of community in small towns, not to mention a belief that families, friends, and neighbours can mediate the reality of the lack of formal services in rural areas. This contradiction resonates with concern for the ability of rural communities and their informal sectors to cope.

IMPLICATIONS FOR NURSING: The researchers concluded that how seniors living in small towns are imagined (or romanticized) remains a fundamental question. They challenge decision makers, researchers, and providers to debunk assumptions about services for seniors in rural Canada. The researchers warn of the very real danger that belief in community will continue to justify health policies and programs, further prejudicing the situation of rural seniors and their caregivers.

Spiritual Domain

The changes in cognition and the ability to communicate that occur in dementia may discourage some nurses from attempting to provide individualized spiritual care. Yet, despite communication impairment, the need to be respected, to have hope, and to connect with others and, perhaps, a higher power does not diminish. If the spiritual domain is neglected in care, the person living with the symptoms of dementia may be denied important comforting and supportive measures. It is important to understand the person's spiritual beliefs as early as possible in the progression of dementia when they may be better able to explain what has spiritual importance for them. Their religious beliefs, rituals, and their participation in a religious community can be explored at this time. The diagnosis of dementia may have brought despair that challenged the person's existing spiritual beliefs. This needs to be recognized and opportunities for the person to express spiritual distress should be created.

Béphage (2009) has outlined strategies for spiritual care with persons with dementia under three categories: communication, religious interventions, and nonreligious interventions. Communication is the foundation for identifying the patient's spiritual disposition. A key action is to look for positive efforts to communicate by the patient. Nurses can be sensitive to the spirituality-related verbal and nonverbal cues from the patient and to the presence of spiritually meaningful items or artefacts (e.g., bible, Koran, prayer wheel). Helping the patient remain connected with religious activities can be accomplished by support from the family and/the patient's religious community and from pastoral care workers. If the patient can no longer attend religious services in person, alternative forms of attendance may be possible, such as via radio or television. The patient may want to share past memories of faith and practices or listen to hymns or spiritual music. Being able to see and touch meaningful symbols may be comforting. Nonreligious interventions that support spiritual well-being include art therapy (e.g., drawing or simply looking at paintings), outdoor activities, meditation, pet therapy, and reminiscence therapy. As well, active efforts to fulfill the patient's need for companionship may relieve the loneliness and social isolation that dementia brings.

For persons with AD (although it may not be appropriate for other forms of dementia, such as Huntington's disease), Procedural and Emotional Religious Activity Therapy (PERAT) is an approach that may provide some spiritual support (Vance, Moore, Farr, & Struzick, 2008). Based on matching the cognitive ability of the person with the cognitive demands of an emotionally meaningful activity, such as a religious or spiritual activity, PERAT involves an assessment of patients' religious and spiritual history and of their cognitive status. Tasks are selected for their procedural memory component and emotional salience to the patient. Materials (i.e., items that have an emotional attachment) for the activities are obtained, usually from family members. Making family photographs, religious pictures, and books available within the patient's setting can be helpful and soothing. Activities can include reciting favourite scripture, engaging in prayer, holding a religious icon, or maintaining a shrine. This is a counterproductive approach if the activities are not spirituality appropriate to the individual patient, and more research is required to develop this approach for patients with AD (Vance et al., 2008).

EVALUATION AND TREATMENT OUTCOMES

The objectives of nursing interventions are to help the patient with dementia remain as independent as possible and to function at the highest cognitive, physical, emotional, spiritual, and social levels. The maximum level of functional ability can be promoted when nursing care is related to and based on the remaining abilities of the patient. Patients who receive diagnoses of AD or other types of dementia have a wide and varying range of functional abilities. As cognitive decline progresses, there is a tendency for caregivers to perform more and more tasks for the patient. It is essential to assess for strengths and to assist in the maintenance of existing skills. Adaptive and appropriate behaviours continue to some degree in people with dementia, even in the presence of an increasing cognitive decline. It is important for nursing interventions to focus on more than the maintenance of optimal physical functional ability; interventions also must focus on meeting psychological, social, and spiritual needs of the patient with dementia.

Nurses can maintain quality of life if they protect a patient's overall well-being by balancing physical, mental, social, and spiritual health. Figure 31-5 illustrates the truly bio/psycho/social/spiritual aspects of the treatment of individuals with dementia by summarizing potential outcomes of nursing care.

Forbes et al. (2008, 2009) studied the role of home care and other agencies in meeting the needs of Canadians with dementia and their unpaid caregivers, such as family members. Service *availability* and *acceptability* were the overarching themes of the study findings. Family caregivers desired an integrated continuing care model that includes the person with dementia and family as partners in care; addresses all the determinants of health, and encompasses sensitivity, flexibility and diversity. Formal care providers (paid professional and nonprofessional caregivers) described challenges to service availability as including service waitlists lack of homecare provider training, lack of community-based dementia care, lack of service infrastructure, and sociocultural and geographical barriers. Agency partnerships, however, facilitated availability. Key to the acceptability of services was comprehensive personal care with adequate service time for such

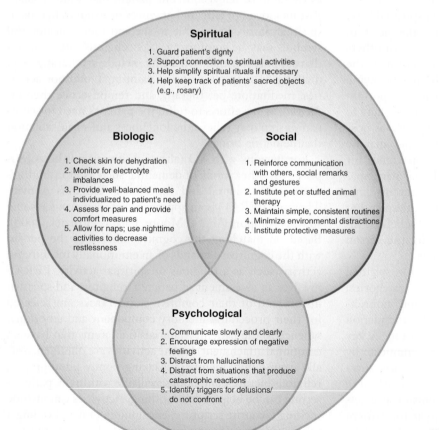

FIGURE 31.5 Bio/psycho/social/spiritual interventions for patients with dementia.

care, as well as for support of the patient, family, and the formal care providers. Difficulty navigating the system was a barrier. This type of research, focused on the voices of those directly affected by, and involved with, dementia care has direct implications for the evolution of services.

CONTINUUM OF CARE

Community Care

In 2003, 566,500 noninstitutionalized seniors received home care. Services included nursing care, general health care, personal care, home help, shopping, and respite care. Women are more likely to receive homecare than men, but this may be because women have a longer life expectancy. fifty-seven percent of seniors who received home care received that care from a formal source; 28% relied on family, friends, and neighbours, while 15% received care from formal sources and family, etc. (Statistics Canada, 2005). Cooperation among health care providers of different disciplines and in various settings is needed to meet the highly individualized needs of patients with deficits.

Inpatient-Focused Care

Comprehensive admission assessment, followed by the development of an individualized (and constantly updated) care plan that involves the patient, significant others, and a variety of health care professionals, is the foundation of an effective and efficient predischarge plan. Attention to all aspects of this process is necessary to ensure that the goal of continuity of care is achieved. The hospital-based nurse may initiate family education and counselling as part of discharge planning. For more information on caring for the patient with dementia, see Nursing Care Plan 31.1.

Nursing Home Care

As the dementia progresses, most patients are placed in a nursing home for care. Nursing care in is usually delivered by nurses' aides, who need support and direction. Interestingly, people with dementia require complex nursing care, but the skill level of people caring for these individuals often is minimal. Education and support of the direct caregiver are the focus of most nursing homes.

Other Dementias

Dementia symptoms may occur as a result of a number of disorders and underlying etiologies. The subsequent sections provide a brief description of some of the dementias listed in the *Diagnostic and Statistical Manual of Mental Disorders*, 4th ed., Text revision (*DSM-IV-TR*; APA, 2000). In each case, the classic symptoms of dementia (e.g., memory impairment with a number of other cognitive deficits) must be present. Nursing interventions for all dementias are similar to those described for individuals with AD.

VASCULAR DEMENTIA

Vascular dementia (VaD) is seen in about 20% of patients with dementia, most commonly people between the ages of 60 and 75 years. Slightly more men than women are affected. VaD results from multiple cerebral infarctions (transient ischemic attacks or TIAs). Infarcts can be either cortical or subcortical. Most often, a blood clot or plaques (fatty deposits) block the vessels that supply blood to the brain, causing a stroke. However, a stroke can also occur when a blood vessel ruptures in the brain.

The primary causes of strokes include high blood cholesterol levels, diabetes, heart disease, and high blood pressure. Of these, high blood pressure is the greatest risk factor for vascular dementia. It is essential that anyone who demonstrates symptoms of dementia or who has a history of stroke should have a complete physical examination that includes neurologic and neuropsychological evaluation, diet and medication history, review of recent stressors, and an array of laboratory tests. Damage to the brain in vascular dementia is usually apparent using computed tomography scans or magnetic resonance imaging. At autopsy, multifocal lesions may be found, rather than the more generalized cortical atrophy characteristic of AD.

The behaviour changes that result from vascular dementia are similar to those found in AD, such as loss of memory, judgment, and reasoning, depression, emotional lability, wandering or getting lost in familiar places, bladder or bowel incontinence, difficulty in following instructions, gait changes such as small shuffling steps, and problems handling daily activities. However, these symptoms usually begin more suddenly, rather than developing slowly, as is the case in AD. Often, the neurologic symptoms associated with a TIA are minimal (slight weakness in an extremity, dizziness, or slurred speech) and may last only a few days. Thus, the clinical progression is often described as step-like deterioration, with the patient's cognitive and functional status plateauing for a period of time, followed by a rapid decline in function after another series of small strokes. The Hachinski Ischemia Score in Box 31-14 may be helpful in differentiating vascular dementia from AD and in summarizing the symptoms more closely related to vascular dementia.

Treatment aims to reduce the primary risk factors for vascular dementia, including hypertension, diabetes, and additional strokes. Interventions that reduce the tendency of the blood to clot and of platelets to aggregate

Patient with Dementia

LW is a 76-year-old widow who lives independently. Recently, her children have noticed that she is becoming more forgetful and seems to have periods of confusion. She has agreed to have someone help her during the day. Her oldest son lives with her and is with her during the evening and night. LW refuses to see a health care provider but did agree to go in for a routine checkup. Her daughter helped her get dressed and took her to the primary health care clinic.

Setting: Primary Health Care Clinic

Baseline Assessment: A well-groomed woman is accompanied by her daughter. LW says there is nothing wrong, but her daughter disagrees. A review of body systems reveals poor hearing and vision but is otherwise unremarkable. MMSE score is 19. Daughter reports that LW has become very suspicious of neighbours and has changed her locks several times.

Associated Psychiatric Diagnosis	Medications
Axis I: Probable dementia of the Alzheimer's type	Galantamine (Reminyl) 4 mg bid, titrate to 8 mg bid over 4 weeks.
Axis II: None	Consider risperidone 0.5–1 mg od, if psychotic symptoms occur.
Axis III: History of breast cancer, unilateral mastectomy, arthritis	
Axis IV: Social problems (suspiciousness)	
GAF = Current 70	
Potential 70	

Nursing Diagnosis 1: Impaired Memory

Defining Characteristics	Related Factors
Inability to recall information	Neurocognitive changes associated with dementia
Inability to recall past events	
Observed instances of forgetfulness	
Forgets to perform daily activities—grooming	

Outcomes

Initial	Long Term
Maintain or improve current memory	Delay cognitive decline associated with dementia

Interventions

Interventions	Rationale	Ongoing Assessment
Develop memory cues in home. Have clocks and calendars well displayed. Make lists for patients.	Maintaining current level of memory involves providing cues that will help patient recall information.	Contact family members for patient's ability to use memory cues.
Teach patient and family about taking an acetylcholinesterase inhibitor. Review expected effects, side effects, and adverse effects. Develop a titration schedule with family to decrease the appearance of side effects.	Confidence and self-esteem improve when a person looks well groomed.	Monitor response to suggestions.
Observe patient for visuospatial impairment. If present, sequence habitual activities, such as eating, dressing, bathing, etc.	Visuospatial impairment is one of the symptoms of dementia.	Observe for appropriate dress, bathing, eating, etc.

Evaluation

Outcomes	Revised Outcomes	Interventions
LW did have some improvement in memory. Suspiciousness and behavioural symptoms improved.	Continue maintaining memory.	Continue with memory cues and galantamine.

BOX 31.14

Hachinski Ischemia Score

Abrupt onset	2
Stepwise progression	1
Fluctuating course	2
Nocturnal confusion	1
Relative preservation of personality	1
Depression	1
Somatic complaints	1
Emotional incontinence	1
History of hypertension	1
History of stroke	2
Evidence of associated atherosclerosis	1
Focal neurologic symptoms	2
Focal neurologic signs	2
AD if scores total	4 or less
Vascular dementias if scores total	7 or more

From Hachinski, V. C. (1983). Differential diagnosis of Alzheimer's dementia: Multi-infarct dementia. In B. Reisberg (Ed.), *Alzheimer's disease* (pp. 188–192). New York, NY: Free Press/Macmillan.

include lifestyle changes (diet, exercise, and smoking cessation) and using medications. Increasingly, physicians are recommending anticoagulants and medication to control hypertension, cholesterol, and glucose. Cholinesterase inhibitors may be ordered to slow the progress of dementia.

DEMENTIA WITH LEWY BODIES (DLB)

Twenty percent of all cases of dementia can be attributed to DLB. DLB can manifest on its own, with Parkinson's disease, or with AD. It generally affects people between 75 and 80 years and is more likely to affect males than females. The prominent features of DLB include fluctuations in cognition, visual hallucinations, delusions, changes in gait with repeated falls, syncope, neuroleptic sensitivity, and REM sleep disorder.

Persons with DLB may spend short periods of time staring off into space and unaware of their surroundings. Unlike AD, visual hallucinations are common. Thoughts may have a delusional content. A shuffling gait, not unlike with Parkinson's disease, may become apparent. Safety becomes a concern with falls and faintness. More than 50% of persons with DLB are sensitive to neuroleptics; therefore, they should be avoided. A hallmark of the possible onset of DLB is REM sleep behaviour disorder (a sleep parasomnia). In REM sleep behaviour disorder, the paralysis that normally occurs during REM sleep is absent allowing the person to physically and vocally act out their dreams. Researchers continue to investigate DLB as to the cause and treatment.

FRONTOTEMPORAL DEMENTIA

FTD incorporates many conditions including long-duration Creutzfeldt-Jakob disease and dysphasic dementia. FTD affects both the frontal and temporal lobes of the brain; therefore, a patient's personality, behaviour, and speech can be altered. FTD can begin to affect people in their younger adult years. A patient with FTD may become socially withdrawn and apathetic or may become disinhibited and impulsive. Disturbances of mood and anxiety are common. It is not unusual for the patient to exhibit ritualistic and obsessive behaviours. The ability to speak may be lost or the patient may have progressive reduction in the ability to carry on a conversation. Echolalia may be present. In the early stages of the dementia, a patient with FTD often remains oriented to all three spheres and retains visuospatial skills and memory.

A person with FTD may have changes in personality but be still able to manage the running of a home. They can still make meals, clean, and go shopping. Just as they can run a home, a person with FTD can still manage all the psychomotor and spatial skills needed to maintain employment, but often lose their position due to changes in personality. They may become easily irritated, loud, and argumentative. This is particularly distressing to a family if they do not understand what is going on for the person with FTD. As with all dementias, eventually all symptoms of brain impairment affect the patient.

DEMENTIA CAUSED BY OTHER GENERAL MEDICAL CONDITIONS

People of any age, race, or gender are at risk for dementia caused by a medical condition known to cause cerebral pathology. Older adults are particularly vulnerable to the development of dementia caused by general medical conditions because so many are affected by one or more chronic medical illnesses. Strong relationships have been reported between the chronic medical illness and the development of dementia.

Dementia Caused by AIDS

Dementia associated with AIDS has been called AIDS dementia complex (ADC). ADC has been observed in nearly two thirds of all patients with AIDS. AIDS is caused by human immunodeficiency virus 1 (HIV-1), which infects and destroys T lymphocytes as well as the CNS. HIV-1 directly invades the CNS and allows opportunistic infections of the CNS and other organ systems. Although there has been a proportional increase in ADC at AIDS diagnosis, survival after ADC has improved markedly in the era of highly active antiretroviral therapy (HAART) (Dore et al., 2003).

Dementia Caused by Head Trauma

When head trauma occurs in the context of a single injury, the resulting dementia is usually not progressive, but repeated head injury (e.g., from the sport of boxing) may lead to a progressive dementia. When the nurse observes progressive decline in intellectual functioning after a single incident of head trauma, the possibility of another superimposed process must be considered. Head injury associated with a prolonged loss of consciousness (days to months) may be followed by delirium, dementia, or a profound alteration in personality. Falls are a common cause of head injury in the older adult. Subarachnoid hemorrhage is often a result of an unwitnessed fall and often gets missed, leading to the potential for permanent brain damage and/or death. Subarachnoid hemorrhage is treatable if caught early.

The degree and type of cognitive impairment or behavioural disturbances demonstrated by a person with head trauma depend on the location and extent of the brain injury (as with other forms of dementia). Repeated head injuries, such as those sustained by young, healthy boxers, may lead to *dementia pugi listica*, or "punch-drunk syndrome." Although the exact mechanism of this disorder is unknown, it appears likely that early damage to neurons and their connections becomes clinically manifest later, when the combination of normal neuronal cell loss and prior damage summates to reach a threshold of impaired cognitive function.

Dementia Caused by Parkinson's Disease

Parkinson's disease is a neurologic syndrome of unknown etiology, which manifests as a disorder of movement, with a slow and progressive course. Clinical manifestations of Parkinson's disease are **bradykinesia** (the slowing of body movements), rigidity, resting tremor, and postural changes. The person's gait is unstable, resulting in frequent falls. Parkinson's disease may appear at any time after a person reaches 30 years of age, but the median age of onset is about 70 years of age. A subcortical dementia can be diagnosed in about 20% to 60% of patients with Parkinson's disease (APA, 2000). Although investigators do not know why, there is considerable pathologic overlap between Parkinson's disease and AD. Medical treatment of Parkinson's disease typically is with anticholinergics and dopamine agonists. It is important for nurses to know that in patients with dementia caused by Parkinson's disease, anticholinergic medications are likely to increase cognitive impairment (Katzenschlager, Sampaio, Costa, & Lees, 2003).

Dementia Caused by Huntington's Disease

Huntington's disease is a progressive, genetically transmitted autosomal dominant disorder characterized by choreiform movements and mental abnormalities.

The onset is usually between the ages of 30 and 50 years, but onset occurs before 5 years of age in the juvenile form or as late as 85 years of age in the late-onset form. The disease affects men and women equally. A person with Huntington's disease usually lives for 15 to 20 years after diagnosis (APA, 2000). The dementia syndrome of Huntington's disease is characterized by insidious changes in behaviour and personality. Typically, the dementia is frontal, which means that the person demonstrates prominent behavioural problems and disruption of attention.

Dementia Caused by Pick's Disease

Pick's disease is a rare form of dementia that is clinically similar to AD. The etiology of Pick's disease is unknown. Pick's disease particularly affects the frontal and temporal lobes of the brain (APA, 2000). The disorder usually manifests in individuals between the ages of 50 and 60 years, although it can occur among older individuals. Pick's disease is not readily distinguishable from AD until autopsy (APA), when the distinctive intraneuronal Pick's bodies can be identified microscopically.

Dementia Caused by Creutzfeldt-Jakob Disease

Creutzfeldt-Jakob disease is a rare, rapidly fatal brain disorder. Many of the symptoms seen in Creutzfeldt-Jakob disease are similar to those found in AD and other dementias. However, changes in the brain tissue are different in Creutzfeldt-Jakob disease and are best differentiated by surgical biopsy or on autopsy. Scientists speculate that Creutzfeldt-Jakob disease is caused by infectious agents known as *prions*, which are misfolded proteins that collect in central nervous tissue and cause nerve cells to die by an, as yet, unknown process, leaving gaps in the tissues (Public Health Agency of Canada, 2007).

At present, there is no effective treatment for the disease, and nothing has been found to slow progression of the illness. Because of its rapid clinical course, an important nursing role is assisting family members to understand and come to terms with the illness and to make decisions related to treatment setting and life-sustaining treatments. Creutzfeldt-Jakob disease progresses much more rapidly than most dementias, and death usually occurs within 1 year after onset, although some evidence suggests that extensive changes in the brain may be present before symptoms appear.

Only about 3,000 cases of Creutzfeldt-Jakob disease have been reported worldwide in the past 70 years, resulting in an annual incidence of about 1 per 1 million population. The disease strikes both men and women, most commonly between the ages of 50 and 75 years. Interestingly, there appears to be a genetic component to Creutzfeldt-Jakob disease (Cummings, 2003). Inhabitants of certain rural areas of the world, such as Slovakia and Chile, and Libyan-born Jews living in Israel have a much higher incidence of the disease.

Person-to-person transmission of Creutzfeldt-Jakob disease is rare (but possible), and it can be transmitted from people to animals and between animals. Evidence indicates that the prions can be introduced into the nervous system of healthy patients during medical procedures, such as corneal transplantation, implantation of contaminated electrodes in the brain, and injection of contaminated growth hormones (a few health care workers, probably exposed to the infectious agent through blood and spinal fluids, have experienced the disease). Because of the transmissible nature of Creutzfeldt-Jakob disease, strict criteria for the handling of infected tissues and other contaminated materials have been developed.

A variant type of Creutzfeldt-Jakob disease (vCJD) now exists that is linked to eating beef products from cattle infected with bovine spongiform encephalopathy (BSE). There has been only one case in Canada, and the person affected had been living in the United Kingdom. There have been no cases of vCJD linked to eating Canadian beef (Public Health Agency of Canada, 2007). Nevertheless, the sixteenth occurrence of BSE in Canadian cattle was confirmed on May 15, 2009 in Alberta (Canadian Food Inspection Agency, 2009). It was detected by Canada's BSE Surveillance system, and no part of the animal's carcass entered the human food (nor animal feed) systems.

Substance-Induced Persisting Dementia

If dementia results from the persisting effects of a substance (e.g., drugs of abuse, a medication, or exposure to toxins), substance-induced persisting dementia is diagnosed. Other causes of dementia (e.g., dementia caused by a general medical condition) must always be considered, even in a person with a dependence on or exposure to a substance. For example, head injuries often result from substance use and may be the underlying cause of the dementia syndrome (APA, 2000).

Drugs of abuse are the most common toxins in young adults, and prescription drugs are the most common toxins in older people. In older patients, dementia results from the use of long-acting benzodiazepines, barbiturates, meprobamate, and a host of other drugs, depending on their dose and the length of time they have been used. Drugs such as flurazepam (Dalmane), with a half-life of more than 120 hours, accumulate rapidly in a person's body. Other drugs accumulate more slowly or require relatively high doses for toxicity to develop. A toxic etiology should be suspected in every patient with a probable diagnosis of dementia. The nurse should inquire about exposure to drugs and toxins (exposure to toxins at work sites, medication use, and recreational drug use) for each

patient with dementia, and any substances known to be potentially injurious to the nervous system should be withdrawn if at all possible.

Most of the dementias in this category are related to chronic alcohol abuse. Understanding the cognitive deficits associated with chronic alcohol consumption is complicated. Alcoholic dementia is directly related to the toxic effects of alcohol, although the vitamin deficiencies associated with alcoholism (thiamine and niacin) are also known to be etiologically related to dementia. Individuals with alcoholism also have a high incidence of systemic illnesses that can affect cognition (e.g., cirrhosis, cardiomyopathy), and they are susceptible to repeated head injuries, which carry cognitive consequences of their own.

Much of our knowledge about cognitive deficits in individuals with alcoholism comes from the study of patients with Korsakoff's syndrome, which is a profound deficit in the ability to form new memories and is associated with a variable deficit in the recall of old memories, despite a clear sensorium. Further careful examination reveals a flattening of drives, unconcern about incapacity, and profound apathy. Nonetheless, Korsakoff's syndrome does not qualify as a dementia; rather, it is considered an amnestic syndrome (or restricted deficit of memory). In alcohol-induced dementia, the cognitive deficits span a wider range of functioning than with Korsakoff's syndrome (see Chapter 24).

Chemicals and organic compounds that impair functioning of the CNS usually have their primary effects on other body systems: the gastrointestinal, renal, hepatic, blood-forming, and peripheral nervous systems. For example, metal poisonings generally produce gastrointestinal symptoms and peripheral neuropathy. Cognitive changes with poisoning tend to be more characteristic of delirium than dementia, with altered levels of consciousness a prominent feature. Table 31-1 lists some of the organic compounds or chemicals that can cause symptoms of dementia; related distinguishing symptoms are also included.

Many adolescents and indigent adults engage in the act of "huffing" because the cost of purchasing spray paint, hair spray, glue, and other aerosol products is relatively inexpensive (compared with illicit street drugs). The nurse is reminded to evaluate people who abuse drugs for signs of cognitive impairment because neural and cognitive symptoms tend to appear before permanent brain damage occurs. It is also important to realize that the patient's cognitive status may not immediately improve after discontinuation of use of the offending agent. The effects of drugs taken for a long period may be long lasting, and improvement may follow discontinuation of drug use only slowly. For example, in dementia associated with chronic alcoholism, cognition may improve only after many months of abstinence.

SUMMARY OF KEY POINTS

❑ Neuropsychiatric disorders, such as delirium and dementia, are characterized clinically by significant deficits in cognition or memory that represent a clear-cut change from a previous level of functioning. In some disorders, the loss of cognitive function is progressive, such as in AD.

❑ Two major syndromes of cognitive impairment in older adults are delirium and chronic cognitive impairments, such as dementia. It is important to recognize the differences because the interventions and expected outcomes of the two syndromes are different.

❑ The symptoms of de.ression can overlap with the symptoms of both delirium and dementia. One individual may have one, two, or three of the conditions in the triad of delirium, dementia, and depression simultaneously.

❑ Delirium is characterized by a disturbance in consciousness and a change in cognition that develops over a short period of time. It requires rapid detection and treatment because in 25% of cases, it is a sign of impending death.

❑ Usually, delirium is caused by a combination of precipitating factors. The most commonly identified causes are medications, infections (particularly urinary tract and upper respiratory tract infections), fluid and electrolyte imbalance, and metabolic disturbances such as electrolyte imbalance or poor nutrition. Other important predisposing factors include advanced age, brain damage, preexisting dementia, and bio/psycho/social/spiritual stressors.

❑ The primary goal of treatment of delirium is prevention or resolution of the acute confusional episode with return to previous cognitive status and interventions focusing on (1) elimination or correction of the underlying cause and (2) symptomatic and safety and supportive measures.

❑ Dementia is characterized by the gradual onset of decline in cognitive function, especially memory, usually accompanied by changes in behaviour and personality. There are numerous causes of the symptoms of dementia, some of which are reversible, such as hypoxia, carbon monoxide poisoning, and vitamin deficiencies.

❑ AD is an example of a progressive, degenerative dementia. Treatment efforts currently focus on the reduction of cognitive symptoms (e.g., memory loss, confusion, and problems with learning, speech, and reasoning) in attempts to improve the quality of life for both patients and their caregivers.

❑ No one cause of dementia or AD has been discovered. Research efforts continue to pinpoint a singular identifiable genetic basis while focusing on other implicated etiologies, including neurochemical (i.e., decreased acetylcholine believed to play a major role in memory impairment), neuropathologic (i.e., degeneration of glutamatergic nerve terminals, head injury causing damage to the blood–brain barrier, defects in the immune system), and even some environmental factors.

❑ Some of the psychosocial stressors known to precipitate delirium and contribute to worsening dementia include sensory overload or underload, immobilization, sleep deprivation, fatigue, pain or hunger, change in routine (pace or caregiver), or demands beyond the patient's ability. Nursing interventions should include reducing the impact of these stressors on patients and educating their families or caregivers.

❑ Educating families and caregivers about what to expect, progressive cognitive decline and behaviour changes, environment safety, and community resources for patients with dementia is essential to ensuring proper care.

❑ Symptoms of dementia may occur as a result of a number of disorders, including vascular and amnestic disorders, head trauma, AIDS, and substance abuse and as a symptom of Parkinson's, Huntington's, Pick's, and Creutzfeldt-Jakob diseases.

CRITICAL THINKING CHALLENGES

1   What factors should the nurse consider in differentiating AD from vascular dementia?

2   Compare the defining characteristics and related risk factors of acute confusion with those for the NANDA diagnoses of impaired thought processes and sensory/perceptual disturbances. What are the differences and similarities between the recommended nursing interventions for delirium and dementia? What is the theoretic base for these similarities and differences?

3   Describe three ways in which medical disease can disrupt brain functioning, and relate these mechanisms to the neuropsychiatric disorders presented in this chapter.

4   Suggest reasons that older adults are particularly vulnerable to the development of neuropsychiatric disorders.

5   In what ways can culture and education influence mental status test scores?

6   The physical environment is particularly important to the patient with dementia. Every effort should be made to modify the physical environment to compensate for the cognitive and functional impairment associated with AD and related disorders, including safety measures and the avoidance of misleading stimuli. Visualize your last experience in a health care setting (hospital, nursing home, day care program, or home care setting). Identify environmental factors that could be misleading or stress producing to a person with impaired cognition (dementia), and identify ways to modify this environment to alleviate some of the stressors or misleading stimuli.

WEB LINKS

www.alz.org This Alzheimer's Association website provides information, resources, and consumer and caregiver support.

www.rnao.org/bestpractices Screening & Selecting Care Strategies for Delerium, Dementia & Depression in Older Adults.

www.pdsg.org.uk This website of the Pick's Disease Support Group provides information on Pick's disease, Lewy bodies, and other dementias.

www.alzheimer.ca This site of the Alzheimer Society of Canada provides information and resources related to the disease.

MOVIES, NOVELS, AND BIOGRAPHIES

Away From Her: 2006. An award winning Canadian movie directed by Sarah Polley and starring Gordon Pinsent and Julie Christie. Based on the short story, The Bear Came Over the Mountain, by Alice Munro, Away From Her invites the audience into the lives of Grant and Fiona. Fiona is diagnosed with AD and goes to live in a nursing home. The movie shows the struggle Grant has in coming to terms with the loss of his wife as she moves away from him and into her dementia.

VIEWING POINTS: How would you react if your spouse of many years no longer recognized you? What were the "tell-tale" signs that Fiona was developing Alzheimer's?

The Notebook: 2004. Every day an older man reads to a woman from his faded notebook. They are in a nursing home, and it is their own love story that he is reading. It is a story about how they met, fell in love, and then spent their lives together. Based on a novel by Nicholas Sparks, the movie reveals the fleeting moments of clarity that Noah's story brings to Allie, his wife, who is suffering from dementia. It shows the hope that keeps him trying to reach her.

VIEWING POINTS: Consider what it might be like to hear your own life story and to recognize it only momentarily and vaguely. Can you think of other ways people cope with the loss of a loved one who remains, at least physically, before them?

Iris: 2001. Based on the book by her husband, John Bayley, this movie (directed by Richard Eyre) tells the story of an influential British woman of letters, Dame Iris Murdoch. Young Iris is played by Kate Winslet, and the older Iris by Dame Judi Dench, in the unfolding of her rich and interesting life. The story reveals the couple's struggle with Iris's AD as her exceptional capabilities are increasingly diminished.

VIEWING POINTS: Consider how the love and friendship of the couple is both strengthened and challenged by AD. Are there any external supports and resources that might have made their situation in living with AD less difficult?

REFERENCES

Alzheimer Society of Canada. (2009). *Alzheimer's disease and risk factors.* Retrieved November 25, 2009, from www.alzheimer.ca/english/disease/causes-riskfac.htm

American Psychiatric Association. (2000). *Diagnostic and statistical manual of mental disorders* (4th ed., Text revision). Washington, DC: Author.

Béphage, G. (2009). Care approaches to dementia. *British Journal of Healthcare Assistants, 3*(1), 43–46.

British Geriatrics Society and Royal College of Physicians Guidelines for the prevention, diagnosis and management of delirium in older people. (2006). *Diagnosis and management of delirium in older people.* London, UK: RCP.

Byszewski, A. M., Graham, I. D., Amos, S., Man-Son-Hing, M., Dalziel, W. B., Marshall, S., Hunt, L., Bush, C., & Guzman, D. (2003). A continuing Medical Education Initiative for Canadian Primary Care Physicians. The Driving and Dementia Tool Kit: A pre and post evaluation of knowledge, confidence gained, and satisfaction. *Journal of the American Geriatrics Society, 51*(10), 1484–1489.

Canadian Food Inspection Agency (2009, May). BSE Case confirmed in Alberta. Retrieved June 18, 2009, from http://www.inspection.gc.ca

Cacchione, P. Z. (2002). Assessment. Four acute confusion assessment instruments: Reliability and validity for use in long-term care facilities. *Journal of Gerontological Nursing, 28*(1), 12–19.

Canadian Study of Health and Aging Working Group. (1994). Canadian study of health and aging: study methods and prevalence of dementia. *Canadian Medical Association Journal, 150,* 899–913.

Carpenito-Moyet, L. (2004). *Nursing diagnosis.* Philadelphia, PA: Lippincott Williams & Wilkins.

Carpenter, B. D., Xiong, C., Porensky, E. K., Lee, M. M., Brown, P. J., Coats, M., Johnson, D. & Morris, J. (2008). Reaction to a dementia diagnosis in individuals with Alzheimer's disease and mild cognitive impairment. *Journal of American Geriatrics Society, 56*(3), 405–412.

Cummings, J. L. (2003). *The neuropsychiatry of Alzheimer's disease and related dementias.* London, UK: Martin Dunitz.

DeJong, R., Osterlund, O. W., & Roy, G. W. (1989). Measurement of quality-of-life changes in patients with Alzheimer's disease. *Clinical Therapeutics, 11,* 545–554.

Dore, G. J., McDonald, A., Li, Y., Kaldor, J. M., Brew, B. J., & National HIV Surveillance Committee. (2003). Marked improvement in survival following AIDS dementia complex in the era of highly active antiretroviral therapy. *AIDS, 17*(10), 1539–1545.

Edwards, N., Davies, B., Ploeg, J., Virani, T., & Skelly, J. (2007). Implementing nursing best practice guidelines: Impact on patient referrals. *BioMed Central, 6*(4).

Fick, D. M., Hodo, D. M., Lawrence, F., & Inouye, S. K. (2007). Recognizing delirium superimposed on dementia. *Journal of Gerontological Nursing, 33*(2), 40–47.

Flaherty, J. H. (1998). Commonly prescribed and over the counter medications: Causes of confusion. *Clinics in Geriatric Medicine, 14*(1), 101–125.

Folstein, M. F., Folstein, S. E., & McHugh, P. R. (1975). Mini-mental state: A practical method for grading the cognitive state of patients for the clinician. *Journal of Psychiatric Research, 12,* 189–198.

Forbes, D. A., & Neufeld, A. (2008). Looming dementia care crisis: Canada needs an integrated model of continuing care now! *Canadian Journal of Nursing Research, 40*(1), 9–16.

Forbes, D.A., Markle-Reid, M., Hawranik, P., Kingston, D., Peacock, S., Henderson, S., et al. (2009). Formal care providers' perceptions of home- and community-based services: Informing dementia care quality. *Home Health Care Services Quarterly, 28,* 1–23.

Forbes, D. A., Markle-Reid, M., Hawranik, P., Peacock, S., Kingston, D., Morgan, D., Henderson, S., Leipert, B. & Jansen, S.L. (2008). Avaialbility and acceptability of Canadian home and community-based services: Perspectives of family caregivers of persons with dementia. *Home Health Care Services Quarterly, 27*(2), 75–99.

Forbes, D. A., Morgan, D., & Janzen, B. L. (2006). Rural and urban Canadians with Dementia: Use of health care services. *Canadian Journal on Aging, 25*(3), 321–330.

Gibson, M., MacLean, J., Barrie, M., & Geiger, J. (2004). Orientation behaviors in residents relocated to a redesigned dementia care unit. *American Journal of Alzheimer's disease, 19*(1), 45–49.

Gill, S. S., Bronskill, S. E., Normand, S.L.T., Anderson, G.M., Sykora, K., Lam. K., Bell, C.M., Lee, P.E., Fischer, H.D., Hermann, N., Gurwitz, J. H. & Rochon, P.A. (2007). Antipsychotic drug use and mortality in older adults with dementia. *Annals of Internal Medicine, 146*(11), 775–786.

Gleason, O. C. (2003). Delirium. *American Family Physician, 67*(5), 1027–1034.

Gotell, E., Brown, S., & Ekman, S-L. (2009). The influence of caregiver singing and background music on vocally expressed emotions and moods in dementia care: A qualitative analysis. *International Journal of Nursing Studies, 46*(4), 422–430.

Hachinski, V. C. (1983). Differential diagnosis of Alzheimer's dementia: Multi-infarct dementia. In B. Reisberg (Ed.), *Alzheimer's disease* (pp. 188–192). New York, NY: Free Press/Macmillan.

Hagen, B., Armstrong-Esther, C., Ikuta, R., Williams, R. J., Le Navenac, C. L., & Aho, M. (2005). Antipsychotic drug use in Canadian long-term care facilities: prevalence and patterns following resident relocation. *International Psychogeriatrics, 17*(2), 179–193.

Health Canada. (2005). *Health Canada advises consumers about important safety information on atypical antipsychotic drugs and dementia. Advisory 2005–63.* June 13, 2005. Ottawa, ON: Author.

Heidrich, D. E. (2007). Delirium: An under-recognized problem. *Clinical Journal of Oncology Nursing, 11*(6), 805–807.

Hicks-Moore, S. L., & Robinson, B. A. (2008). Favorite music and hand massage: Two interventions to decrease agitation in residents with dementia. *Dementia, 7*(1), 95–108.

Inouye, S. K. (2000). Prevention of delirium in hospitalized older patients: Risk factors and targeted intervention strategies. *Annals of Medicine, 32*(4), 257–263.

Inouye, S. K., van Dyck, C. H., Alessi, C. A., Balkin, S., Siegal, A. P., & Horwitz, R. I. (1990). Clarifying confusion: The confusion assessment method. *Annals of Internal Medicine, 113*, 941–948.

Jansen, L., Forbes, D.A., Markle-Reid, M., Hawranik, P., Kingston, D., Peacock, S., Henderson, S., & Leipert, B. (2009). Formal care providers' perceptions of home and community-based services: Informing dementia care quality. *Home Health Care Services Quarterly, 28*(1),1–23.

Katzenschlager, R., Sampaio, C., Costa, J., & Lees, A. (2003). Anticholinergics for symptomatic management of Parkinson's disease. *Cochrane Database of Systematic Reviews, 2*, CD003735.

Keren, R. (2006). Dementia drugs: When should they be stopped? *The Canadian Journal of Diagnosis, 23*(10), 90–94.

Kwasny, P., Hagen, B., & Armstrong-Esther, C. (2006). Use of major and minor tranquilizers with older patients in an acute care hospital: An exploratory study. *Journal of Advanced Nursing, 55*(2), 135–141.

Levkoff, S., Liptzin, B., Cleary, P., Reilly, C. H., & Evans, D. (1991). Review of research instruments and techniques used to detect delirium. *International Psychogeriatrics, 3*, 253–271.

McCloskey, J. C., & Bulechek, G. M. (2000). *Nursing interventions classification (NIC).* St. Louis, MO: Mosby.

McCusker, J., Cole, M., Dendukuri, N., Han, L., & Belzile, E. (2003). The course of delirium in older medical inpatients: A prospective study. *Journal of General Internal Medicine, 18*, 696–704.

Metzger, E. (2008). Depression among older adults with dementia: Double trouble. *Geriatrics & Aging, 11*(1), 31–36.

Morgan, D., Funk, M., Crossley, M., Basran, J., Kirk, A., & Dal Bello-Haas, V. (2007). The potential of gait analysis to contribute to differential diagnosis of early stage dementia: Current research and future directions. *Canadian Journal on Aging, 26*(1), 19–32.

Mosconi, L., Herholz, K., Prohovnik, I., Nacmias, B., De Cristofaro, M. T., Fayyaz, M., Bracco, S., Sorbi, S. Pupi, A. & Nacimas, M.T. R. (2005). Metabolic interaction between ApoE genotype and onset age in Alzheimer's disease: Implications for brain reserve. *Journal of Neurology, Neurosurgery & Psychiatry, 76*(1), 15–23.

National Advisory Council on Aging. (2004). The NACA position on Alzheimer's disease and related dementias, No. 23. Minister of Public Works and Government Services Canada. Available at: http://www.naca.ca [on-line].

Neal, M., & Briggs, M. (2003). *Validation therapy for dementia.* Oxford, UK: The Cochrane Library, 2, CD001394.

North American Nursing Diagnosis Association (NANDA). (2006). *Nursing diagnoses: Definition and Classification 2005–2006.* Philadelphia, PA: NANDA International.

Omelan, C. (2006). Approach to managing behavioural disturbances in dementia. *Canadian Family Physician, 52*, 191–199.

Parsons-Suhl, K., Johnson, M. E., McCann, J. L., & Solberg, S. (2008). Losing one's memory in early Alzheimer's disease. *Qualitative Health Research, 18*(1), 31–42.

Perry, J., Galloway, S., Bottorff, J. L., & Nixon, S. (2005). Nurse-patient communication in dementia: Improving the odds. *Journal of Gerontological Nursing, 31*(4), 43–52.

Public Health Agency of Canada. (2007). Variant Creutzfeldt-Jakob disease (vCJD) in Canada. Retrieved May, 2008, from htpc://www.phac-aspc.gc.ca

Raina, P., Santaguida, P., Ismaila, A., Patterson, C., Cowan, D., Levine, M., Booker, L. & Oremus, M. (2008). Effectiveness of cholinesterase inhibitors and memantine for treating dementia: Evidence review for a clinical practice guideline. *Annals of Internal Medicine, 148*(5), 379–397.

Rapoport, M., Verhoeff, N. P., & van Reekum, R. (2004). Traumatic brain injury and dementia. *The Canadian Alzheimer Disease Review*, September, 4–8.

Registered Nurses Association of Ontario. (2003). *Screening for delirium, dementia and depression in older adults.* Toronto, ON: Author.

Registered Nurses Association of Ontario. (2004). *Caregiving strategies for older adults with delirium, dementia, and depression.* Toronto, ON: Author.

Reisberg, B., Schneck, M. K., & Ferris, S. H. (1983). The Brief Cognitive Rating Scale (BCRS): Findings in primary degenerative dementia. *Psychopharmacology Bulletin, 19*, 47.

Rogaeva, E. (2002). The solved and unsolved mysteries of the genetics of early-onset Alzheimer's disease. *Neuromolecular Medicine, 2*(1), 1–10.

Rosen, J., Burgio, L., Kollar, M., Cain, M., Allison, M., Fogleman, M., Michael, M. & Zubenko, G. S. (1994). The Pittsburg agitation scale: User-friendly instrument for rating agitation in dementia patients. *The American Journal of Geriatric Psychiatry, 2*(1), 52–59.

Schwartz, G. E. (1983). Development and validation of the Geriatric Evaluation by Relatives Rating Instrument (GERRI). *Psychological Reports, 53*, 478–488.

Skinner, M. W., Rosenberg, M. W., Lovell, S. A., Dunn, J. R., Everitt, J. C., Hanlon, N., & Rothwell, T. A. (2008). Services for seniors in small-town Canada: The paradox of community. *Canadian Journal of Nursing Research, 40*(1), 80–101.

Staal, J. A., Sacks, A., Matheis, R., Collier, L., Calia, T., Hanif, H., & Kofman, E.S. (2007). The effects of Snoezelen (multi-sensory behavior therapy) and psychiatric care on agitation, apathy, and activities of daily living in dementia patients on a short term geriatric psychiatric inpatient unit. *The International Journal of Psychiatry in Medicine, 37*(4), 357–370.

Stahl, S. M. (2000). *Essential psychopharmacology: Neuroscientific basis and practical applications* (2nd ed.) New York, NY: Cambridge University Press.

Statistics Canada. (2005, February) Senior's health care use. Retrieved April, 2008, from http://www.statcan.ca/english/freepub/82-003-SIE/2005000/pdf/82-003-SIE20050007449.pdf

Statistics Canada. (2007, July). 2006 censusus: Age and sex. *The Daily.* Ottawa, ON: Author. Retrieved April, 2008, from http://www.statcan.ca/Daily/English/070717/d070717a.htm

Stern, Y., Albert, S. M., Sano, M., Richards, M., Miller, L., Folstein, M. Albert, M. Bylsma, F. W. & Lafleche, G. (1994). Assessing patient dependence in Alzheimer's disease. *Journal of Gerontology, 49*, M216–M222.

Suh, Y. H., & Checler, F. (2002). Amyloid precursor protein, presenilins, and alpha-synuclein: Molecular pathogenesis and pharmacological applications in Alzheimer's disease. *Pharmacological Reviews, 54*(3), 469–525.

Taddei, K., Fisher, C., Laws, S. M., Martins, G., Paton, A., Clarnette, R. M., Chung, C., Brooks, W. S., Hallmayer, J., Miklossy, J. Relkin, N., Saint-George-Hyslop, P.H., Gandy, S. E. & Martins, R. N. (2002). Association between presenilin-I Glu318Gly mutation and familial Alzheimer's disease in the Australian population. *Molecular Psychiatry, 7*(7), 776–781.

Tanzi, R. & Bertram, L. (2008). Alzheimer's disease: The latest suspect. *Nature, 454*(7205), 706–708.

Tarkowski, E., Andreasen, N., Tarkowski, A., & Blennow, K. (2003). Intrathecal inflammation precedes development of Alzheimer's disease. *Journal of Neurology, Neurosurgery, and Psychiatry, 74*(4), 1200–1205.

Trzepacz, P. T., Baker, R. W., & Greenhouse, J. (1988). A symptom rating scale for delirium. *Psychiatry Research, 23*, 89–97.

Tune, L. (2000). Delirium. In C. E. Coffey & J. L. Cummings (Eds.), *American Psychiatric Press textbook of geriatric neuropsychiatry* (2nd ed., pp. 441–462). Washington, DC: American Psychiatric Press.

United States Department of Health and Human Services (U.S. DHHS). (2003). *National Institute on Aging, 2001–2002. Alzheimer's Disease Progress Report*. National Institutes of Health Publication No. 03–533.

Vance, D., Moore, B., Farr, K. & Struzick, T. (2008). Procedural memory and emotional attachment in Alzheimer disease: Implications for meaningful and engaging activities. *Journal of Neuroscience Nursing, 40*(2), 96–102.

Vollmer, C., Rich, C., & Robinson, S. (2007). How to prevent delirium: A practical protocol. *Nursing 2007, 37*(8), 26–28.

Werezak, L., & Stewart, N. (2002). Learning to live with early dementia. *Canadian Journal of Nursing Research, 34*(1), 67–85.

White, S., & Bayer, A. (2007). Delirium-a clinical overview. *Reviews in Clinical Gerontology, 17*, 45–62.

Williams, M. A., Ward, S. E., & Campbell, E. B. (1988). Confusion: Testing versus observation. *Journal of Gerontological Nursing, 14*(1), 25–30.

Wolkove, N., Elkholy, O., Baltzan, M., & Palayew, M. (2007). Sleep and aging: Sleep disorders commonly found in older people. *Canadian Medical Association Journal, 176*(9), 1299–1304.

Zieber, C. G., Hagen, B., Armstrong-Esther, C., & Aho, M. (2005). Pain and agitation in long-term care residents with dementia: Use of the Pittsburgh Agitation Scale. *International Journal of Palliative Nursing, 11*(2), 71–78.

UNIT *VII*

Care of Special Populations

CHAPTER 32

Issues in Dual Diagnosis

Brad F. Hagen

Adapted from the chapter "Issues in Dual Diagnosis" by Barbara G. Faltz and Sandra C. Sellin

LEARNING OBJECTIVES

After studying this chapter, you will be able to:

- Define the term *dual disorders*.
- Discuss the epidemiology of dual disorders.
- Describe the cycle of relapse.
- Describe the effects of alcohol and other drugs on mental illness.
- Analyze the barriers to the treatment of patients with dual disorders.
- Discuss the four etiologies of dual disorders.
- Integrate relapse prevention concepts into the care of a patient with dual disorders.

KEY CONCEPT

- relapse cycle

KEY TERMS

- alcohol-induced persisting amnestic disorder • deinstitutionalization • dual disorders • Korsakoff's psychosis • motivational interviewing • substance use • 12-step programs • Wernicke's syndrome

We drank for joy and became miserable;
We drank for exhilaration and became depressed;
We drank for friendship and became enemies;
We drank to diminish our problems and saw them multiply.

Anonymous

Dual disorders, defined here as the coexistence of a substance use disorder and a mental health disorder, pose many issues for the psychiatric and mental health (PMH) nurse (Cleary, Walter, Hunt, Clancy, & Horsfall, 2008). Other terms that may be used to describe dual disorders include "comorbidity," "concurrent disorders," and "dual diagnosis," although in Canada, the term "dual diagnosis" often refers to a person with both a mental illness and a developmental disability. Traditionally, substance use and mental health treatment providers have attempted to treat only one aspect of a dual problem. This approach can lead to recurrent relapses into drug or alcohol use and to successive psychiatric hospitalizations.

The relapse cycle becomes continuous unless both the mental illness and the substance use disorder are treated.

> **KEY CONCEPT** In the **relapse cycle**, reemerging psychiatric symptoms lead to ineffective coping strategies, increased anxiety, substance use to avoid painful feelings, adverse consequences, and attempted abstinence, until psychiatric symptoms emerge once more and the cycle repeats itself.

Figure 32-1 shows the relationship between increased psychiatric symptoms and the use of substances as a coping strategy. Without alternative effective coping behaviours,

793

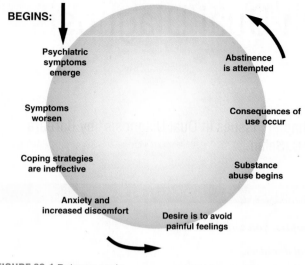

BEGINS:

Psychiatric
symptoms
emerge

Symptoms
worsen

Coping strategies
are ineffective

Anxiety and
increased discomfort

Abstinence
is attempted

Consequences of
use occur

Substance
abuse begins

Desire is to avoid
painful feelings

FIGURE 32.1 Relapse cycle.

the patient will continue to experience this cycle of relapse and abstinence. The goal of the treatment for patients with dual disorders is a comprehensive recovery plan for the complex problems presented—one that offers the patient a way out of what can be a downward spiral of debilitation.

This chapter highlights the methods of assessing dual disorders, explores the psychodynamics of their development, and discusses specific mental illnesses and the adverse effects of concurrent substance use. It offers treatment strategies and nursing interventions to address the complex yet common presentation in psychiatric and substance use treatment settings. A complete discussion of related substance use disorders is provided in Chapter 24.

RELATIONSHIP OF SUBSTANCE USE TO MENTAL ILLNESS

Although it has been prevalent throughout the history of mental illness treatment, the problem of dual disorders has been inadvertently magnified by the community mental health reform movement that began in the 1950s. One major facet of this reform was a rational movement toward **deinstitutionalization** of people with mental illness, which resulted in a large number of them being homeless and living on the streets (Joseph, 1997). Along with homelessness came the increased use of drugs and alcohol and increased incidence of mental illness (Hwang, 2001).

It is impossible to make any meaningful distinction between simple recreational use of a substance and actual **substance use** with this population because even small amounts of alcohol or other drugs can be damaging to people who have concurrent psychiatric problems. All substances of abuse exert profound effects on mental states, perception, psychomotor function, cognition, and

behaviour. The specific neurochemical and other biologic mechanisms that evoke these psychological features are discussed in Chapter 24. Table 32-1 lists the psychological effects of substances of abuse.

The pattern of alcohol and illicit drug use by the mentally ill varies. Some individuals with mental illness use alcohol and drugs recreationally, whereas others experience severe problems from the use of these substances. Individuals can become caught in a "revolving door" of repeated hospitalizations because of the distressing symptoms of mental illness that are exacerbated by substance use. When the presenting symptoms are stabilized and the patient is released, perhaps with new medications or a new discharge plan in place, the patient may be unable to follow the therapeutic regimen. The patient may resume or increase his or her use of alcohol or drugs as a way of coping with difficulties, only to find that the substance abuse results in an exacerbation of his or her emotional problems or interferes with the metabolization of medication and leads to rehospitalization. This cyclic pattern of mental health or substance use decompensation, hospitalization, stabilization, discharge, and decompensation can make it challenging for nurses to provide care for persons suffering from dual disorders (Coombs & Wratten, 2007).

MANIFESTATIONS OF DUAL DISORDERS

The four possible manifestations of dual disorders and a clinical example describing each follow. For additional information, see Table 32-2.

- *A primary mental illness with subsequent substance use.* In this manifestation, a primary mental illness leads to addictive behaviour when the patient self-medicates to cope with the symptoms of the illness. It includes abuse resulting from impaired judgment, poor impulse control, impaired social skills, and ineffective coping strategies.

  When she was 18 years old, Sylvia G. was raped and held by her assailant for 2 days. She has frequent nightmares, relives the experience almost daily, and is extremely anxious around men whom she does not know. She began drinking heavily after this incident and states that it provides some relief from her anxiety. Although Sylvia finds that drinking helps her to block out the terrifying memories and feelings associated with the rape, it also has numerous adverse consequences. For example, Sylvia was threatened with the loss of her job after she came to work with alcohol on her breath. Sylvia has received diagnoses of posttraumatic stress disorder (PTSD) and alcohol dependence.

- *A primary substance use disorder with psychopathologic sequelae.* Psychiatric symptoms are consequences of drug or alcohol intoxication, of withdrawal symptoms

Table 32.1	Psychological Effects of Substances of Abuse
Substance	**Psychological Effects**
Alcohol	Organic brain disorders—alcohol amnestic syndrome; dementia Agitation, anxiety disorders, sleep disorders Ataxia, slurred speech Withdrawal symptoms, which may include hallucinations, confusion, illusions, delusions; protracted withdrawal delirium can occur Depression, increased rate of suicide, disinhibition
Cocaine	Anxiety, agitation, hyperactivity, sleep disorders, delusions, paranoia, euphoria, internal sense of interest and excitement Rebound withdrawal symptoms, such as prolonged depression, somnolence, anhedonia
Amphetamines	Similar to cocaine but more prolonged Hyperactivity, agitation, anxiety, increased energy
Hallucinogens (MOMA Ecstasy) and phencyclidine	Hallucinations, delusions, paranoia, confusion Withdrawal can produce severe depression, somnolence Hallucinations, illusions, delusions, perceptual distortions, paranoia, rage, anxiety, agitation, confusion
Marijuana	Acute reactions: panic, anxiety, paranoia, sensory distortions, rare psychotic episodes; patients with schizophrenia use these reactions to distance themselves from painful symptoms and to gain control over symptoms Antimotivational syndrome: apathy, diminished interest in activities and goals, poor job or school performance, memory and cognitive deficits
Opiates	Confusion, somnolence Withdrawal can produce anxiety, irritability, and depression and can trigger suicidal ideation
Sedative-hypnotics	Confusion, slurred speech, ataxia, stupor, sleep disorders, withdrawal delirium, dementia, amnestic disorder, sleep disorders
Volatile solvents	Hallucinations, delusions, hyperactivity, sensory distortions, dementia

Adapted from Beauchamp, J. K., & Olson, K. R. (2000). Drug overdoses and dependence. In R. M. Wachter, L. Goldman, & H. Hollander (Eds.), *Hospital medicine*. Philadelphia, PA: Lippincott Williams & Wilkins.

Table 32.2	Assessment and Classification of Dual Disorder Conditions			
Assessment Issue	**Primary Mental Illness With Substance Use**	**Substance Use With Psychiatric Sequelae**	**Dual Primary Disorders**	**Common Etiology**
Are dual syndromes present?	Yes	Yes	Yes	Yes
Which came first?	Mental illness	Substance use	None	None
What is the family history?	Mental illness, if any	Substance use, if any	Mental illness, substance use, or both	Mental illness, substance use, or both, if any
What are the psychosocial factors?	Vulnerable to victimization by peers because of primary mental illness	Often can maintain family and employment during periods of sobriety	Prognosis is less favourable; may often be incarcerated or hospitalized	Common risk factor possible (e.g., homelessness)
What is the treatment and response to treatment?	Treatment for mental illness alleviates both syndromes; discharge plan focuses on mental health maintenance	Treatment for substance use alleviates both syndromes; discharge plan focuses on maintenance of sobriety	Treatment for both mental illness and substance use required	Treatment for common risk factor alleviates both mental illness and substance use

Adapted from Lehman, A. F., Myers, C. P., & Corty, E. (1989). Assessment and classification of patients with psychiatric and substance abuse syndromes. *Hospital and Community Psychiatry, 40*(10), 1019–1024.

(such as severe depression after cessation of prolonged cocaine abuse), or of cognitive impairments related to chronic alcohol or drug use.

Ralph D. has been smoking crack cocaine for 3 years. In the last year, Ralph has been unable to hold a job, been forced by his wife to move out, and is now living on the streets. Ralph recently attempted suicide after a prolonged cocaine binge, and claims he feels powerless and hopeless about his addiction to cocaine.

• *Dual primary diagnoses.* Psychiatric and substance use diagnoses interact to exacerbate each other.

Joan K. has been given a diagnosis of bipolar type II disorder. For many years, she has engaged in heavy drinking, which began in early adolescence after the death of her father. When she is binge drinking, she often forgets to take her medications, despite experiencing manic episodes and deep depressions. Joan has succeeded in being sober in the past, but always seems to start drinking again, particularly when she becomes socially isolated and/or she stops her treatment plan.

• *A common etiology.* A common factor that might be causing both disorders. While no definite causes have been attributed to mental health and/or substance abuse problems, there are several proposed factors that may have a causal role, such as genetics, and alterations in dopaminergic and/or cholinergic neurotransmitter activity (Lehman, Myers, & Corty, 1989). In addition, childhood abuse and adverse experiences have been shown to have a strong association with subsequent development of adult mental health and/or substance abuse problems (Kendler et al., 2000; MacMillan et al., 2001).

Frank L. received a diagnosis of attention deficit hyperactivity disorder as a child. His parents, both of whom struggled with alcohol abuse, had difficulty parenting him and would give him alcohol to attempt to "calm him down." Frank continues to have difficulty concentrating, is hyperactive, and has developed numerous medical problems related to his alcohol abuse as an adult.

EPIDEMIOLOGY

It can be difficult to know precisely how many people have a dual or concurrent disorder, although it is generally accepted that people suffering from a mental illness have much higher rates of substance abuse than those without a mental illness. For example, a recent national Canadian study found that approximately 20% of people who suffer from a mental disorder also have a substance abuse problem (Rush et al., 2008). A British Columbia study found an even higher rate, with 55% of mental health service clients also having substance abuse issues with their first episode of mental illness (B.C. Partners for Mental Health and Addictions Information, 2003).

IN A LIFE

Michael J. Fox (1961–)
Famous Canadian Actor

Public Persona

Michael J. Fox is one of the most famous Canadian-born actors, and he has charmed audiences with his wit, sensitivity, and charisma in such movies and TV series as *Back to the Future, Family Ties, The Secret of My Success, and Spin City.* Born as the son of a Canadian army officer, Michael J. Fox, like many other Canadian kids, originally wanted to play hockey for a living. He decided to pursue acting instead, however, and moved to Hollywood at the age of 18. An Emmy Award winner, Michael J. Fox first became well known for the hit TV series *Family Ties,* and proceeded to enjoy a successful career involving a number of hit movies and TV series. In 1998, he publicly announced that he was suffering from Parkinson's disease, a condition he had managed to keep hidden from the public for 7 years.

Personal Realities

In his autobiography, *Lucky Man: A Memoir,* Michael J. Fox describes how he was heavily addicted to alcohol in his early celebrity years, an addiction that continued as he struggled with the increasing disability associated with Parkinson's disease. In his memoir, Fox describes his climbing up from his periods of depression and addiction, how he has begun to deal with his Parkinson's disease, and the opportunity he now has to help search for a cure for Parkinson's disease and to raise public awareness of the disease.

Source: Fox, M. J. (2002). *Lucky man: A memoir.* New York, NY: Hyperion.

Similarly, a high proportion of people experiencing substance abuse problems also face mental health challenges. For example, Rush and colleagues (2008) found that just under 16% of people with substance use problems also had a mental disorder in the last year, and Canadian researchers have found that lifetime drug and alcohol use is particularly high among persons suffering from psychoses (Margolese, Malchy, Carlos Negrete, Tempier, & Gill, 2004).

Given these Canadian and other U.S. studies, there is strong epidemiologic evidence for the widespread coexistence of mental health issues and substance abuse problems. Therefore, nurses need to incorporate thorough assessment and screening techniques into their care of clients with mental health or substance abuse issues, to ensure that complete and appropriate treatment is provided.

PSYCHODYNAMIC MODEL OF DUAL DISORDERS

Confusion and professional disagreement exist about the etiology of dual disorders. Differing views of the etiology affect the proposed treatment strategies. Biologic aspects

BOX 32.1

Research for Best Practice: Psychosocial Treatments of Co-occurring Severe Mental Illness and Substance Use Disorder

Cleary, M., Hunt, G.E., Matheson S., & Walter G. (2009). Psychosocial treatments for people with co-occurring severe mental illness and substance misuse: systematic review. Journal of Advanced Nursing, 65*(2), 238–258.*

THE QUESTIONS: (1) How effective are psychosocial (nonpharmaceutical) interventions for reducing substance use, as well as improving mental health and encouraging treatment retention, among people with dual diagnosis? (2) Are some psychosocial treatments more effective than others?

METHODS: A systematic review was conducted of 54 studies published between January 1990 and February 2008, which included one systematic review with meta-analysis, 30 randomized control trials, and 23 nonexperimental studies. The data presented in these studies were compiled and cross-compared to determine the current evidence for the efficacy of the several psychosocial interventions undertaken in practice, which were grouped under cognitive behavioural therapy, motivational interviewing, group therapies,

contingency management, integrated assertive community treatment, intensive case management, residential programs, and forensic settings.

FINDINGS: The diversity of psychosocial interventions and the means of their evaluation made comparisons difficult. Some support was found for the effectiveness of motivational interviewing for the reduction of substance use, at least in the short term and, when combined with cognitive behavioural therapy over longer periods, improvements in mental health were apparent.

IMPLICATIONS FOR NURSING PRACTICE: Review of the literature indicates that motivational interviewing in psychiatric settings can in the short term be effective for the reduction of substance abuse. Further research should target particular diagnoses and substance use in order to determine whether some interventions work better for some groups than others.

and theories of mental illness have been integrated into each chapter of this book. Chapter 24 examines several different models of substance use etiology. The psychodynamic model is particularly relevant to dual disorders. This section examines this model of chemical dependency and dual disorders.

Current psychodynamic thought views substance use as an attempt by a person to return to homeostasis after experiencing psychological suffering (Brehm & Khantzian, 1997). The person attempts to alleviate or control disturbing feelings such as anxiety, depression, or anger through use of alcohol or drugs. The patient's inability to achieve homeostasis or relief from those feelings without substance use results from "self-regulatory deficiencies" (Brehm & Khantzian).

Ineffective self-regulation leads to the use of substances to achieve emotional homeostasis. Addicts often do not seek a "high" but rather desire to feel "normal" or comfortable in their lives. The purpose of psychotherapy is to help the patient acquire insight into the reasons for the psychological suffering, increase tolerance and modulation of painful feelings, learn skills to care for and nurture the self, and adopt a reality that is not based on childhood illusions (Brehm & Khantzian, 1997).

Searches have been numerous for an addictive personality or other personality traits associated with substance use. A person's problematic chemical use may also be viewed as a symptom of or a response to family dysfunction. Models that regard alcohol and drug abuse as symptoms of another primary psychiatric or family dysfunctional problem are problematic. If these models offered the only explanation for dual disorders, the logical

treatment would be to seek insight into substance-abusing behaviour through psychotherapy. The goal would be to decrease substance use as insight emerges. This model of addiction is helpful in viewing the possible etiologies of dual disorders, but it is narrowly focused and is only one of many models (see Chapter 24).

Because of the barriers to treatment (described below) and differing views on the etiology of addiction, completing a careful and thorough assessment is essential in mental health, chemical dependency, and medical settings. Comprehensive assessment will help ensure that interventions meet patients' needs. Current research trends in dual disorders are empirical studies to test the validity of cherished treatment beliefs and efficacy studies of treatment approaches (see Box 32-1).

■■ BARRIERS TO TREATMENT

High comorbidity rates point to the need for effective treatment of dual disorders. However, patients with dual disorders often face barriers to obtaining proper treatment because of specific cultural, economic, and health-related issues. These include the nature of substance use, countertransference and the position of substance users in society, misunderstandings about and stigmatization of mental illness, and related health issues.

Nature of Substance Use

Substance users may not recognize the need to seek mental health treatment because they may dismiss disturbing emotions as unrelated to their drug or alcohol abuse or to withdrawal symptoms. They may view the disturbing emotions as just a "bad trip," viewing drugs and alcohol as the "cure," rather than the cause of their distress. Conversely, patients who are substance users may seek mental health treatment for problems associated with the consequences of their abuse but may fail to mention their substance use. In addition, they may seek medications to alleviate symptoms that are caused by their abuse, such as anxiety, depression, and insomnia. Beeder and Millman (1997) pointed out the dilemma facing these patients. The patient with dual disorder must choose between two equally unsatisfactory options:

1. Take the substance of choice to experience fleeting moments of joy and escape, even though doing so will prompt a decline in overall function and worsen psychiatric symptoms.
2. Accept prescribed treatments, such as neuroleptics or antidepressants, which promote a better level of functioning and a better treatment outcome, but are not intoxicating and can often cause uncomfortable side effects of their own.

Countertransference

PMH professionals in psychiatric treatment programs can experience frustration when caring for patients with substance use disorders. Behaviour often associated with addiction—such as denial of a substance use problem, challenging behaviour, and the inability to follow health-related protocols—is often regarded as a sign of treatment failure. This type of behaviour can provoke hostility from the staff and can make planning for mental health recovery difficult. Drug-dependent patients may have the additional stigma of being regarded as criminals because they commit illegal acts every time they purchase, use, or distribute illicit drugs. Strong public feelings about alcohol-related motor vehicle crashes, negative experiences with family members or friends with drinking problems, and cultural biases against public intoxication can prejudice interactions with patients who are alcohol dependent.

PMH professionals may have difficulty understanding the compelling nature of drug or alcohol cravings, may not understand differences in drug use patterns and behaviours associated with particular drugs of abuse, and may overdiagnose personality disorders in those who take drugs and commit crimes (Churchill, 2003). Nurses who work with persons with dual diagnosis may also find that the work is very time-consuming, may not have the proper skills, knowledge, and support to work with dual diagnosis clients, may experience difficulty trying to coordinate care, and may find the medical model inadequate

for working with clients with a dual diagnosis (Coombs & Wratten, 2007).

Misunderstandings about and Stigmatization of Mental Illness

Some health care providers who treat substance dependence regard mental illness as outside their area of interest or expertise and may not accept patients with mental health disorders into addiction treatment programs. They may lack a general understanding of the nature of mental illness or fear unpredictable behaviour, recurrent substance use relapses, and the inability of some patients with dual disorders to understand or use 12-step programs. Sometimes, counsellors may mistakenly view patients as unmotivated by not recognizing possible cognitive impairments.

Such common symptoms of mental illness as depression, anxiety, and sleep disturbances are often attributed to substance use or withdrawal (Beeder & Millman, 1997). Thus, underlying or concurrent mental health disorders may remain undiagnosed and untreated. Providers may also misunderstand the second step of the Alcoholics Anonymous (AA) program, which states, "We came to believe that a power greater than ourselves could restore us to sanity," thinking that mental health-related symptoms will abate if a patient "works the program" (Wallen & Weiner, 1989). In addition, confusion exists about the use of psychoactive medication to treat these common psychiatric symptoms.

Health Issues

Numerous health hazards are associated with alcohol and drug abuse (see Chapter 24). Patients with dual disorders are more likely than others to use emergency departments for primary health care and are less aware of other available forms of health care. They may also more likely to be unclear about the treatment plans offered to them, and therefore may be less likely or motivated to follow these plans. The use of alcohol and other substances in addition to medications prescribed for mental illness can lead to drug interactions and may exacerbate side effects of these medications. Homelessness can increase patients' medical problems (Hwang, 2002), with inadequate nutrition, poor hygiene, and the adverse effects of exposure to the elements adding to their difficulties. Health care providers often become frustrated with patients' inability to follow treatment plans and with what they perceive as difficult behaviours. Their frustration may negatively affect the way they treat patients with dual disorders. Because of providers' biases against patients with dual disorders, the nature of these patients' behaviour, and confusion about what is the primary and most immediate problem to treat, these patients are often underserved and only partially treated.

DISORDER-SPECIFIC ASSESSMENT AND INTERVENTIONS

It is crucial for patients with dual disorders to receive a thorough assessment of both psychiatric and substance use disorders (Petrakis, Gonzalez, Rosenheck, & Krystal, 2002). An important part of assessment is to delineate the relative contribution of each diagnosis to the severity of the current symptoms presented and to determine treatment priorities accordingly. Because patients with dual disorders may have difficulty remembering their past or may downplay their mental health problems and/or the severity of their substance use, obtaining objective data is especially important. Ideally, one should obtain an objective history of the patient from the family, significant others, board and care operators, other health care providers, or anyone familiar enough with the patient to provide an accurate history. Box 32-2 lists basic assessment tools and methods used for patients with dual disorders.

BOX 32.2

Methods of Assessment of Dual Disorders

History and physical examination, laboratory tests (e.g., liver function tests, complete blood count, early detection of alcohol consumption) to confirm medical indicators related to substance use and also to rule out medical disorders with psychiatric presentations

- Substance use history and severity of consequences, and physical symptoms
- Mental status examination and severity of symptoms (e.g., suicidal, homicidal, florid psychosis)
  Interview with and assessment of family members, to verify or determine: (1) the accuracy of the patient's self-reported substance use or mental health history; (2) the patient's history of past mental health problems during periods of abstinence; and if possible; (3) the sequence of the diagnoses (i.e., what symptoms appeared first)
- Interviews with partner, friends, social worker, and other significant people in the patient's life
- Review of court records, medical records, and previous psychiatric and substance use treatment
- Urine and blood toxicity screens; use of breath analyzer to test blood alcohol level
  Revision of initial assessment by observation of the patient in the clinical setting; full assessment of the underlying psychiatric problem may not be possible until there is a long (up to 6 months) period of total abstinence
- Observation of patient for reappearance of psychiatric symptoms after a period of sobriety
- Assessment of patient's motivation to seek treatment, desire to change behaviour, and understanding of diagnoses

The following concepts are paramount to diagnosis and assessment of dual disorders (Drake et al., 2001):

CRNENOTE

Patients with both mental illness and substance abuse disorders respond to both disorders. Prioritizing nursing care will depend upon the immediate issue, but responses to both disorders should be assessed.

- Substance use can cause psychiatric symptoms and mimic psychiatric syndromes.
- Substance use can initiate or exacerbate a psychiatric disorder.
- Substance use can mask psychiatric symptoms and syndromes.
- Withdrawal from alcohol, tobacco, and other drugs can cause psychiatric symptoms and mimic psychiatric syndromes.
- Psychiatric and substance use disorders can coexist.
- Psychiatric behaviours can mimic alcohol and other drug use problems.

PSYCHOTIC ILLNESSES AND SUBSTANCE USE

Approximately 45% of persons with psychosis have a lifetime history of substance abuse (Margolese et al., 2004). The diagnosis of schizophrenia can be made only if the symptoms, as described in the *Diagnostic and Statistical Manual of Mental Disorders*, 4th ed., Text revision (*DSM-IV-TR*) (American Psychiatric Association [APA], 2000), last at least 6 months. A diagnosis of schizophrenia can be made accurately only without the added complication of substance use. The patient with a psychotic disorder may have an altered thought process or delusional thinking and may experience auditory hallucinations. He or she may also be cognitively impaired and have poor memory. These patients can have negative symptoms, such as poor motivation and poor hygiene. They often have low self-esteem and poor social skills, and may have a general sense of not belonging to a community. Their sense of self in relation to the world may be altered. These symptoms also can result from intoxication with or withdrawal from substances of abuse (Olson, 2004).

Acute and chronic psychotic disorders may be precipitated in predisposed people by the use of cocaine, amphetamines, marijuana, and the hallucinogens, as well as during severe withdrawal states (Beeder & Millman, 1997). Whereas all people are vulnerable to experiencing psychotic episodes from the use of various drugs, one psychotic episode renders a person more susceptible to subsequent episodes (Olson, 2004). Rosenthal and Westreich (1999) caution that the default diagnosis for patients presenting with substance use disorders and psychotic symptoms should be that these symptoms are related to substance use until proved otherwise.

Assessing the needs of people with schizophrenia who are also chemically dependent is complicated by the changing interaction among psychotic symptoms, the antipsychotic effects of medications, and the side effects of medications. Management and treatment of the psychotic substance user may vary according to the severity of symptoms. Drake (2001) suggested the following as the dual-focus approach for assessment and treatment:

- Initial focus on severity of presenting symptoms, not on diagnosis of one disorder or another
- Acute crisis intervention and crisis management
- Acute, subacute, and long-term stabilization of the patient
- Ongoing diagnostic efforts
- Multiple-contact longitudinal treatment.

The confrontational approach of addressing a patient's denial of his or her problems would not benefit this population (see Chapter 24 for additional discussion of confrontation) and could alienate a patient. A more supportive approach is appropriate, in which relapses are treated as an expected part of the recovery process. Addressing relapse risk is part of treatment planning, and nurses should explore with patients the behaviour, feelings, thoughts, and circumstances that led to the relapse. The nurse must avoid blame and guilt-inducing statements.

Bellack and Gearon (1998) suggest a multifaceted approach for treating the patient with concurrent schizophrenia and substance use. Their treatment approach, behaviour treatment for substance abuse in schizophrenia (BTSAS), consists of four parts:

1. Social skills training to help the patient learn ways to interact in a sober living situation and problem-solving training to review and refine his or her behaviour
2. Education about the nature of substance use, including triggers and cravings
3. **Motivational interviewing**, which helps the patient clarify personal goals and increase commitment to recovery (see Chapter 24)
4. Education regarding relapse prevention techniques.

Another important intervention is to integrate the administration of antipsychotic medication into the chemical dependency treatment plan to reduce the chances of relapse. Relapse may be partly due to patients' inability or unwillingness to take medications, which can often be related to the many undesirable side effects of neuroleptics (Beeder & Millman, 1997).

ANXIETY DISORDERS AND SUBSTANCE USE

The *DSM-IV-TR* (APA, 2000) includes acute distress disorder, generalized anxiety disorder, agoraphobia, obsessive-compulsive disorder, panic disorder, PTSD, social phobia, and other specific phobias as some of the anxiety disorders. Twenty-one percent of patients with anxiety disorder have had a substance abuse problem in the last year (Rush et al., 2008). PTSD increases the risk for substance use relapse and is associated with poor treatment outcome (Rosenthal & Westreich, 1999). Among patients with substance use disorders, coexisting anxiety disorder is likely (Drake et al., 2001).

The symptoms of anxiety may result from an anxiety disorder, such as panic attack, and may be secondary to drug or alcohol use, as part of a withdrawal syndrome. The symptoms are so subjectively disturbing that they can lead to drug or alcohol abuse as self-medication for the emotional pain; therefore, they require prompt evaluation and treatment. Pharmacologic treatment of anxiety is difficult because the traditional medications used, the benzodiazepines, are themselves addicting. Kushner, Abrams, and Borchardt (2000) found in their review of the literature regarding whether anxiety causes or is caused by alcohol use that both are true: that anxiety can cause alcohol dependence through self-medication, as well as be caused by the chronic drinking and withdrawal associated with alcohol abuse.

Patients with anxiety disorders should also pay particular attention to their physical health. Regular, balanced meals, exercise, and sleep are ways to decrease and manage stress levels. Patients should avoid excessive consumption of caffeine and sugars. If the patient has a fear of crowds, he or she may benefit from gradual desensitization techniques. Ries (1995) suggests the following guidelines for treating anxiety and coexisting substance use disorders:

- Treatment of anxiety can be postponed unless the anxiety interferes with substance use treatment.
- Anxiety symptoms may resolve with abstinence and substance use treatment.
- Affect-liberating therapies should be postponed until the patient is stable.
- Psychotherapy, when required, should be recovery oriented.
- Nonpsychoactive medications are preferred when medication is required.
- Antianxiety treatments such as relaxation techniques can be used with and without medications.
- A healthy diet, aerobic exercise, and avoiding caffeine can reduce anxiety.

MOOD DISORDERS AND SUBSTANCE USE

The term *mood disorder* describes various mood disturbances, including major depressive disorder, dysthymic disorder, bipolar I and bipolar II disorders, and cyclothymic disorder (APA, 2000). Thirty-two percent of patients with a mood disorder have a comorbid substance use disorder, whereas 56% of patients with a bipolar disorder have a comorbid substance use disorder (Regier et al., 1990). Substance use is more common in patients with a bipolar disorder than in those with any other Axis I diagnosis and may also contribute to challenges following treatment plans and less positive outcomes (Goldberg et al., 1999). Mood disorders may be more prevalent among patients using opiates than among other drug users (Drake et al., 2001). During the first few months of sobriety, symptoms of depression may persist. Initiation of pharmacologic interventions may be delayed until the diagnosis of underlying depression or other mood disorder can be made.

A study of the Canadian National Population Health Survey found that nearly 20% of participants who were alcohol dependent also reported suffering at least one major depressive episode within the past year (Wang & El-Guebaly, 2004). The same study found that being young (aged 12 to 24 years), being divorced, separated, or widowed, and having low family income were all positively associated with major depressive episodes, alcohol dependence, and their comorbidity (Wang & El-Guebaly).

In 2005, there were 3,743 suicides in Canada, resulting in a national rate of 11.6 suicides per 100,000 of population (Statistics Canada, 2009). In Canada, suicide is the leading cause of death for men aged 25 to 29 and 40 to 44, and for women aged 30 to 34 (Senate Committee on Social Affairs, Science and Technology, 2004). In addition, certain groups experience higher suicide rates than others. For example, Aboriginal adolescents have a suicide rate roughly five to six times greater than that of their non-Aboriginal counterparts (Royal Commission on Aboriginal Persons, 1996). More than 90% of completed suicides are associated with psychiatric disorders and substance abuse. The most common psychiatric disorders associated with completed suicide are major depression and alcohol abuse. Depression during withdrawal from alcohol, cocaine, opiates, and amphetamines puts patients at severe risk for suicide.

As with anxiety disorders, determining whether mood disorders are the cause or the effect of protracted substance use is difficult (Table 32-3). One important assessment is to determine whether drug use relates to mood states. Patients may be attempting to alleviate uncomfortable symptoms, such as depression or agitation, or to enhance a mood state, such as hypomania. Symptoms that persist during periods of abstinence are a clue to the degree that the mood disorder contributes to the presenting symptoms. When possible, the use of medication for mood disorders should be initiated after a period of abstinence (Beeder & Millman, 1997) so that indications are clear as to whether the alcohol or other drug use was not the sole cause of the symptoms.

Patients with bipolar disorders can benefit from chemical dependency treatment if their medications are stabilized and they can tolerate group treatment approaches, focus on and complete simple goals, and follow simple ground rules in a treatment program. Evans and Sullivan (2001) suggest these guidelines for treatment:

- Limit responses in group sessions (e.g., to less than 5 minutes of total group time).
- Limit the length of responses to simple exercises.
- Work with patients to heal interpersonal relationships that may have become impaired as a result of manic episodes.
- Relate patients' substance use and manic episodes to out-of-control behaviour for which ongoing treatment (recovery) plans are needed.

For patients who have depression and a substance use disorder, employing interventions centred on examining cognitive distortions (e.g., "I'll never get better, no one likes me, alcohol is my only friend") and cognitive therapy techniques can help improve mood. Use of positive self-talk can be helpful for both the depression and the substance use disorders. Working on unresolved grief can be appropriate. However, assignments that deal with

Table 32.3 Drugs That Precipitate or Mimic Mood Disorders		
Mood Disorders	**During Use (Intoxication)**	**After Use (Withdrawal)**
Depression and dysthymia	Alcohol, benzodiazepines, opioids, barbiturates, cannabis, steroids (chronic use), stimulants (chronic use)	Alcohol, benzodiazepines, opioids, barbiturates, cannabis, steroids (chronic use), stimulants (chronic use)
Mania and cyclothymia	Stimulants, alcohol, hallucinogens, inhalants, steroids (chronic and acute use)	Alcohol, benzodiazepines, barbiturates, opiates, steroids (chronic use)

patients' previous actions can evoke guilt, self-blame, and expressions of low self-esteem, thereby increasing depression (Evans & Sullivan, 2001).

ORGANIC MENTAL DISORDERS AND SUBSTANCE USE

Current terminology refers to cognitive impairment and deficits related to alcohol use as **alcohol-induced persisting amnestic disorder. Wernicke's syndrome** is a reversible alcohol-induced amnestic disorder caused by a thiamine-deficient diet. Thiamine is an essential element in producing fatty acids for synthesis and maintaining cerebral myelin. Wernicke's syndrome is marked by diplopia from palsy of the third or fourth cranial nerves, hyperactivity and delirium from stimulation of cortical brain and thalamic lesions, and coma caused by lesions in cranial nerve nuclei and in the mesencephalon and diencephalon of the brain (Goodwin, 1997). Thiamine treatment can reverse this process if initiated rapidly. All the B vitamins are essential for myelination. Deficiencies can lead to the development of lesions in distal peripheral nerves, causing neuropathies.

A second syndrome, which can occur concurrently with Wernicke's, is **Korsakoff's psychosis**. It is characterized by a loss of recent memory and confabulation (or filling in the blanks in memory by making up facts to cover this deficit). The patient with this condition is highly suggestible, has poor judgment, and cannot reason critically. Korsakoff's psychosis often follows Wernicke's encephalopathy and is also associated with prior peripheral neuropathy (Goodwin, 1997). It is treated with thiamine and can often be partially reversed.

Patients with alcohol-induced persisting amnestic disorder usually have histories of many years of heavy alcohol abuse, are generally older than 40 years, can experience sudden onset of symptoms, or may have had symptoms develop during a period of many years (APA, 2000). Impairment can be severe, and once the disorder is established, it can persist indefinitely (APA). Sedative-hypnotics, anxiolytic agents, and anticonvulsants are also known to cause a persisting amnestic disorder.

Cerebellar degeneration can occur from increased levels of acetaldehyde, a toxic by-product of alcohol metabolism, resulting from years of alcohol abuse. Symptoms are impaired coordination, a broad-based unsteady gait, and fine tremors. Alcohol is directly toxic to the brain, causing atrophy of the frontal cortex and eventually, chronic brain syndrome. Sedative-hypnotic effects of long-term alcohol abuse lead to disturbances in rapid–eye-movement sleep and chronic sleep disorders.

Organic brain disorders resulting from head trauma are more common in substance users than in the general population. This discrepancy is largely attributable to motor vehicle crashes, fights, physical abuse, and other trauma.

COGNITIVE IMPAIRMENT IN EARLY STAGES OF RECOVERY FROM SUBSTANCE USE

Most cognitive impairment in the population of patients seeking alcohol or drug abuse treatment is transitory and resolves within the first month of abstinence. Patients often experience difficulties with disorientation, clouding of consciousness, incoherent thoughts, memory loss, and delirium, which may hinder their ability to learn new concepts (Miller, 1998). In addition to the biologically based etiologies discussed, psychosocial factors can have a negative influence on cognitive ability. Fear of legal or relationship difficulties, depression, grief, and feelings of guilt and shame all may contribute to cognitive impairment (Petrakis et al., 2002). Psychological testing and other methods of assessment are necessary to determine whether the patient's cognitive functioning can improve and whether chemical dependency treatment can be used (Shivani, Goldsmith, & Anthenelli, 2002). The nurse must assess the patient's abilities for self-care, independent living, impulse control, control of assaultiveness, direction taking, and development of new responses to new situations and ideas. The nurse must also evaluate changes in mental status during the past 6 months and examine previous treatment outcomes (Evans & Sullivan, 2001).

Intervention for patients with cognitive or memory impairment must consist of clear, direct, simple messages. The following points (Evans & Sullivan, 2001) illustrate this approach:

- Use reading material that is relevant to recovery and that can be referred to in short study sessions.
- For patients who have trouble grasping abstract concepts, read first-person accounts of addiction and recovery found in AA and Narcotics Anonymous (NA) literature.
- Concentrate on basic concepts of recovery, such as those in AA slogans, and on patients' need for continuing care after discharge.
- Show films with scenes illustrating relevant family problems or other problems related to substance use. Movies can be more effective than lectures.
- Avoid discussing extraneous issues and avoid theoretic or technical discussions.

PERSONALITY DISORDERS AND SUBSTANCE USE

Personality disorders are frequently diagnosed in alcohol and other drug abusers. Regier and colleagues (1990) noted that 14.3% of people with an alcohol-related disorder and 17.8% of those with a drug-related disorder had a lifetime prevalence rate of antisocial personality disorder.

Conversely, people with an antisocial personality disorder had a lifetime prevalence rate of 83.6% for any substance use disorder. Those with borderline personality disorder had a 28% rate of substance dependence (Thomas, Melchert, & Banker, 1999).

Another study suggested a 40% to 50% concurrent diagnosis of antisocial personality disorder and substance dependence. In addition, the study reported that 90% of patients with antisocial personality disorders who are criminal offenders are substance users (Messina, Wish, & Nemes, 1999). Thomas and colleagues (1999) noted that this population has a higher rate of involuntary hospital admissions, greater resistance to treatment, poor coping skills, poorer interpersonal relationships, and a higher level of impulsivity.

Beeder and Millman (1997) noted that the label *personality disorder* is often incorrectly applied to patients who seek treatment because of legal problems, interpersonal violence, or other difficulties. Chronic drug use can cause personality changes and even psychiatric illness. Alcohol and other drug use in patients with personality disorders are often secondary to these disorders. For example, people with antisocial personality disorder may use alcohol and other drugs to enhance their view of the world as fast-paced and dramatic and may be involved in crime and other sensation-seeking, high-risk behaviour (Ball & McCann, 2001).

Addiction treatment based on tight structure, peer support, and appropriate confrontation that addresses the significant destructive behaviour on the part of patients with personality disorders appears to be the most useful approach (Beeder & Millman, 1997). Formally structured groups may improve patients' ability to learn new and more appropriate behaviours and to develop new perceptions that may help them in relating to others. Cognitive therapy approaches may help these patients examine the cognitive distortions that contribute to their substance use.

�as GENERAL TREATMENT ELEMENTS

Patients with dual disorders enter treatment at various stages of recovery. Flexible treatment programs that can meet each patient's needs are the most effective. Regardless of the patient's primary diagnosis or degree of recovery, some common elements exist in the treatment of dual disorders. The following discussion highlights these essential components of treatment.

Setting Priorities When Hospitalization Is Necessary

Often, patients with dual disorders can be treated effectively in community mental health settings if their symptoms are stable, they are following their treatment plan, and they remain alcohol and drug free. Dackis and Gold (1997) specified that patients who meet any of the following criteria should be admitted to the hospital for treatment:

- Serious medical needs, such as the need for detoxification
- An exacerbated medical disorder or an illness that prevents abstinence or outpatient treatment
- Suicidal or homicidal ideation, psychotic disorganization, or other serious psychiatric illnesses
- Failed outpatient treatment
- Addiction severity that prevents any significant period of abstinence
- Serious psychosocial problems, such as immediate risk for incarceration, homelessness, or abusive relationships
- Continued abuse of substances during pregnancy.

Crisis Stabilization

Setting priorities is essential for hospitalized patients with dual disorders. The first priorities are gathering data from nursing assessments, stabilizing psychiatric symptoms, and treating withdrawal symptoms (Beeder & Millman, 1997) (see Chapter 24). After these issues have been addressed, the patient can enter the rehabilitation phase of treatment for both diagnoses. Rehabilitative therapy is appropriate if the patient (1) can participate in a group process, (2) can focus attention on groups or reading material, (3) does not engage in behaviour that is detrimental to the group process, (4) can listen to and receive feedback from others, and (5) can benefit from the group process.

Engagement

Engagement entails establishing a treatment relationship and enhancing motivation to make behaviour changes and a commitment to treatment (Miller, 1995). Patients who are abusing substances may experience repeated cycles of detoxification and relapse. Mentally ill patients may have prolonged cycles of "revolving-door" admissions before they are able to engage in continuous treatment (Kertesz, Horton, Friedmena, & Samet, 2003). Each admission is a "window of opportunity." Relapse does not mean that a treatment intervention, the health care provider, or the patient has failed. Readmission and clear, realistic goals can further the patient's engagement in the treatment process. Effective programs emphasize a combination of empathic, long-term relationship building and the use of leverage and possible confrontation by family, other caregivers, or the legal system.

Engaging patients with dual disorders in treatment presents two main challenges. The first is developing relationships with people who tend to have difficulties in their relationships and with trusting authority figures. The second is patients' lack of motivation and the need to encourage them to enter drug and alcohol treatment programs.

Possible social barriers to patients becoming motivated to seek treatment are homelessness, unemployment, and lack of social support for abstinence. In addition, patients or their therapists may excuse substance use because of the patients' psychiatric symptoms. Patients who deny a problem with substances do not seek treatment because they do not view themselves as needing it. These patients do not fully understand their mental illness or the effect of substance use on their mood or behaviour.

Engagement in treatment is a process that may take many contacts with a patient and requires patience. The treatment team members may need to gain the trust of patients who have had poor experiences with authority figures or being controlled. The engagement process is enhanced if the staff members can deal with presenting crises concretely (e.g., provide help in avoiding legal penalties and obtaining food, housing, entitlements, relief from psychiatric symptoms, vocational opportunities, recreation, and socialization). Harm reduction may be a first step toward a goal of abstinence.

The process of engagement is often characterized by approach–avoidance behaviour by the patient. Intake and assessment procedures may discourage the patient from engagement or be intolerable if they are protracted and begin with asking the patient numerous pointed personal questions. These procedures may have to be adjusted to tailor treatment and accommodate the needs or reactions of the patient with dual disorders.

Medication Management

One essential feature of dual disorder treatment is medication management. A person's inability or unwillingness to take prescribed medications can lead to increased problems after discharge, and may be a significant contributing factor for relapse and rehospitalization. Impulsive behaviour in response to transient exacerbations of psychotic symptoms, depressed mood, or anxiety symptoms may lead to relapse. Treating a patient with dual disorders can be as complex as the presenting symptoms. Errors in treatment can include treating temporary psychiatric symptoms resulting from withdrawal as if they were a permanent feature of the individual, withholding needed medication for a psychiatric disorder, or setting arbitrary limits on medication based on a belief that medication for all psychiatric symptoms should be suspended for a time.

Collaboration between the patient's prescriber and other treatment providers is important to minimize the possible misuse of prescription drugs. In addition, caution is essential in prescribing medications that can increase the patient's potential for relapse into abusing the drug of choice. The patient in recovery is often reluctant to use potentially mind-altering drugs, and the nurse should explore any concerns the person may have.

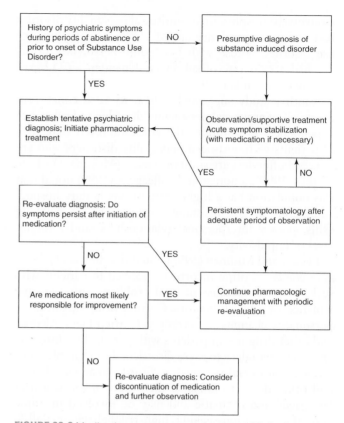

FIGURE 32.2 Medication management of patient with dual diagnosis. From Sowers, W., & Golden, S. (1999). Psychotropic medication management in persons with co-occurring psychiatric and substance use disorders. *Journal of Psychoactive Drugs, 32*(1), 59–70. Used with permission.

Figure 32-2 presents an algorithm, developed by Sowers and Golden (1999). A cooperative partnership between the health care provider and the patient will help determine which medication is most effective and offers the greatest chance of patient compliance.

The term *abuse* can be applied to the improper use of prescription drugs. Portenoy and Payne (1997) listed the following as clear examples of abuse: (1) prescription forgery; (2) selling of prescription drugs by unauthorized people; (3) acquisition of drugs from nonmedical sources; (4) use of illicit opiates to supplement therapy; (5) unsanctioned drug dose escalation; (6) use of drugs to treat symptoms other than those targeted by the therapy; (7) frequent visits to emergency departments to obtain drugs; (8) contacts with multiple prescribers to obtain drug prescriptions; and (9) drug hoarding.

Patient Education

Patient education is an essential element in treating dual disorders. Topics for group sessions should encourage interaction among patients. By sharing their experiences with their peers, patients can enhance these presentations. Topics should be clear, relevant to the group members, and illustrated with charts, handouts, or appropriate films.

Topics for Education Groups for Patients with Dual Disorder

The effects of alcohol and drugs on the body Alcohol, drugs, and medication—what can go wrong

- What is a healthy lifestyle?
- Triggers for relapse
- What is Alcoholics (or Narcotics) Anonymous?
- What is a sponsor in Alcoholics (or Narcotics) Anonymous?
- What is the recovery from mental illness and substance abuse?
- What are the tools of recovery?
- The disease of addiction
- The relapse cycle
- How to cope with feelings without using alcohol or other drugs
- Relapse prevention: what works?
- What are cognitive distortions?
- HIV prevention and education
- Leisure time management
- How to manage stress
- Relaxation training
- Assertiveness and recovery
- Common slogans to live by
- Pitfalls in treatment
- The process of recovery
- Creating a relapse prevention plan
- What are my goals? How does the use of alcohol and drugs affect them? Coping with thoughts about alcohol and drugs
- Problem-solving basics
- Coping with anger
- Negative thinking and how to manage it
- Enhancing social support networks

Each lecture or discussion group should be relatively short and should not contain too many new or difficult concepts. Reinforcing and reviewing previous discussions can be helpful to remind patients of particularly relevant concepts. Box 32-3 lists some suitable topics for nurse-led discussion groups. Individual patient education can focus on areas of knowledge deficits and reinforce topics discussed in group settings. Group sessions can also assist patients in learning interpersonal skills (e.g., assertiveness) and problem-solving skills and in relapse prevention planning.

Mutual Self-Help Groups

Several mutual self-help groups are appropriate for many patients with dual disorders. The most common groups are **12-step programs**, such as AA and NA (see Chapter 24). Zweben (1987) raised the issue of whether a patient who is taking psychotropic medications may participate in a 12-step program. AA published a landmark report by a group of physicians in AA that addressed this issue. In it, the physicians gave guidelines to the members for the sensible use of medications and indicated pitfalls that can occur with psychoactive prescription drug use. The report presented the members' stories of abuse and discussed the benefits some members derived from the judicious use of appropriately prescribed medications. The authors concluded "It becomes clear that just as it is wrong to enable or support any alcoholic to become readdicted to any drug, it's equally wrong to deprive any alcoholic of medication which can alleviate or control other disabling physical and/or emotional problems" (Alcoholics Anonymous World Services, 1984, p. 300).

For patients who are concerned that they might not be accepted into AA because of their use of psychiatric medications, this AA literature can be helpful. The advisability of a patient enrolling in a 12-step program needs to be evaluated on an individual basis. A health care provider familiar with 12-step concepts can often facilitate patients' attempts to use these programs. The numerous advantages of self-help groups make them a potentially powerful support for continued recovery. Alternative mutual self-help programs similar to 12-step programs are available in some geographic areas. Rational Recovery and Secular Organization for Sobriety are groups that downplay the concept of powerlessness and the spiritual aspects associated with 12-step programs.

Relapse Prevention: Creating A New Lifestyle

Relapse is the failure to maintain the behaviours needed to remain abstinent (Annis & Davis, 1995). One model of relapse prevention is based on the self-efficacy theory. It proposes that when a patient enters a situation in which the risk for resuming drinking or drug use is high, his or her expectations of the ability to cope with the situation without substances will predict his or her substance use (Annis & Davis). If a patient feels confident that he or she can cope with an emotionally charged situation, his or her likelihood of using substances in that situation is lower. See Box 32-4 for a list of common situations in which relapse often occurs.

Relapse prevention groups can be valuable sources of support for patients. These groups help patients to (1) analyze which situations are most likely to trigger relapses; (2) examine cognitive, emotional, and behavioural components of high-risk situations; and (3) develop cognitive, behavioural, and effective coping strategies and environmental supports. Role playing ways out of high-risk situations is a technique that these groups often use (Annis & Davis, 1995; Marlatt & Gordon, 1985). Homework assignments help patients create relapse prevention plans that address new coping strategies for these high-risk situations.

The relapse prevention model uses cognitive-behavioural techniques to help patients plan for stressors that can

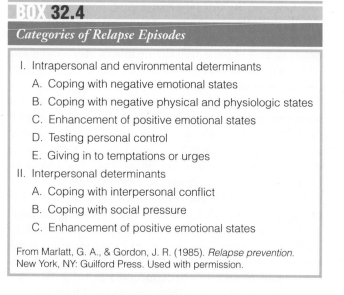

lead to relapse. The methods highlighted are practical, emphasize and strengthen patients' coping skills, and can be adapted to the needs of individual patients. Relapse prevention plans initiated in treatment are just pieces of paper if they are not implemented after discharge. The following section discusses elements in effective discharge planning for patients with dual disorders.

■ CONTINUUM OF CARE AND DISCHARGE PLANNING

Early intervention in crises is important for patients with dual disorders, but equally important is a focus beyond medication management and inpatient treatment episodes. Social interaction skills and coping skills learned in treatment need to be reinforced in community settings to create or enhance a stable living situation and possible vocational opportunities. Active planning and intervention are needed for housing and employment, or deterioration may occur, despite gains made during hospitalization.

Establishing a positive social network is a critical function of any program intended to treat dual disorders. Isolation and alienation from prior sources of support is a problem that most chronically mentally ill substance users share. Some patients relate poorly to their families, others are overly dependent on them, and others have difficulty establishing and maintaining social relationships. Some patients' only "families" are peers within the drug subculture who reinforce substance-abusing behaviour.

Opportunities to socialize, access to positive recreational activities, and a supportive peer group are stabilizing influences on patients who may otherwise drop out of treatment altogether. Part of a comprehensive relapse prevention plan is to establish or reinforce the patient's social support network so that he or she can obtain (1) opportunities for substance-free socializing, (2) crisis counselling to prevent readmission to a hospital, and (3) support for sobriety.

Supportive housing is also essential for patients with dual disorders. Supportive housing is especially crucial for patients who are being discharged from the hospital because the risk for relapse is greatest during the first few months after discharge. Halfway houses for substance users may not offer enough support for clients to follow their treatment plans, and housing designed for the chronically mentally ill may not emphasize abstinence enough. Thus, an important part of the multidisciplinary team approach to discharge planning for patients with dual disorders is to help them find the best possible living situation.

Younger patients with severe mental illness may want and expect to find appropriate employment, but some of these patients may be unrealistic about potential professions. However, the desire to find meaningful work can be a significant motivator and a useful tool in a treatment program. Referring patients to halfway houses or residential substance use treatment programs that stress vocational skill training can be beneficial. Use of community vocational rehabilitation services and of educational opportunities can be an important part of a discharge plan.

Case Management

Case managers are responsible for conducting outreach activities, linking patients with direct services, monitoring patients' progress through various milieus, educating patients about psychiatric and substance use disorders, reiterating treatment recommendations, and coordinating treatment planning across programs (Segal, 1988). Case managers can use four approaches for delivering services to patients with dual disorders (Segal):

- *Brokerage-generalist.* This short-term model seeks to identify the patient's needs and helps gain access to appropriate resources.
- *Assertive community treatment.* This model involves assertive advocacy, making contact with patients in their homes and natural settings, with the focus on practical problems of daily living.
- *Strength-based perspective.* This model emphasizes providing support for patients to assert direct control over their search for resources and to examine the patients' own strengths in acquiring these resources.
- *Clinical rehabilitation.* In this model, the clinician provides counselling and is responsible for resource acquisition.

Table 32-4 lists how these models of case management address case management activities for the patient with dual disorders.

Table 32.4	Models of Case Management for Patients with Dual Disorders				
Primary Case Management Activities	Brokerage-Generalist	Strengths Perspective	Assertive Community Treatment	Clinical Rehabilitation
Engages in outreach and case finding	No	Depends on agency mission and structure	Depends on agency mission and structure	Depends on agency mission and structure
Provides assessment and reassessment	Specific to immediate resource acquisition needs	Strength-based, applicable to any area of need	Broad-based, comprehensive assessment	Broad-based, comprehensive assessment
Assists in goal planning	Brief, related to acquiring resources	Patient driven, teaches specific ways to set and achieve goals	Comprehensive and may include any area of patient's life	Comprehensive and may include any area of patient's life
Makes referrals to needed resources	Patient or case manager may make contact	Patient or case manager may make contact	As needed; resources may be integrated in services	Patient or case manager may make contact
Provides additional services such as therapy, skills teaching	Referral to others for these	Limited; teaches patient to identify strengths and about self-help groups	Provides many services in comprehensive package	Provides services consistent with model
Responds to crisis	Related to resource needs	Related to resource and mental health concerns: active in stabilization and referral	Assertive advocacy on several levels	Assertive advocacy on several levels
Provides direct services related to resource acquisition as part of case management (e.g., drop-in centre; employment counselling)	Referral to resources that provide direct services	Provides services to prepare patient to gain own resources (e.g., role playing, accompanying patient to services)	Provides many direct services as part of comprehensive package	Provides services as part of a rehabilitation services plan; skill teaching

---

BOX 32.5

Features of a Dual Disorder Outpatient Program

COMMUNITY MEETING AND GOAL SETTING: Patients set small, realistic goals for themselves for the day, which aids them in their ultimate goal of better living in recovery.

ANGER MANAGEMENT AND SOCIAL COMMUNICATION: Patients learn appropriate ways to express anger and how to socialize with others.

GROUP THERAPY: Patients discuss interpersonal issues, get feedback from their peers, and learn problem-solving skills.

DUAL RECOVERY ANONYMOUS MEETINGS: Patient-run meeting (a modified AA meeting) addresses the specific needs of the patient with dual disorders.

LEISURE PLANNING: Patients learn skills to enjoy leisure involving clean and sober fun.

GARDENING, ART THERAPY, MUSIC THERAPY, SWIMMING: These methods provide alternatives to the use of alcohol and other drugs.

HEALTH EDUCATION: Patients learn about the effects of drugs and alcohol on the body and about other relevant medical topics.

MEDICATION EDUCATION: Patients learn about psychiatric medications, their uses, the side effects, and interactions with drugs or alcohol.

RELAPSE PREVENTION PLANNING: Patients talk about their last relapse; triggers, feelings, and stresses that contributed to the relapse and the consequences and formulate relapse prevention plans.

INDIVIDUAL COUNSELLING: Patients receive individual counselling to develop goals and work on problem-solving techniques.

PSYCHIATRIC CONSULTATION: Patients are evaluated and followed up for medication and other psychiatric interventions.

Note: Patients are *not* discharged from the program if they are intoxicated. They are asked not to come to the program intoxicated but to return when they are sober to continue work on their recovery.

Family Support and Education

The families of patients with dual disorders need education and support. The focus of family support groups, such as those under the auspices of the National Alliance for the Mentally Ill, has been both to educate and to help the family cope with a mentally ill relative. Al Anon and Nar Anon take a similar approach to providing peer support to families of substance users. These self-help groups aid family members in balancing confrontation of the problem, detachment from forcing a solution to it, and support of the treatment process.

Comprehensive Concurrent Treatment

Several traditional approaches are possible for treating dual disorders:

- Treat the mental illness first.
- Treat the substance use disorder first.
- Treat both conditions concurrently.

Recent literature suggests that a comprehensive concurrent approach is often beneficial once the presenting problem has been stabilized. Box 32-5 presents features of a dual disorder outpatient program.

◼◼◼ PLANNING FOR NURSING CARE

Numerous challenges face the nurse who provides care to patients with dual disorders. Comprehensive planning within a multidisciplinary team approach has been highly successful in the care of such patients. Community organizations can be valuable sources of support as well.

SUMMARY OF KEY POINTS

❑ The incidence of substance-related disorders and one or more comorbid mental health disorders is very high.

❑ Dual disorders can consist of a primary mental illness and subsequent substance use, a primary substance use disorder and psychopathologic sequelae, dual primary diagnoses, or two disorders resulting from a common cause.

❑ In patients with dual disorders, relapse is common if both the substance use disorder and the mental health disorder are not addressed concurrently.

❑ Barriers to effective treatment of dual disorders include the nature of substance use, countertransference and the position of substance users in society, misunderstandings about and the stigmatization of mental illness, and underlying health issues.

❑ Assessment of dual disorders often depends on objective data obtained from interviews with family members, reviews of court records, laboratory test results, and physical examination findings.

❑ Alcohol and drug use can cause numerous mental health problems, including organic brain disorders, depression, hallucinations, agitation, confusion, and stupor. These substances interact with common prescription and over-the-counter drugs to cause adverse reactions.

❑ Alcohol and other drugs often exacerbate existing mental health disorders and can make it difficult for patients to follow treatment plans.

❑ Elements of treatment for patients with dual disorders include possible hospitalization, crisis stabilization, engagement in long-term treatment, medication management, patient education, use of self-help groups, relapse prevention, continuation of care, case management, and family support.

❑ Relapse prevention is crucial in treating patients with dual disorders and entails analyzing high-risk situations for relapse; examining the cognitive, emotional, and behavioural components of high-risk situations; and using effective coping strategies and available environmental supports.

CRITICAL THINKING CHALLENGES

1 What criteria would you use to refer an intoxicated and depressed patient in a psychiatric emergency department to the following?
   a. An alcohol detoxification centre
   b. An inpatient psychiatric unit
   c. An outpatient alcohol-treatment program
   d. An outpatient community mental health clinic
2 How would you respond to a patient with dual disorders who states, "Once my medication is stable, I will be able to drink again."
3 In your opinion, what are the five most important concepts to cover in educating a patient with dual disorders?

WEB LINKS

www.camh.net   This website of the Centre for Addiction and Mental Health, which is Canada's leading addiction and mental health teaching hospital, in Toronto, provides many links to education, research, treatment, policy, and so forth.

www.hc-sc.gc.ca   The Health Canada site has links to best practices for concurrent mental health and substance abuse disorders. It also provides a National program directory listing programs that address concurrent mental health and substance abuse disorders.

www.ccsa.ca   The website of the Canadian Centre on Substance Abuse includes information, policy material, and research on dual disorders.

www.corp.aadac.com   The website of the Alberta Alcohol and Drug Abuse Commission provides basic information related to dual diagnosis.

www.heretohelp.bc.ca   The website of the B.C. Partners for Mental Health and Addictions Information provides information, support, resources, and links related to dual diagnosis issues.

MOVIES, NOVELS, AND BIOGRAPHIES

Patrick's Story: 1999. *The National Film Board of Canada.* Patrick Bird was a "casualty of colonialism," having walked a dark boyhood journey of sexual abuse, neglect, foster homes, detention centres, loss, abandonment, drugs, alcohol, and self-mutilation. Through no fault of his own, Patrick was disconnected from his family, his childhood, and his Cree culture and left with few resources to cope with the pain and powerlessness. *Patrick's Story* explores what brought a young man to attempt suicide and what turned his life around.

VIEWING POINTS: In your opinion, how does this film highlight the relationship between substance abuse and mental health issues? What were your feelings as you watched this movie? In what ways does this movie offer a message of inspiration and hope?

Poundmaker's Lodge: A Healing Place: 1987. *The National Film Board of Canada. Poundmaker's Lodge*, named after a 19th century Aboriginal leader, is a treatment centre in St. Albert, Alberta, where Aboriginal people troubled by addiction to drugs and alcohol can come together for mutual support, to partake of healing rituals like the sweat lodge, and to rediscover their traditions. The film places Aboriginal alcoholism and mental health issues in historical and sociocultural contexts. It shows the despair of people dispossessed of land, culture, language, and dignity and their strength and courage in overcoming substance abuse.

VIEWING POINTS: In your opinion, what are some of the steps that nurses could take to help ensure that multicultural groups of all kinds receive more culturally appropriate treatment for difficulties with addictions and mental health issues?

REFERENCES

Alcoholics Anonymous World Services, Inc. (1984). *The A. A. member-medications and other drugs: A report from a group of physicians in A. A.* New York, NY: Author.

American Psychiatric Association. (2000). *Diagnostic and statistical manual of mental disorders* (4th ed., Text revision). Washington, DC: Author.

Annis, H. M., & Davis, C. S. (1995). Relapse prevention. In R. K. Hester & W. R. Miller (Eds.), *Handbook of alcoholism treatment approaches* (2nd ed., pp. 170–181). Boston, MA: Allyn & Bacon.

Ball, E. M., & McCann, R. A. (2001). Antisocial personality disorder. In J. L. Jacobson & A. M. Jacobson (Eds.), *Psychiatric secrets* (2nd ed.). Philadelphia, PA: Hanley & Belfus.

B.C. Partners for Mental Health and Addictions Information. (2003). *Concurrenet disorders: Addictions and mental disorders.* Vancouver, BC: Author.

Beauchamp, J. K., & Olson, K. R. (2000). Drug overdoses and dependence. In R. M. Wachter, L. Goldman, & H. Hollander (Eds.), *Hospital medicine.* Philadelphia, PA: Lippincott Williams & Wilkins.

Beeder, A. B., & Millman, R. B. (1997). Treatment of patients with psychopathology and substance abuse. In J. H. Lowinson, P. Ruiz, R. B. Millman, & J. G. Langrod (Eds.), *Substance abuse: A comprehensive textbook* (3rd ed., pp. 675–690). Baltimore, MD: Williams & Wilkins.

Bellack, A., & Gearon, J. (1998). Substance abuse treatment for people with schizophrenia. *Addictive Behaviors, 23*(6), 749–766.

Brehm, N. M., & Khantzian, E. J. (1997). A psychodynamic perspective. In J. H. Lowinson, P. Ruiz, R. B. Millman, & J. G. Langrod (Eds.), *Substance abuse: A comprehensive textbook* (3rd ed., pp. 106–117). Baltimore, MD: Williams & Wilkins.

Churchill, D. M. (2003). Toward an integrative approach to substance abuse: An inquiry into the recognition, diagnosis and treatment of substance abuse by social workers. *Dissertation Abstracts International, 63*(8-A), US: University Microfilms International.

Cleary, M., Hunt, G.E., Matheson S., & Walter G. (2009). Psychosocial treatments for people with co-occurring severe mental illness and substance misuse: systematic review. *Journal of Advanced Nursing, 65*(2), 238–258.

Cleary, M., Walter, G., Hunt, G. E., Clancy, R., & Horsfall, J. (2008). Promoting dual diagnosis awareness in everyday clinical practice. *Journal of Psychosocial Nursing, 46*(12), 43–49.

Coombs, L., & Wratten, A. (2007). The lived experience of community mental health nurses working with people who have dual diagnosis: A phenomenological study. *Journal of Psychiatric and Mental Health Nursing, 14*, 382–392.

Dackis, C., & Gold, M. S. (1997). Psychiatric hospitals for treatment of dual diagnosis. In J. H. Lowinson, P. Ruiz, R. B. Millman, & J. G. Langrod (Eds.), *Substance abuse: A comprehensive textbook* (3rd ed., pp. 467–485). Baltimore, MD: Williams & Wilkins.

Drake, R. E., Essock, S. M., Shaner, A., Cary, K. B., Minkoff, K., Kola, L., et al. (2001). Implementing dual diagnosis services for clients with severe mental illness. *Psychiatric Services, 52*(4), 469–476.

Evans, K., & Sullivan, J. (2001). *Dual diagnosis: Counselling the mentally ill substance abuser.* New York, NY: Guilford Press.

Goldberg, J., Garno, J., Leon, A., et al. (1999). A history of substance abuse complicates remission from acute mania in bipolar disorder. *Journal of Clinical Psychiatry, 60*(11), 733–739.

Goodwin, D. W. (1997). Alcohol: Clinical aspects. In J. H. Lowinson, P. Ruiz, R. B. Millman, & J. G. Langrod (Eds.), *Substance abuse: A comprehensive textbook* (3rd ed., pp. 144–151). Baltimore, MD: Williams & Wilkins.

Hwang, S. (2001). Mental illness and mentality among homeless people. *Acta Psychiatrica Scandinavicca, 103*(2), 81–82.

Hwang, S. (2002). Is homelessness hazardous to your health? Obstacles to the demonstration of a causal relationship. *Canadian Journal of Public Health, 93*(6), 407–410.

Joseph, H. (1997). Substance abuse and homelessness within the inner cities. In J. H. Lowinson, P. Ruiz, R. B. Millman, & J. G. Langrod (Eds.), *Substance abuse: A comprehensive textbook* (3rd ed., pp. 875–889). Baltimore, MD: Williams & Wilkins.

Kendler, K. S., Bulik, C. M., Sillberg, J., Hettema, J. M., Myers, J., & Prescott, C. A. (2000). Childhood sexual abuse and adult psychiatric and substance use disorders in women. *Archives of General Psychiatry, 57*(10), 953–959.

Kertesz, S. G., Horton, N. J., Friedmena, P. D., & Samet, J. H. (2003). Slowing the revolving door: Stabilization programs reduce homeless persons' substance use after detoxification. *Journal of Substance Abuse Treatment, 24*(3), 197–207.

Kushner, M. G., Abrams, K., & Borchardt, C. (2000). The relationship between anxiety disorders and alcohol use disorders: A review of major perspectives and findings. *Clinical Psychology Review, 20*(2), 149–171.

Lehman, A. F., Myers, C. P., & Corty, E. (1989). Assessment and classification of patients with psychiatric and substance abuse syndromes. *Hospital and Community Psychiatry, 40*(10), 1019–1024.

MacMillan, H. L., Fleming, J. E., Streiner, D. L., Lin, E., Boyle, M. H., Jamieson, E., et al. (2001). Childhood abuse and lifetime psychopathology in a community sample. *American Journal of Psychiatry, 158*, 1878–1883.

Marlatt, G. A., & Gordon, J. R. (1985). *Relapse prevention.* New York, NY: Guilford Press.

Margolese, H. C., Malchy, L., Carlos Negrete, J., Tempier, R., & Gill, K. (2004). Drug and alcohol use among patients with schizophrenia and related psychoses: Levels and consequences. *Schizophrenia Research, 67*, 157–166.

Messina, N., Wish, E., & Nemes, S. (1999). Therapeutic community treatment for substance abusers with antisocial personality disorder. *Journal of Substance Abuse Treatment, 17*(1–2), 121–128.

Miller, N. S. (1995). *Addiction psychiatry: Current diagnosis and treatment* (p. 112). New York, NY: Wiley-Liss.

Miller, N. S. (1998). Management of withdrawal syndromes and relapse prevention in drug and alcohol dependence. *American Family Physician, 58*(1), 139–146.

Olson, W. (2004). Delirium tremens. In F. Ferri (Ed.), *Ferri's clinical advisor, 2004: Instant diagnosis and treatment*. St. Louis, MO: Mosby.

Petrakis, I., Gonzalez, G., Rosenheck, R., & Krystal, J. (2002). Comorbidity of alcoholism and psychiatric disorders: An overview. *Alcohol Research and Health, 26*(2), 81–89.

Portenoy, R. K., & Payne, R. (1997). Acute and chronic pain. In J. H. Lowinson, P. Ruiz, R. B. Millman, & J. G. Langrod (Eds.), *Substance abuse: A comprehensive textbook* (3rd ed., pp. 236–246). Baltimore, MD: Williams & Wilkins.

Regier, D. A., Farmer, M. E., Rae, D. S., et al. (1990). Comorbidity of mental disorders with alcohol and other drug abuse: Results from the epidemiologic catchment area (ECA) study. *Journal of the American Medical Association, 264*, 2511–2518.

Ries, R. (1995). *Assessment and treatment of patients with coexisting mental illness and alcohol and other drug abuse* (pp. 29–89). Rockville, MD: U.S. Department of Health and Human Services.

Rosenthal, R. N., & Westreich, L. (1999). Treatment of persons with dual diagnosis of substance use disorders and other psychological problems. In *Addictions: A comprehensive guide* (pp. 439–476). New York, NY: Oxford University Press.

Royal Commission on Aboriginal Persons. (1996). *Report of the Royal Commission on Aboriginal Persons*. Ottawa, ON: Author.

Rush, B., Urbanoski, K., Bassani, D., Castel, S., Cameron Wild, T., Strike, C., et al. (2008). Prevalence of co-occurring substance use and other mental disorders in the Canadian Population. *The Canadian Journal of Psychiatry, 53*(12), 800–809.

Segal, B. (1988). *Drugs and behavior*. New York, NY: Gardner Press.

Senate Committee on Social Affairs, Science and Technology. (2004). *Mental health, mental illness and addiction: Issues and options for Canada*. Ottawa, ON: Author.

Shivani, R., Goldsmith, R., & Anthenelli, R. (2002). Alcoholism and psychiatric disorders: Diagnostic challenges. *Alcohol Research and Health, 26*(2), 90–98.

Sowers, W., & Golden, S. (1999). Psychotropic medication management in persons with co-occurring psychiatric and substance use disorders. *Journal of Psychoactive Drugs, 31*(1), 59–70.

Statistics Canada. (2009). *Mortality, Summary List of Causes (2005)*. Retrieved May 18, 2009 from http://www.statcan.gc.ca/pub/84f0209x/84f0209x2005000-eng.pdf

Thomas, V., Melchert, T., & Banker, J. (1999). Substance dependence and personality disorders: Comorbidity and treatment outcome in an inpatient treatment population. *Journal of Studies of Alcohol, 60*, 271–277.

Wallen, M. C., & Weiner, H. D. (1989). Impediments to effective treatment of the dually diagnosed patient. *Journal of Psychoactive Drugs, 21*(2), 161–168.

Wang, J. L., & El-Guebaly, N. (2004). Sociodemographic factors associated with comorbid major depressive episodes and alcohol dependence in the general population. *Canadian Journal of Psychiatry, 49*(1), 37–44.

Zweben, J. E. (1987). Can patients on medication be sent to 12-step programs? *Journal of Psychoactive Drugs, 19*(3), 299–300.

Psychosocial Aspects of Medically Compromised Persons

Michel A. Tarko

Adapted from the chapter "Psychosocial Aspects of Medically Compromised Persons" by Gail L. Kongable

$\mathscr{P}$sychiatric illness often accompanies medical illness and is a significant health care problem in the medically ill population. People who have chronic medical illnesses have a nearly 41% higher rate of psychiatric disorders than do people without chronic medical illness. In addition, the chronically medically ill have a 28% higher lifetime prevalence of psychiatric disorders than do people without psychiatric disorders. Studies spanning decades indicate that diabetes mellitus, cardiac disease, and associated metabolic disorders are more common among clients with psychiatric disorders than among the general population (Joffe, Brasche, & MacQueen, 2003). As many as 80% of chronically mentally ill clients have significant medical illness, which may or may not be related to psychopharmacologic therapy (Dixon, Postrado, Delahanty, Fischer, & Lehman, 1999; Goldsmith, 1999). Mood, anxiety, and substance use disorders are the most prevalent psychiatric conditions of clients with chronic or terminal illnesses, such as chronic pain, acquired immunodeficiency syndrome (AIDS), acute trauma, stroke, and cancer (Ford, Trestman, Steinberg, Tennen, & Allen, 2004). Because most medically ill people are elderly, biologic, psychological, social, and spiritual changes may place them at greater risk for mental illness and increased potential mortality and morbidity.

Psychological Illness Related to Specific Physiologic Disorders

The biologic basis of mental disorders that are preceded by comorbid medical disorders is thought to be similar to the biologic basis of primary psychiatric disorders, in which neurochemical changes occur in the process of catecholamine metabolism (Arnsten, 1997). The neurochemicals (transmitters) that orchestrate thinking, learning, speaking, and motor responses also influence mood, perception, and emotional interpretation. Neurochemical modulation maintains a balance in the essential levels of these transmitters. When modulation is disrupted, either mechanically or chemically, disorder occurs.

 KEY CONCEPT **Neurochemical modulation** maintains a balance in the essential levels of the neurotransmitters that influence mood, perceptions, and emotional interpretation.

Unfortunately, mental illness is not commonly recognized or treated in general medical settings. Psychiatric symptoms may be masked by medical symptoms or misdiagnosed as somatoform disorders. The treatment regimen may contribute to psychosocial dysfunction because many medications prescribed for chronic illness alter affect (Goldsmith, 1999; Neese, 1991). Generally, health care providers expect clients to exhibit depressed mood and anxiety as a normal response to illness. In fact, it is considered abnormal if a client does not grieve over the loss of health or does not express discouragement or anxiety about treatment and the possibility of death.

When psychosocial dysfunction remains unexamined and untreated, the course and outcome of associated medical illness may be affected. Mental illness may weaken the motivation for self-care, impair symptom reporting, and delay the search for treatment (Katon & Schulberg, 1992). These symptoms may precede or occur during acute hospitalization and continue after discharge and apparent physical recovery. As a result, hospitalization may be prolonged and recovery delayed, or impaired, at increased emotional and financial cost to the client and the family (Levenson, 1992). In severe cases, mood disorders associated with medical illness increase morbidity and mortality (Eriksson et al., 2004; Hill, Kelleher, & Shumaker, 1992;

Paten, 1999; Polsky et al., 2005). Careful assessment to identify and evaluate symptoms of concomitant mental illness separately from those of medical illness is required, together with appropriate treatment, to achieve the client's best psychological and medical outcome.

Another aspect of psychiatric disorders and medical illness is the common **comorbidity** of physical disorders among people who require primary psychiatric care. Factors associated with increased hospital stays of psychiatric clients include physical disability and concomitant medical illness (Bressi, Marcus, & Solomon, 2006; Cohen & Cosimer, 1989; Collins, 1991). Mental health care professionals must carefully evaluate and monitor changes in coexisting medical conditions to prevent their exacerbation or serious complications that would necessitate acute medical treatment or prolonged hospital stay.

This chapter reviews issues related to mental illness in the medically ill population and common comorbid medical disorders in the psychiatric population. The psychosocial disturbances associated with chronic pain, human immunodeficiency virus (HIV), trauma, neurologic disorders, stroke, and chronic medical illnesses such as heart disease and cancer are presented. Suggestions for diagnostic appraisal and appropriate intervention are given. These medical conditions were chosen because they are responsible for most hospital admissions and frequently are associated with psychiatric comorbidity. The content of this chapter underscores the need for all nurses to have adequate preparation and support in attending to the mental health needs of clients and for effective collaboration between primary care clinicians and clinicians practicing in psychiatric and mental health settings (WHO & Wonca, 2008).

Psychological Impact of Pain

Physiologic pain is a protective response to noxious stimuli that serves as a warning of injury. Clinical pain related to inflammation and pathologic processes is characterized by low-threshold sensitization. Despite major advances in treatments that lessen its force, pain remains one of the most powerful and complex human experiences. Assessing and treating pain are difficult because the pain response is subjective and a client's degree of pain cannot be observed directly. A client's complaints may be difficult to localize. Moreover, the person's discomfort may seem out of proportion to the observed conditions or influenced by disordered emotions, personality, or environmental conditioning. Severe or chronic pain may affect mentally healthy people in adverse ways. The prevalence and impact of pain have led to numerous approaches to therapy, including the use of antipsychotic drugs, antidepressants, antianxiety agents, and stimulants. Considerable evidence suggests that psychiatric medications and interventions can be effective in treating acute and chronic pain.

The **gate-control model** of pain response is based on physiologic evidence that pain perception (**nociception**) involves pathways in the dorsal horn of the spinal cord that relay noxious stimuli to the brain. In addition, certain other nerve fibers function as an antagonistic "gate" to augment or dampen the subjective experience of pain (Melzack, 1993; Robinson, 2003). The cognitive-biobehavioural model (see Chapter 15) considers not only the client's emotive and cognitive perception of pain but also the interaction of environmental influences, physical factors, and pain perceptions over time. From this perspective, clients' interpretation of pain, their coping resources, and their emotive psychological processes interact with the experience of pain and can influence the physiologic activities that characterize pain (Turk, 2004). Some pain theorists believe that the gate-control theory has been largely discredited (McCaffery & Pasero, 1999); others are working to refine the theory as more knowledge of pain becomes available.

> **KEY CONCEPT** The **cognitive-behavioural model** is the model of perception that includes emotion, cognition, environment, and physical and psychological factors.

BIOLOGIC BASIS OF THE PAIN RESPONSE

Pain is transmitted through specific neural pathways that carry information about touch and temperature (Fig. 33-1). Recent physiologic evidence obtained from magnetic resonance imaging and positron emission tomography has demonstrated that painful stimuli also cause significant activation in areas of the brain responsible for memory, emotion, and personality (Talbot & Marrett, 1991) (Fig. 33-2). Pain receptors may be activated by mechanical, thermal, or chemical stimuli. **Neurotransmitters** are chemicals circulating in the synaptic areas of neurons. They serve to initiate, block, or modulate nerve signal transmission and ultimately control neural function. Several neurotransmitters within primary pain pathways are involved in pain transmission (Box 33-1). When these neurochemicals are released, they initiate local inflammatory reactions and sensitize and stimulate central pain receptors. **Substance P** and prostaglandins are the most common nociceptive transmitters that are released and transported along the central and peripheral pain synapses in the presence of noxious stimuli. **Endorphins**, neurotransmitters that have opiate-like behaviour, produce an inhibitory effect at opiate receptor sites and probably are responsible for pain tolerance. The release of endorphins is centrally mediated by serotonin (Zangen, Nakash, & Yadid, 1999). Serotonin, histamine, and bradykinin sensitize and stimulate the pain receptors to generate the experienced pain. Direct demonstrations of changes in endorphin levels during pain and relief from pain are being reported (Ren, 1994; Sosnowski, 1994). The role of endorphins may go beyond pain modulation to include mood enhancement behaviour modification and influence the development of tolerance or dependence on narcotics.

Acute pain, one of the most common symptoms of clients in emergency and acute care settings, can result from a variety of physiologic abnormalities and trauma. It is characterized by sudden, severe onset and generally subsides as the injury heals. Postoperative incisional pain is an iatrogenic (physician-induced) tissue injury most often seen in medical settings. Careful assessment and treatment of pain in these settings have a great impact on healing and recovery.

Chronic pain, defined as pain on a daily basis or pain that is constant for more than 6 months (Atkinson & Slater, 1989), can be related to various pathologies and takes the form of syndromes, such as headache, temporomandibular pain disorders, back pain, arthritis, and can further be conceptualized multidimensionaly in terms of future pain course and outcomes (Von Koff & Dunn, 2008). Clinical syndromes with chronic pain symptoms include neoplasia (cancer), thalamic stroke (central pain), neuropathies (diabetes), and reflex sympathetic dystrophy (Box 33-2). Nervous tissue injury leads to neuropathic pain that may be described as burning, aching, pricking, or lancinating. This central or neuropathic pain is the underlying mechanism for most chronic pain and leads to **hyperalgia** (increased sensation of pain), **allodynia** (lowered pain threshold), and **hyperesthesia** (increased nociceptor sensitivity). Permanent change in central pain interpretation frequently

Motor action system   Sensory discrimination

Thalamus (nociception)

Corpus callosum

Limbic area

Medial surface of frontal lobe (Motivational and affective)

FIGURE 33.1 Pain stimuli activate regions of the brain that influence memory, emotion, and personality.

FIGURE 33.2 Ascending sensory pathways: anterior spinothalamic tract with a schematic diagram of the gate-control theory of pain mechanism.

BOX **33.1**

Neurotransmitters Active in Pain Sensation and Induced Plasticity

C-Fiber Neuropeptides Released By Noxious Stimulation Peripherally

Substance P
Neurokinin A
Somatostatin
Calcitonin gene-related peptide (CGRP)
Prostaglandins
Galanin
Vasoactive intestinal polypeptide (VIP)
Cholecystokinin

Excitatory Amino Acids With Widespread Activity In The CNS (Thalamus And Somatosensory Cortices)

L-Glutamate
N-methyl-D-aspartate (NMDA)

Pain-Modulating Neurotransmitters

Endorphins
Enkephalin
Serotonin

Note: Many of these same neurotransmitters are released in large amounts during brain injury and contribute to neuronal cell death in a variety of neurologic and psychological disease processes.

results in abnormal physiologic, biochemical, cellular, and molecular responses that misinterpret nonpainful sensations as painful (**plasticity**; Melzack, Coderre, Katz, & Vaccarino, 2001). This neural plasticity contributes to the development of errant firing and the pain syndromes of referred pain (pain felt in a part other than where it was produced) and phantom pain (pain that feels as though its source is a missing [amputated] limb).

▪ PSYCHOLOGICAL ASPECTS OF THE PAIN RESPONSE

Pain is not only a sensation but also a perceptual phenomenon with an important affective component. When a client's pain persists for an extended period, a range of psychosocial and spiritual influences, such as the client's mood, fears, expectancies, coping efforts, and financial, social, and spiritual resources, and the responses of significant others begin to influence the client's perception of the pain. Affective and anxiety disorders are prevalent among people with chronic pain. They may be a symptom of or a defence against psychological stress caused by continuous nociceptive input (Koob, 1999). Bio/psycho/social/spiritual stimuli and responses may cause the client

BOX **33.2**

Pain Syndromes Seen in the Primary Care Setting

MIGRAINE HEADACHE: a cerebrovasomotor disorder in which a focal reduction of cerebral blood flow initiates an ischemic headache. May be preceded by a visual aura and followed by nausea, vomiting, and incapacitating head pain.

LOW BACK PAIN: pain arising from the vertebral column or surrounding muscles, tendons, ligaments, or fascia. Causes range from simple muscle strain to arthritis, fracture, or nerve compression from a ruptured disk.

CHRONIC BENIGN OROFACIAL PAIN: temporomandibular joint pain.

RHEUMATOID ARTHRITIS: more than 100 different types of joint disease produce inflammation of the joints. Associated with varying degrees of pain and stiffness and eventual loss of use of the affected joints.

REFLEX SYMPATHETIC DYSTROPHY: causalgia. A painful burning syndrome that occurs after peripheral nerve injury. Associated with hyperesthesia, vasomotor disturbances, and dystrophic changes due to sympathetic hyperactivity.

CANCER PAIN: pain from malignant tumors that is caused by local infiltration or metastatic spread involving specific organs, bones, peripheral or cranial nerves, or the spinal cord. Pain therapy is aimed at providing sufficient relief to allow maximum possible daily functioning and a relatively pain-free death.

NEUROPATHIC PAIN

POLYNEUROPATHY: neuropathy involving multiple peripheral nerves

DIABETIC NEUROPATHY: neuropathy due to diabetes mellitus; marked by diminished sensation secondary to vascular changes

INFLAMMATORY NEUROPATHY: neuropathy related to the presence of chemical or microorganic pathogens

TRAUMATIC NEUROPATHY: neuropathy caused by avulsion or compression

PLEXOPATHY: neuropathy involving a peripheral nerve plexus

PERIPHERAL OR CENTRAL NEURALGIA: abrupt, intense, paroxysmal pain due to intrinsic nerve injury or extrinsic nerve compression

HERPETIC NEURALGIA: pain associated with the dermatomal rash of acute herpes zoster

RADICULOPATHY: pain radiating along a peripheral nerve tract, such as sciatica

VASOOCCLUSIVE PAIN: thrombotic crisis of sickle cell anemia in joints and peripheral muscles that is caused by ischemia

MYOFASCIAL PAIN: pain in palpable bands (trigger points) of muscle. Associated with stiffness, limitation of motion, and weakness with chronic pain to become preoccupied with the pain and can contribute to depression. In addition, the presence of persistent noxious sensations contributes to neurochemical and neurohormonal imbalances that lead to

---

IN A LIFE

Sue Rodriguez (1950–1994)
Amyotrophic Lateral Sclerosis (ALS)

Public Persona

After being diagnosed in 1991 with ALS (also known as Lou Gehrig's disease), Sue Rodriguez realized that she might want to end her life once she was severely incapacitated with the disease. She also recognized that, if this time came, she would be physically incapable of killing herself and would need assistance. Assisting a person to die is illegal, however, under Section 241(b) of the Canadian Criminal Code. Euthanasia (i.e., deliberately ending the life of a suffering person) is also illegal. Sue Rodriguez challenged these laws all the way to the Supreme Court but failed to change them. Ultimately, she defied the law in 1994 by deciding the time and the method of her death. She had an unnamed physician and a friend, Sven Robinson (who was a Member of Parliament at the time), by her side.

Personal Realities

One can only imagine how Sue Rodriguez struggled with the anguish of her terminal illness, the anxiety and despair of leaving behind a teenage son, and her desire to end her life with respect and dignity. The stress of going public with her beliefs and fighting for them was great, but she hoped that her actions would help others living with similar illnesses. She also wanted her son to respect the law and didn't want her last act on earth to be illegal. She asserted that if she could not obey the law in the end, at least she would know that she had done all that she could to change it… as would her son.

See http://archives.cbc.ca/IDD-1–69–1135/life_society/sue_rodriguez/

---

depressed mood and anxiety. Whether the psychological pain is primary or secondary may be difficult to determine because the neurovegetative symptoms of depression may resemble the client's attempts to control the pain or the concomitant medical-physical conditions. Anorexia, sleep disturbance, and agitation or psychomotor retardation may be present. In addition, affective disturbances, such as sadness, loss of interest in life, feelings of worthlessness, self-reproach, excessive guilt, indecisiveness, and suicidal ideation, are all symptoms reported by clients with chronic pain (Turk, 2004). Substance use disorder may arise from the client's search for relief through overuse of drugs that lessen the pain sensation. A formal psychiatric assessment is essential when these symptoms exist.

■ ASSESSMENT OF THE CLIENT WITH CHRONIC PAIN

Appropriate diagnosis and treatment of pain as a primary presenting symptom must begin with a comprehensive history and physical examination. In talking with the nurse about the pain, a client will not only describe its characteristics, location, and severity but may also provide information about possible psychosocial and behavioural factors that are influencing the pain experience. No direct relationship may be evident between the severity or extent of detectable disease and the intensity of the client's pain.

A number of assessment instruments have been developed to aid in evaluation, but a fundamental approach is necessary to determine the impact of pain on the client's life. All systems must be examined in the client to determine

---

BOX 33.3

Assessing Clients Who Report Pain

A. What is the extent of the client's disease or injury (physical impairment)?

B. What is the magnitude of the illness? That is, to what extent is the client suffering, disabled, and unable to enjoy usual activities?

C. Does the client's behaviour seem appropriate to the disease or injury, or is there any evidence of amplification of symptoms for any of a variety of psychological or social reasons or purposes?

D. How often and for how long does the client perform specific behaviours, such as reclining, sitting, standing, and walking?

E. How often does the client seek health care and take analgesic medication (frequency and quantity)?

The Multiaxial Assessment of Pain (MAP) (Rudy & Turk, 1991) includes evaluation of three axes: biomedical, psychosocial, and behavioural.

PAIN BEHAVIOUR CHECKLIST

Pain behaviours have been characterized as interpersonal communications of pain, distress, or suffering. Pain behaviour may be a more accurate indication of intensity and tolerance than verbal reports. Check the box of each behaviour you observe or infer from the client's comments.

- Facial grimacing, clenched teeth
- Holding or supporting of affected body area
- Questions such as, "Why did this happen to me?"
- Distorted gait, limping
- Frequent shifting of posture or position
- Requests to be excused from tasks or activities; avoidance of physical activity
- Taking of medication as often as possible
- Moving extremely slowly
- Sitting with rigid posture
- Moving in a guarded or protective fashion
- Moaning or sighing
- Using a cane, cervical collar, or other prosthetic device
- Requesting help in ambulation; frequent stopping while walking
- Lying down during the day
- Irritability

BOX 33.4

Research for Best Practice: Nursing Students' Experiences of Pain and of Imagining Pain

Bergh, I., Jakobsson, E. & Sjöström, B. (2008). Worst experiences of pain and conceptions of worst pain imaginable among student nurses. Journal of Advanced Nursing, 61(5), 484–491.

THE QUESTION: What are nursing students' own worst experiences of pain and their conceptions of worst pain imaginable?

METHODS: Nursing students (n = 529) completed a questionnaire with two main questions: What is the worst experience of hurt, ache, or pain you have had?; What is the worst pain imaginable for you? Their answers were analyzed using content analysis.

FINDINGS: Students' own worst experiences of pain were primarily related to acute or traumatic painful conditions, inflicted pain, pain associated with female physiology, chronic pain conditions, as well as psychological suffering. The worst pain imaginable for these students were pain related

to particular conditions, overwhelming pain, deliberately inflicted pain, pain related to loss and to psychological suffering, and vicarious pain. Students were able to imagine pain in ways that included the dimensions of grief, control over the situation, and powerlessness. They imagined hope of relief and empathy for others, and suffering related to others' pain. While their own worst experiences were primarily related to concrete bodily pain, they were capable of describing pain as involving emotional and existential distress, as well.

IMPLICATIONS FOR NURSING: The researchers note that their findings show that students bring a personal competence to nursing that includes the ability to imagine another's pain. As professional nurses' ability to do so has been questioned in the literature, these researchers pose as a potential research question: Do nurses' powers of imagination change as a result of professional experience? If so, why?

---

the degree to which biomedical, psychosocial, and behavioural factors interact to influence the nature, severity, and persistence of the client's pain and disability. Box 33-3 presents a pain assessment tool (see also Box 33-4).

 SENSORY AND PHARMACOLOGIC MODULATION OF PAIN

Chronic pain occurs with a wide variety of medical illnesses. Proper diagnosis of the underlying condition determines primary treatment, which could eliminate or significantly reduce the need for analgesic drugs. Unsuspected medical conditions, such as alcoholism, autoimmune disease, or cancer, must be considered if pain develops in the absence of a known cause. Caregivers must know the mechanisms of action of analgesic drugs to administer them safely and monitor their effects. Clients' responses to individual drugs vary, and many agents at different doses may be tried before pain relief is achieved. Table 33-1 presents treatment approaches to pain. The use of physical and psychological modulation techniques, as well as pharmacotherapy or physical therapy, is more successful than the latter therapies alone (Turk, 2004). Combination treatment often affects mood and anxiety levels as well. Clients educated to use cognitive strategies such as biofeedback, a positive emotional state, relaxation, physical therapy or exercise, meditation, guided imagery, suggestion, hypnosis, placebos, and positive self-talk are able to tolerate higher levels of pain than are clients without specific coping strategies (Turk & Feldman, 1992). Most of these techniques involve redirecting the client's attention away from the pain and helping the client learn strategies of **self-efficacy** (self-effectiveness). Some

of the bio/psycho/social/spiritual outcomes that can be measured to determine effectiveness of prescribed therapies include improvements in biologic, psychological, sociocultural, and spiritual well-being (Fig. 33-3). The biologic basis for the effectiveness of these strategies may be their ability to increase brain endorphin production (Bandura, O'Leary, & Taylor, 1987).

Many barriers exist to effective pain management (Box 33-5). Reluctance on the part of health professionals and the client may contribute to persistent pain, which ultimately can adversely affect the client's quality of life. Clients with chronic pain experience not only decreased functional capability but also diminished strength and endurance, nausea, poor appetite, and poor, interrupted sleep. The psychological impact includes diminished leisure and enjoyment, anxiety and fear, depression, somatic preoccupation, and difficulty concentrating. Social impairment may exist in the form of diminished social and sexual relationships, altered appearance, and increased dependence on others. While persons living with chronic pain can find that their suffering helps them to understand the "real value of life," they may wonder why they deserve such suffering (Dušová & Cseszárová, 2008, p. 29). All these contribute to the misery caused by the pain experience.

Maladaptive coping by clients with chronic pain leads them to fear pain and to acquire a negative attitude about pain and how it affects their lives. These negative views can adversely influence biopsychological and physiologic processes, thereby sustaining or even exacerbating the pain. Nonadherence by these clients with sequential prescription changes and combined treatments also can be problematic. Strategies to assess adherence are regular self-report, assessment of behavioural change, biochemical assay, clinical improvement, and outcome assessment.

| Table 33.1 | Treatment Approaches to Pain |

Principles of Pain Treatment	Second Step	Third Step	Fourth Step

• Establish the correct diagnosis
• Recognize that pain reduction, rather than complete pain control, is a reasonable goal
• Control other symptoms besides pain. This includes treating the symptoms that were present before treatment (such as depression and anxiety) and the adverse effects associated with the pain therapy.
• Treat physical conditions that may initiate or exacerbate the pain
 	
First Step
Analgesics for treatment of pain and:
Nonsteroidal anti-inflammatory drugs (NSAIDs)
    Acetaminophen
    Acetylsalicylic acid
    Ibuprofen
Oral local anesthetics
    Flecainide
    Mexiletine
    Tocainide
Topical agents
    Capsaicin
    EMLA
    Lidocaine gel
    Baclofen
    Neuroleptics
    Pimozide
    Corticosteroids
    Calcitonin
    Benzodiazepines
    Clonazepam
Drugs for sympathetically maintained pain
    Nifedipine
    Phenoxybenzamine
    Prazosin
    Propranolol
	Antidepressants, TENS, and psychosocial support, and/or:
	Tricyclic and tetracyclic antidepressants
	    Amitriptyline
	    Clomipramine
	    Desipramine
	    Doxepin
	    Imipramine
	    Maprotiline
	    Nortriptyline
	    Mirtazapine
	Selective and nonselective serotonin reuptake Inhibitors
	    Buproprione
	    Fluoxetine
	    Fluvoxamine
	    Nefazodone
	    Olanzopine
	    Paroxetine
	    Sertraline
	    Trazodone
	    Venlafaxine
	Anticonvulsants
	    Carbamazepine
	    Neurontin
	    Phenytoin
	Opioid analgesics
	    Codeine
	    Meperidine
	    Morphine
	Monoamine oxidase inhibitors
	    Isocarboxazid
	    Phenelzine sulfate
	    Tranylcypromine
	Herbal and alternative medicine
	    SamE
	    Ginseng
	    Swedish massage
	    Acupressure
	    Acupuncture
	    Zero balancing
	    Reflexology
	    Meditation
	    Prayer
	Note: Treat the adverse effects of all the agents used.
		Adrenergic agents, TENS, and psychosocial support, and/or:
		Clonidine
		Naloxone infusion, and/or:
		Other agents (mexiletine, diphenhydramine)
		Note: Add the third-step agents to partially helpful agents used in first step, or use alone and treat the adverse effects of all the agents used.
			Psychiatric intervention
			Psychotherapy with pain clients:
			
			Cognitive
			• Explain the nature of the pain sensation.
			• Describe realistic expectations about the degree and course of pain.
			• Describe realistic expectations of treatment and side effects.
			• Use the placebo effect by supporting the treatment efficacy.
			• Relieve anxiety.
			
			Behavioural
			• Make the initial doses large rather than small, to effect some relief.
			• Reassure that medication will be available, not contingent on proof of need.
			• Reinforce healthy behaviour/adaptation; do not reinforce obsession with pain.
			• Assure of regular evaluation not contingent on presence of pain.
			
			Ablative Procedure for Selected Clients
			Neuroblockade
			• Trigger point injection (TPI)
			• Epidural steroid injection (ESI)
			• Facet joint injection (FJI)
			• Nerve root blocks
			• Medical branch blocks
			• Peripheral nerve block
			• Sympathetic nerve block
			
			Spinal Cord Stimulation
			• Neurostimulator implants
			• TENS
			• Thalamic stimulation

Note: If the client has failed to experience response to all standard pharmacologic treatments, psychiatric evaluation for underlying problems (such as severe depression and risk for suicide) should be emphasized.

TENS, transcutaneous electrical nerve stimulation.

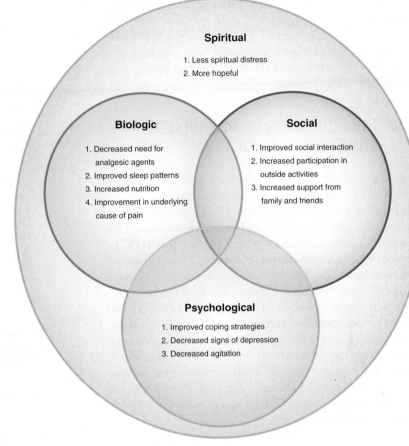

FIGURE 33.3 Bio/psycho/social/spiritual outcomes for clients with pain.

Barriers to Pain Management

PROBLEMS OF HEALTH CARE PROFESSIONALS
- Inadequate knowledge and experience with pain management
- Poor assessment of pain
- Concern about regulation of controlled substances
- Fear of client tolerance and addiction
- Concern about side effects of analgesics

PROBLEMS OF CLIENTS
- Reluctance to report pain
- Concern about primary treatment of underlying disease
- Fear that pain means the disease is worse
- Concern about being a good client and not a complainer
- Reluctance to take pain medications
- Fear of tolerance and addiction, fear of "addict" label
- Fear of unmanageable side effects

PROBLEMS OF HEALTH CARE SYSTEM
- Restrictive regulation of controlled substances
- Problems with availability of treatment or access to it

The nurse can enhance adherence to the intervention plan by closely monitoring the therapeutic efficacy and untoward effects of the treatments being used, involving the client and family in treatment planning, educating the client and family about self-care, and instructing the client in noninvasive approaches to pain control. Effective communication with the client and family is of prime importance (Mackintosh & Elson, 2008).

CRNENOTE

In the assessment of a client's pain, it is important to determine a baseline measure of the person's experience of pain against which changes can be noted. Changes in the words used by a client to describe his or her pain (e.g., from "sharp" to "shooting") should alert the nurse to possible changes in client status.

Psychopathologic Complications of AIDS

The medical syndrome of AIDS is characterized by multiple opportunistic infections and is associated with malignancy. People with AIDS are often overwhelmed by devastating disorders that cause profound fatigue, insomnia, anorexia, emaciation, pain, and disfigurement. The psychological impact of AIDS is considerably worsened by the social stigma associated with the infection and the special affinity of HIV for brain and central nervous system (CNS) tissue.

BIOLOGIC BASIS OF NEUROLOGIC MANIFESTATIONS OF HIV

In as many as 60% of those who have AIDS, neurologic complications occur that are directly attributable to infection of the brain. Important clinical manifestations include impaired cognitive and motor functions. This aspect of the syndrome is referred to as the **HIV-1–associated cognitive-motor complex**. Neuronal injury and frank nerve cell loss probably contribute to the neurologic deficits (Manji & Miller, 2004). Evidence suggests that the presence of HIV stimulates brain cells to release neurotoxins and excitatory amino acids in excess. The resultant neurochemical changes and disrupted cell membrane integrity cause cell death similar to that which occurs with other types of brain injury. These neurochemical changes and eventual catecholamine depletion contribute to the cognitive, motor, and psychiatric manifestations of HIV infection.

PSYCHOLOGICAL ASPECTS OF AIDS

The most common initial signs and symptoms of the AIDS dementia complex are changes in mentation and personality, followed by delirium, dementia, organic mood disorder, and organic delusional disorder. The onset of major depression and uncomplicated bereavement soon after diagnosis is common. Comorbid neurologic infections such as encephalitis and meningitis can predispose the client with AIDS to delirium. The clinical picture reflects the areas of the brain invaded by HIV; however, physiologic conditions such as addiction to alcohol or drugs, brain damage, chronic illness, hypoxia related to pneumonia, infections, space-occupying brain lesions, and systemic reactions to medications may contribute to the progression of mental changes. Loss of normal cortical function may lead to abnormal social behaviour, depression, psychosis, and anxiety. The psychological influences of stress and sleep and sensory deprivation can further contribute to the altered perception and mentation. Figure 33-4 shows the possible pathologic progression of HIV neuronal injury.

Psychiatric disorders contribute to the course of AIDS in several ways. Mood disorder may be reflected

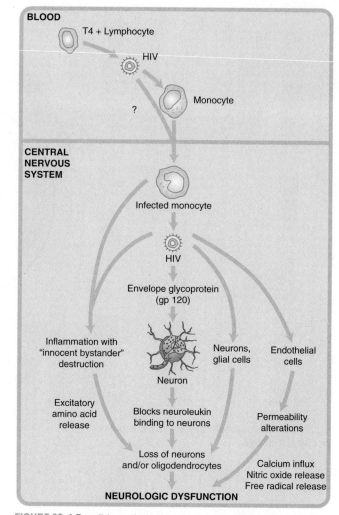

FIGURE 33.4 Possible pathologic progression of HIV neuronal injury.

in the client who has an initial substance use disorder or an antisocial personality that predisposes him or her to a lifestyle that increases his or her risk for exposure to HIV. The neuropathology associated with the presence of HIV then contributes to the progression of the disease and deterioration. AIDS-associated psychopathology frequently is unrecognized, misdiagnosed, and incorrectly treated. Diagnosis can be difficult when risk factors are not known or when cognitive or psychiatric symptoms precede the onset of other manifestations of HIV infection. Early CNS involvement is detected through neuropsychological testing and magnetic resonance imaging. The degree of cognitive dysfunction may not be a valid indication of the degree of organic involvement. In addition, diagnostic findings on computed tomography scans, such as cerebral atrophy and prominent basal ganglia calcification, may not correlate with the severity of the client's dementia (Gabuzda & Hirsch, 1987).

BOX 33.6

Psychiatric Disorders Associated With HIV Infection

ORGANIC MENTAL DISORDER
Dementia
    HIV dementia or AIDS–dementia complex
    Dementia associated with opportunistic infection
      Fungal
        Cryptococcoma
        Cryptococcal meningitis
        Candidal abscesses
      Protozoal
        Toxoplasmosis
      Bacterial
        Mycobacterium avium–intracellulare
      Viral
        Cytomegalovirus
        Herpesvirus
        Papovavirus progressive multifocal
        leukoencephalopathy
    Dementia associated with cancer
      Primary cerebral lymphoma
      Disseminated Kaposi's sarcoma
    Delirium

Organic delusional disorder
Organic mood disorder
    Depression
    Mania
    Mixed
Affective disorders
    Major depression
    Dysthymic disorder
Adjustment disorders
    Adjustment disorder with
    depressed mood
    Adjustment disorder with anxious mood
Substance abuse disorder
Borderline personality disorder
Antisocial personality disorder
Bereavement
Anxiety disorders
    Obsessive-compulsive disorder
    Panic

ASSESSMENT OF THE CLIENT WITH AIDS

Early recognition of psychiatric disorders associated with AIDS is important to enhance our understanding of the behaviour of people with AIDS. Mental status changes and altered affect should be investigated through formal neurologic and psychological testing to determine the extent of impairment. Successful coping and cognitive adaptation are often further hindered by the presence of psychiatric disorders associated with HIV (Box 33-6). These mental illnesses include mood disorders, adjustment disorders, anxiety disorders, substance use disorders, and personality disorders. Organic mood disorder may be characterized by symptoms of a major depressive or manic episode. The depressed mood, feelings of guilt, anhedonia, and hopelessness can be accompanied by insomnia or hypersomnia, psychomotor retardation or agitation, and suicidal ideation. Low self-esteem, feelings of worthlessness and hopelessness, and impaired thinking or concentration are other likely findings. It is important to differentiate between major depression and complicated or uncomplicated grieving over the loss of health or of significant others to premature death because of HIV. When a client receives a diagnosis of AIDS, he or she may face social isolation, severe life-threatening complications, unfamiliar and perhaps ineffective treatments, and the prospect of premature death. As with any life crisis, the client and family members experience severe anxiety, fear, and depression. They may develop obsessive-compulsive rituals to allay anxiety related to the infection. In addition, these clients may experience panic disorders.

People who do not engage in high-risk behaviour and who are unlikely to have been exposed to HIV may nevertheless report physical and psychological manifestations associated with HIV. Anxiety about the disease can produce symptoms not unlike those of HIV infection. Phobias, delusions, and factitious (Munchausen syndrome) AIDS disorders have all been reported in uninfected people. In many cases, psychotherapy for the underlying psychological disorder is effective.

BIO/PSYCHO/SOCIAL/SPIRITUAL INTERVENTIONS

Treatment of AIDS should attempt to maintain normal hydration, electrolyte balance, and nutrition, as well as a safe, comfortable environment promoting a sense of peace, love, and creativity. Antiviral agents, such as zidovudine, ribavirin, and phosphonoformate, and recently approved antiviral agents such as maraviroc, raltegravir, and etravirine, cross the blood–brain barrier and achieve adequate anti-HIV concentrations in cerebrospinal fluid after systemic administration (Hammer et al., 2008).

In addition, it is important to provide the client and the client's family, friends, and caregivers with emotional and educational support. Their sense of competence and control in relation to living with AIDS should be promoted

(Littrell, 1996; Mo & Coulson, 2008). Those close to the client may especially need psychotherapy if the client is young. Treatment of psychiatric disorders should include the individual and family, as well as psychotropic medications, in a manner similar to the treatment of primary psychiatric disorders.

Early diagnosis and treatment are imperative to maximize the client's adherence to risk reduction regimens and to prevent the transmission of infection. Treatment plans can often be tailored to meet the needs of the client and family. The consultation–liaison psychiatric professional can recommend appropriate multidisciplinary interventions to meet the challenge of AIDS with compassion and dignity.

Psychological Illness Related to Trauma

Physiologic trauma activates the overall stress response of the autonomic nervous system (see Chapter 35). Massive catecholamine release causes certain cardiovascular, muscular, gastrointestinal, and respiratory symptoms that release energy stores and support survival. Tissue destruction, musculoskeletal pain, physical disability, and body image changes all contribute to the physiologic and psychological stress response, which continues long after the injury is sustained. The overwhelming behavioural responses are hypervigilance, fear, and anxiety; psychological sequelae may include social isolation, agitation, personality disorders, posttraumatic stress disorder, and depression or, in extreme cases, dissociative identity disorders.

▬▬ BIOLOGIC BASIS OF THE TRAUMA RESPONSE

The neurotransmitters responsible for behavioural responses to fear and anxiety are usually held in balance to maintain a level of arousal appropriate for environmental threat. Information from the sensory processing areas in the thalamus and cortex alerts the amygdala (the lateral and central nucleus). Events that are interpreted as threatening activate the **hypothalamic–pituitary–adrenal (HPA) axis**, initiating the stress response. Adrenal steroids are released and trigger the physiologic reactions just described. Complex neurochemical processes involving norepinephrine, γ-aminobutyric acid (GABA), and serotonin are overwhelmed by the catecholamine release. For example, norepinephrine receptors adjust to the increased level of hyperstimulation. Then, as the catecholamines are depleted, the norepinephrine receptors react to the relative catecholamine shortage. This response alters cognitive and affective functions similar

to the altered function that occurs in anxiety disorders. Persistent, severe distress leads to a general dysregulation of the HPA axis and inappropriate and prolonged secretion of high levels of catecholamines. This chronic stress disorder has been linked to increased susceptibility to immunosuppressive medical illness, such as certain cancers, as well as to infection, myocardial disease, and neurologic degenerative disorders (Radley et al., 2004).

Adaptation to trauma is related to such factors as the severity of the trauma, the person's maturity and age when the trauma occurs, available social support, and the person's ability to mobilize coping strategies (Heim et al., 2000). During adaptation to prolonged stress, the client's cognitive thought processes and coping behaviours cause dopamine to be released in the prefrontal cortex of the brain. These dopaminergic systems are presumed to play a major role in physiologic and emotional coping responses, storage of the trauma experience into memory, and possibly the development of posttraumatic stress disorder (McAllister, Flashman, Sparling, & Saykin, 2004). **Serotonin** is also thought to influence adaptation and mobilize coping strategies.

▬▬ PSYCHOLOGICAL ASPECTS OF THE TRAUMA RESPONSE

Individual behaviour and perception are essential components of the stress reaction. Response to the challenge depends on prior experience, developmental history, and physical status. Individual differences in the extent of endocrine and autonomic activity also occur during stress. Psychological sequelae of sustained stress and trauma may be manifested as flashbacks, intrusive recurring thoughts, panic or anxiety attacks, paranoia, inappropriate startle reactions, nightmares, or the extreme of posttraumatic stress disorder. Catecholamine depletion and activation of the dopamine pathways may contribute to deterioration in social and intellectual functioning after severe physical or emotional trauma. The client may become so withdrawn and depressed that he or she stops participating in activities of daily living (ADLs). Toward the other extreme, the client may become agitated and combative, perceiving any treatment as a continued threat.

Extreme forms of maladaptation are manifested in kindling and dissociative identity disorder. **Kindling** is thought to be responsible for the spontaneous recurrence of depressive illness that is associated with loss and trauma at an early age. Permanent biochemical changes from the early trauma response precipitate the sudden onset of affective disorder in the absence of any present stressor (Nemeroff, 2004). Dissociation disorders are rare but take the form of somatization (physical symptoms), agnosia, multiple personalities, or amnestic fugue states in which the client escapes the stressor by subconscious loss of identity or adoption of a new identity. Although these disorders are not common, mood and anxiety disorders may occur after a trauma event. They are associated with slowed rehabilitation and deterioration in social functioning and ADLs after the trauma period has passed (Jorge et al., 2004).

ASSESSMENT OF THE TRAUMATIZED CLIENT

Complete physical assessment after physical traumatic injury is imperative in life-threatening circumstances. Multiple trauma and head injury are the major causes of death and disability in young adults. Emergency care and intensive care providers are highly trained to recognize signs and symptoms of physiologic injury and to intervene to stabilize primary and secondary trauma in the general medical setting. Trauma scales and triage models have been developed to assist in immediate assessment and to measure neurologic and physical conditions (Fig. 33-5) (Burkle, 1991). They have also been used to predict long-term outcome in clients for whom permanent cognitive and physical disability may limit recovery and challenge adaptive responses.

Psychological injury must be evaluated thoroughly through observation and interview to determine prevalent signs and symptoms of accompanying psychological disorders. This process includes evaluating the client's adjustment and coping skills, personal way of dealing with the trauma, social circumstances, and environmental and life stressors. Assessment must be ongoing to help the client deal with disfigurement, sudden disability, and changes in self-care. The evaluation should include assessment of the client's perception of experienced stress, feelings related to the stress, dominant mood, cognitive functioning, defence and coping mechanisms, and available support systems. In addition, assessment of the risk for self-inflicted injury or suicide is critical.

BIO/PSYCHO/SOCIAL/SPIRITUAL INTERVENTIONS

Psychiatric clinicians provide an important aspect of emergency care. Interventions that establish trust, reduce anxiety, promote adaptive coping, and cultivate a sense of control help the client to begin recovery and maintain emotional health. Crisis intervention methods, stress management, cognitive-behavioural therapies, psychotherapy, and psychotropic medications, alone or in combination, may be useful in achieving the best possible outcome.

When trauma causes the client's death, the family must be informed of the death and allowed to grieve, to prevent the development of a pathologic or prolonged grief response. Traumatic death is sudden and unexpected, and often the victim is young. Surviving family members usually have a severe emotional reaction to the death. Dysfunctional family dynamics may become evident during this period. The psychiatric liaison nurse can use family intervention strategies to enhance or improve relationships, while the family's motivation to do all that is possible is high.

Psychological Illness Related to CNS Disorders

Neurologic impairment is most often related to brain cell (neuron) destruction. The primary causes of neuronal damage are traumatic injury, ischemia, infarction (cerebrovascular accident), abnormal neuron growth (brain tumor), and metabolic poisoning associated with systemic disease. Brain cell loss may also be the result of degenerative processes, such as those that occur in Alzheimer's or Parkinson's disease. Psychological illness often is a complication of organic neurologic disease and may be difficult to distinguish from the neuropathology itself. Therefore, appropriate intervention depends on skilled assessment to discriminate and detect mental status changes related to organic brain injury, as well as disorders of mood and thought.

BIOLOGIC BASIS OF NEUROLOGIC IMPAIRMENT

All mechanisms of brain cell injury destroy brain cells directly or initiate a cascade of cell breakdown from ischemia. This **ischemic cascade** begins with hypoxia and is followed by paralysis of the ion exchange across the cell membrane, edema, calcium influx, free-radical production, and lipid peroxidation (Fig. 33-6). The severity of brain injury is related to the degree and duration of ischemia. Complete ischemia results in brain infarction, commonly known as stroke. The resulting neurologic impairment is related to the size and location of the affected brain area (Fig. 33-7). More eloquent areas of the brain, such as the internal capsule, are extremely sensitive to ischemia. They are typically injured first and contribute to more generalized impairment, such as memory loss or altered judgment.

The primary psychological disorder experienced by people with brain injury is depression (Astrom, Adolfsson, & Asplund, 1993). Depressive symptoms related to organic brain injury are generated by altered biochemical neurotransmitter systems. Hyperactivity and dysregulation of the HPA axis probably contribute to the elevated cortisol and catecholamine levels after a

FIGURE 33.5 Triage algorithm for the primary casualty: neuropsychiatric guidelines. (Adapted from Burkle, F. M. Jr. [1991]. Triage of disaster-related neuropsychiatric casualties. *Psychiatric Aspects of Emergency Medicine, 9*[1], 87–105.)

PRIMARY CASUALTY

T₁

Triage risks
- Behaviour disturbance; loss of limb function or cosmetic change

Immediate interventions
- Rule out occult hypoxia, postconcussion syndrome; neuropsych consult
- Mental health team consult; clergy

Considerations
- Mental health team consult; clergy

T₂₋₃

Triage risks
- Behaviour disturbance; potential for loss of function or cosmetic change

Immediate interventions
- Rule out occult injury, postconcussion syndrome; mental health team consult

Considerations
- Assess response to ventilation; reassurance and support; assess losses, preimpact and impact responses, relocation risks, survivor guilt; psych profile; rating scales

T₄

Triage risks
- Family unable to accept triage decision; multiple injuries; mangled, deformed remains

Immediate interventions
- Mental health team, clergy, social worker

Considerations
- Ongoing grief counselling; assist in paperwork, morgue visit and disposition of remains

Panel A. Triage algorithm for the primary casualty: neuropsychiatric (NP) guidelines.

PRIMARY CASUALTY

T₁₋₄

Triage risks
- Same as adult plus: occult injury more elusive: behaviour may relate to separation

Immediate interventions
- Same plus: re-triage upgrade; pediatric consult; avoid separation from family

Considerations
- Same plus: review high-risk stressors, question prolonged entrapment, question compromised nutrition, question intensity of impact; parent substitute with strong communication with mental health team; play encouraged; parental counselling

T_NP (Child)

SECONDARY CASUALTY

High-Risk Stressors
- Sudden loss of parent, sibling, relative.
- Disruptive family separation
- Developmental phase risks
- New and prolonged behaviours reported.
- Handicapped
- Fails to respond to reassurance and support.
- Regressive symptoms
- Communicated parental anxiety.

Panel C. Neuropsychiatric (NP) algorithm supplement for the pediatric casualty.

PRIMARY CASUALTY

T₁₋₄

Triage risks
- Same as adult plus: organic brain syndrome; occult hypoxia

Immediate interventions
- Same plus: neuropsych consult; early medical and psych profile

Considerations
- Same plus: review high-risk stressors, possible compromised nutrition, possible medication delay; rating scales; rule out depersonalized and devalued communication

SECONDARY CASUALTY

High-Risk Stressors
- Sudden loss of dependent spouse, pet.
- May be more disturbed by property loss, relocation.
- Sense of time loss
- Handicapped.
- Medication or health equipment loss.
- Neuropsychiatric disorder
- Positive psych profile
- Sleep deprivation, poor nutrition.
- Fails to respond to reassurance and support.
- Regression

Panel B. Neuropsychiatric (NP) algorithm supplement for the elderly casualty.

T_NP (Adult)

SECONDARY CASUALTY

High-Risk Stressors
- All family, friends perished; possible survivor guilt.
- Fails to respond to ventilation, support.
- Intense anger, self-destructive or defeating behaviours.
- Positive psych profile
- Fatigue; unable to find or indentify family victims.
- Dependent

Interventions
- Crisis information resources
- Social work and/or mental health team consult.
- Rating scales
- Rest, comfort, support
- Medicate only if necessary

TERTIARY CASUALTY

High-Risk Stressors
- Inexperienced, young
- Immature
- Nonprofessional
- Task of recovering and identifying human remains.
- Reports disturbed coping at scene
- Predisaster emotional and health risks.
- Fatigue, exhaustion

Interventions
- Early critical incident stress debriefing
- Buddy system
- Sleep, task relief
- Avoid alcohol and unnecessary sedation.

Panel D. Neuropsychiatric (NP) algorithm supplement for the adult secondary and tertiary casualty.

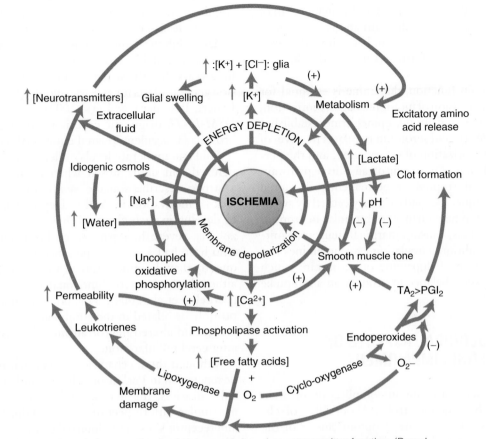

FIGURE 33.6 Ischemic cascade causes secondary brain injury and altered neurotransmitter function. (Based on Raichle, M. E. [1983]. The pathophysiology of brain ischemia. *Annals of Neurology, 13*[1], 2–10.)

FIGURE 33.7 Functional cerebral anatomy and stroke.

cerebral insult. In addition, changes in the metabolism of biogenic amines after brain cell death and ischemia may mediate both mood disturbances and cognitive dysfunction in clients who have had stroke (Luis, Vanderploeg, & Curtiss, 2003).

In cognitive brain function, dopamine is essential for normal neurotransmission of motor messages, motivation, and level of anxiety and mood; epinephrine establishes learning and memory; and serotonin regulates the level of alertness, the categorization of information, and the perception of well-being. These neurotransmitter pathways are temporarily interrupted or permanently disrupted during the acute injury. Secondary injury caused by swelling and compression may further compromise neurons in the surrounding areas, causing marginal neurotransmitter function. In addition, circulating catecholamines can lead to oversecretion of dopamine or serotonin, which disrupts the necessary balance in production and uptake of the transmitters.

PSYCHOLOGICAL ASPECTS OF NEUROLOGIC IMPAIRMENT

Depressive disorder is a common complication of brain injury, particularly ischemic stroke. About 20% of clients with acute stroke have the symptom cluster of the (*Diagnostic and Statistical Manual of Mental Disorders*, 4th ed., Text revision [*DSM-IV-TR*]; American Psychiatric Association, 2000) criteria for major depression (see Chapter 20). Other symptoms, such as sleep disturbances, cognitive dysfunction, poor concentration, difficulty making decisions, somatic discomfort, poor appetite, social withdrawal, and fatigue or agitation, often accompany the mood disturbance. The high-risk period extends for 2 years after the stroke, and left untreated, the depression generally lasts for at least 6 months (Verdelko, Henon, Lebert, Pasquiere, & Leys, 2004). Table 33-2 compares *DSM-IV-TR* diagnostic criteria for depression and cerebrovascular accident–related emotional sequelae.

Mild and moderate levels of depression may go unrecognized and undiagnosed when clients who have had a stroke describe somatic symptoms and demonstrate lack of motivation in ADLs. Depression is more likely to develop in such clients if they have altered speech or aphasia, severe hemiparesis, or both. However, clients who have had a stroke experience depression more frequently than do other disabled and chronically ill clients, although the level of functional disability is the same (Verdelko et al., 2004). This phenomenon is thought to possibly be related to the combination of permanent disability and altered neurotransmitter systems that persist after cerebral infarction.

Although the mechanism of neuronal injury is one of degeneration in Parkinson's disease and other neuromuscular diseases, the neurochemical changes in the brain are similar with respect to the loss of dopamine secretion and receptor sites in the internal capsule motor pathways. About 40% of clients with Parkinson's disease experience depression (Rojo et al., 2003). Although major depression may occur, most have less severe forms that contribute to impairment in daily functioning possibly as much as does

Table 33.2	Comparison of *DSM-IV-TR* Diagnostic Criteria for Depression and Stroke-Related Affective Sequelae		
Major Depression	**Dysthymia***	**Stroke Residual Sequelae**	**Other Symptoms Associated With Depression**
Depressed mood	Depressed mood	Depressed mood	Decreased sexual desire or sexual functioning
Anhedonia	Appetite change	Anhedonia	Loss of insight
Weight change	Sleep disturbance	Weight loss	Autonomic symptoms (e.g., sweating, tachycardia)
Low energy or fatigue	Low energy or fatigue	Low energy or fatigue	Somatic anxiety symptoms
Motor disturbance	Low self-esteem	Paralysis or paresis	Psychic anxiety symptoms
Sleep disturbance	Decreased concentration	Sleep disturbance	Somatic preoccupation (hypochondriasis)
Feelings of worthlessness or guilt	Hopelessness	Feelings of guilt	Pain, especially chronic pain
Decreased concentration		Decreased concentration	Diminished self-care
Thoughts of death or suicide		No psychotic symptoms	Social incapacitation
No independent psychosis		Diminished self-care	
Some psychotic symptoms		Pain, usually chronic	
		Social withdrawal	
		Isolation	
		Hopelessness	
		Somatic preoccupation	

*Cameron, O. G. (1990). Guidelines for diagnosis and treatment of depression in patients with medical illness. *Journal of Clinical Psychiatry, 51,* 7(Suppl.), 49–54.

the underlying disease. Depression is the main factor negatively affecting quality of life and is a source of distress for the client and the family and caregivers. There is evidence suggesting that altered serotonergic function may be responsible, at least in part, for the depressive symptoms in Parkinson's disease and that altered noradrenergic function may underlie some of the associated anxiety symptoms. Clinical trials have demonstrated that selective serotonin reuptake inhibitors (SSRIs) and combined selective serotonin and norepinephrine reuptake inhibitors (SNRIs) are more effective than traditional tricyclic antidepressants in reducing or relieving depression and anxiety in clients with neurologic disease (Murai et al., 2001). In addition, the serotonergic system is disrupted as the neuronal synapses are destroyed or injured. This generalized loss of dopaminergic activity and decreasing functional ability also probably contribute to depressed mood in clients who have had a stroke.

Mental illness related to organic brain injury is consistently dependent on the degree of functional impairment, particularly loss of the ability to communicate and administer self-care. Depressed mood may become evident in the acute recovery phase or during rehabilitation. Depression often negatively affects survival and recovery. It impedes progress throughout the rehabilitation process and ultimately prevents an optimal outcome. Early evaluation assists in the detection of mental illness after brain injury.

■ ASSESSMENT OF THE CLIENT WITH NEUROLOGIC PROBLEMS

A thorough neurologic examination is important in determining the location and degree of disability but is even more critical in establishing the locus of the retained function. Many scales exist that accurately assess neurologic function and that are easy to administer and generally accepted as reliable tools to detect the degree and limitations of disability. Cognition and mentation can be more discretely measured by the Folstein Mini-Mental State examination (Folstein, Folstein, & McHugh, 1975), and functionability for self-care can be measured using the Barthel Index (Mahoney & Barthel, 1965). The evaluation of mood using the Centre for Epidemiological Studies Depression Scale (CES-D) or the Beck Depression Inventory (Beck, Ward, Mendelson, Mock, & Erbaugh, 1961) provides important information for designing intervention strategies for the at-risk client who has had a stroke. Findings of depressive symptoms indicate the need for a more definitive neuropsychological referral. The dexamethasone suppression test (DST) has also been used to diagnose clinical depression. However, it is not completely reliable, and frequent false-positive test results limit its clinical utility (Carroll et al., 1981).

■ BIO/PSYCHO/SOCIAL/SPIRITUAL INTERVENTIONS

Isolation, lack of companionship, bereavement, and poverty are associated with depressive symptoms in the general population and compound the relative risk of depression developing after brain damage. In addition, a personal or family history of major depression increases the risk for depressed mood. Prevention strategies should be used as early as possible for clients known to have these risks. These strategies include the assessment and provision of social support resources while the client is hospitalized as an important component of discharge planning to rehabilitation services; the prescription of therapies to enhance competence in the performance of ADLs, with a focus on the use of retained function, rather than on adaptation to disabilities only; and formal psychosocial testing and psychopharmacologic treatment when appropriate (Palomaki et al., 1999; Robinson et al., 2000). Assessment and support of the client's own spiritual resources should be addressed, particularly related to change in life meaning for the client that may have occurred due to the neurological impairment. There needs to be education of the client and family to increase their awareness of signs and symptoms of depressed mood so that they will know when to seek medical attention and treatment to avert major depression, if possible. In addition, the presence of depressed mood and other symptoms of the depressive cluster indicate the need for cognitive, behavioural, biologic, social, and spiritual interventions to support appropriate psychopharmacologic treatment.

Psychological Illness Related to Acute and Chronic Medical Illness

Systemic medical illness is associated with a higher prevalence of concurrent psychiatric disorders. Disorders such as cancer, heart disease, endocrine abnormalities, and organ failure are often associated with more functional disabilities than most chronic medical illnesses and may be the basis of medically unexplained somatic symptoms. Among the psychiatric disorders, substance use disorder, anxiety, and depressive disorder occur most frequently in clients with chronic medical illnesses. Within the anxiety disorders, phobias are most common, with panic disorder and obsessive-compulsive disorder less common (Härter, Conway, & Merikangas, 2003). Table 33-3 compares the prevalence rates of depressive and anxiety disorders in people who are medically ill with the rates in people who are not.

Table 33.3	Prevalence of Psychiatric Disorders in Medically Ill Compared With People Who Are Not Medically Ill	
Prevalence of Psychiatric Disorders*	**Medically Ill (%)**	**Not Medically Ill (%)**
6-month prevalence	24.7	17.5
Substance abuse	8.5	
Anxiety	11.9	
Affective disorder	9.4	
Lifetime prevalence	42.4	33.0
Substance use	26.2	
Anxiety	18.2	
Phobias	12.1	
Panic disorder	1.5	
Obsessive-compulsive disorder	2.4	
Affective disorder	12.9	

*Prevalence rates are sex- and age-adjusted.

Adapted from National Institute of Mental Health Epidemiologic Catchment Area Program, & Burkle, F. M. Jr. (1991). Triage of disaster-related neuropsychiatric casualties. *Psychiatric Aspects of Emergency Medicine, 9*(1), 87–104.

■ BIOLOGIC ASPECTS OF MENTAL ILLNESS RELATED TO MEDICAL DISEASE

The nervous, endocrine, and immune systems and their components are designed to communicate and interact through biochemical means. The cerebral cortex and limbic system initiate neuroendocrine HPA axis activity by thought processes in response to environmental stimuli. Various hormonal messengers travel between the hypothalamic, pituitary, and adrenal systems to initiate secondary peripheral responses. The immune system responds to signals from the HPA axis and returns messages as well.

Its protective activities rely on neurochemicals to initiate the infection defence and stress response. At all levels, the circulating hormone levels serve as feedback messengers to inhibit HPA activity after sufficient response has occurred.

Dysregulation of the hypothalamic, pituitary, and adrenal systems at all levels leads to malfunction of the other systems. Abnormal nervous system firing in the hippocampus alerts the adrenal and immune systems unnecessarily and vice versa. The principal neurochemical messengers in this regulation are thought to be norepinephrine, endorphins, cortisol, and dopamine. This trio of systems detects metabolic and cellular disease processes that eventually cause signs and symptoms of medical diseases, and body resources are activated to stop these pathologic processes. Psychiatric conditions occur during the course of these medical illnesses and in some instances may contribute to the genesis of the physiologic disease.

A psychiatric disorder may be the first manifestation of a primary disease, such as depressive syndrome in Huntington's chorea, multiple sclerosis, Parkinson's disease, HIV, Cushing's disease, and systemic lupus erythematosus. Depressive symptoms are an intrinsic part of the primary pathophysiology of endocrine disorders, metabolic disturbances, malignancies, viral infections, inflammatory disorders, and cardiopulmonary conditions. Tables 33-4 and 33-5 list medical conditions associated with anxiety disorders and depression, respectively.

Endocrine system pathologic processes involve abnormal HPA axis function, which affects neurotransmitter balance (Stratakis & Chrousos, 1995). Depression and anxiety are often present in clients with hyperthyroidism and hypothyroidism, Cushing's disease (hyperadrenalism), and Addison's disease (hypoadrenalism).

Malignancies have also been associated with anxiety and depression. Depressive syndromes have been associated with cancer, and biologic relationships between the

Table 33.4	Medical Conditions Associated With Anxiety Disorders	
Psychiatric Disorder	**Medical Illness**	**Incidence (%)**
Panic disorder	Parkinson's disease	20
	Primary biliary cirrhosis	10
	Chronic obstructive pulmonary diseases	24
	Cardiomyopathy	83
	Post-MI	16
	Chronic pain	16
	Focal seizures	*
Social phobia	Parkinson's disease	17
Obsessive-compulsive disorder	Sydenham's chorea	13
Phobia	Multiple sclerosis	*
Generalized anxiety	Primary biliary cirrhosis	10
	Graves' disease	62

*Incidence not significant but reportable.

Table 33.5	Medical Illnesses Associated With Symptoms of Depression
Endocrinopathies	Hypothyroidism and hyperthyroidism Hypoparathyroidism and hyperparathyroidism Cushing's syndrome (steroid excess) Adrenal insufficiency (Addison's disease) Hyperaldosteronism
Malignancies	Abdominal carcinomas, especially pancreatic Brain tumors (temporal lobe) Breast cancer Gastrointestinal cancer Lung cancer Prostate cancer Metastases
Neurologic disorders	Ischemic stroke Subarachnoid hemorrhage Parkinson's disease Normal-pressure hydrocephalus Multiple sclerosis Closed head injury Epilepsy
Metabolic imbalance	Serum sodium and potassium reductions Vitamin B_{12}, niacin, vitamin C deficiencies; iron deficiency (anemias) Metal intoxication (thallium and mercury) Uremia
Viral/bacterial infection	Infectious hepatitis Encephalitis Tuberculosis AIDS
Hormonal imbalance	Premenstrual, premenopausal, postpartum periods
Cardiopulmonary	Acute MI Post–cardiac arrest Post–coronary artery bypass graft Post–heart transplantation Cardiomyopathy
Inflammatory disorders	Rheumatoid arthritis

related to metabolic imbalances and neuropsychiatric side effects from treatment.

Cardiac disease deserves special attention because it has been associated with precipitated depressive syndromes and anxiety disorders. The fact that more than 70% of clients who have an acute myocardial infarction (MI) remain depressed for as long as 1 year after the event indicates that the mental illness may not be simply an adjustment disorder. Gender differences in risk for anxiety and depression after MI have been found. In a 5-year prospective study, women had increased risk for both anxiety and depression in the first 2 years after MI, whereas men had increased risk for depression that began 2 years after MI (Bjerkeset, Nordahl, Mykletun, Holmen, & Dahl, 2005). The incidence of depression is also high in cardiac transplant recipients (54%) but is much lower in clients who undergo cardiac bypass surgery (6% to 15%). In a study of clients with coronary heart disease, 75% of cardiac clients who received therapy for their depression experienced response to treatment (Hill et al., 1992).

In addition to the disease process contributing to psychological complications, the drugs used to treat chronic disease may induce mental illness. Psychotropic and nonpsychotropic medications can be potent generators of depression and anxiety (Table 33-6). The indications and pharmacologic activity of these medications often have bio/psycho/social/spiritual implications. In addition, medically ill elderly clients are particularly susceptible to medication effects at lower doses. Depressive and anxiety-related symptoms may in fact have an additive effect on client function, well-being, and recovery when combined with medical illness. When a drug is suspected of causing mental changes, the recommended course of action is to withdraw the drug and find an effective alternative. When an alternative is not available, the dosage should be decreased to an effective level at which symptoms resolve.

PSYCHOLOGICAL ASPECTS OF MEDICAL ILLNESS

In all cases of medical illness, it is natural for clients to respond to the loss of health with hopelessness, particularly when the illness is demoralizing, life threatening, and without a clear prognosis. People who are chronically ill are distressed by loss of function and limitations on their daily activities. They are often forced to comply with treatments that add discomfort but no apparent benefit. Medical clients commonly experience weight loss, insomnia, and motor retardation but perhaps not to the degree of "conspicuous" psychiatric illness. In addition, chronic life stress and mental illness may have set in motion a series of biologic processes ultimately resulting in the medical disorder, which may be further exacerbated

two disorders may exist such that the onset of depression may herald undetected carcinoma. Diagnoses range from major depression to adjustment disorder with depressed mood.

Systemic infections and generalized inflammatory disorders such as rheumatoid arthritis that acutely and chronically stress the immune system or that may be the result of immune dysfunction are associated with psychological disorders. In addition, renal, pancreatic, and hepatic transplant recipients, who are artificially immunosuppressed because of treatment with prophylactic anti-infectious agents, experience primary neuropsychiatric symptoms

Table 33.6	Medications Associated With Mental Illness in Medically III Clients
Analgesics and NSAIDs	Ibuprofen
	Indomethacin
	Opiates
	Pentazocine
	Phenacetin
	Phenylbutazone
Antihypertensives	Clonidine
	Hydralazine
	Methyldopa
	Propranolol
	Reserpine
Antimicrobials	Ampicillin (Gram-negative agents)
	Clotrimazole
	Cycloserine
	Griseofulvin
	Metronidazole
	Nitrofurantoin
	Streptomycin
	Sulfamethoxazole (sulfonamides)
Neurologic agents	l-Dopa
	Levodopa
Antiparkinsonian drugs	Amantadine
Anticonvulsants	Carbamazepine
	Phenytoin
Antispasmodics	Baclofen
	Bromocriptine
Cardiac drugs	Digitalis
	Guanethidine
	Lidocaine
	Oxprenolol
	Procainamide
Psychotropic drugs	Benzodiazepines
Stimulants/sedatives	Amphetamines
	Barbiturates
	Chloral hydrate
	Clorazepate
	Diethylpropion
	Ethanol
	Fenfluramine
	Haloperidol
Steroids and hormones	Adrenocorticotropic hormone
	Corticosteroids
	Estrogen
	Oral contraceptives
	Prednisone
	Progesterone
	Triamcinolone
Antineoplastic drugs	Bleomycin
	C-Asparaginase
	Trimethoprim
	Vincristine
Other miscellaneous drugs	Anticholinesterases
	Cimetidine
	Diuretics
	Metoclopramide

by the stress of hospital admittance. A vicious cycle of medical and mental disorders may arise.

Mental illness in medically ill people is potentially lethal because normal affects and cognitive functioning may be essential to recovery and adherence to the medical treatment plan. In addition, the use of excessive analgesics and reluctance to perform self-care and rehabilitative activities hinder recovery and expose the person to other potential complications. The detection and diagnosis of any secondary mental illnesses in clients with medical illnesses are critical. The physiologic and pharmacologic factors that contribute to the mental illness must be explored and ruled out before effective intervention can begin.

ASSESSMENT OF THE CLIENT WITH MEDICAL ILLNESS

Unfortunately, it may be very difficult for the clinician, evaluating a medically ill client in whom psychiatric symptoms develop, to ascertain whether these symptoms are the result of direct psychobiologic changes brought about by the illness. The psychosocial impact of the medical illness can influence the illness experience in such ways as frustration, fear, loss, fatigue, isolation, and confusion about the future (Costello & Boblin, 2004). People at obvious risk have a family history or personal history of mental illness or were experiencing psychological problems before symptoms of the medical illness were present. The main problem for the clinician is to determine which signs and symptoms are part of the medical illness and its treatment and which signify the presence of a psychological disorder. A complete health assessment and physical examination, including a psychological examination and a cognitive-affective assessment, will help determine the priority and severity of symptoms and interventions. In some instances, the primary diagnosis may be depression, although the symptoms may be similar to those of medical illness in the absence of diagnostic findings. Factors to be considered in diagnosing mental illness in medical clients are outlined in Box 33-7.

Several important cognitive-affective symptoms best differentiate the effects of depression from those of medical illness. These include feelings of failure, low self-esteem, guilt feelings, loss of interest in people, feelings of being punished, suicidal ideation, dissatisfaction, difficulty with decisions, and crying (Neese, 1991). The severity of the vegetative symptoms generally increases with the severity of the depressive disorder as well as the severity of the medical illness. Decreased appetite, sleep disturbances, and loss of energy are not considered indicators of depression in the medically ill client because these symptoms are common in medical illness as well. The Beck Depression Inventory and the CES-D are easy to administer and may indicate the need for a psychiatric referral.

Factors to Consider in Diagnosing Depression in Medical Clients

- One or more specific medical illnesses
- Defining criteria for one of the depressive syndromes
- Family psychiatric history
- Past psychiatric history of the client
- Client's response to treatment, if any, for any prior depressive episode
- Sex of the client
- Client's age at onset of depression
- Depression that preceded the medical illness
- Psychosocial precipitants before onset of depression
- Duration of depressive illness
- Biologic markers of depression
- Relative frequence in the population of diagnoses under consideration
- Diagnosis by commission, not omission

CLINICAL FEATURES OF SPECIAL SIGNIFICANCE

Two problems of special significance, psychosis and suicidal thoughts, are related in that clients with delusions or hallucinations tend to be at greater risk for suicide attempts or more likely to resist treatment (e.g., to refuse to eat or take medication) for their medical condition. It is important to distinguish between a mentally competent client's right to refuse life-saving medical treatment and a depressed client's desire to die. A clinical evaluation of the effect of depression on the client's capacity to make competent decisions is imperative. If optimal medical and psychiatric treatments have been provided and the client has been found competent enough to make decisions about further medical care, it may be appropriate to honour the client's desire to die.

Clients with chronic medical illness and clients with primary mental illness may pose similar problems in psychiatric hospitals when their medical condition fails. The use of advance directives helps in addressing these problems.

BIO/PSYCHO/SOCIAL/SPIRITUAL INTERVENTIONS

It is essential to provide optimal treatment of clients' medical illnesses without neglecting their mental distress. Most reports suggest that clinicians should be more aggressive in the pharmacologic treatment of mental illness in the medically ill. The basic rules for medicating clients include using the minimum dose initially, advancing the dose slowly, and performing frequent blood level monitoring. The doses required to achieve therapeutic blood levels may be lower or even half the usual therapeutic dose and take longer to titrate. It is important to understand the

pharmacokinetics (absorption, distribution, metabolism, and elimination) of the treatment of choice, to prevent further systemic effects. SSRIs and SNRIs are used equally as the treatment for depression in the medically ill client population. Because the side effects of psychopharmacologic agents can be especially troublesome in medically ill people, treatment must be changed or stopped if drug or illness interactions occur or if treatment of the mental illness appears to be unsuccessful. SSRIs are increasingly popular in treating medically ill clients because their side effect profile is more tolerable within a wider therapeutic range. Most clients experience response to antidepressant therapy with a decrease in the severity of their vegetative symptoms in 4 to 8 days.

Both supportive individual psychotherapy and family therapy are helpful. Assisting the client and family in understanding the nature and relationship of the medical and psychiatric diagnoses may strengthen the support system, alter the perception of caregiver burden, and identify appropriate coping strategies. Mutually agreed-upon goals and therapy actively involve the client in progress toward recovery. At some point, the clinician may need to help the client identify psychodynamic conflicts, maladaptive coping strategies, and, perhaps, spiritual concerns related to being ill that may be contributing to his or her distress. Cognitive intervention should address those areas of the client's life that can be controlled, despite major lifestyle changes, to reinforce a feeling of competence. It also is important to convey the fact that although medical and mental illnesses are difficult to prevent, they are often treatable.

Intervening in Mental and Medical Illnesses

The relationship between stress and illness is becoming more apparent as studies increasingly disclose the effects of stress on the body. Chronic illness is viewed as a stressor and is associated with increased psychological distress, and interventions can minimize that distress. Nurses are committed to preventing illness and promoting healthy living. Thus, it is essential that they be aware of the physiologic and psychological impact of chronic stress, understand the coping process, and know appropriate alternative strategies for coping with illness. In addition, nurses can evaluate the effectiveness of strategies being used and revise care plans to improve outcomes for the client.

Clients, with primary mental illness, in need of medical care are at particular risk when somatic complaints are viewed as part of the primary process. Undiagnosed pathophysiologic processes may become advanced while being attributed to somatization. As well, comorbid medical conditions can affect the psychiatric illness. For instance, a study of depressed geriatric inpatients found that 62% reported chronic pain; those with chronic pain were more likely to report suicidal ideation (Meeks et al., 2008). A thorough medical history and physical examination are standard practice for clients in all settings. Ideally, a multidisciplinary team of care providers that includes a psychiatric and mental health liaison nurse should work together to deliver optimum treatment of complex medical and mental illnesses. All clients with chronic medical illnesses are at risk for psychological distress and should be approached with this understanding. Clinicians should include a general cognitive-affective status evaluation in their assessment of all medically ill clients and make appropriate psychiatric liaison consultation to offset the negative impact of mental illness on recovery.

A psychosocial review of systems is useful in admission assessment to detect psychosocial stress or risk. This review provides the minimum information needed for each client—neglect of even one area could compromise client care. Information on substance use, stressful life events, expectations, fears, meanings, social support, sexual concerns, work, finances, education, psychiatric history, mood, cognition, culture, and functional status is obtained from the review. This information is useful in determining relevant nursing diagnoses and developing the plan of care.

Stress management training, systematic relaxation, supportive education, and stress monitoring should be built into the plan of care, regardless of the medical diagnosis. Assessment of anxiety and depression is ongoing, and crisis intervention with psychotherapy may be necessary to reduce the severity of mental distress. Physiologic stress factors, such as increased heart rate, blood pressure, and respiration, and signs of restlessness and sadness can be measured to determine the effectiveness of the intervention. Secondary mental illness can be approached using the same strategies that are effective for primary mental dysfunction. Interventions overlap across criteria, and all interventions provide some element of supportive therapy or social support.

Mental health can and should be monitored in clients who have physical illnesses. This monitoring may need to be long-term. Research is suggesting that survivors of life-threatening illness can have psychological problems or distress that persist over time (Mitka, 2009). Certain kinds of pathologic processes place clients at greater risk for mental illness. These processes can be identified and interventions prescribed to prevent psychiatric disorders from developing or to minimize their severity. Cognitive and behavioural strategies have a place in the treatment regimen and offer the practitioner an opportunity to expand the boundaries of traditional client-oriented practice in effective ways.

Alternatives to traditional medical intervention are increasingly employed as adjunct therapy in clients with pain related to cancer, neuropathy, or degenerative disorders. Natural and herbal therapies, therapeutic massage, zero balancing, thought field therapy, imaging, prayer, and meditation have all been found to be useful in easing the mental and physical discomfort of the client with medical illness. In addition, these therapies are more satisfying to clients who otherwise must receive toxic medication as part of their conventional medical treatment (see Table 33-1).

SUMMARY OF KEY POINTS

☐ Psychiatric disorders are more common in people with systemic or chronic medical illnesses than in other people. Comorbid depression is common in certain medical diseases, such as endocrine and metabolic disturbances, viral infections, inflammatory disorders, and cardiopulmonary diseases. Specific anxiety disorders are associated with other medical conditions, such as Parkinson's disease, focal seizures, primary binary cirrhosis, and chronic pain.

☐ Psychiatric illness that accompanies medical illness is seldom recognized and treated. Psychiatric symptoms may precede the onset of disease symptoms, and it may be difficult to distinguish between the symptoms of the two conditions.

☐ The biologic basis of mental illness associated with medical illness (e.g., catecholamine depletion, disorders in metabolism or production of neurotransmitters) is similar to that of primary psychiatric illness, and bio/psycho/social/spiritual interventions are effective.

☐ Mental illness in medically ill people is potentially lethal because normal affective-cognitive function may be critical to recovery and adherence to the medical treatment plan. Therefore, it is imperative that mental health is included in the standard health assessment of all medically ill people and that appropriate referrals be made.

CRITICAL THINKING CHALLENGES

1 You are caring for a client who has had a stroke and who refuses breakfast and a morning bath. Applying what you know about the neurologic damage caused by stroke and the frequency of depression in such clients, develop a care plan addressing the client's bio/psycho/social/spiritual needs.

2 As you care for a client with AIDS, you notice that his partner is pacing and hyperventilating. Using your knowledge of relationships, systems, and the interconnectedness of physical and psychological illness, how would you approach him?

3 Discuss pain syndromes you may see in the primary care setting.

4 A client is being seen for chronic pain. Discuss how you would go about assessing barriers to pain management with this client.

5 You are a psychiatric and mental health liaison nurse and have been asked to prepare a program for the

medical-surgical nursing staff on psychiatric aspects of medical illnesses. What topics would you include, and what would be your rationale for including each?

MOVIES, NOVELS, AND BIOGRAPHIES

The Barbarian Invasions (Restricted, in French With English subtitles): 2003. This movie, a sequel to The Decline of the American Empire, deals with a universal topic: mortality from cancer. The ethos of impending death hovers across the entire film, yet it is neither a grim nor a depressing experience. The Director, Denis Arcand, has infused a great deal of wit throughout the film, and it meshes well with the anticipated pathos.

VIEWING POINTS: As one watches the film, one could easily make the argument that *The Barbarian Invasions* is as much about life (love, despair, humour) as it is about death. Does thinking about death help us live in a better way?

Philadelphia: 1993. This is the story of Andy Beckett, played by Tom Hanks. Beckett is an exceptionally gifted and successful Philadelphia lawyer who is gay. Beckett did not declare his sexual orientation to the law firm that aggressively recruited and employed him. When he becomes HIV positive and develops AIDS, he is fired by the firm, allegedly for incompetence. Beckett sues them for wrongful dismissal.

VIEWING POINTS: As you observe the film, consider the dynamics of his trials and tribulations as a gay man living with AIDS in a heterosexist corporate world. Take note of prejudice and discrimination but also of tolerance, understanding, and compassion. The movie was criticized for providing its main character with a much more understanding family than is typically the case for peoples with AIDS. What do you think about this? The movie *Philadelphia* may be seen as a modern-day David and Goliath story. Do you think it is essentially a story of hope?

REFERENCES

American Psychiatric Association. (2000). *Diagnostic and statistical manual of mental disorders* (4th ed., Text revision). Washington, DC: Author.

Arnsten, A. F. (1997). Catecholamine regulation of the pre-frontal cortex. *Journal of Psychopharmacology, 11,* 151–162.

Astrom, M., Adolfsson, R., & Asplund, K. (1993). Major depression in stroke patients: A 3-year longitudinal study. *Stroke, 24,* 976–982.

Atkinson, J. H. Jr., & Slater, M. A. (1989). Psychiatric medications and pain management in emergency medicine. *Topics in Emergency Medicine, 11*(3), 1–110.

Bandura, A., O'Leary, A., & Taylor, C. B. (1987). Perceived selfefficacy and pain control-opioid and nonopioid mechanisms. *Journal of Personality and Social Psychology, 53,* 563–571.

Beck, A. T., Ward, C. H., Mendelson, M., Mock, J., & Erbaugh, J. (1961). An inventory for measuring depression. *Archives of General Psychiatry, 4,* 561–571.

Bergh, I., Jakobsson, E. & Sjöström, B. (2008). Worst experiences of pain and conceptions of worst pain imaginable among student nurses. *Journal of Advanced Nursing, 61*(5), 484–491.

Bjerkeset, O., Nordahl, H., Mykletun, A., Holmen, J., & Dahl, A. (2005). Anxiety and depression following myocardial infarction: Gender differences in a 5-year prospective study. *Journal of Psychosomatic Research, 58,* 153–161.

Bressi, S., Marcus, S., & Solomon, P. (2006). The impact of psychiatric comorbidity on general hospital length of stay. *The Psychiatric Quarterly, 77*(3), 203–209.

Burkle, F. M. Jr. (1991). Triage of disaster-related neuropsychiatric casualties. *Emergency Medicine Clinics of North America, 9*(1), 87–105

Cameron, O. G. (1990). Guidelines for diagnosis and treatment of depression in patients with medical illness. *Journal of Clinical Psychiatry, 51*(7 Suppl.), 49–54.

Carroll, B. J., Feinberg, M., Greden, J. F., Tarika, J., Albala, A. A., Haskett, R., et al. (1981). A specific laboratory test for the diagnosis of melancholia: Standardization, validation and clinical utility. *Archives of Clinical Psychiatry, 38,* 15–22.

Cohen, C., & Cosimer, G. (1989). Factors associated with increased hospital stay by elderly psychiatric patients. *Hospital and Community Psychiatry, 40*(7), 741–743.

Collins, J. G. (1991). Acute pain management. *International Anesthesiology Clinics, 29*(1), 23–36.

Costello, J., & Boblin, S. (2004). What is the experience of men and women with congestive heart failure? *Canadian Journal of Cardiovascular Nursing, 14*(3), 9–20.

Dixon, L., Postrado, L., Delahanty, J., Fischer, P. J., & Lehman, A. (1999). The association of medical comorbidity in schizophrenia with poor physical and mental health. *Journal of Nervous and Mental Disease, 187*(8), 496–502.

Dušová, B., & Cseszárová, M. (2008). An overview of the quality of life of clients with chronic pain. *Primary Health care, 18*(1), 25–29.

Eriksson, M., Asplund, K., Glader, E.L., Norrving, B., Stegmayr, B., Terent, A., et al. (2004). Self-reported depression and use of antidepressants after stroke: A national survey. *Stroke: A Journal of Cerebral Circulation, 35*(4), 936–941.

Folstein, M. F., Folstein, S. E., & McHugh, P. R. (1975). Mini-Mental state: A practical method for grading the cognitive state of patients for the clinician. *Journal of Psychiatric Research, 12,* 189–198.

Ford, J. D., Trestman R. L., Steinberg, K., Tennen, H., & Allen, S. (2004). Prospective association of anxiety, depressive, and addictive disorders with high utilization of primary, specialty, and emergency medical care. *Social Science & Medicine, 58*(11), 2145–2148.

Gabuzda, D. H., & Hirsch, M. S. (1987). Neurologic manifestations of infection with human immunodeficiency virus: Clinical features and pathogenesis. *Annals of Internal Medicine, 107,* 383–391.

Goldsmith, R. J. (1999). Overview of psychiatric comorbidity: Practical and theoretical considerations. *Psychiatric Clinics of North America, 22*(2), 331–349.

Hammer, S. M., Eron, J. J., Reiss, P., Schooley, R. T., Thompsn, M. A., Walmsley, S., et al. (2008). Antiretroviral treatment of adult HIV infection: 2008 recommendations of the Internatioal AIDS Society-USA panel. *The Journal of the Americam Medical Association, 300*(5), 555–570.

Heim, C., Newport, D. J., Heit, S., Graham, Y., Wilcox, M. Bonsall, R., et al. (2000). Pituitary-adrenal and autonomic responses to stress in women after sexual and physical injury in childhood. *Journal of the American Medical Association, 284*(5), 592–597.

Hill, D. R., Kelleher, K., & Shumaker, S. A. (1992). Psychosocial interventions in adult patients with coronary heart disease and cancer: A literature review. *General Hospital Psychiatry, 14*(6 Suppl.), 28S–42S.

Härter, M. C., Conway, K. P., & Merikangas, K. R. (2003). Associations between anxiety disorders and physical illness. *European Archives of Psychiatry and Clinical Neuroscience, 253*(6), 313–320.

Joffe, R. T., Brasche, J. S., & MacQueen, G. M. (2003). Psychiatric aspects of endocrine disorders in women. *Psychiatric Clinics of North America, 261*(3), 683–691.

Jorge, R. E., Robinson, R. G., Moser, D., Tateno, A., Crespo-Facorro, B., & Arndt, S. (2004). Major depression following traumatic brain injury. *Archieves of General Psychiatry, 61*(1), 42–50.

Katon, W., & Schulberg, H. (1992). Epidemiology of depression in primary care. *General Hospital Psychiatry, 14,* 237–247.

Koob, G. F. (1999). Corticotrophin-releasing factor, norepinephrine and stress. *Biological Psychiatry, 46*, 1167–1180.

Levenson, J. L. (1992). Psychosocial interventions in chronic medical illness: An overview of outcome research. *General Hospital Psychiatry, 14*(6 Suppl.), 43S–49S.

Littrell, J. (1996). How psychological states affect the immune system: Implications for interventions in the context of HIV. *Health & Social Work, 21*(4), 287–296.

Luis, C. A., Vanderploeg, R. D., & Curtiss, G. (2003). Predictors of postconcussion symptom complex in community dwelling male veterans. *Journal of the International Neuropsychological Society, 9*(7), 1001–1015.

Mackintosh, C., & Elson, S. (2008). Chronic pain: Clinical features, assessment and treatment. *Nursing Standard, 23*(5), 48–56.

Mahoney, F. T., & Barthel, D. W. (1965). Functional evaluation: Barthel index. *Maryland Medical Journal, 14*, 61–65.

Manji, H., & Miller, R. (2004). The neurology of HIV infection. *Journal of Neurology Neurosurgery and Psychiatry, 75*(Suppl.), 29–38.

McAllister, J. W., Flashman, L. A., Sparling, M. B., & Saykin, A. J. (2004). Working memory deficits after traumatic brain injury: Catecholeminergic mechanisms and prospects for treatment. *Brain Injury, 18*(4), 331–350.

McCaffery, M., & Pasero, C. (1999). *Pain clinical manual* (2nd ed.). St. Louis, MO: Mosby.

Meeks, T., Dunn, L., Kim, D., Golshan, S., Sewell, D., Atkinson, J., et al. (2008). Chronic pain and depressin among geriatric psychiatry inpatients. *International Journal of Geriatric Psychiatry, 23*, 637–642.

Melzack, R. (1993). Pain: Past, present and future. *Canadian Journal of Experimental Psychology, 47*(4), 615–629.

Melzack, R., Coderre, T. J., Katz, J., & Vaccarino, A. L. (2001). Central neuroplasticity and pathological pain. *Annals of New York Academy of Science, 933*, 157–174.

Mitka, M. (2009). New focus on long-term mental health of patients who survive serious illness. *Journal of the American Medical Association, 302*(13), 1408–1409.

Mo, P. K., & Coulson, N. S. (2008). Exploring the communication of social support within virtual communities: A content analysis of messages posted to an online HIV/AIDS support group. *Cyberpsychology & Behavior: The Impact of the Internet, Multimedia and Virtual Reality On Behavior and Society, 11*(3), 371–374.

Murai, T., Muller, U., Werheid, K., Sorger, D., Reuter, M., Becker, T., et al. (2001). In vivo evidence for differential association of striatal dopamine and midbrain serotonin systems with neuropsychiatric symptoms in Parkinson's disease. *Journal of Clinical Neuroscience, 13*, 222–228.

Neese, J. B. (1991). Depression in the general hospital. *Nursing Clinics of North America, 26*(3), 613–622.

Nemeroff, C. B. (2004). Neurobiological consequences of childhood trauma. *Journal of Clinical Psychiatry, 65*(Suppl. 1) 18–28.

Palomaki, H., Kaste, M., Berg, A., Lonnqvist, R., Lonnqvist, J., Lehtihalmes, M., et al. (1999). Prevention of poststroke depression: 1 Year randomised placebo controlled double blind trial of mianserin with 6 month follow up after therapy. *Journal of Neurology, Neurosurgery and Psychiatry, 66*, 490–494.

Paten, S. B. (1999). Long-term medical conditions and major depression in the Canadian population. *Canadian Journal of Psychiatry, 44*(2), 151–157.

Polsky, D., Doshi, J. A., Marcus, S., Oslin, D., Rothbard, A., Thomas, N., et al. (2005). Long-term risk for depressive symptoms after a medical diagnosis. *Archives of Internal Medicine, 165*(11), 1260–1266.

Radley, J. J., Sisti, H. M., Has, J., Rocker, A. B., McCall, T., Hef, P. R., et al. (2004). Chronic behaviour stress induces apical dendritic reorganization in pyramidal neurons of the medial prefrontal cortex. *Neuroscience, 125*(1), 1–6.

Ren, K. (1994). Wind-up and the NMDA receptor: From animal studies to human pain. *Pain, 59*, 157–158.

Robinson, R. G. (2003). Poststroke depression: Prevalence, diagnosis, treatment, and disease progression. *Biological Psychiatry, 54*(3), 376–387.

Robinson, R, Schultz, S., Castillo, C., Kopel, T., Kosier, J.T., Newman, M. et al. (2000). Nortriptyline versus fluoxetine in the treatment of depression and in short-term recovery after stroke: A placebo controlled, double-blind study. *American Journal of Psychiatry, 157*, 351–359.

Rojo, A., Aguilar, M., Garolera, M. T., Cubo, E., Navas, I., & Quintano, S. (2003). Depression in Parkinson's disease: Clinical correlates and outcomes. *Parkinsonism Related Disorders, 10*(1), 23–28.

Rudy, T. E., & Turk, D. C. (1991). Psychological aspects of pain. *International Anesthesiology Clinics, 29*(1), 9–21.

Sosnowski, M. (1994). Pathophysiology of acute pain. *Pain Digest, 4*, 100–105.

Stratakis, C., & Chrousos, G. (1995). Neuro-endocrinology and pathophysiology of the stress system. *Annals of New York Academy of Science, 771*, 1–18.

Talbot, J. D., & Marrett, S. (1991). Multiple representations of pain in human cerebral cortex. *Science, 251*(4999), 1355–1358.

Turk, D. C. (2004). Understanding pain sufferers: The role of cognitive successes. *Spine Journal, 4*(1), 1–7.

Turk, D. C., & Feldman, C. S. (1992). Facilitating the use of non-invasive pain management strategies with the terminally ill. *Hospice Journal, 8*(1–12), 193–214.

Verdelko, A., Henon, H., Lebert, F., Pasquiere, F., & Leys, D. (2004). Depressive symptoms after stroke and relationship with dementia: A three year follow-up study. *Neurology, 62*(6), 905–911.

Von Korff, M., & Dunn, K. M. (2008). Chronic pain reconsidered. *Pain, 138*(2), 267–276.

World Health Organization, & World Organization of Family Doctors (2008). *Integrating mental health into primary care: a global perspective.* Geneva, Switzerland: WHO Press.

Zangen, A., Nakash, R., & Yadid, G. (1999). Serotonin-mediated increases in the extracellular levels of beta-endorphins in the arcuate nucleus and nucleus accumbens: A microdialysis study. *Journal of Neurochemistry, 73*(6), 2569–2574.

Forensic Psychiatric and Mental Health Nursing

Cindy Peternelj-Taylor

LEARNING OBJECTIVES

After studying this chapter, you will be able to:

- Describe the complexity of mental health challenges experienced by the forensic population.
- Examine the issues that are critical to the development of therapeutic relationships with forensic clients.
- Consider the challenges and opportunities that exist for nursing given the diversity of settings in which forensic nurses practice.
- Analyze the issues inherent in professional role development for nurses practicing with forensic clients.
- Evaluate the societal norms that affect contemporary care and treatment of forensic clients.
- Discuss the strategies for ongoing education, research, and practice development in forensic nursing.

KEY CONCEPTS

- custody and caring
- manipulation
- othering
- vulnerable

KEY TERMS

- boundary violations • compassionate release • dynamic security • forensic nursing • static security

---

*F*orensic nurses practice at the shifting interface of the criminal justice system and the health care system, and their ability to provide competent and ethical care is often compromised by social and political animosities regarding crime, criminality, and mental disorder. Regrettably, for a variety of reasons and life circumstances, a large number of vulnerable and at-risk individuals find themselves seeking health care under the auspices of the criminal justice system. It is no wonder that forensic nurses have been described as pioneers, exploring new horizons for nursing (Holmes, 2005).

As members of an emergent specialty of nursing, forensic nurses are responsible for providing care and treatment to forensic clients in a variety of secure institutional facilities, including jails, prisons, correctional facilities, young offender institutions, forensic psychiatric hospitals, and forensic psychiatric units within general hospitals. They are also involved in community-based court diversion schemes and CTOs, and they assist forensic clients with

reintegration into the community. This chapter, therefore, focuses on nursing care of individuals who have violated the law in some way: those remanded in custody while awaiting trial (charged but not yet sentenced); those who have been remanded in custody for a psychiatric evaluation; those who are found unfit to stand trial (UST) or not criminally responsible on account of a mental disorder; and those who have been charged, remanded in custody, and sentenced by the courts. A variety of terms are used to refer to this evolving specialty area of practice, including forensic psychiatric nursing, community forensic mental health nursing, and correctional or prison nursing. For simplicity, **forensic nursing** is used throughout this chapter and refers to nurses who integrate psychiatric and mental health nursing "philosophy and practice within a sociocultural context that includes the criminal justice system to provide comprehensive care to clients, families, and communities" (Peternelj-Taylor & Hufft, 2006, p. 379).

CRIMINALIZATION OF THE MENTALLY ILL

Throughout Canada, jails, prisons, and custodial facilities for youth in conflict with the law have become, by default, repositories for individuals with mental illness. In the past decade alone, the number of individuals with significant mental health needs within the federal correctional system in Canada has more than doubled. When compared to the general Canadian population, mental health problems are up to three times more common among federal correctional populations. Mental health services within correctional facilities have not kept up with this dramatic increase, and in many facilities, treatment is often non-existent or unsatisfactory when compared with the community standard (Office of the Correctional Investigator [OCI], 2005, 2007). This trend is also noted in the United States, where correctional institutions are commonly referred to as "primary mental health facilities" (Human Rights Watch, 2003) or the "new psychiatric hospitals" (Aufderheide & Brown, 2005). The criminalization of the mentally ill has frequently been attributed to the deinstitutionalization movement that occurred in the 1960s and the 1970s, and it continues today (Canadian Institute for Health Information [CIHI], 2008; Sealy & Whitehead, 2004; Statistics Canada, 2003). Unfortunately, the ongoing failure of provincial and federal governments to provide sufficient mental health funding to fully realize the goals of deinstitutionalization (e.g., independent living within the community) has resulted in a fragmented mental health system. Individuals who experience chronic mental illness are often well known by the police, the courts, jails, and correctional facilities. Critics conclude that for many individuals caught up in this web, their only crime is that they are "guilty of mental illness" (Kanapaux, 2004).

In the final report of the Standing Senate Committee on Social Affairs, Science, and Technology (2006), entitled *Out of the shadows at last: Transforming mental health, mental illness, and addiction services in Canada*, a mother whose son has bipolar disorder poignantly called the incarceration of mentally ill people in jails and prisons "cruel, unjust and ineffective"(p. 300). She stated:

> Prisons do not have adequate or appropriate facility resources or medical care to deal with the mentally ill. Poorly trained staff is unable to handle the difficulties of mental illness. The mentally ill suffer from illogical thinking, delusions, auditory hallucinations, paranoia, and severe mood swings. They do not always comprehend the rules of jails and prisons. They are highly vulnerable and prone to bizarre behavior that prison staff must deal with and inmates must tolerate (p. 300).

Her concerns regarding the lack of mental health services in Canadian jails and prisons are shared by many forensic health professionals.

THE PARADOX OF CUSTODY AND CARING

Forensic settings are controversial. They arouse strong convictions from various sectors who debate their proper place in society. Nursing practice within this domain is particularly complex because it brings together the "coupling of two contradictory socio-professional mandates: to punish and to provide care" (Holmes, 2005, p. 3). This paradox is disconcerting because a clear distinction between these two mandates is not always easily demarcated. Forensic settings provide society with two fundamental services: social necessities and social goods. Social necessities are considered essential to a community's existence; conversely, social goods are perceived as kindnesses, and although not necessarily essential, they are of benefit to the community nonetheless. Forensic settings meet their social necessity mandate through social control of those in their care. The protection of the community at large is perceived as a direct consequence of the processes of confinement and control. Forensic settings also provide social goods in the form of health care to those who are confined. In essence, forensic nurses are charged with the predicament of providing social good (e.g., health care) within institutions dedicated to the provision of social necessities (e.g., confinement) (Osborne, 1995; Peternelj-Taylor, 2004; Peternelj-Taylor & Johnson, 1995).

KEY CONCEPT Nurses in forensic settings must meet the competing demands of **custody** (confinement and security) **and caring** (nursing care).

This coexistence of social control and nursing care creates a paradox for nurses (Holmes, 2005, 2007), one that is laden with clinical issues and moral dilemmas not commonly encountered in more traditional health care settings. This paradox requires special attention and discernment because it permeates every aspect of forensic nursing. It is likely the single factor that differentiates forensic nursing from mental health nursing in a more general sense (Peternelj-Taylor, 2000) (Box 34-1). It is within this paradox, where the competing demands for custody and caring are embraced, that the moral climate of forensic institutions is shaped (Austin, 2001) (Fig. 34-1).

FORENSIC NURSING: A MODEL FOR CARE

Nurses working with forensic clients will find a familiar psychiatric and mental health nursing role, one that is "like 'stepping through the looking glass'—everything is the same, yet different" (Smith, 2005, p. 54). To illustrate

BOX 34.1

Research for Best Practice Nursing in Corrections: Comparing Canada and France

Holmes, D., Perron, A., & Michaud, G. (2007). Nursing in corrections: Lessons from France. Journal of Forensic Nursing, 4(3&4), 126–131.

THE PURPOSE: To compare nursing practice in corrections in France and Canada, particularly nurses' perceptions of their roles and ethical responsibilities toward inmates in their care and the ways in which nursing practice was balanced with security imperatives.

METHODS: Grounded theory, an inductive qualitative approach, was selected for this study. Data were obtained from RNs (employed in a correctional facility for at least 6 months) through semistructured interviews (23 in Canada; 15 in France). A continuous, systematic, constant comparative analysis was employed.

FINDINGS: Data analysis identified four categories: (1) Logics, (2) Socio-professional identity of nursing staff, (3) Description of prisoners, and (4) Interpersonal relationships among staff members. Although all categories were conceptually distinct, the researchers focused on "logics" as the core category. Logics represents the sociological scene evident in the data. In Canada, nurses work as both agents of care and agents of social control and, like all other socio-professional correctional employees, are responsible

for enforcing regulations. This lack of differentiation between health care and penal custody expresses itself daily in the attitudes and responsibilities of nurses. In contrast, French legislation separates the responsibilities of health care and corrections, making correctional nursing radically different in France. Although French nurses concluded that the paradoxical aims of health care and correctional ideologies make conflicts inevitable, optimum health care is achievable when one is independent, answering to only one hierarchy. In France, correctional nurses are answerable to a regional hospital versus correctional administration as is the case in Canada.

IMPLICATIONS FOR NURSING: This research reveals the ideological differences that exist in correctional health care between Canada and France. For French nurses, the distinct separation between correctional and health care ideologies and mandates facilitates the preservation of a professional nursing identity. The French model offers important insights regarding the restructuring of correctional health care services in Canada. The researchers conclude that, regardless of the ideological underpinnings of health care in corrections, ethical reflection is necessary to all milieus where issues of security (power and control) and the health care of vulnerable individuals coexist.

FIGURE 34.1 Custody and caring. (Courtesy of the Division of Media and Technology, University of Saskatchewan.)

the uniqueness of forensic nursing, a model of care is presented. It highlights the contextual and clinical practice issues affecting the articulation of a professional nursing role with forensic clients, regardless of setting. The five components of this model are the forensic client, nurse–client relationship, professional role development, treatment setting, and societal norms. Although each component of the model is discussed separately, in reality, the components are dynamic and interactive in nature. Peternelj-Taylor and Hufft (2006) conclude that health care goals must be consistent with the reality of

FIGURE 34.2 Forensic nursing: a model for care. (From Peternelj-Taylor, C. (2004). *NURS 486—Forensic Nursing in Secure Environments.* College of Nursing, University of Saskatchewan.)

the client's life circumstances, as well as the realities and the limitations of the setting in which nursing practice takes place. It may well be that not all forensic nurses will engage fully with each component of the model of care presented. However, the model as presented herein reflects the nature and scope of forensic nursing in Canada (Fig. 34-2).

Determinants of Health and the Forensic Client

As a group, forensic clients present with a multitude of long-neglected physical and mental health care challenges, often complicated by significant substance abuse problems. The health and psychosocial issues that they experience are often complex and multifaceted, contributing to the challenges encountered in their attempts to engage in treatment, relapse prevention, and reintegration. Frequently, their lives have been marked by illiteracy, poverty, and homelessness. Cultural minorities, in particular, are overrepresented in correctional institutions (Anno, Graham, Lawrence, & Shansky, 2004; Canadian Public Health Association [CPHA], 2004). Morbidity and mortality data suggest that those who are incarcerated experience higher rates of disease and disability when compared with nonincarcerated populations, which highlights the need for nursing leadership in primary, secondary, and tertiary levels of intervention (Box 34-2). As individuals, forensic clients often experience discrimination, stigmatization, and marginalization; they often lack supportive relationships commonly associated with emotional and mental well-being. And, they are totally dependent on the system (whether it is the correctional system or the health care system) to meet their health care needs. Given the magnitude of these commingling issues, many forensic clients are at risk for dual, multiple, and overlapping sources of vulnerability. Yet, referring to those who have committed crimes against society as "vulnerable" seems somewhat contrary to conventional wisdom (Peternelj-Taylor, 2005a).

Vulnerability and Vulnerable Populations

Broadly defined, vulnerability refers to a multifaceted concept that represents the commingling of resources, risk factors, and health status among a particular population or aggregate of people, which places them at risk for altered health status (de Chesnay, 2008). As a concept, vulnerability is generally understood in one of two ways, from an:

- Individual focus (vulnerability)—which is concerned with such notions as "susceptibility" or "at risk for health problems"; and from an

---

BOX 34.2

Health Status of Federally Incarcerated Individuals in Comparison to the General Canadian Population

CHARACTERISTICS OF INCARCERATED INDIVIDUALS

SOCIOECONOMIC MEASURES
- Twice as likely not to have finished high school
- Nine times as likely to have been unemployed

HEALTH BEHAVIOURS
- More than twice as likely to smoke
- Thirty times more likely to inject drugs
- Two to 10 times more likely to have an alcohol or substance abuse disorder

CHRONIC CONDITIONS
- 40% more likely to be treated for diabetes if male and three times more likely if female
- 68% more likely to be treated for cardiovascular conditions if male and more than two times more likely if female
- 43% more likely to be treated for asthma if male and almost three times more likely if female
- 50% more likely to need the use of mechanical aids

INFECTIOUS DISEASES
- More than twice as likely to have been infected with hepatitis B virus
- More than 20 times more likely to have been infected with hepatitis C virus
- More than 10 times more likely to have been infected with human immunodeficiency virus
- Much more likely to be infected with tuberculosis

MENTAL HEALTH DISORDERS
- More than twice as likely to have had a mental disorder
- Three times more likely to have schizophrenia in males and 20 times more likely in females
- Four times more likely to have a mood disorder

MORTALITY
- At a 45% increased risk for death
- Eight times more likely to die of homicide
- Almost four times more likely to die of suicide

From Canadian Public Health Association. (2004). *A health care needs assessment of federal inmates, 95*(Suppl.1), S49. Copyright 2004 by the Canadian Public Health Association. Reprinted with permission.

- Aggregate view (vulnerable populations)—which focuses on those with a greater than average risk of developing physical, psychological, or social health challenges by virtue of their marginalized status, limited access to resources, and personal characteristics (de Chesnay, 2008).

KEY CONCEPT Persons or populations are considered **vulnerable** when attributes, factors, or assigned status places them at greater risk for injury or poor health when compared with others.

Clearly, forensic clients represent a significant portion of society's at-risk population. As such, understanding the concepts of vulnerability and vulnerable populations is essential to contemporary forensic nursing practice. Nurses are positioned at the interface of vulnerability and as such are challenged to engage in partnerships that encourage growth in their clients (Michaels & Moffett, 2008).

Clients Experiencing Mental Illness

There is a great variation in the nature and severity of mental illnesses experienced by individuals who come into conflict with the law. In 1992, the Corrections and Conditional Release Act (Bill C-30) was proclaimed. This ended the Lieutenant Governor's Warrant System, whereby clients who were found "not guilty by reason of insanity" were held at the pleasure of the Lieutenant Governor for an unspecified period of time. It created review boards that are mandated to oversee the care and disposition of persons found UST or not criminally responsible on account of mental disorder (NCRMD; Statistics Canada, 2003). Under current Canadian law, an individual who comes into conflict with the law and is mentally ill can be found as follows:

- UST, when it is recognized that the accused is not fully capable of instructing legal counsel, or not capable of understanding the nature and the consequences of a trial (can later be found "fit" and tried in court and convicted, or deemed NCRMD).
- NCRMD, based on the accused person's mental state at the time the offence was committed. Although it is not a finding of guilt, the court may give the following dispositions: detention in hospital, conditional discharge, or an absolute discharge. Individuals detained in a hospital are not required to submit to treatment; the disposition is meant to detain the person and make care available. If treatment is required, owing to the individual's deteriorating mental status, treatment is then provided as per provincial or territorial mental health policies.
- In some jurisdictions, CTOs and Court Diversion are options that may be exercised to treatment programs

through community or provincial mechanisms, instead of going to trial (Statistics Canada, 2003).

In all cases, the mentally disordered offender challenges the collective wisdom of both the health care system and the criminal justice system, creating a "crossover" of sorts, particularly when the individual has been found responsible for his or her crimes despite the mental illness. The incarceration experience represents a significant stressful life event, even for those who do not have a mental disorder; separation from family and friends, limitations on privacy, overcrowding, and fear of assault severely affect the individual's quality of life. For those with mental illness, prisons are dangerous places; they are often victimized by other offenders; they are at greater risk for attempting suicide (including self-harming); and they are confined to segregation for their own protection. Unfortunately, such experiences can completely overwhelm the resources of individuals with mental illness. When compared with the individuals in the community, offenders experience greater rates of schizophrenia, depression, bipolar disorder, anxiety disorders, and substance abuse disorders (CIHI, 2008; CPHA, 2004; Phillips & Caplan, 2003).

In the 2005 report of the Correctional Investigator, a major overhaul of the existing mental health services provided by federal corrections was recommended, including: (1) comprehensive clinical intake assessment; (2) improvement to the existing treatment centres; (3) intermediate mental health units within existing penitentiaries to provide ongoing assessment and treatment; and (4) community mental health services to support offenders on conditional release (OCI, 2005). Although the Correctional Service of Canada has made strides in meeting these recommendations, failure to fully implement their approved mental health strategy continues to be identified as a major area of concern in the most recent report of the Correctional Investigator (OCI, 2007). Investing in assessment, treatment, and community supervision will not only contribute to the mental well-being of individual clients but also enhance public safety by maximizing safe reintegration into the community (OCI, 2007).

Not meeting this goal is to condemn far too many offenders to a life of going through a revolving door, repeatedly in and out of prison. If the goal of incarcerations is rehabilitation as well as public safety, this goal must be met (Standing Senate Committee on Social Affairs, Science, and Technology, 2006, p. 311).

Special Populations in the Forensic Setting

Although it could be argued that all forensic clients have special needs requiring the attention of special services and interventions by forensic nurses, groups more likely to require unique approaches include women, older adults, youth, cultural minorities, and families.

Female Forensic Clients

The past decade has seen a marked increase in the number of women confined to forensic settings; and even though women represent a small percentage of the overall forensic population, they currently account for its largest growth in Canada and other Western nations (Blanchette & Brown, 2006; CPHA, 2004). In general, the literature consistently reports that women most likely to find themselves within forensic settings are those who have grown up in poor communities, have limited education and job skills, and are the primary caregivers for dependent children. For many women, the fear of losing custody of their children is ever present (Blanchard, 2004; Blanchette & Brown, 2006; Harner, 2004; Maeve, 2003). Female forensic clients are frequently victims as well as perpetrators of crime, having experienced physical, emotional, and sexual abuse, as children and as adults, at the hands of fathers, husbands, boyfriends, acquaintances, and strangers (Green et al., 2005; Maeve, 2003; Peternelj-Taylor, 2005c). Aboriginal women are overrepresented within correctional systems. Nationally, Aboriginal people make up less than 3% of the Canadian population, but 32% of women in federal penitentiaries are Aboriginal (OCI, 2007). Unfortunately, their adaptation is complicated by forced separation from their family and community, creating significant barriers to timely reintegration into their home communities.

Common health concerns of incarcerated women include significant substance abuse problems; higher rates of blood-borne infections such as HIV, AIDS, and hepatitis B and C viruses; significant mental health concerns including anxiety-related disorders (e.g., posttraumatic stress disorder), concerns related to personality disorders (e.g., poor interpersonal functioning and self-injurious behaviours), and serious mental illness (including depression and schizophrenia); pregnancy and gynaecologic problems; obesity; and chronic disorders such as diabetes, hypertension, epilepsy, and respiratory diseases (CPHA, 2004; Green et al., 2005; Maeve, 2003; Peternelj-Taylor, 2005c; Roth & Pressé, 2003).

The Older Forensic Client

For an increasing number of older Canadians, growing old in a prison or in a forensic psychiatric facility is a harsh reality. Forensic clients are considered to be "older" (sometimes still termed, "elderly") if aged 50 or more years. The transformation to being "older" or "elderly" is thought to be accelerated by 10 to 12 years within this group of clients (Anno et al., 2004; Gallagher, 2001).

Depending on the nature of imprisonment or hospitalization, the individual may experience stressors related to general survival (particularly those who are incarcerated), coping with financial pressures, and withdrawal from drugs or alcohol, as well as the cumulative impact of high-risk behaviours, negative lifestyle practices, and inadequate health care, coupled with psychosocial issues related to confinement and isolation (Anno et al., 2004; Beckett, Peternelj-Taylor, & Johnson, 2003). Older forensic clients experience both physical and mental health care needs that set them apart from their younger counterparts, as well as those typical age-related problems experienced by their nonincarcerated peers. Common physical concerns evident in this population include cardiovascular diseases, pulmonary disorders, diabetes, arthritis, cancer, and Alzheimer's disease and other dementias. Common mental health needs include stress, social isolation, depression, and suicide (Beckett et al., 2003; CPHA, 2004; Correctional Services of Canada [CSC], 2005; World Health Organization, 2007).

The health care needs of older forensic clients clearly challenge traditional correctional resources and budgets, and questions related to the ability of correctional facilities to adequately care for older offenders are real (Beckett et al., 2003; Gallagher, 2001). For increasing numbers of older and infirm forensic clients, the fear of dying while confined is a terse reality. Although **compassionate release** to community-based long-term care facilities, known as *parole by exception* in Canada, is allowed under the Corrections and Conditional Release Act, ongoing fears about community safety, bed shortages in long-term care facilities, and the stigma surrounding the circumstances of the forensic client's hospitalization or incarceration are considered on an individual basis. This option, however, is available to only a very few long-term and infirm forensic clients, and palliative care within forensic settings is a poignant reality (Beckett et al.; Duggleby, 2005; Fowler-Kerry, 2003).

Youth

Youth who come into conflict with the law are a vastly underserved population with greater than average health care needs, and because of this, they are particularly vulnerable to adverse outcomes. Studies consistently show that rates of anxiety disorders, attention-deficit hyperactivity disorder (ADHD), depression, and substance abuse disorders are higher among youth in custody when compared to youth in the general population (CIHI, 2008). Frequently, their behavioural problems associated with their criminal charges mask their overall health care needs and thwart treatment efforts. It is not uncommon for youth who find themselves in custody to experience symptoms consistent with a wide array of mental health disorders, even though they may not have a formal diagnosis as such. Additionally, youth frequently demonstrate health patterns related to their family environments, as families commonly struggle with mental and physical health problems and substance abuse issues, and present with criminal histories and records (Shelton, 2000, 2001, 2004; Shelton & Pearson, 2005).

Canada holds the dubious honour of incarcerating more youth per capita than any other country in the Western world, including the United States (Department of Justice Canada, 2008). Aboriginal youth in particular are overrepresented among youth in custody at every stage of the Canadian criminal justice system. Latimer and Foss (2004) report that Aboriginal youth are almost eight times more likely to be in custody than their non-Aboriginal counterparts. Using a 1-day snapshot approach to data collection, the incarceration rate for Aboriginal youth during the data collection period was 64.5 per 10,000 population, whereas the incarceration rate for non-Aboriginal youth was 8.2 per 10,000. These figures are particularly alarming when one considers that Aboriginal youth represent about 5% of the Canadian population.

The mental health care concerns reported by Latimer and Foss (2004) are equally alarming and include high rates of fetal alcohol spectrum disorder, significant substance use issues, suicidal ideation, self-harm, and histories of attempted suicide and high rates of physical, sexual, and emotional abuse contributing to a large portion of the youth being involved with a child protection agency at the time of their admission.

Tragically, most forensic nurses will come into contact with youth through the criminal justice system because very few hospitals are set up to deal with the complexity of needs experienced by youth who come into conflict with the law. However, confinement in and of itself will not facilitate improvement in the mental health of this vulnerable group (Shelton, 2001), and intersectoral approaches, which bring together justice, law, social services, education, and health care, are necessary to address the complexity of issues facing at-risk youth.

Culturally Diverse Clients

The ethnic diversity of Canada as a whole is reflected in the demographic profile of Canadian forensic facilities. However, as might be predicted, clients representing ethnic and racial minorities are disproportionately represented (CPHA, 2004). Although Aboriginal people make up only 3% of Canada's adult population, they represent about 19% of the federal incarcerated population (OCI, 2007). Comparable rates of hospitalization in forensic settings operated by the health care system are unavailable.

Overrepresentation of Aboriginal people within the criminal justice system is attributed to a number of complex factors related to the effects of rapid culture change, cultural oppression, and marginalization (Kirmayer, Brass, & Tait, 2000), resulting in high rates of poverty, substance abuse, and victimization within families and communities of origin (CSC, 2005; Latimer & Foss, 2004). There has been a growing awareness among the health care and criminal justice systems of the need to provide culturally sensitive and appropriate programming. In the past, programs were developed on the assumption of sameness; this approach not only negated the forensic client's ethnic identity and culture of origin but also created barriers in the formation of therapeutic relationships and treatment programs, which ultimately interfered with successful community rehabilitation (Amellal, 2005; Hufft & Kite, 2003).

Families

In recent years, the needs of family members, the "forgotten clients" (Goldkuhle, 1999), have necessitated expanded roles for forensic nurses and community-based partnerships. Family members, children, and friends are a hidden forensic population; they are not accounted for and are rarely discussed by policy makers or health service providers. Incarceration has unintended consequences on families: higher rates of female-headed households, family disruption, family breakup, forced kinship care, and foster care (Freudenberg, Daniels, Crum, Perkins & Richie, 2005). The legacy of family violence is profound. Family members have often experienced various types of violence (e.g., child abuse, domestic violence, elder abuse), and children in particular are more likely to experience physical, emotional, and cognitive problems and engage in self-destructive patterns that increase their likelihood of spending time within the forensic system (i.e., prisons) when compared with children of nonincarcerated parents.

All too often, forensic nurses assess their clients in isolation of their support systems, home environments, and daily routines. This is problematic (Peternelj-Taylor, 2008). Creating a forensic family genogram is helpful when working with forensic clients (Kent-Wilkinson, 1999). A genogram is both an assessment and an intervention tool, one that can assist nurses in identifying individual and family patterns (e.g., mental health history, criminal behaviour, substance abuse) and contribute to more comprehensive assessments, interventions, and appropriate community referrals for family members (see Chapter 17 for information regarding genograms).

Collaborating with family members is critical to the safe reintegration of the forensic client into the community and is a role that is increasingly being embraced by forensic nurses, particularly those affiliated with community-based mental health programs. For instance, family caregivers can play a vital role in the provision of community care of older offenders with dementia (Encinares, 2007). Many factors affect the forensic client's care in, and readjustment to, the community, including family dynamics, stress, and the family's degree of involvement. It is not uncommon for families to experience guilt and remorse regarding the forensic client's criminal acts (Encinares & Lorbergs, 2001). In some cases, the behaviours of family members can sabotage treatment and reintegration plans, and nursing staff members often bear the brunt of sarcasm and hostility (Encinares & Golea, 2005).

Nurse–Client Relationship

Nursing by its very nature is relational; it is through the nurse–client relationship that nurses gain a deeper understanding and appreciation of the human condition. In fact, the ability to establish and maintain a therapeutic relationship with a forensic client is among the most important competencies required by forensic nurses (Peternelj-Taylor, 2002, 2004). In the forensic milieu, the emphasis of the therapeutic relationship as a primary intervention strategy is dependent on how the nurse's role is defined and on the context of the setting in which nursing practice takes place. For example, for forensic nurses practicing in an inpatient forensic psychiatric unit, working at a sex offender treatment program, or counselling HIV positive clients in a prison setting, the therapeutic relationship is fundamental to the identification and resolution of problems. In other areas of forensic nursing practice, for example, in an ambulatory care clinic in a correctional facility, the therapeutic relationship may be more in the background (Registered Nurses Association of Ontario, 2002, 2006). Regardless of the setting or the nature of the relationship, it cannot be assumed that a therapeutic relationship will be present, simply by virtue of one's nursing role (Peternelj-Taylor, 2004; Schafer & Peternelj-Taylor, 2003).

Engagement in a therapeutic relationship can be especially difficult for nurses when the client is accused (or convicted) of committing a morally reprehensible act. Clearly, some forensic clients possess characteristics that could easily evoke negative responses from their caregivers. They engage in threatening behaviours, they break rules and test boundaries, and they are unappreciative of nurses' efforts in providing health care (Austin, 2001; Schafer, 2002). Nurses, as members of society, are not immune to attitudes, beliefs, and stereotypes, and these may negatively colour their perceptions, their therapeutic responses, and their professional roles with forensic clients. The belief that every client has the potential to change and the right to treatment is one not shared by all forensic nurses (Peternelj-Taylor & Johnson, 1995; Rose, 2005). Martin (2001) warns that nurses "need to be cautious that their approach to patients does not reinforce the stigma and discrimination of the wider community" (p. 29).

To be successful, forensic nurses need to honestly and candidly explore their own preconceived ideas, attitudes, beliefs, and stereotypes regarding the forensic client. All too often, nurses can get caught up in the sensationalism that surrounds a particular forensic client (often fuelled by media hype), or the setting in which practice takes place, and ultimately they can lose sight of the person in need of care. Furthermore, it is not uncommon for nurses who are employed in forensic settings to experience additional stressors unique to their work, which ultimately affect their ability to establish and maintain therapeutic relationships with the clients in their care. Some examples are issues related to personal safety (i.e., threat of violence by forensic clients), ethical dilemmas, understaffing, secondary trauma and related posttraumatic stress disorder, and competing and conflicting expectations held between health care and correctional authorities (Holmes, 2005, 2007; Peternelj-Taylor, 2004).

Common Relationship Issues Experienced by Forensic Nurses

Although barriers to therapeutic relationships can be found in all areas of nursing, it is the "special circumstance" (Austin, 2001) of forensic settings, where the moral climate is shaped by the divergent and competing demands for custody and caring, that contributes to forensic settings being described as "hotbeds" for potential problems. This is in part due to the complexity of health care needs experienced by forensic clients, the seductive pull of helping and the intensity of relationships that can develop, the professional isolation experienced by forensic nurses, and the cultural and philosophical differences that exist between forensic clients, forensic nurses, and other members of the treatment team (Hufft & Kite, 2003; Peternelj-Taylor, 2002, 2005a; Schafer & Peternelj-Taylor, 2003). Forensic nurses, like all nurses, are moral agents, and as such, they are responsible for practicing ethically with the clients in their care, regardless of the setting in which care is provided (Canadian Nurses Association [CNA], 2008).

Othering

It is within these habitats of special circumstance that nurses meet forensic clients, and how the client is perceived is often illustrated by how nurses "language" their care. For example, are the clients seen as inmates, cons, psychopaths, murderers, psychos, or borderlines? Such labels not only evoke stereotypical images but also, more importantly, cast the individual into the role of the "other" (Peternelj-Taylor, 2004, 2005b). This negative form of engagement, known as *exclusionary othering*, can affect all aspects of nursing care and promote underinvolvement in a client's care. *Inclusionary othering*, on the other hand, is promoted as a way of learning about the other, as an individual, and not simply a crime or a label. One way of coming to know the forensic client is through role taking and trying to understand the world from the client's perspective. Although this may be a tall order when working with forensic clients, nurses can learn about othering by gaining an appreciation for what it means to be othered (Canales, 2000).

KEY CONCEPT Othering is about the way one perceives and engages with another person. It can be exclusionary and negative (i.e., the other is different from and thus "less than" me) or inclusionary and tolerant or accepting (i.e., the other is different from me, so I need to learn about his or her world view).

Boundary Violations

The complexities and uncertainties surrounding boundaries and **boundary violations** in practice can be difficult for forensic nurses to manage, leading to ongoing confusion in practice. The inability to differentiate the professional relationship from a social relationship by attempting to have one's personal needs met through the nurse–client relationship is consistently discussed as a precursor to boundary violations in the nursing literature (Peternelj-Taylor & Schafer, in press; Peternelj-Taylor & Yonge, 2003; Pilette, Berck, & Achber, 1995) (see Chapter 9). In forensic settings, nurses are often warned about getting "too close" to their patients, while at the same time painted as "victims of circumstances" when boundaries are transgressed with a forensic client. However, it is important to remember that, from an ethical perspective, the nurse is the one responsible for managing boundaries within the nurse–client relationship, not the client. Mixed messages regarding treatment boundaries can be especially disconcerting for forensic clients, who frequently have problems with boundaries in general.

Manipulation

The potential for manipulation is a very real factor in secure environments, one that requires thoughtful consideration by nurses in the provision of nursing care. In some cases, individuals in forensic settings will attempt to manipulate health care services for some secondary gain (e.g., medication, escape from the prison environment, social diversion), and issues pertaining to safety cannot be ignored (Peternelj-Taylor, 2004). As Austin (2001) notes, "cautioning, scepticism, and the questioning of patients' motives and actions, are part of the daily experience of forensic nurses" (Austin, p. 13).

KEY CONCEPT Manipulation is a concern in secure environments because it can involve the use of deceit to reach a goal that could not be pursued openly (e.g., escape).

However, when a forensic client is labelled a manipulator, nurses and others will generally respond more punitively and fail to engage the client in a therapeutic dialogue surrounding the meaning of his or her behaviours; as such, the opportunity for mutual problem solving, around the manipulative behaviours, is lost to the relationship (Peternelj-Taylor, 2004; Schafer, 2002). In short, forensic nurses need to be astutely aware that there exists the potential for manipulation in all interactions with forensic clients, and they need to find the right balance between assuming the worst and knowing that it can always happen (Smith, 2005).

Professional Role Development

Historically, role development for forensic nurses has been difficult, owing to the myth that nurses who work with forensic clients are "second class nurses" unable to secure employment elsewhere (Peternelj-Taylor & Johnson, 1995; Pullan & Lorbergs, 2001). During this time of a global nursing shortage, recruitment and retention of forensic nurses can be particularly challenging for both mental health care and correctional administrators (American Nurses Association, 2007; Pullan & Lorbergs, 2001). Given the breadth and scope of forensic nursing as illustrated within this chapter, it should be evident that forensic nurses are highly skilled and knowledgeable professionals, committed to the health and well-being of the clients in their charge, as well as the community at large.

Professional Nursing Identity

One of the greatest challenges that nurses experience when working in forensic environments is to remain true to their professional nursing roles and avoid being seduced or co-opted into assuming custodial roles, where expectations and responsibilities are more clearly defined (Holmes, 2007; Holmes & Federman, 2003, 2006; Maeve, 2003; Peternelj-Taylor & Johnson, 1995; Smith, 2005). In forensic settings operated by the criminal justice system, forensic nurses must have a strong nursing identity in order to maintain their professional authority and responsibility, without succumbing to the temptation to align themselves with the correctional staff. However, forensic nurses who work within the health care system should also heed this lesson, for they too can assume a more custodial stance, especially when they believe that CTOs or dispositions in hospital are lenient forms of punishment. So, even when the care of forensic clients is the responsibility of the health care system, incongruent attitudes among health care staff *may* prevail (Rose, 2005). Lawson (2005) states that when we "set ourselves up as judge and jury" (p. 149) we minimize our ability to be therapeutic.

Professional Development for Forensic Nurses

Petryshen (1981) published a classic paper entitled "Nursing the Mentally Disordered Offender." Since then, forensic nursing in Canada has undergone significant transformations in education, research, and practice developments related to the provision of nursing care to forensic clients.

Education

Forensic nursing content is slowly finding its way into undergraduate and graduate nursing curricula across the country, primarily through existing courses in psychiatric mental health or community health nursing. Kent-Wilkinson (2006) concludes that successful programs have often been pioneered by forensic nurse experts, based on their clinical and teaching experiences. Furthermore, technologic advances in nursing education have

contributed to the growth of this specialty as a result of opportunities inherent through online learning. For example, the College of Nursing, University of Saskatchewan, offers an online elective nursing course entitled *Forensic Nursing in Secure Environments* in its undergraduate baccalaureate program. Smith (2005) also supports the need for continuing professional development for nurses who practice in forensic settings, as a way of reinforcing the therapeutic identity of nurses, and thereby assisting them with nursing policy development.

Research

Canadian nurses have been writing about forensic nursing issues for many years, yet the literature remains largely theoretical and anecdotal, and forensic nursing research in Canada remains largely underdeveloped at this time. Embracing a research agenda with forensic clients will guide nursing practice in this highly specialized area; provide new insights into primary, secondary, and tertiary health care (including reintegration into the community); and contribute to nursing science through the advancement of nursing knowledge regarding vulnerable populations in general. The pursuit of an active research agenda is fundamental to keeping forensic nursing as a specialty alive and well (Peternelj-Taylor, 2000, 2005a).

Practice Developments

Although forensic nurses can find guidance in the Canadian Federation of Mental Health Nurses' (2006) *Canadian standards for psychiatric-mental health nursing*, standards to guide the unique needs of Canadian forensic mental health nurses are nonexistent. In July 2007, the Forensic Nurses Society of Canada was approved as an emerging special interest group by the CNA (see Web Links). The mandate of the Society is twofold: to provide a network for forensic nurses and to provide a forum to discuss evidence-based practice within the broad subspecialty areas of forensic nursing (such as interpersonal violence/sexual assault, legal nurse consulting, and death investigation) in addition to forensic mental health. Such recognition by the CNA is a formal recognition of forensic nursing as a specialty area; however, certification as a designated specialty remains uncertain (see Chapter 7).

Treatment Setting

Unlike more traditional practice settings, the interpersonal climate, organizational culture, and social context of forensic settings result in forensic environments being identified among the most severe and extreme environments known to society. Power, control, and implicit authority are manifested in the physical and interpersonal environments of both correctional systems and health care systems and can be incompatible with the achievement of treatment goals (Austin, 2001; Holmes, 2005; Phillips & Caplan, 2003).

Security Awareness

When working with forensic clients, issues surrounding safety and security are considered critical competencies, and nurses often struggle to find the right balance between their caring and custodial roles. The therapeutic treatment needs of their clients must always be considered within the context of maintaining security. Forensic settings (apart from community-based programs) are typically highly controlled environments, with the whereabouts of clients constantly monitored through a variety of institutional routines, mechanisms, rules, and regulations (Austin, 2001; Peternelj-Taylor & Johnson, 1995). Surveillance of staff and clients is deemed critical to the safe operation of all forensic facilities. Because of this, however, nursing staff members often experience additional stressors because they too are subject to the judgment of others: those who watch over are watched over in turn (Holmes, 2005). For example, in correctional environments, health care is not generally viewed as a priority, and nursing interventions are often poorly understood and viewed with suspicion (Smith, 2005).

Forensic nurses quickly become aware of two forms of security awareness: **static security** and **dynamic security**. Static security awareness includes such things as the structural or environmental artefacts common to secure environments, for example, the use of two-way radios, personal protection alarms, video monitoring, electronic door locks, internal barriers, and perimeter fences or walls. Dynamic security awareness, on the other hand, is concerned with institutional policies, staffing patterns, methods of operation, and relational security. Finding the right balance between the security needs of the forensic setting (and the community at large) and the client's treatment needs is a balancing act at best. Practical points for competent and safe practice are found in Box 34-3.

In forensic settings operated under the jurisdiction of the health care system (e.g., forensic psychiatric hospitals and forensic psychiatric units), forensic nurses assume broader roles in the maintenance of security. This can be particularly disconcerting because they may be expected to handcuff clients before a court visit, or search them for contraband before and after personal visits (or absences from the unit), while at the same time engage them in a therapeutic nurse–client relationship. This overt attention to custodial roles can jeopardize the fragility of the developing therapeutic relationship, and systems often need to be in place that see nurses from other units, or those not responsible for direct nursing care, to assist with these necessary custodial measures (Woods, 2004).

BOX 34.3

Tips for Security Awareness in Forensic Settings

- When working in institutional settings, never bring anything in or take anything out for a client, regardless of how insignificant the request may seem.
- Always let coworkers know your whereabouts at all times; interview clients in designated interview rooms, or in places visible to other staff members. When working in the community, always leave your itinerary, the anticipated length of your visits, and how you can be reached.
- Observe policies and procedures related to security awareness specific to the forensic setting in which you are working. Ask questions in order to understand the rationale behind the policies.
- Do not share personal information about yourself, or other staff members, with clients.
- Clients will sometimes engage in sexually inappropriate banter or gestures. Report this immediately, no matter how embarrassed you may be.
- Be aware of the location of staff members in relation to clients. Use a buddy system (e.g., another staff member) when uncomfortable approaching a client, especially when entering the client's living space.
- In all cases, open communication is critical to safe and competent nursing practice. Report all suspicious behaviours as soon as possible.

Risk Assessment and Management

Forensic nurses practicing in forensic settings work with clients with a proven capacity for violence. In recent years, risk assessment and management have become increasingly important competencies required of forensic nurses. Risk assessment is critical because it guides intervention and treatment. Simply stated, the greater the assessed risk, the higher the levels of intervention and supervision that are required; conversely, the lower the assessed risk, the lower the levels of intervention and supervision that are required, regardless of whether the forensic client is seeking treatment within a secure environment or a community treatment program (Woods, 2004). Although a detailed discussion of risk assessment and management is beyond the scope of this chapter, it is mentioned here because increasingly forensic nurses, with additional training and experience, are using actuarial (or statistical) tools and structured clinical judgment to formulate treatment plans that increasingly include risk assessment and management (Encinares & Golea, 2005; Encinares & Lorbergs, 2001; Encinares, McMaster, & McNamee, 2005). In a recent review of the literature, Woods and Lasiuk (2008) conclude that forensic nurses should integrate the use of empirically guided approaches to risk, including actuarial measures and structured clinical approaches, along with their own subjective qualitative clinical assessments.

◼◖ SOCIETAL NORMS

Humane care is defined by society, including the public, politicians, and the media (Mason, Lovell, & Coyle, 2008). The continual expansion of correctional facilities, however, reveals society's failure to address complex health and social issues. The Canadian Association of Elizabeth Fry Societies has declared "Women don't belong in cages: Prisons are the real crime" (see Web Links). There is a societal expectation that imprisonment will deter others from committing crimes, as well as contribute to community safety. This can mean that prisons are more readily funded than other strategies to deal with poverty, homelessness, and mental illness. The impact of interpersonal violence and illicit drug–related activities on individuals and communities is not sufficiently addressed, nor is the lack of health care services available to vulnerable and marginalized groups (Peternelj-Taylor, 2005c).

To understand the comprehensive needs of individuals whose lives have become enmeshed within the criminal justice system requires an understanding of both the individual and the social determinants of health that are associated with mental health, mental illness and delinquency, and criminal activity. Such an understanding provides for greater opportunities for the development of interventions and policies that may be effective at promoting mental health, preventing crime, and reducing the risk of repeat offending among those with a mental illness (CIHI, 2008; Foot, 2008). "Nursing is uniquely positioned to intervene with the socially significant health issues associated with crime, incarceration, and release" (Maeve, 2003, p. 39). Such interventions must be grounded in the conviction that caring for forensic clients as vulnerable members of society is the appropriate and decent thing to do.

SUMMARY OF KEY POINTS

▢ The provision of nursing care to individuals who have transgressed the law is a challenging and rewarding psychiatric and mental health nursing experience, one that balances the conflicting convictions of custody and caring.

▢ Components of care in forensic nursing include the forensic client, nurse–client relationship, professional role development, treatment setting, and societal norms.

▢ The ability to engage the forensic client in a therapeutic relationship is critical to competent forensic nursing care. Relationship issues experienced by forensic nurses include othering, boundary violations, and manipulation.

▢ Forensic nurses are uniquely situated to provide nursing care to forensic clients in a variety of community- and institution-based treatment settings.

▢ Intersectoral approaches, which bring together justice, law, social services, education, and health care, are deemed necessary to address the multitude of issues facing forensic clients, their families, and their communities.

CRITICAL THINKING CHALLENGES

1 In recent years, correctional facilities have experienced great challenges in caring for older and infirm forensic clients, and on occasion, clients are transferred to community-based long-term care facilities for compassionate reasons. What challenges might accompany the implementation of such a policy?

2 Canada has the dubious honour of incarcerating more youth than any other Western country. What are the implications of this phenomenon for forensic nurses?

3 The ability to engage the forensic client in a therapeutic relationship is a critical competency for forensic nurses. How might nurses overcome their negative reactions to a client who has committed a heinous crime?

4 The nursing profession as a whole has become more attune to the importance of boundaries in the therapeutic relationship. How would you approach a colleague who you suspected was struggling to maintain professional boundaries with a forensic client?

5 Working with forensic populations often brings nurses face to face with many complex health and social issues previously not considered. Given the fact that each and every forensic nurse is a member of many communities, how might a forensic nurse effect change at the community level?

WEB LINKS

www.ccsd.ca/cpsd/ccsd/index.htm "When kids flourish, crime doesn't" is the motto of Children and Youth: Crime Prevention Through Social Development, hosted by the Canadian Council on Social Development. The theory and practice of crime prevention through social development, current projects in this field, and opportunities for getting involved are presented.

www.csc-scc.gc.ca The Correctional Service of Canada (CSC) contributes to the protection of society by actively assisting offenders (with sentences of over two years) to become law-abiding citizens, while exercising safe, secure, and humane control. CSC's website is an excellent resource for policy, legislation, and research. There is access to various publications, including *Forum on Corrections Research*, and the corporate magazine *Let's Talk*.

www.usask.ca/nursing/custodycaring/index.htm
Since 1989, the College of Nursing, University of Saskatchewan, with the Regional Psychiatric Centre, CSC, has hosted a biennial, international nursing conference showcasing the contributions and concerns of forensic nurses.

www.elizabethfry.ca The Canadian Association of Elizabeth Fry Societies (CAEFS) is made up of 26 self-governing, community-based societies from across Canada that work with, and for, women and girls in the justice system, particularly those who are, or may be, criminalized. Through public education, research, and legislative reform, the CAEFS attempts to meet women's needs in the community and promote alternatives to incarceration.

www.forensicnurse.ca The Forensic Nurses' Society of Canada, an emerging special interest group of CNA, aims to provide a network for forensic nurses in Canada and a forum to discuss evidence-based practice unique to the diverse areas of forensic nursing in Canada.

www.iafn.org The International Association of Forensic Nurses (IAFN), founded in 1992, brought together nurses whose practice interfaced in someway with the law. In 1995, forensic nursing was officially recognized as a specialty area by the American Nurses Association (ANA) and, in 1997, the IAFN and the ANA published the *Scope and Standards of Forensic Nursing*. In 2005, the IAFN launched the *Journal of Forensic Nursing*.

www.johnhoward.ca The John Howard Society of Canada is an organization of provincial and territorial societies aimed at understanding and responding to problems of crime and the criminal justice system. Their motto "Effective, just and humane responses to the causes and consequences of crime" is actualized by advocacy, research, and community education.

www.justequipping.org/ Just.Equipping is a not-for-profit organization created in 2006/07, committed to educating, training, and equipping prison chaplains and workers in Restorative Justice. With Queens University, it offers an international diploma in Restorative Justice.

www.prisonersofage.com This website features photographs, interviews, and documentaries with older inmates and correctional personnel, conducted in Canadian and American prisons since 1996, providing a glimpse into their lives, crimes, and the challenges that they experience.

www.sfu.ca/crj/ The Centre for Restorative Justice at Simon Fraser University provides a wealth of information on restorative justice, including examples applicable to forensic nursing.

MOVIES, NOVELS, AND BIOGRAPHIES

100 Days of Freedom: 2006. This 1-hour documentary introduces three Canadian offenders released into the community after many years of incarceration: David, a former cocaine addict; Gloria, a former sex-trade worker and an addict; and Wayne, a former drug dealer and gang banger. This painful story illustrates the stark reality of their hopes and fears and their struggle to succeed.

VIEWING POINTS: Assisting clients with reintegration into the community is a forensic nursing role, but one that is not actualized in all forensic settings. What "red flags of caution" in relation to relapse are evident in their stories? How might risk assessment and risk management be used to facilitate successful reintegration?

Gothika: 2003. This supernatural thriller features Dr. Miranda Grey (Halle Berry), a respected criminal psychologist, who finds herself as a patient on the psychiatric unit of the penitentiary where she practices. Accused of killing her husband, her claims of innocence and loss of memory are seen by her former coworkers as a descent into madness. Although the tagline "You can't trust someone who thinks you're crazy" held promise for revealing aspects of therapeutic relationships in prison, portrayals of clients and settings are very stereotypical. The movie will no doubt contribute to the public's impression that individuals who are mentally ill are violent.

VIEWING POINTS: How do the nurses and other health care professionals interact with Dr. Grey and the other clients? What static and dynamic security measures are illustrated within the forensic psychiatric unit at Woodward Penitentiary for Women?

Dead Man Walking: 1995. This acclaimed film features the relationship between a death-row inmate, Matthew Poncelet (Sean Penn), and a local nun, Sister Helen Prejean (Susan Sarandon), whom he consults with for spiritual guidance in the days before his execution. The viewer experiences Prejean's personal distress as she attempts to reconcile her anti–death penalty views with the truth of Poncelet's brutal crimes and the pain of the victims' families and communities.

VIEWING POINTS: Although capital punishment was abolished in Canada in 1976, the film illustrates the conflicting convictions and dilemmas that nurses often experience when working with clients who have committed reprehensible crimes.

The Shawshank Redemption: 1994. This is a thought-provoking movie about prison life in the 1940s. The lead character, Andy Dufresne (Tim Robbins), is wrongfully convicted of killing his wife and her lover and is sentenced to two consecutive life terms. Although the harsh realities of prison culture, including the abuse of power, are brutally portrayed in this film, *The Shawshank Redemption* is really about the human spirit, friendship, and the redeeming nature of hope, as illustrated in the movie's tagline, "Fear can hold you prisoner. Hope can set you free."

VIEWING POINTS: Observe how the concept of institutionalization is illustrated within the movie. How might a forensic nurse use "hope" as an intervention strategy within his or her practice?

REFERENCES

Amellal, D. (2005, October). A diversified correctional approach. *Let's Talk*, *30*(2), 9–10. Retrieved August 1, 2008, from http://www.csc-scc.gc.ca/text/pblct/lt-en/2005/30–2/pdf/letstalk_30–2_e.pdf

American Nurses Association. (2007). *Corrections nursing: Scope & standards of practice*. Silver Spring, MD: Nursesbooks.org.

Anno, B. J., Graham, C., Lawrence, J. E., & Shansky, R. (2004). *Correctional health care: Addressing the needs of elderly, chronically ill, and terminally ill inmates* (Accession No. 018735). Washington, DC: National Institute of Corrections.

Aufderheide, D. H., & Brown, P. H. (2005, February). Crisis in corrections: The mentally ill in America's prisons. *Corrections Today*, *67*(1), 30–33.

Austin, W. (2001). Relational ethics in forensic psychiatric settings. *Journal of Psychosocial Nursing and Mental Health Services*, *39*(9), 12–17.

Beckett, J., Peternelj-Taylor, C., & Johnson, R. (2003). Growing old in the correctional system. *Journal of Psychosocial Nursing and Mental Health Services*, *41*(9), 12–18.

Blanchard, B. (2004). Incarcerated mothers and their children: A complex issue. *Forum on Correctional Research*, *16*(1), 45–46.

Blanchette, K., & Brown, S. L. (2006). *The assessment and treatment of women offenders: An integrative perspective*. Chichester, UK: John Wiley & Sons.

Canadian Federation of Mental Health Nurses. (2006). *Canadian standards for psychiatric-mental health nursing* (3rd ed.). Toronto, ON: Author.

Canadian Institute for Health Information. (2008). *Improving the health of Canadians: Mental health, delinquency and criminal activity*. Ottawa, ON: Author. Retrieved August 7, 2008, from http://www.cmha.ca/data/1/rec_docs/1771_mh_crime_full_report_apr11_08_e.pdf

Canadian Public Health Association. (2004). *A health care needs assessment of federal inmates*, *95*(Suppl. 1), S1–S63.

Canales, M. K. (2000). Othering: Toward an understanding of difference. *Advances in Nursing Science*, *22*(4), 16–31.

Correctional Services of Canada. (2005, February). *Issues and challenges facing CSC*. Retrieved August 1, 2008, from http://www.csc-scc.gc.ca/text/pblct/sb-go/pdf/sb-go-eng.pdf

de Chesnay, M. (2008). Vulnerable populations: Vulnerable people. In M. de Chesnay & B. A. Anderson (Eds.), *Caring for the vulnerable: Perspectives in nursing theory, practice and research* (2nd ed., pp. 3–14). Sudbury, MA: Jones & Bartlett.

Department of Justice Canada. (2008). *Why did the government introduce new youth justice legislation?* Retrieved August 1, 2008, from http://www.justice.gc.ca/eng/pi/yj-jj/ycja-lsjpa/why-pourq.html

Duggleby, W. (2005). Fostering hope in incarcerated older adults. *Journal of Psychosocial Nursing and Mental Health Services*, *43*(9), 15–20.

Encinares, M. (2007). Mental health forum: Community care of elderly offenders with dementia. *Journal of Chinese Clinical Medicine*, *2*(1), 34–41.

Encinares, M., & Golea, G. (2005). Client centered-care for individuals with dual diagnoses in the justice system. *Journal of Psychosocial Nursing and Mental Health Services*, *43*(9), 29–36.

Encinares, M., & Lorbergs, K. (2001). Framing nursing practice within a forensic outpatient service. *Journal of Psychosocial Nursing and Mental Health Services*, *39*(9), 35–41.

Encinares, M., McMaster, J. J., & McNamee, J. (2005). Risk assessment of forensic patients: Nurses' role. *Journal of Psychosocial Nursing and Mental Health Services*, *43*(3), 30–36.

Foot, R. (2008, January). Inmates lack services, training before being released: report. *Canwest News Services*. Retrieved August 25, 2008, from http://www.canada.com/topics/news/national/story.html?id=51626f1c-83bf-4585-be28–82a88aa73f05

Fowler-Kerry, S. (2003). Palliative care within secure forensic environments. *Journal of Psychiatric and Mental Health Nursing*, *10*, 367–369.

Freudenberg, N., Daniels, J., Crum, M., Perkins, T., & Ritchie, B. E. (2005). Coming home from jail: The social and health consequences of community reentry for women, male adolescents, and their families. *American Journal of Public Health*, *95*(10), 1725–1726.

Gallagher, E. M. (2001). Elders in prison: Health and well-being of older inmates. *International Journal of Law and Psychiatry*, *24*, 325–333.

Goldkuhle, U. (1999). Professional education for correctional nurses: A community-based partnership model. *Journal of Psychosocial Nursing and Mental Health Services*, *37*(9), 38–44.

Green, B. L., Miranda, J., Daroowalla, A., & Siddique, J. (2005). Trauma exposure, mental health functioning, and program needs of women in jail. *Crime & Delinquency*, *51*, 133–151.

Harner, H. M. (2004). Relationships between incarcerated women: Moving beyond stereotypes. *Journal of Psychosocial Nursing*, *42*(1), 38–46.

Holmes, D. (2005). Governing the captives: Forensic psychiatric nursing in corrections. *Perspectives in Psychiatric Care*, *41*(1), 3–13.

Holmes, D. (2007). Nursing in corrections: Lessons from France. *Journal of Forensic Nursing*, *3*(3&4), 126–131.

Holmes, D., & Federman, C. (2003). Constructing monsters: Correctional discourse and nursing practice. *International Journal of Psychiatric Nursing*, *8*(1), 942–962.

Holmes, D., & Federman, C. (2006). Organizations as evil structures. In T. Mason (Ed.), *Forensic psychiatry: Influences of evil* (pp. 15–30). Totowa, NJ: Humana Press.

Hufft, A., & Kite, M. M. (2003). Vulnerable and cultural perspectives for nursing care in correctional systems. *Journal of Multicultural Nursing & Health*, *9*(1), 18–26.

Human Rights Watch. (2003). *Ill equipped: U.S. prisons and offenders with mental illness*. New York, NY: Author. Retrieved August 1, 2008, from http://www.hrw.org/reports/2003/usa1003

Kanapaux, W. (2004). Guilty of mental illness. *Psychiatric Times*, *XXI* (1). Retrieved October 17, 2005, from http://www.psychiatrictimes.com/p040101a.html

Kent-Wilkinson, A. (1999). Forensic family genogram: An assessment and intervention tool. *Journal of Psychosocial Nursing and Mental Health Services*, *37*(9), 52–56.

Kent-Wilkinson, A. (2006). Forensic nursing education: Developments, theoretical conceptualizations, and practical applications for curriculum. In R. M. Hammer, B. Moynihan, & E. M. Pagliaro (Eds.), *Forensic nursing: A handbook for practice* (pp. 781–820). Sudbury, MA: Jones & Bartlett.

Kirmayer, L. J., Brass, G. M., & Tait, C. L. (2000). The mental health of Aboriginal peoples: Transformations of identity and community. *Canadian Journal of Psychiatry*, *45*(7), 607–616.

Latimer, J., & Foss, L. C. (2004, February). *A One-Day Snapshot of Aboriginal Youth in Custody Across Canada: Phase II*. Ottawa, ON: Department of Justice Canada. Retrieved August 1, 2008, from http://canada.justice.gc.ca/eng/pi/rs/rep-rap/2004/yj2-jj2/yj2.pdf

Lawson, L. (2005). Furthering the search for truth and justice. *Journal of Forensic Nursing*, *1*(4), 149–150.

Maeve, K. M. (2003). Nursing care partnerships with women leaving jail: Effects on health and crime. *Journal of Psychosocial Nursing and Mental Health Services*, *41*(9), 30–40.

Martin, T. (2001). Something special: Forensic psychiatric nursing. *Journal of Psychiatric and Mental Health Nursing*, *8*, 25–32.

Mason, T., Lovell, A., & Coyle, D. (2008). Forensic psychiatric nursing: Skills and competencies: I role dimensions. *Journal of Forensic and Mental Health Nursing*, *15*, 118–130.

Michaels, C., & Moffett, C. (2008). Rethinking vulnerability. In M. de Chesnay & B. A. Anderson (Eds.), *Caring for the vulnerable: Perspectives in nursing theory, practice and research* (2nd ed., pp. 15–24). Sudbury, MA: Jones & Bartlett.

Office of the Correctional Investigator. (2005). *Annual report of the Correctional Investigator 2004–2005*. Retrieved August 1, 2008, from http://www.oci-bec.gc.ca/reports/pdf/AR200405_e.pdf

Office of the Correctional Investigator. (2007). *Annual report of the Correctional Investigator 2006–2007*. Retrieved August 7, 2008, from http://www.oci-bec.gc.ca/reports/pdf/AR200607_e.pdf

Osborne, O. (1995). Public sector psychosocial nursing. *Journal of Psychosocial Nursing and Mental Health Services*, *33*(8), 4–6.

Peternelj-Taylor, C. (2000). The role of the forensic nurse in Canada: An evolving specialty. In D. Robinson & A. Kettles (Eds.), *Forensic nursing and multidisciplinary care of the mentally disordered offender* (pp. 192–212). London, UK: Jessica Kingsley Publishers.

Peternelj-Taylor, C. (2002). Professional boundaries: A matter of therapeutic integrity. *Journal of Psychosocial Nursing and Mental Health Services, 40*(4), 22–29.

Peternelj-Taylor, C. (2004). An exploration of othering in forensic psychiatric and correctional nursing. *Canadian Journal of Nursing Research, 36*(4), 130–146.

Peternelj-Taylor, C. (2005a). Conceptualizing nursing research with offenders: Another look at vulnerability. *International Journal of Law and Psychiatry, 28*, 348–359.

Peternelj-Taylor, C. (2005b). Engaging the "other." *Journal of Forensic Nursing, 1*(4), 179, 191.

Peternelj-Taylor, C. (2005c). "Ordinary" women, extraordinary life circumstances. *Journal of Forensic Nursing, 1*(2), 84–85.

Peternelj-Taylor, C. (2008). Pregnancy, childbirth and mothering: A forensic nursing response. *Journal of Forensic Nursing, 4*(2), 53–54.

Peternelj-Taylor, C. A., & Hufft, A. G. (2006). Forensic nursing. In W. K. Mohr (Ed.), *Psychiatric-mental health nursing* (6th ed., pp. 377–393). Philadelphia, PA: Lippincott Williams & Wilkins.

Peternelj-Taylor, C., & Johnson, R. (1995). Serving time: Psychiatric mental health nursing in corrections. *Journal of Psychosocial Nursing and Mental Health Services, 33*(8), 12–19.

Peternelj-Taylor, C., & Schafer, P. (2008). Management of therapeutic boundaries. In A. Kettles, P. Woods, & R. Byrt (Eds.), *Forensic mental health nursing: Capabilities, roles and responsibilities* (pp. 309–331). London, UK: Quay Books.

Peternelj-Taylor, C., & Yonge, O. (2003). Exploring boundaries in the nurse-client relationship: Professional roles and responsibilities. *Perspectives in Psychiatric Care, 39*(2), 55–66.

Petryshen, P. (1981). Nursing the mentally disordered offender. *Canadian Nurse, 77*(6), 26–28.

Phillips, R. T. M., & Caplan, C. (2003). Administrative and staffing problems for psychiatric services in correctional and forensic settings. In R. Rosner (Ed.), *Principles and practice of forensic psychiatry* (2nd ed., pp. 505–512). New York, NY: Chapman & Hall.

Pilette, P. C., Berck, C. B., & Achber, L. C. (1995). Therapeutic management of helping boundaries. *Journal of Psychosocial Nursing and Mental Health Services, 33*(1), 40–47.

Pullan, S. E., & Lorbergs, K. A. (2001). Recruitment and retention: A successful model in forensic psychiatric nursing. *Journal of Psychosocial Nursing and Mental Health Services, 39*(9), 18–25.

Registered Nurses Association of Ontario. (2002). *Establishing therapeutic relationships*. Toronto, ON: Author. Retrieved August 1, 2008, from http://www.rnao.org/Storage/15/936_BPG_TR_Rev06.pdf

Registered Nurses Association of Ontario. (2006). *Establishing therapeutic relationships: Supplement*. Toronto, ON: Author. Retrieved August 1, 2008, from http://www.rnao.org/Storage/15/936_BPG_TR_Rev06.pdf

Rose, D. (2005). Respect for patient autonomy. *Journal of Forensic Nursing, 1*(1), 23–27.

Roth, B., & Pressé, L. (2003). Nursing interventions for parasuicidal behaviors in female offenders. *Journal of Psychosocial Nursing and Mental Health Services, 41*(9), 20–29.

Schafer, P. E. (2002). Nursing interventions and future directions with patients who constantly *break rules and test boundaries*. In A. M. Kettles, P. Woods, & M. Collins (Eds.), *Therapeutic interventions for forensic mental health nurses* (pp. 56–71). London, UK: Jessica Kingsley Publishers.

Schafer, P. E., & Peternelj-Taylor, C. (2003). Therapeutic relationships and boundary maintenance: The perspective of forensic patients enrolled in a treatment program for violent offenders. *Issues in Mental Health Nursing, 24*, 605–625.

Sealy, P., & Whitehead, P. C. (2004). Forty years of deinstitutionalization of psychiatric services in Canada: An empirical assessment. *Canadian Journal of Psychiatry, 49*(4), 249–257.

Shelton, D. (2000). Health status of young offenders and their families. *Journal of Nursing Scholarship, 32*(2), 173–178.

Shelton, D. (2001). Emotional disorders in young offenders. *Journal of Nursing Scholarship, 33*(3), 259–263.

Shelton, D. (2004). Experiences of detained young offenders in need of mental health care. *Journal of Nursing Scholarship, 36*(2), 129–133.

Shelton, D., & Pearson, G. (2005). ADHD in juvenile offenders: Treatment issues nurses need to know. *Journal of Psychosocial Nursing and Mental Health Services, 43*(9), 38–46.

Smith, S. (2005, February). Stepping through the looking glass: Professional autonomy in correctional nursing. *Corrections Today*, 54–56, 70.

Standing Senate Committee on Social Affairs, Science and Technology. (2006, May). *Out of the shadows at last: Transforming mental, mental illness and addiction services in Canada*. Retrieved August 7, 2008, from http://www.parl.gc.ca/39/1/parlbus/commbus/senate/com-e/soci-e/rep-e/rep02may06-e.htm

Statistics Canada. (2003). *Special study on mentally disordered accused and the criminal justice system*. Canadian Centre for Justice Studies (no. 85-559-XIE). Ottawa, ON: Ministry of Industry. Retrieved August 1, 2008, from http://www.statcan.ca/english/freepub/85-559-XIE/85-559-XIE2002001.pdf

Woods, P. (2004). The person who uses forensic mental health services. In I. Norman & I. Ryrie (Eds.), *The art and science of mental health nursing: A textbook of principles and practice* (pp. 594–623). Maidenhead, UK: Open University Press.

Woods, P., & Lasiuk, G. (2008). Risk prediction: A review of the literature. *Journal of Forensic Nursing, 4*(1), 1–11.

World Health Organization. (2007). *Preventing suicide in jails and prisons*. Retrieved August 11, 2008, from http://www.who.int/mental_health/prevention/suicide/resource_jails_prisons.pdf

UNIT *VIII*

Care Challenges in Psychiatric and Mental Health Nursing

Stress, Crisis, and Disaster Management

Gerri Lasiuk

Adapted from the chapter "Stress, Crisis, and Disaster Managment" by Lorraine D. Williams and Mary Ann Boyd

LEARNING OBJECTIVES

After studying this chapter, you will be able to:

- Discuss the evolution of our current understanding of stress as a response, as a stimulus, and as a transaction.
- Use the transactional model to assess individuals' stress, adaptation, and coping abilities.
- Differentiate problem-focused and emotion-focused coping.
- Define *stress, crisis,* and *disaster*; compare and contrast each of these with a psychiatric emergency.

KEY CONCEPTS

- coping
- crisis
- disaster
- stress

KEY TERMS

•allostasis •allostatic load •bereavement •cognitive appraisal •dissupport •emotion-focused coping •emotions •grief •homeostasis •mourning •person-environment relationship •problem-focused coping •reappraisal •social functioning •social network •social support •stress-diathesis model •stressors

*A*lthough stress has been the focus of considerable scientific, clinical, and general interest over the past century, most of us would be hard-pressed to explain what it is. As Selye (1980, p. 127) quipped, "stress, like relativity, is a scientific concept which has suffered the mixed blessing of being too well known, and too little understood." This chapter explores the concepts of stress, crisis, and disaster and describes how nurses can use the nursing process to identify and address the needs of individuals experiencing these events.

STRESS

Evolving Understandings of the Concept of Stress

The word *stress* has its roots in the Latin word *stringere*, meaning to draw tight (Cooper & Dewe, 2004), and the Middle English word *stresse*, which refers to hardship or distress (Harper, 2001). Some believe that the idea of stress as hardship evolved through the 18th and 19th centuries to mean force, pressure, or strain; this may explain why, prior to the middle of the last century, stress was a term used almost solely by engineers. The early decades of the 20th century saw the rise of *psychosomatic medicine*, a movement fuelled by a reaction to the prevailing view of the body as a machine (Cooper & Dewe). Proponents of psychosomatic medicine believed that a mechanistic model was too reductionistic and could not explain the role of the mind and spirit in health and illness. It was in this context that the concept of stress as hardship was taken up by biological and social scientists as a possible explanation of disease and illness (Bartlett, 1998). Throughout the last century, our understanding of stress evolved through three distinct periods in which it was conceptualized as a physiological response, as a stimulus, and finally, as a transaction.

853

Stress as a Response

Walter Cannon and Hans Selye, two pioneers in the study of stress, both conceptualized stress as a response to changing environmental conditions. Cannon (1939), a noted Harvard physiologist, is considered by many to be the father of modern stress research. In his book *The Wisdom of the Body*, he coined the term **homeostasis** to describe the body's ability to maintain a stable internal environment despite changing environmental conditions. His thesis was that environmental changes are perceived as threats to personal integrity or safety and signal a compensatory response mediated by the sympathetic branch of the autonomic nervous system (ANS). He also believed that strong **emotions** like fear and anger are fundamental to the stress response and have evolved because of their high survival value. "Fear," he wrote, "has become associated with the instinct to run, to escape; and anger or aggressive feeling, with the instinct to attack" (p. 227). This notion, later dubbed the *fight or flight* response, remains a key concept in any discussion of stress.

Working at McGill University in Montreal, Selye (1956, 1974) developed his general adaptation syndrome (GAS). Selye differentiated stress (a nonspecific response of the body to any demand placed on it) from **stressors** (events that initiate the response) and argued that stressors can be physical (e.g., infection, intense heat or cold, surgery, debilitating illnesses), psychological (e.g., psychological trauma, interpersonal problems), or social (e.g., lack of social support). They can also be short-term (acute) or long-term (chronic). According to Selye, the perception of a stressor triggers an automatic, total-body response. The first stage of this response is the *alarm reaction*, during which virtually all body systems (e.g., sense organs, brain, heart and blood vessels, lungs, digestive system, immune system) respond in a coordinated effort to mediate the stressor. If this effort is successful, the body returns to its normal state. If, on the other hand, the stressor continues for hours or days, the organism moves into the *stage of resistance*, and efforts to adapt to the stressor continue. In circumstances in which the stressor is ongoing or extreme, the body moves into the *stage of exhaustion*, during which the individual's resources deplete, and exhaustion and death ensue. Selye hypothesized that many diseases, including hypertension, peptic ulcer, and autoimmune illnesses, are caused by prolonged adaptive reactions in which corticosteroids play a pathogenic role.

Although Selye made significant contributions to our understanding of human stress, he was criticized for his notion that stress is a nonspecific response to diverse environmental stimuli. Selye's challengers (e.g., Mason, 1971; Mikhail, 1981) pointed out that many neuroendocrine responses are not general at all but very specific.

They further argued that all stressors do not necessarily produce the same response in every individual; what is a stressor for one person may not be a stressor for another (Lazarus & Folkman, 1984). The conceptualization of stress solely as a response was also criticized for its circular reasoning (i.e., an event is stressful because it elicits a stress response).

Stress as a Stimulus

Those who conceptualized stress as a stimulus (e.g., Dohrenwend & Dohrenwend, 1974; Holmes & Rahe, 1967) viewed it as an event that elicits a stress response (however that is defined). In this approach to understanding stress, researchers looked for associations between significant life events (e.g., marriage, divorce, relocation, death) and stress. One of the most widely used tools in this type of research is the Recent Life Changes Questionnaire (RLCQ; Holmes & Rahe; see Table 35-1). A major problem with this conceptualization of stress is that stimuli (i.e., stressors) can be identified only in retrospect, that is, only after a response occurs. Other criticisms are that it does not take into consideration the meaning an individual assigns to an item, their coping abilities, or the implications of chronic or recurrent events (see Jones & Kinman, 2001).

The mid-1970s to the early 1990s was a critical period in stress research. During this time, a debate raged in the literature between two camps of stress researchers. One group favoured the view that critical life events (i.e., the presence of an objective event) mediate the experience of stress. Supporters "urged researchers to measure pure events, uncontaminated by perceptions, appraisals, or reactions" (Dohrenwend & Shrout, 1985, p. 782). On the other side, Richard Lazarus and his colleagues (Lazarus, DeLongis, Folkman, & Gruen, 1985) maintained that it is the appraisal of an event (i.e., the subjective evaluation of an event or situation) that is critical to the stress experience. Although the debate centred on measurement and other methodological problems, Lazarus (1999) later wrote that what was at issue was the fundamental nature of stress and the **person–environment relationship**. In the end, the latter group prevailed, and the view of stress as a relationship between the person and his or her environment has become the dominant explanatory model.

Stress as a Transaction between Person and Environment

In their seminal work, *Appraisal and Coping*, Lazarus and Folkman (1984) conceptualized stress as resulting from a perceived imbalance between an individual's resources and the demands placed on them. In their

Table 35.1	Recent Life Changes Questionnaire	
Social Area	**Life Changes**	**LCU Values***
Family	Death of spouse	105
	Marital separation	65
	Death of close family member	65
	Divorce	62
	Pregnancy	60
	Change in health of family member	52
	Marriage	50
	Gain of new family member	50
	Marital reconciliation	42
	Spouse begins or stops work	37
	Son or daughter leaving home	29
	In-law trouble	29
	Change in number of family get-togethers	26
Personal	Jail term	56
	Sex difficulties	49
	Death of a close friend	46
	Personal injury or illness	42
	Change in living conditions	39
	Outstanding personal achievement	33
	Change in residence	33
	Minor violations of the law	32
	Begin or end school	32
	Change in sleeping habits	31
	Revision of personal habits	31
	Change in eating habits	29
	Change in church activities	29
	Vacation	29
	Change in school	28
	Change in recreation	28
	Christmas	26
Work	Fired at work	64
	Retirement from work	49
	Trouble with boss	39
	Business readjustment	38
	Change to different line of work	38
	Change in work responsibilities	33
	Change in work hours or conditions	30
Financial	Foreclosure of mortgage or loan	57
	Change in financial state	43
	Mortgage (home, car, etc)	39
	Mortgage or loan less than $10,000 (stereo, etc)	26

Directions: Total the LCUs for your life change events during the past 12 months.

250 to 400 LCUs per year: Minor life crisis

More than 400 LCUs per year: Major life crisis

*LCU, Life change unit. The number of LCUs reflects the average degree or intensity of the life change.

Source: From Rahe, R. H. (2000). Recent Life Changes Questionnaire (RLCQ) (1997). In T. H. Holmes, American Psychiatric Association. Task Force for the Handbook of Psychiatric Measures. *Handbook of psychiatric measures* (pp. 235–237). Washington, DC: American Psychiatric Association,

transactional model, stress depends on how a stressor is appraised in relation to the individual's resources for coping with it. The central premise is that stress is "neither an environmental stimulus, a characteristic of the person, nor a response, but a relationship between demands and the power to deal with them without unreasonable or destructive costs" (Coyne & Holroyd, 1982, p. 108).

Cognitive Appraisal

Lazarus and Folkman (1984) use the term **cognitive appraisal** to describe the process an individual uses to examine the demands and constraints of a situation in relation to his or her personal resources. Cognitive appraisal has two levels—primary and secondary. In primary appraisal, the individual evaluates the situation and

A.   Demands   Resources

A good balance between demands and resources implies modest amounts of stress or not stress.

B.   Demands

Resources

High demands with few resources can result in a high stress balance.

Resources

C.

Demands

A low stress balance, which could imply boredom.

FIGURE 35.1 Lazarus's (1999) seesaw analogy of stress (with permission).

determines whether he or she is in danger. If the answer is yes, the individual goes on to secondary appraisal, during which he or she considers the options for dealing with the situation. As stated earlier, in this model, stress is the perception of threat or harm (primary appraisal) for which an individual has no effective response (secondary appraisal). Figure 35-1 depicts Lazarus's (1999, p. 59) seesaw analogy illustrating stress as a balance between environmental demands and personal resources.

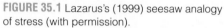

KEY CONCEPT   Stress is the relationship between the person and the environment that is appraised as exceeding the person's resources and endangering his or her well-being.

Environment and Person Variables That Influence Appraisal

A strength of the transactional model of stress (Lazarus & Folkman, 1984) is its ability to account for why individuals will react differently to the same situation or event. According to Lazarus (1999), this is because appraisal is influenced by unique interactions of environment and person variables. *Environment variables* include demands, constraints, opportunity, and culture. Demands are all of the stated and unstated rules that define acceptable behaviour, social conventions, expressing correct attitudes, and enacting role expectations. While demands prescribe what we should do, constraints delineate what we must not do. A third environment variable that affects appraisal is opportunity, that is, the insight or wisdom that enables us to recognize "the right action at the right moment" (Lazarus, p. 63). Finally, because culture imbues all aspects of life with meaning, it is a major influence in how we perceive and interpret our environment. *Individual variables* shaping appraisal are our goals and our level of commitment to those goals, beliefs about our self and the world, and personal resources (e.g., intelligence, interpersonal skills, education, social support, health, energy, money).

Person–Environment Relationship

Overall, the *person–environment relationship* is a dynamic interaction between a person and his or her environment. It is assumed that an individual brings to every event or situation beliefs, values, attitudes, and behaviours developed over a lifetime under the influence of genetic, personal, social, and environmental factors. These contribute to a worldview and shape the meaning, value, and significance ascribed to a particular situation or event. This explains why two individuals may perceive and react very differently to the same circumstances.

The Role of Positive Self-Perceptions

As discussed earlier, an individual's beliefs about himself or herself and the world are personal variables that influence stress. Research suggests that an individual's sense of self as well as his or her social and emotional resources can protect against the negative effects of stress (Taylor, Kemeny, Reed, Bower, & Gruenewald, 2000). One of these resources is termed *positive illusions*, a form of overly positive self-perceptions, illusions of personal control, and unrealistic optimism about the future. In a study that examined the relationship between positive beliefs and disease progression among a group of men infected with HIV, it was found that even unrealistically optimistic beliefs about the future and the ability to find meaning in the experience were associated with a less rapid course of illness (Taylor et al., 2000). These and other findings suggest that beliefs have an important role in the stress response by mitigating the meaning we assign to experience.

Personality and Behaviour Patterns

As well as values, beliefs, and goals, individuals have characteristic patterns of response to similar situations. These attitudes and behaviours develop over time and become almost reflexive. In the mid-1970s, cardiologists Friedman and Rosenman (1974) observed an association between what they called *type A* personality characteristics and the development of cardiovascular disease. They suggested that the person with type A personality characteristics is typically competitive, aggressive, ambitious, and impatient. Alert, tense, and restless, these individuals think, speak, and act quickly. Such individuals also tend to be aggressive, hostile, and have a sense of time urgency that keeps them in a chronic state of physiologic arousal. These individuals have a high need to control events around them and are frustrated when they are unsuccessful in doing so. In contrast, individuals with *type B* personality characteristics are more relaxed, easygoing, and content. They take minor irritations in their stride and approach challenges as problems to be solved. Individuals who exhibit type B characteristics move through life at a comfortable pace and have realistic expectations of what they can achieve in a given period.

Although early research seemed to support a link between type A personality characteristics and atherosclerosis leading to coronary heart disease (CHD), later research did not bear this out. There were failures to replicate earlier findings and even negative results. For example, Dimsdale (1988) reported lower post–myocardial infarction mortality rate among individuals with type A characteristics than those with type B characteristics. Wright's (1988) research later identified five factors that contribute to CHD: inherited risk, risks associated with lifestyle choices (e.g., smoking, overeating), anger directed inward, anger directed outward (i.e., time urgency and chronic autonomic arousal), and classic type A characteristics. The current consensus seems to be that although the type A trait cluster has some heuristic value, chronic negative emotions are probably the most significant predictors of CHD (Williams et al., 2000).

Other research in the area examined what was called *hardiness*, a cluster of personality traits that buffer or moderate the effects of stress (Kobasa, 1979). In her study of a large group of individuals undergoing the same stressful event, Suzanne Kobasa identified three factors that separated those who became ill from those who did not. These factors were control, commitment, and expectancy of change. That is, individuals who have some sense of being able to control events in their life, who are committed to something (e.g., values, goals, other people), and who view change as a part of life are less likely to become ill than individuals who do not demonstrate these things. Kobasa's notion of control as conferring protection against stress relates closely to Rotter's (1966) concept of internal locus of control.

Rotter, a social learning theorist, proposed that there are two dimensions of locus of control—internal and external. Individuals with an internal locus of control believe that they can influence the outcome of events in the world. They accept that they are responsible for their behaviour, appraise situations rationally, and choose a course of action that will have favourable consequences. By contrast, individuals who have an external locus of control believe that their fate is under the control of some external agent (e.g., fate, luck, authority figures). The latter tend to be passive and do not see themselves as having the agency to affect desired outcomes. Not surprisingly, individuals with an internal locus of control perceive stressful events differently than those who have an external locus of control. Individuals with an internal locus of control perceive situations less catastrophically and assess their coping resources as being more effective than those who have an external locus of control. As we shall see later, a person's appraisal of a situation and of his or her coping abilities directly influences the experience of stress.

Interpersonal Relationships

The external is everything outside of the person, including both physical surroundings and social interactions. Things such as crowding, temperature, and noise are all aspects of the physical environment, as is exposure to hazardous material in the soil, air, and water (Matthies, Höger, & Guski, 2000). Social aspects of the environment include living arrangements and interpersonal relationships.

Social Networks

We all live within networks of relationships among a defined set of people with whom we have regular face-to-face contact (Clegg, 2001). It is through these relationships that we are socialized and acquire emotional support, material aid, services, and information (Majer, Jason, Ferrarie, Venable, & Olson, 2002). An individual's **social network** can be a resource, enhance the ability to cope with change, and influence the course of illness (Jones & Johnston, 2000).

Contacts within a social network are categorized into three levels:

1. *Level I*—6 to 12 people with whom the person has intimate contact (e.g., one's closest family and friends)
2. *Level II*—30 to 40 people whom the person sees regularly (e.g., more distant family and friends, neighbours, coworkers)
3. *Level III*—the several hundred people with whom an individual has direct contact, but incidental contact in the course of their day-to-day life (e.g., acquaintances, the grocer, mail carrier)

The various levels of an individual's social network often intersect with each other; for example, a friend may be a confidant, a neighbour, and a workout buddy. Generally speaking, the larger and more interconnected a social network is, the more support that is available to its members. An ideal network is dense and interconnected so that each individual within the network relates to the other at various levels. Dense networks are typically better able to respond in times of stress and crisis because they represent a large reservoir of social, emotional, and instrumental resources.

Intensity and reciprocity are two concepts important to understanding social networks. *Intensity* is the degree or closeness of a relationship. Some relationships are naturally more intense than others, and ideally, an individual's social network reflects a balance between intense and less intense relationships. Intense relationships can restrict a person's opportunity to interact with other network members, but without at least a few intense relationships, a person lacks intimacy. *Reciprocity* is the extent to which there is balanced give-and-take in a relationship. Network members provide and receive support, aid, services, and information from each other; sometimes members are on the giving side; at other times, they receive. Reciprocity represents a necessary equilibrium between the two states.

Social Support

Broadly defined as resources provided to us by others (Cohen & Wills, 1985), **social support** has been shown to moderate the adverse effects of stress (Haslam, O'Brien, Jetten, Vormedal, & Penna, 2005; Park, 2007). Although it takes various forms, social support is broadly categorized as either *functional* or *structural* (Cropley & Steptoe, 2005). Functional support refers to the quality of the relationships and the degree to which an individual believes that help is available; structural support relates to the quantitative characteristics of a social support network (e.g., size, number of interconnections).

Much of the research on how social support mediates the effects of stress has focused on two hypotheses (Cohen & Wills, 1985). As its name suggests, the *direct effect hypothesis* proposes that social support enhances health directly by providing an individual with positive experiences and a set of stable, socially rewarding roles regardless of stress levels. The second hypothesis (the *buffering* or *moderating hypothesis*) holds that the positive effects of social support are apparent only during periods of high stress. In a study of the relationships between life stress, social support, and physical symptom reporting, Cropley and Steptoe (2005) found that social support had no general beneficial effects on the symptom reporting (i.e., health) of individuals who had not experienced recent stress. It did, however, have a moderating effect on the health of individuals reporting recent high stress, which lends credence to the stress-buffering hypothesis. The same study found that social support did not moderate the effects of chronic stress. The authors concluded that chronically stressed individuals (even those who had high levels of social support) may habituate to chronic stress exposure.

From this, we may conclude that social support is a dynamic process that is in constant flux and varies with life events and health status (Yeager & Roberts, 2003). It is also important to keep in mind that not all interpersonal interactions within a network are supportive; an individual can have a large, complex social network but little social support. The concept of **dissupport** (Malone, 1988) derives from the observation that some relationships can be harmful, stressful, and even damaging to an individual's self-esteem. Examples of dissupport include verbal, physical, or emotional abuse; discounting an individual's opinions, feelings, behaviours, or values; blocking access to resources; or consuming an individual's material resources. As one might expect, social dissupport can hinder growth, is emotionally destructive, and depletes resources. Even more complex are those relationships that are both supportive and dissupportive, such as those that provide tangible support (e.g., money) but are emotionally destructive at the same time.

Physiologic Stress Responses

The appraisal of a situation as dangerous or threatening to one's personal integrity triggers an automatic, total-body response. Structures in the brain receive and integrate simultaneous inputs from a number of sources and coordinate a series of physiologic and behavioural responses that enhance an individual's chances of survival.

The physiologic response to stress begins in the central nervous system (CNS) but quickly involves all body systems, as Table 35-2 illustrates. The hypothalamus is responsible for maintaining the body's internal environment and for initiating the body's stress response, which

Table 35.2	Physiologic Stress-Related Symptoms
System	**Symptom**
Cardiovascular	Headache
	Chest pain
	Increased pulse
	Palpitations
	Fainting (blackouts, spells)
	Increased blood pressure
Respiratory	Shortness of breath
	Smoking history
	Increased rate and depth of breathing
	Chest discomfort (pain, tightness, ache)
Gastrointestinal	Nausea
	Vomiting
	Abdominal pain (cramps, stomach ache)
	Change in appetite
	Change in stool
	Obesity/frequent weight changes
Musculoskeletal	Pain
	Weakness
	Fatigue
Genitourinary	Menstrual changes
	Urinary discomforts (pain, burning, urgency, hesitancy)
	Sexual difficulty (pain, impotence, altered libido, anorgasmia)
Dermatologic	Itching
	Rash
	"Sweats"
	Eczema

Adapted from Carpenito-Moyet, L. (2009). *Nursing diagnosis: Application to clinical practice* (13th ed.). Philadelphia, PA: Lippincott Williams & Wilkins.

it orchestrates through its dense neural connections with the posterior pituitary gland, brain stem, and spinal cord and through its endocrine links with the anterior pituitary gland (Kindlen, 2003). The hypothalamus activates the sympathetic branch of the ANS, which mediates vigilance, arousal, activation, and mobilization (Sapolsky, 2004; see Fig. 35-2). It also secretes corticotropin-releasing hormone (CRH) to signal the anterior pituitary gland to release adrenocorticotropic hormone (ACTH), which stimulates the adrenal medulla to secrete catecholamines. Also through CRH, the hypothalamus excites firing of the locus coeruleus (LC) in the brainstem to increase norepinephrine in the CNS. The hypothalamus also synthesizes arginine vasopressin or antidiuretic hormone (AVP/ADH), which is released by the posterior pituitary gland and increases blood pressure by causing vasoconstriction and water retention.

The activities of the hypothalamic–pituitary–adrenocortical (HPA) axis and the sympathetic-adrenal medullary system operate within different time frames to provide the body with a wide range of defensive responses. Because the neural response of the ANS is instantaneous, it is the body's first line of defence against stressors. The release of AVP/ADH and catecholamines is slightly slower and augments ANS effects. In the short term, these responses mobilize energy reserves (mainly in the form of glucose) and prepare the body to deal with the stressor by running away or fighting it off. If the stressor is prolonged, the body must make longer-term metabolic adjustments that ensure a sufficient supply of energy. Through the release of growth hormone–releasing hormone (GH-RH) and CRH, the hypothalamus stimulates the release of growth hormone (GH) and ACTH from the anterior pituitary and the secretion of glucocorticoids (e.g., cortisol) from the adrenal cortex. Cortisol is essential to the body's sustained stress response because it mobilizes lipid stores and skeletal protein for energy, which allows the conservation of glucose energy for neural tissue. It also acts on the liver to elevate and stabilize blood glucose levels through gluconeogenesis and lipolysis. As well as having these metabolic effects, cortisol is an antiinflammatory. By reducing the dilation and permeability of blood vessels, which is part of the inflammatory response, cortisol aids in the maintenance of blood pressure and minimizes fluid loss to the tissue. At the same time, chronically elevated cortisol prolongs healing and leaves the body vulnerable to infection.

Allostasis

A recent refinement in our understanding of stress is the concept of **allostasis**. The word, which literally means *maintaining stability through change*, was coined by Sterling and Eyer (1988) to describe how the cardiovascular system adjusts to resting and active states of the

FIGURE 35.2 Physiologic responses to stress.

body. Unlike the concept of homeostasis, which posits a single optimum state, allostasis reflects the notion that different environmental circumstances or conditions require different set points. For instance, individuals' ideal blood pressure when asleep is very different from their ideal blood pressure if they are bungee jumping (Sapolsky, 2004). Maintaining an allostatic balance in wide-ranging circumstances calls for continuous systemic adjustments throughout the whole body. For example, the hypothalamus regulates sleep and wakefulness and the production of adrenocortical hormones in response to the light–dark cycle that occurs as the earth rotates on its axis every day. When the light–dark cycle is altered (e.g., long flights across several time zones), the production

of adrenocortical hormones is disrupted and alterations occur in the usual patterns of sleep, activity, appetite, and cognitive function (i.e., jet lag).

The term **allostatic load** (McEwen, 1998) refers to the cumulative negative effects on the body of continually having to adapt to changing environmental conditions and psychosocial challenges. It is mediated by the efficiency of the body's response to these changing conditions and to the number of stressors an individual experiences throughout his or her lifetime. Allostatic load is more than "chronic stress"; it is the sum total of the "wear and tear" on the body that accumulates from the constant effort required to maintain normal body rhythms in the face of changing environmental conditions, the challenges

Table 35.3	15 Basic Emotions
Emotion	**Relational Meaning**
Anger	A demeaning offense against me and mine
Anxiety	Facing an uncertain, existential threat
Fright	Facing an immediate, concrete, and overwhelming physical danger
Guilt	Having transgressed a moral imperative
Shame	Having failed to live up to an ego ideal
Sadness	Having experienced an irrevocable loss
Envy	Wanting what someone else has
Jealousy	Resenting a third party for the loss of or a threat to another's affection
Disgust	Taking in or being too close to an indigestible object or idea (metaphorically speaking)
Happiness	Making reasonable progress toward the realization of a goal
Pride	Enhancement of one's ego identity by taking credit for a valued object or achievement, either our own or that of someone or a group with whom we identify
Relief	A distressing goal-incongruent condition that has changed for the better or gone away
Hope	Fearing the worst but yearning for better
Love	Desiring or participating in affection, usually but not necessarily reciprocated
Compassion	Being moved by another's suffering and wanting to help

Source: Adapted from Lazarus, R. S. (1999). *Stress and emotion: A new synthesis.* New York, NY: Springer.

of daily life, and the adverse physiologic consequences of harmful lifestyle choices (e.g., fat-rich diet, excessive alcohol, smoking).

Emotional Responses to Stress

Although it is clear that emotion is key to the human stress response, there is still debate about the relationship between emotion and cognition. On one side is the argument that emotions are primary and influence both the form and content of our perceptions, while opponents believe that cognition is primary and gives rise to emotion. Consistent with his transactional view of stress, Lazarus (1991) takes a more integrative approach and contends that cognition and emotion are essentially simultaneous and interdependent. He and his colleagues define emotion as "complex, organized psychophysiological reactions consisting of cognitive appraisals, action impulses, and patterned somatic reactions" (cited in Folkman & Lazarus, 1991, p. 209).

Cognitive appraisal is fundamental to the experience of emotion because it colours the meaning of a situation or an event. Based on their research, Lazarus and colleagues believe that there are 15 basic emotions, each of which is elicited in response to a particular perception of what a situation or an event means to the individual (see Table 35-3). Anxiety, for example, is typically associated with the perception of a nonspecific threat or some uncertainty, whereas happiness reflects an appraisal of the person–environment condition that is beneficial. Patterned somatic reactions are the individual's own, unique experience of the physiologic changes associated with an emotion. For one person, a rush of energy is the salient feature of anger, whereas for another person, it is trembling and a feeling of weakness. These physical reactions motivate or inhibit action impulses. For example, the person who feels energized may attack an aggressor, whereas the person who experiences trembling and weakness is likely to withdraw.

Coping

According to Lazarus (1998), the following three principles are vital to an understanding of *coping*: (1) it continually changes over the course of an encounter, (2) it must be assessed independently of its outcomes, and (3) it consists of what an individual thinks and does in response to the perceived demands of a situation. With those principles in mind, coping is defined as "the efforts we take to manage situations we have appraised as being potentially harmful or stressful" (Kleinke, 2007, pp. 290–291). Coping reflects an individual's continual reappraisal of the person–environment relationship in light of changing conditions, as well as the success of his or her efforts to mitigate the situation. Those who evaluate their coping responses as effective are likely to feel competent and to repeat those responses in the future. Conversely, individuals who see their efforts as ineffective are likely to feel helpless and overwhelmed. Positive coping leads to adaptation, which is characterized by well-being and maximum social functioning. The inability to cope leads to maladaptation and contributes to ill health, a diminished self-concept, and deterioration in **social functioning**. These ideas are captured in the stress, coping, and adaptation model presented in Figures 35-3 and 35-4.

FIGURE 35.3 Stress, coping, and adaptation model.

FIGURE 35.4 Bio/psycho/social/spiritual adaptation.

Table 35.4	Ways of Coping: Problem-Focused Versus Emotion-Focused
Problem-Focused Coping	**Emotion-Focused Coping**
Outer-directed When noise from the television in the apartment next door interrupts a student's studying, she experiences anxiety about being ready for an important exam the next day. She responds by asking her neighbour to turn the volume down. *Inner-directed* When an abused woman feels guilt about leaving her husband, she reminds herself that her children are much happier and doing well in school.	A man dislikes visiting his wife's mother because she has two cats that roam her house freely, and the cat hair on all of the furniture irritates him. Rather than refusing to visit his mother-in-law, which causes conflict in his marriage, the man plans strategies that help him manage his distress during visits (e.g., long walks, a good book to distract him, thinking about how pleased his wife is).

KEY CONCEPT Coping is an individual's constantly changing cognitive and behavioural efforts to manage specific external or internal demands that are appraised as taxing or exceeding the individual's resources.

There are two general approaches to coping: problem-focused and emotion-focused. As Kleinke (2007) explains, **problem-focused coping** may be inner- or outer-directed. Outer-directed strategies attempt to eliminate or alter a situation or another's behaviour, while inner-directed strategies aim at altering one's own beliefs, attitudes, skills, responses, and so forth. In **emotion-focused coping,** the individual seeks to manage his or her emotional distress (e.g., through exercise, prayer/meditation, expressing emotions, talking to friends). Table 35-4 contrasts problem-focused and emotion-focused coping.

Coping involves the continuous reevaluation or reappraisal of the changing person–environment relationship. **Reappraisal** incorporates feedback about the effects of coping and allows for continual processing of new information. No single coping strategy is effective in all situations. Throughout life a repertoire of coping strategies is developed and adapted to suit different situations, and these strategies become ingrained into patterned responses. Well-adapted individuals are realistic in their appraisal of the demands upon them, are flexible in their use of coping resources, and remain open to learning new coping strategies. Poor reality testing, impaired judgment, inflexibility, and an unwillingness to acquire new resources can render individuals vulnerable to stress-related problems and illness.

Stress and Health Illness

There is more than 50 years of accumulated research demonstrating a relationship between stress and illness. Animal experiments in the 1950s and 1960s demonstrated that a number of stressors (e.g., isolation, crowding, exposure to predators, electrical shock) increased morbidity and mortality from tumours and infections (Saddock & Saddock, 2003). In humans, acute academic-exam stress is linked to a reduction in natural killer cells and increased activation of latent viruses (Glaser, Rice, Sherridan, & Fertel, 1987). Other studies demonstrate a correlation between exam stress and an increase in cytokines—proteins (produced by lymphocytes and other cells) that promote or inhibit an immune response (Lui et al., 2002). As well, Segerstrom and Miller's (2003) meta-analysis of 30 years of research on the effects of chronic stress associated with caring for a relative with dementia found a reduction in most measures of immune function.

The **stress-diathesis model** offers one explanation about the relationship between stress and mental health illness (Stanley & Burrows, 2005). This model proposes that preexisting genetic, biologic, and psychological vulnerabilities interact with negative or stressful life events to cause illness. Further, the model predicts an inverse relationship between vulnerability and stress such that the more vulnerable the individual, the smaller the stressor required to cause illness. Several lines of research conclude that the tendency to "nervousness, emotionality, 'neuroticism,' negative affect, anxiety, and being 'high strung' runs in families and has a high genetic component, with 50% of these characteristics arising from genetic or biologic vulnerability" (Stanley & Burrows, p. 90). In a large community-based study, Kendler, Neale, Kessler, Heath, and Eaves (1992) found that generalized anxiety disorder and depression share a common genetic predisposition and that episodes of illness are related to environmental stressors.

Ineffective coping has other implications for health. For instance, if emotion-focused coping is used when a problem-focused approach is appropriate, stress is not relieved. In addition, if a coping strategy violates gender, ethnic, or cultural norms, stress is often exaggerated. Some coping strategies actually increase the risk for mortality and morbidity, such as the excessive use of alcohol, drugs, tobacco, or overeating. Although these strategies may provide some short-term stress relief, they often cause long-term secondary stress. The corollary is that healthy coping strategies such as exercising, adequate sleep, leisure activities, and good nutrition reduce the negative effects of stress and promote health and well-being.

Posttraumatic Stress Disorder

Although historical and literary documents dating back to the 3rd century BC describe human responses to extreme stress (e.g., natural disasters, combat, physical/sexual assault; Birmes, Hatton, Brunet, & Schmitt, 2003), modern psychiatry did not officially recognize them until 1980, when posttraumatic stress disorder (PTSD) appeared in the *Diagnostic and Statistical Manual of Mental Disorders (DSM*; American Psychiatric Association [APA], 1980).

PTSD (APA, 2000) is an anxiety disorder that develops following direct or indirect exposure to an extreme stressor to which an individual responds with feelings of intense fear, helplessness, or horror. The APA defines an extreme stressor as (1) direct exposure to events that threaten death or serious injury to oneself or others (e.g., physical, sexual, or emotional abuse or assault; motor vehicle crash; a natural disaster; combat or military experience), (2) witnessing an event that involves death or injury to another, or (3) learning about the unexpected or violent death or serious harm to a loved one or close associate.

In the aftermath of an extremely stressful event, many people experience symptoms that are typically grouped into one of three clusters: reexperiencing, avoidance/emotional numbing, and arousal/hypervigilance. Reexperiencing includes recurring and persistent thoughts and images, nightmares, or flashbacks (i.e., vivid reliving) of the stressful event. Symptoms of avoidance/emotional numbing are manifested as attempts to block out all reminders of the stressful event and may involve avoiding people, places, or activities associated with the event; inability to remember some or all aspects of the event; feeling detached from others; and/or a lack of interest or participation in usual activities. In an effort to numb or block out their thoughts and feelings, some individuals may turn to alcohol or drugs. Arousal/hypervigilance symptoms reflect ANS arousal and may include startling easily, difficulty concentrating, sleep disruption, irritability, and feeling "keyed up" and "on guard." These PTSD symptom clusters typically begin immediately after the stressful event and usually disappear without treatment within a few weeks. The *Diagnostic and Statistical Manual of Mental Disorders, Fourth Edition–Text Revision (DSM-IV-TR*; APA, 2000) specifies that these symptom clusters must persist for at least 1 month for a diagnosis of PTSD to be made. It also describes various courses of the disorder: *acute* (symptoms last <3 months), *chronic*

(symptoms last ≥3 months), and *delayed onset* (symptoms do not appear until at least 6 months after the stressful event).

According to the National Comorbidity Study (Kessler, Sonnega, Bromet, Hughes, & Nelson, 1995), a large U.S. population–based study, 60.7% of men and 51.2% of women reported being exposed to at least one traumatic event during their lifetime. This estimate increases to 80% when clinical populations are surveyed. Factors that predict the development of PTSD include female gender, type and severity of the trauma, past trauma (including childhood physical, sexual, and emotional abuse), and availability of support at the time of the stressful event (Richardson, Naifeh, & Elhai, 2007). Treatments include cognitive-behavioural therapy (CBT), psychotherapy, and medication.

Nursing Care of Individuals Affected by Stress

Nursing assessment of individuals experiencing stress attends to biologic, psychological, emotional, and environmental (physical and social), as well as coping, resources. In particular, the nurse should explore recent

---

IN A LIFE

Maria Campbell (1940–)

Maria Campbell is a Métis woman and the eldest daughter of seven children. She was born in Park Valley, Saskatchewan, to parents of Scottish, Indian, and French descent. Her autobiography, *Halfbreed* (1973), recounts the first 33 years of her life and tells of how Maria lost her mother when she was only 12 years old, leaving her to care for her younger siblings. In an effort to keep her family together, young Maria married an abusive white man who reported her to child welfare authorities, and her siblings were placed in foster homes. Devastated, Maria moved to Vancouver, where her husband deserted her, and she turned to a life of drugs and prostitution. Alone and desperate, she attempted suicide twice and was hospitalized for psychiatric care. It is in the hospital that Maria joined Alcoholics Anonymous and began a journey of healing.

In the book, Maria Campbell not only tells her own story, but she speaks of the discrimination and racism that affect all Métis people. In the book's introduction, she says, "I write this for all of you, to tell you what it is like to be a half-breed woman in this country. I want to tell you about the joys and sorrows, the oppressing poverty, the frustrations and the dreams" (p. 8). Although Maria's story is one of stress and crises, it is also a story of courage and resilience. She is no longer a scared little girl but a strong, independent woman full of hope for herself and her people.

Today, Maria continues to write, teaches at the University of Saskatchewan, and is a political activist for Métis rights. She is the recipient of many writing awards and has Honorary Doctorate degrees from the University of Regina and York University.

Campbell, M. (1973). *Halfbreed*. Halifax, NS: Goodread Biographies.

Table 35.5 Key Diagnostic Characteristics of Adjustment Disorder

Diagnostic Criteria	Target Symptoms and Associated Findings
• Emotional or behavioural symptoms in response to an identifiable stressor occurring within 3 months of the onset of the stressors. • Clinically significant symptoms or behaviours (1) are characterized by distress that is in excess of what would be expected from exposure to the stressor or (2) cause a significant impairment in social or occupational (academic) functioning. • Stress-related disturbance does not meet the criteria for another specific Axis I disorder and is not merely an exacerbation of a pre-existing Axis I or Axis II disorder. • Symptoms do not represent bereavement. • Symptoms do not persist for more than 6 months after the stressor has terminated.	• Subjective distress or impairment in functioning • Decreased performance at work or school • Temporary changes in relationships • Associated physical examination findings • Decreased compliance with recommended medical regimen

Acute: disturbance lasts no more than 6 months
Chronic: disturbance lasts for 6 months or longer
309.0   With depressed mood
309.24   With anxiety
309.28   With mixed anxiety and depressed mood
309.3   With disturbance of conduct
309.4   With mixed disturbance of emotions and conduct
309.9   Unspecified

changes (positive or negative) in the individual's life (e.g., trauma, loss, developmental milestones).

If an individual's signs and symptoms meet the diagnostic criteria for an Axis I or II disorder (APA, 2000), the stress response is considered as part of that disorder. However, if he or she is experiencing significant emotional or behavioural symptoms in response to an identifiable stressful situation and the diagnostic criteria do not account for the response, a diagnosis of adjustment disorder (APA) may be appropriate (see Table 35-5).

This residual category captures responses to a stressful situation that do not meet the criteria for an Axis I disorder. There are six subtypes: with depressed mood, with anxiety, with anxiety and depressed mood, with disturbance of conduct, with mixed disturbance of emotions and conduct, and unspecified. The diagnosis of adjustment disorder specifies that the onset of the emotional or behavioural disturbances must begin within 3 months of the stressful situation and cannot last for more than 6 months after the stressor abates.

The overall goals of care for those individuals actively experiencing a stress response are to eliminate or moderate the stressor (if possible), to reduce untoward effects of the stress response, and to facilitate the maintenance or development of positive coping skills. The goals of care for individuals who are at high risk for stress (e.g., are experiencing significant life changes, have preexisting vulnerabilities, have limited coping mechanisms) are to

recognize the potential for stress and to strengthen or develop positive coping skills.

Biologic Domain

Biologic Assessment

Biologic data are essential for analyzing an individual's physical responses to stress, coping efforts, and adaptation. This information comes from the health history, physical examination, and diagnostic testing (as indicated; see Chapter 11). Nurses should pay particular attention to

• Signs and symptoms of sympathetic arousal (Table 35-6)
• Alterations in vegetative functions (e.g., appetite and eating patterns, sleep, energy level, sexual activity)
• Chronic illness or conditions with a strong stress component (e.g., hypertension, migraine, chronic pain syndromes, irritable bowel syndrome)
• Evidence of immune system suppression (e.g., frequent infections)
• Physical appearance (e.g., deficits in grooming and hygiene; nonverbal indications of muscle tension, anxiety, or depression)
• Alterations in activity and exercise patterns

As well, the biologic assessment of stress and coping considers the use of pharmacologic agents, including prescribed and nonprescribed medications, over-the-counter

Table 35.6	Effects of Sympathetic Nervous System Arousal		
Organ	**Effect of Sympathetic Stimulation**	**Organ**	**Effect of Sympathetic Stimulation**
Eye		Kidney	Decreased output and renin secretion
Pupil	Dilated		
Ciliary muscle	Slight relaxation (far vision)	Bladder	
Glands	Vasoconstriction and slight secretion	Detrusor	Relaxed (slight)
Nasal		Trigone	Contracted
Lacrimal		Penis	Ejaculation
Parotid		Systemic arterioles	
Submandibular		Abdominal viscera	Constricted
Gastric		Muscle	Constricted (adrenergic α)
Pancreatic			Dilated (adrenergic β_2)
Sweat glands	Copious sweating		Dilated (cholinergic)
Apocrine glands	Thick, odoriferous secretions	Skin	Constricted
Heart		Blood	
Muscle	Increased rate	Coagulation	Increased
	Increased force of contraction	Glucose	Increased
		Lipids	Increased
Coronaries	Dilated (β_2); constricted (α)	Basal metabolism	Increased up to 100%
Lungs		Adrenal medullary secretion	Increased
Bronchi	Dilated	Mental activity	Increased
Blood vessels	Mildly constricted	Piloerector muscles	Contracted
Gut			Increased glycogenolysis
Lumen	Decreased peristalsis and tone	Skeletal muscle	Increased strength
Sphincter	Increased tone (most times)	Fat cells	Lipolysis
Liver	Glucose released		
Gallbladder and bile ducts	Relaxed		

Source: From Guyton, A. C., & Hall, J. E. (2000). *Textbook of medical physiology* (10th ed., p. 775). Philadelphia, PA: WB Saunders.

and herbal preparations, alcohol, tobacco, and illicit drugs. As noted previously, some individuals begin or increase the frequency of using these agents as a way of coping with stress. At the same time, however, reliance on relaxants or mood-altering substances can become a secondary stressor and contribute to maladaptation. Understanding patterns of use (e.g., frequency, dose, circumstances, effects) is important to assessing their role in stress management. The more important the substances are to a person's handling of stress, the greater the potential for abuse and addiction. Box 35-1 lists some potential nursing diagnoses within the North American Nursing Diagnosis Association (NANDA; 2005) taxonomy for individuals experiencing or at risk for stress response.

Interventions for the Biologic Domain

Individuals experiencing or at risk for untoward stress responses may benefit from a number of biologic interventions.

- The importance of (re)establishing regular routines for activities of daily living (e.g., eating, sleeping, self-care, leisure time) cannot be overstated. As well

as ensuring adequate nutrition, sleep and rest, and hygiene, a routine may help to structure an individual's time and give him or her a sense of personal control or mastery.

- Exercise can reduce the emotional and behavioural responses to stress. In addition to the physical benefits of exercise, regular exercise can provide structure to a person's life, enhance self-confidence, and increase feelings of well-being. Under stress, many individuals are not receptive to the idea of exercise, particularly if it has not been a part of their life. Exploration of usual activity patterns, as well as knowledge and beliefs about the value of exercise, will help to identify where the nurse may intervene.

- Activities such as yoga, meditation, deep breathing, and progressive muscle relaxation can help individuals mediate the physical stress response, improve sleep, and reduce pain. Nurses should also consider referring clients for hypnosis or biofeedback when indicated.

- Health teaching in such areas as nutrition, sleep hygiene, and medication management may also be a part of nursing interventions in this domain.

BOX 35.1

Potential Nursing Diagnoses in the Biologic Domain

Within the NANDA taxonomy, the following are some potential nursing diagnoses for individuals experiencing or at risk for stress response:

- Anxiety
- Body image, disturbed
- Comfort, impaired
- Constipation
- Diarrhea
- Energy field, disturbed
- Fatigue
- Fear
- Fluid volume, deficit/risk for deficient
- Health maintenance, ineffective
- Infection, risk for
- Knowledge, deficit
- Noncompliance
- Nutrition, more/less than body requirements
- Pain, acute/chronic
- Posttrauma syndrome
- Self-care deficit, hygiene/feeding
- Sexual dysfunction
- Sleep pattern, disrupted
- Therapeutic regime management, ineffective

From North American Nursing Diagnosis Association. (2005). *NANDA nursing diagnoses: Definitions and classification, 2005–2006.* Philadelphia, PA: Author.

BOX 35.2

Potential Nursing Diagnoses in the Psychological Domain

From North American Nursing Diagnosis Association. (2005). *NANDA nursing diagnoses: Definitions and classification, 2005–2006.* Philadelphia, PA: Author. Adjustment, impaired

- Anxiety
- Body image, disturbed
- Conflict, decisional
- Confusion, acute/chronic
- Coping, ineffective/defensive
- Denial, ineffective
- Development, risk for delayed
- Diversional activity, deficit
- Environmental interpretation, impaired
- Failure to thrive
- Growth and development, delayed
- Hopelessness
- Identity, disturbed
- Knowledge, deficit
- Memory, impaired
- Posttrauma syndrome
- Powerlessness
- Relocation syndrome
- Role performance, ineffective
- Self-esteem, chronic low/situational low
- Self-mutilation
- Sensory perception, disturbed
- Sexual dysfunction
- Spiritual distress
- Suicide, risk for
- Thought process, disturbed
- Violence, self/other directed

Psychological Domain

Psychological Assessment

Information about the psychological and emotional dimensions of stress may be forthcoming throughout the assessment process. In particular, the nurse should do the following:

- Observe for behavioural and affective indicators of stress response (e.g., energy level and general presentation; appearance, grooming, and hygiene; psychomotor agitation and retardation; facial expression; speech characteristics).
- Explore reports of recent changes in mood or current emotional distress (e.g., anxiety, fear, irritability, anger, tension, pressure, depression).
- Note alterations or impairment in mental status (e.g., suicidal ideation; self-deprecatory thoughts; impulsivity; ruminations; impaired concentration, problem solving, or memory).
- Explore the individual's appraisal of significant life events (e.g., losses, physical or sexual abuse or assault, motor vehicle crashes, natural disasters, combat experience), the effect of those experiences, and the commitment to particular outcomes.
- Ask about alterations in day-to-day function or inability to fulfill responsibilities (e.g., family, work, school).

- Explore the individual's current resources and effectiveness of usual coping strategies. (see Table 35-7).

Box 35-2 lists potential nursing diagnoses in the psychological domain.

Interventions for the Psychological Domain

The Nursing Interventions Classification (NIC; Johnson et al., 2006) provides interventions in the behavioural domain that support psychological functioning and facilitate lifestyle changes. NIC includes six classes of useful nursing interventions: behaviour therapy, cognitive therapy, communication enhancement, coping assistance, patient education, and psychological comfort promotion. The interventions are listed in Table 35-8.

Social Domain

Social Assessment

Information from a social assessment is invaluable to understanding an individual's coping resources. The ability to make healthy lifestyle changes is strongly influenced

Table 35.7   Problem-Focused and Emotion-Focused Behaviours

Behaviour	Focused Type	Definition	Effective	Ineffective
Goal setting	Problem focused	The conscious process of setting time limitations on behaviour	When goals are attainable and manageable (e.g., making an appointment with boss to discuss pay raise)	When the appraisal of the situation is missed or inaccurately evaluated
Information seeking	Problem focused	Process of learning about all aspects of a problem that provides perspective and reinforces self-control	When situations are complex and additional information is needed (e.g., attending a parent effectiveness class because of being unsure about discipline techniques)	When the needed information is already obtained and the activity delays action
Mastery	Problem focused	Learning of new procedures or skills that facilitate self-esteem and reinforce self-control	When there are new procedures to learn (e.g., self-care activities, insulin injection, catheter care)	When the situation does not require learning new procedures, or they have nothing to do with the stressful situation
Help seeking	Problem focused	Reaching out to others for support; sharing feelings provides an emotional release, reassurance, and comfort	When similar problems are shared by others (e.g., in Alcoholics Anonymous, weight-loss programs, psychosocial programs)	When using help seeking to avoid action in the current situation
Minimization	Emotion focused	The seriousness of the problem is minimized	Useful way of providing needed time for appraisal (e.g., a person is told that her child is in an automobile accident and forces herself to think the accident is minor until additional information is received)	When the appraisal of the situation is missed or inaccurately evaluated
Projection, displacement, and suppression of anger	Emotion focused	When anger is attributed to or expressed toward a less-threatening person or thing	When threat is reduced, the individual can deal with the situation (e.g., the boss reprimands a worker for submitting a report late—the worker in turn hits his fist on the copying machine as he walks by)	When reality is distorted and relationships disturbed, which further compound the problem; suppression of anger may result in stress-related physical symptoms
Anticipatory preparation	Emotion focused	Mental rehearsal of possible consequences of behaviour or outcomes of stressful situations	Provides the opportunity to develop perspective as well as to prepare for the worst (e.g., when waiting for exam results, the client develops a plan of action if the results are negative)	When anticipation creates unmanageable stress as in anticipatory mourning
Attribution	Emotion focused	Finding personal meaning in the problem situation, which may be through religious faith or individual belief	May offer consolation (e.g., fate, the will of the divine; luck)	When all sense of self-responsibility is lost

Source: Adapted from Carpenito-Moyet, L. (2009). *Nursing diagnosis: Application to clinical practice* (13th ed.). Philadelphia, PA: Lippincott Williams & Wilkins.

Table 35.8	Interventions for Stress Reduction and Coping Enhancement					
Behaviour Therapy*	**Cognitive Therapy**	**Communication Enhancement**	**Coping Assistance Interventions**	**Client Education**	**Psychological Comfort Promotion**
Reinforce or promote desirable behaviours or alter undesirable behaviours	Reinforce or promote desirable cognitive functioning or alter undesirable functioning	Facilitate effective verbal and nonverbal interactions	Help build on existing strengths, foster adaptation to change, achieve a higher level of function	Facilitate new learning	Promote comfort using psychological techniques
Generalist Interventions					
Assertiveness training Behaviour management Behaviour modification Limit setting Client contracting Self-modification assistance Self-responsibility assistance Smoking cessation assistance Substance use prevention Activity therapy	Anger management Bibliotherapy Reality orientation	Active listening skills Communication enhancement Socialization enhancement	Anticipatory guidance Body image enhancement Counselling Grief work facilitation Decision-making support Care of the dying Emotional support Hope instillation Humour Role enhancement Recreation therapy Self-awareness enhancement Self-esteem enhancement Spiritual support Support system enhancement Values clarifications	Learning facilitation Learning readiness enhancement Parent education Teaching: disease process Teaching: group individual Teaching: activity exercise, diet, medication, procedure/ treatment, psychomotor skills, safe sex	Anxiety reduction Calming technique Distraction Simple guided imagery Simple relaxation therapy
Specialist (Advanced Practice) Interventions†					
Psychotherapy Consultation Animal-assisted therapy Substance use treatment Art therapy	Psychotherapy Consultation Cognitive restructuring Cognitive stimulation Memory training Reminiscence therapy	Psychotherapy Consultation Complex relationship building Music therapy Art therapy Play therapy Animal-assisted therapy	Psychotherapy, individual and group Consultation Genetic counselling Grief therapy Guilt work Sexual counselling Touch therapy	Same as generalist	Psychopharmacologic agents prescribed Autogenic training Biofeedback Hypnosis Meditation

*Behavioural interventions: care that supports psychological functioning and facilitates lifestyle changes.

†Specialist interventions require additional training. Specialist interventions are in addition to those at the generalist level.

Source: McCloskey, J., & Bulechek, G. (2004). *Nursing interventions classification (NIC)* (4th ed.). St. Louis, MO: Mosby–Year Book.

by one's social support system. Even the expression of stress is related to social factors, particularly ethnic and cultural expectations and values.

Social assessment also includes identification of the person's social network. The nurse should elicit the following information:

- Size and extent of the network, both relatives and nonrelatives, and the length and quality of the relationships

- Functions the network serves (e.g., intimacy, social integration, nurturance, reassurance of worth, guidance and advice, access to new contacts)
- Degree of reciprocity between the individual and others in the network (i.e., Who provides support to the client? Who does the client support?)
- Degree of interconnectedness among network members

Box 35-3 lists potential nursing diagnoses within the social domain.

BOX 35.3

Potential Diagnoses in the Social Domain

Potential nursing diagnoses within the social domain include:

- Anxiety, death
- Attachment, impaired or risk for impaired
- Caregiver role strain
- Communication, impaired
- Conflict
- Coping, ineffective
- Family processes: alcoholism, dysfunctional
- Grieving
- Loneliness
- Parenting, impaired
- Role performance, ineffective
- Sexual dysfunction
- Sexuality patterns, ineffective
- Social interaction, impaired
- Sorrow, chronic
- Violence, other directed

From North American Nursing Diagnosis Association. (2005). *NANDA nursing diagnoses: Definitions and classification, 2005–2006.* Philadelphia, PA: Author.

Interventions for the Social Domain

Individuals who are coping with stressful situations often benefit from interventions that facilitate social functioning and promote the health and welfare of social network members. NIC (Johnson et al., 2006) includes the following generalist interventions in family care: caregiver support, family integrity promotion, family involvement, family mobilization, family process maintenance, family support, respite care, and home maintenance assistance. Parenting education can also be useful to effective family functioning. The nurse should also consider referring the client to family therapy when that is indicated.

Spiritual Domain

The challenges faced by individuals in times of stress and crisis can lead to an acute questioning about one's life choices and situation, about one's relationships, and about the meaning of one's very existence. Making sense of what is happening to you is fundamental to being human. If we want to believe in a "just world," one response may be to search for reasons that one deserves to be "punished" (Hafer & Bègue, 2005). In his book, *When Bad Things Happen to Good People*, Rabbi Harold Kushner (1981) describes how a personal tragedy compelled him to "rethink everything"

that he had been taught about God and God's ways (p. 1). He couldn't make sense of what was happening to his family and felt "a deep aching sense of unfairness" (p. 2). Ultimately, Rabbi Kushner concluded that suffering happens in our natural world and that there are no exceptions for nice people; God gives humans strength to cope with their misfortunes and does not leave them to suffer alone. While his book reveals the search for meaning a life crisis can inspire, his conclusions are his own. Others, even those in very similar circumstances, may choose a different resolution. For instance, lasting anger at the sacred power in which one believes may be the response if one feels totally abandoned, or one may view the crisis situation as revealing direction for personal growth.

Nurses attending to the spiritual domain of their practice need to recognize that such searching on the part of clients under duress or in crisis is likely to occur. Nurses need to refrain from providing their own answers to questions of meaning but, rather, through listening, provide support. Thoughtful questions may be helpful in understanding the client's perspective: Has your current stressful situation influenced the way you understand the world? Have your beliefs been affected? If so, in what way? What is sustaining you through this time? Are there spiritual acts, such as prayer or ritual, which you are finding helpful? What, if anything, can you take from this experience to help you in the future?

When a traumatic or crisis event is catastrophic in its scope (see Characteristics of Disasters section later in this chapter), entire communities can struggle to understand the cause of what has happened and the meaning of the loss suffered. At one time in Western societies, disasters were understood as evidence of the wrath of the gods or God (Grandjean, Rendu, MacNamee, & Scherer, 2008). The Lisbon earthquake of 1755 is used to mark the beginnings of change in societal attitudes toward disaster: it is called the first modern disaster as it was attributed to "natural" rather than "supernatural" causes. The type of disaster influences this struggle, of course, and can affect the community's recovery (Furedi, 2007).

Spirituality can positively influence the response to disaster. In a study of psychiatric morbidity following a tsunami in a community with diverse religious beliefs, it was found that altruistic behaviour on the part of community leaders, religious faith, and spirituality (along with family systems and social support) were factors that positively affected the early coping of survivors (Math et al., 2008). Nurses responding to a disaster in their own community will have to address, in addition to professional challenges, their personal reaction as members of the community with their own spiritual questions.

EVALUATION AND TREATMENT OUTCOMES

The treatment goals established in the plan of care guide evaluation. The goals of individual care relate to improved health, well-being, and social function. Depending on the level of intervention, there may also be goals for the family and other members of the client's social network. Family outcomes may relate to improved communication or social support (e.g., reduced caregiver stress). Social network outcomes focus on strengthening the social network and improving its function.

CRISIS

Our current understanding of the bio/psycho/social/spiritual implications of a crisis has its roots in Lindeman's (1944) study of **bereavement** among friends and relatives of the Coconut Grove nightclub fire in Boston in 1942. Four hundred and thirty-nine individuals died in that fire, which at the time was the worst single building fire in U.S. history. In the course of his research, Lindeman learned that family and friends of those who died experienced somatic symptoms, feelings of anger and guilt, and preoccupation with the deceased. From this work, he developed a model that describes **grief** as progressing through three stages: shock and disbelief, acute **mourning,** and resolution. Lindeman concluded that grief is both a natural response to loss and necessary to survivors' mental health. He later extended his ideas about crisis to more common, yet significant, life events (e.g., the birth of a child, marriage, death) and hypothesized that the changes associated with these events cause emotional strain and require individuals to adapt to a new reality (Lindeman, 1956). These adaptive efforts either lead to mastery (psychological growth) or impaired functioning. Lindeman was convinced that by helping individuals through the bereavement process, mental health professionals could prevent later psychological and emotional problems. This thinking reflected two important trends that were germinating in psychiatry around the globe: the recognition of the potential for and the value of early intervention to prevent emotional and psychological problems and the movement from hospital-based to community-based psychiatric treatment.

Although Lindeman did much of the foundational work in the area of crisis, Gerald Caplan is widely acknowledged as the master architect of crisis intervention. A psychiatrist and close colleague of Lindeman's, Caplan (1961) equated mental health with a strong, mature ego, which he defined as: (1) the capacity to withstand stress and maintain equilibrium, (2) an accurate perception of reality, and (3) a balanced repertoire of coping strategies based on sound reality testing. Under the aegis of the Harvard School of Public Health, Caplan established the Harvard Family Guidance Centre, an interdisciplinary crisis research and consultation project that studied the impact of four stressors: premature birth, birth of children with congenital abnormalities, birth of twins, and tuberculosis. Caplan is believed to be the first to apply the term *crisis* in psychiatry, to relate the concept of homeostasis to crisis intervention, and to describe the stages of a crisis.

Caplan defined crisis as occurring "when a person faces an obstacle to important life goals, that is, for a time, insurmountable through the utilization of customary methods of problem solving" (1961, p. 18). More specifically, a crisis is a response in which psychological equilibrium is disrupted, usual coping methods are ineffective in restoring that equilibrium, and there is evidence of functional impairment (Caplan, 1961; Flannery & Everly, 2000). This disequilibrium causes a rise in inner tension and anxiety that, if it continues, engenders emotional upset and an inability to function (Caplan). Figure 35-5 summarizes the phases of crisis.

Although crises force individuals into uncharted territory, Caplan (1961) recognized that most individuals achieve resolution without professional help within 4 to 6 weeks. He viewed this time as a period of transition in which the individual, family, or group is more vulnerable to harm and at the same time more open to outside intervention. This prompted him to advocate for community-based crisis services aimed at identifying maladaptive responses and intervening early to assist those involved to transform problems into opportunities for personal growth and new learning.

> **KEY CONCEPT** A **crisis** response occurs when an individual encounters an obstacle or problem that might affect his or her life goals that cannot be solved by customary problem-solving methods. It is acute, time limited and may be developmental, situational, or interpersonal in nature.

Types of Crises

Situational Crisis

A situational crisis is any event that overwhelms an individual's coping resources and upsets his or her equilibrium. The precipitating event may be positive or negative, physiological, psychological, or social in nature. Examples of situational crises include illness, the death of a loved one, separation or divorce, job loss, school problems, physical or sexual assault, or an unplanned

A problem arises that contributes to increase in anxiety levels. The anxiety stimulates the implementation of usual problem-solving techniques of the person.

The usual problem-solving techniques are ineffective. Anxiety levels continue to rise. Trial-and-error attempts are made to restore balance.

The trial-and-error attempts fail. The anxiety escalates to severe or panic levels. The person adopts automatic relief behaviours.

When these measures do not reduce anxiety, anxiety can overwhelm the person and lead to serious personality disorganization, which signals the person is in crisis.

FIGURE 35.5 Phases of crisis response.

pregnancy. Situational crises also result from less common occurrences such as accidents, natural or human-caused disasters, and acts of terrorism. Box 35-4 discusses the death of a loved one, a situational crisis that each of us will encounter in our lifetime.

Developmental Crisis

Theorists such as Erik Erikson propose that human development proceeds sequentially through a series of stages, each with a new set of social roles and responsibilities. Stage theorists hold that demands from the social environment exert pressure on an individual to move on to the next developmental stage and that a failure to meet these new expectations precipitates a developmental crisis. Successful resolution of this crisis is necessary for movement into the next stage. Developmental crises are an expected part of maturation and are a time during which individuals acquire new skills and resources.

The concept of developmental crisis assumes that psychosocial development progresses in an orderly, easily identifiable process. Other developmental theories, for example those proposed by Miller (1994) and Gilligan (1994), refute the notion that human development advances in stages (see Chapter 8). That being said, the concept of developmental crisis is useful for describing unfavourable person–environment relationships that relate to maturational events, such as leaving home for the first time, completing school, or the birth of one's first child.

Crisis or Not? The Effects of Balancing Factors

Aguilera (1998) believes that whether or not a stressful event evolves into a crisis depends on three interdependent *balancing factors*: perception of the event,

available situational supports, and coping mechanisms. As Figure 35-6 illustrates, the timely and successful resolution of a crisis is more likely if an individual has a realistic view of the situation, adequate supports available, and effective coping mechanisms.

Nursing Care of Individuals Experiencing Crisis

Crisis Intervention

Crisis intervention is the provision of emergency psychological care to assist victims in returning to an adaptive level of functioning and to prevent or moderate the potentially negative effects of psychological trauma (Everly & Mitchell, 1999). Although there are several models of crisis intervention, virtually all of them incorporate the following principles (Flannery & Everly, 2000):

1. **Early intervention.** By their nature, crises are acute and distressing events that overwhelm an individual's coping resources. Inability to resolve a crisis in a timely manner renders those affected at higher risk for long-term health problems. Crisis intervention services are typically community based and operate 24 hours per day. Crisis teams provide telephone triage and counselling but may also travel to the scene of the crisis, where they work closely with other emergency service personnel (e.g., police officers, firefighters, hospital emergency staff).
2. **Stabilization.** An immediate goal of all crisis intervention efforts is to prevent the situation from worsening. Stabilization involves mobilizing resources and support networks with the aim of minimizing harm and quickly restoring some semblance of order and routine.

BOX 35.4

Death of a Loved One: A Crisis Event

One of the most common crisis-provoking events is the loss of a loved one through death. Although death is a certainty for all of us, Western culture "denies and defies death. Death is often seen as a defeat, a failure, and an outcome to be avoided at all costs. As a result, the bereaved often feel profoundly isolated" (Roberts & Berry, 2002, p. 53).

DEFINITION OF TERMS

Bereavement is typically understood to be the objective event or occurrence of having suffered a loss (Rando, 1993).

Grief is the subjective experience (e.g., thoughts, feelings, behaviours, body sensations) that accompanies the perception of a loss (Rando, 1993).

Mourning is the external manifestation of grief, which is highly influenced by gender, ethnicity, culture, religion, and the cause of death (Wolfelt, 1999).

TASKS OF MOURNING

Worden (2003) describes the four tasks of mourning, which are necessary to the process of adapting to loss and reestablishing equilibrium. Unlike other theorists who conceptualize mourning in terms of *stages* or *phases*, which connote linearity, Worden emphasizes the issues that bereaved individuals must face and successfully negotiate as they come to terms with their new reality:

1. *Accepting the reality of the loss.* The first task of grieving is to accept the reality and full consequence of the loss. A part of this is recognizing the permanence of death and that life as it was is over forever.

2. *Working through the pain of grief.* It is important for the bereaved individual to experience and acknowledge the pain of grief. Denial or suppression of this pain prolongs grieving.

3. *Adapting to an environment in which the deceased is absent.* This adaptation requires the bereaved individual to adjust to a new reality, which involves developing a new self-identity (e.g., as a widow or single person) and taking on new social roles and responsibilities.

4. *Developing a new relationship with the deceased and reengaging with life.* In coming to terms with the loss, the bereaved individual does not forget the deceased but rather establishes a new relationship with the deceased. This involves healing the wound of the severed attachment so that new attachments can be formed.

Resolution of grief is manifested by the gradual return of feelings of well-being and the ability to continue with life. The bereaved person does not deny his or her former life or forget the loved one but finds a way to weave memories of the past into the current reality.

It is important to keep in mind that although the experience of loss is universal, individual responses vary widely, and there is no one clearly defined course or process of bereavement or grieving. Grief is influenced by age, development, gender, history of loss and/or trauma, history of depression, the nature and quality of the relationship with the deceased, and the type of loss (e.g., anticipated, violent, traumatic). Research underscores that the experience and expressions of grief are influenced by such factors as familial relationships and expectations, social and cultural factors, and religion (Center for the Advancement of Health, 2003).

COMPLICATED GRIEF

Complicated grief is also termed abnormal, pathologic, chronic, or exaggerated grief. It refers to grief that does not seem to be advancing the bereaved individual toward acceptance and reorganization. Grief is complicated when an individual does not accomplish one or more of the tasks of mourning. Examples of this include denying the reality of one's loss; prolonged and intense emotions that do not seem to lessen over time; the apparent absence of mourning; and the inability to reinvest in life.

ROLE OF HEALTH CARE TEAMS IN SUPPORTING GRIEF

As members of the health care team, nurses participate in supporting bereaved individuals through the process of grieving. The goals of this care are to assist bereaved individuals with the tasks of mourning and to prevent complicated grief. Activities may include sitting in silence with the bereaved, active listening, assistance with practical needs, and referral for ongoing support.

---

3. **Facilitating understanding.** An important part of crisis intervention is helping individuals to develop an accurate understanding of the situation and its potential consequences. This usually involves listening to individuals' accounts of their experience and assisting them to identify and articulate their feelings about what is happening. Facilitating a clear understanding of a situation helps individuals to develop a realistic appraisal of the demands on them and aids the integration of the crisis into their cognitive schema.

4. **Focusing on problem solving.** A primary task of crisis intervention is the identification and prioritization of immediate problems. Once achieved, interventions focus on assisting those involved to find short-term solutions.

5. **Encouraging self-reliance.** Encouraging and supporting individuals to participate in identifying and solving problems facilitate their return to independent function and the development of a sense of mastery.

CRNENOTE

The goals of crisis intervention are to assist individuals to return to an adaptive level of functioning and to prevent or moderate the potentially negative effects of extreme stress. Principles of crisis intervention include early intervention, stabilization, facilitating understanding, a focus on problem solving, and encouragement of self-reliance.

FIGURE 35.6 The effect of balancing factors in a stressful event (From Aguilera, D. C. (1998). *Crisis intervention: Theory and methodology.* St. Louis, MO: Mosby.).

The case study in Box 35-5 uses Roberts' Seven-Stage Crisis Intervention Model (Fig. 35-7; Roberts, 1991) to illustrate the application of these principles to a clinical situation.

Telephone Help Lines

Many health authorities now have telephone help lines, typically staffed by mental health professionals or trained volunteers, which offer support for problems such as child abuse, suicide, and family stress. These lines permit immediate access to a spectrum of support and intervention services for individuals who are experiencing a crisis or need help to manage life stressors.

Short-Stay Hospitalization and Community-Based Emergency Housing

Some health authorities also designate a few beds on their psychiatric units for short-stay crisis stabilization. Individuals are admitted to these beds for a brief period of inpatient care (typically 72 hours) when they have no supports in the community, need to have their medications assessed or stabilized, or require some other health service. There is also often community-based emergency housing, such as shelters for children and youth who cannot remain at home, shelters for victims of domestic violence, and short- and long-term accommodations for individuals with serious and persistent mental illness. These settings provide

Case Study Demonstrating Roberts' Seven-Stage Crisis Intervention Model

The mobile mental health crisis unit in a large Canadian city receives a call from Theresa, the maternal aunt of 19-year-old Billy, an Aboriginal male whose 12-year-old brother died 4 months ago from sniffing gasoline. On hearing of his brother's death, Billy quit college and went on a 5-day drinking binge. At the time of the call, he is lying on his bed in the dark. Theresa tells the crisis nurse that Billy has been eating very little for the past several weeks and has been sleeping 12–14 hours/day. He rarely leaves his room and speaks only when addressed directly. What little conversation he does offer is preoccupied with his brother and their parents, who died in a car crash a number of years earlier. Theresa has tried everything she can think of to convince Billy to get help; she is worried about leaving him alone for fear he will harm himself.

STAGE 1: Conduct Crisis And Bio/Psycho/Social/Spiritual Assessment (Including Lethality Assessment). Joanne, the crisis intervention nurse, performs a focused assessment and, using direct questions, ascertains important details about the situation (e.g., caller name, address, and telephone number; nature of emergency; presence of/ potential for injury or loss of life; availability of weapons or other potentially dangerous items). Within 2 or 3 minutes she determines that Billy has experienced major losses (one of them very recently), that his behaviour is suggestive of acute mourning and/or depression; that he is at high risk for self-harm; and that his aunt, who is his primary social support, has exhausted her resources for dealing with the situation. The nurse tells Theresa that she and a colleague are on their way to talk with Billy and that they will be bringing police assistance. The nurse decides to involve the police for two reasons. The first is that by their nature, crises are unpredictable situations and have some potential for violence; a police presence sometimes deters aggressive acting out; and if it does not, it ensures that there are trained personnel to effectively contain it. The second reason is that the police have authority, under provincial mental health legislation, to transport individuals for psychiatric assessment, even against their will. In order to do this, they must have evidence that the individual is in imminent danger to himself or herself or someone else.

STAGE 2: Establish Rapport and a Working Therapeutic Relationship. Joanne establishes rapport with Theresa on the telephone by listening carefully to her, validating her

concerns, and offering concrete and specific assistance. When the nurse and other members of the crisis team arrive at the home, Joanne stays with Theresa while her colleague Don begins talking with Billy through his locked bedroom door. Don uses his well-developed interpersonal skills (see Chapter 8) to make a connection with the young man and to convince him to come out of his room and talk face to face. When it becomes apparent that Billy is not a danger to himself or others, the police leave.

STAGE 3: Identify Dimensions of Presenting Problem. Fortunately, when the crisis team speaks with Billy, they learn that he has not done anything to harm himself. He is experiencing a great deal of emotional pain for which he has few words, has lost his sense of meaning in life, and has only a vague plan of shooting himself. He does not have immediate access to a firearm. In his conversation with Don, Billy acknowledges that the loss of his parents was devastating, but it is his brother's death that caused his "world to crash apart."

STAGE 4: Explore Feelings and Emotions. Don encourages Billy to talk about his experience and offers him words for the things he is feeling. Eventually, Billy agrees to include his aunt and Joanne in the conversation.

STAGE 5: Generate and Explore Alternatives. Billy, Theresa, Don, and Joanne sit around the kitchen table with cups of tea discussing the supports available to the family.

STAGE 6: Develop a Plan. Theresa states that praying to the Creator everyday and speaking to a local elder help her to get through many difficult times. Billy says that he will pray with her every day, signs a written safety contract, and agrees to see an intake worker at the mental health centre for an assessment the next day. The safety contract specifies a number of things that Billy will do if he begins to feel overwhelmed again, including praying, talking to Theresa, and calling the crisis line.

STAGE 7: Develop a Follow-up Plan. Joanne calls Theresa the next afternoon and learns that she and Billy had spent the evening talking and praying together. He had eaten breakfast and showered this morning before attending his appointment at the mental health centre. The intake worker referred Billy to a men's grief support group and was going to speak with the student counselling service at his college to arrange one-to-one counselling.

users with food, a place to stay, emotional support, and referrals to other community services.

■ DISASTER: NATURAL AND HUMAN-CAUSED

A natural or human-caused disaster strikes with little warning. Examples of natural disasters include hurricanes, tsunamis, and earthquakes; examples of human-caused

disasters include transportation accidents, chemical or nuclear waste spills, and acts of terrorism. Often, it is the unpredictability of such events that causes fear, confusion, and a sense of helplessness that can have lasting effects on the health and well-being of those involved. Individuals exposed to disasters experience multiple stressors, including threats to personal safety and integrity, loss of property, exposure to suffering and death, economic devastation, lawlessness, and social disorganization. By definition, disasters overwhelm institutions, health

FIGURE 35.7 Roberts' (1991) Seven-Stage Crisis Intervention Model.

care, and social services and require months or years for individuals and communities to recover (Fullerton, Ursano, Norwood, & Holloway, 2003).

KEY CONCEPT A **disaster** is a sudden, overwhelming, and catastrophic event that causes widespread damage, social disorganization, mass casualties, and human suffering.

Characteristics of Disasters

Disasters are not alike; each is defined by a constellation of characteristics that has implications for surviving individuals and communities. These include natural versus human causation, proximity and degree of personal impact, magnitude and scope, visible end or "low point," and probability of recurrence (DeWolfe, 2000). Individually and collectively, these characteristics affect the nature, intensity, and duration of the stress associated with a disaster.

Natural Versus Human Causation

The research is not clear as to whether it is natural or human-caused disasters that have the greater impact on the psychological well-being of those affected. What seems to be the case is that there are cognitive, emotional, psychological, and social reactions unique to each (DeWolfe, 2000; Weisaeth, 1994). In disasters with a human element (e.g., suicide bombings and other acts of terrorism, chemical or nuclear spills, transportation disasters), survivors struggle to come to terms with the deliberate intent to harm and with human error. The belief that an event was both senseless and preventable, a sense of betrayal by another human being, and an identifiable agent who is the target of anger and blame can complicate and prolong survivors' recovery period.

Such delayed healing was evident in the events following the bombing of Air India Flight 182, which occurred on June 23, 1985 over the Atlantic Ocean south of Ireland (Canadian Broadcasting Corporation [CBC], 2006). All 329 passengers and crew died, including 82 children. The explosion, caused by a bomb planted in checked baggage, was the single largest terrorist attack before those of September 11, 2001 and the largest mass murder in Canadian history. The Canadian government's trial of those accused of the bombing ended in March 2005, with the acquittal of Ripudaman Singh Malik and Ajaib Singh

Bagri. The trial lasted almost two decades and cost nearly $130 million. The only person convicted of any involvement in the bombing was Inderjit Singh Reyat, who pled guilty in 2003 to building the explosive device used on Flight 182; he was sentenced to 10 years in jail. Many of the surviving families say publicly that they are still searching for answers and a sense that justice has been served.

Although their results may be devastating, natural disasters are usually seen as being without evil intent and beyond human control. Some survivors find it easier to accept the destruction and loss of life as a random occurrence or an *act of God*. In all disasters, no matter what the cause, individuals' belief in the world as safe and predictable is irrevocably changed. A central part of the recovery process involves reconstructing a sense of self and a set of beliefs about how the world operates within this new reality.

Degree of Personal Impact

Research evidence consistently demonstrates that the greater the exposure individuals have to a disaster and its effects, the greater the postdisaster response (DeWolfe, 2000; Solomon & Green, 1992). Injury and death of loved ones, the loss of one's home and belongings, and widespread destruction of one's community all affect an individual's postdisaster response. The complex interaction of grief and trauma exacerbate the effects of each and can prolong recovery (Kohn & Levav, 1990). Individuals directly exposed to the devastation associated with disaster tend to experience more anxiety; depression; sadness; posttrauma symptoms; somatic symptoms; and, in some studies, substance abuse.

Magnitude and Scope of the Disaster

As with the degree of personal impact, there is a *dose–response relationship* between the magnitude of devastation and psychological impact (DeWolfe, 2000). When a disaster destroys an entire community, all semblance of normalcy disappears, and survivors' lives are turned upside down. Not surprisingly, there are higher levels of anxiety, depression, PTSD, somatic symptoms, and generalized distress associated with widespread community destruction (Solomon & Green, 1992). When at least some elements of community life remain intact (e.g., schools, churches, businesses), they serve as a foundation for the recovery process. Social networks establish or reestablish more readily when gathering places remain standing and institutional structures are functional.

Compare, for example, the effects of hurricane Katrina with the ice storm that affected parts of Ontario, Quebec, and New Brunswick in January 1998 (CBC, n. d.). Katrina, a category-4 hurricane, made landfall along the Central Gulf Coast near New Orleans, Louisiana, on August 29, 2005. Its storm surge soon breached the levee system that protected New Orleans from Lake Pontchartrain, and areas of the city were subsequently flooded. More than 1,100 individuals died in Katrina's wake; whole communities were razed, and thousands of individuals were displaced. Although the Canadian ice storm caused massive power outages lasting for several weeks in some areas, the infrastructure remained intact.

Visible End or "Low Point"

When disasters have a clearly identifiable ending, it signals to survivors that the threat has passed and that the situation has reached its low point (DeWolfe, 2000). A clear end point enables the community to begin tallying its losses and marks the beginning of the recovery process. When the end point of a disaster is ambiguous (e.g., as it was with hurricane Katrina or with the 2005 Canadian National train derailment near Squamish, British Columbia, that spilled toxic sodium hydroxide into the Cheakamus River [CBC, 2005]), it may take weeks or months before survivors feel that the disaster is over. In disasters involving chemical or nuclear contamination, the impact period is even more uncertain and protracted because visible evidence of damage (e.g., birth defects, increased rates of cancer and other diseases, implications for the natural environment) may not be apparent for decades (Green & Solomon, 1995). This prolonged impact period with no clear end impedes survivors' recovery.

Probability of Recurrence

When a disaster has a seasonal pattern (e.g., forest fires, floods, hurricanes, tornadoes) survivors may worry that they will be hit again before the season ends. During the off-season, communities rebuild, vegetation grows back, and visual reminders of the disaster gradually recede, all of which facilitate recovery. When the probability of a recurrence is perceived as high (e.g., following earthquakes and floods), recovery can be slowed. For example, aftershocks following an earthquake and media coverage of the increased risk for flooding due to high water tables or overwhelmed sewage systems can keep affected individuals anxious and preoccupied. As well, delays in disaster relief payments or insurance settlements can frustrate survivors and hinder rebuilding.

Individual Survivor Characteristics

Although disasters indiscriminately affect everyone and everything in their path, the experience will be slightly different for every individual. The meaning assigned to the disaster, personality characteristics, worldview, social supports, and spiritual beliefs all affect individuals' appraisals

BOX 35.6

Research for Best Practice: Positive Responses to Traumatic Events

Davis, C. G., & Macdonald, S. L. (2004). Threat appraisals, distress and the development of positive life changes after September 11th in a Canadian sample. Cognitive Behaviour Therapy, 33(2), 63–78.

QUESTION: Does the magnitude of perceived threat and the intensity of resultant emotional distress predict positive life changes?

METHOD: Adults in Ottawa, Ontario, were surveyed to determine whether the magnitude of perceived personal threat in response to the terrorist attacks of September 11, 2001 correlated with the intensity of their emotional distress and whether stronger first-day emotional reactions would predict positive life changes.

FINDINGS: Although the participants in this study were not directly harmed by the attacks of September 11, participants appraised the events as personally threatening and reported feeling significantly distressed. This study found that the higher the appraisal of personal threat and the more distress an individual reported immediately after the attacks, the more likely the individual was to report having made positive life changes (e.g., closer to family, refocused priorities) several weeks later. Initial distress and greater perceived threat also correlated positively with whether people provided help after the disaster. Follow-up data 11 months later revealed significant stability of these positive life changes.

IMPLICATION FOR PRACTICE: Although stress, crises, and disaster affect all of us, human beings have an innate capacity to rebound and recover from traumatic events. Many trauma experts (e.g., United States Department of Veterans' Affairs [n. d.]) agree that for most of us, adversity fosters resilience not psychopathology. Research on individuals with positive responses after a traumatic event indicates that their preferred coping mechanisms are to (1) focus on brief time intervals (e.g., think only about the next step), (2) maintain a view of oneself as competent and a view of others as willing and able to provide support, and (3) focus on the current implications of the trauma and avoid regretting past decisions and actions.

---

of the situation, their coping abilities, and their recovery. Previous trauma and losses can either enhance coping or compromise it. Well-developed personal coping resources, an intact and dense social network, and timely and adequate disaster relief all greatly assist recovery. By contrast, preexisting health problems, concurrent stressors, and weak social support all increase vulnerability to the negative effects of disaster (van der Kolk & McFarlane, 1996).

Once again, research findings are inconsistent with regard to who fares worse during a disaster. There is some evidence that individuals in the 40- to 60-year-old range (the so-called *sandwich generation*) may be at higher risk for stress-related illness because of the competing demands of parenting, employment, and caring for aging parents (Green & Solomon, 1995). Although those individuals who are not in long-term relationships may be more vulnerable to some aspects of stress, marital conflict often escalates following a disaster. On the other hand, as Box 35-6 demonstrates, a distressing event can motivate positive life changes.

Phases of Disaster

Although the experience of disaster is unique to each individual and community, there are some identifiable phases, influenced by interacting elements of the person–environment relationship (DeWolfe, 2000). Disasters may or may not include all of the following phases.

Warning or Threat Phase

Disasters vary with respect to the amount of warning that communities have before they occur. For instance, earthquakes usually strike without warning, whereas floods and hurricanes may have hours to days of warning. The lack of warning before an impending disaster is associated with greater feelings of vulnerability and lack of control, which may exacerbate subsequent psychological trauma. Also, individuals may feel guilt or blame themselves if they do not respond adequately to warnings and suffer losses as a result.

Impact Phase

Depending on the nature of the disaster, the impact phase can be short or protracted. Moreover, the greater the magnitude of personal loss associated with the disaster, the greater the psychosocial effects. Typically, individuals are initially immobilized by shock and confusion and cannot fully comprehend what is happening to the world around them. This quickly abates as they turn their attention to the immediate survival needs of themselves and their loved ones.

Rescue or Heroic Phase

During the first minutes and hours of a disaster, the preservation of life and property is paramount. For some individuals, the epinephrine-driven autonomic arousal enables heroic rescue efforts, and altruism is evident among survivors and emergency personnel alike. There are two potentially negative aspects associated with this phase of disaster. The first is that although activity levels may be high, actual productivity is often low. Second, stress impairs cognitive function and the ability to appraise risk, which can result in injury and death.

Remedy or Honeymoon Phase

In the days and weeks following a disaster, government and volunteer assistance may be readily available. The relief of having survived and the camaraderie of sharing a life-threatening experience can draw individuals and communities closer together. When this happens, survivors experience a short-lived sense of optimism that life will soon return to normal.

Inventory Phase

As time passes and the reality of the situation settles in, individuals begin to realize the full impact of their losses and the limits of disaster assistance. At the same time, most individuals are suffering the effects of lack of sleep compounded by the enormous demands of moment-by-moment survival. The unrealistic optimism of the honeymoon phase fades into discouragement and fatigue.

Disillusionment Phase

When the immediate danger passes and disaster relief agencies and volunteers begin to leave, survivors may feel abandoned and angry. If parts of a community are not affected by the disaster, they quickly return to *business as usual*, which further discourages and alienates survivors. As well, resentments flare up if survivors believe that they have not received the same amount of assistance or compensation as others. Issues like this foster divisiveness, jealousy, and hostility in communities and undermine community cohesion and support. As disaster survivors begin to accept the loss of life as it was, stressors accumulate in the forms of family conflict, financial hardship, bureaucratic red tape, rebuilding and relocation, and a lack of recreation or leisure time. As the wear and tear takes its toll, stress-related health problems emerge.

Reconstruction and Recovery Phase

The postdisaster reconstruction and recovery phase goes on for years. Eventually survivors realize that they are primarily responsible to solve the problems associated with rebuilding their homes, their businesses, and their lives. New buildings and roads serve as permanent reminders of loss. At the point that individuals can begin to see meaning, personal growth, and opportunity in relation to their disaster experience, they are well on the road to recovery.

Individuals and communities recover from disaster at different rates depending on the nature of the disaster and the degree of exposure. This process is never linear or sequential because of the many interacting variables involved. In Canada, all levels of government participate in preparing for and responding to disasters. Health-service agencies work closely with municipal governments to develop, update, and practice disaster response plans. Because of the vital role that nurses play in health care delivery, nurses make important contributions in every aspect of disaster relief, both at home and abroad.

CRNENOTE

Disasters are defined by a number of interacting factors, including natural versus human causation, proximity and degree of personal impact, magnitude and scope, visible end or low point, and probability of recurrence. Individually and collectively, these factors influence the nature, intensity, and duration of the stress associated with a disaster.

SUMMARY OF KEY POINTS

- Many personal factors, such as personality patterns, beliefs, values, and commitment to an outcome, interact with environmental demands and constraints that produce a person–environment relationship.
- Stress occurs when a person–environment relationship is appraised as being unfavourable. Stress responses are simultaneously emotional and physiologic, leading to an innate tendency to act.
- Within the social network, social support can help a person cope with stress.
- Effective coping can be either problem-focused or emotion-focused. The outcome of successful coping is enhanced health, psychological well-being, and social functioning.
- A crisis is a severely stressful situation that causes exaggerated stress responses. The nursing process is similar for the person experiencing a stress response, except that increased attention is paid to safety issues.
- Disaster is a sudden, overwhelming catastrophic event that causes great damage, destruction, mass casualties, and human suffering that require assistance from all available resources.

CRITICAL THINKING CHALLENGES

1 Compare and contrast Selye's stress response to Lazarus and Folkman's model of stress, coping, and adaptation.
2 Explain why two individuals may experience the same stressful event or situation very differently.
3 Briefly explain the physiologic stress response.
4 An 18-year-old man is admitted to a psychiatric unit for psychotic behaviour and is eventually given the diagnosis of schizophrenia. His parents refuse to accept this and take him all over the country seeking

other opinions. Is this an example of problem-focused or emotion-focused coping? Explain your answer.

5   After the death of his mother, a 24-year-old single man with schizophrenia moves into an apartment. He continues to take his medication but feels sad about his mother's death. He is not adjusting well to living alone and tells his nurse that he no longer wants to go to work. In tears, he admits that he is lonely and can no longer manage the day-to-day demands of his apartment. The nurse generates the following nursing diagnosis: Ineffective coping related to inadequate support system. Develop a plan of care for this young man.

6   Define *stress*, *crisis*, and *disaster*. Compare and contrast each of these with a psychiatric emergency.

7   Identify Worden's (1991) tasks of mourning and discuss the nurse's role in relation to them.

8   You are a nurse working with a mobile mental-health crisis team. An elderly woman calls to say that she has just been robbed at knifepoint on her way home from shopping. What assessment questions would you ask her? Explain your answer.

WEB LINKS

cehs.unl.edu/stress/workshop/tableofcontents.html This document, "Stress Management: A Review of Principles," presents the core concepts of stress management education.

www.hc-sc.gc.ca/ed-ud/prepar/index_e.html This is Health Canada's website on emergency and disaster readiness.

www.healthnet.org/disasterhealthpaper.php This site has a number of resources on disaster preparedness from the International Council of Nurses.

www.isma.org.uk This is the site of the U.K.'s International Stress Management Association (ISMA), a leading professional body for stress management. This site has articles from the *ISMA* journal.

www.pep.bc.ca This site contains a 26-step *to-do list* for emergency preparedness published by the government of British Columbia.

www.stress-management-isma.org This is the site of the ISMA, which seeks to advance the education of professionals and students and to facilitate methodically sound research in several professional interdisciplinary stress management fields.

www.yorku.ca This York University site contains a report, *Ethics and SARS: Learning Lessons from the Toronto Experience*, by a working group of the University of Toronto Joint Centre for Bioethics and discusses ethical concerns that nurses face during crisis and disaster situations, including the duty to care.

MOVIES, NOVELS, AND BIOGRAPHIES

Blindness: 2008. Based on the 1995 novel, *Blindness*, authored by José Saramago, winner of the Nobel Prize for Literature, the movie tells the story of a small group of people, including an ophthalmologist, his wife, and some of his patients, whose city is faced with an epidemic of "White Sickness." This sickness of unknown origin strikes suddenly, causing blindness and inspiring panic and terror. The city and its society flounders as the government tries to contain the outbreak and maintain order.

VIEWING POINTS: During disasters, such as epidemics, decision makers need to balance individual freedoms against the common good. Identify some of the key health and social issues that must be addressed during an epidemic. Discuss the ethical dilemmas and concerns that will arise. Imagine being a nurse living in this city during the blindness epidemic. What might be your personal challenges at such a time?

Paradise Road: 1997. Based on a true story, this movie chronicles the experiences of a group of women from different countries and social levels in a Japanese concentration camp. Adrienne Pargiter, a graduate of the Royal Academy of Music, organizes a vocal band in spite of their captors' resistance.

VIEWING POINTS: Resilience refers to human capacity to adapt and even thrive in the face of adversity and trauma. What factors contributed to the women's resilience in this film? At what points in the story did the different women transform from victim to survivor?

Schindler's List: 1993. The film presents the true story of Oskar Schindler, a member of the Nazi party, womanizer, and war profiteer, who saved the lives of more than 1,000 Jews during the Holocaust. The movie shows how during long periods of political turmoil and terror, life can become somewhat normalized. Yet, fear underlies people's daily lives. Crises erupt at different times during the very long period of chronic stress.

VIEWING POINTS: Differentiate the periods of chronic stress from crisis in this film. Observe the reactions of different characters under stress. Is the behaviour different from what you would expect? Observe your own feelings throughout the movie. Did you experience stress?

REFERENCES

Aguilera, D. C. (1998). *Crisis intervention: Theory and methodology*. St. Louis, MO: Mosby.

American Psychiatric Association. (1980). *Diagnostic and statistical manual of mental disorders* (3rd ed.). Washington, DC: Author.

American Psychiatric Association. (2000). *Diagnostic and statistical manual of mental disorders* (4th ed., Text revision). Washington, DC: Author.

Bartlett, D. (1998). *Stress: Perspectives and processes*. Philadelphia, PA: Open University Press.

Birmes, P., Hatton, L., Brunet, A., & Schmitt, L. (2003). Early historical literature for post-traumatic symptomatology. *Stress and Health, 19*, 17–26.

Campbell, M. (1973). *Halfbreed*. Halifax, Nova Scotia, Canada: Goodread Biographies.

Canadian Broadcasting Corporation. (n.d.). *The ice storm of 1998*. Retrieved November 25, 2009, from http://archives.cbc.ca/environment/extreme_weather/clips/1437

Canadian Broadcasting Corporation. (2005, November). *Train derails near Squamish, sparking safety calls*. Retrieved May 24, 2008, from http://www.cbc.ca/canada/story/2005/11/03/bctrain051103.html

Canadian Broadcasting Corporation. (2006, September). *The bombing of Air India flight 182*. Retrieved November 25, 2009, from http://www.cbc.ca/news/background/airindia/bombing.html

Cannon, W. B. (1939). *The wisdom of the body*. New York, NY: WW Norton.

Caplan, G. (1961). *An approach to community mental health*. New York, NY: Grune & Stratton.

Carpenito-Moyet, L. (2009). *Nursing diagnosis: Application to clinical practice* (13th ed.). Philadelphia, PA: Lippincott Williams & Wilkins.

Center for the Advancement of Health. (2003). *Report on bereavement and grief research*. Retrieved May 24, 2008, from http://www.cfah.org/pdfs/griefreport.pdf

Clegg, A. (2001). Occupational stress in nursing: A review of the literature. *Journal of Nursing Management, 9*(2), 101–106.

Cohen, S., & Wills, T. A. (1985). Stress, social support, and the buffering hypothesis. *Psychological Bulletin, 98*(2), 310–357.

Cooper, G. L., & Dewe, P. (2004). *Stress: A brief history*. Malden, MA: Blackwell Publishing.

Coyne, J. C., & Holroyd, K. (1982). Stress, coping and illness: A transactional perspective. In T. Milton, C. Green, & R. Meagher (Eds.), *Handbook of clinical health psychology* (pp. 103–127). New York, NY: Plenum Press.

Cropley, M., & Steptoe, A. (2005). Social support, life events and physical symptoms: A prospective study of chronic and recent life stress in men and women. *Psychology, Health and Medicine, 10*(4), 317–325.

Davis, C. G., & Macdonald, S. L. (2004). Threat appraisals, distress and the development of positive life changes after September 11th in a Canadian sample. *Cognitive Behaviour Therapy, 33*(2), 68–78.

DeWolfe, D. J. (2000). *Training manual for mental health and human service workers in major disasters* (2nd ed.). Rockville, MD: Substance Abuse and Mental Health Services Administration (DHHS/PHS).

Dimsdale, J. E. (1988). A perspective on Type A behavior and coronary disease. *New England Journal of Medicine, 318*(2), 110–112.

Dohrenwend, B. S., & Dohrenwend, B. P. (1974). *Stressful life events: Their nature and their effects*. New York, NY: Wiley & Sons.

Dohrenwend, B. P., & Shrout, P. E. (1985). "Hassles" in the conceptualization and measurement of stress variables. *American Psychologist, 40*(7), 780–785.

Everly, G. S., & Mitchell, J. T. (1999). *Critical incident stress management: A new era and standard of care in crisis intervention* (2nd ed.). Ellicott City, MD: Chevron.

Flannery, R, B., & Everly, G. S. (2000). Crisis intervention: A review. *International Journal of Emergency Mental Health, 2*(2), 119–125.

Folkman, S., & Lazarus, R. S. (1991). The concept of coping. In A. Monat and & R. S. Lazarus (Eds.), *Stress and coping: An anthology* (3rd ed., pp. 209–227). New York, NY: Columbia University Press.

Friedman, M., & Rosenman, R. (1974). *Type A and your heart*. New York, NY: Knopf.

Fullerton, C. S., Ursano, R. J., Norwood, A. E., & Holloway, H. H. (2003). Trauma, terrorism, and disaster. In R. J. Ursano, C. S. Fullerton, & A. E. Norwood (Eds.), *Terrorism and disaster* (pp. 1–20). Cambridge, MA: Cambridge University Press.

Furedi, F. (2007). The changing meaning of disaster. *Area, 39*(4), 482–489.

Gilligan, C. (1994). Joining the resistance: Psychology, politics, girls and women. In M. Berger (Ed.), *Women beyond Freud: New concept of feminine psychology* (pp. 99–145). New York, NY: Brunner Mozel.

Glaser, R., Rice, J., Sherridan, J., & Fertel, R. (1987). Stress-related immune suppression: Health implications. *Brain, Behavior and Immunity, 1*(1), 7–20.

Grandjean, D., Rendu, A.-C., MacNamee, T., & Scherer, K. R. (2008). The wrath of the gods: Appraising the meaning of disaster. *Social Science Information, 47*(2), 187–204.

Green, B. L., & Solomon, S. D. (1995). The mental health impact of natural and technological disasters. In J. R. Freedy & S. E. Hobfoll (Eds.), *Traumatic stress: From theory to practice*. New York, NY: Plenum Press.

Guyton, A. C., & Hall, J. E. (2000). *Textbook of medical physiology* (10th ed.). Philadelphia, PA: WB Saunders.

Hafer, C., & Bègue, L. (2005). Experimental research on just-world theory: Problems, developments, and future challenges. *Psychological Bulletin, 131*(1), 128–167.

Harper, D. (2001). *Online etymology dictionary*. Retrieved November 25, 2009, from http://www.etymonline.com

Haslam, S. A., O'Brien, A., Jetten, J., Vormedal, K., & Penna, S. (2005). Taking the strain: Social identity, social support, and the experience of stress. *British Journal of Social Psychology, 44*(Pt 3), 355–370.

Holmes, T., & Rahe, R. (1967). The Social Readjustment Patient Scale. *Journal of Psychosomatic Research, 11*(2), 213–218.

Johnson, M., Bulechek, G. M., McCloskey-Dochterman, J., Maas, M. L., Moorhead, S., Swanson, S., et al. (2006). *Nursing diagnoses, outcomes, and interventions: NANDA, NOC, and NIC linkages*. St. Louis, MO: Mosby.

Jones, F., & Kinman, G. (2001). Approaches to studying stress. In F. Jones & J. Bright (Eds.), *Stress: Myth, theory & research* (pp. 17–44). London, UK: Prentice Hall.

Jones, M. C., & Johnston, D. W. (2000). Reducing distress in first level and student nurses: A review of the applied stress management literature. *Journal of Advanced Nursing, 32*(1), 66–74.

Kendler, K. S., Neale, M. C., Kessler, R. C., Heath, A. C., & Eaves, L. G. (1992). Major depression and generalized anxiety disorder. Same genes, (partly) different environments. *Archives of General Psychiatry, 49*(9), 716–722.

Kessler, R. C., Sonnega, A., Bromet, E., Hughes, M., & Nelson, C. B. (1995). Posttraumatic stress disorder in the National Comorbidity Survey. *Archives of General Psychiatry, 52*(12), 1048–1060.

Kindlen, S. (2003). Injury and illness. In S. Kindlen (Ed.), *Physiology for health care and nursing* (2nd ed.). Edinburgh, UK: Churchill Livingstone.

Kleinke, C. L. (2007). What does it mean to cope? In A. Monat, R. S. Lazarus, & G. Reevy (Eds.), *The Praeger handbook on stress and coping* (pp. 289–308). Westport, CT: Praeger.

Kobasa, S. C. (1979). Stressful life events, personality and health: An inquiry into hardiness. *Journal of Personality and Social Psychology, 37*(1), 1–11.

Kohn, R., & Levav, I. (1990). Bereavement in disaster: An overview of the research. *International Journal of Mental Health, 19*(2), 61–76.

Kushner, H. (1981). *When bad things happen to good people*. New York, NY: Random House Inc.

Lazarus, R. (1991). *Emotion and adaptation*. New York, NY: Oxford University Press.

Lazarus, R., & Folkman, S. (1984). *Stress, appraisal and coping*. New York, NY: Springer.

Lazarus, R. S. (1998). *The life and work of an eminent psychologist: An autobiography of Richard S. Lazarus*. New York, NY: Springer.

Lazarus, R. S. (1999). *Stress and emotion: A new synthesis*. New York, NY: Springer.

Lazarus, R. S., DeLongis, A., Folkman, S., & Gruen, R. (1985). Stress and adaptation outcomes: The problem of confounded measures. *American Psychologist, 40*(7), 770–779.

Lindeman, E. (1944). Symptomatology and management of acute grief. *American Journal of Psychiatry, 151*(6 Suppl.), 155–160.

Lindeman, E. (1956). The meaning of crisis in individual and family. *Teachers College Record, 57*, 310.

Lui, L. Y., Coe, C. L., Swenson, C. A., Kelly, E. A., Kita, H., & Busse, W. W. (2002). School examinations enhance airway inflammation to antigen challenge. *American Journal of Critical Care Medicine, 165*(8), 1062–1067.

Majer, J. M., Jason, L. A., Ferrarie, J. R., Venable, L. B., & Olson, B. D. (2002). Social support and self-efficacy for abstinence: Is peer identification an issue? *Journal of Substance Abuse Treatment, 23*(3), 209–215.

Malone, J. (1988). The social support and dissupport continuum. *Journal of Psychosocial Nursing and Mental Health Services, 26*(12), 18–22.

Mason, J. W. (1971). A re-evaluation of the concept of 'non-specificity' in stress theory. *Journal of Psychiatric Research, 8*(3), 323–333.

Math, S., John, J., Girimaji, S., Benegal, V., Sunny, B., Krishnakanth, K., et al. (2008). Comparative study of psychiatric morbidity among the displaced and non-displaced populations in the Andaman and Nicobar Islands following the tsunami. *Prehospital and Disaster Medicine, 23*(1), 29–34.

Matthies, E., Höger, R., & Guski, R. (2000). Living on polluted soil: Determinants of stress symptoms. *Environment and Behavior, 32*(2), 270–286.

McCloskey, J., & Bulechek, G. (2004). *Nursing interventions classification (NIC)* (4th ed.). St. Louis, MO: Mosby–Year Book.

McEwen, B. S. (1998). Protective and damaging effects of stress mediators. *The New England Journal of Medicine, 338*(3), 171–179.

Mikhail, A. (1981). Stress: A psychophysiological conception. *Journal of Human Stress, 7*(2), 9–15.

Miller, J. (1994). Women's psychological development: Connections, disconnections, and violations. In M. Berger (Ed.), *Women beyond Freud: New concept of feminine psychology* (pp. 79–97). New York, NY: Brunner Mozel.

North American Nursing Diagnosis Association. (2005). *NANDA nursing diagnoses: Definitions and classification, 2005–2006.* Philadelphia, PA: Author.

Park, K. O. (2007). Social support for stress prevention in hospital settings. *Journal of the Royal Society of Health, 127*(6), 260–264.

Rahe, R. H. (2000). Recent Life Changes Questionnaire [RLCQ] [1997]. Holmes, T. H. American Psychiatric Association. Task Force for the Handbook of Psychiatric Measures. *Handbook of psychiatric measures* (pp. 235–237). Washington, DC: American Psychiatric Association.

Rando, T. (1993). *Treatment of complicated mourning.* Champaign, IL: Research Press.

Richardson, J. D., Naifeh, J. A., & Elhai, J. D. (2007). Posttraumatic stress disorder and associated risk factors in Canadian peacekeeping veterans with health-related disabilities. *Canadian Journal of Psychiatry, 52*(8), 510–518.

Roberts, A. R. (1991). Conceptualizing crisis theory and the crisis model. In A. R. Roberts (Ed.), *Contemporary perspectives on crisis intervention and prevention* (pp. 3–17). Englewood Cliffs, NJ: Prentice-Hall.

Roberts, K. F., & Berry, P. H. (2002). Grief and bereavements. In K. K. Kuebler, P. H. Berry, & D. E. Heidrich (Eds.), *End of life care: Clinical practice guidelines,* (pp. 53–63). Philadelphia, PA: WB Saunders.

Rotter, J. B. (1966). Generalized expectancies for internal versus external control reinforcement. *Psychological Monographs, 80*(whole no. 609).

Saddock, B. J., & Saddock, V. A. (2003). *Kaplan & Saddock's synopsis of psychiatry* (9th ed.). Philadelphia, PA: Lippincott Williams & Wilkins.

Sapolsky, R. M. (2004). *Why zebras don't get ulcers* (3rd ed.). New York, NY: Henry Holt.

Segerstrom, S. C., & Miller, G. E. (2003). Psychological stress and the immune system in humans: A meta-analytic view of 30 years of inquiry. *Psychological Bulletin, 130*(4), 601–630.

Selye, H. (1956). *The stress of life.* New York, NY: McGraw-Hill.

Selye, H. (1974). *Stress without distress.* Philadelphia, PA: JB Lippincott.

Selye, H. (1980). The stress concept today. In I. L. Kutash, L. B. Schlesinger, and Associates (Eds.), *Handbook on stress and anxiety* (pp. 127–143). San Francisco, CA: Jossey-Bass.

Solomon, S. D., & Green, B. L. (1992). Mental health effects of natural and human-made disasters. *PTSD Research Quarterly, 3*(1), 1–8.

Stanley, R. O., & Burrows, G. D. (2005). The role of stress in mental illness: The practice. In C. L. Cooper (Ed.), *Handbook of stress medicine and health* (2nd ed., pp. 87–100). Boca Raton, FL: CRC Press.

Sterling, P., & Eyer, J. (1988). Allostasis: A new paradigm to explain arousal pathology. In S. Fisher, & J. Reason (Eds.), *Handbook of life stress, cognition and health* (pp. 629–649). New York, NY: John Wiley & Sons.

Taylor, S. E., Kemeny, M. E., Reed, G. M., Bower, J. E., & Gruenewald, T. L. (2000). Psychological resources, positive illusions, and health. *American Psychologist, 55*(1), 99–109.

United States Department of Veterans' Affairs. (n. d.). *National Center for PTSD Fact Sheet: Self-care and self-help following disasters.* Washington, DC: Author. Retrieved March 10, 2009, from http://www.ncptsd.va.gov/ncmain/ncdocs/fact_shts/fs_self_care_disaster.html

van der Kolk, B. A., & McFarlane, A. (1996). The black hole of trauma. In B. A. van der Kolk, A. McFarlane, & L. Weisaeth (Eds.), *Traumatic stress: The effects of overwhelming experience on mind, body, and society* (pp. 3–23). New York, NY: Guilford Press.

Weisaeth, L. (1994). Psychological and psychiatric aspects of technological disasters. In R. J. Ursano, B. G. McCaughey, & C. S. Fullerton (Eds.), *Individual and community responses to trauma and disaster: The structure of human chaos.* New York, NY: Cambridge University Press.

Williams, J. E., Paton, C. C., Siegler, I. C., Eigenbrodt, M. L., Nieto, F. J., & Tyroler, H. A. (2000). Anger proneness predicts coronary heart disease risk. *Circulation, 101*(17), 2034–2039.

Wolfelt, A. D. (1999). Dispelling 5 common myths about grief. Retrieved November 25, 2009, from http://www.griefwords.com/index.cgi?action=page&page=articles%2Fhelping7.html&site_id=2

Worden, J. W. (1991). *Grief counselling and grief therapy* (2nd ed.). New York, NY: Springer.

Worden, J. W. (2003). *Grief counseling and grief therapy: A handbook for the mental health practitioner* (electronic edition). New York, NY: Brunner-Routledge.

Wright, L. (1988). The Type A behavior pattern and coronary artery disease. *American Psychologist, 43*(1), 2–14.

Yeager, K. R., & Roberts, A. R. (2003). Differentiating among stress, acute stress disorder, crisis episodes, trauma, and PTSD: Paradigm and treatment goals. *Brief Treatment and Crisis Intervention, 3*(1), 145–167.

Management of Aggression and Violence

Yvonne Savard

Adapted from the chapter "Management of Aggression and Violence" by Sandy Harper-Jaques and Marlene Reimer

After studying this chapter, you will be able to:

- Explore feelings about the experience and expression of anger.
- Discuss the bio/psycho/social/spiritual factors that influence the expression of aggressive and violent behaviour.
- Discuss the theories used to explain anger, aggression, and violence.
- Identify the behaviour or actions that escalate and de-escalate violent behaviour.
- Recognize the risk for "nurse abuse" (attacks on nurses).
- Generate options for responding to the expression of anger and violent behaviour in clinical nursing practice.
- Apply the nursing process to the management of anger, aggression, and violence in clients.

KEY CONCEPTS

- aggression
- anger
- assertiveness

KEY TERMS

• catharsis • emotional circuit • mindfulness • restraint • seclusion • violence

*A*nger is considered a universal human emotion by theorists who believe that prototypical emotions exist (DiGiuseppe & Tafrate, 2007). We get our knowledge about emotion in several ways: personal knowledge, knowledge about others' emotions, social norms, and conceptual knowledge that is evolving as we study emotion (Faucher & Tappolet, 2008). Definitions of anger, aggression, and violence vary and are influenced by experience, beliefs, culture, and gender. Individuals and groups develop their own views of acceptable and unacceptable words and actions. Theoretic distinctions can be made among anger, aggression, and violence, but clinically, their expression may be blurred. Each phenomenon may occur alone or in combination with one or both of the others.

Most societies develop norms for acceptable and unacceptable behaviour; some groups at some point in time have accepted all forms of aggression and violence. Today, images and stories about aggressive and violent acts throughout the world are rampant. Like other places, health care settings are not immune to expressions of anger, aggression, and violence.

In any setting, aggression and violence are a reflection of the values of the individual, family, community, and society. Many people tend to minimize the frequency and severity of aggressive and violent acts; for example, couples who interact violently downplay the severity and effects of the episodes (Belknap, 2003). The expression of anger, aggression, and violence by clients and, sometimes, their families is a tremendous challenge for nurses. This chapter discusses prominent theories about the nature of these phenomena and offers varying, sometimes controversial, models, theories, and evidence, with each discussion attempting to explain the phenomena of anger, aggression, and violence. Clinicians can use a particular model as a basis for assessment, nursing diagnosis, planning, intervention, and evaluation. The chapter also explores how the nurse can apply the nursing process in managing angry, aggressive, or violent clients and in preventing or de-escalating situations that may lead to aggression or violence.

Anger

Anger is "a strong, uncomfortable emotional response to a provocation that is unwanted and incongruent with one's values, beliefs or rights" (Thomas, 1998). Anger is usually described as a temporary state of emotional arousal, in contrast to hostility, which is associated with a more enduring negative attitude (Thomas, 2001; see Chapter 37). Although anger is portrayed as a bad emotion that always leads to aggression, this is often not the case. Thomas (2001) asserts that the expression of anger may prevent aggression and help to resolve a situation.

Language pertaining to anger is imprecise and confusing. The word *anger* is used to describe a wide range of feelings, from annoyance at having to wait at a red light when in a hurry to a severe emotional reaction to the news that a family member has been physically assaulted. Some of the words used interchangeably with anger include annoyance, frustration, temper, resentment, hostility, hatred, and rage. In addition, the word *angry* is used to describe both a transient emotional state and a personality trait (Thomas, 1993). This imprecision is related to varying beliefs and theories, including the following (Gerloff, 1997; Novaco, 2007; Shannon, 2000):

- Anger is a fixed quantity that either dams up or floods the system.
- Anger and aggression are linked. Anger is the feeling, and aggression is the behaviour; both result from an innate instinct.
- Anger is the instinctive response to a threat or to the inability to meet goals or desires.
- If outward expression of anger is blocked, then it turns inward and develops into depression.
- Anger arises out of feelings of hurt or anxiety.

Box 36-1 invites the reader to explore variations in responses to anger through the use of an experiential exercise.

KEY CONCEPT **Anger** is an affective state experienced as the motivation to act in ways that warn, intimidate, or attack those who are perceived as challenging or threatening. It occurs when there is a threat, delay, thwarting of a goal, or conflict between goals.

■◖ EXPERIENCE OF ANGER

Thomas (2001) suggests that the experience of anger can serve as a warning that demands are greater than available resources. If one accepts that human beings are rational

---

BOX 36.1

Self-Awareness Exercise: Personal Experience of Anger

People's reactions differ when they experience anger. Some people report a sense of power, control, and calmness different from their usual experience; others report feeling shaky, tearful, and on the verge of collapse. Still others describe physical sensations of nausea and dizziness.

Think about the last time that you felt angry. List the body sensations and other emotions that you experienced. Now ask a friend, colleague, or family member to do the same. Compare lists. What are the similarities and differences between you? How will awareness of these differences help you in your clinical practice?

---

and capable of appraising situations, the subjective component of the experience of anger becomes an important area for study. With the exception of anger that arises from specific neurologic damage or biochemical imbalances, angry episodes can be viewed as social events (Thomas, 1998). The meaning of angry episodes develops from the beliefs held about anger and the interpretation given to the episode (Shannon, 2000). According to Ellis (1977), people choose to experience anger, basing this choice on the related thinking processes. Following Ellis's model, the thinking process would be as follows:

- I wanted something.
- I didn't get what I wanted, and I feel frustrated.
- It's awful not to get what I want.
- Others should not frustrate me.
- Others are bad for frustrating me.
- Bad people should be punished.

The experience of anger is a normal human emotion; it is the inappropriate expression of anger that may be threatening to the self or others.

■ EXPRESSION OF ANGER

Difficulties in expressing anger have often been associated with psychiatric health problems. Anger turned inward has been implicated as a contributor to mood disorders, especially depression (Koh, Kim, & Park, 2002). Several medical disorders have also been positively correlated with the suppression of anger, including essential hypertension, migraine headaches, psoriasis, rheumatoid arthritis, and Raynaud's disease.

Behavioural expressions of anger vary. In the 19th century, anger was viewed as sinful, dangerous, and destructive—an emotion to be contained, controlled, and denied. This negatively viewed emotion was to be dominated and conquered, and an ideal family life was free of anger. Husbands and wives were discouraged from expressing anger toward each other; parenting manuals promoted the suppression of anger in children (Thomas, 1993). This view contributed to the development of a powerful taboo against feeling and expressing anger. People who have accepted this persistent taboo may have difficulty even knowing when they are angry (Shannon, 2000).

During the early 20th century, Freud and Lorenz advocated the use of **catharsis**, the release of ideas through talking and expressing appropriate emotion, in the expression of anger. However, catharsis has been shown empirically to promote, not reduce, anger (Thomas, 1998). There is an old joke that expresses what research has shown: "How do you become a great performer?" Answer: "Practice, practice, practice." "How do you become a really angry person?" Answer: "Practice, practice, practice" (DiGiuseppe & Tafrate, 2007). In recent years, interest has grown in developing communication techniques that promote the expression of anger in nondestructive ways (Gerloff, 1997; Shannon, 2000). These varying beliefs have added to the confusion about anger. Differences in expectations about how men and women should express anger also contribute to the confusion. Table 36-1 gives examples of different styles of anger expression.

Varying beliefs about appropriate ways to express anger become apparent when a client and a nurse enter into a therapeutic relationship. Genetic predisposition, emotional development during infancy and childhood, and family environment influence the variations in expression for both the nurse and the client (Thomas, 2001, 2009). Previous experiences in expressing anger and reactions from others are also influential. Frequency, duration, intensity, and mode of expression are aspects of anger that can be explored and considered (Novaco, 2007).

Aggression and Violence

While anger is an emotion, aggression and violence are actions. In this chapter, aggression is defined as "verbal statements against someone that are intended to intimidate or threaten the recipient." **Violence** is defined as "a physical act of force intended to cause harm to a person or an object

Table 36.1	Styles of Anger Expression	
Style	**Characteristic**	**Gender Socialization**
Anger suppression	Emphasizing the need to keep angry feelings to oneself	In North America, girls are discouraged from expressing anger.
Anger expression	Expressing anger in an attacking or blaming way	In North America, boys are encouraged to express their anger, to not "lie down" or "give in" to others.
Anger discussion	Discussing the anger with a friend or family member. Approaching a person with whom one is angry and discussing the concern directly	Popular and professional literature offers techniques in assertive expression.

Table 36.2	Examples of Behaviours on the Continuum of Aggression and Violence	
Term	**Description**	**Clinical Example**
Suspicious behaviour	Hypervigilance to external cues. Attends more to cues that fit with current thinking patterns	A female client with a long history of delusional disorder (including the belief that her family wants to "lock her away") questions the motives of a community mental health nurse when she asks the client about her medication regimen. The client misperceives the nurse's inquiry as evidence of a conspiracy against her.
Verbal hostility	Verbal comments that are sarcastic or blaming and often expressed with the intent to hurt others. May be used as a means of getting attention or inviting others to take action	When administration of PRN medication is delayed, a client's mother comes to the nursing station and starts to yell. She states that the nurses do not care, are lazy, and should work harder. She also demands that someone give her daughter the analgesic. (Family members have been previously reported as using demanding behaviours to have needs met.)
Physical violence	Act of striking out, throwing an object, pushing, etc., that appears to be intended to cause harm to a person or object	A young man attending a mental health clinic has missed his appointment with the psychiatrist. When he finds out he cannot be scheduled to see her for another week, he yells at the receptionist, bangs his fist on the desk, and then picks up a chair and throws it at her.

FIGURE 36.1 Etiologies for clients with aggression.

and to convey the message that the perpetrator's point of view is correct and not the victim's" (Harper-Jaques & Reimer, 1992, p. 312). Aggression and violent behaviour reflect a continuum from suspicious behaviour to extreme actions that threaten the safety of others or result in injury or death (see Table 36-2 for examples).

KEY CONCEPT **Aggression** is defined as verbal statements and/or physical actions that are intended to threaten.

Aggression does not occur in a vacuum. Both the client and the context must be considered. Therefore, a multi-dimensional framework (Fig. 36-1) is essential for understanding and responding to these behaviours (Morrison & Carney Love, 2003).

Models of Anger, Aggression, and Violence

The field of affective science is rapidly evolving. This section discusses some of the dominant theoretical explanations for anger, aggression, and violence. As yet, a single model or theory cannot fully explain anger, aggression,

and violence; instead, the nurse must choose the most useful models for explaining a particular client's experience and for planning interventions.

BIOLOGIC THEORIES

From a biologic viewpoint, a tendency to have more frequent angry episodes may partially originate from developmental deficits, anoxia, malnutrition, toxins, tumours, or neurodegenerative diseases or trauma affecting the brain. Clients with a history of damage to the cerebral cortex are more likely to exhibit increased impulsivity, decreased inhibition, and decreased judgment than are those who have not experienced such damage. The interaction of neurocognitive impairment and social history of abuse or family violence increases the risk for violent behaviour (Scarpa & Raine, 1997). The odds of violent behaviour also increase when separate risk factors, such as schizophrenia, substance abuse, and not taking prescribed medications, coexist in the same person (Citrome & Volavka, 1999). Before reading additional research evidence, try the anger exercise in Box 36-2. What does daily experience suggest about biologically based aspects of the experience and expression of anger? (See Chapter 10.)

Self-Awareness Exercise: Intensity of Anger

IMAGINE THIS SCENE:

You are coming home late at night. You've been at the library studying for midterm examinations and are tired. As you come up the front walk, you trip over a skateboard, probably left by one of the neighbourhood children. Before you know it, you are sprawled across the front step.

What emotions threaten to overwhelm you at that moment? What contributes to the intensity of the anger that you feel?

- The pain where you scraped your leg across the cement?
- Your general state of tiredness?
- The fact that you skipped dinner?
- The five cups of coffee you had today?
- The careless children who left a toy in your way?

If the same thing had happened when you were well rested and feeling good, would the feeling and the intensity be the same?

Cognitive Neuroassociation Model

The cognitive neuroassociation model is one explanation for the interplay of biologic and other internal influences (Berkowitz, 1989; Miller, Pedersen, Earleywine, & Pollock, 2003). Initially, an adverse event (e.g., pain from tripping over a skateboard) triggers a primitive negative response. Peripheral receptors communicate this response to the spinal cord through the spinothalamic tract to the hypothalamus. The hypothalamus, which synthesizes input from throughout the nervous system, is part of the limbic system. The limbic system mediates primitive emotion and basic drives to produce behaviours for survival, such as the fight-or-flight response (Harper-Jaques & Reimer, 1992).

At first, cognitive appraisal is not involved in these rudimentary feelings of fear or anger, other than identifying the stimulus as aversive; however, higher order cognitive processing quickly begins to take over. The brain associates the current experience of physiologic sensations with memories, ideas, and previously experienced expressive motor reactions. It then interprets and differentiates the experience. Depending on prior experience and associations, the response may be intensified or suppressed. It is this latter part of the process that is most amenable to modification through psychotherapy.

· CRNENOTE

In caring for a potentially aggressive client, the nurse should recognize that biochemical imbalance contributes to the person's inability to control aggression.

Neurostructural Model and the Emotional Circuit

The brain structures most frequently associated with aggressive behaviour are the limbic system and the cerebral cortex, particularly the frontal and temporal lobes. Harper-Jaques and Reimer (1992) propose the phrase **emotional circuit** to describe the interrelationship between the emotional processes of the limbic system and the neurocognitive processes of the frontal lobe and other parts of the cortex. They hypothesize that the functioning of this system determines the meaning a person gives to a particular situation. Thus, meaning is influenced by physiologic capability to perceive incoming messages, prioritize among competing stimuli, and interpret these messages in relation to stored ideas, beliefs, and memories.

NEUROCHEMICAL MODEL AND LOW SEROTONIN SYNDROME

In recent decades, knowledge has exploded about the complex role of neurotransmitters in human behaviour. Serotonin is a major neurotransmitter involved in mood, sleep, and appetite. Low serotonin levels are associated not only with depression but also with irritability, increased pain sensitivity, impulsiveness, aggression, vulnerability to alcoholism, and obsessive-compulsive behaviour (Heinz, Mann, Weinberger, & Goldman, 2001).

Serotonin is sensitive to fluctuations in dietary intake of its precursor, tryptophan, which is found in high-carbohydrate foods. Once it crosses the blood–brain barrier, tryptophan is synthesized into serotonin within the 5-hydroxytryptophan (5-HTP) neurons by interaction with the enzyme tryptophan hydroxylase. Normally, the amount of tryptophan available in the plasma is below saturation (i.e., below the amount that could be used if available). Tryptophan intake and the availability of binding sites on the plasma proteins affect the synthesis of serotonin. Thus, assessing overall dietary intake is relevant, particularly of good tryptophan sources, such as wheat, flour, corn, milk, and eggs. Preliminary research evidence suggests that tryptophan depletion may increase anger levels in individuals already prone to aggressive behaviour (Schmeck et al., 2002).

People with a history of aggressive behaviour have been found to have a lower-than-average level of serotonin. Studies of humans with known aggressive tendencies, such as violent offenders, have repeatedly shown lower-than-average concentrations of 5-hydroxyindoleacetic acid (5-HIAA), the major metabolite for serotonin (Soloff, Lynch, & Moss, 2000) and prefrontal cortex dysfunction (Best, Williams, & Coccaro, 2002). Similarly, the plasma concentration of tryptophan is lower in people with alcoholism who have a history of aggressive behaviour than in people with alcoholism and no such history. Criminals whose acts of violence were committed impulsively have lower levels of 5-HIAA than do criminals whose acts of violence were premeditated. Impulsivity and difficulty controlling anger are characteristic of borderline personality disorder, another condition associated with lower-than-normal serotonin levels (Paris, 2005). Hyperarousal, such as may occur through being constantly vigilant against possible attack (e.g., in guerrilla warfare), also may contribute to aggressive behaviour.

This evidence for a biologic component to aggressive behaviour does not mean that only biologic means of treatment can be effective. Feedback between human behaviour and biochemistry is continuous; verbal suggestions and even early life stressors can affect biochemistry, just as biochemistry affects behaviour (Heinz et al., 2001; Pardo, Pardo, & Raichle, 1993). Environmental and learned behaviours influence the type and degree of aggression expressed, even by those for whom there is a biologic component (Soloff et al., 2000).

■■■ PSYCHOLOGICAL THEORIES

Several psychological explanations exist for aggressive and violent behaviours. This section discusses psychoanalytic, behavioural, and cognitive theories.

Psychoanalytic Theories

Psychoanalytic theorists view emotions as instinctual urges. They view suppression of these urges as unhealthy and as possible contributors to the development of psychosomatic or psychological disorders (Thomas, 1998). Freud struggled to understand the nature and expression of human aggressive behaviour. In his early works, he linked aggression with libidinal factors; however, this association did not explain destructive actions during wars and armed conflict. In his later writings, Freud identified aggression as a separate instinct, like the sexual instinct. He viewed aggression as an innate human quality that could be expressed when a person is provoked or abused. In doing so, he challenged the commonly held belief that human beings are essentially good.

Freud explained aggressive or violent behaviour as a combination of instinctual impulses and events in the environment that stimulated release of the instinctual urge. Freud's view fostered the use of catharsis. Therapeutic approaches, such as primal scream and nursing interventions that direct the client to "let it out" by pounding a pillow, find their origins in this theory (Tavris, 1989; Thomas, 1990). However, recent studies have not shown catharsis to be helpful in reducing anger. Venting can

also have negative consequences when the action taken is hurtful to or blaming of others or damages property.

Erich Fromm (1900–1980), an American psychoanalyst best known for his application of psychoanalytic theory to social and cultural problems, believed that animals and humans share a form of aggression he called *benign*. This genetically programmed response was designed as a defence to protect oneself against a threat. The distinction between humans and animals is that human beings could reason. This capability provided them with options that are not available to animals. Thus, unlike animals, human beings are capable of behaving aggressively for reasons other than self-preservation. Fromm (1973) defined aggression in humans as any behaviour that causes or intends to cause damage to another person, animal, or object. Humans may foresee both real and perceived threats. Perceived threats that are based on distorted perceptions may lead to aggressive and violent behaviours; for example, the cognitive and information-processing deficits of clients with psychosis or schizophrenia (see Chapter 18) are frequently implicated in episodes of aggression and violence.

Behavioural Theories

The goal of behaviourists is to predict and control behaviour. Introspection has no role in these theories. One behavioural theory, drive theory, suggests that violent behaviour originates externally. A person experiences anger and acts violently in response to interference with or blocking of a goal. Laboratory experiments and the reality of everyday experience have proved the limitations of this theory (Thomas, 1990). Not all situations in which one's goal is blocked lead to anger or violence.

Another behavioural theory is social learning theory. In his research, Bandura (1973) drew attention to the role of learning and rewards in the expression of anger and violence. He studied interactions between mothers and children. The children learned that anger and aggressive behaviour helped them get what they wanted from their mothers. The children learned aggressive behaviour in a context that may have made them understand aggressive behaviour as appropriate. According to this view, people learn to be aggressive by participating in an aggressive environment.

Cognitive Theories

Cognitive theorists are interested in how people transform internal and external stimuli into useful information. They emphasize understanding how a person takes new information and fits it into an already developed schema. Beck (1976) proposed that cognitive schema such as judgments, self-esteem, and expectations influence angry responses. In a situation perceived as intentional, dangerous, and unprovoked, the recipient's reaction will be intensified. The person's reaction will be further intensified if he or she views the offender as undesirable. In psychological disorders, cognitive processing may be compromised (Rubinsztein, Sahakian, & Dolan, 2002; Sergi & Green, 2003).

Rational-emotive theory, a type of cognitive theory, considers cognition, affect, and behaviour to be interrelated psychological processes (Ellis, 1977). This theory regards anger as an inappropriate negative emotion because it stems from irrational beliefs. Change is directed at altering irrational beliefs by identifying and working to change them and their associated psychological processes. Cognitive theories inform us about how not to get angry in the first place not about what to do when we become angry (Novaco, 2007).

SOCIOCULTURAL THEORIES

Sociocultural theories suggest violent behaviour has multiple determinants, including social experiences in family and peer settings and the social consequences (positive and negative) of physical aggression. These determinants can be influenced by the gender of the individual and the way that gender differences are conceived and enacted within a society (Snyder, Schrepferman, Brooker, & Stoolmiller, 2007).

Western society often is characterized by a competitive, success-oriented ideology that values the individual and individual accomplishments over collaboration and a sense of community. Self-esteem, particularly for men, may be based on social and economic status and influence over others and the environment (Thomas, 2003). The pursuit of status produces inequities in relationships, whereby one person is superior and the other is subordinate. A hazard inherent in the pursuit of status is the view that a person is entitled to have influence and control, and that the "entitled person" has the right to use whatever means necessary to obtain status (Jenkins, 1990). These means may include force or disregarding the rights and needs of others. The entitled person may also begin to consider other people responsible for his or her thoughts, feelings, or actions. Such a belief in entitlement can be used to justify such actions as threatening, hurting, or murdering less powerful individuals.

Violence against women is a pressing global health issue. In 2001, the United Nations (UN) Commission on Human Rights issued a resolution toward eliminating it, asking countries to develop policies and provide funding for violence prevention and treatment programs. This resolution provides governments with a rationale to challenge men's position of entitlement and calls for societies to view women as equal partners with men. It has had an impact: women now have greater access to education,

increased economic independence, and opportunities to control the frequency and number of pregnancies. Some believe, however, that these changes have led to a backlash against women's efforts to be equal, evident in continuing violence toward women (Tajaden & Thoennes, 2000).

A World Health Organization (WHO) study in 2005 revealed that the incidence of violence against women varies considerably across countries. For instance, the percentage of violence against a woman by a male partner ranged from 13% in Japan to 61% in Peru. Social factors related to violence against women included degree of economic inequality between males and females, level of women's mobility and autonomy, societal attitudes toward gender and toward violence, whether extended family or neighbours would intervene, and the level of crime and male-to-male violence (WHO, 2005).

INTERACTIONAL THEORY

Morrison (1998) challenges research and theories suggesting that aggression and violence are biologically or psychologically based. She asserts that these views lead to excusing the person's behaviour. She proposes that violence among people in psychiatric settings is the same as violence in other settings. Therefore, the client's behaviour should be considered a social problem and responded to on that basis. This challenge is grounded in several studies that examined the interactional style of the aggressive and violent individual. People with interactional styles that were argumentative or coercive were more likely to engage in aggressive or violent interchanges. Such people are often described as having a "chip on their shoulders." Morrison clearly states her view that the antecedent variables (e.g., history of violence, psychiatric diagnosis, length of hospitalization) and the mediating variable of interactional style are the primary reasons for the behaviour.

NURSING MANAGEMENT: HUMAN RESPONSE TO ANGER AND AGGRESSION

Aggression and violence often arise from an individual's belief that his or her view of a situation is the only correct one. The first party considers other views wrong and in need of change. A second party's refusal to give in to the view of the first may lead to violence (Capra, 2002). Box 36-3 illustrates such a scenario in the clinical setting.

Contrary to popular belief, many clients who have mental health problems do not behave aggressively or violently. To develop a means of predicting aggressive and violent behaviours, some researchers have

BOX 36.3

Clinical Vignette: *Paul's Anger*

Paul, a new client on the unit, appears to be experiencing auditory hallucinations. The nurse approaches Paul, careful not to invade his personal space, and begins to walk with him. In an attempt to assess his current mental status, the nurse points out that he seems restless and asks if the voices have returned. Paul responds, "They are telling me this place isn't safe. The angel in the corner is signaling to me. She wants me to leave!" Paul starts to walk toward the door. In an attempt to offer an alternative point of view and orient him to the present, the nurse understands that what the client is seeing and hearing are hallucinations. The nurse attempts to increase Paul's feeling of safety by identifying his perceptions as hallucinations and reassuring him of his safety. "No I won't stay and you can't make me." Paul pushes the nurse aside and runs to the door.

WHAT DO YOU THINK?

If you were the nurse in this situation, what would be your next response? How would you acknowledge Paul's concerns and encourage him to stay?

---

attempted to determine the relationship between medical diagnosis and violence. Others have focused on the role of a person's history in predicting violence or examined demographics, client characteristics, and unit climate.

Although media attention highlights violence related to mental illness, the American Psychiatric Association (APA; 2000) concludes individuals suffering from schizophrenia pose no more of a danger to others than the rest of the population. Citrome and Volavka (2002) have identified many possible causes for aggressive behaviours in individuals experiencing a psychiatric disorder, including the presence of comorbid substance abuse, dependence, and intoxication. As well, individuals experiencing symptom manifestation of hallucinations or delusions or those with neuropsychiatric deficits are identified as posing an increased risk for violence. Individuals with underlying antisocial personality traits may use violent acts as a means to achieve specific goals. Finally, environmental factors that are associated with aggressive behaviours are identified, including a chaotic or unstable home or hospital situation, which may further encourage maladaptive aggressive behaviours (Citrome & Volavka). A description of psychiatric diagnosis and patterns of aggression are identified in Table 36-3. An important consideration for the nurse is the course of violence related to changes in symptomatology (Bernstein & Saladino, 2007).

Research suggests that particular characteristics are predictive of violent behaviours. Low self-esteem that may be further eroded during hospitalization or treatment may influence a client to use force to meet his or her needs or to experience some sense of empowerment. Many people who have chronic mental health problems "fight" the experience and have difficulty accepting medical treatment. When admitted to the hospital, they may experience turmoil from both the illness and the anger at the additional loss of control that hospitalization mandates. Clients may resort to violence to force change or to regain or maintain control. Rewards from violence include attention from nursing staff and/or status and prestige among the client group (Harris & Morrison, 1995). For example, the client who behaves violently is observed more frequently and has more opportunities to discuss concerns with nurses. Impaired communication, disorientation, and depression have been found to be consistently associated with aggressive behaviour among nursing home residents with dementia (Talerico, Evans, & Strumpf, 2002).

Nurses bring their own perceptions and reactions to clinical settings. They respond to the behaviours of the clients and families for whom they care. Clients and families, in turn, react to nurses (Leahey & Harper-Jaques, 1996). Nurses' beliefs about themselves as individuals and professionals will influence their responses to aggressive behaviours. For example, the nurse who considers any expression of anger or aggression inappropriate will approach an agitated client in a manner different from that used by the nurse who considers agitated behaviour to be meaningful. In a phenomenological study of patient experiences of violent encounters (Carlsson, Dahlberg, Ekebergh, & Dahlberg, 2006), participants described wanting caregivers who were calm and confident and who did not respond to client anger by disconnecting (e.g., becoming cool and distant). They said that such reactions on the part of caregivers increased their despair and with it, their aggression. When a caregiver genuinely related to the client as a person and seemed to recognize the suffering being experienced, the client's anger was diffused. The researchers found the clients to be "longing for authentic personal care" (p. 287).

Duxbury and Whittington (2005) studied clients' (N = 80) and nurses' (N = 82) perspectives on inpatient aggression and violence. Clients believed poor communication on the part of staff played a significant role; nurses believed it was clients' mental illness that was most significant. Both noted that environmental conditions (e.g., restrictive and underresourced) play a role. Clients advocated for communication training for staff, while nurses looked for organizational deficits to be addressed.

The nurse's ability to maintain personal control is challenged when faced with angry, provoking clients. Some clients who are experiencing emotional problems have an uncanny ability to verbally target a nurse's vulnerable characteristics. It is a usual response to become

Table 36.3   Psychiatric Diagnosis and Patterns of Aggression and/or Violence

Child and Adolescent Population-Specific Disorder

Diagnosis	Attention deficit/hyperactivity disorder	Oppositional defiant disorder	Conduct disorder
Patterns of aggression or violence	Predominantly hyperactive-impulsive type with low frustration tolerance, temper outbursts, intrusive, oppositional behaviour (may continue to adulthood)	Primarily by verbal aggression with negativistic, hostile, defiant, spiteful, blaming behaviour directed at adults or peers	Aggressive conduct that threatens or causes physical harm to other people or animals

Personality Disorder

Diagnosis	Antisocial personality disorder	Paranoid personality disorder	Borderline personality disorder
Patterns of aggression or violence	Contemptuous of the feelings and rights of others, cynical, irresponsible, exploitative, lacks empathy, often violent	Pervasive distrust and suspiciousness of others, exploitative, harms or deceives oneself even with no evidence of such, vigilant, holds grudges, may attack others suddenly	Inappropriate, intense anger or difficulty controlling anger (e.g., frequent displays of temper, constant anger, recurrent physical fights)

General Psychiatric Disorder

Diagnosis	Schizophrenia	Posttraumatic stress disorder	Bipolar disorder	Substance-related disorder	Delusional disorder	Intermittent explosive disorder
Patterns of aggression or violence	Paranoid type with persecutory delusions or commending hallucination may predispose the person to suicidal behaviour or anger and aggression toward others	Irritability, hypervigilance, and outbursts of anger, feeling of detachment or estrangement from others, restricted range of affect	Irritability, agitation, and violent behaviour during manic or psychotic episodes; highly comorbid with substance use, which worsens the prognosis	Aggressive episodes during intoxication, withdrawal, and while seeking substance of abuse	Primarily persecutory type (e.g., being conspired against, cheated, spied on, maliciously maligned, poisoned, or drugged); often resentful and angry	Discrete episode of failure to resist aggressive impulses resulting in serious injury to self, assaults on others, or destruction of property

Geriatric Population-Specific Disorder

Diagnosis	Dementia
Patterns of aggression or violence	Generalized irritability and low frustration tolerance, confusion, destructive attempts at self-protection

Source: Adapted from American Psychiatric Association. (2000). *Diagnostic and statistical manual of mental disorders* (4th ed., Text revision). Washington, DC: Author.

defensive when one feels vulnerable. However, when nurses lose control of their own responses, the potential for punitive interventions or the use of threats or sarcasm is greater.

Nurses in all areas of clinical practice need to understand angry emotions, know how to prevent aggression and violence, and respond assertively. To better prepare themselves to respond to different types of behaviour, many nurses take assertiveness training courses and workshops. Many nursing schools also teach assertiveness. Nurses should understand the phenomena of anger, aggression, and violence as meaningful behaviours that warrant attention rather than as disruptive behaviours to control.

> **KEY CONCEPT** **Assertiveness** is a set of behaviours and a communication style that is open, honest, direct, and confident. Assertiveness enables the expression of emotions, including anger, in a manner that assumes responsibility. It allows placement of boundaries and prevents acceptance of inappropriate aggression from others.

Predictors of Violence

When assessing a client, his or her history is probably the most important predictor of potential for violence. Important markers include previous episodes of rage and violent behaviour, escalating irritability, intruding angry thoughts, and fear of losing control. Brain injury, substance use or abuse, and temporal lobe epilepsy have also been discussed as possible predictors of violence (Harper-Jaques & Reimer, 1992; Mesulam, 2000). Whether a relationship exists between temporal lobe epilepsy and aggressive behaviour remains a matter of controversy (Citrome & Volavka, 1999). Aggressive behaviour that occurs in the interictal period (i.e., between seizures) may also be related to the intense frustration that people who have epilepsy often experience and could lead to violent behaviour.

Certain antiepileptic drugs, particularly barbiturates, may contribute to irritability and aggressive behaviour. However, mood-stabilizing medications such as carbamazepine (Tegretol) and divalproex sodium (Depakote) have reduced aggressive behaviour. The nurse should include any history of seizures, current medications, and compliance with pharmacotherapy in client assessments. Some physiologic and behavioural cues to anger are listed in Table 36-4.

Analysis and Outcome Identification

The nurse analyzes all assessment data across the biologic, psychological, and social domains to understand the dangers that the client's behaviour poses for self or others. The most common nursing diagnoses for clients experiencing intense anger and aggression are Risk for Self-Directed Violence and Risk for Other-Directed Violence (North American Nursing Diagnosis Association [NANDA], 2005). Outcomes focus on aggression control.

Planning and Implementing Interventions

This section emphasizes the development of a partnership between the nurse and client, who work together to find solutions to prevent the recurrence of explosive episodes and to de-escalate volatile situations. However, sometimes the client's condition (e.g., advanced dementia) or the situation will prevent the development of a partnership. In such instances, the nurse must take charge. The nurse who intervenes from within the context of the therapeutic relationship must be cognizant of the fit of a particular intervention. The nurse's action is based on his or her response to the client. The client's affective, behavioural, and cognitive responses to the intervention provides information about its effects and guides the nurse's next response (Wright & Leahey, 2005; Fig. 36-2).

Table 36.4	Physiologic and Behavioural Cues to Anger
Internal Signs	**External Signs**
• Increased pulse, respirations, and blood pressure • Chills and shudders • Prickly sensations • Numbness • Choking sensations • Nausea • Vertigo	• Increased muscle tone • Changes in body posture, clenched fists, set jaw • Changes to the eyes: eyebrows lower and draw together, eyelids tense, eyes assume a "hard" appearance • Lips pressed together to form a thin line, or in a square shape • Flushing or pallor • Goose bumps • Twitching • Sweating

Spiritual
1. Support consideration of spiritual issues
2. Support spiritual activities
3. Support hope for change

Biologic
1. Administer psychotropic agents
2. Monitor hepatic function
3. Encourage proper nutrition
4. Administer vitamins, such as thiamine and niacin
5. Reduce intake of caffeinated beverages
6. Modify environmental stimuli
7. Anticipate need for bladder and bowel elimination

Social
1. Develop family support groups
2. Use restraints and seclusion only as a last resort
3. Encourage use of resources for information and support

Psychological
1. Use past experiences to normalize and validate client's experiences
2. Explore beliefs about expressing aggression
3. Assist with taking charge of situation
4. Explain behavioural limits and consequences clearly
5. Develop written contracts
6. Plan to prevent escalation
7. Allow choices if possible

FIGURE 36.2 Interventions for clients with aggression.

The following assumptions are important to consider in planning interventions with this client population (Harper-Jaques & Masters, 1994):

- The nurse and client collaborate to find solutions and alternatives to aggressive and violent outbursts.
- Anger is a normal emotion. All people have the right to express their anger. All people have a responsibility to express their anger in a way that does not, emotionally or physically, threaten or harm others.
- In most instances, the person who behaves aggressively or violently can assume responsibility for the behaviour.
- The nurse views the client from the perspective of acknowledging that the client has solved problems before and is only temporarily in need of help.
- The nurse understands that norms for behaviour are created within the context of a particular environment and are influenced by the client's history and culture.

Nurses who work collaboratively with potentially violent clients must also keep in mind that they can take certain actions to minimize personal risk:

- Using nonthreatening body language.
- Respecting the client's personal space and boundaries.

- Positioning themselves so that they have immediate access to the door of the room in case they need to leave the room.
- Choosing to leave the door open to an office while talking to a client.
- Knowing where colleagues are and making sure those colleagues know where they are.
- Removing or not wearing clothing or accessories that could be used to harm them, such as scarves, necklaces, or dangling earrings.

When a violent outburst appears imminent or occurs, immediate intervention is required and should be directed by a designated leader (see Box 36-4 for guidelines).

Preassigning a leader according to organization protocols (e.g., Code White Leader) helps to maintain clarity and focus should a crisis arise. The leader assumes responsibility to collaborate in assessing the situation, planning safe and practiced interventions, and, thereafter, to lead in organizing and implementing these interventions. It is also important that the leader is involved in facilitating resolutions between the client and the staff, as well as in ensuring team members are provided the opportunity to debrief amongst themselves (Carpenito-Moyet, 2002).

BOX 36.4

🕐

Emergency: Guidelines for Crisis Intervention

1. Call for assistance (e.g., other nurses, security staff).
2. Brief all staff; plan intervention.
3. Assign staff to limbs should physical restraint or movement of the client become necessary.
4. Remove other clients from the area. Also, remove any items that may impede the staff's movement.
5. The crisis intervention leader talks to the client firmly and calmly. Other staff members are present.
6. Leader gives client choices (e.g., go to room to calm down, talk with someone, lose privileges, take medication).
7. If the client continues to argue, the leader tells the client that staff will escort him or her to his or her room. If the client refuses to walk, staff carry the client to the room.

From Carpenito-Moyet, L. J. (2002). Guidelines for code white response: A component of prevention and management of aggressive behaviour in health care. Occupational Health and Safety Agency for Health Care in British Columbia (BC), Workmen's Compensation of BC, Health Association in BC.

The nurse who works with potentially aggressive clients does so with respect and concern. The goal is to work with clients to find solutions. The nurse approaches these clients calmly, being mindful to use nonthreatening body language and to avoid violation of boundaries. In dealing with aggression, as in other aspects of nursing practice, the nurse will find that at times the best intervention is silence. It is easy to equate intervention with activity, the sense that "I must do something." But quiet calmness on the nurse's part may be enough to help a client regain control of his or her behaviour and perspective on the situation.

Trying to clarify what has upset the client is important. The nurse can use therapeutic communication techniques to prevent a crisis or defuse a critical situation (see Box 36-5). During daily interactions with clients, nurses intervene in many creative and useful ways. The intervention alone does not serve as the solution; it is the process or art of offering the intervention within the context of the nurse–client relationship that is successful. These interventions will not be successful with all clients all the time. However, it is not the nurse or client's fault when an intervention is ineffective. The intervention simply did not fit the situation at that particular time.

BOX 36.5

Anger Control Assistance

DEFINITION: Facilitation of the expression of anger adaptively and nonviolently

ACTIVITIES

- Establish basic trust and rapport with the client.
- Use a calm, reassuring approach.
- Determine appropriate behaviour expectations for expression of anger, given the client's level of cognitive and physical functioning.
- Limit the client's access to frustrating situations until he or she can express anger adaptively.
- Encourage the client to seek assistance of nursing staff or responsible others during periods of increasing tension.
- Monitor the client's potential for inappropriate aggression and intervene before its expression.
- Prevent physical harm (e.g., apply restraint, remove potential weapons) if the client directs anger at self or others.
- Provide reassurance to the client that nursing staff will intervene to prevent him or her from losing control.
- Use external controls (e.g., physical or manual restraint, time-outs, seclusion) as needed to calm a client who is expressing anger destructively.
- Provide feedback on behaviour to help the client identify anger.
- Assist the client in identifying the source of anger.
- Identify the function that anger, frustration, and rage serve for the client.
- Identify consequences of inappropriate expressions of anger.
- Assist the client in planning strategies to prevent the inappropriate expression of anger.
- Identify with the client the benefits of expressing anger adaptively and nonviolently.
- Establish expectation that the client can control his or her behaviour.
- Instruct the client on the use of calming measures (e.g., time-outs, deep breaths).
- Assist the client to develop appropriate methods of expressing anger to others (e.g., assertiveness, use of statements).
- Provide role models who express anger appropriately.
- Support the client in implementing anger-control strategies and appropriately expressing anger.
- Provide reinforcement for appropriate expression of anger.

Adapted from McCloskey, J., & Bulechek, G. (2000). *Nursing interventions classification (NIC)* (3rd ed.). St. Louis, MO: Mosby.

Biologic Domain

Biologic Assessment

The nurse may encounter clients whose aggressive tendencies have been exacerbated by a biochemical imbalance. However, nurses must recognize that biologic alterations are neither necessary nor sufficient to account for most aggressive behaviours. In taking the client's history, the nurse listens for evidence of industrial exposure to toxic chemicals, missed doses of medications, alcohol intoxication, and withdrawal or premenstrual dysphoric disorder. Similarly, a history of even minor structural changes resulting in trauma, hemorrhage, or tumour may contribute to lowering a client's anger threshold, and thus requires investigation.

Aggressive episodes that are mainly biologic in origin share certain characteristics (Corrigan, Yudofsky, & Silver, 1993):

- The client has a history or evidence of central nervous system (CNS) lesion or dysfunction.
- Onset of the episode is sudden and relatively unprovoked.
- The outburst is less controlled than those associated with external influences.
- The episode has a clear beginning and ending.
- The client expresses remorse after the episode.

Sensory Impairment

The most common impairments are hearing loss and reduced visual acuity. A common component of nursing assessment documents is visual and hearing impairments. If a client cannot provide information about his or her hearing and vision, the nurse should ask a family member or friend. If there are impairments, the nurse should ensure that hearing aids are working for clients who use them and assess clients for access to glasses or contact lenses.

Interventions for the Biologic Domain

Administering and Monitoring Medications

Several classes of drugs are used in the management of aggressive behaviour. Important points for the nurse to consider in making decisions about client and family teaching, medication administration, and consultation with physicians and pharmacists are as follows:

- Evidence supports the use of *atypical antipsychotics*, such as clozapine (Clozaril), risperidone (Risperdal), and olanzapine (Zyprexa), in reducing agitation (Chakos & Lieberman, 2001). As with other psychotropic medications, the action of atypical antipsychotics is not fully understood. It is thought that they block dopamine and serotonin receptors. Extrapyramidal side effects are few, which makes these drugs easier to tolerate than the typical antipsychotics (see the drug profile on risperidone [Risperdal] in Chapter 18 for more information).

- *Selective serotonin reuptake inhibitors* (SSRIs; e.g., fluoxetine [Prozac], paroxetine [Paxil]) are increasingly being used for their antiaggressive effects, as well as for their antidepressant effects. Their effects on aggressive behaviour usually occur before their effects on depression.

- *β-Adrenergic receptor blockers*, such as propranolol (Inderal), may be used for their effect in decreasing the peripheral manifestations of rage that are associated with excitement of the sympathetic nervous system (Silver et al., 2000).

- *Lithium carbonate* has been effective in treating aggressive behaviour associated with brain injury (Burke, Loeber, & Birmaher, 2002).

- *Divalproex sodium* and *carbamazepine* have been shown to reduce aggressive behaviour.

- Psychotropic drugs often interact with antiepileptic and antispasmodic agents, altering pharmacokinetics. For example, chlorpromazine may increase the risk for seizures in clients taking antiepileptic drugs (Fahs, Potiron, Senon, & Perivier, 1999).

- The liver metabolizes most psychotropic drugs (except lithium). The nurse should be alert to possible hepatic dysfunction in clients with a history of alcohol or drug abuse.

Managing Nutrition

Clients with long-standing poor dietary habits (e.g., indigent clients, clients with alcoholism) often have deficiencies of thiamine, niacin, and folic acid (Young, 2002). Prolonged use of alcohol can block as much as 70% of thiamine uptake. Increased irritability, disorientation, and paranoia may result. Encouraging clients to eat more whole grains, nuts, fruits, vegetables, organ meats, and milk, instead of "junk" foods, is important. The nurse may need to help clients with obtaining the resources needed to buy and prepare healthier food choices.

Caffeine is a potent stimulant (Lorist & Tops, 2003). Some inpatient psychiatric units have reduced clients' accessibility to coffee and other caffeinated beverages as a means of trying to reduce aggressive behaviour. Results have been mixed.

Psychological Domain

Psychological Assessment

The nurse interested in working with clients to prevent and manage aggressive and violent behaviours should observe them for disturbances in thought processing. Clients may have disordered thoughts for various reasons, including associated psychiatric diagnoses. Some common diagnostic categories that the nurse needs to look for in the client's history are major depressive episode, bipolar disorder, delusional disorders, posttraumatic stress disorder, schizophrenia, and depersonalization. The nurse should also look for a current or past history of substance abuse because clients who abuse drugs, alcohol, or solvents may also exhibit disordered thought processing. Intoxication can trigger erratic thought processes and unpredicted violence. Some form of thought disorder may remain after a person is detoxified, becoming a permanent feature of the person's way of processing ideas. In addition, the nurse must look for acute and chronic medical conditions, such as brain tumour, encephalitis, electrolyte imbalance, and hepatic failure, which may also alter thought processing (Citrome & Volavka, 1999). The thought processes of greatest interest to the nurse in assessing a client's potential for aggression and violence are perception and delusion.

Perception

Perception is awareness of events and sensations and the ability to make distinctions between them. Clients with disordered perceptions may misinterpret objects or events. Such misperception is called an *illusion*. For example, a client may assume that a person walking toward him or her is going to strike out and thus take action to defend against this illusionary foe. The nurse can explore a client's perception by asking such questions as, "I noticed you were looking very cautious as I approached you. I wonder what you are thinking."

Delusions

Clients may maintain false or unreasonable beliefs, known as delusions, despite attempts to dissuade them from their point of view. The nurse may not notice any abnormalities in the client's behaviour or appearance until the client begins to discuss delusional ideas. Discussion of the delusions may precipitate aggressive or violent behaviour. To explore these false beliefs, the nurse could, with the client's consent, ask questions respectfully. The nurse should match the pacing of such questions to the client's responses. Attempts to dissuade the client from his or her beliefs are usually ineffective.

Interventions for the Psychological Domain

Psychological interventions help clients gain control over their expression of anger and aggressive behaviour. In some instances, these interventions eliminate the need for chemical (medications) or mechanical restraints. De-escalating potential aggression is always preferable to challenging or provoking a client. Anger control assistance, as set forth in the *Nursing Interventions Classification* (NIC; McCloskey & Bulechek, 2000), is useful and can prevent deterioration of a client's control of behaviour (Box 36-6).

Affective Interventions

Affective interventions are designed to reduce or increase intense emotions that may hinder the client from finding alternatives to the use of aggression or violence (Wright & Leahey, 2005). They include validating, listening to the client's illness experience, and exploring beliefs.

Validating

Clients who experience intense anger and rage can feel isolated. The nurse can reduce the client's feelings of isolation by acknowledging these intense feelings. By drawing on past experience with other client's, the nurse can also reassure the client that others have felt the same way.

Listening to the Client's Illness Experience

Often, clients and their family members are invited to provide details about past medical treatments, medications, hospitalizations, and therapies. What is overlooked is the experience of the health problem or the experience of interactions with professionals. Inviting clients and families to talk about their previous experience with the health care system may highlight both their concerns and resources. See Box 36-7 for an example of how a nurse uses this intervention to improve a client's care.

Exploring Beliefs

Exploring the client's beliefs about the expression of angry feelings can be useful. Discussion of beliefs that prevent the client from seeking alternate ways of handling distressing emotions and situations may help him or her to take charge of the situation.

Cognitive Interventions

Cognitive interventions are usually those that provide new ideas, opinions, information, or education about a particular problem. The nurse offers a cognitive intervention with the goal of inviting the client to consider other possibilities (Wright & Leahey, 2005). Examples include giving commendations, offering information, providing education, and using thought stopping and contracting.

> **CRNENOTE**
> The best time to teach the client techniques for managing anger and aggression is when the client is not experiencing the provoking event. Cognitive therapy approaches are useful and can be prioritized according to responses.

BOX 36.6

Therapeutic Dialogue: **The Potentially Aggressive Client**

Paul is a 23-year-old client in the high observation area of an inpatient unit. He is pacing back and forth. He is pounding one fist into his other hand. In the past 24 hours, Paul has been more cooperative and less agitated. The behaviour the nurse observes now is more like the behaviour that Paul displayed 2 days ago. Yesterday, the psychiatrist told Paul that he would be granted more freedom in the unit if his behaviour improved. The psychiatrist has just seen Paul and refused to change the restrictions on Paul's activities.

INEFFECTIVE APPROACH

Nurse: Paul, I can understand this is frustrating for you.

Paul: How can you understand? Have you ever been held like a prisoner?

Nurse: I do understand Paul. Now you must calm down or more privileges will be removed.

Paul: [voice gets louder] But I was told that calm behaviour would mean more privileges. Now you are telling me calm behaviour only gets me what I have got! Can't you talk to the doctor for me?

Nurse: No, Paul. I can't talk to the doctor. [Paul appears more frustrated and agitated as the conversation continues.]

EFFECTIVE APPROACH

Nurse: Paul, you look upset (observation). What happened in your conversation with the psychiatrist? (seeking information)

Paul: Yesterday, he said calmer behaviour would mean more freedom in the unit. I have tried to be calmer and not to swear. You said you noticed the difference. But today he says "no" to more freedom.

Nurse: Some people might feel cheated if this happened to them (validation). Is that how you feel?

Paul: Yeah, I feel real cheated. Nothing I do makes a difference. That's the way it is here and that's the way it is when I am out of the hospital.

Nurse: Sounds like experiences like this leave you feeling pretty powerless (validation).

Paul: I don't have any power, anywhere. Sometimes when I have no power I get mean. At least then people pay attention to me.

Nurse: In this situation with your doctor, what would help you feel that you had some power? (Inviting client partnership).

Paul: Well if he would listen to me; if he would read my chart.

Nurse: I am a bit confused by the psychiatrist's decision. I won't make promises that your privileges will change but would it be okay with you if I talk with him?

Paul: That would make me feel like someone is on my side.

CRITICAL THINKING CHALLENGE

- In the first scenario, how did the nurse escalate the situation?
- Compare the first scenario with the second. How are they different?

BOX 36.7

Clinical Vignette: **Mary's Rage**

Mary, a 22-year-old single woman, was a regular client at the crisis centre. During previous visits, she came alone or with her mother and demanded immediate attention. This time she comes with her mother. The receptionist groans and rolls her eyes as she describes this family to the new intake nurse. "They are obnoxious. It is best to handle them fast and get them out of here!"

Before the interview, the nurse reviews Mary's extensive file. She notes that on many occasions Mary was aggressive and violent while in the centre. The mother has complained to the local health authority about the centre on at least two occasions.

During the interview, the nurse asks the mother and daughter the following questions:

- What was the most useful thing that has happened during previous contacts at the centre?
- What was the least useful thing about previous contacts at the centre?

The family looks surprised to be asked these questions. They state that previous visits were useful only in providing them with written proof that Mary could not work. That information required by the social service agency ensured continuation of Mary's disability checks. Furthermore, Mary and her mother state that they often left the centre feeling that the nurses were not interested in their concerns and believed that if Mary tried harder, her hallucinations would decrease. They add that they often waited 1 to 2 hours to be seen, whereas other clients were seen more quickly. Mary admits that she sometimes made a lot of noise in the waiting room to be seen sooner.

The nurse then asks, "What would need to happen during your visit today to make you feel that coming here was worthwhile?" The mother expresses interest in receiving information about hallucinations and how she could help Mary when she experiences them. Mary says she wants to know how to handle angry feelings.

Giving Commendations

A commendation focuses on the client's behaviour pattern over time and highlights his or her strengths and resources (Limacher & Wright, 2003). For example, commending a client's decision to request medication or to remove herself from an overstimulating environment highlights the woman's ability to assume responsibility for thoughts and feelings that have previously invited aggressive behaviour.

Offering Information

Nurses can offer information or arrange opportunities for clients to receive information from other professionals. Clients may sometimes become agitated and threaten to harm the nurse because they do not know what is expected of them or they do not remember why they need to be in treatment. The nurse can tell them about unit expectations or the reasons for hospitalization. The nurse can also determine the client's information needs by asking questions. One option in providing information, education, and support is to develop a family support group, which can provide a forum for responding to general concerns and questions at the same time.

In the mental health setting, the nurse must make behavioural limits and consequences clear. When possible, the nurse should match consequences to the client's interests and desires. For example, Jane was slamming doors and banging down dishes in the kitchen of the group home. The nurse approached her to discuss other means of expressing her anger. During the conversation, the nurse reminded Jane that further agitated behaviour would mean that Jane would not participate in a shopping trip planned that day. The trip was important to Jane, so she chose to discuss her concern with the nurse.

Providing Education

Nurses can offer education to clients and families about various topics, including anger management and strategies to control aggressive behaviours. Greater understanding about mental health problems and altered mental status may help to prevent aggression by clarifying misunderstandings. Effective use of debriefing techniques following a crisis situation can also provide nurses and clients insights to ineffective coping and further allow for client learning in the development of strategies for future behavioural change.

Thought Stopping

In thought stopping, the nurse asks the client to identify thoughts that heighten feelings of anger and invites the client to "turn the thoughts off" by focusing on other thoughts or activities (Burns, 1999). Ideas of other activities include talking to someone, reading, baking, or thinking about a future event.

Contracting

A contract is a written document that the nurse and client develop. The document clearly states acceptable and unacceptable behaviours, consequences and rewards, and the role of both the client and nurse in preventing and managing aggressive behaviour (Morrison, 1998).

Behavioural Interventions

Behavioural interventions are designed to assist the client to behave differently (Wright & Leahey, 2005). Examples of such interventions include assigning behavioural tasks, using bibliotherapy, interrupting patterns, and providing choices.

Assigning Behavioural Tasks

Sometimes, the nurse may assign a behavioural task as a way to help the client maintain or regain control over aggressive behaviours. Behavioural tasks might include writing down a list of grievances that the client will discuss with the nurse or observing how other people take charge of anger and aggression. For example, the nurse may ask the client to observe clients or staff on the unit, people at a shopping mall, or particular movies or television shows to evaluate how other people in real or fictitious situations handle anger.

Using Bibliotherapy

In bibliotherapy, the nurse may ask the client to read a particular pamphlet or article on anger management. The nurse and client then discuss what the client read to decide which, if any, of the ideas the client can use when angry.

Interrupting Patterns

Although clients are not usually aware of it, escalation of feelings, thoughts, and behaviour from calmness to violence usually follows a particular pattern. Disruption of the pattern can sometimes be a useful means for preventing escalation and can help the client regain composure. Nurses can suggest several strategies to interrupt patterns:

- Counting to 10 or using a mantra (sacred name repetition).
- Removing oneself from interactions or stimuli that may contribute to increased distress.
- Doing something different (e.g., reading, exercising, watching television).

Providing Choices

When possible, the nurse should provide the client with choices, particularly clients who have little control over their situation because of their condition. For example, the client who is experiencing a manic episode and is confined to her room may have few options in her daily schedule. However, she may be allowed to make choices about food, personal hygiene, and which pyjamas to wear.

Social Domain

Social Assessment

The nurse should evaluate factors related to the social domain that may be contributing to aggression or violence in a client. For example, are conditions in the client's home, family, or community leading to aggression or violent episodes? Are financial or legal troubles placing stress on the client that places him or her at risk?

Interventions for the Social Domain

Reducing Stimulation

Normally, people adjust their environments to suit their needs: some people like their music loud, whereas others want it soft; some people seek out the thrill of high-risk sports, whereas others prefer to be spectators. Within the context of a brain disorder or an unusually restrictive environment, such adjustments may not be within the client's control. A client with a brain injury, progressive dementia, or distorted vision may be experiencing intense and highly confusing stimulation, even though the environment, from the nurse or family's perspective, seems calm and orderly.

For people whose perceptions or thoughts are disordered from brain damage, degeneration, or other thought-processing difficulties, modification of the environment may be one of the main interventions.

Likewise, introducing more structure into a chaotic environment can help decrease the risk for aggressive behaviour (Citrome & Volavka, 1999). The nurse can make stimuli meaningful or can simplify and interpret the environment in many practical ways, such as by identifying people or equipment that may be unfamiliar, providing cues as to what is expected (e.g., posting signs with directions, putting toothbrush and toothpaste by the sink), and removing or silencing unnecessary stimuli (e.g., turning off paging systems). A good place to start is with the NIC environmental management interventions (Box 36-8).

Considering the environment from the client's viewpoint is essential. For instance, if the surroundings are unfamiliar, the client will need to process more information. Lack of a recognizable pattern or structure further taxes the client's capacity to encode information. Appropriate interventions include clarifying the meaning and purpose of people and objects in the environment, enhancing the client's sense of control and the predictability of the environment, and reducing other stimuli as much as possible (Stolley, Gerdner, & Buckwalter, 1999).

Anticipating Needs

The nurse can anticipate many needs of clients. In assuming responsibility for clients with cognitive impairment, the nurse needs to know when the client

---

BOX 36.8

Environmental Management: Violence Prevention

DEFINITION: Monitoring and manipulating the physical environment to decrease the potential of violent behaviour directed toward self, others, or environment

ACTIVITIES

- Remove potential weapons (e.g., sharps, rope-like objects) from the environment.
- Search the environment routinely to maintain it as hazard free.
- Search the client and his or her belongings for weapons or potential weapons during inpatient admission procedures as appropriate.
- Monitor the safety of items that visitors bring to the environment.
- Instruct visitors and other caregivers about relevant client safety issues.
- Limit the client's use of potential weapons.
- Monitor the client during the use of potential weapons (e.g., razors).
- Place the client with potential for self-harm with a roommate to decrease isolation and opportunity to act on self-harm thoughts, as appropriate.

- Assign a single room to the client with potential for violence toward others.
- Place the client in a bedroom located near a nursing station.
- Limit access to windows, unless locked and shatterproof, as appropriate.
- Lock utility and storage rooms.
- Provide paper dishes and plastic utensils at meals.
- Place the client in the least restrictive environment that still allows for the necessary level of observation.
- Provide ongoing surveillance of all client access areas to maintain client safety and therapeutically intervene, as needed.
- Remove other individuals from the vicinity of a violent or potentially violent client.
- Maintain a designated safe area (e.g., seclusion room) for the client to be placed when violent.
- Provide plastic, rather than metal, clothes hangers, as appropriate.

Adapted from McCloskey, J., & Bulechek, G. (2000). *Nursing interventions classification (NIC)* (3rd ed.). St. Louis, MO: Mosby.

last voided and the pattern of bowel movements. Regular toileting routines are not just interventions to prevent incontinence. Similarly, the anticipation of basic needs such as thirst and hunger is important, especially when working with adults or children who cannot readily express their needs. Other discomforts can arise from such conditions as ingrown toenails and adverse medication reactions.

The urge to void can be a powerful stimulus to agitated behaviour. It is not uncommon in a neurologic observation unit to see a young man with a recent head injury become violent just before spontaneously voiding. From a biologic perspective, such a client is probably normally sensitive or even hypersensitive to a full bladder. He probably also has sufficient cognitive function to recognize his need to void. Even some level of social inhibition may be operational in that he recognizes that voiding while lying on his back in bed, with strangers around, is inappropriate. But if he cannot speak or ask for help, he may become increasingly panic stricken. Thrashing around in bed, unable to communicate his need, he may strike out at staff.

The following scenario is the true account of how one graduate student dealt with another common situation. A 75-year-old woman was pacing around the nursing station of a psychogeriatric unit in a nursing home, crying for her mother. Various people spoke kindly to her, trying to explain that her mother was not there. Donna, a graduate student, was studying the wandering behaviours of clients with Alzheimer's disease on the unit. Hypothesizing that there is purpose behind these actions, she walked alongside the woman. After talking a bit with her about the client's mother, Donna asked the client what she would like to do if her mother were there. Gradually the client confided that she needed her mother to help her find the bathroom. Donna then offered to help the woman, walking her to the bathroom. After voiding copiously, the client seemed greatly relieved and settled down.

Using Seclusion and Restraint

Seclusion and **restraint** are controversial interventions to be used judiciously and only when other interventions have failed to control the client's behaviour. The availability of effective psychotropic medications since the 1950s has reduced the need for these interventions of last resort. Reasons usually cited for using them are to protect the client from injury to self or others, to help the client re-establish behavioural control, and to minimize disruption of unit treatment regimens. The controversy over these interventions and their potential to be applied punitively heightens the need for clear institutional standards for their use. The development and use of clear practice standards can reduce

the likelihood that these interventions will be misused (College of Registered Psychiatric Nurses of British Columbia, 2008). Lewis (2002) challenges the use of restraint as a primary intervention in forensic settings. Lewis presents nontouch interventions as an alternative to restraint. In contrast, Hibbs (2000) proposes the use of cognitive interventions with clients while they are restrained. These interventions are designed to challenge thought patterns that contribute to aggressive behaviours.

Evaluation is also important in tracking the use of seclusion and restraint. In a Quebec audit study of the use of a secure room/security guard in a rural hospital, it was found that only 1.1/1,000 emergency room visits occasioned such use, most commonly indicated by physicians' perception of client risk for suicide or self-harm (Brock, Gurekas, Gelinas, & Rollin, 2009). Only 10% of use of these measures was related to staff safety. Most stays in the secure room were less than two nights. An interdisciplinary approach is reported by Hancock et al. (2001) and Morrison et al. (2000). Through a process of joint planning and implementation with health professionals from several disciplines, use of restraint was reduced by 83%.

Spiritual Domain

In addressing the spiritual domain of care for the client who is experiencing anger and aggression issues, contemplative practices, such as **mindfulness,** may be valuable to both the client and nurse. Mindfulness is being fully attentive in the "here and now" moment (Marlatt & Kristeller, 1999). The process of paying attention (without judgment) to what is happening can promote a connection to one's inner being and spirit. Acknowledging the present moment of reality is the beginning of transforming that reality (Kabat-Zinn, 1993). Mindfulness is similar to meditation: awareness of breathing and of the body is central to it. As well, it is about acting with attentiveness and concentration as one walks, eats, looks about, and carries out daily tasks of living. It is about being consciously aware of our body and mind, rather than thinking "about" experience (Sherman & Siporin, 2008). This meditative act can bring a sense of calmness within minutes.

Mindfulness can be found within most religious and spiritual traditions (Sherman & Siporin, 2008). It is a way to recognize one's connection with something beyond oneself, to realize that one is not separate nor alone, to experience serenity (Kreitzer, Gross, Waleekhachonloet, Reilly-Spong, & Byrd, 2009), and/or to search for meaning and purpose (Reed, 1992). Shapiro (2008, p. 3), who researches mindfulness, finds that individuals "often find their faith is deepened as a result of becoming more mindful".

Mindfulness in the health literature, however, is most often discussed as a cognitive behavioural technique. This practice tends to utilize a brief, structured format called Mindfulness Based-Stress Reduction (MBSR). MBSR programs, initially designed by Kabat-Zinn (1990, 1994), involve three basic techniques: meditation, body scan (involves directing one's attention through the entire body), and yoga. In addition to the resource of health care team members trained to teach mindfulness to clients, there are local community programs and educational tools, such as books and videos, that are available to learn about this contemplative practice.

Lown (2007) calls for mindfulness on clinicians' part when addressing anger in the clinician–client/family relationship. He notes that mindfulness in such an encounter allows one to be both a participant and an observer. In taking a moment to assess one's own response to the situation (e.g., anxiety; anger) and to focus on being present in a genuine way to the client/family member, one is better able to respond.

■ INTERACTIONAL PROCESSES

When the nurse develops a collaborative relationship with the client, he or she can assist the client to not exhibit aggressive behaviour. Johnson, Martin, Guha, and Montgomery (1997) explored the experience of thought-disordered individuals before an aggressive incident. Three themes emerged from interviews with 12 clients who had a diagnosis of a thought disorder and a history of aggressive incidents:

- The strong influence of the external environment.
- The use of aggressive behaviours to feel empowered briefly in a situation.
- The occurrence of aggressive incidents, despite knowledge of strategies to control anger.

A 2009 review of the research by Hamrin, Iennaco, and Olsen (2009) regarding factors affecting violence on psychiatric units showed that violence is influenced by complex interactions among clients, staff, and unit culture. A positive culture has appropriate levels of stimulation and meaningful client activities, as well as positive staff attitudes and values toward client care. Good assessment of client factors, including violence history, plays an important role. Therapeutic relationship strategies, including being available, being a client advocate, providing client education, and collaborating with the client in treatment planning, can decrease the potential for violence. An emerging theme in the literature is client and staff power struggles as precipitants for violence.

The skills the nurse uses in interactions with the client may invite escalation or de-escalation of a tense situation (Morrison, 1998). When the nurse uses communication skills to draw out the client's experience, together the nurse and client coevolve an alternative view of the problem. Some nursing writers (Leahey & Harper-Jaques, 1996; Wright & Leahey, 2005) have highlighted the importance of attending to notions of reciprocity and circularity when providing nursing care. For example, the nurse explores the meaning of the expression of aggressive behaviours with the client and the client's beliefs about the ability to control aggressive impulses. Or the nurse and client could discuss the effects of the nurse's behaviours on the client and the effects of the client's behaviours on the nurse. Such an approach facilitates the development of an accepting and equal nurse–client relationship. The client is a partner invited to assume responsibility for inappropriate actions. This approach is in contrast to a hierarchical nurse–client relationship that emphasizes the nurse's role in controlling the client's behaviours and defining changes the client must make. In a collaborative approach, the nurse values the client's experience and acknowledges his or her strengths. The nurse asks the client to use those strengths to either maintain or resume control of behaviour.

In Western cultures, events are typically thought of in a linear fashion (Wright & Leahey, 2005). The nurse who uses a linear causality frame of reference to think about client aggression and violence will view the problem as follows:

PACING → leads to → THREATENING
                                         BEHAVIOURS
(Event A)   (Event B)

From this linear perspective, the nurse labels the client as the problem, and other factors assume secondary importance. The nurse might decide, first, to gain control over the client's behaviour. The nurse may base this decision on his or her affective response and previous experience (e.g., that threatening behaviours frighten other clients and disrupt the unit routine). The nurse's response to a client's behaviour could be to ask the client to stop yelling, to inform the client that the behaviour is inappropriate, or to suggest the use of medication if the client does not calm down. When one thinks based on linear causality, he or she assumes that event A (pacing) causes event B (threatening behaviour).

When one thinks using circular causality, he or she attempts to understand the link between behaviours and to determine how the threatening behaviour will influence a continuation or cessation of pacing. The nurse who engages in circular thinking will also know that his or her responses to the client will influence the situation. The nurse's responses will be in the domains of cognition (ideas, concepts, and beliefs), affect (emotional state), and behaviour (Tomm, 1980). The nurse will be aware of the reciprocal influences of the nurse and client's behaviours (Wright & Leahey, 2005). In viewing the situation from a circular perspective, the nurse is interested in understanding how people are involved, rather than in discovering who is to blame. This perspective does not ignore individual responsibility for aggressive or violent actions, and it does not blame the victim. It does invite the nurse to consider the multiple influences on the expression of aggressive and violent behaviour (Robinson, Wright, & Watson, 1994).

◼◼◼ RESPONDING TO ASSAULT

In recent years, compelling scientific evidence that violence portrayed in the media is harmful to children has fostered debate about violence and its effects. As a result, television networks have taken both voluntary and legislated actions to limit violent programming during hours when children are generally watching programs. However, these gains in limiting access to violence have been countered by the growing availability of violent video games and websites.

Given today's societal context, it is not surprising that aggression and violence directed toward nurses are often ignored. Close proximity to clients by health care workers presents a higher risk to experience acts of violence. Approximately 40% of time loss claims-related violence is from health care workers (Rotin, 2005). Aggression and violence by clients can threaten the safety of nurses, other clients, other health care professionals, family members, and visitors. Family members may also direct aggression and violence toward nurses, especially if family members have increased stress levels and ineffective coping skills and/or experience long wait times and/or use substances (Ferns, 2007). Ineffective communication between nurses and families can contribute to increased aggression (Ferns).

In health care settings, nurses assume an active role in preventing and managing aggressive and violent behaviours. Involuntary (as opposed to voluntary) admission to a psychiatric facility or altered mental status in any setting may constrain the development of a trusting relationship between the nurse and client. Nurses are more likely than physicians to be involved with clients who are aggressive or potentially violent because of the amount of time they are in close contact with clients. Nurses also have a major role in setting limits and defining boundaries (Bostrom, Boyd, & White, 2006).

Concern and investigation of assaults on nurses have been growing. Research shows that the incidence and severity of violence directed toward nurses are on the rise with the most common form of violence being verbal abuse followed by threatening behaviours (Luck, Jackson, & Usher, 2006). The Nova Scotia Department of Health (2006) indicated that 32% of nurses reported being physically assaulted by clients within the past year. Nurses commonly report emotional abuse, with 44%

experiencing emotional abuse from a client (Canadian Institute for Health Information, 2005). Reported violence is higher in long-term care, general hospitals, and psychiatric facilities, but nurses who work in ambulatory care settings or community clinics are not immune to assault (Gerberich et al., 2004). Banerjee et al. (2008) report Canadian personal support workers in long-term care facilities to be seven times more likely to experience violence directed toward them than their Nordic counterparts. The most common injury experienced by health care workers due to violence include strains to the body, such as the back (65%) and bruises/contusions (18%; WCB Statistical Services, 2005).

Variations in statistics can result from differences in definitions of violence, reporting practices, data collection and analysis, and underreporting. Rationale for underreporting is common and includes time constraints, staff attitudes, conflict between the traditional caring role and reporting the violence, belief that an individual will be blamed or perceived as inadequate, minimization of the event by the nurses involved or by their colleagues, and lack of understanding in the importance of data collection (Munro, 2002). Data, as identified by WHO (2002), provide important information in the development of strategies to minimize violence. Lack of data limits health care facilities' ability to enact measures to protect their workers and others. Data collected should include information about gender (Ferns, 2006).

Assaults on nurses by clients can have immediate and long-term consequences (Henderson, 2003). Reported assaults range from verbal threats and minor altercations to severe injuries, rape, and murder. Any assault can produce severe consequences for the victim. Nonphysical violence toward nurses by clients or others can have long-lasting effects on nurses, such as posttraumatic stress disorder (Gerberich et al., 2005).

Lanza's research (1992) indicates that nurses experience a wide range of responses (Table 36-5) similar to those of victims of any other type of trauma. However, because of their role as caregivers, nurses may suppress the normal range of feelings after an assault, believing that it is wrong to experience strong feelings of anger and fear in this situation. This belief may relate to the conflict nurses experience in having to care for clients who have hurt them.

Steps can be taken at a clinical and management level to reduce the risk for assaults on nurses by clients. Clinically, nurses must be provided with training programs in the prevention and management of aggressive behaviour. These programs, like courses on cardiopulmonary resuscitation (CPR), impart both knowledge and skills. Like CPR training, the courses need to be made available to nurses and students regularly so that they have opportunities to reinforce and update what they have learned. Nurses who have participated in preventive

Table 36.5	Nurses' Responses to Assault	
Response Type	Personal	Professional
Affective	• Irritability • Depression • Anger • Anxiety • Apathy	• Erosion of feelings of competence, leading to increased anxiety and fear • Feelings of guilt or self-blame • Fear of potentially violent clients
Cognitive	• Suppressed or intrusive thoughts of assault	• Reduced confidence in judgment • Consideration of job change
Behavioural	• Social withdrawal	• Possible hesitation in responding to other violent situations • Possible overcontrolling • Possible hesitation to report future assaults • Possible withdrawal from colleagues • Questioning of capabilities by coworkers
Physiologic	• Disturbed sleep • Headaches • Stomach aches • Tension	• Increased absenteeism from somatic complaints

training programs as students or as professionals are more likely to effectively manage and reduce aggressive or violent situations. Additionally, training programs can raise awareness as to the nature of the problem, develop the nurses' knowledge and skills, and improve attitudes toward clients who have a propensity for violence (Deans, 2004). Less experienced staff with poor communication skills are at higher risk for assault (Wright, Dixon, & Tompkins, 2003).

EVALUATION AND TREATMENT OUTCOMES

Treatment outcomes can be considered at both individual and aggregate levels. The desired outcome at the individual level is for the client to regain or maintain control over aggressive or potentially aggressive thoughts, feelings, and actions. *Aggression control* is the term used in the *Nursing Outcomes Classification* (NOC; Moorhead, Johnson, & Maas, 2003). The nurse may observe that the client shows decreased psychomotor activity (e.g., less pacing), has a more relaxed posture, speaks more directly about feelings of anger and personal needs, requires less sedating medication, shows increased tolerance for frustration and the ability to consider alternatives, and makes effective use of other coping strategies. Evidence of a reduction in risk factors may include decreased noise and confusion in the immediate environment, calmness on the part of nursing staff and others, and a climate of clear expectations and mutual acceptance and respect. In units, day hospitals, or group home settings, indicators of

positive treatment outcomes might be a reduction in the number and severity of assaults on staff and other clients, fewer incident reports, and increased staff competency in de-escalating potentially violent situations.

CONTINUUM OF CARE

Anger and aggression occur in all settings. During periods of extreme aggression, in which people are a danger to themselves or others because of a mental disorder, they are admitted to an acute psychiatric unit. Removing individuals from their environment and hospitalizing them in a locked psychiatric unit provide enough safety that the aggressive behaviour dissipates. Because uncontrolled anger and aggression interfere with their ability to function, people who have problems in these areas require referral to appropriate resources before these destructive behaviours erupt.

Additional understanding of the phenomena of anger, aggression, and violence as they occur in the clinical setting is needed. Research studies that have illuminated this problem from a nursing perspective need to be continued and expanded. Specific areas of study need to examine the links among biology, neurology, and psychology. In addition, further explorations of the reciprocal influence of client interactional style and treatment setting culture will assist in the development and management of humane treatment settings. Finally, and perhaps most importantly, nurses must research the effectiveness of particular nursing interventions (see Box 36-9).

BOX 36.9

Research for Best Practice: Key Factors With Aggression on Inpatient Psychiatric Units

Bowers, L., Allan, T., Simpson, A. Jones, J., Van Der Merwe, M., & Jeffery, D. (2009). Identifying key factors associated with aggression on acute inpatient psychiatric wards. Issues in Mental Health Nursing, 30, 260–271.

QUESTION: What is the relationship of patient aggression to the use of containment methods, environment, routines, and staff variables?

METHOD: A multivariate cross-sectional design was used. The sample included 136 acute care psychiatric units in England. The Patient-Staff Conflict Checklist, an end-of-shift report on the frequency of conflict and containment, was collected over 6 months on all participating units. The Bongar Lethality Scale was used to assess the severity of all incidents of self-harm or attempted suicide. Other measures included the Ward Atmosphere Scale, the Climate Team Inventory, and the Attitudes to Containment Measures Questionnaire, as well as measures related to leadership and to burnout. Analysis ascertained factors most strongly associated with verbal and physical aggression against objects and against others.

FINDINGS: High levels of aggression were associated with patients detained under mental health legislation, high patient turnover, unit doors being locked, and higher staffing ratios. The reasons that more nursing resources (professional staff) were associated with increased adverse (aggressive) events could not be ascertained from the evidence. The researchers postulate that more staff and thus more violence may result from greater patient–staff interaction, and possibly more restrictions on patients as an outcome. Although there is some indication that staff psychosocial functioning influences aggressive incidents, the evidence is not strong.

IMPLICATIONS FOR PRACTICE: The imposition of restrictions on patients is associated with increased rather than reduced aggression on acute care inpatient units. Further research is needed to determine the direction of the influence: Does an increase in potential for aggression on a unit cause increased restrictions or vice versa?

SUMMARY OF KEY POINTS

☐ Theories used to explain anger, aggression, and violence include the following types:

- Neurobiologic, including the cognitive neuroassociation model, the neurostructural model (the emotional circuit), and the neurochemical model (low serotonin syndrome).
- Psychological, including psychoanalytic theories, behavioural theories (e.g., drive theory, social learning theory), and cognitive theories (e.g., rational-emotive theory).
- Sociocultural theories.
- Interactional theory.

☐ Biologic factors to assess in clients who display aggressive and violent behaviours include exposure to toxic chemicals, use of medications, substance abuse, premenstrual dysphoric disorder, trauma, hemorrhage, and tumour.

☐ Biologic intervention choices include administering medications and managing nutrition.

☐ Psychological factors to assess in clients who display aggressive and violent behaviours include thought processing (e.g., perception, delusion) and sensory impairment.

☐ Psychological intervention choices can be affective (e.g., validating, listening, exploring beliefs), cognitive (e.g., giving commendations, offering information, providing education, using thought stopping, contracting), or behavioural (e.g., assigning tasks, using bibliotherapy, interrupting patterns, providing choices).

☐ Social intervention choices include reducing stimulation, anticipating needs, and using seclusion or restraints.

☐ Mindfulness can be a component of addressing the spiritual domain of care. It is a contemplative practice that both clients and nurses may find useful in dealing with anger and situations involving aggression.

☐ Client aggression and violence are serious concerns for nurses in all areas of clinical practice. Training in and policies and procedures for the prevention and management of aggressive episodes should be available in all work settings.

CRITICAL THINKING CHALLENGES

1 Mary Jane, a 24-year-old single woman, has just been admitted to an inpatient psychiatry unit. She was transferred to the unit from the emergency room, where she was treated for a drug overdose. She is sullen when she is introduced to her roommate and refuses to answer the questions the nurse has that are part of the admission procedure. The nurse tells Mary Jane that he will come back later to see how she is. A few minutes later, Mary Jane approaches the nursing station and asks in a demanding tone to talk with someone and complains that she has been completely ignored since she came into the unit. What frameworks can the nurse use to understand Mary Jane's behaviour? At this point in time, what data does

he have to develop a plan of care? What interventions might the nurse choose to use to help Mary Jane behave in a manner that is consistent with the norms of this inpatient unit?

2 Discuss the influence of gender and cultural norms on the expression of anger. When a nurse is caring for a client from a culture that the nurse is not familiar with, what could the nurse ask to ensure that his or her expectations of the client's behaviour are consistent with the gender and cultural norms of the client?

3 Under what circumstances should people who are aggressive or violent be held accountable for their behaviour? Are there any exceptions?

4 When a nurse minimizes verbally abusive behaviour by a client, family member, or healthcare colleague, what implicit message does he or she send?

5 In what way does our understanding of sociocultural theories influence the relationships that we, as nurses, develop with clients and families? Does this understanding also influence the relationships between nurses and other health professionals?

6 Paul is sitting quietly reading a newspaper. Jane sits down next to him and starts talking to him about the weather. Paul responds by pushing Jane off the couch. How do you understand Paul's behaviour? Could Paul's action have been prevented?

WEB LINKS

www.ccmhi.ca/en/resources/links.html This is the resources section of the Canadian Collaborative Mental Health Initiative site, which provides references and articles as well as numerous additional links of interest to mental health practices.

www.cna-nurses.ca This is a link to the Canadian Nurses Association Position Statement on Violence, which discusses the important role nurses play in dealing with and eliminating violence.

www.crpnbc.ca/worksafe_links.html This site provides additional links to the College of Registered Psychiatric Nurses of British Columbia's report on client safety in mental health settings.

www.phac-aspc.gc.ca/chn-rcs/index-eng.php This is the site of the Public Health Agency of Canada, which provides useful web-based information on many health-related topics, including information on violence and its impact on health.

www.who.int/mediacentre/events/violence_health The World Health Organization World Report on Violence and Health describes the magnitude and impact of violence throughout the world. A broad spectrum of violence is examined, with a separate chapter of the report devoted to each of the following seven topics: child abuse, youth violence, violence by intimate partners, sexual violence, elder abuse, suicide, and collective violence. There are also country and regional data available.

MOVIES, NOVELS, AND BIOGRAPHIES

Anger Management: 2003. Adam Sandler stars as Dave, a mild-mannered businessman wrongly court mandated to attend anger management therapy. Jack Nicholson plays the role of Buddy, a psychiatrist and anger management expert whose unorthodox means of therapy may be just what Dave needs.

VIEWING POINTS: What are some of the ways anger may be expressed by a client? Can you identify differences between appropriate anger and inappropriate anger? What are some of the "management" techniques utilized in this movie? Would any of these techniques be appropriate to use with a client? What physiological symptoms of anger are evident?

Girl Interrupted: 2000. The story is told through a teenage girl's (Winona Ryder) eyes about being committed to psychiatric unit where she comes into contact with another teen (Angelina Jolie) who suffers from volatile borderline personality disorder.

VIEWING POINTS: In what way do the behaviours of the staff encourage aggression and violence? How do nurses intervene to help the clients regain or maintain control of aggressive behaviours? How do the nurses manage clients' personal verbal outbursts?

What About Bob: 1991. Richard Dreyfess plays the role of Dr. Leo Marvin, a staunched psychiatrist who takes on a new client named Bob. Bob suffers from OCD and is highly dependent. The movie unravels as Bob insinuates himself into his psychiatrist's life.

VIEWING POINTS: What do you think of the psychiatrist's initial assessment techniques? What communication techniques were or were not employed to assist the client in telling his story? What do you think about the psychiatrist's comment "I don't get upset?" Is this possible? How would you assist the psychiatrist in decreasing his anger initially when it was only frustration? (This is a common factor for many clients as they grow in their anger. There are multiple contributing factors compounding a problem, and frequently, the final straw has nothing to do with the root of the problem.)

REFERENCES

American Psychiatric Association. (2000). Diagnostic and statistical manual of mental disorders (4th ed., Text revision). Washington, DC: Author.

Bandura, A. (1973). *Aggression: A social learning analysis*. New York, NY: Prentice-Hall.

Banerjee, A., Daly, A., Armstrong, H., Armstrong, P., Lafrance, S., & Szebehely, M. (2008). "Out of control": Violence against personal support workers in long-term care. York University/Carlton University. Retrieved June 4, 2008, from http://www.yorku.ca/mediar/special/out_of_control___english.pdf

Beck, A. T. (1976). *Cognitive therapy and emotional disorders.* New York, NY: International Universities Press.

Belknap, R. A. (2003). Understanding abuse and violence against women: A two-day immersion course. *Nurse Educator, 28*(4), 170–174.

Berkowitz, L. (1989). Frustration-aggression hypothesis: Examination and reformulation. *Psychological Bulletin, 106*(1), 59–73.

Bernstein, K. S., & Saladino, J. P. (2007). Clinical assessment and management of psychiatric patients' violent and aggressive behaviours in general hospital. *MEDSURG Nursing, 16*(5), 301–331.

Best, M., Williams, J. M., & Coccaro, E. F. (2002). Evidence for a dysfunctional prefrontal circuit in clients with an impulsive aggressive disorder. *Proceedings of the National Academy of Sciences, 99*(12), 8448–8453.

Bostrom, A. C., Boyd, M., & White, D. (2006). Coping with aggressive behavior in patients with schizophrenia. *Psychiatric Nurse: Counseling Points, 1*(2), 4–12.

Bowers, L., Allan, T., Simpson, A., Jones, J., Van Der Merwe, M., & Jeffery, D. (2009). Identifying key factors associated with aggression on acute inpatient psychiatric wards. *Issues in Mental Health Nursing, 30,* 260–271.

Brock. G., Gurekas, V., Gelinas, A-F., & Rollin, K. (2009). Use of a "secure room" and a security guard in the management of the violent, aggressive or suicidal patient in a rural hospital: A 3-year audit. *Canadian Journal of Rural Medicine, 14*(1), 16–20.

Burke, J. D., Loeber, R., & Birmaher, B. (2002). Oppositional defiant disorder and conduct disorder: A review of the past 10 years, Part II. *Journal of American Academy of Adolescent Psychiatry, 41*(11), 1275–1293.

Burns, D. (1999). *Feeling good: The new mood therapy.* New York, NY: Avon Books.

Canadian Institute for Health Information. (2005). *A summary of highlights from the 2005 national survey of the work and health of nurses.* Ottawa, ON: Statistics Canada.

Capra, F. (2002). *The hidden connections: Integrating the biological, cognitive and social dimensions of life into a science of sustainability.* New York, NY: Doubleday.

Carlsson, G., Dahlberg, K., Ekebergh, M., & Dahlberg, H. (2006). Patients longing for authentic personal care: A phenomenological study of violent encounters in psychiatric setting. *Issues in Mental Health Nursing, 27*(3), 287–305.

Carpenito-Moyet, L. J. (2002). *Guidelines for code white response: A component of prevention & management of aggressive behaviour in health care.* Occupational Health & Safety Agency for Health Care in British Columbia (BC), Workmen's Compensation of BC, Health Association in BC.

Chakos, M., & Lieberman, J. A. (2001). Effects of clozapine, olanzapine, risperidone, and haloperidol on hostility among clients with schizophrenia. *Psychiatric Services, 52*(11), 1510–1514.

Citrome, L., & Volavka, J. (1999). Violent clients in the emergency setting. *Psychiatric Clinics of North America, 22*(4), 789–801.

Citrome, L., & Volavka, J. (2002). *Aggression.* Retrieved June 3, 2008, from http://www.emedicine.com/Med/topic3005.htm

College of Registered Psychiatric Nurses of British Columbia. (2008). *The use of physical restraint & seclusion as psychiatric nursing interventions: Position statement.* Port Moody, BC: Author.

Corrigan, P. W., Yudofsky, S. C., & Silver, J. M. (1993). Pharmacological and behavioral treatment for aggressive psychiatric in-patients. *Hospital and Community Psychiatry, 44*(3), 125–133.

Deans, C. (2004). The effectiveness of a training program for emergency department nurses in managing violent situations. *Australian Journal of Advanced Nursing, 21*(4), 17–22.

DiGiuseppe, R., & Tafrate, R. (2007). *Understanding anger disorders.* Oxford, UK: Oxford University Press.

Duxbury, J., & Whittington, R. (2005). Causes and management of patient aggression and violence: Staff and patient perspectives. *Journal of Advanced Nursing, 50*(5), 469–478.

Ellis, A. (1977). *Anger: How to live with and without it.* Secaucus, NJ: Citadel Press.

Fahs, H., Potiron, G., Senon, J. L., & Perivier, E. (1999). Anticonvulsants in agitation and behavior disorders in demented subjects. *Encephale, 25*(2), 169–174.

Faucher, L., & Tappolet, C. (2008). *The Modularity of Emotions.* Calgary, AB: University of Calgary Press.

Ferns, T. (2006). Underreporting of violent incidents against nursing staff. *Nursing Standard, 21*(40), 41–45.

Ferns, T. (2007). Factors that influence aggressive behaviours in acute care settings. *Nursing Standard, 21*(33), 41–45.

Fromm, E. (1973). *The anatomy of human destructiveness.* New York, NY: Holt, Rinehart and Winston.

Gerberich, S. G., Church, T. R., McGovern, P. M., Hansen, H. E., Nachreiner, N. M., Geisser, M. S., et al. (2004). An epidemiological study of the magnitude and consequences of work related violence: The Minnesota nurses' study. *Occupational Environmental Medicine, 61,* 495–503.

Gerberich, S. G., Church, T. R., McGovern, P. M., Hansen, H., Nachreiner, N. M., Geisser, M. S., et al. (2005). Risk factors for work-related assaults on nurses. *Epidemiology, 16,* 704–709.

Gerloff, L. (1997). Anger management. *Arkansas Nursing News, 14*(1), 5–7.

Hamrin, V., Iennaco, J., & Olsen, D. (2009). A review of ecological factors affecting inpatient psychiatric unit violence: Implications for relational and unit culture improvements. *Issues in Mental Health Nursing, 30,* 214–226.

Hancock, C. K., Buster, P. A., Oliver, M. S., Fox, S. W., Morrison, E., & Burger, S. L. (2001). Restraint reduction in acute care: An interdisciplinary approach. *Journal of Nursing Administration, 31*(2), 74–77.

Harper-Jaques, S., & Masters, A. (1994). Powerful words: The use of letters with sexual abuse survivors. *Journal of Psychosocial Nursing and Mental Health Services, 32*(8), 11–16.

Harper-Jaques, S., & Reimer, M. (1992). Aggressive behavior and the brain: A different perspective for the mental health nurse. *Archives of Psychiatric Nursing, 6*(5), 312–320.

Harris, D., & Morrison, E. F. (1995). Managing violence without coercion. *Archives of Psychiatric Nursing, 9*(4), 203–210.

Heinz, A., Mann, K., Weinberger, D. R., & Goldman, D. (2001). Serotonergic dysfunction, negative mood states, and response to alcohol. *Alcoholism: Clinical and Experimental Research, 25*(4), 487–495.

Henderson, A. D. (2003). Nurses and workplace violence: Nurses' experiences of verbal and physical abuse at work. *Canadian Journal of Nursing Leadership, 16*(4), 82–98.

Hibbs, A. (2000). Cognitive therapy: A complementary strategy for expressed anger during the restraint of an aggressive individual. *British Journal of Forensic Practice, 2*(2), 19–29.

Jenkins, A. (1990). *Invitations to responsibility.* Adelaide, New South Whales, Australia: Dulwich Centre Publications.

Johnson, B., Martin, M. L., Guha, M., & Montgomery, P. (1997). The experience of thought disordered individuals preceding an aggressive incident. *Journal of Psychiatric and Mental Health Nursing, 4,* 213–220.

Kabat-Zinn, J. (1990). *Full catastrophe living: Using the wisdom of your body and mind to face stress, pain, and illness.* New York, NY: Dell.

Kabat-Zinn, J. (1993). Mindfulness meditation: Health benefits of an ancient Buddhist practice. In D. Goleman & J. Gurin (Eds.), *Mind/body medicine* (pp. 259–276). New York, NY: Consumer Reports Books.

Kabat-Zinn, J. (1994). *Wherever you go, there you are: Mindfulness meditation in everyday life.* New York, NY: Hyperion.

Koh, K. B., Kim, C. H., & Park, J. K. (2002). Predominance of anger in depressive disorders compared with anxiety disorders and somatoform disorders. *Journal of Clinical Psychiatry, 63*(6), 486–492.

Kreitzer, M. J., Gross, C. R., Waleekhachonloet, O. A., Reilly-Spong, M., & Byrd, M. (2009). The brief serenity scale: A psychometric analysis of a measure of spirituality and well-being. *Journal of Holistic Nursing, 27*(1), 7–16.

Lanza, M. L. (1992). Nurses as client assault victims: An update, synthesis, and recommendations. *Archives of Psychiatric Nursing, 6*(3), 163–171.

Leahey, M., & Harper-Jaques, S. (1996). Family–nurse relationship: Core assumptions and clinical implications. *Journal of Family Nursing, 2*(2), 133–151.

Lewis, D. M. (2002). Responding to a violent incident: Physical restraint or anger management as therapeutic interventions. *Journal of Psychiatry and Mental Health Nursing, 9*(1), 57–63.

Limacher, L. H., & Wright, L. M. (2003). Commendations: Listening to the silent side of a family intervention. *Journal of Family Nursing, 9*(2), 130–150.

Lorist, M. M., & Tops, M. (2003). Caffeine, fatigue, and cognition. *Brain and Cognition, 53*(1), 82–94.

Lown, B. (2007). Difficult conversations: Anger in the clinician-patient/family relationship. *Southern Medical Journal, 100*(1), 34–39.

Luck, L., Jackson, D., & Usher, K. (2006). Survival of the fittest, or socially constructed phenomena? Theoretical understandings of aggression & violence towards nurses. *Contemporary Nurse, 21*(2), 251–263.

Marlatt, G. A., & Kristeller, J. L. (1999). Mindfulness and meditation. In W. R. Miller, (Ed.), *Integrating spirituality into treatment*. Washington, DC: American Psychological Association.

McCloskey, J., & Bulechek, G. (2000). *Nursing interventions classification (NIC)* (3rd ed.). St. Louis, M.: Mosby.

Mesulam, M. (2000). *Principles of behavioral and cognitive neurology* (2nd ed.). Oxford: Oxford University Press.

Miller, N., Pedersen, W. C., Earleywine, M., & Pollock, V. E. (2003). Artificial theoretical model of triggered displaced aggression. *Personality Social Psychology Review, 7*(1), 57–97.

Moorhead, S., Johnson, M., & Maas, M. (2003). *Nursing outcomes classification* (3rd ed.). Philadelphia, PA: Elsevier.

Morrison, E. F. (1998). The culture of caregiving and aggression in psychiatric settings. *Archives of Psychiatric Nursing, 12*(1), 21–31.

Morrison, E. F., & Carney Love, C. (2003). An evaluation of four programs for the management of aggression in psychiatric settings. *Archives of Psychiatric Nursing, 17*(4), 146–155.

Morrison, E. F., Fox, S., Burger, S., Goodloe, L., Blosser, J., & Gitter, K. (2000). A nurse led, unit based program to reduce restraint use in acute care. *Journal of Nursing Care Quality, 14*(3), 72–80.

Munro V. (2002). 'Why Do Nurses Neglect to Report Violent Incidents?'. *Nursing Times, 98*(17): 38–40.

North American Nursing Diagnosis Association. (2005). *Nursing diagnoses: Definitions and classification 2005–2006*. Philadelphia, PA: Author.

Novaco, R. (2007). Anger dysregulation. In T. Cavell & K. Malcolm (Eds.), *Anger, aggression, and interventions for interpersonal violence* (pp. 3–54). London: Lawrence Erlbaum Associates.

Nova Scotia Department of Health. (2006). *The National Survey of the Work and Health of Nurses, 2005*. Halifax, Nova Scotia, Canada: Author.

Pardo, J. V., Pardo, P. J., & Raichle, M. E. (1993). Neural correlates of self-induced dysphoria. *American Journal of Psychiatry, 150*(5), 713–719.

Paris, J. (2005). Borderline personality disorder. *Canadian Medical Association Journal, 172*(12), 1579–1583.

Reed, P. G. (1992). An emerging paradigm for the investigation of spirituality in nursing. *Research in Nursing & Health, 15*, 349–357.

Robinson, C., Wright, L., & Watson, W. (1994). A non-traditional approach to family violence. *Archives of Psychiatric Nursing, 8*(1), 30–37.

Rotin, J. (2005). Preventing workplace violence. *WorkSafe Magazine, 4*, 12–14.

Rubinsztein, E. R., Sahakian, B. J., & Dolan, R. J. (2002). The neural basis of mood congruent processing biases in depression. *Archives of General Psychiatry, 59*(7), 597–604.

Scarpa, A., & Raine, A. (1997). Psychophysiology of anger and violent behavior. *Psychiatric Clinics of North America, 20*(2), 375–394.

Schmeck, K., Sadigorsky, S., Englert, E., Demisch, L., Dierks, T., Barta, S., et al. (2002). Mood changes following acute tryptophan depletion in healthy adults. *Psychopathology, 35*(4), 234–240.

Sergi, M. J., & Green, M. F. (2003). Social perception and early visual processing in schizophrenia. *Schizophrenia Research, 59*(2–3), 233–241.

Shannon, J. W. (2000). *Understanding and managing anger: Diagnosis, treatment and prevention*. Presentation by Mind Matters Seminar, April 2000, Calgary, Alberta, Canada.

Shapiro, S.L. (2008). Exploring the effects of mindfulness meditation on health, well-being, and spirituality. *Spirituality in Higher Education, 4*(2), 1–5.

Sherman, E., & Siporin, M. (2008). Contemplative theory and practice for social work. *Journal of Religion & Spirituality in Social Work, 27*(3), 259–274.

Silver, J. M., Yudofsky, S. C., Slater, J. A., Gold, R. K., Stryer, B. L., Williams, D. T., et al. (2000). Propranolol treatment of chronically hospitalized aggressive clients. *Journal of Neuropsychiatry & Clinical Neuroscience, 12*(3), 413.

Snyder, K., Schrepferman, L., Brooker, M., & Stoolmiller, M. (2007). The roles of anger, conflict with parents and peers, and social reinforcement in the early development of physical aggression. In T. Cavell & K. Malcolm (Eds.), *Anger, aggression, and interventions for interpersonal violence* (pp. 187–214). London: Lawrence Erlbaum Associates.

Soloff, P. H., Lynch, K. G., & Moss, H. B. (2000). Serotonin, impulsivity, and alcohol use disorders in the older adolescent: A psychobiological study. *Alcoholism: Clinical and Experimental Research, 24*(11), 1609–1619.

Stolley, J. M., Gerdner, L. A., & Buckwalter, K. C. (1999). Dementia management. In G. M. Bulechek & J. C. McCloskey (Eds.), *Nursing interventions: Effective nursing treatments* (3rd ed., pp. 533–548). Philadelphia, PA: WB Saunders.

Tajaden, P., & Thoennes, N. (2000). *Findings from national violence against women survey*. Washington, DC: U.S. Department of Justice.

Talerico, K. A., Evans, L. K., & Strumpf, N. E. (2002). Mental health correlates of aggression in nursing home residents with dementia. *Gerontologist, 42*(2), 169–177.

Tavris, C. (1989). *Anger: The misunderstood emotion*. New York, NY: Simon & Schuster.

Thomas, S. P. (1990). Theoretical and empirical perspectives on anger. *Issues in Mental Health Nursing, 11*, 203–216.

Thomas, S. P. (1993). *Women and anger*. New York, NY: Springer.

Thomas, S. P. (1998). Assessing and intervening with anger disorders. *Nursing Clinics of North America, 33*(1), 121–133.

Thomas, S. P. (2001). Teaching healthy anger management. *Perspectives in Psychiatric Care, 37*(2), 41–48.

Thomas, S. (2003). Men's anger: A phenomenological exploration of its meaning in a middle class sample of American men. *Psychology of Men & Masculinity, 4*(2), 163–175.

Thomas, S. (2009). *Transforming nurses' stress and anger: Steps toward healing* (3rd ed.). New York, NY: Springer.

Tomm, K. (1980). Towards a cybernetic systems approach to family therapy at the University of Calgary. In D. Freeman (Ed.), *Diagnosis and assessment in family therapy* (pp. 101–122). London: Aspen.

United Nations High Commission on Human Rights. (2001). Human rights resolution 2001.49. *Elimination of violence against women*. Retrieved November 25, 2009, from http://www.unhchr.ch/huridocda/huridoca.nsf/(symbol)/a.res.48.104.en

WCB Statistical Services. (2005). *Fact sheet: Violence in health care and social assistance provincial overview*. Vancouver, BC: Author

World Health Organization. (2002). *World report on violence and health*. Geneva, Switzerland: WHO Press.

World Health Organization. (2005). *Multi-country study on women's health and domestic violence against women*. Geneva, Switzerland: WHO Press.

Wright, L. M., & Leahey, M. (2005). *Nurses and families: A guide to family assessment and intervention* (3rd ed.). Philadelphia, PA: FA Davis.

Wright, N. M. J., Dixon, A. J., & Tompkins, C. N. E. (2003). Managing violence in primary care: An evidence-based approach. *British Journal of General Practice, 53*, 557–562.

Young, S. N. (2002). Clinical nutrition. 3. The fuzzy boundary between nutrition and psychopharmacology. *Canadian Medical Association Journal, 166*(2), 205–209.

CHAPTER 37

Caring for Abused Persons

Elizabeth A. McCay

Adapted from the chapter "Caring for Abused Persons"
by Mary R. Boyd

LEARNING OBJECTIVES

After studying this chapter, you will be able to:

- Describe the bio/psycho/social/spiritual theories of abuse.
- Discuss theories explaining why some persons become abusive and why some persons remain in violent relationships.
- Describe the bio/psycho/social/spiritual consequences of abuse.
- Describe the diagnostic criteria for posttraumatic stress disorder (PTSD).
- Discuss the three major symptom categories found in PTSD and their associated etiologic factors.
- Describe the diagnostic criteria for dissociative identity disorder (DID).
- Integrate bio/psycho/social/spiritual theories into the analysis of human responses to abuse.
- Formulate nursing care plans for survivors of abuse.

KEY CONCEPTS

- resilience
- self-esteem

KEY TERMS

- acute stress disorder (ASD) • alexithymia • behavioural sensitization • complex posttraumatic stress disorder (C-PTSD) • cycle of violence • dissociation • dissociative identity disorder (DID) • emotional abuse • extinction • factitious disorder by proxy (Munchausen's syndrome by proxy) • fear conditioning • intergenerational transmission • neglect • physical abuse • posttraumatic stress disorder (PTSD) • sexual abuse • traumatic bonding

$\mathcal{V}$iolence demonstrated in the abuse of women, men, children, and elders is a national health problem that causes significant impairment in survivors. Abuse of any type permanently changes the survivor's construction of reality and the meaning of his or her life. It wounds deeply, endangering core beliefs about self, others, and the world. It usually destroys the survivor's self-esteem.

Nurses encounter survivors of abuse in all health care settings. For this reason, they must be knowledgeable about abuse. They must understand its indicators, causes, assessment techniques, and effective nursing interventions. The importance of assessing for abuse in health care settings is being increasingly recognized (Gallop, McCay, Austin, Bayer, & Peternelji-Taylore, 1998; Hollingsworth & Ford-Gilboe, 2006). It requires nurses to possess the necessary educational background to ask questions about abuse that will ultimately prevent further abuse (Yonaka, Yoder, Darrow, & Sherck, 2007) and facilitate recovery. Protection and recovery from abuse require survivors to remember and discuss terrible events. However, secrecy and silence protect perpetrators and seriously endanger survivors. Failure to assess for abuse communicates a powerfully disturbing message: that the most traumatic event of a patient's life is too upsetting for others to hear. If nurses do not allow and encourage survivors to tell their stories, the abuse experiences will continue to haunt patients as symptoms of mental disorders.

This chapter focuses on the nursing process with women, men, children, and elders who are survivors of abuse. It provides basic nursing information needed to address the multiple, complex problems of these patients.

> **KEY CONCEPT** **Self-esteem** is how one feels about oneself. Its components are self-acceptance, self-worth, self-love, and self-nurturing.

■■■ TYPES OF ABUSE

Most abuse that women, men, children, and elders experience is intimate violence; that is, the perpetrator is a loved and trusted partner or family member. As a result, the world and home may no longer be safe, people seem dangerous, and life may become a tortured existence of warding off ever-present threats. However, for some resilient individuals, healthy relationships across the lifespan appear to be protective; such that minimal psychological sequela occurs in adult life in spite of childhood abuse (Collishaw et al., 2007).

> **KEY CONCEPT** **Resilience** is the capacity to overcome adversity in spite of extreme stress and involves the balancing of risk and protective factors.

Woman Abuse

Woman abuse, domestic violence, spousal abuse, partner abuse, and battered wives are all terms used interchangeably to denote violence directed toward women. However, some of these terms do not specifically refer to the abuse of a woman by an intimate partner. For example, the term *domestic violence* may be used in cases in which one person directs abuse against an entire family. The terms *spouse abuse* and *partner abuse* could indicate that the couple in whom abuse occurs, either heterosexual or homosexual, lives together but is unmarried. According to Statistics Canada, females account for 83% of spousal violence that is reported to police compared to 17% for men (Canadian Centre for Justice Statistics, 2009). When women use force against their male partners, they often do so in self-defence, and the injuries they receive are more severe than those they inflict (Swann, 2001).

For these reasons, *woman abuse* has been chosen as the most appropriate term to use in this chapter in designating violence, including rape, directed toward a woman by an intimate partner.

Woman abuse is a significant health problem that crosses all ethnic, racial, and socioeconomic lines. Estimates of the annual prevalence of woman abuse range from 2 million to approximately 4 million cases (Brady & Dansky, 2002). Specific rates of victimization were assessed in the 2004 General Social Survey (GSS) on Victimization of 25,000 women and men. Survey results indicated that 7% of women and 6% of men reported being the victim of violence in the relationship with their intimate partner (Canadian Centre for Justice Statistics, 2005). Specifically, it is estimated that 653,000 women and 546,000 men were the victims of intimate partner violence (IPV) at the time of the 2004 GSS survey (Canadian Centre for Justice Statistics). It is possible that these figures may be low because underreporting contributes to conservative estimates. Many women are afraid or reluctant to identify their abusers. In some cases, they fear retaliation against themselves or their children. In other cases, they continue to hold strong feelings for their partners, despite the abuse. Men, given the societal expectation of male strength, may not want to admit to being victims of violence.

It is important to recognize that women of all ages and sociocultural backgrounds may have experienced abuse. Regardless, certain factors have been found to be associated with increased risk for violence in women. Women who are at higher risk of abuse are younger (18 to 24 years of age), elders (65 years of age or older), or pregnant and have a history of childhood victimization or of witnessing maternal abuse (Statistics Canada, 1993; as cited in Health Canada, 2002). Women living with disabilities may also be at higher risk for abuse than nondisabled women because these women frequently depend on others to assist with a wide range of activities, which increases vulnerability (Health Canada).

Evidence suggests that single, divorced, and separated women may actually be at greater risk for abuse than are married women (Fishwick, Campbell, & Taylor, 2004). Moreover, this group is at particularly high risk for severe violence. Danger assessments show that abusive ex-partners often exhibit obsessive threatening behaviour after their relationships end and pose significant dangers to women. Forty-three percent of women seen in emergency departments (EDs) attributed their abuse to a past partner. These findings emphasize that ending a relationship often does not end violence (Fishwick et al.). This information is important for health care providers, who frequently pressure women to end abusive relationships.

Rates of woman abuse vary among women of different racial backgrounds. Research supports that Aboriginal women are at high risk for violence in their intimate relationships. The GSS data indicate that 24%

of Aboriginal women had experienced IPV within the 5-year period before the 2004 survey (Canadian Centre for Justice Statistics, 2005). Even higher rates of woman abuse have been reported for Aboriginal women by other studies. For example, a study in Ontario documents that 8 of 10 Aboriginal women experienced violence at the hands of their intimate partner (Health Canada, 1996, as cited in Health Canada, 2002). Specifically, 87% reported physical abuse, and 55% reported sexual abuse. Further, physical abuse of women in Northern Aboriginal communities is thought to be pervasive, with estimates ranging from 75% to 90% (Health Canada, 1996, as cited in Health Canada).

The perpetuation of violence begins early in dating relationships. The prevalence of dating violence is unknown because, as with other forms of violence, it usually takes place in private and is not reported. A few studies provide some data on the extent of the problem. One study found that of 1,870 cases of domestic assaults, 51.5% were classified as boyfriend or girlfriend violence. About 20% to 50% of men and women in dating relationships have admitted physically abusing a dating partner. These figures do not include date rape. One study found that behaviours that would qualify as date rape or sexual assault occurred at a rate of 15.4%, or 38 per 1,000 women (Barnett, Miller-Perrin, & Perrin, 1997). More recent sources suggest that the prevalence of dating violence ranges from 9% to 46% of adolescent females and males involved as victims or perpetrators (King & Ryan, 2004). Some studies report that dating violence is mutual and reciprocal. One study conducted in an ethnically and economically diverse urban community found that dating violence affected 45.5% of participating girls and boys (Watson, Cascardi, Avery-Leaf, & O'Leary, 2001). A qualitative study of 40 adolescent girls aged 15 and 16 years provides some insight into these high rates of dating violence (Banister, Jakubec, & Stein, 2003). The study findings highlight the tremendous power imbalance that exists in dating relationships for adolescent girls, which frequently results in a tolerance of violence simply to maintain the relationship (Banister et al.). A longitudinal study of dating violence in adolescent boys residing in Montreal (LaVoie et al., 2002) illustrates the importance of familial factors for adolescent boys in dating violence. Specifically, harsh parenting and antisocial behaviour were found to be predictive of dating violence in 717 boys aged 16 to 17 years living in a less affluent area of Montreal (LaVoie et al.).

Battering

Battering is the single greatest cause of serious injury to women. Estimates of injury related to battering seen in EDs range from 14% to 50% (Campbell, Torres, McKenna, Sheridan, & Landenburger, 2004). In a cross-sectional survey of 3,287 Canadian women living in

shelters, 73% had gone to the shelter as a consequence of abuse (Statistics Canada, 2003a). GSS data indicate that women are three times more likely to be physically injured than men in the context of IPV (Health Canada, 2002). Woman abuse contributes to a high rate of completed and attempted suicides in women; 81% of women reporting suicide attempts have experienced abuse by an intimate partner (Thompson M. P., Kaslow, Kingree, Thompson N. J., & Meadows, 1999). Moreover, many women who experience abuse experience posttraumatic stress disorder (PTSD; Norris, Foster, & Weisshaar, 2002). In a study of 65 women receiving treatment from three Canadian urban mental health centres, women reporting early-onset sexual abuse were more likely to meet the criteria for complex PTSD than women reporting late-onset PTSD (McLean & Gallop, 2003). In addition, individuals with PTSD are 15 times more likely to attempt suicide than are individuals in the general population (Thompson et al., 1999).

In some instances, battered women may even be killed by their abusers (Health Canada, 2002), especially when they take deliberate action to leave an abusive relationship. In 1996, 75% of 1,800 homicides perpetrated by intimate partners had female victims (Sisley, Jacobs, Poole, Campbell, & Esposito, 1999).

Indeed, the realistic fear of being killed is one factor that keeps many women from leaving abusive partners, even after years of severe abuse.

Battering also poses a significant danger to unborn children. The literature suggests that there is an increased risk of violence for women who are pregnant, although this observation may be related to increased opportunities for detection of abuse at health clinics during pregnancy (Cook & Dickens, 2009). Estimates of the prevalence of battering during pregnancy vary from 4% (Sisley, Jacobs, Poole, Campbell, & Esposito, 1999) to as high as 22% (Parker, Bullock, Bohn, & Curry, 2004). Differences in prevalence rates may be attributed to differences in definitions of abuse used by study authors. According to a Statistics Canada survey, 21% of women who were battered by a former or existing partner were pregnant (Statistics Canada, 1993, as cited in Health Canada, 2002). Abuse during pregnancy is a significant risk factor for several foetal and maternal complications, including low birth weight, low maternal weight gain, infections, and anaemia. Moreover, abuse of women often results in their use of alcohol and other drugs (AOD), which, in turn, may harm unborn children (Parker et al.).

Rape and Sexual Assault

Rape and sexual assault are common in Canada, with 24,049 sexual assaults being reported in 2000 and women constituting the majority (86%) of sexual assault victims (Statistics Canada, 2001). Younger women are at increased risk for sexual assault: in 2000, 54% of female victims of sexual assault were younger than 18 years of age. In a study of sexual assault among undergraduate women attending Canadian Universities, 28% of women reported that they had been sexually victimized in a dating relationship (DeKeseredy & Schwartz, 1998). Sexual assault includes any form of nonconsenting sexual activity, ranging from fondling to penetration. Most sexual assaults are underreported for the same reason that domestic violence is underreported—women are embarrassed and ashamed and fear being blamed for the assault. These reactions to sexual assault persist, even though rape is a felony (Abbey, Zawacki, Buck, Clinton, & McAuslan, 2003).

Sex and Increased Risk for Human Immunodeficiency Virus

Woman abuse is also a risk factor for human immunodeficiency virus (HIV) infection among women. Among women who test positive for HIV, the lifetime prevalence of adult coerced sexual activity perpetrated by a male partner has been estimated to be 74% or higher (Morrill, Kasten, Urato, & Larson, 2001). In an earlier study of women in treatment for AOD use and at high risk for HIV infection, 42% reported that their sexual partner physically abused them, 45% reported that sexual partners threatened them with violence, and 21% reported that they had sex because they were afraid that they would be hurt if they refused (Brown, Recupero, & Stout, 1995).

An abusive partner may increase the risk for HIV infection in several ways. Women who have abusive partners may not be able to avoid sexual contact. Fear of a partner's violent behaviour may prevent women from insisting on the use of condoms. A woman's insistence on condom use can imply that either partner is being unfaithful and can result in abuse. Victimized women are also four times more likely to have sex with a risky partner than are women who have not been abused (Morrill et al., 2001).

The rate of HIV infection has grown in Aboriginal women living in northern Alberta (Mill, 1997). A qualitative study of eight Aboriginal women infected with HIV indicates that these women endured abusive familial relationships that lead to the adoption of high-risk life on the street, which frequently included prostitution, intravenous drug use, and revictimization, increasing the risk for HIV infection (Mill). Similar findings are reported by McKeown, Reid, and Orr (2004) in a sample of 18 First Nations women, further supporting the relationship between childhood abuse and the risk for HIV infection in this population. Further, high rates of sexual abuse documented among Aboriginal youth (48% of 543 surveyed) are clearly linked to an increased risk for HIV infection through injection drug use and/or ongoing sexual contact (Cedar Project Partnership et al., 2008).

Stalking

Stalking is a crime of intimidation. Stalkers intimidate and terrorize their victims through threatening behaviours, which include waiting, watching, and calling, that cause fear or substantial emotional distress (Canadian Centre for Justice Statistics, 2005). In the 2004 GSS of 2,50,000 women and men, 11% of women and 7% of men aged 15 years and older reported that they were stalked to the extent that the experience evoked fear for themselves or someone else close to them (Canadian Centre for Justice Statistics). As with other abuse, most knew the stalker, whereas one fourth were stalked by strangers (Canadian Centre for Justice Statistics). Women were more likely than men to be harassed by an ex-spouse, ex-boyfriend, or ex-partner. Individuals who were stalked by an intimate ex-partner were stalked for longer periods of time. For example, those who were stalked by an ex-spouse were pursued for well over 1 year, and women were stalked by an ex-spouse two times more often than men (Canadian Centre for Justice Statistics).

In Canada, stalking, or in legal terms criminal harassment, is against the law (Canadian Centre for Justice Statistics, 2005). It is notable that in 2001, charges were laid for 57% of reported stalking incidents involving women, whereas charges were laid for only 39% of stalking incidents involving men (Statistics Canada, 2003a). The Department of Justice, Canada, is involved in an ongoing process of review to strengthen the laws pertaining to violence and sexual assault, including criminal harassment (Department of Justice, Canada, 2005).

Abuse of Men

Although sexual assault and violence have typically focused on women, the literature is now indicating that the rate of violence and sexual assault is now higher in men than traditionally believed (Stermac, Del Bove, & Addison, 2004). As noted earlier, the GSS data indicated that 6% of men are the victims of IPV, only 1% less than the rate of IPV reported for women (Department of Justice, Canada, 2005). The consequences of violence and sexual assault can also be devastating for men. For example, more than half of a sample of male rape victims referred to a forensic setting met the criteria for PTSD, and many male victims reported profound emotional distress and sexual dysfunction (Huckle, 1995). A recent study examined 141 cases from a sexual assault database located in a large urban Ontario city (Stermac et al.). The data suggest that male victims of sexual assault are more likely to be young, street involved, with an increased vulnerability such as either a cognitive or a physical disability (Stermac et al.). The authors suggest that future research is needed to understand better this previously unrecognized vulnerable group.

Child Abuse

Child abuse can take several forms, and the definition of each type varies by state. All forms of child abuse rob children of rights they should have. Those rights include the rights to be and behave like a child; to be safe and protected from harm; and to be fed, clothed, and nurtured so that the child can grow, develop, and fulfill his or her unique potential.

The prevalence of child abuse is unknown. The Canadian Incidence Study of Reported Child Abuse and Neglect of 7,000 child welfare investigations over a 3-month period in 1998 estimated that there were 1,35,573 child maltreatment investigations in 1998. Child welfare workers confirmed abuse in 45% of the reported cases of maltreatment (Trocme & Wolfe, 2001, as cited in Department of Justice Canada, 2003). Of course, this figure does not include cases that were unreported. Of the total number of reported child abuse cases, estimates are that 43% represent neglect, 31% physical abuse, and 10% sexual abuse (Trocme & Wolfe, 2001, as cited in Department of Justice Canada). Emotional maltreatment was the primary reason for the investigation in 19% of cases, and emotional maltreatment was confirmed in 54% of those reported. Police statistics also provide valuable information about the prevalence of violence against children and youth. Specifically, the Incident-based Uniform Crime Reporting Survey (UCR2) documents the number of physical and sexual assaults reported to the police in a designated period of time. In 2003, data from 122 police units compiled in the UCR2 indicated that 25% of reported physical and sexual assaults pertained to children and youth younger than 18 years of age, who compose 21% of Canada's population (Canadian Centre for Justice Statistics, 2005).

It is also extremely important to acknowledge the child abuse that occurred in the residential schools for Aboriginal children within the last century (Law Commission of Canada, 2000). The Law Commission of Canada noted that Aboriginal children were the only children who were designated to live in an institution, away from their families and communities, because of their race. Frequently these children were prohibited from speaking their mother tongue and were deliberately deprived of all connections with their culture and identity, placing this group of children at high risk for abuse (Law Commission of Canada). The report acknowledges the profound level of harm to the children, families, and communities that occurred as a result of these children being displaced and mistreated.

Child Neglect

Child neglect is the most common form of child abuse reported (Gary, Campbell, & Humphreys, 2004; Gary &

Humphreys, 2004) and frequently is chronic (Department of Justice, Canada, 2003). There are several types of **neglect**, such as failure to protect a child, physical neglect, and medical neglect. Failure to protect a child includes failure to prevent various kinds of accidental injury, such as ingestion of poison, electric shocks, falls, and burns (Barnett et al., 1997). Physical neglect includes failure to provide food, clothing, shelter, or cleanliness (Department of Justice, Canada). Indicators of physical neglect include diaper dermatitis, lice, scabies, dirty appearance, clothes inappropriate for the weather, and unclean and unsafe living environment. Medical neglect includes failure to provide for the child's medical needs, including failure to seek appropriate care or to comply with the prescribed treatments (Wallace, 1999).

Physical Abuse

Physical abuse may include severe spanking, hitting, biting, burning, kicking, shoving, choking, or any other type of physical action directed toward the child that results in nonaccidental injury (Department of Justice, Canada, 2003). Injuries to children caused by physical abuse range from mild to severe and life threatening. Types of injuries include skin and soft tissue injuries; internal injuries; dislocations and fractures; tooth loss; burns; abrasions or bruises made by fists or belts; hair loss from pulling the hair; wounds from guns, knives, razors, or other sharp objects; retinal haemorrhage; and conjunctival haemorrhage (Gary et al., 2004; Gary & Humphreys, 2004; Wallace, 1999). Often, clothing hides these injuries, and practitioners must look for other signs of abuse, such as fear, aggressive or withdrawn behaviour, poor social relations, learning problems, delinquent behaviour, and wearing clothing that is meant to cover injuries but is inappropriate for the weather. In addition, when treating a child with such injuries, professionals should suspect abuse when explanations are implausible and inconsistent with injuries, involved parties give different versions of the incident, or treatment seeking is delayed (Wallace).

Sexual Abuse

Behaviours that constitute child **sexual abuse** range from mild, covert behaviours to overt sexual acts. Examples of sexual abuse include exhibitionism; voyeurism; touching the child's sexual organs; and oral, anal, and vaginal sex (Department of Justice, Canada, 2003; Gary et al., 2004; Gary & Humphreys, 2004; Urbancic, 2004; Wallace, 1999). Childhood sexual exploitation is also included with the discussion of childhood sexual abuse, specifically, using children for the purpose of pornography or prostitution (Department of Justice, Canada).

There are three categories of sexual abuse: incest, sexual abuse perpetrated by a nonfamily member, and pedophilia. Incest is defined in the Criminal Code of Canada (1985) in this way: Everyone commits incest who, "Knowing that another person by blood relationship is his or her parent, child, brother, sister, grand parent or grand child, as the case may be, has sexual intercourse with that person" (5.155). This definition limits the illegal sexual activity to sexual intercourse; it does not include fondling, oral sex, and masturbation. These acts, when committed against children, are covered under other laws not restricted to blood relatives. Pedophilia describes those who have a sexual fixation on young children that usually translates into sexual acts with the victims. The following conditions qualify as pedophilia:

- For at least 6 months, the person has recurrent intense sexual urges and sexually arousing fantasies involving sexual activity with a prepubescent child.
- The person has acted on or is extremely distressed by these urges.
- The person is at least 16 years old and at least 5 years older than the child (Wallace, 1999).

Research shows that about 8% to 10% of child sexual abuse offenders are strangers; 47% are family members; 40% are acquaintances. The high-risk years for child sexual abuse are ages 4 to 9 years (Wallace, 1999).

Several factors may mediate the effects of child sexual abuse. In general, younger children with a history of emotional difficulties may be more traumatized than will be older and more stable children. Repeated abuse for long periods with more violence and bodily penetration results in greater traumatization. Sexual abuse by someone that the child knows and trusts causes more severe trauma. The child abused by a family member experiences a devastating breach of trust, loss of a safe home, and threats to fundamental survival requirements (Boyd & Mackey, 2000a). Finally, negative reactions by significant others, health care professionals, or others may exacerbate the effects of trauma (Wallace, 1999).

Emotional Abuse

Emotional abuse includes acts or omissions that psychologically damage the child (Gary et al., 2004). The emotionally abused child does not have visible injuries to alert others. Nevertheless, emotional abuse severely affects a child's self-esteem and often leaves permanent emotional scars. Survivors of abuse frequently report that emotional abuse is worse than physical abuse (Wallace, 1999).

There are several types of emotional abuse. *Rejecting* involves refusing to acknowledge the child's worth and the legitimacy of his or her needs. The child receives the message that he or she is no good and is unwanted.

Isolating involves cutting the child off from normal social experiences, preventing the child from forming friendships, and hindering the development of social skills. *Terrorizing* involves creating a climate of fear and making the child believe that the world is a capricious and hostile place. *Ignoring* means being psychologically unavailable to the child and, therefore, starving him or her emotionally. Normal self-development depends on an emotional connection to others. *Corrupting* involves mis-socializing the child to engage in destructive and antisocial behaviours and reinforcing deviance. This type of abuse makes the child unfit for normal social experiences and sets him or her up for additional rejection (Barnett et al., 1997; Wallace, 1999).

Factitious Disorder by Proxy: Munchausen's Syndrome by Proxy

Factitious disorder by proxy is another form of child abuse (see Chapter 22). This disorder includes "the intentional production or feigning of physical or psychological signs or symptoms in another person who is under the individual's care for the purpose of indirectly assuming the sick role" (American Psychiatric Association [APA], 2000, p. 781). The signs of this disorder include repeated hospitalizations and medical evaluations of the child without definitive diagnosis; symptoms or medical signs that are inappropriate or inconsistent; symptoms that disappear when the child is away from the parent; a parent who encourages medical tests for the child; parental uneasiness as the child recovers; and a parent who is less concerned with the child's health than with spending time with caregivers (Bartsch, Risse, Schutz, Weigand, & Weiler, 2003). One source estimates that approximately 10% of children who are the victims of factitious disorder by proxy will die at the hands of their parents (Wallace, 1999).

Secondary Abuse: Children of Battered Women

Research on children of battered women has become more evident over the past 25 years (Clements, Oxtoby, & Ogle, 2008). These children often show signs of PTSD (Berman, Hardesty, & Humphreys, 2004; Campbell & Lewandowski, 1997). Children may witness their mother being choked, threatened with a weapon, or threatened with death (Berman et al.; Boyd & Mackey, 2000a; Campbell & Lewandowski). These children fear for both their own and their mother's safety (Boyd & Mackey). The 2004 GSS data indicate that children witnessed spousal violence in 33% of cases (Canadian Centre for Justice Statistics, 2005). Research has substantiated the traumatic long-term effects of witnessing violence. For example, children who have witnessed violence in the home were more likely to demonstrate increased levels of depression, emotional problems, and delinquency (Fitzgerald, 2004, as cited in Canadian Centre for Justice Statistics, 2005). In addition, children who grow up in violent families experience living with secrecy, relocations as the mother leaves home to seek safety, economic hardship, maternal depression that may reduce her ability to nurture, and frightening interactions with the police and court systems (Berman et al.; Boyd & Mackey; Campbell & Lewandowski). Moreover, many children who witness violence begin to accept it as a normal part of relationships and a way to deal with problems (Sisley, Jacobs, Poole, Campbell, & Esposito, 1999). A National Longitudinal Survey of Children and Youth in 1994 to 1995 found that children who witnessed violence in the home were more likely to be physically aggressive 2 to 4 years later (Statistics Canada, 2003b).

Elder Abuse

Elder abuse is increasingly recognized as a serious problem in Canada and other countries. However, more recent statistics (based on police reports) identify that seniors over the age of 65 years are the group least likely to be a victim of violence (Canadian Centre for Justice Statistics, 2009). Seniors over the age of 65 years were more likely to be victimized by someone that they knew; most likely an adult child (34 per 100,000). Over half of the violent incidents reported to the police did not result in physical injury. Estimated rates of neglect are not available in Canada, whereas in the United States, the estimated prevalence rate of neglect is the most frequent type of mistreatment (Comijs, Pot, Smit, Bouter, & Jonker, 1998; Wallace, 1999). The nature of neglect and of physical, sexual, and emotional abuse is similar to that described for women and children. Financial or material mistreatment may include improper or illegal acts to obtain and use an elder's resources for personal benefit (Wallace).

Risk factors for elder abuse include older age, impairment in the activities of daily living (ADLs), cognitive disability or other mental illness, dependency on the caregiver, isolation, stressful events, and a history of intergenerational conflict between the elder and the caregiver (Sengstock, Ulrich, & Barrett, 2004).

▇▇▇ THEORIES OF ABUSE

Many theories have attempted to explain violence between intimate partners and in the family. The theories reviewed here have been categorized as biologic, psychological, and social. In all likelihood, family violence is truly a bio/psycho/social/spiritual phenomenon that no one of these theories can fully explain (Fig. 37-1). A separate section presents additional theories that are more specific to the phenomenon of woman abuse.

Biologic Theories

Neurologic Problems

Aggressive behaviour may be associated with several neurologic conditions, including traumatic brain injury, seizure disorder, and dementia (see Chapter 36). Neurodevelopmental factors and traumatic brain injury can produce seizure disorders, attentional dysfunction, or focal neurobehavioural syndromes, all of which are associated with aggressive behaviour. The most common association between seizures and aggressive behaviour occurs during the postictal period (the period immediately after the seizure), during which the individual may be confused and react aggressively.

Damage to the orbitofrontal cortex often causes impulsive, labile, irritable, and socially inappropriate behaviour. Individuals with such damage often respond aggressively to trivial stimuli. In addition, damage to the neocortex, limbic system, and hypothalamus may result in aggressive behaviour. These systems have hierarchic control over one another. Damage to higher centres may disinhibit aggression from lower centres. Aggressive behaviour also may be related to disruptions in neurotransmitter systems. Disruption in serotonin, dopamine, and gamma-aminobutyric acid (GABA) systems has been linked with several psychiatric disorders, including depression, schizophrenia, impulsive behaviour, suicide, and aggression (Rosenbaum, Geffner, & Benjamin, 1997).

Links With Substance Abuse

The use of AOD is commonly associated with violent incidents. Alcohol has been found to be present in approximately one half to two thirds of sexual assaults (Ulman, 2003). Although AOD use alone is rarely sufficient to account for violence, the Ontario Mental Health Supplement indicated that parental substance use is significantly associated with an increased risk for childhood physical and sexual abuse (Walsh, MacMillan, & Jamieson, 2003). Other factors, such as low family income, stress, and abuse in the family of origin, are often more important (Collins & Messerschmidt, 1993; Wallace, 1999). The relationship of AOD to violence may result from three factors: (1) AOD-induced cognitive impairment, (2) the user's expectations that AOD increases the tendency toward aggression, and (3) socioculturally grounded beliefs that people are unaccountable for their behaviour while intoxicated (Abbey et al., 2003).

Studies have demonstrated that drinking alcohol may change perceptions about accountability for behaviour (Abbey et al., 2003). The belief that intoxicated behaviour will be judged less harshly may encourage and provide an excuse for those who abuse substances to engage in normally unacceptable behaviours. Research shows that people attempt to justify their criminal behaviour by

FIGURE 37.1 Bio/psycho/social/spiritual etiologies for violent behaviour.

blaming alcohol after the fact (Abbey et al.). There has been increasing concern about the growing number of drug-facilitated sexual assault. In particular, flunitrazepam has become known as the date rape drug (Du Mont et al., 2009). A recent Canadian study of primarily female sexual assault victims receiving care at hospital-based treatment centres found that 21% of the sample ($n = 882$) met the criteria for suspected drug-facilitated assault. The researchers conclude that treatment centres need to be prepared to respond to "date rape" victims, since it is a common problem (Du Mont et al.).

Psychosocial Theories

Psychopathology Theory

Psychopathology theory seeks to understand violence by examining the characteristics of individual men and women (Wallace, 1999). Theorists from this perspective focus on personality traits, internal defence systems, and mental disorders. An outdated theory that was particularly damaging labelled women as masochistic, paranoid, or depressed (Bograd, 1999). One underlying assumption of this labelling was that some women enjoy abuse and deliberately provoke attacks because they need to suffer.

Research on batterers has shown that there is not a common profile or a typical batterer. Studies have found evidence of personality disorders, including antisocial, borderline, narcissistic, and dependent. A Canadian study of 997 men who were recruited from outpatient forensic settings and the community indicated that abusive or severely abusive men were more likely to have antisocial personality disorders, demonstrate impulsive behaviour, and have dysfunctional attitudes regarding spousal abuse compared with nonabusive men (Hanson, Cadsky, Harris, & Lalonde, 1997). Abusive men were also more likely to have a history of violence during childhood.

Although research has not consistently found one common mental disorder or set of characteristics in violent individuals, there is a typology of men who batter that shows promise (Emery & Laumann-Billings, 1998). Type I batterers are violent in many situations, have many victims, and display antisocial characteristics. Type II batterers abuse only their family, commit less severe violence, are generally less aggressive, and demonstrate remorse. These men tend to be dependent, jealous, and unlikely to have personality or other disorders. Type III batterers display dysphoric-borderline or schizoid characteristics, such as emotional volatility, depression, feelings of inadequacy, and social isolation (Emery & Laumann-Billings).

Type III batterers also tend to be violent only within their families.

Social Learning Theory

Violent families create an atmosphere of tension, fear, intimidation, and tremendous confusion about intimate relationships (Boyd & Mackey, 2000a). Children in violent homes often learn violent behaviour as an approved and legitimate way to solve problems, especially within intimate relationships. Social learning theory posits that men who witness violence in their homes often perpetuate violent behaviour in their families as adults (Dewey, 2004; Emery & Laumann-Billings, 1998; Wallace, 1999). Moreover, women who grow up in violent homes learn to accept violence and expect it in their own adult relationships (Boyd & Mackey). These concepts are often referred to as the **intergenerational transmission** of violence. Consistent with the theory of intergenerational transmission of violence, research findings from a telephone survey of 1,249 adults living in the city of Vancouver provide evidence that all forms of violence occurring in families of origin are predictive of relationship violence (Kwong, Bartholomew, Henderson, & Trinke, 2003).

Findings of extreme violence in the parental homes of battered individuals and individuals who grew up witnessing violence are common and support the intergenerational transmission of violence theory (Dewey, 2004). However, not all those who batter or are abused come from violent homes. Estimates are that approximately 40% of those who experienced abuse or witnessed abuse in childhood will consequently abuse their wives or children (Dutton, 1998).

Social Theories

Covering the many sociologic theories of violence is beyond the scope of this chapter. Sociologic theories posit that abuse occurs because of cultural norms that permit and even glamorize violent behaviour (Dewey, 2004). From a societal perspective, the acceptance of violence as normal appears widespread among young people. In one study, as many as 70% of a group of female college students listed at least one form of violence as acceptable in dating relationships. Even more disturbing is that 80% of these women mentioned situations in which physical force between partners was tolerable. Slapping was cited most often (49%), whereas punching was seen as acceptable by 21% of these women (Girshick, 1993). In addition, as many as 34% of women marry someone who abused them in a dating relationship (Barnett et al., 1997). In keeping with these findings, a qualitative study by Canadian researchers

revealed that young adolescent girls (15 and 16 years of age) were so eager to have a male dating partner that they were willing to tolerate physical violence and verbal abuse, just to "keep the guy" (Banister, Jakubec, & Stein, 2003).

Family violence is also related to qualities of the community in which the family is embedded. Poverty, absence of family services, social isolation, lack of cohesion in the community, and stress contribute to family violence (Dewey, 2004). The relationship of poverty, social isolation, and child abuse has been well established (Emery & Laumann-Billings, 1998; Health Canada, 1998). Economic disadvantage creates tremendous stress for families, increasing the risk for child abuse and maltreatment. It should be kept in mind that economically impoverished families may seek social services more frequently, and as such, the reporting of abuse may be increased in these families (Health Canada). However, not all poor families abuse their children. One difference between poor families who do and do not abuse their children lies in the degree of social cohesion and mutual caring found in their communities (Emery & Laumann-Billings). Neighbourhoods with high levels of child abuse frequently have severe social disorganization and lack of community identity. In addition, they have higher rates of juvenile delinquency, drug trafficking, and violent crime (Emery & Laumann-Billings).

One of the most accepted theories of elder abuse is the family stress theory. The theory hypothesizes that providing care for an elder induces stress within the family. Family stress includes economic hardship, loss of sleep, and intrusions into family activities and routines. Moreover, caring for a dependent elder takes an enormous physical toll on the caregiver. If there is no relief, the caregiver may become overwhelmed, lose control, and abuse the elder (Sengstock et al., 2004; Wallace, 1999). With the aging of the Canadian population, the demands on family members to provide care are rising, as are the associated stress of caregiving and the increased risk for elder abuse (Canadian Centre for Justice Statistics, 2005). Other characteristics of caregivers that may predispose them to abuse elderly parents include alcohol or drug abuse, dementia, restricted outside activities, unrealistic expectations, and a blaming, hypercritical personality.

Theoretic Dynamics Specific to Woman Abuse

Feminist Theories

Feminist theory focuses on issues of gender, inequality, power and privilege, patriarchy, and the subordination of women as explanations for woman abuse (Landenburger,

Campbell, & Rodriguez, 2004). According to the feminist perspective, woman abuse results from a patriarchal society that perpetuates attitudes that support violence against women (Lloyd & Emery, 2000; Wallace, 1999). Three major characteristics of such a patriarchal society are the devaluation of women, power inequities, and the view of women as property (Barnett et al., 1997; Wallace).

Feminists also point to a power inequity in society as a contributing factor to woman abuse. Women have made many advances in recent years; however, men continue to control most institutions (Lloyd & Emery, 2000). Women continue to earn less than men for paid work and are less likely to advance to positions of authority and power (Nolen-Hoeksema, 2002; Sampselle et al., 1992). Moreover, marriage often victimizes women in ways other than through violence. Although men now contribute to household work, most women who hold jobs outside the home continue to perform most household and child care tasks (Lloyd & Emery). This power inequity is reflected in higher depression rates among married women than among married men (Nolen-Hoeksema). In cases of divorce, most women become single parents with a standard of living significantly lower than that of their former spouse (Wallace, 1999). The study findings from a feminist grounded theory study of 40 single mothers who recently left abusive partners in Ontario and New Brunswick reveal that the majority of participants continued to experience ongoing harassment, even though these single mothers had left their abusive partners (Ford-Gilboe, Wuest, & Merritt-Gray, 2005). The central challenges faced by these women included decreased resources, persistent persecution, and ongoing chronic health problems that were, in fact, a consequence of leaving the abusive relationship (Ford-Gilboe et al.).

Women are viewed as property in many parts of the world. The entertainment and advertising industries perpetuate the image of women as property by depicting them as objects and often portraying the dismembering of women's bodies (Kilbourne, 1987, 1999). The focus on women's body parts in advertising dehumanizes women, and that dehumanization is often the first step in making women acceptable targets of violence. For example, a 3-month study of newspaper coverage of disabled men and women in Canada and Israel indicated that women received less media coverage then men, yet the media coverage of women demonstrated a higher level of victimization and violence, overall (Gold & Auslander, 1999). Moreover, the explicit portrayal in the media of women in various states of undress and in seductive postures suggests that they are vulnerable and openly welcome sexual advances. Frequently, the message is, "Buy the product and get the woman" (Kilbourne, 1987).

Theory of Borderline Personality Organization and Violence

Dr. Donald Dutton, a professor at the University of British Columbia, is an international expert in the field of domestic violence, who has advocated extensively for more comprehensive interventions to respond to domestic violence. His 1998 book, *The Abusive Personality*, is a seminal work that addresses the relationship of borderline personality organization (BPO) to the type of batterer who is chronically and intermittently abusive but abusive only within his family (see Chapter 25). Dutton's work combines aspects from social learning theory, reinforcement principles from learning theory, and evidence that early trauma can alter personality through changes that occur biologically or through learning. He bases his theory on his own research and that of others, such as Bandura (social learning theory; 1977) and van der Kolk, McFarlane, and Weisaeth (traumatic stress and its consequences; 1996).

Dutton (1998) describes three characteristics or cycles of BPO that shift with time and seem to coincide with the cycle of violence first proposed by Walker in 1979 and described later in this chapter. These characteristics can apply to men or women with BPO; however, because this discussion focuses on men's aggression toward their female partners, it addresses the individual with BPO as male. Phase I of the male borderline personality, or "cyclic personality," consists of an internal buildup of tensions, in which the man feels depressed and irritable but does not know how to verbalize his inner dysphoria. In fact, he may not even be able to recognize or label the painful feelings, a condition called **alexithymia** (Dutton). The inability to recognize or express painful feelings and ask for what he needs traps the man in a downward spiral of bad feelings, compounded by an inability to maintain his own self-integrity. He is dependent on his partner for his sense of self. Therefore, the loss of the partner carries the risk that he will lose himself. According to Dutton, the reason that men with BPO become so abusive in their intimate relationships, but not in other relationships, is linked to their extreme dependency on their partners for a sense of self and their inability to tolerate aloneness. This type of dependency is often called a "masked or hostile dependency." To maintain this relationship, the man with BPO must control his partner; therefore, his controlling behaviour masks his dependency. The man with BPO expects his partner to do the impossible. When she fails, he erupts in extreme anger because his sense of self is threatened. He converts dysphoria into abuse through (1) the belief that the partner should be able to soothe the bad feelings and (2) the conversion of feelings of terror into rage. His use of projection, a defence mechanism, leads him to believe that it is her fault. The explosive combination of ego needs, an inability to communicate them, chronic irritability, jealousy, and projective blaming ensures a violent relationship (Dutton).

As this phase continues, the man with BPO becomes verbally abusive, and the partner withdraws. The man wants closeness, not withdrawal, but he does not have the skills to ask for it. In addition to increasing anger, the man with BPO becomes increasingly demanding. At this stage, the dichotomous thinking or splitting characteristic of BPO is evident, and the man sees the partner as "all bad"—unfaithful, unloving, and malevolent. The unexpressed rage builds until the man with BPO erupts with violence. The violence drives the partner further away, increasing the man's feelings of abandonment. As a result, the abusive man promises anything to get the partner back. (This phase coincides with Walker's contrition phase in the cycle of violence.) The opposite side of splitting is now in evidence, as the man describes his partner as "all good"—"a madonna" (Dutton, 1998, p. 96). This example of splitting is sometimes referred to as "madonna/whore."

It is hypothesized that the abuser's BPO results from early physical abuse. Researchers suggest that early physical abuse causes long-term problems in modulating emotions and aggression and may lead to chronic anger (Dutton, 1998). The difficulty in modulating emotions often manifests first in affective numbing and constriction or in alexithymia. Hyperarousal follows emotional numbing, a process that culminates in violence (Dutton). These symptoms are manifestations of PTSD, described later in this chapter. Abusive men also score higher than do control subjects on other measures of trauma, such as depression, anxiety, sleep disturbances, and dissociation (Dutton). However, the form that the violence takes appears to be learned. That is, boys tend to identify with the aggressor and act out, whereas girls often identify with the victim and turn to self-destructive acts, such as substance abuse and self-mutilation (Dutton).

One other aspect of this cycle appears to ensure its continuation—that of positive reinforcement. The type of violence perpetrated by men with BPO has been labelled "deindividuated violence"; that is, the violence is responsive only to internal cues from the perpetrator and unresponsive to cues from the victim (Dutton, 1998). The violence feeds on itself because it is rewarding; it reduces the perpetrator's aversive arousal and tension. As a result, batterers often continue the assault until they are exhausted. Expressing rage through violent acts is the only way they know to reduce their tension or aversive arousal, and it becomes addictive (Dutton).

The cycle described by Dutton helps explain the descriptions of violent men provided by more than 200 women with whom he has worked. The following are the examples of their descriptions of violent partners: "He's like Jekyll and Hyde," "He's completely different sometimes," and "His friends never see the other side of him; they think he's just a nice guy, just one of the boys" (Dutton, 1998, p. 53).

Theories of Why Women Stay in Violent Relationships

A more appropriate question than "Why do women stay in violent relationships?" is "How does she ever manage to leave given all the strikes against her?" (Anderson & Saunders, 2003). There are many reasons why women stay in violent relationships. One of the strongest reasons is economic (Wallace, 1999). Despite years of progress, women still earn less than men for equal work. Many women lack the education or skills that would allow them to earn an adequate living outside the home. For these women, leaving their abusive partners means that they and their children would be homeless and without any source of support for even basic necessities. Furthermore, many shelters for battered women have long waiting lists and provide only temporary housing.

The socialization of women to assume major responsibility for marriages and child rearing is often another barrier to leaving abusive relationships. Society teaches women that their proper place is at home and their primary responsibility is caring for their husbands and children (Chodorow, 1974; Gilligan, 1982; Wallace, 1999). Many women believe that making their marriage a success is their responsibility. Therefore, when they are abused, they assume that it is their fault and that their duty is to remain and try harder for their children's sakes (Boyd & Mackey, 2000a; Lloyd & Emery, 2000). Moreover, many women who were abused in childhood or witnessed abuse of their mothers think that abuse is part of a normal relationship (Boyd & Mackey).

Women also face political and legal obstacles in leaving abusive partners. If a man is arrested for assault and no action is taken to prevent future violence, he may be released shortly and retaliate against his partner. Fear for their lives and the lives of their children and other relatives often keeps women from attempting to leave abusive relationships (Anderson & Saunders, 2003; Boyd & Mackey, 2000a).

Even more difficult to understand is why some women stay in violent dating relationships. About 30% to 50% of dating couples continue their relationships despite violence (Barnett et al., 1997). One factor is that dating violence often does not occur until the relationship has been sustained for a long time. By then, many women feel that they have invested too much in the relationship to end it. Research has shown that the length of the relationship and the commitment level are positively correlated with physical and sexual abuse. Similarly, an analysis of the Canadian National Survey on woman abuse in universities and colleges demonstrates that deference (the degree of conformity to social norms) and availability (the time spent in the relationship) are important concepts that predict woman abuse in dating relationships (Alvi & Selbee, 1997).

Survivors may go though a process consisting of several phases in leaving an abusive relationship (Anderson & Saunders, 2003). Women may leave and return several times as they are learning new coping skills. The phases may involve cognitive and emotional "leaving" before actually leaving the relationship. The phases may include (1) enduring and managing the violence while disconnecting from self and others; (2) acknowledging the abuse, reframing it, and counteracting it; and (3) disengaging and focusing on her own needs (Anderson & Saunders). The phase immediately following separation from an abusive partner is extremely important as the woman attempts to establish a new life. Based on the findings from a qualitative study of 15 women residing in eastern Canada, a four-stage process of "reclaiming the self" emerged as the main psychological process central to leaving an abusive partner (Wuest & Merritt-Gray, 2001), which is consistent with the stages described by Anderson and Saunders (Box 37-1).

Cycle of Violence

Many cases of woman abuse reflect a recognized **cycle of violence** (Wallace, 1999). The cycle consists of three recurring phases that often increase in frequency and severity (Walker, 1979). The cycle is fully described in Figure 37-2.

Traumatic Bonding

The formation of strong emotional bonds under conditions of intermittent maltreatment has been reported in several studies with human and animal subjects. For example, people taken hostage may show positive regard for their captors. Abused children often show strong attachment to their abusing parents. Cult members show strong loyalty to malevolent cult leaders (Dutton, 1995). Therefore, the relationship between battered women and their partners may be just one example of traumatic bonding—the development of strong emotional ties between two people, one of whom intermittently abuses the other. **Traumatic bonding** suggests that a power imbalance and intermittent abuse help to form extremely strong emotional attachments. Traumatic bonding theory (Dutton & Painter, 1993) explains why the cycle of violence is so powerful in entrapping a woman in a violent relationship. Researchers from British Columbia generated hypotheses based on Dutton's theory of traumatic bonding and attachment theory to assess the relevance of attachment theory to 63 women who had recently left abusive relationships (Henderson, Bartholomew, & Dutton, 1997). As predicted, women who demonstrated attachment patterns consistent with a negative view of the self composed the majority of the sample (88%).

BOX 37.1

Research for Best Practice: Understanding Strategies Used by Rural Women to Stop, Avoid, or Escape from IPV

Riddell, T., Ford-Gilboe, M., & Leipert, B. (2009). Strategies used by rural women to stop, avoid or escape from intimate partner violence. Health Care for Women International, 30, 134–159.

THE QUESTION: What are the strategies used by rural women to stop, avoid, or escape from violence in a relationship with an abusive partner?

METHODS: The researchers used a mixed-methods approach employing two quantitative measures, as well as qualitative interviews to identify the frequency and helpfulness of strategies used to cope with IPV. Forty-three rural Canadian women (13 from Ontario and 30 from New Brunswick) enrolled in an ongoing longitudinal study were included in the analysis. In order to gain further understanding of the quantitative findings, interactive collaborative qualitative interviews were conducted with 9 of the 43 participants. Audiotaped interviews were transcribed verbatim, and the data were analyzed initially using a line-by-line approach to identify strategies used by women to deal with IPV. Conceptual-based patterns and themes were developed and integrated with the quantitative findings.

FINDINGS: Quantitative findings revealed that placating and resistance strategies were used most frequently by the women in the study to deal with IPV, even though these strategies were rated as least helpful. On the other hand, only half of the women in the study identified that they used safety planning, seeking legal counsel, and seeking help from networks (formal and informal) even though these strategies were rated as most effective in dealing with IPV. The qualitative findings further explicated the quantitative findings. Specifically, the women in the study deliberately used placating and resistance strategies to keep their children and themselves safe while ultimately planning to leave the abusive relationship. Further, numerous barriers exist in rural settings to seeking help for IPV, including physical and social isolation, limited resources, and patriarchal attitudes. The integration of the quantitative and qualitative findings revealed the critical role of safety planning in living with IPV.

IMPLICATIONS FOR NURSING: Nurses providing care for women in rural communities need to be cognizant of the many factors that may impede women from seeking help for IPV. These factors include physical and social isolation, limited economic resources, controlling patriarchal attitudes, and limited access to services. The researchers suggest that nurses create opportunities to speak privately with women living in rural settings in an open and direct manner to facilitate disclosure and access to much needed help. Nurses practicing in rural communities are in an ideal position to advocate for social change and to enhance existing resources in rural communities for women dealing with IPV.

Phase 1. Tension Building
* Minor incidents
* Perpetrator establishes total control of victim by psychological and emotional means
* Perpetrator demands total acquiescence of victim. Verbal abuse and accusations follow
* Perpetrator isolates victim by approving/disapproving social contacts
* Perpetrator monitors victim's activities, phone calls, mail, and travels and demands explanations
* Perpetrator degrades and demoralizes victim by scrutinizing victim's physical and mental characteristics (unattractive, stupid) and functions and assaulting victim's self-esteem (worthless, "no good")

Phase 2. Violence Erupts
* Severe injury to victim and children
* Victim may incite violence as a way to control mounting terror
* Period of relative calm follows battering

Phase 3. Remorse Ensues
* Perpetrator becomes kind, contrite, and loving—begging for forgiveness and promising never to inflict abuse again (until the next time)
* Tension builds; the cycle repeats.

FIGURE 37.2 The cycle of violence.

The woman in a power imbalance perceives herself to be in a powerless position in relation to her partner, whom she perceives as extremely powerful. As the power imbalance intensifies, she feels increasingly worthless, less capable of fending for herself, and, therefore, more in need of her partner. This cycle of dependency and lowered self-esteem is continually repeated, eventually creating a strong affective bond to the partner (Dutton, 1995).

Intermittent reinforcement or punishment is one of the strongest learning paradigms in behavioural theory, especially in maintaining a particular behaviour (Dutton, 1995). An example that is often used to illustrate this concept is the gambler who persistently puts coins in a slot machine. Despite substantial losses, the gambler persists because the next time just might be the big payoff.

Therefore, the gambler is not rewarded every time, but intermittently. To apply this to battered women, women may stay because this time the man may actually mean what he says and stop the abuse. After all, he has been kind and loving intermittently.

Research suggests that traumatic bonding is especially important when a woman attempts to leave her abusive partner (Dutton, 1995). When a woman leaves an abusive relationship, especially after a battering incident, she is emotionally drained and vulnerable. As time passes, her fear of her abuser diminishes, and needs supplied by the partner become evident. At this time, she is particularly susceptible to the abuser's attempts to persuade her to return to the relationship (Dutton & Painter, 1993).

SURVIVORS OF ABUSE: HUMAN RESPONSES TO TRAUMA

The experience of violence and abuse is overwhelming for most survivors and often has devastating long-term consequences (Wilson, 2001; Wilson, Friedman, & Lindy, 2001). Victimization does not produce a single uniform syndrome or response. Research on the effects of victimization reflects considerable consistency in the bio/psycho/social/spiritual responses to overwhelming trauma, whether the victim is a child, an adult, or an elder (Hendricks-Matthews, 1993).

Biologic Responses

Victims of violence experience mild to severe physical consequences. Mild injuries may include bruises and abrasions of the head, neck, face, trunk, and extremities. Severe injuries include multiple traumas, major fractures, major lacerations, and internal injuries, including chest and abdominal injuries and subdural haematomas (Campbell et al., 2004; Health Canada, 2002). Loss of vision and hearing can result from blows to the head. Physical or sexual violence may result in head injuries that can produce changes in cognition, affect, motivation, and behaviour. Victims of sexual abuse may have vaginal and perineal trauma that is sufficient to require surgical repair (Barnett et al., 1997; Health Canada). Anorectal injuries may also be present, including the disruption of anal sphincters, retained foreign bodies, and mucosal lacerations. The following section covers the most common responses to violence and abuse:

- Depression (the dysregulated stress response theory of depression)
- Acute stress disorder (ASD)
- Posttraumatic stress disorder (PTSD)
- Dissociative identity disorder (DID)

Depression

Depression, one of the most common responses to abuse, is a biologically based disorder that can result from the effects of chronic stress on neurotransmitter and neuroendocrine systems. The body's response to stress is a complex, integrated system of reactions, encompassing the body and mind. Threat or stress engages the stress system, which consists of the hypothalamic–pituitary–adrenal (HPA) axis and the sympathetic nervous system (Thase, Jindal, & Howland, 2002; Wong & Yehuda, 2002). Engagement of the HPA axis is associated with the release of corticotropin-releasing hormone (CRH) from the pituitary gland. CRH stimulates the pituitary gland to secrete adrenocorticotropic hormone (corticotropin), which stimulates the adrenal cortex to secrete cortisol.

Stress also engages the sympathetic nervous system, causing the locus ceruleus and the adrenal medulla to release norepinephrine.

The CRH and locus ceruleus and norepinephrine systems participate in a mutually reinforcing feedback loop (Thase et al., 2002; Wong & Yehuda, 2002). That is, increases in CRH stimulate increased firing of the locus ceruleus and increased release of norepinephrine. Similarly, stressors that activate norepinephrine neurons increase CRH concentrations in the locus ceruleus (Charney, Deutch, Krystal, & Southwick, 1993). These systems prepare the threatened person to respond to danger by enhancing the person's arousal, attention, perception, energy, and emotion and by suppressing the immune response (Wong & Yehuda).

The stress response is meant to be of limited duration (Thase et al., 2002). However, when resistance or escape is impossible, the human stress system becomes overwhelmed and disorganized (Herman, 1997). Exposure to severe stressors early in life has been shown to compromise the regulation of HPA activity for a lifetime (Carter-Snell & Hegadoren, 2003; Thase et al.). Accordingly, Carter-Snell and Hegadoren theorize that the increased occurrence of sexual abuse in girls may contribute to the increased prevalence of stress disorders reported in women. Most types of abuse are extreme forms of chronic stress. A protracted or dysregulated stress response has been associated with the development of major depression, especially the melancholic type (Chrousos & Gold, 1992; Henry, 1992). Melancholic features include dysphoric hyperarousal that is reflected in agitation, early morning awakening, anorexia, anxiety, excessive guilt, and hypervigilance (APA, 2000). Survivors of abuse report many of these symptoms.

Acute Stress Disorder and Posttraumatic Stress Disorder

The experience of trauma exerts tremendous physical and psychological stress on survivors. The cluster of signs and symptoms that frequently occur after major trauma is now labelled **acute stress disorder** (ASD) and **posttraumatic stress disorder** (PTSD; for a comprehensive discussion of PTSD and ASD, see Chapter 21). Lasiuk and Hegadoren (2006a) in their historical overview of the PTSD concept describe the often misunderstood link between the condition "hysteria" described in early 19th century Europe, war trauma, and PTSD. Subsequent research has demonstrated that symptoms of ASD and PTSD occur not only after war but also after many types of severe trauma, including physical abuse, sexual abuse, and rape.

A comprehensive review of research on the epidemiology of PTSD suggests several gender differences (Norris et al., 2002). Men are more exposed to traumatic events than are women. However, women are about twice as likely as men to experience PTSD, and the median time from onset to remission for women is 4 years, compared with 1 year for men (Lasiuk & Hegadoren, 2006b). Several factors may contribute to these differences. One factor is that men and women experience different types of traumatic events. More men report exposure to events such as fire or disaster, life-threatening accidents, physical assault, combat, being threatened with a weapon, and being held captive. More women report child abuse, sexual molestation, and sexual assault. Sexual violence is associated with a high risk for the development of PTSD. Another factor is differing reactions to traumatic events. To meet the criteria for a diagnosis of PTSD, the traumatized individual must experience terror, horror, or helplessness in response to the trauma (Criterion A2 in *DSM-IV-TR*; APA, 2000, p. 467). More women than men meet this criterion, suggesting that women may be more distressed than men by traumatic events. However, neither types of events nor perceptions of threat fully account for the difference in prevalence rates of PTSD in men and women (Norris et al.).

Other factors that may contribute to a higher prevalence of PTSD in women include higher rates of anxiety and depressive disorders and traumatic events before the age of 15 years (Breslau, Davis, Andreski, Peterson, & Schultz, 1997; Carter-Snell & Hegadoren, 2003; Orsillo, Raja, & Hammond, 2002).

In one study of childhood exposure to trauma, a greater percentage of women (27%) than men (8%) reported rape, assault, or ongoing physical or sexual abuse. More men (28%) than women (11%) with childhood trauma reported serious accidents or injury. Exposure to accidents or injury in childhood did not lead to PTSD in the respondents of either gender; whereas, rape and abuse resulted in a high rate of early PTSD in women (63%), but no cases in men (Breslau, Davis, Andreski, Peterson, & Schultz, 1997).

PTSD may develop any time after the trauma. The delay may be as short as 1 week or as long as 30 years (Kaplan & Sadock, 1998). Symptoms may fluctuate in intensity with time and usually are worse during periods of stress. Some 30% of patients with PTSD recover completely, 40% continue to have mild symptoms, 20% continue to have moderate symptoms, and 10% remain unchanged or become worse (Kaplan & Sadock).

Young children and elderly people have special difficulty with traumatic events. Young children may not have developed adequate coping mechanisms to deal with severe stressors, and older people are likely to have rigid coping mechanisms, making successful coping with the trauma more difficult (Kaplan & Sadock, 1998).

Women with PTSD frequently have comorbid anxiety, depressive disorders, or both, and the association among childhood abuse, PTSD, and substance abuse is also becoming well established (Boyd, 2000, 2003;

Boyd & Mackey, 2000b; Brady & Dansky, 2002; Stewart, Ouimette, & Brown, 2002).

Hyperarousal

After a traumatic experience, the stress system seems to go on permanent alert, as if the danger might return at any time (Rasmusson & Friedman, 2002; Wong & Yehuda, 2002). In this state of physiologic hyperarousal, the traumatized person is hypervigilant for signs of danger, startles easily, reacts irritably to small annoyances, and sleeps poorly. These symptoms are characteristic of increased noradrenergic function (O'Donnell, Hegadoren, & Coupland, 2004), particularly in the locus ceruleus and limbic system (hypothalamus, hippocampus, and amygdala), and of increased dopamine activity, particularly in the prefrontal cortical dopamine system (Rasmusson & Friedman; Wong & Yehuda). Dopamine hyperactivity is associated with the hypervigilance seen in PTSD. Many people with PTSD do not return to their normal baseline level of alertness. Instead, they seem to have a new baseline of elevated arousal, as if their "thermostat" had been reset (Bremner, Southwick, & Charney, 1999). Based on advances in neuroscience, however, a sensorimotor approach to therapy is evolving that shows promise for helping persons with PTSD to restore normal arousal levels (Ogden, Minton, & Pain, 2006).

Behavioural sensitization may be one mechanism underlying the hyperarousal seen in PTSD. This phenomenon, sometimes referred to as *kindling*, occurs after an exposure to severe, uncontrollable stressors. The sensitized person reacts with a magnified stress response to later, milder stressors (Bremner, Southwick, et al., 1999; Charney, Deutch, Krystal, & Southwick, 1993; Krystal et al., 1989).

Research shows that a single or repeated exposure to a severe stressor potentiates the capacity of a subsequent stressor to increase synaptic levels of norepinephrine and dopamine in the forebrain (Charney, Deutch, Krystal, & Southwick, 1993). This finding would account for the fact that some survivors with PTSD experience intense fear, anxiety, and panic in response to minor stimuli. One example of behavioural sensitization is that PTSD after combat exposure is more likely to develop in veterans who are survivors of childhood abuse than in those who have not experienced prior trauma (Southwick, Bremner, Krystal, & Charney, 1994).

The state of hyperarousal causes other problems for survivors. The loss of neuromodulation leads to a loss of affect regulation, so that the survivor is irritable and overreacts to others (van der Kolk & Fisler, 1993). This type of behaviour may cause others to avoid the survivor. The continual arousal may desensitize the survivor to real threat and decrease the probability that he or she will respond to perceived danger (Messman-Moore & Long, 2003). This development may cause the person to miss clues of danger and place himself or herself in situations that can lead to revictimization.

Intrusion

Long after abuse has stopped, survivors relive it as though it were continually recurring. Flashbacks and nightmares, which the survivor experiences with terrifying immediacy, are vivid and often include fragments of traumatic events exactly as they happened (Bremner, Southwick, et al., 1999). Moreover, a wide variety of stimuli that may have been associated with the trauma can elicit flashbacks and dreams. Consequently, survivors avoid such stimuli (Bremner, Southwick, et al.).

Three related but somewhat different explanations may account for the vivid, disturbing flashbacks and dreams that individuals with PTSD have: disturbances of memory, classic conditioning (fear conditioning), and extinction.

Memory function is altered in PTSD. Memory deficits include short-term memory and potentiation of recall of traumatic experiences and dissociative flashbacks. Human beings are bombarded constantly by sensory stimuli yet attend to and remember only a fraction of it (Bremner, Southwick, et al., 1999; Southwick et al., 1994). People seem to remember best those events that have emotional effects and occur when they are alert, aroused, and responsive to their internal and external environments. Because noradrenergic activity is elevated in individuals with PTSD when exposed to emotional and traumatic stimuli, memory encoding may be improved, leading to intrusive thoughts and memories (O'Donnell, Hegadoren, & Coupland, 2004).

During stress, there is a massive release of neurotransmitters, particularly norepinephrine, epinephrine, and opioid peptides. This flood of "stress hormones" may lead to structural changes in the brain that potentiate long-term memory. In most situations, this type of memory has survival value: remembering events that occur during danger may protect oneself during similar future situations. However, in PTSD, the memories occur when the individual is not in danger. Research supporting this hypothesis demonstrated that if norepinephrine is administered to animals immediately after training, long-term memory is enhanced. Epinephrine and endogenous opioids may influence memory consolidation (transforming short-term memory to long-term memory) by affecting norepinephrine (Bremner, Southwick, et al., 1999; Southwick et al., 1994).

The hippocampus and amygdala are involved in memory consolidation. The hippocampus is involved in object memory and placement of memory traces in space and time (Bremner, Southwick, et al., 1999; Cohen, Perel, DeBellis, Friedman, & Putnam, 2002). High levels of stress have been shown to damage the hippocampus and decrease its volume, producing memory deficits such as amnesia and deficits in autobiographical memory

(memory of one's life story; Bremner, Southwick, et al.). The amygdala integrates sensory information for storage in and retrieval from memory. The amygdala also attaches emotional significance to sensory information and transmits this information to all the other systems involved in the stress response. Overreactivity of the amygdala might explain the recurrent and intrusive traumatic memories and the excessive fear associated with traumatic reminders characteristic of PTSD (Cohen et al., 2002). Moreover, electrical stimulation of the amygdala and hippocampal area has been associated with dream-like and memory-like hallucinations that are similar to flashbacks reported by patients with PTSD (Bremner, Narayan, et al., 1999).

Classic conditioning, or **fear conditioning**, occurs when a neutral stimulus (the conditioned stimulus [CS]) is paired with an aversive unconditioned stimulus (US) that elicits an unconditioned fear response (UR). After repeated pairing, the CS alone will elicit the fear response, which is now the conditioned response (CR). For example, certain sights, sounds, or smells that occurred in close proximity to the traumatic event may elicit a fear response in the future. The result of this process is that an individual becomes fearful and anxious in response to a wide variety of stimuli (Bremner, Southwick, et al., 1999; Southwick et al., 1994); therefore, a wide variety of stimuli can elicit symptoms of PTSD.

The amygdala and hippocampus also appear to be important players in fear conditioning (Bremner, Southwick, et al., 1999; O'Donnell et al., 2004; Southwick et al., 1994). Other important brain sites include the thalamus, locus ceruleus, and sensory cortex. Interaction between the cortex and the amygdala may be necessary for specific stimuli to elicit traumatic memories (Bremner, Southwick, et al.; Charney, Deutch, Krystal, & Southwick, 1993).

Several neurochemical systems are involved in regulating fear conditioning, including norepinephrine, dopamine (DA), opiate, and corticotropin-releasing systems. In addition, *N*-methyl-D-aspartate (NMDA), one of the major excitatory neurotransmitters in the brain, appears necessary for this type of learning to occur. NMDA antagonists applied to the amygdala prevent the development of fear-CRs (Bremner, Southwick, et al., 1999; Charney, Deutch, Krystal, & Southwick, 1993).

Extinction is the loss of a learned conditioned emotional response after repeated presentations of the conditioned fear stimulus without a contiguous traumatic event. In other words, the individual no longer responds with fear to the CR. For example, many children are afraid of the dark; however, after many uneventful nights, children gradually lose their fear. Failure of the neuronal mechanisms involved in extinction also may explain the continued ability of conditioned stimuli to elicit traumatic memories and flashbacks in PTSD (Bremner, Southwick, et al., 1999; Charney, Deutch, Krystal, & Southwick, 1993). Recent research on brain dysfunction associated with PTSD resulting from childhood abuse of women has shown that damage to the medial prefrontal cortex interferes with extinguishing fear responses. In addition, individuals with damage to the medial prefrontal cortex show emotional dysfunction and an inability to relate in social situations that require correct interpretation of the emotional expressions of others. These findings suggest that dysfunction of this area of the brain may play a role in pathologic emotions that follow exposure to extreme stressors, such as childhood sexual abuse (Bremner, Narayan, et al., 1999).

Avoidance and Numbing (Dissociative Symptoms)

Survivors try to avoid people or situations that might provoke memories of the trauma. This restriction in their activities may interfere with normal functioning. Survivors also report anhedonia (loss of ability to sense pleasure) and may report that they feel as if parts of themselves have died. These disturbing symptoms may lead them to engage in acts of self-mutilation to feel alive or ultimately to suicide (van der Kolk & Fisler, 1993).

A person who is completely powerless may go into a state of surrender. In that state, the person escapes the situation by altering his or her state of consciousness, that is, by dissociating (Herman, 1997). **Dissociation** is defined as a disruption in the normally occurring linkages between subjective awareness, feelings, thoughts, behaviours, and memories (APA, 2000; Briere & Elliott, 1994).

Dissociation is a complex psychophysiologic process that produces alterations in sense of self, accessibility of memory and knowledge, and integration of behaviour (Putnam, 1994; Rothschild, 1998). In simpler words, a person who dissociates is making himself or herself "disappear." That is, the person has the feeling of leaving his or her body and observing what happens to him or her from a distance. During trauma, dissociation enables a person to observe the event while experiencing no pain, or only limited pain, and to protect himself or herself from awareness of the full impact of the traumatic event (van der Kolk, 1996). A study of Montreal school-aged girls indicates that sexual abuse was associated with eight times the level of dissociation and four times the level of PTSD in the girls who had been sexually abused compared with matched controls without sexual abuse (Collin-Vezina & Herbert, 2005). Examples of dissociation include (1) derealization and depersonalization (the experience of self or the environment as strange or unreal); (2) periods of disengagement from the immediate environment during stress, such as "spacing out"; (3) alterations in bodily perceptions; (4) emotional numbing; (5) out-of-body experiences; and (6) amnesia for abuse-related memories (Briere & Elliott, 1994; Rothschild). Fear activates the endogenous opioid system, producing stress-induced analgesia (SIA; Bremner,

Southwick, et al., 1999; van der Kolk). SIA may be associated with avoidance and numbing. The purpose of SIA is to protect against pain in dangerous situations so that the individual (animal or human) can defend itself (fight) or escape the situation (flight). In severely stressed animals, opiate withdrawal symptoms can be produced by removing the stressor or by injecting naloxone, an opiate antagonist. In people with PTSD, SIA can become conditioned to stimuli resembling the original trauma. Research with humans showed that as long as 20 years after the original trauma, people with PTSD developed SIA equivalent to 8 mg of morphine in response to such stimuli. Excessive opioid and norepinephrine secretion can interfere with memory. Freezing or numbing responses may prevent animals from remembering situations of overwhelming stress. Trauma-related dissociative reactions after prolonged exposure to severe, uncontrollable stress may be analogous to this effect in animals (van der Kolk).

Dissociative Identity Disorder

Dissociation exists on a continuum, with most people experiencing short, situation-specific episodes, such as daydreaming (Putnam, 1994). Among survivors of abuse, dissociative symptoms may be part of the symptom picture of ASD and PTSD, or they may be the predominant symptom (Lasiuk & Hegadoren, 2006b). In such cases, the disorder is **dissociative identity disorder** (DID) (formerly multiple personality disorder) (Rothschild, 1998). The hallmarks of DID are two or more distinct identities with unique personality characteristics and an inability to recall important information about self or events that is too extensive to be explained by ordinary forgetfulness (APA, 2000). Other memory disturbances linked with dissociation include intermittent and disruptive intrusions of traumatic memories into awareness and difficulties in determining whether a given memory reflects an actual event or information acquired through another source (Putnam). The diagnostic criteria for DID are found in Table 37-1.

Two other dimensions of dissociation that are associated with DID include passive influence experiences and hallucinatory experiences. A passive influence experience is a situation in which a person feels as if he or she were controlled by a force from within. These experiences may include a sense that one is being made to do something against one's will that may be distasteful or harmful to self and others (Putnam, 1994).

Many survivors of abuse report dissociative perceptual disturbances, such as visual hallucinations, extrasensory perceptions, and peculiar time distortions (Anderson, Yasenik, & Ross, 1993; Hendricks-Matthews, 1993). The hallucinatory experiences in dissociative disorders are distinct in several ways from those that occur in psychotic disorders. They are often experienced as internalized,

Table 37.1 Key Diagnostic Characteristics for DID	DSM IV
Diagnostic Criteria	**Target Symptoms and Associated Findings**
• Presence of two or more distinct personality states or identities • At least two identities or personality states recurrently take control of the person's behaviour • Inability to recall important information that is too extensive to be explained by ordinary forgetfulness • Not due to direct physiologic effects of substances or a general medical condition • In children, symptoms not attributable to imaginary playmates or other fantasy play	• Posttraumatic symptoms (nightmares, flashbacks, startle responses) • PTSD • Self-mutilation • Suicidal behaviour • Aggressive behaviour • Repetitive relationships characterized by physical and sexual abuse *Associated Physical Examination Findings* • Scars from self-inflicted injuries or physical abuse • Migraine and other types of headaches, irritable bowel syndrome, and asthma *Associated Laboratory Findings* • Physiologic functioning may vary across personality states • High scores on measures of hypnotizability and dissociative capacity

rather than externalized, voices and may be associated with specific experiences or people. The affected person hears the voices distinctly; the voices often have particular attributes such as gender, age, and affect. The voices may be supportive and comforting or berating (Putnam, 1994). Hallucinatory experiences may also involve the appearance of "shadowy figures," ghosts or spirits, or rapidly moving objects. The person is generally aware that the voices or images are not real (Putnam).

The overall prevalence of DID is unknown. Estimates are that 1% of the American population may be affected and as many as 5% to 20% of people in psychiatric hospitals (National Women's Health Information Center [NWHIC], 2003). The cause of DID is unknown. However, the patient history invariably involves a traumatic event in childhood. Four types of causative factors have been identified: a traumatic event, a psychological or genetic vulnerability to develop the disorder, formative environmental factors, and the absence of external support (Kaplan & Sadock, 1998). Examples of psychological vulnerability include being suggestible or easily hypnotized. Formative environmental events may include a lack of role models who demonstrate healthy problem solving or practices to relieve anxiety or stress. Many who experience DID lack supportive others, such as parents, siblings, other relatives, and supportive people outside the family (e.g., teachers; Kaplan & Sadock).

Complex Trauma

In her book *Trauma and Recovery*, Herman proposed a new diagnosis: "**complex posttraumatic stress disorder**" (1997, p. 119). Her proposal was based on experience that none of the diagnostic categories in the APA's *Diag-*

nostic and Statistical Manual (3rd ed., Revision.; APA, 1987) were appropriate for survivors of extreme, prolonged trauma, especially interpersonal trauma (i.e., severe, prolonged child abuse), including the diagnosis of PTSD. She noted that survivors of prolonged, repeated trauma experience characteristic personality changes, including problems of relatedness, identity, and vulnerability to repeated harm, inflicted by others or self. C-PTSD was considered for inclusion in the fourth edition of the *DSM* as "disorders of extreme stress not otherwise specified (DESNOS)" (van der Kolk, 1996, p. 203). DESNOS was eventually incorporated into the *DSM-IV-TR* under the "Associated Features and Disorders" section. The symptoms include impaired affect modulation (difficulty modulating anger or sexual behaviours; self-destructive and suicidal behaviours); impulsive/risk-taking behaviour; alterations in attention and consciousness (amnesia, dissociation); somatization; chronic characterologic changes, including alterations in relations with others (an inability to trust or maintain relationships, a tendency to be revictimized or to victimize others); and alterations in systems of meaning (e.g., despair, hopelessness, loss of previously sustaining beliefs; APA, 2000; van der Kolk).

These symptoms are similar to those of borderline personality disorder (BPD). Many people with BPD were severely abused in childhood. Splitting self and others into "all good" or "all bad" may result from a developmental arrest: a fragmentation of self, based on modes of organizing experience that were common in earlier developmental stages. Self-mutilation, often labelled as masochism or manipulative behaviour, may be a way of regulating psychological and biologic equilibrium when ordinary means of self-regulation have been disturbed by trauma. Psychotic episodes in patients with BPD are similar to flashbacks, intrusive recollections of traumatic memories that were stored on a somatosensory level (van der Kolk, 1996). Research findings demonstrate that the diagnoses of both BPD and C-PTSD were significantly higher in a group of women with early-onset sexual abuse compared with late-onset sexual abuse, suggesting that women with a history of childhood sexual abuse might be better understood within the rubric of C-PTSD (McLean & Gallop, 2003).

Substance Abuse and Dependence

Childhood abuse, PTSD, and substance abuse are known to be associated. Investigators have reported that as many as 84% of female inpatient substance abusers had a history of sexual or physical assault (Brady & Dansky, 2002; Stewart et al., 2002). High rates of abuse have also been found in samples of outpatient, rural women (Boyd, 2000, 2003). The Vancouver Injection Drug User Study of sexual violence among intravenous drug users indicates that 68% of women and 19% of men had a lifetime history of sexual violence (Braitstein et al., 2003).

Survivors who experience PTSD, depression, and other forms of dysphoric hyperarousal or emotional distress often abuse substances, including alcohol and other sedative drugs that lessen stress and reduce hyperarousal and distress by inhibiting noradrenergic activity (Brady & Dansky, 2002; Stewart et al., 2002). Sexually abused adolescents and adults may use AOD as alternatives to psychological dissociation (Roesler & Dafler, 1993). Increasing numbers of women reportedly abuse cocaine to wipe out dysphoric feelings caused by abuse. These women report that the intense high of cocaine totally obliterates painful feelings, if only for a short time (Boyd, 2000). Substance abuse in a person with PTSD is particularly problematic. The comorbidity worsens the symptoms and courses of both disorders, increases suicidality, and makes treatment more difficult (Boyd; Hana & Grant, 1997).

Psychological Responses

Low Self-Esteem

The consequences of abuse are devastating, and the term "low self-esteem" seems inadequate. Women who are abused as children often experience "alienation from self and others" (Boyd & Mackey, 2000a). Alienation from self includes painful feelings that go to the "core of a woman being"—experiencing self as fundamentally flawed and having no purpose in life. Alienation from others, especially significant others, is associated with painful feelings of loneliness, depression, anger, shame, and guilt and with feeling hurt, unloved, and unwanted (Boyd & Mackey). Women who experience alienation from self and others

often turn to substance abuse to cope with their intense pain (Boyd & Mackey, 2000b).

Low self-esteem or alienation may be attributable to the direct effects of physical or sexual abuse or to the accompanying psychological abuse. One technique that perpetrators use to control and disempower women is to erode their sense of self-worth with a constant barrage of criticism. Perpetrators frequently tell women that they are stupid, ugly, inadequate wives and mothers, inadequate sexually, and incompetent. Other contributing factors include a sense of being different from other people, the need to maintain secrecy, lack of trust, and self-blame (Boyd & Mackey, 2000a).

Low self-esteem may be one factor contributing to a battered woman's reluctance to disclose her abuse. Because of low self-esteem, battered women, even many who are successful outside the home, underestimate their ability to do anything about the abuse (Boyd & Mackey, 2000a). As such, it is not surprising that "reclaiming the self" was identified as the main psychological process central to leaving an abusive partner in a qualitative study of women who had recently left abusive male partners (Wuest & Merritt-Gray, 2001).

Guilt and Shame

A history of abuse is often associated with excessive guilt and shame. These feelings stem from survivors' mistaken beliefs that they are somehow to blame for their abuse (Boyd & Mackey, 2000a; Campbell et al., 2004; Long & Smyth, 1998). Feelings of humiliation and shame may prevent women from seeking medical care and reporting abuse to authorities. The experience of being battered is so degrading and humiliating that women are often afraid to disclose it. Many women fear that they will not be taken seriously or will be blamed for inciting the abuse or for staying with their abusers (Boyd & Mackey; Campbell et al.; Long & Smyth). In keeping with this observation, research findings indicate that resilient women with a history of childhood sexual abuse and no history of substance abuse felt less blame and stigma associated with being sexually abused compared with women with a history of childhood sexual abuse who were currently receiving treatment for substance abuse (Dufour & Nadeau, 2001).

Anger

Chronic irritability, unexpected or uncontrollable feelings of anger, and difficulties with the expression of anger are frequent experiences for survivors of abuse (Campbell et al., 2004). They may express anger toward the perpetrator, fate, those who have been spared the suffering, or someone whom the victim believes could have prevented the abuse (Barnett et al., 1997). However, some incest survivors have difficulty expressing anger and mask it with compliance and perfectionism (Campbell et al.; Hendricks-Matthews, 1993).

Social and Interpersonal Responses

Problems With Intimacy

The abused child experiences intrusion, abandonment, devaluation, or pain in the relationship with the abuser, instead of the closeness and nurturing that are normal for intimate relationships, such as those between the parent and the child (Briere & Elliott, 1994; Long & Smyth, 1998; Urbancic, 2004). As a result, many survivors have difficulty trusting and forming intimate relationships.

Sexual problems are common among survivors of abuse. Among the most common and chronic problems are fear of intimate sexual relationships, feelings of repulsion toward sex, lack of enjoyment of sex, dysfunctions of desire and arousal, and failure to achieve orgasm. Some survivors engage in compulsive promiscuity and prostitution, reflecting their internalization of the message that the only thing that they are good for is sex (Hendricks-Matthews, 1993; Long & Smyth, 1998; Urbancic, 2004).

Revictimization

Many women who have been sexually abused as children are revictimized on multiple occasions later in life. Among women with a history of sexual assault, rates of revictimization range from 15% to 79% (Arata, 2002; Breitenbecher, 2001; Messman-Moore & Long, 2003). A community-based Toronto study of sexual violence surveyed 420 women and found that 26.4% had an experience of sexual assault in childhood and adulthood (Randall & Haskell, 1995). Numerous factors have been related to revictimization, including PTSD symptoms, dissociation, alexithymia, the use of AOD, boundary issues, and sexual behaviour (Breitenbecher; Messman-Moore & Long). Proneness to revictimization may result from a general vulnerability in dangerous situations that may be associated with dissociation. Dissociation makes women unaware of their environment and also may make them look confused or distracted. Thus, women in a dissociative state may be easy targets (Cloitre, Scarvalone, & Difede, 1997; Messman-Moore & Long).

Alexithymia may also add to a woman's risk for revictimization. Difficulty in labelling and communicating feelings may make it difficult for a woman to set limits on sexual advances. Moreover, these women may not be able to read accurately the emotional cues of others, which diminishes their ability to respond effectively in interpersonally dangerous situations (Cloitre et al., 1997).

Women with abuse histories frequently have difficulty with boundaries. During childhood abuse, they experienced boundary violations as normal and connected with their expectations of intimate relationships. Confusion over boundaries may result in confusion about appropriate behaviour in adult intimate relationships (Cloitre et al., 1997; Messman-Moore & Long, 2003).

The sexual behaviour pattern of survivors may place them at risk for revictimization. One effect of sexual victimization is that the child's sexuality is shaped by "traumatic sexualization." Traumatic sexualization occurs when a child is rewarded for sexual behaviour with affection, attention, privileges, and gifts. As a result, the child may learn that her self-worth is tied to her sexuality, and she may use sexual behaviour to manipulate others (Breitenbecher, 2001; Messman-Moore & Long, 2003).

■ NURSING MANAGEMENT: HUMAN RESPONSE TO ABUSE

Nurses encounter survivors of abuse in many health care settings. The percentage of ED visits that are attributed to domestic violence ranges from 4% to 18% (Campbell et al., 2004); however, reports have been as high as 80% (McGrath et al., 1997). A critical ethnographic study of 30 nurses working in the EDs of two urban hospitals in Canada provides direction for the care of abused women in the ED (Varcoe, 2001). Specifically, issues that obscure the needs of abused women, such as the perceived need to focus on rapid processing of patients and stereotypical judgments, were identified (Varcoe). As well, the importance of supporting a developing sense of efficacy for nurses working in EDs has been identified by Canadian researchers (Hollingsworth & Ford-Gilboe, 2006). Approximately 50% of female patients admitted to psychiatric facilities are victims of either child or adult abuse (Seeman, 2002). Other settings in which the nurse encounters battered women include primary care settings, obstetric-gynecology settings, paediatric units, well-child clinics, geriatric units, and nursing homes.

The paediatric ED provides a unique opportunity to identify and respond to child survivors, as well as battered mothers (Campbell et al., 2004). As many as 59% of mothers of child abuse victims are battered women, and child abuse occurs disproportionately in homes with woman abuse (Wright, Wright, & Isaac, 1997). Identifying battered mothers may be the most important means of identifying child abuse. Conversely, when a nurse suspects child abuse, he or she cannot ignore the possibility that the mother is also a victim. Identifying children who are traumatized by witnessing the battering of their mothers also is essential. However, despite the opportunity the paediatric ED affords, disturbingly few battered women are identified there.

Health care providers in paediatric EDs have reported several obstacles to identification, including lack of training, time constraints, powerlessness, lack of comfort, lack of control over the victim's circumstances, and fear of offending the patient (Wright et al.). Another important setting for an effective identification of battered women is in the postpartum setting. Researchers implemented a domestic violence assessment in two hospitals in the city of Vancouver and found that the screening rate for domestic violence increased from 42% to 60% for a period of 18 months (Janssen, Holt, & Sugg, 2002).

Nurses may encounter elder abuse in virtually any setting. Examples include EDs, medical-surgical units, psychiatric units, and homes during home care visits. In addition, nurses may encounter elder abuse in nursing homes. Events such as unnecessary chemical (medications) or physical restraints used to control an elder's behaviour may be abusive and should be investigated.

Although some aspects of care are specific to adult, child, or elderly survivors of abuse, many elements are common in the nursing care of all survivors, regardless of age or setting. The goals of all nursing interventions in cases of abuse are to stop the violence and to ensure the survivor's safety. Victimization removes all power and control from a woman, child, or elder. Therefore, as appropriate for age and ability, all nursing interventions should empower survivors to act on their own behalf and must be done in a collaborative partnership. To that end, nurses must be willing to offer support and information and not impose their own values on survivors by encouraging them to leave abusive relationships. Strong psychological and economic bonds tie many women to their perpetrators. Moreover, adult survivors who are capable of making decisions are the experts on their situations. They are the best judges of when leaving the relationship is appropriate (Canadian Nurses Association [CNA], 1992; Walker, 1994).

However, removing children and elders from their families or caregivers often is necessary to ensure immediate safety. If the home of an abused or neglected child or elder cannot be made safe, the nurse must support other professionals involved in placing the child or elder in a foster or nursing home (Gary & Humphreys, 2004; Sengstock et al., 2004). However, intervening in cases of elder abuse is not a clear-cut issue. Nurses must allow elders whose decision making is not impaired (*competence* is a legal term) an appropriate degree of autonomy in deciding how to manage the problem, even if they choose to remain in the abusive situation (Allan, 1998). Forcing an elder to do something against his or her wishes is itself a form of victimization.

Intervention strategies for elders depend on whether the elder accepts or refuses assistance and whether he or she can make decisions. If the elder refuses treatment, the nurse must remain nonjudgmental and provide information about available services and emergency numbers. The Canadian approach to adult protection legislation, concerned with preventing abuse and neglect, has been guided by reforms in adult guardianship and substitute decision making. There are three adult protection models now in existence across Canada. Please see Gordon's (2001) article for a comprehensive review of adult protection legislation in Canada.

Biologic Domain

Biologic Assessment

Research indicates that health care providers often fail to respond therapeutically to survivors of abuse. In many instances, they neglect to identify abuse as the cause of traumatic injuries or mental health problems (Blakely & Ribeiro, 1997; Campbell et al., 2004; Henderson, 2001). Even more damaging, many health care professionals treat abuse survivors derogatorily, blaming them for the abuse or for staying in abusive situations. Unfortunately, nursing staff may revictimize survivors with BPD. Often, these women have been severely traumatized, and their behaviour is difficult and disruptive. In some cases, caregivers react negatively, labelling this behaviour as attention seeking and manipulative. When nurses react to the patient in a negative, punitive manner, they retraumatize these women (Gallop, McCay, Guha, & Khan, 1999). It is not uncommon to see this behaviour punished by staff avoidance, time in seclusion rooms, and overmedication. BPD symptoms should be interpreted as ineffective coping strategies, developed in response to severe trauma, rather than as deliberate attempts to manipulate staff (Hattendorf & Tollerud, 1997).

To improve providers' responses, the CNA recommends that students acquire the necessary knowledge and skill acquisition to prevent violence, as well as to detect and intervene with individuals who are survivors of abuse and violence. The CNA (1992) states that nurses can play a significant role in addressing family violence because nurses are frequently the first professionals to interact with individuals affected by family violence. Nurses should assess everyone for violence—both women and men, no matter what age or presenting problem. An awareness of violence and a high index of suspicion are the most important elements in assessing the problem (Campbell et al., 2004). If suspected abuse is never assessed, it will never be uncovered.

Establishing a trusting nurse–patient relationship is one of the most important steps in assessing any type of abuse. Survivors are unlikely to disclose sensitive information unless they perceive the nurse to be

IN A LIFE

Sheldon Kennedy (1970–)
Professional Hockey Player

Public Persona

Canadian-born Sheldon Kennedy played professional hockey in the National Hockey League (NHL). He was an outstanding and talented hockey player who began training in the Canadian Hockey League (CHL) at a young age. As a junior-level hockey player in Winnipeg, he was coached by Graham James, one of the most nationally famous and highly respected coaches.

Personal Realities

In 1996, Kennedy came forward with sexual abuse allegations against his former CHL coach, Graham James. Kennedy said that the assaults took place between the ages of 14 and 19 and occurred on a weekly basis. On September 3, 1996, Kennedy reported the sexual abuse by James to the Calgary city police. In January 1997, Graham James was sentenced to 3½ years in prison for the sexual abuse. Kennedy then went public with his story, including the revelation of the many times he contemplated suicide. Shortly afterward, the NHL sponsored Kennedy to enroll in a substance abuse program for his drinking and drug problems.

Kennedy's courage has brought hope to many. He has created the Sheldon Kennedy Foundation that helps increase awareness of sexual abuse, raises money through events such as a cross-country skate, and contributes to programs such as the Anaphe Ranch in British Columbia, a healing place for Canadian children who have been abused. In honour of his efforts, the government of Saskatchewan declared August 21, 1998, Sheldon Kennedy Day.

From information gathered at http://www.silent-edge.org/, http://www.gov.sk.ca/, and http://www.snn-rdr.ca/

trustworthy and nonjudgmental. Important considerations in establishing open communication are ensuring confidentiality and providing a quiet, private place in which to conduct assessment. The law mandates that nurses report child abuse to the authorities, and nurses must make that responsibility clear before beginning the assessment. Child abuse is usually reported to the children aid society.

Lethality Assessment First. The most important assessment and the one to be done first is a lethality assessment (CNA, 1992; Walker, 1994). The nurse must ascertain whether the survivor is in danger for his or her life, either from homicide or suicide, and, if children are in the home, whether they are in danger (Campbell et al., 2004). The nurse should take immediate steps to ensure the survivor's safety. In the case of suspected child abuse assessed in a health care agency, an interdisciplinary team consisting of physicians, psychologists, nurses, and social workers usually makes this decision. In other settings, the nurse may be the person to make that decision. Nurses do not have to obtain proof of abuse, only a reasonable suspicion. The Danger Assessment Screen developed by Jacquelyn Campbell and colleagues is a useful tool for assessing the risk that either the adult survivor or the perpetrator will commit homicide (Box 37-2).

Most survivors do not report abuse to health care workers without being asked specifically about it. Only 13% of women seen in the ED after a battering incident

BOX 37.2

Danger Assessment

Several risk factors have been associated with homicides (murders) of both batterers and battered women in research that has been conducted after the killings have taken place. We cannot predict what will happen in your case, but we would like you to be aware of the danger of homicide in situations of severe battering and to see how many of the risk factors apply to your situation. (The "he" in the questions refers to your husband, partner, ex-husband, ex-partner, or whoever is currently physically hurting you.)

1. Has the physical violence increased in frequency during the past year?
2. Has the physical violence increased in severity during the past year, or has a weapon or threat with weapon been used?
3. Does he ever try to choke you?
4. Is there a gun in the house?
5. Has he ever forced you into sex when you did not wish to do so?
6. Does he use drugs? By drugs, I mean "uppers" or amphetamines, speed, angel dust, cocaine, "crack," street drugs, heroin, or mixtures.
7. Does he threaten to kill you, or do you believe he is capable of killing you?
8. Is he drunk every day or almost every day? (In terms of quantity of alcohol.)
9. Does he control most or all of your daily activities? For instance, does he tell you whom you can be friends with,

how much money you can take with you shopping, or when you can take the car? (If he tries, but you do not let him, check here___.)
10. Has he ever beaten you while you were pregnant? (If never pregnant by him, check here___.)
11. Is he violently and constantly jealous of you? (For instance, does he say, "If I can't have you, no one can.")
12. Have you ever threatened or tried to commit suicide?
13. Has he ever threatened or tried to commit suicide?
14. Is he violent toward the children?
15. Is he violent outside the home?

TOTAL YES ANSWERS:___.

THANK YOU. PLEASE TALK TO YOUR NURSE, ADVOCATE, OR COUNSELLOR ABOUT WHAT THE DANGER ASSESSMENT MEANS IN TERMS OF YOUR SITUATION.

Adapted from Campbell, J., & Humphreys, J. (Eds.). (1993). *Nursing care of survivors of family violence* (p. 259). St. Louis, MO: Mosby.

either told or were asked by staff about abuse (Sisley, Jacobs, Poole, Campbell, & Esposito, 1999). A survey of the ED in 230 Canadian hospitals indicated that the implementation of domestic violence policies may be as low as 10% or 20% (Hotch, Grunfeld, Mackay, & Ritch, 1996). Survivors may be reluctant to report abuse because of shame and fear of retaliation, especially if the victim depends on the abuser as caregiver. In addition, children may be afraid that they will not be believed. Asking specific abuse screening questions has been shown to increase the detection of abuse substantially (from 3% to 15%) (Sisley et al.). For that reason, nurses must develop a repertoire of age-appropriate, culturally sensitive abuse-related questions.

Appropriate questions to ask in assessing abuse in women are found in the Abuse Assessment Screen in Box 37-3. Other questions that might be useful in eliciting disclosure are "When there are fights at home, have you ever been hurt or afraid?" "It looks like someone has hurt you. Tell me about it." "Some women have described problems like yours and have told me that their partner has hurt them. Is that happening to you?" (Campbell et al., 2004) When survivors are disclosing abuse, they need privacy and time to tell their story. They need to know that the nurse is listening, believes them, and is concerned for their safety and well-being (Long & Smyth).

Most survivors are not offended when health care workers ask about abuse directly, as long as they conduct the interview nonjudgmentally. Survivors may perceive failure to ask about abuse as evidence of lack of concern, adding to the feelings of entrapment and helplessness. The high prevalence of abuse and the reluctance of survivors to volunteer information about

it mandate routine screening of every patient for abuse by explicit questioning. Perhaps even more important, the nurse must complete such screening in privacy, away from the woman's partner, the child's parents or legal guardians, or the elderly person's relative or companion (Campbell et al., 2004; Sisley, Jacobs, Poole, Campbell, & Esposito, 1999). If a partner, parent, other relative, or companion accompanies the patient to the health care facility, protocols should be in place to separate the patient from these individuals until the assessment is completed. One approach is to ask the other person to wait in the reception area, explaining that assessments are always done in private.

After the assessment is completed in a health care agency, the nurse should offer the adult survivor use of the telephone. The agency appointment may be the only time that the survivor can make calls in private to family, who might offer support, or to the police, lawyers, or shelters. Scheduling future appointments may provide the survivor with a legitimate reason to leave the perpetrator temporarily and continue to explore her options.

History and Physical Examination. All survivors who report or for whom the nurse suspects abuse should receive a complete history and physical examination. Throughout, the nurse must remain nonjudgmental and communicate openly and honestly (CNA, 1992; Campbell et al., 2004; Long & Smyth, 1998). A Canadian grounded theory study of woman survivors of child sexual abuse indicates that feeling safe with a health care provider who is sensitive and willing to listen can facilitate disclosure (Schachter, Radomsky, Stalker, & Teram, 2004). It is not the nurse's responsibility to judge any situation, whether that is a woman's decision to remain in an abusive relationship, the abusive actions of children's parents, or abuse perpetrated by caregivers of the elderly. Therefore, nurses must continually monitor their own feelings toward the abuser and survivor, especially in cases of child abuse. Working with child survivors often causes distress and feelings of anger and inadequacy. Seeking supervision may prevent negative feelings from influencing the nurse–patient relationship in a nontherapeutic manner and perhaps retraumatizing the survivor (Long & Smyth).

The history should include past and present medical histories, ADLs, and social and financial supports. The nurse should obtain a detailed history of how injuries occurred. As with any history, the nurse begins with the complaint that brought the patient to the health care agency. The nurse assesses whether the explanation for the injuries or symptoms is plausible, given their nature. Discrepancies between the history and the physical examination findings may suggest abuse or neglect. The nurse moves from safe to more sensitive

---

BOX 37.3

Abuse Assessment Screen

1. Have you ever been emotionally or physically abused by your partner or someone important to you?
   YES _____
   NO _____
2. Within the past year, have you been hit, slapped, kicked, or otherwise physically hurt by someone?
   YES _____
   NO _____
   If YES, by whom: _____
   Number of times: _____
   Mark the area of injury on body map.
3. Within the past year, has anyone forced you to have sexual activities?
   If YES, who: _____
   Number of times: _____
4. Are you afraid of your partner or anyone you listed above?
   YES _____
   NO _____

topics, such as the nature of the injuries. Walker (1994) suggests using what she calls the "four-incident technique" to elicit a complete abuse history. The nurse asks the survivor to describe four battering incidents: the first incident that she remembers, the most recent incident, the worst incident, and a typical incident. This series of questions is designed to elicit a complete picture of the cycle of violence and its progression. If the child is too young or an elder is too impaired to give a history, the nurse should interview one or both parents of the child or the caregiver of the elder. If the survivor is a child or dependent elder who cannot describe what happened or make decisions about personal safety and care, the health care team may take steps to place the survivor in protective custody and defer additional assessment to the appropriate agency. The physical examination should include a neurologic examination, radiographs to identify any old or new fractures, and an examination for sexual abuse. Nurses assessing the elderly need to be familiar with normal aging and with the signs and symptoms of common illnesses in the elderly to distinguish those conditions from abuse (Allan, 1998). Similarly, nurses need to know healthy child development to detect deviations that abuse or neglect may cause. For children, assessing developmental milestones, school history, and relationships with siblings and friends is important (Walker). Any discrepancies between the history and the physical examination and implausible explanations for injuries and other symptoms should alert the nurse to the possibility of abuse. Box 37-4 lists indicators of actual or potential abuse that need to be thoroughly assessed for all survivors.

The nurse should thoroughly document all findings. Injuries should be photographed if possible, but this can be done only with written permission from an adult survivor or one of the child's parents. If the survivor will not permit photographing, the nurse should document the injuries on a body map. Survivors may need assurance that their medical records will not be released to anyone without written permission and that documentation of injuries will be important if legal action is taken. If the survivor does not admit abuse, the nurse cannot note abuse in the record. However, the nurse can document that the description of injuries is inconsistent with the injury pattern.

Biologic indicators, such as elevated pulse and blood pressure, sleep and appetite disturbances, exaggerated startle responses, flashbacks, and nightmares, may suggest PTSD or depression. Signs and symptoms of dissociation include memory difficulties, a feeling of unreality about oneself or events, a feeling that a familiar place is strange and unfamiliar, auditory or visual hallucinations, and evidence of having done things without remembering them (Carlson & Putnam, 1993). If any of these signs or symptoms is present, the survivor requires a thorough diagnostic workup for PTSD and DID.

· CRNENOTE

In accordance with the Canadian Standards of Psychiatric and Mental Health Nursing, people in abusive relationships have a right to self-determination. Care involves offering choice and respecting individual preference.

BOX 37.4

History and Physical Findings Suggestive of Abuse

PRESENTING PROBLEM
- Vague information about the cause of the problem
- Delay between occurrence of injury and seeking of treatment
- Inappropriate reactions of significant other or family
- Denial or minimizing of seriousness of injury
- Discrepancy between the history and the physical examination findings

FAMILY HISTORY
- Past family violence
- Physical punishment of children
- Children who are fearful of parent(s)
- Father and/or mother who demands unquestioning obedience
- Alcohol or drug abuse
- Violence outside the home
- Unemployment or underemployment

- Financial difficulties or poverty
- Use of elder's finances for other family members
- Finances rigidly controlled by one member

HEALTH AND PSYCHIATRIC HISTORY
- Fractures at various stages of healing
- Spontaneous abortions
- Injuries during pregnancy
- Multiple visits to the ED
- Elimination disturbances (e.g., constipation, diarrhoea)
- Multiple somatic complaints
- Eating disorders
- Substance abuse
- Depression
- PTSD
- Self-mutilation
- Suicide attempts

Continued

BOX 37.4

History and Physical Findings Suggestive of Abuse (Continued)

- Feelings of helplessness or hopelessness
- Low self-esteem
- Chronic fatigue
- Apathy
- Sleep disturbances (e.g., hypersomnia, hyposomnia)
- Psychiatric hospitalizations

PERSONAL AND SOCIAL HISTORY
- Feelings of powerlessness
- Feelings of being trapped
- Lack of trust
- Traditional values about home, partner, and children's behaviour
- Major decisions in family controlled by one person
- Few social supports (isolated from family, friends)
- Little activity outside the home
- Unwanted or unplanned pregnancy
- Dependency on caregivers
- Extreme jealousy by partner
- Difficulties at school or work
- Short attention span
- Running away
- Promiscuity
- Child who has knowledge of sexual matters beyond that appropriate for age
- Sexualized play with self, peers, dolls, toys
- Masturbation
- Excessive fears and clinging in children

NEUROLOGIC SYSTEM
- Difficulty with speech or swallowing
- Hyperactive reflexes
- Developmental delays
- Areas of numbness
- Tremors

MENTAL STATUS
- Anxiety, fear
- Depression
- Suicidal ideation
- Difficulty concentrating
- Memory loss
- Verbal aggression
- Themes of violence in artwork and school work

DISTORTED BODY IMAGE
- History of chronic physical or psychological disability
- Inability to perform ADLs
- Delayed language development

PHYSICAL EXAMINATION FINDINGS
General Appearance
- Fearful, anxious, hyperactive, hypoactive
- Watching partner, parent, or caregiver for approval of answers to questions
- Poor grooming or inappropriate dress
- Malnourishment
- Signs of stress or fatigue

- Flinching when approached or touched
- Inappropriate or anxious nonverbal behaviour
- Wearing clothing inappropriate to the season or occasion to cover body parts

Vital Statistics
- Elevated pulse or blood pressure
- Other signs of autonomic arousal (exaggerated startle response, excessive sweating)
- Underweight or overweight

Skin
- Bruises, welts, edema, scars
- Burns (cigarette, immersion, friction from ropes, a pattern like electric iron or stove)
- Subdural haematoma
- Missing hair
- Poor skin integrity: dehydration, decubitus ulcers, untreated wounds, urine burns or excoriation

Eyes
- Orbital swelling
- Conjunctival haemorrhage
- Retinal haemorrhage
- Black eyes
- No glasses to accommodate poor eyesight

Ears
- Hearing loss
- No prosthetic device to accommodate poor hearing

Mouth
- Bruising
- Lacerations
- Missing or broken teeth
- Untreated dental problems

Abdomen
- Abdominal injuries during pregnancy
- Intra-abdominal injuries

Genitourinary System or Rectum
- Bruising, lacerations, bleeding, edema, tenderness
- Untreated infections

Musculoskeletal System
- Fractures or old fractures in various stages of healing
- Dislocations
- Limited range of motion in extremities
- Contractures

MEDICATIONS
- Medications not indicated by physical condition
- Overdose of drugs or medications (prescribed or over the counter)
- Medications not taken as prescribed

COMMUNICATION PATTERNS/RELATIONS
- Verbal hostility, arguments
- Negative nonverbal communication, lack of visible affection
- One person answers questions and looks to the other person for approval
- Extreme dependency of family members

The nurse should assess every adult or adolescent who discloses victimization for substance abuse. The Michigan Alcoholism Screening Test (MAST; Selzer, 1971) and the Drug Abuse Screening Test (DAST; Skinner, 1982) are two screening instruments for use in any health assessment. An adolescent version of the MAST is available. If the results of these tests or the answers to any alcohol-related or drug-related questions are positive, the nurse should evaluate the survivor further for an alcohol or drug disorder.

Nursing Diagnoses for the Biologic Domain Selected nursing diagnoses focusing on the human responses that nurses manage in the biologic domain may include posttrauma syndrome, delayed growth and development, impaired memory, and rape-trauma syndrome.

Interventions for the Biologic Domain Restoring health is a primary concern for survivors of abuse. When injuries are severe and surgery is required, the survivor may require hospital admittance.

Treating Physical Symptoms. Treatment of trauma symptoms may include cleaning and dressing burns or other wounds and assisting with casting of broken bones (see Box 37-5 for more information). Malnourished and dehydrated children and elders may require nursing interventions such as intravenous therapy or nutritional supplements that alleviate the alteration in nutrition and fluid and electrolyte balance.

CRNENOTE

CRNENOTE
It is essential to assess the risk for danger to people who are experiencing abusive relationships. Remember that their basic needs must be met (safety, housing, food, child care) before their psychological traumas can be addressed.

Promoting Healthy Daily Activity. Teaching sleep hygiene and promoting exercise, leisure time, and nutrition will help battered survivors regain a healthy physical state and learn self-care. Taking care of oneself may be difficult, yet important, for survivors who have spent years trying to separate themselves from their bodies (dissociate) to survive years of abuse (Walker, 1994). A history of IPV threatens the physical and mental health of women and children in many ways (Ford-Gilboe, Wuest, & Merritt-Gray, 2005). Techniques such as going to bed and arising at consistent times, avoiding naps and caffeine, and scheduling periods for relaxation just before retiring may be useful in promoting sleep. Aerobic exercise is a useful technique for relieving anxiety and depression and promoting sleep.

Administering and Monitoring Medications. Survivors with a comorbid mood or anxiety disorder including PTSD may require pharmacologic interventions. Although only nurses with advanced preparation and prescriptive authority may prescribe medications, all

---

BOX 37.5

Special Concerns for Victims of Sexual Assault

ASSESSMENT FOCUS
The history and physical examination of the survivor of sexual assault differ significantly from other assessment routines because the evidence obtained may be used in prosecuting the perpetrator (Sheridan, 2004). Therefore, the purpose is twofold:

- To assess the patient for injuries
- To collect evidence for forensic evaluation and proceedings

Usually, someone with special training, such as a nurse practitioner who has taken special courses, examines a rape or sexual assault victim. Generalist nurses may be involved in treating the injuries that result from the assault, including genital trauma, such as vaginal and anal lacerations, and extragenital trauma, such as injury to the mouth, throat, wrists, arms, breasts, and thighs (Sheridan, 2004).

KEY INTERVENTIONS
Nursing intervention to prevent short- or long-term psychopathology after sexual assault is crucial. Psychological trauma following rape and sexual assault includes immediate anxiety and distress and the development of PTSD,

depression, panic, and substance abuse (Resnick, Acierno, Holmes, Kilpatrick, & Jager, 1999).

Key interventions include

- Early treatment because initial levels of distress are strongly related to later levels of PTSD, panic, and anxiety (Resnick et al., 1999).
- Supportive, caring, and nonjudgmental nursing interventions during the forensic rape examination are also crucial. This examination often increases survivors' immediate distress because they must recount the assault in detail and submit to an invasive pelvic or anal examination.
- Anxiety-reducing education, counselling, and emotional support, particularly in regard to unwanted pregnancies and sexually transmitted diseases, including HIV. All survivors should be tested for these possibilities. Treatment may include terminating a pregnancy; administering medications to treat gonorrhoea, chlamydia, trichomoniasis, and syphilis; and administering medications that may decrease the likelihood of contracting HIV infection.
- Interventions that are helpful for survivors of domestic violence; these also apply to the survivors of sexual assault.

nurses must be familiar with medications used to treat mood and anxiety disorders and the side effects of these drugs. Medications may be contraindicated for young and elderly survivors.

The autonomic nervous system is involved in many of the symptoms of depression and PTSD. Therefore, the use of agents that decrease its activity, such as the benzodiazepines, β-blockers, and antidepressants, can help treat these symptoms (Friedman, 2001; Sutherland & Davidson, 1999). Tricyclics and other antidepressants are effective in treating depression and some symptoms of PTSD, such as nightmares, sleep disorders, and startle reactions. They are less effective in treating other PTSD symptoms, such as numbing (Friedman; Sutherland & Davidson). The benzodiazepines are useful in treating anxiety and sleep disturbances in PTSD, but because they can cause dependence, they are contraindicated in women who also have a substance abuse disorder.

Approved for treating PTSD, the selective serotonin reuptake inhibitor (SSRI) sertraline (Zoloft) has improved PTSD symptoms in women but not in men (Henney, 2000; see Chapters 19 and 20 for information on monitoring medications and their side effects).

Managing Care of Patients With Comorbid Substance Abuse.

Survivors who have a comorbid substance abuse disorder need referral to a treatment centre for alcohol and drug disorders. The treatment centre should have programs that address the special needs of survivors. Alcohol-dependent and drug-dependent survivors frequently stop treatment and return to alcohol and drug abuse if their abuse-related problems are not addressed appropriately (Boyd, 2000; Ouimette, Moos, & Brown, 2003). As might be expected, research findings suggest that attitudes, such as self-blame and stigmatization, seem to be important variables related to substance abuse for women with a history of childhood sexual abuse (Dufour & Nadeau, 2001).

Survivors, especially those with substance abuse problems, are at high risk for HIV infection and AIDS. If women do not know their HIV status, they should be encouraged to get tested. Those with positive test results should receive counselling and begin taking appropriate medications. Those without HIV need to be taught about the high-risk behaviours for HIV infection and how to protect themselves from contracting HIV infection.

Psychological Domain

Psychological Assessment

A mental status evaluation should be part of every health assessment. Symptoms such as anhedonia, difficulties concentrating, feelings of worthlessness or guilt, and thoughts of death or suicide suggest depression or PTSD. A thorough assessment of suicidal intent is crucial.

Nursing Diagnoses for the Psychological Domain

Selected nursing diagnoses focusing on the human responses that nurses manage in the psychological domain may include ineffective coping, hopelessness, chronic low self-esteem, anxiety, risk for self-directed violence, and risk for other-directed violence.

Interventions for the Psychological Domain

Assisting With Psychotherapy for Counselling. Psychotherapy may include individual, group, family, or marital therapy. Only psychiatric nurse specialists at the master's or doctoral levels who have had training in these therapeutic methods may conduct psychotherapy. In addition, the nurse therapist should have training in conducting therapy specifically with survivors of abuse. That training should include care of PTSD, DID, depression, and substance abuse. The goals of the therapy are to integrate the patient's traumatic memories with the remainder of the patient's personal history and identity, manage painful affect, and restructure the meaning of the traumatic experiences (Wilson, 2001). The ultimate goal is for the survivor to integrate the trauma in memory as a past event that no longer has the power to terrorize.

Family or marital therapy may be unwise unless the perpetrator of abuse has obtained therapy for himself or herself and demonstrated change. Otherwise, survivors are placed in a very difficult situation. If they disclose abuse in family or marital therapy, perpetrators may retaliate with violence, but if they do not disclose the abuse, the crucial issue will not be addressed (Landenburger et al., 2004).

Several issues must be addressed for all survivors in psychotherapy or counselling (Campbell et al., 2004). All nurses can implement these interventions, using skills appropriate to their educational level and training. Nurses must address the guilt, shame, and stigmatization that survivors experience. They can approach these issues in several ways. Assisting survivors to verbalize their experience in an accepting, nonjudgmental atmosphere is the first step. Nurses must challenge directly attributions of self-blame for the abuse and feelings of being dirty and different. Helping survivors to identify their strengths and validating thoughts and feelings may help to increase self-esteem. An anonymous case report by a nursing student describes the importance of therapy for nurses who have a history of childhood sexual abuse in promoting their own healing journey and ultimately their capacity to help others (Anonymous, 1998).

Working With Children. Children may need to learn a "violence vocabulary" that allows them to talk about their abuse and assign responsibility for abusive behaviour. Children also need to learn that violence is not okay, and it is not their fault (Berman et al., 2004). Allowing children to discuss their abuse in the safety of a supportive, caring relationship may alleviate anxiety and fear (Berman et al.).

Reenacting the abuse through play is another technique that may be helpful in assisting children to express and work through their anxiety and fear. Play therapy uses dolls, human or animal figures, or puppets to work through anxieties or fears (Hill, 2003). Other techniques used with children to reduce fear include reading stories about recovery from abusive experiences (literal or metaphoric), using art or music to express feelings, and psychodrama. In addition, teaching strategies to manage fear and anxiety, such as relaxation techniques, coping skills, and imagery, may give the child an added sense of mastering his or her fear (Barnett et al., 1997). In a comprehensive review of child maltreatment literature, MacMillian (2000) indicates that research supports the use of abuse-specific cognitive-behavioural therapy as a treatment to improve the outcome for school-aged children.

Managing Anger. Anger and rage are part of the healing process for survivors (Walker, 1994). Expression of intense anger is uncomfortable for many nurses. However, they should expect anger expression and develop comfortable ways to respond. Moreover, an important nursing intervention is teaching and modelling anger expression appropriately. Inappropriate expressions of anger might drive supportive people away. Anger management techniques include appropriately recognizing and labelling anger and expressing it assertively, rather than aggressively or passive-aggressively. Assertive ways of expressing anger include owning the feeling by using "I feel" statements and avoiding blaming others. Teaching anger management and conflict resolution may be especially important for children who have seen nothing but violence to resolve problems (Lowenthal, 2001).

Teaching Skills and Clarifying Identity. Other nursing interventions include teaching self-protection skills, healthy relationship skills, and healthy sexuality. Again, this teaching may be especially important for children who have no role models for healthy relationships. Children also need to know what constitutes controlling and abusive behaviour and how to get help for abuse.

Children who have been sexually abused may become confused about their sexuality. They may regard sex as dirty and as something that can be used against other people. Discussions about healthy sexuality and feelings about sex may help these children regain a healthy perspective on sex-related matters (Peled, Jaffe, & Edleson, 1995).

Group therapy with survivors offers a powerful method to counter self-denigrating beliefs and to confront issues of secrecy and stigmatization (Urbancic, 2004). Moreover, one of the therapeutic factors in group therapy—universality, or the discovery that others have had similar experiences—may be a tremendous relief, especially to child survivors.

Providing Education. Education is a key nursing intervention for survivors. As appropriate to age or condition, survivors must understand the cycle of violence and the danger of homicide that increases as violence escalates or the survivor attempts to leave the relationship. Survivors also need information about resources, such as shelters for battered women, legal services, government benefits, and support networks (CNA, 1992; Walker, 1994). Before giving the survivor any written material, the nurse must discuss the possibility that if the perpetrator were to find the information in the survivor's possession, he or she might use it as an excuse for battering.

Survivors also need education appropriate for age and cognitive ability about the symptoms of anxiety, depression, dissociation, and PTSD. They must understand that these symptoms are common in anyone who has sustained significant stressors and are not signs of being "crazy" or weak. If survivors require medications for these symptoms, they must know how to monitor symptoms so that the effectiveness of pharmacologic management can be determined (Box 37-6).

One of the most important teaching goals is to help survivors develop a safety plan (CNA, 1992; Walker, 1994). The first step in developing such a plan is helping the survivor recognize the signs of danger. Changes in tone of voice, drinking and drug use, and increased criticism may indicate that the perpetrator is losing control. Detecting early warning signs helps survivors to escape before battering begins (Campbell et al., 2004; Urbancic, 2004; Walker).

The next step is to devise an escape route (CNA, 1992; Walker, 1994). This involves mapping the house and identifying where the battering usually occurs and what exits are available. The survivor needs to have a bag packed and hidden, but readily accessible, that has what is needed to get away. Important things to pack are clothes, a set of car and house keys, bank account numbers, birth certificate, insurance policies and numbers, marriage license, valuable jewelry, important telephone numbers, and money (CNA; Walker). The survivor must carefully hide the bag so that the perpetrator cannot find it and use it as an excuse for assault. If children are involved, the adult survivor should make arrangements

BOX **37.6**

BOX 37.6

Psychoeducation Checklist: Abuse

When caring for the patient who has been abused, be sure to address the following topics in the teaching plan:

- Cycle of violence
- Access to shelters
- Legal services
- Government benefits
- Support network
- Symptoms of anxiety, dissociation, and PTSD
- Safety or escape plan
- Relaxation
- Adequate nutrition and exercise
- Sleep hygiene
- HIV testing/counselling

to get them out safely. That might include arranging a signal to indicate when it is safe for them to leave the house and to meet at a prearranged place (Walker). A safety plan for a child or dependent elder might include safe places to hide and important telephone numbers, including 911 and those of the police and fire departments and other family members and friends.

Finding Strength and Hope. Providing hope and a sense of control is important for survivors of trauma (Campbell et al., 2004). Nurses can help survivors find hope and view themselves as survivors by assisting them to identify specific strengths and aspects of their lives that are under their control. This type of intervention may empower women to find options to remaining in an abusive relationship. The research by Ford-Gilboe et al. (2005) indicates that women were able to promote the health of their families after leaving an abusive partner, offering hope and a means of understanding for nurses working with women who are struggling to find the strength to choose health.

Using Behavioural Interventions. Treatment for depression, anxiety, and PTSD symptoms can be divided into two categories: exposure therapy and anxiety management training (Rothbaum & Foa, 1996). Only professionals trained in exposure therapy techniques can use them; however, nurses need to be familiar with this approach. The goal of exposure therapy, which includes flooding and systematic desensitization, is to promote the processing of the traumatic memory by exposing the survivor to the traumatic event through memories or some cue that reactivates trauma memories. Through repeated exposure, the event loses its ability to cause intense anxiety (Coffey, Dansky, & Brady, 2003).

Coping With Anxiety. Anxiety management is a crucial intervention for all survivors. There is a high comorbidity among trauma, PTSD, and anxiety disorders (Orsillo et al., 2002). During treatment, survivors will experience situations and memories that provoke intense anxiety and must know how to soothe themselves when they experience painful feelings. Moreover, most survivors struggle with control issues, especially involving their bodies. Anxiety management skills offer one way to maintain some control over their bodies (Lundberg-Love, 1997).

Anxiety management training may include progressive relaxation, deep breathing, imagery techniques, and cognitive restructuring. Progressive relaxation entails systematically tensing and then relaxing the major muscle groups. Visualization consists of imagining a scene that is especially relaxing (e.g., spending a day at the beach), while practicing relaxation and deep breathing. Any interventions that reduce dysphoric symptoms can help survivors feel more in control of their situation.

Anxiety disorders, including PTSD and depression, are associated with cognitive distortions that cognitive therapy techniques can challenge (Zust, 2000). Self-defeating thoughts in anxiety disorders involve perceptions of threat and danger, and those in depression involve negative self-perceptions (Blackburn & Davidson, 1990). Nurses can teach survivors how to identify and challenge these self-defeating thought patterns. Cognitive therapy techniques may be especially useful in helping survivors to stop blaming themselves for their abuse.

Nurses must become accustomed to measuring gains in small steps when working with survivors. Making any changes in significant relationships has serious consequences, and it can be done only when the adult survivor is ready. Carter-Snell and Hegadoren (2003) point out that women are frequently the primary caregiver and, as such, may have limited resources to devout to therapy. Therefore, the context of each individual woman's life needs to be kept in mind. It is easy for nurses to become angry or discouraged, and they must be careful not to communicate these feelings to survivors (Campbell et al., 2004; Urbancic, 2004). Discussing such feelings with other staff provides a way of dealing with them appropriately. In such discussions with supervisors or other staff members, the nurse must protect the patient's confidentiality by discussing feelings around issues, not particular patients. The nurse should frame the discussion in such a way that individual patients cannot be identified.

Social Domain

Social Assessment

An evaluation of social networks and daily activities may provide additional clues of psychological abuse and controlling behaviour (Gary & Humphreys, 2004;

Wallace, 1999). When a nurse assesses social isolation, evaluating the reasons behind it is crucial. Many perpetrators isolate their family from all social contacts, including other relatives. Some survivors isolate themselves because they are ashamed of the abuse or fear nonsupportive responses. An evaluation of social support is important for other reasons. Having supportive family or friends is crucial in short-term planning for developing a safety plan and is also important to long-term recovery. A survivor cannot leave an abusive situation if she has nowhere to go. Supportive family and friends may be willing to provide shelter and safety.

Nurses can assess restrictions on freedom that may suggest abuse and control by asking such questions as "Are you free to go where you want?"; "Is staying home your choice?"; and "Is there anything that you would like to do that you cannot?"

The degree of dependency on the relationship is another important variable to assess. Women who have young children and are economically dependent on the perpetrator may feel that they cannot leave the abusive relationship. Those who are emotionally dependent on the perpetrator may experience an intense grief reaction that further complicates their leaving (Campbell et al., 2004; Wallace, 1999). Elders and children are often dependent on the abuser and cannot leave the abusive situation without alternatives.

Nursing Diagnoses for the Social Domain

Selected nursing diagnoses focusing on the human responses that nurses manage in the social domain may include hopelessness, powerlessness, and ineffective role performance.

Interventions for the Social Domain

Working With Abusive Families. Family interventions in cases of child abuse focus on behavioural approaches to improve parenting skills (Gary & Humphreys, 2004). A behavioural approach has multiple components. *Child management skills* help parents manage maladaptive behaviours and reward appropriate behaviours. *Parenting skills* teach parents how to be more effective and nurturing with their children. *Leisure skills* training is important to reduce stress in the household and promote healthy family time. *Household organization* training is another way to reduce stress by teaching effective ways to manage the multiple tasks that families have to perform. Such tasks include meal planning, cooking, shopping, keeping physician's appointments, and planning family activities (Gary & Humphreys).

Anger control and stress management skills are important parts of behavioural programs for families.

Anger control programs teach parents to identify events that increase anger and stress and to replace anger-producing thoughts with more appropriate ones. Parents learn self-control skills to reduce the expression of uncontrolled anger. Stress-reduction techniques include relaxation techniques and methods for coping with stressful interactions with their children (Lowenthal, 2001). These skills may be especially important in families in which elder abuse is occurring. Both caregivers and abused elders may need to learn assertive ways to express their anger and healthy ways to manage their stress. Helping caregivers find ways to get some relief from their caregiving burdens may be crucial in reducing abuse that comes from exhaustion in trying to manage multiple roles. Examples might be to identify agencies that offer respite care or agencies that offer day care for elders and support groups in which caregivers can share experiences and gain support from others dealing with similar issues.

Working in the Community. Nurses may be involved in interventions to reduce violence at the community level. Many abusive parents and battered women are socially isolated. Assistance in developing support networks may help reduce stress and, therefore, reduce abuse. Community contacts vary for each survivor but might include crisis hot lines, support groups, and education classes (Gary & Humphreys, 2004).

Community health nurses may play a vital role in the detection, treatment, and referral of child sexual abuse (Blakeley & Ribeiro, 1997). Specifically, nurses may make home visits to abusive parents. Home visits provide support to families and provide them with knowledge about child development and management (Barnett et al., 1997). Abuse of any kind is a volatile situation, and nurses may place themselves or the survivor in danger if they make home visits. Nurses should carefully assess this possibility before proceeding. If necessary, the nurse and the adult survivor may need to arrange a safe place to meet.

Spiritual Domain

Although abuse and violence can devastate one's understanding of life and one's relationship with the sacred, spirituality can be a source of great strength. It can be a significant personal coping resource (Humphreys, 2000). A spiritual response to violence and abuse begins with a sense of connection to a higher power (or with an attempt to connect) that allows a healing journey to begin (Knapik, Martsolf, & Draucker, 2008). Some individuals find that the struggle to recover and rebuild after abuse has made them stronger; it has helped them to grow spiritually, to have greater self-acceptance, and to express greater compassion towards others (Wright, Crawford, & Sebastian, 2007). For many individuals, however, abuse shatters any sense of a just, benevolent, and meaningful world. It becomes incredibly challenging for them to evolve a new sense of personal spirituality.

When abuse is perpetrated by a religious leader, it can be particularly devastating. The person is violated spirituality as well as physically (Guido, 2008). Women sexually abused by members of the clergy have described their survival as involving a reorientation away from structured traditional religious practice toward a form of spirituality that is more relationally grounded (Flynn, 2008).

Nurses and other health professionals have, in the past, tended to focus primarily on the bio/psycho/social domains of patients who have been abused. It is important to understand how spirituality affects both the impact of abuse and the healing from it (Pargament, Murray-Swank, & Mahoney, 2008). Such understanding can inform discussions with patients about spirituality and can point to ways of support for patients who want to explore spirituality as a means of healing (Knapik, Martsolf & Draucker, 2008). Nurses can offer patients an environment in which spiritual concerns can be expressed and compassionate responses expected (Humphreys, 2000).

▪ EVALUATION AND TREATMENT OUTCOMES

Evaluation and outcome criteria depend on the setting for interventions. For instance, if the nurse encounters a survivor in the ED, successful outcomes might be that injuries are appropriately managed and the patient's immediate safety is ensured. For long-term care, outcome criteria and evaluation might centre on ending abusive relationships. Examples of other outcome criteria that would indicate successful nursing intervention are recognizing that one is not to blame for the violence, demonstrating knowledge of strengths and coping skills, and reestablishing social networks.

The evaluation of nursing care for abused children depends on attaining goals mutually set with the parents. An end to all violence is the optimal outcome criterion; however, attainment of smaller goals indicates progress toward that end. Outcomes such as increased problem-solving and communication skills within the family, increased self-esteem in both children and parents, and increased use of nonphysical forms of discipline may all indicate progress toward the total elimination of child abuse.

Follow-up efforts are important in evaluating the outcomes of elder abuse. The optimal outcome is to end all abuse and keep the elderly person in his or her own living environment, if appropriate. Although the abuse may have been resolved temporarily, it may flare up again. Ongoing support for the caregiver and assistance with caregiving tasks may be necessary if the elder person is to remain at home. Nursing home or assisted living may be the most desirable option if the burden is too great for the family and the likelihood of ongoing abuse or neglect is high.

Another important outcome of nursing intervention with survivors is appropriate treatment of any disorder resulting from abuse (e.g., ASD, PTSD and other anxiety disorders, DID, major depression, substance abuse). Follow-up nursing assessments should monitor symptom reduction or exacerbation, adherence to any medication regimen, and side effects of medication. The ultimate outcome is to end violence and enable the survivor to return to a more productive, safe, and nurturing life without being continually haunted by memories of the abuse.

Treatment for the Batterer

Participants in programs that treat batterers are usually there because the court has mandated the treatment. Programs are often outpatient groups that meet weekly for an extended period of time, often 36 to 48 weeks. Some advocate longer programs, believing that chronic offenders require 1 to 5 years of treatment to change abusive behaviour.

Groups often use cognitive-behavioural techniques or a psychoeducational, skill-building approach (Healey, Smith, & O'Sullivan, 1998). This approach offers the batterer tools that help him see that his violent acts are not uncontrollable outbursts but rather foreseeable behaviour patterns that he can learn to interrupt. Cognitive-behavioural interventions target three elements: (1) what the batterer thinks about just before a battering incident; (2) the batterer's physical and emotional responses to these thoughts; and (3) what the batterer does that progresses to violence (e.g., yelling, throwing things). The group teaches members to recognize and interrupt negative feelings about their partners and to reduce physiologic arousal through relaxation techniques.

Psychoeducational topics are often similar to those covered by the Duluth Curriculum, which is a model program. Topics may include nonviolence; nonthreatening behaviour; respect; support and trust; honesty and accountability; sexual respect; and partnership, negotiation, and fairness. Other programs also offer more in-depth counselling, arguing that psychoeducational approaches do not address the true problem (Healey et al., 1998). If the problem were simply a deficit in skills, the batterer would be dysfunctional in work or relationships outside the family. Batterers need resocialization that convinces them that they do not have the right to abuse their partners. Other programs add a moral aspect by taking a value-laden approach against violence and confronting the batterer's behaviour as unacceptable and illegal.

Accountability for violent acts is an important early goal in treating batterers (Healey et al., 1998). Most batterers deny responsibility for their actions and refuse to look at battering as a choice. Therefore, it is important that batterers become accountable for their actions. Interventions aim at getting the batterer to acknowledge his violence across the full range of abusive acts that he has committed, for example, verbal abuse, intimidation, controlling behaviour, and sexual abuse. Batterers may use several tactics to avoid accountability, and all must be addressed. Those tactics include denying the abuse ever happened ("I never touched her"); minimizing the abuse by downplaying the violent acts or underestimating its effects ("It was just a slap" or "she bruises easily"); and blaming the abuse on the victim ("she pushed me too far"), alcohol or other drugs ("I was high"), or other life circumstances ("I had too many pressures at work").

A recent qualitative study conducted in Nova Scotia of six group facilitators engaged in providing programs to men who batter revealed the many complexities of providing effective treatment for these men (Augusta-Scott & Dankwort, 2002). Discussions with the group facilitators suggested that a form of narrative therapy, in which the men were invited to discover what would be personally meaningful about engaging in treatment, might be a necessary prerequisite to effective treatment (Augusta-Scott & Dankwort).

Because batterers typically minimize or deny their violent behaviour, it is often necessary to interview the survivor to gain a complete picture of the batterer's behaviour. A trained victim advocate usually contacts partners. There are other reasons for contacting partners. This may be the first contact the partner has had with professionals, and she may benefit by telling her story. Many partners do not know that services are available to them, and this is an opportunity to tell her what is available. In addition, advocates often explain the batterer program and emphasize that it takes a long time and requires the batterer to take responsibility for his violent behaviour. Partners need to hear that many batterers are not willing to change their behaviour. Another important point that partners need to know and discuss with professionals is that batterers often use entry into treatment as a justification for pressuring partners to remain in the relationship, but that this behaviour is a good indicator that abuse will continue.

There are four points in treating batterers when it is essential to contact the partner for safety reasons: (1) when the batterer begins attending the program; (2) if and when he is terminated from treatment for noncompliance; (3) when he has completed treatment; and (4) if he is an imminent threat to the partner's safety (Healey et al., 1998).

Batterer intervention must be culturally competent (Healey et al., 1998). Many factors can affect violence against women, including socioeconomic status, racial or ethnic identity, country of origin, and sexual orientation, and those differences must be addressed. Another factor that must be addressed is AOD use. Intervention programs may require batterers to undergo substance abuse treatment concurrently, and batterers are required to remain sober and submit to random drug testing.

Treatment programs alone are not sufficient to stop many batterers (Healey et al., 1998). To be effective, programs must operate within a comprehensive intervention effort that includes criminal justice support. The criminal justice response includes arrest, incarceration, adjudication, and probation supervision that includes issuing a warrant if the batterer does not attend the batterer program or supervision. The combination of criminal justice response and batterer treatment may convey a more powerful message to the batterer about the seriousness of his actions than a batterer program alone. Unfortunately, many offenders never show up for batterer intervention, and arrests for violation of probation may be rare because of overload and staffing shortages. Inaction by the criminal justice system is serious; it sends the message that there is little concern for violence against women and that batterers can get away with it. Several approaches to batterer intervention are controversial (Healey et al.).

Anger management attributes battering to out-of-control anger and teaches anger management techniques. There are several arguments against this approach. It does not address the real issue—batterers' desire to control their partners. Batterers are able to control their behaviour in other difficult situations but choose anger and intimidation to control their partners. Anger management may merely teach batterers nonviolent methods to exert control. Couples counselling may endanger the survivor. Women will not be free to disclose, and any disclosures may give the batterer reason to retaliate. Self-help groups modelled on Alcoholics Anonymous are inappropriate for initial intervention for several reasons. Without trained facilitators who will confront denial and excuses, batterers may never accept accountability for their violence. On the other hand, an untrained facilitator may use an excessively confrontational approach that is abusive and models antagonistic behaviour.

How effective is batterer treatment? Results from an extended follow-up of court-ordered batterer intervention programs show that many men continue to be assaultive during or on completion of treatment. Based on partners' reports, 32% had reassaulted their partners by 15 months after treatment, 38% had done so by 30 months, and 42% had done so at 48 months. Twenty-five percent of the men repeatedly reassaulted their partners through 48 months of follow-up. However, the results did show that reassaults de-escalated somewhat with time (Gondolf, 2001).

SUMMARY OF KEY POINTS

▢   The abuse of women, men, children, and elders is a national health problem that requires awareness and sensitivity from nurses.

▢   The abuse of women may be physical, emotional and psychological, or social.

▢   Child abuse may be neglectful, physical, sexual, or emotional. Other forms of child abuse include Munchausen's syndrome by proxy and witnessing abuse of their mothers or significant caregivers.

▢   The abuse of Aboriginal children in residential schools was particularly harmful because these children were segregated from their families and communities, frequently for years at a time.

▢   Elder abuse may be physical, emotional, neglectful, or financial.

▢   Among the many theories that have been proposed to explain abuse are psychopathology, social learning, sociologic, feminist, neurobiologic, BPD, and substance abuse.

▢   A well-documented cycle of violence consists of three phases of increasing frequency and severity.

▢   Child abuse leaves many scars that can lead to such problems in adulthood as depression, anxiety, self-destructive behaviour, poor self-esteem, and lack of trust.

▢   Responses to abuse include depression, ASD, PTSD, and DID.

▢   Nurses need to be familiar with the signs and symptoms of abuse and to be vigilant when assessing patients.

▢   Nurses can help victims of abuse to view themselves as survivors.

CRITICAL THINKING CHALLENGES

1   Abuse is a pervasive problem, and anyone can be a victim (women, men, children, elders, gays, lesbians). Why do so few nursing units and nurses make it a routine to ask questions about abuse?

2   Abuse is not just a "women's issue." The prevalence of abuse might decrease if men make it a "men's issue" as well. What is preventing this from happening?

3   What are your thoughts and feelings about women who are victims of abuse in which both partners (victim and perpetrator) abuse AOD?

4   What are your thoughts and feelings about women who will not leave an abusive relationship?

5   What are some reasons that women remain in abusive relationships?

6   Why do some women become involved in more than one abusive relationship?

7   How do you handle your feelings toward abusive parents or relatives who abuse elders?

8   What are the issues in mandatory reporting of violence toward women, particularly violence that occurs in the home?

WEB LINKS

www.phac-aspc.gc.ca/ncfv-cnivf/familyviolence/ refer_e.html   The National Clearinghouse on Family Violence (NCFV) is Canada's national resource centre for information about family violence. The NCFV collects, develops, and disseminates resources on prevention, protection, and treatment. By increasing awareness, the NCFV encourages Canadian communities to become involved in reducing the occurrence of family violence. This website includes provincial, national, local, and international links.

www.hc-sc.gc.ca/   The website of the Canada Health Portal, a public health agency of Canada, provides a listing of services and programs to meet the needs of older adult victims of violence in Canada. Two hundred and eighty programs and services are listed by province, from the east to the west coast.

www.canada.justice.gc.ca   The website of the Department of Justice, Canada, provides a comprehensive overview of violence in Canada, including family violence, spousal abuse, child abuse, abuse of older adults, and dating violence. The site includes Canadian statistics, relevant literature, and policies and legal implications, as well as links to additional sites.

www.cnpea.ca/   The web site of the Canadian Network for the Prevention of Elder Abuse, providing information about issues related to abuse and neglect in later life, and the strategies being used to address them.

MOVIES, NOVELS, AND BIOGRAPHIES

Marion Bridge: 2002. Winner of the 2002 best Canadian film at the Toronto International Film Festival, Marion Bridge is the story of Agnes' return home to the Maritimes to help care for her dying mother. The audience shares the tension as family secrets emerge and Agnes and her two sisters, Theresa and Louise, struggle with their past and present.

VIEWING POINTS: What are the ways that the members of this family have used to cope with the abuse in their lives? What does their story reveal about both positive and negative ways of coping? Do you think that ideal images of love, such as the one Agnes treasured in the song, "Marion Bridge," are helpful or harmful?

Once Were Warriors: 1994. A mother of five reevaluates her 18-year marriage to her alcoholic, hot-tempered husband when his barroom violence tragically encroaches into their home life. Produced and filmed in New Zealand, this film also presents how urbanization has undermined the culture and strength of the indigenous Maori people.

VIEWING POINTS: What evidence can you find in this film that may reflect intergenerational transmission of violence? In what ways do you think that culture can influence attitudes toward abuse (both positive and negative)? What are positive and negative cultural influences in this film?

Loyalties: 1987. In this critically acclaimed movie set in Alberta, the friendship between an English physician's wife and her children's Aboriginal "nanny" sets the scene for a conflict of loyalties. This story captures well the shame, hope, and fear of a family living with a dark secret.

VIEWING POINTS: Consider the alternative ways in which the situation of these two families could have evolved differently. What factors influence the outcome of such a situation?

REFERENCES

Abbey, A., Zawacki, T., Buck, P., Clinton, A., & McAuslan, P. (2003). Sexual assault and alcohol consumption. What do we know about their relationship and what types of research are needed? *Aggression & Violent Behaviour,* 277, 1–33.

Allan, M. A. (1998). Elder abuse: A challenge for home care nurses. *Home Health Care Nurse,* 16(2), 103–110.

Alvi, S., & Selbee, K. (1997). Dating status variations and woman abuse: A test of the dependence, availability and deterrence (DAD) model. *Violence Against Women,* 3(6), 610–628.

American Psychiatric Association. (1987). *Diagnostic and statistical manual of mental disorders* (3rd ed., Revised.). Washington, DC: Author.

American Psychiatric Association. (2000). *Diagnostic and statistical manual of mental disorders* (4th ed., Text revision). Washington, DC: Author.

Anderson, D. K., & Saunders, D. G. (2003). Leaving an abusive partner: An empirical review of predictors, the process of leaving, and psychological well-being. *Trauma, Violence, & Abuse,* 4(2), 163–191.

Anderson, G., Yasenik, L., & Ross, C. A. (1993). Dissociative experiences and disorders among women who identify themselves as sexual abuse survivors. *Child Abuse and Neglect,* 17(5), 677–686.

Anonymous. (1998). Battling back from childhood sexual abuse and surviving the journey. *Journal of Psychosocial Nursing & Mental Health Services,* 36(12), 13–17.

Arata, C. M. (2002). Child sexual abuse and sexual revictimization. *Clinical Psychological: Science and Practice,* 9, 135–164.

Augusta-Scott, T., & Dankwort, J. (2002). Partner abuse groups interventions: Lessons from educational and narrative therapy approaches. *Journal of Interpersonal Violence,* 17(7), 783–805.

Bandura, A. (1977). *Social learning theory.* New York, NY: General Learning Press.

Banister, E. M., Jakubec, S. L., & Stein, J. A. (2003). "Like what am I supposed to do?" Adolescent girls' health concerns in their dating relationships. *Canadian Journal of Nursing Research,* 35(2), 16–33.

Barnett, O. W., Miller-Perrin, C. L., & Perrin, R. D. (1997). *Family violence across the lifespan: An introduction.* Thousand Oaks, CA: Sage.

Bartsch, C., Risse, M., Schutz, H., Weigand, N., & Weiler, G. (2003). Munchausen syndrome by proxy (MSBP): An extreme form of child abuse with a special forensic challenge. *Forensic Science International,* 137(2–3), 147–151.

Berman, H., Hardesty, J., & Humphreys, J. C. (2004). Children of abused women. In J. C. Campbell & J. C. Humphreys (Eds.), *Family violence and nursing practice* (pp. 160–185). Philadelphia, PA: Lippincott Williams & Wilkins.

Blackburn, I., & Davidson, K. (1990). *Cognitive therapy for depression and anxiety.* Boston, MA: Blackwell Scientific Publications.

Blakeley, J., & Ribeiro, V. (1997). Community health and pediatric nurses' knowledge, attitudes, and behaviors regarding child sexual abuse. *Public Health Nursing,* 14(6), 339–345.

Bograd, M. (1999). Strengthening domestic violence theories: Intersections of race, class, sexual orientation, and gender. *Journal of Marital and Family Therapy,* 25(3), 275–289.

Boyd, M. R. (2000). Predicting substance abuse and comorbidity in rural women. *Archives of Psychiatric Nursing,* 14(2), 64–72.

Boyd, M. R. (2003). Vulnerability to alcohol and other drug disorders in rural women. *Archives of Psychiatric Nursing,* 17(1), 33–41.

Boyd, M. R., & Mackey, M. (2000a). Alienation from self and others: The psychosocial problem of rural alcoholic women. *Archives of Psychiatric Nursing,* 14(3), 134–141.

Boyd, M. R., & Mackey, M. (2000b). Running away to nowhere: Rural women's experience of becoming alcohol dependent. *Archives of Psychiatric Nursing,* 14(3), 142–149.

Brady, K. T., & Dansky, B. S. (2002). Effects of victimization and posttraumatic stress disorder on substance use disorders in women. In F. L. Hall, T. S. Williams, J. A. Panetta, & J. M. Herrera (Eds.), *Psychiatric illnesses in women* (pp. 449–466). Washington, DC: American Psychiatric Publishing.

Braitstein, P., Li, K., Tyndall, M., Spittal, P., O'Shaughnessy, M., Schilder, A., Johnston, C., Hogg, R. S., & Schechfer, M. T. (2003). Sexual violence among a cohort of injection drug users. *Social Science & Medicine,* 57(3), 561–570.

Breitenbecher, K. H. (2001). Sexual victimization among women: A review of the literature focusing on empirical investigations. *Aggression and Violent Behavior,* 6, 415–432.

Bremner, J. D., Narayan, M., Staib, L. H., Southwick, S. M., McGlashan, T., & Charney, D. S. (1999). Neural correlates of memories of childhood sexual abuse in women with and without posttraumatic stress disorder. *American Journal of Psychiatry,* 156, 1787–1795.

Bremner, J. D., Southwick, S. M., & Charney, D. S. (1999). The neurobiology of posttraumatic stress disorder: An integration of animal and human research. In P. A. Saigh & J. D. Bremner (Eds.), *Posttraumatic stress disorder: A comprehensive text.* Boston, MA: Allyn and Bacon.

Breslau, N., Davis, G. C., Andreski, P., Peterson, E. L. & Schultz, L. R. (1997). Sex differences in posttraumatic stress disorder. *Archives of General Psychiatry,* 54(11), 1044–1048.

Briere, J. N., & Elliott, D. M. (1994). Immediate and long-term impacts of child sexual abuse. *The Future of Children,* 4(2), 54–69.

Brown, P. J., Recupero, P. R., & Stout, R. (1995). PTSD substance abuse comorbidity and treatment utilization. *Addictive Behaviors,* 20, 251–254.

Campbell, J. C., & Lewandowski, L. A. (1997). Mental and physical effects of intimate partner violence on women and children. *Psychiatric Clinics of North America,* 20(2), 353–354.

Campbell, J. C., McKenna, L. S., Torres, S., Sheridan, D. & Landenburger, K. (1993). Nursing care of abused women. In J. C. Campbell & J. C. Humphreys (Eds.), *Nursing care of survivors of family violence* (pp. 248–289). St. Louis, MO: Mosby.

Campbell, J. C., Torres, S., McKenna, L. S., Sheridan, D. J., & Landenburger, K. (2004). Nursing care of survivors of intimate partner violence. In J. C. Campbell & J. C. Humphreys (Eds.), *Family violence and nursing practice* (pp. 307–360). Philadelphia, PA: Lippincott Williams & Wilkins.

Canadian Centre for Justice Statistics. (2005). *Family violence in Canada: A statistical profile 2005.* Ottawa, ON: Statistics Canada.

Canadian Centre for Justice Statistics. (2009). *Family violence in Canada: A statistical profile 2009.* Ottawa, ON: Statistics Canada.

Canadian Nurses Association. (1992). *Family violence clinical guidelines for nurses.* Ottawa, ON: National Clearing House on Family Violence.

Carlson, E. B., & Putnam, F. W. (1993). An update on the Dissociative Experiences Scale. *Dissociation,* 6(1), 16–27.

Carter-Snell C., & Hegadoren K. (2003). Stress disorders and gender: Implications for theory and research. *Canadian Journal of Nursing Research,* 35(2), 34–55.

Cedar Project Partnership, Mehrabadi, A., Peterson, K., Pearce, M., Patel, S., Craub, K., Moniruzzaman, A., Schechter, M. & Spittal, P. (2008). Gender differences in HIV and Hepatitis C related vulnerabilities among Aboriginal young people who use street drugs in two Canadian cities. *Women & Health,* 48(3), 235–260.

Charney, D. S., Deutch, A. Y., Krystal, J. H., & Southwick, M. (1993). Psychobiologic mechanisms of posttraumatic stress disorder. *Archives of General Psychiatry, 50*(4), 294–305.

Chodorow, N. (1974). Family structure and feminine personality. In M. R. Rosaldo & L. Lamphere (Eds.), *Woman, culture, and society* (pp. 43–66). Stanford, CA: Stanford University Press.

Chrousos, G. P., & Gold, P. W. (1992). The concepts of stress and stress system disorders. *Journal of the American Medical Association, 267*(9), 1244–1252.

Clements, M., Oxtoby, C. & Ogle, R. L. (2008). Methodological issues in assessing psychological adjustment in child witnesses of intimate partner violence. *Trauma, Violence, & Abuse, 9*(2), 114–127.

Cloitre, M., Scarvalone, P., & Difede, J. (1997). Posttraumatic stress disorder, self- and interpersonal dysfunction among sexually retraumatized women. *Journal of Traumatic Stress, 10*(3), 437–452.

Coffey, S. F., Dansky, B. S., & Brady, K. T. (2003). Exposure-based, trauma-focused therapy for comorbid posttraumatic stress disorder-substance use disorder. In P. Ouimette & P. J. Brown (Eds.), *Trauma and substance abuse: Causes, consequences, and treatment of comorbid disorders* (pp. 127–146). Washington, DC: American Psychiatric Association.

Cohen, J. A., Perel, J. M., DeBellis, M. D., Friedman, M. J., & Putnam, F. W. (2002). Treating traumatized children: Clinical implications of the psychobiology of posttraumatic stress disorder. *Trauma, Violence, & Abuse, 3*(2), 91–108.

Collin-Vezina, D., & Hebert, M. (2005). Comparing dissociation and PTSD in sexually abused school-aged girls. *Journal of Nervous & Mental Disease, 193*(1), 47–52.

Collins, J. J., & Messerschmidt, P. M. (1993). Epidemiology of alcohol-related violence. *Alcohol Health and Research World, 17*(2), 93–100.

Collishaw, S., Pickles, A., Messer, J., Rutter, M., Shearer, C., & Maughan, B. (2007). Resilience to adult psychopathology following childhood maltreatment: Evidence from a community sample. *Child Abuse & Neglect, 31*(3), 211–229.

Comijs, H. C., Pot, A. M., Smit, J. H., Bouter, L. M., & Jonker, C. (1998). Elder abuse in the community: Prevalence and consequences. *Journal of the American Geriatric Society, 46*(7), 885–888.

Cook, R., & Dickens, B. (2009). Dilemmas in intimate partner violence. *International Journal of Gynecology & Obstetrics, 106*(1), 72–75.

Criminal Code of Canada, r.s.c. (1985). c–C-46, s/55.

DeKeseredy, W. S., & Schwartz, M. D. (1998). Woman abuse on campus: Results from the Canadian National Survey. London, UK: Thousand Oaks Sage Publications.

Department of Justice, Canada. (2003). *Child Abuse: A fact sheet from the Department of Justice*. Ottawa, ON: Author.

Department of Justice, Canada. (2005). *Abuse of older adults: A fact sheet from the Department of Justice*. Ottawa, ON: Author.

Dewey, J. (2004). Theories of aggression and family violence. In J. C. Campbell & J. C. Humphreys (Eds.), *Family violence and nursing practice* (pp. 3–28). Philadelphia, PA: Lippincott Williams & Wilkins.

Dufour, M. H., & Nadeau, L. (2001). Sexual abuse: A comparison between resilient victims and drug-addicted victims. *Violence and Victim, 16*(6), 655–672.

Du Mont, J., Macdonald, S., Rotbard, N., Asllani, E., Bainbridge, D., & Cohen, M.M. (2009). Factors associated with suspected drug-facilitated sexual assault. *CMAJ, 180*(5), 513–519.

Dutton, D. G. (1995). *The domestic assault of women*. Vancouver, BC: UBC Press.

Dutton, D. G. (1998). *The abusive personality*. New York, NY: Guilford.

Dutton, D. G., & Painter, S. (1993). Emotional attachments in abusive relationships: A test of traumatic bonding theory. *Violence and Victims, 8*(2), 105–120.

Emery, R. E., & Laumann-Billings, L. (1998). An overview of the nature, causes, and consequences of abusive family relationships: Toward differentiating maltreatment and violence. *American Psychologist, 53*(2), 121–135.

Fishwick, N. J., Campbell, J. C., & Taylor, J. Y. (2004). Theories of intimate partner violence. In J. C. Campbell & J. C. Humphreys (Eds.), *Family violence and nursing practice* (pp. 29–57). Philadelphia, PA: Lippincott Williams & Wilkins.

Flynn, K. (2008). In their own voices: Women who were sexually abused by members of the clergy. *Journal of Child Sexual Abuse, 17*(3–4), 216–237.

Ford-Gilboe, M., Wuest, J., & Merritt-Gray, M. (2005). Strengthening the capacity to limit intrusion: Theorizing family health promotion in the aftermath of women abuse. *Qualitative Health Research, 15*(4), 477–501.

Friedman, M. J. (2001). Allostatic versus empirical perspective in pharmacotherapy for PTSD. In J. P. Wilson, M. J. Friedman, & J. Lindy (Eds.), *Treating psychological trauma and PTSD* (pp. 94–124). New York, NY: Guilford.

Gallop, R., McCay, E., Austin, W., Bayer, M., & Peternelji-Taylor, C. (1998). Working with psychiatric clients who have been sexually abused. *Journal of the American Psychiatric Nursing Association, 4*, 9–17.

Gallop, R., McCay, E., Guha, M., & Khan. P. (1999). The experience of hospitalization and restraint of women who have a history of childhood sexual abuse. *Health Care Women International, 20*(4), 401–416.

Gary, F. A., Campbell, D. W., & Humphreys, J. (2004). Theories of child abuse. In J. C. Campbell & J. C. Humphreys (Eds.), *Family violence and nursing practice* (pp. 58–73). Philadelphia, PA: Lippincott Williams & Wilkins.

Gary, F. A., & Humphreys, J. C. (2004). Nursing care of abused children. In J. C. Campbell & J. C. Humphreys (Eds.), *Family violence and nursing practice* (pp. 252–287). Philadelphia, PA: Lippincott Williams & Wilkins.

Gilligan, C. (1982). In a different voice: Psychological theory and women's development. Cambridge, MA: Harvard University Press.

Girshick, L. B. (1993). *Teen dating violence. Violence update*. Thousand Oaks, CA: Sage.

Gold, N., & Auslander, G. (1999). Gender issues in newspaper coverage of people with disabilities: A Canada-Israel comparison. *Women and Health, 29*(4), 75–96.

Gondolf, E. W. (2001). *An extended follow-up of batterers and their partners*. Atlanta, GA: Centers for Disease Control and Prevention. Available at http://www.iup.edu

Gordon, R. M. (2001). Adult protection legislation in Canada: Models, issues, and problems. *International Journal of Law and Psychiatry. 24*(2–3), 117–134.

Guido, J. (2008). A unique betrayal: Clergy sexual abuse in the context of the Catholic religious tradition. *Journal of Child Sexual Abuse, 17*(3–4), 255–269.

Hana, E. Z., & Grant, B. F. (1997). Gender differences in DSM-IV alcohol use disorders and major depression as distributed in the general population: Clinical implications. *Comprehensive Psychiatry, 38*(4), 202–212.

Hanson, R. K., Cadsky, O., Harris A., & Lalonde, C. (1997). Correlates of battering among 997 men: Family history, adjustment and attitudinal differences. *Violence and Victims, 12*(3), 191–208.

Hattendorf, J., & Tollerud, T. R. (1997). Domestic violence: Counseling strategies that minimize the impact of secondary victimization. *Perspectives in Psychiatric Care, 33*(1), 14–23.

Healey, K., Smith, C., & O'Sullivan, C. (1998). *Batterer intervention: Program approaches and criminal justice strategies*. Washington, DC: U.S. Department of Justice, National Institute of Justice. Available at: http://www.ojp.usdoj.gov

Health Canada. (1998). *The consequences of child maltreatment: A reference guide for health practitioners*. Ottawa, ON: Family Violence Prevention Unit, Health Canada.

Health Canada. (2002). *Woman abuse: Information from the National Clearing House on family violence*. Ottawa, ON: Health Canada.

Henderson, A. (2001). Factors influencing nurses' responses to abused women: What they say they do and why they say they do it. *Journal of Interpersonal Violence, 16*(12), 1284–1306.

Henderson, A. J. Z., Bartholomew, K., & Dutton, D. G. (1997). He loves me; he loves me not: Attachment and separation resolution of abused women. *Journal of Family Violence, 12*(2), 169–191.

Hendricks-Matthews, M. K. (1993). Survivors of abuse: Health care issues. *Primary Care, 20*(2), 391–406.

Henney, J. E. (2000). Sertraline approved for posttraumatic stress disorder. *Journal of the American Medical Association, 283*(5), 596.

Henry, J. P. (1992). Biological basis of the stress response. *Integrative Physiological and Behavioral Science, 1*, 66–83.

Herman, J. (1997). *Trauma and recovery: The aftermath of violence-from domestic abuse to political terror*. New York, NY: Basic Books.

Hill, A. (2003). Issues facing brothers of sexually abused children: Implication for professional practice. *Child & Family Social Work, 8*(3), 281–291.

Hollingsworth, E., & Ford-Gilboe, M. (2006). Registered nurses' self-efficacy for assessing and responding to woman abuse in emergency department settings. *Canadian Journal of Nursing Research, 38*(4), 54–77.

Hotch, D., Grunfeld, A., Mackay, K., & Ritch, L. (1996). Policy and procedures for domestic violence patients in Canadian emergency departments: A national survey. *Journal of Emergency Nursing, 22*(4), 278–282.

Huckle, P. L. (1995). Male rape victims referred to a forensic psychiatric service. *Medicine Science & Law, 35*(3), 187–192.

Humphreys, J. (2000). Spirituality and distress in sheltered battered women. *Journal of Nursing Scholarship, 32*(3), 273–278.

Janssen, P. A., Holt, V. L., & Sugg, N. K. (2002). Introducing domestic violence assessment in a postpartum clinical setting. *Maternal Child Health Journal, 6*(3), 195–203.

Kaplan, H. I., & Sadock, B. J. (1998). *Kaplan and Sadock's synopsis of psychiatry.* New York, NY: Williams & Wilkins.

Kilbourne, J. (1987). *Still killing us softly.* Cambridge, MA: Cambridge Documentary Films.

Kilbourne, J. (1999). *Can't buy my love: How advertising changes the way we think and feel.* New York, NY: Simon & Schuster.

King, M. C., & Ryan, J. M. (2004). Nursing care and adolescent dating violence. In J. C. Campbell & J. C. Humphreys (Eds.), *Family violence and nursing practice* (pp. 288–306). Philadelphia, PA: Lippincott Williams & Wilkins.

Knapik, G., Martsolf, D. & Draucker, C. (2008). Being delivered: spirituality in survivors of sexual violence. *Issues in Mental Health Nursing, 29,* 335–350.

Krystal, J. H., Kosten, T. R., Southwick, S., Mason, J. W., Perry, B. D., & Giller, E. L. (1989). Neurobiological aspects of PTSD: Review of clinical and preclinical studies. *Behavior Therapy, 20*(2), 177–198.

Kwong, M. J., Bartholomew, K., Henderson, A. J. Z., & Trinke, S. J. (2003). The intergenerational transmission of relationship violence. *Journal of Family Psychology, 17*(3), 288–301.

Landenburger, K., Campbell, D. W., & Rodriguez, R. (2004). Nursing care of families using violence. In J. C. Campbell & J. C. Humphreys (Eds.), *Family violence and nursing practice* (pp. 220–251). Philadelphia, PA: Lippincott Williams & Wilkins.

Lasiuk, G., & Hegadoren, K. (2006a). Posttraumatic stress disorder. Part 1: Historical development of the concept. *Perspectives in Psychiatric Care, 42*(1), 13–20.

Lasiuk, G., & Hegadoren, K. (2006b). Posttraumatic stress disorder. Part 2: Development of the construct within the North American Psychiatric Taxonomy. *Perspectives in Psychiatric Care, 42*(2), 72–81.

LaVoie, F., Herbert, M., Tremblay, R., Vitaro, F., Vezina, L., & McDuff, P. (2002). History of family dysfunction and perpetuation of dating violence by adolescent boys: A Longitudinal study. *Journal of Adolescent Health, 30,* 375–383.

Law Commission of Canada. (2000). *Restoring dignity: Responding to child abuse in Canadian institutions.* Ottawa, ON: Minister of Public Works and Government Services.

Lloyd, S. A., & Emery, B. C. (2000). The context and dynamics of intimate aggression against women. *Journal of Social and Personal Relationships, 17*(4–5), 503–521.

Long, A., & Smyth, A. (1998). The role of mental health nursing in the prevention of child sexual abuse and the therapeutic care of survivors. *Journal of Psychiatric and Mental Health Nursing, 5,* 129–136.

Lowenthal, B. (2001). Teaching resilience to maltreated children. *Reclaiming Children and Youth, 3,* 169–173.

Lundberg-Love, P. K. (1997). Current treatment strategies of adult incest survivors and their partners. In R. Geffner, S. B. Sorenson, & P. K. Lundberg-Love (Eds.), *Violence and sexual abuse at home: Current issues in spousal battering and child maltreatment* (pp. 293–311). New York, NY: Haworth Maltreatment & Trauma Press.

MacMillan, H. L. (2000). Child maltreatment: What we know in the year 2000. *Canadian Journal of Psychiatry, 45*(8), 702–709.

McGrath, M. E., Bettacchi, A., Duffy, S. J., Peipert, J. F., Becker, B. M. & St. Angelo, L. (1997). Violence against women: Provider barriers to intervention in emergency departments. *Academic Emergency Medicine, 4,* 297–300.

McLean, L. M., & Gallop, R. (2003). Implications of childhood sexual abuse for adult borderline personality disorder and complex posttraumatic stress disorder. *American Journal of Psychiatry, 160*(2), 369–371.

McKeown, I., Reid, S., & Orr, P. (2004). Experiences of sexual violence and relocation in the lives of HIV infected Canadian women. *International Journal of Circumpolar Health, 63*(Suppl. 2), 399–404.

Messman-Moore, T. L., & Long, P. J. (2003). The role of childhood sexual abuse sequelae in the sexual revictimization of women: An empirical review and theoretical reformulation. *Clinical Psychology Review, 23,* 237–571.

Mill, J. E. (1997). HIV risk behaviors become survival techniques for aboriginal women. *Western Journal of Nursing Research, 19*(4), 466–489.

Morrill, A. C., Kasten, L., Urato, M., & Larson, M. J. (2001). Abuse, addiction, and depression as pathways to sexual risk in women and men with a history of substance abuse. *Journal of Substance Abuse, 13,* 169–184.

National Women's Health Information Center. (2003). Women with disabilities: Dissociative disorders. Available at: http://www.4woman.gov

Nolen-Hoeksema, S. (2002). Gender differences in depression. In I. H. Gotlib & C. L. Hammen (Eds.), *Handbook of depression* (pp. 492–509). New York, NY: Guilford.

Norris, F. H., Foster, J. D., & Weisshaar, D. L. (2002). The epidemiology of sex differences in PTSD across developmental, social, and research contexts. In R. Kimmerling, P. Ouimette, & J. Wolfe (Eds.), *Gender and PTSD* (pp. 3–42). New York, NY: Guilford.

O'Donnell, T., Hegadoren, K., & Coupland, N. (2004). Noradrenergic mechanisms in the pathophysiology of post-traumatic stress disorder. *Neuropsychobiology, 50*(4), 273–283.

Ogden, P., Minton, K. & Pain, C. (2006). *Trauma and the body: A sensorimotor approach to psychotherapy.* New York, NY: W.W. Norton & Company.

Orsillo, S. M., Raja, S., & Hammond, C. (2002). Gender issues in PTSD with comorbid mental health disorders. In R. Kimerling, P. Ouimette, & J. Wolfe (Eds.), *Gender and PTSD* (pp. 207–231). New York, NY: Guilford.

Ouimette, P., Moos, R. H., & Brown, P. J. (2003). Substance use disorder—posttraumatic stress disorder comorbidity: A survey of treatments and proposed practice guidelines. In P. Ouimette & P. J. Brown (Eds.), *Trauma and substance abuse: Causes, consequences, and treatment of comorbid disorders* (pp. 91–110). Washington, DC: American Psychiatric Association.

Pargament, K., Murray-Swank, N., & Mahoney, A. (2008). Problem and solution: The spiritual dimension of clergy sexual abuse and its impact on survivors. *Journal of Child Sexual Abuse, 17*(3–4), 397–420.

Parker, B., Bullock, L., Bohn, D., & Curry, M. A. (2004). In J. C. Campbell & J. C. Humphreys (Eds.), *Family violence and nursing practice* (pp. 77–96). Philadelphia, PA: Lippincott Williams & Wilkins.

Peled, E., Jaffe, P. G., & Edleson, J. L. (1995). *Ending the cycle of violence.* Thousand Oaks, CA: Sage.

Putnam, F. W. (1994). Dissociative disorders in children and adolescents. In S. J. Lynn & J. W. Rhue (Eds.), *Dissociation: Clinical and theoretical perspectives* (pp. 175–189). New York, NY: Guilford.

Randall, M., & Haskell, L. (1995). Sexual violence in women's lives. Findings from the Women's Safety Project, a community-based survey. *Violence Against Women, 1*(1), 6–31.

Rasmusson, A. M., & Friedman, M. J. (2002). Gender issues in the neurobiology of PTSD. In R. Kimerling, P. Ouimette, & J. Wolfe (Eds.), *Gender and PTSD* (pp. 43–75). New York, NY: Guilford.

Resnick, H., Acierno, R., Holmes, M., Kilpatrick, D. G., & Jager, N. (1999). Prevention of post-rape psychopathology: Preliminary findings of a controlled acute rate treatment study. *Journal of Anxiety Disorders, 13*(4), 359–370.

Riddell, T., Ford-Gilboe, M. & Leipert, B. (2009). Strategies used by rural women to stop, avoid or escape from intimate partner violence. *Health Care for Women International, 30*(1), 134–159.

Roesler, T. A., & Dafler, C. A. (1993). Chemical dissociation in adults sexually victimized as children: Alcohol and drug use in adult survivors. *Journal of Substance Abuse Treatment, 10,* 537–543.

Rosenbaum, A., Geffner, R., & Benjamin, S. (1977). A biopsychosocial model for understanding relationship aggression. In R. Geffner, S. B. Sorenson, & R. K. Lundburg-Love (Eds.), *Violence and sexual abuse at home* (pp. 57–80). New York, NY: Haworth Maltreatment & Trauma Press.

Rothbaum, B. O., & Foa, E. B. (1996). Cognitive-behavioral therapy for posttraumatic stress disorder. In B. A. van der Kolk, A. C. McFarlane, & L. Weisaeth (Eds.), *Traumatic stress: The effects of overwhelming experience on mind, body, and society* (pp. 491–509). New York, NY: Guilford.

Rothschild, B. (1998). Post-traumatic stress disorder: Identification and diagnosis. *Swiss Journal of Social Work.* Available at: http://www.healing-arts.org

Sampselle, C. M., Bernhard, L., Kerr, R. B., Opie, N., Perley, M. J., & Pitzer, M. (1992). Violence against women: The scope and significance of the problem. In C. M. Sampselle (Ed.), *Violence against women: Nursing research, education, and practice issues* (pp. 3–16). New York, NY: Hemisphere.

Schachter, C. L., Radomsky, N. A., Stalker, C. A., & Teram, E. (2004). Women survivors of child sexual abuse. How can health professionals promote healing? *Canadian Family Physician, 50,* 405–412.

Seeman, M. V. (2002). Single-sex psychiatric services to protect women. *Medscape General Medicine, 4*(3) [formerly published in Medscape *Women's Health eJournal* 7(4), 2002]. Available at: http://www.medscape.com

Selzer, M. L. (1971). The Michigan Alcoholism Screening Test: The quest for a new diagnostic instrument. *American Journal of Psychiatry, 127,* 89–94.

Sengstock, M. C., Ulrich, Y. C., & Barrett, S. A. (2004). Abuse and neglect of the elderly. In J. C. Campbell & J. C. Humphreys (Eds.), *Family violence and nursing practice* (pp. 97–149). Philadelphia, PA: Lippincott Williams & Wilkins.

Sheridan, D. (2004). Legal and forensic nursing responses to family violence. In J. C. Campbell & J. C. Humphreys (Eds.), *Family violence and nursing practice* (pp. 386–406). Philadelphia, PA: Lippincott Williams & Wilkins.

Sisley, A., Jacobs, L. M., Poole, G., Campbell, S., & Esposito, T. (1999). Violence in America: A public health crisis–domestic violence. *Journal of Trauma, Injury, Infection, and Critical Care, 46*(6), 1105–1112.

Skinner, H. A. (1982). The drug abuse screening test. *Addictive Behavior, 7,* 363–371.

Southwick, S. M., Bremner, D., Krystal, J. H., & Charney, D. S. (1994). Psychobiologic research in post-traumatic stress disorder. *Psychiatric Clinics of North America, 17*(2), 251–264.

Statistics Canada. (2001). *Canadian Crime Statistics 2000.* Ottawa, ON: Canadian Centre for Justice Statistics, Statistics Canada.

Statistics Canada. (2003a). *Family violence in Canada: A statistical profile.* Ottawa, ON: Federal Family Violence Initiative, Statistics Canada.

Statistics Canada. (2003b). *The Daily. Witnessing violence: Aggression & anxiety in young children.* Ottawa, ON: Health Reports, Statistics Canada.

Stermac, L., Del Bove, G., & Addison, M. (2004). Stranger and acquaintance sexual assault of adult males. *Journal of Interpersonal Violence, 19*(8), 901–915.

Stewart, S. H., Ouimette, P., & Brown, P. J. (2002). Gender and the comorbidity of PTSD with substance use disorders. In R. Kimerling, P. Ouimette, & J. Wolfe (Eds.), *Gender and PTSD* (pp. 232–270). New York, NY: Guilford.

Sutherland, S. M., & Davidson, J. T. (1999). Pharmacological treatment of posttraumatic stress disorder. In P. A. Saigh & J. D. Bremner (Eds.), *Post-traumatic stress disorder: A comprehensive text* (pp. 327–353). Boston, MA: Allyn & Bacon.

Swann, S. C. (2001). Women's use of violence in intimate relationships: Myths and facts. Paper presented at the Effects of Domestic Violence in Children: A Fathers Role Conference, Southern Connecticut State University, New Haven, Connecticut.

Thase, M. E., Jindal, R., & Howland, R. H. (2002). Biological aspects of depression. In I. H. Gotlib & C. L. Hammen (Eds.), *Handbook of depression* (pp. 192–218). New York, NY: Guilford.

Thompson, M. P., Kaslow, N. J., Kingree, J. B., Thompson, N. J., & Meadows, L. (1999). Partner abuse and posttraumatic stress disorder as risk factors for suicide attempts in a sample of low-income, inner-city women. *Journal of Traumatic Stress, 12*(1), 59–71.

Ulman, S. E. (2003). A critical review of field studies on the link of alcohol and adult sexual assault in women. *Aggression and Violent Behavior, 8,* 471–486.

Urbancic, J. C. (2004). Sexual abuse in families. In J. C. Campbell & J. C. Humphreys (Eds.), *Family violence and nursing practice* (pp. 186–219). Philadelphia, PA: Lippincott Williams & Wilkins.

Van der Kolk, B. A. (1996). The complexity of adaptation to trauma self-regulation, stimulus discrimination, and characterological development. In B. A. van der Kolk, A. C. McFarlane, & L. Weisaeth (Eds.), *Traumatic stress: The effects of overwhelming experience on mind, body, and society.* New York, NY: Guilford.

Van der Kolk, B. A., & Fisler, R. E. (1993). The biologic basis of posttraumatic stress. *Primary Care, 20*(2), 417–432.

Van der Kolk, B. A., McFarlane, A. C., & Weisaeth, L. (Eds.). (1996). *Traumatic stress: The effects of overwhelming experience on mind, body, and society.* New York, NY: Guilford.

Varcoe, C. (2001). Abuse obscured: An ethnographic account of emergency nursing in relation to violence against women. *Canadian Journal of Nursing Research, 32*(4), 95–115.

Walker, L. (1979). *The battered woman.* New York, NY: Harper & Row.

Walker, L. (1994). The abused women: A survivor therapy approach [Film]. Available from Newbridge Communications, Inc., 333 East Street, New York, NY 10016.

Wallace, H. (1999). *Family violence: Legal, medical, and social perspectives* (2nd ed.). Boston, MA: Allyn & Bacon.

Walsh, C., MacMillan, H. L., & Jamieson, E. (2003). The relationship between parental substance abuse and child maltreatment: Findings from the Ontario Health Supplement. *Child Abuse & Neglect, 27*(12), 1409–1425.

Watson, J. M., Cascardi, M., Avery-Leaf, S., & O'Leary, K. D. (2001). High school students' responses to dating aggression. *Violence and Victims, 16,* 339–348.

Wilson, J. P. (2001). An overview of clinical considerations and principles in the treatment of PTSD. In J. P. Wilson, M. J. Friedman, & J. Lindy (Eds.), *Treating psychological trauma and PTSD* (pp. 59–93). New York, NY: Guilford.

Wilson, J. P., Friedman, M. J., & Lindy, J. D. (2001). A holistic, organismic approach to healing trauma and PTSD. In J. P. Wilson, M. J. Friedman, & J. Lindy (Eds.), *Treating psychological trauma and PTSD* (pp. 28–56). New York, NY: Guilford.

Wong, C. M., & Yehuda, R. (2002). Sex differences in posttraumatic stress disorder. In F. Lewis-Hall, T. S. Williams, J. A. Panetta, & J. M. Herrera (Eds.), *Psychiatric illnesses in women* (pp. 57–96). Washington, DC: American Psychiatric Press.

Wright, M. O., Crawford, E., & Sebastian, K. (2007). Positive resolution of childhood sexual abuse experiences: The role of coping, benefit-finding and meaning-making. *Journal of Family Violence, 22,* 597–608.

Wright, R. J., Wright, R. O., & Isaac, N. E. (1997). Response to battered mothers in the pediatric emergency department: A call for an interdisciplinary approach to family violence. *Pediatrics, 99*(2), 186–192.

Wuest, J., & Merritt-Gray, M. (2001). While leaving abusive male partners, women engaged in a 4 stage process of reclaiming self. *Canadian Journal of Nursing Research, 32,* 79–94.

Yonaka, L., Yoder, M. K., Darrow, J. B. & Sherck, J. P. (2007). Barriers to screening for domestic violence in the emergency department. *The Journal of Continuing Education in Nursing, 38*(1), 37–46.

Zust, B. L. (2000). Effect of cognitive therapy on depression in rural battered women. *Archives of Psychiatric Nursing, 14*(2), 51–63.

Care for Self-Harm and Suicidal Behaviour: Children, Adolescents, and Adults

B. Lee Murray

Adapted from the chapter "Self-harm and Suicidal Behaviour: Children, Adolescents and Adults" by Emily J. Hauenstein

KEY CONCEPTS

- helplessness
- hopelessness
- lethality
- powerlessness
- risk/rescue ratio

LEARNING OBJECTIVES

After studying this chapter, you will be able to:

- Define suicide, suicidal ideation, self-harm, parasuicide, and suicidal behaviour.
- Describe population groups that have high rates of suicide.
- Discuss the rights of patients and other legal issues in the care of suicidal patients.
- Determine factors that affect the nurse's responsibility in assessment and intervention with suicidal individuals, including adolescents.
- List screening measures for depression, suicide intent, and psychiatric diagnostic measures.
- Discuss the process of a comprehensive suicide risk assessment.
- Describe factors that increase the risk for suicide completion.
- Describe the no self-harm contract (contracting for safety).
- Describe the nurse's responsibilities in promoting short- and long-term recovery in suicidal adult inpatients.
- Discuss the patient's and nurse's responsibilities in discharging the patient to the community.

KEY TERMS

- confidentiality • informed consent • involuntary hospitalization
- least restrictive environment • no self-harm contract • parasuicide • self-harm
- suicidal behaviour • suicidal ideation • suicide • suicide contagion
- voluntary hospitalization

The definition of **suicide** is simple: the voluntary and intentional act of killing oneself. The complexities associated with suicide, however, are grounded in an individual's perceptions and experiences of life, specifically those relating to sexuality, mental health, family factors, age, and gender. Two dimensions of suicide that need to be considered are attempt of suicide and completed suicide. An *attempt of suicide* can be

945

characterized as living through an experience of suicide despite having expected or intended to die. Though the individual may receive support, help, and hospitalization and be grateful for such services, the intent to end life was present. Conversely, a *completed suicide* is the engagement of suicidal behaviour that results in death. Acts of suicide, despite the actual outcome, are defined as **suicidal behaviour**. Likewise, the thought of suicide is known as *suicide ideation*. **Parasuicide** is self-injurious behaviour or self-harm that may mimic suicidal behaviour, but the primary motivating force of action is not to kill oneself (Kreitman, 1970; Zor et al., 2005). Death, however, may occur as a result of parasuicidal actions (Welch, 2001; Zor et al.). It is important to understand that parasuicide is *not* suicide (Kreitman, Philip, Greer, & Bagley, 1969), where the wish is to kill oneself intentionally. Researchers' understanding of parasuicide is incomplete, and its prevalence is believed to be grossly underestimated because most studies report only hospital contacts (Meehan, Lamb, Saltzman, & O'Carroll, 1992). As well, research studies on suicide and parasuicide have not clearly defined these phenomena (Guo, Scott, & Bowker, 2003), and parasuicide may not be distinguished from attempted suicide.

Self-harm exists in the suicide and parasuicide paradigms. **Self-harm** is characterized as any behaviour or act that causes harm to the body. The nature of the self-harm itself is dependent on the intent of the individual.

Many lives are deeply affected by suicide and the struggle to know what to do when a patient, colleague, friend, or loved one is suicidal. Self-harm and suicidal behaviours are very challenging for nurses and other health care professionals to address. It is important to try to understand the meaning of the self-harm and suicidal behaviours, particularly because such behaviours can be understood as a means of communicating one's despair to others.

Suicide, like mental illness, is stigmatized in contemporary society. The stigma against suicide has deep roots in some religions, such as Christianity, and in our collective thinking, and until a few decades ago, it was considered a crime in Western nations. Such stigma can prevent people from voicing their suicidal thoughts or asking for help: they are afraid they will be seen as weak, insane, or coming from bad families (Tadros & Jolley, 2001). When a suicidal act is unsuccessful, the visibility of medical intervention can trigger stigmatization by others (Joachim & Acorn, 2000). Stigma may be also experienced by the survivors of someone who completed suicide if blame for the loss is affixed to them; such stigma can significantly complicate their bereavement (Cvinar, 2005). Reports and portrayals of suicide in the media may further contribute to stigmatization (Coverdale, Naim, & Claasen, 2002).

Suicide remains a significant public health problem in Canada, despite efforts at both policy and clinical levels (e.g., to identify risk and protective factors, as well as appropriate interventions). Suicide prevention is difficult because suicide is "the outcome of complex interactions among neurobiological, genetic, psychobiological, social, cultural, and environmental risk and protective factors" (Guo et al., 2003, p. 2), and our knowledge about it remains limited (Tondo & Baldessarini, 2001). Parasuicide further complicates understanding the prevalence of suicide. Suicide also places significant demands on the health care system (Stewart, Manion, Davidson, & Cloutier, 2001).

Nurses are in a unique position to contribute to preventive efforts. With knowledge of early risk assessment and interventions—understood within the context of a person's family, social world, and broader community—as well as knowledge of how to engage with and respond to the actively suicidal person, nurses can make a difference. They can prevent the escalation or chronicity of the behaviour (Murray, 2003). Nurses can do much to demystify suicide and prevent the stigmatization of those at risk through individual and public education. The content of this chapter provides the information needed to understand suicidal and parasuicidal behaviours, as well as the tools to respond appropriately to them.

▰▰ EPIDEMIOLOGY OF SUICIDAL BEHAVIOUR

Suicide occurs in all age groups, social classes, and cultures. The World Health Organization (WHO, 2002) reports that 815,000 people killed themselves in 2000. This suggests that one death by suicide occurs every 40 seconds worldwide. As attempted suicides are estimated to occur 10 to 20 times more often than completed suicides, there is about one attempt every 3 seconds. In Canada, suicide is the fifth leading cause of death overall. It is, however, the leading cause of death for men aged 25 to 29 years and 40 to 49 years and for women aged 30 to 34 years. It is also the second leading cause of death for those aged 10 to 24 years. The rate of suicide in 2004 was 11.3 per 100,000 (Statistics Canada, 2007), greater than accidents and homicides combined (Cutcliffe, 2003), with rates in the mid-to-high range when compared worldwide (WHO, 2002). The most common means of death were by hanging (39%), poisoning (26%), and firearms (22%) (Statistics Canada, 2006). Prevalence rates may be still underestimated: suicide can be disguised as a motor vehicle collision or homicide, especially in young people (Kohlmeier, McMahan, & DiMaio, 2001; Ohberg & Lonnqvist, 1998).

Suicide is more common among groups with specific risk factors and has been associated with loss, unemployment, transience, recent life events (e.g., divorce, moving, problems with children), interpersonal distress, and earlier attempts (Appleby, Cooper, Amos, & Faragher,

1999). Research indicates that, universally, suicide is strongly associated with depression (O'Connell, Chin, Cunningham, & Lawlor, 2004). The best predictor for suicide is a previous attempt (Nemeroff, Compton, & Berger, 2001), whereas a significant protective factor is being married with dependent children (Tondo & Baldessarini, 2001). See Box 38-1 for a list of risk and protective factors.

> **KEY CONCEPT Hopelessness** is a perception of having no hope that one's life situation or circumstance will change or improve. It is characterized by feelings of inadequacy and an inability to act on one's own behalf.
>
> **Helplessness** is the perception of having limited ability or ambition to change one's current life situation. It is characterized by a sense of being unable to help oneself and a sense that there is a lack of support or protection.
>
> **Powerlessness** is the perception of having no power or control over one's life circumstance; feeling that the world will never be fair; feeling helpless and totally ineffectual; or feeling one lacks legal or other authority.

Age

Prepubertal Children

Suicide is rare among children who are younger than 10 years of age. There were no reports of self-harm resulting in completed suicide in Canadian children this age in 2002, and only two completed suicides were reported from 1993 to 1997 (Statistics Canada, 2008). However, suicides by children this age may be significantly underestimated. Mishara (1999) reported that medical examiners were reluctant to categorize self-inflicted death as suicide because of the belief that children do not fully understand the ramifications of their self-harm behaviour. Mishara, however, found that by grade 3, children have a comprehensive understanding of suicide, and younger children understand what it means to kill themselves.

Preadolescents and Adolescents

More teenagers die from suicide than from cancer, heart disease, birth defects, stroke, pneumonia, influenza, and chronic lung disease combined. In 2002, 35 Canadian children aged 10 to 14 years (10.5% of all deaths within

---

BOX 38.1

Risk and Protective Factors for Suicide

RISK FACTORS

Demographic or social factors
- Being an older adult
- Being male
- Poverty
- Being Aboriginal
- Being single (widow > divorced > separated > single)
- Social isolation, including new or worsening estrangement, and rural location
- Economic or occupational stress, loss, or humiliation
- New incarceration
- History of gambling
- Easy access to firearms

Clinical factors
- Past and current major psychiatric illness (especially depression)
- Personality disorder (borderline, narcissistic, antisocial)
- Impulsive or violent traits by history
- Current medical illness
- Family history of suicide
- Previous suicide attempts or other self-injurious or impulsive acts
- Current anger, agitation, or constricted preoccupation
- Current abuse of alcohol or drugs
- Easy access to lethal toxins (including prescribed medication)

- Formulated plan, preparations for death or suicide note
- Low ambivalence about dying versus living

Factors specific to youth
- All of the above
- Lack of family support
- History of abuse
- School problems
- Social ostracism, humiliation
- Conduct disorder
- Struggle with sexual orientation
- Recent marriage, unwanted pregnancy

Precipitants
- Recent stressors (especially losses of emotional, social, physical, or financial security)

PROTECTIVE FACTORS
- Intact social supports
- Active religious affiliation or faith (may also be a risk factor if shame/guilt about behaviour is involved)
- Marriage and presence of dependent children
- Ongoing supportive relationship with a caregiver
- Absence of depression or substance abuse
- Access to medical and mental health resources
- Impulse control
- Proven problem-solving and coping skills

Presence of risk and protective factors should be noted in the patient's chart as part of the risk assessment.

Adapted from http://www.medceu.com/course-no-test.cfm?CID=308

this age group) died due to intentional self-harm (Statistics Canada, 2005). The Public Health Agency of Canada (2000) reported suicide to be the second leading cause of death for youth aged 15 to 24 years (585 deaths), that is, 24% of all deaths in this age group. In 2002, 215 youth aged 15 to 19 years and 277 aged 20 to 24 years died as a result of self-harm (Statistics Canada, 2005). Preadolescent and adolescent males are nearly twice as likely to complete suicide than their female counterparts.

Although the number of completed suicides may seem disturbingly high, the rate of attempted suicide is equally alarming. Langlois and Morrison (2002) reported that in 1999, 40.8, 152.2, and 117.9 per 100,000 Canadian youth aged 10 to 14, 15 to 19, and 20 to 29 years, respectively, attempted suicide.

Adults

Worldwide trends indicate that the suicide rate increases with age. Rates among those aged 60 years and older are about three times higher than for people aged 15 to 29 years (Statistics Canada, 2005). By age 55 to 64 years, suicide is the eighth leading cause of death (Public Health Agency of Canada, 2000). Although suicide is the second leading cause of death for individuals 25 to 34 years old (21.8% of deaths; Statistics Canada, 2008), it is the fourth leading cause for those aged 35 to 54 (8.5% of deaths). As age increases, suicide rates as a cause of death within the age group decline, indicative of an increase in pathologic deaths occurring from cancers, heart attacks, and so on.

Many young adults who complete suicide have a psychiatric diagnosis (Brieger, Ehrt, Bloeink, & Marneros, 2002; Kishi, Robinson, Kosier, 2001). Other factors linked to suicide include childhood physical and sexual abuse and other psychosocial issues (Appleby, Cooper, et al., 1999; Foster, Gillespie, McClelland, & Patterson, 1999; Gunnell et al., 1999). Recent data show high suicide risk in young widowed men (Luoma & Pearson, 2002).

Older Adults

Although other causes of death are more prominent, suicide risk is high among older adults (O'Connell et al., 2004). Unfortunately, suicidal older adults have received far less attention in the scientific literature than their younger counterparts (Conwell & Duberstein, 2001). Nationally, the ratio of suicide attempts to completions in older adults is 4:1. Older adults generally have a stronger intent to die, plan their suicide more carefully, and are more likely to use more lethal means of killing themselves than are younger people (Conwell & Duberstein). The often frail health of older adults may contribute to the rate of completed suicides, and because many older adults live alone, the chance of a suicide being thwarted is often less than among younger people.

Although Canadian older adults have a higher rate of completing suicide, they have the lowest rate of suicide other than children aged 5 to 14 years (WHO, 2002). Of all suicides in Canada in 2001, 11.8% were by people older than 65 years of age. Suicide is less stigmatized for this age group and may be viewed as more acceptable.

For older adults, suicide is associated with less education, widowhood, previous attempts, depressive disorder, social isolation, financial difficulties, and substance abuse (Conwell & Duberstein, 2001; Conwell, Duberstein, & Caine, 2002; Kishi et al., 2001). Specifically, elderly widowed men have the highest risk for suicide (Tondo & Baldessarini, 2001). As in other age groups, major depressive disorder (MDD) is a significant factor in suicide. In 2001, Conwell and Duberstein reported that 71% to 95% of elderly people who completed suicide had a major psychiatric disorder at the time of death. However, comorbid physical illnesses often make recognition of MDD difficult.

> **KEY CONCEPT Lethality** refers to the probability that a person will complete suicide. Lethality is determined by the seriousness of the person's intent and the likelihood that the planned method will result in death. High lethality includes firearms, hanging, carbon monoxide poisoning, drowning, suffocation, or jumping from a great height.
>
> **Risk/rescue ratio** refers to the lethality of means and the likelihood of rescue. Suicidal risk carries with it a progression of seriousness from suicidal ideation to completed suicide. Risk is lowest when intent is weak and the method used has low lethality. The likelihood of rescue is dependent on communication of intent and lower lethality of means.

Gender

Worldwide, males complete suicide at a rate three times that of females, although women are four times more likely to attempt suicide than men (Health Canada, 2003). In Canada in 2002, 2,849 men died of intentional self-harm compared to 799 women; a ratio of 3.5:1. Suicide is the seventh leading cause of death for all ages of males; it is not in the top 10 causes of death for all ages of females. As a cause of death, suicide is ranked second for males aged 10 to 34 and fourth for males aged 35 to 54. In comparison, it is ranked second for females aged 15 to 19, third for females aged 20 to 34, and fourth for females aged 35 to 54 (Public Health Agency of Canada, 2000).

The reasons for the differences are not entirely understood. One hypothesis contends that completion rates differ because men are more likely to use highly lethal methods such as firearms (Tondo & Baldessarini, 2001).

In fact, men are 4.5 times more likely to use firearms than women, whereas women are twice as likely to die by poisoning. In a study of marital status and suicide risk among men and women, O'Connor and Noel (1997) found that single men were more likely to attempt suicide than their married counterparts; conversely, married women were suicidal more frequently than single women. Similarly, Quan, Arboleda-Flórez, Fick, Stuart, and Love (2002) reported that widowers had a five times higher risk for suicide than did married males, whereas the rates for suicide among married and widowed women remained similar. In an epidemiologic study of relationships and suicides, Eng, Rimm, Fitzmaurice, and Kawachi (2002) found that unmarried, unsociable men between 42 and 77 years with minimal social networks and no close relatives were at significantly greater risk for suicide.

Psychiatric disorders and unemployment are precipitating factors for risk for suicide in both men and women; however, they affect each gender differently. MDD is often comorbid with substance abuse in men, and as many as 33% of patients with alcoholism commit suicide (Angst, Angst, & Stassen, 1999; Berglund & Ojehagen, 1998). Aggression, hopelessness, emotion-focused coping, and having little purpose in life also have been associated with suicidal behaviour in men (Edwards & Holden, 2001; Prigerson & Slimack, 1999), as has social isolation (Alexander, 2001) and less participation in religious activities (Nisbet, Duberstein, Conwell, & Seidlitz, 2000). Economic deprivation and unemployment are more likely to precipitate suicide in men, but not necessarily in women (Hawton, Harriss, Hodder, Simkin, & Gunnell, 2001; Kposowa, 2001). Conversely, women who complete suicide often have several comorbid psychiatric disorders (Hall, Platt, & Hall, 1999). Women who have MDD and comorbid schizophrenia or anxiety and those with bipolar disorder are at high risk for suicide (Rihmer & Pestality, 1999; Saarinen, Lehtonen, & Lonnqvist, 1999). Current or previous exposure to violence, sexual assault, or both also increases women's risk for suicide (Koplin & Agathen, 2002; Nelson et al., 2002), and having a small child reduces it (Qin, Agerbo, Westergård-Nielson, Erikson, & Mortenson, 2000). Although unemployment has long been associated with suicide in men, research has shown that for the long term, unemployed women also are at serious risk for suicide: unemployed women had a suicide rate three times that of employed women in a follow-up study of 9 years (Kposowa, 2001).

Aboriginal Peoples

"I am here today because my ancestors, starving as they often were, fought to survive. Why did the old people strive to live... and the young people now want to die?" (NANYouth, 2004).

It is believed that before Aboriginal people's first contact with Europeans, suicide was rare (White & Jodoin, 2003). Since 1999, suicide and self-harm have been the leading cause of death of Aboriginal people in Canada up to the age of 44 years (Health Canada, First Nations and Inuit Health Branch, 2003). In 2000, the Aboriginal suicide rate was twice the national rate (White & Jodoin), and, from 1999 to 2003 in Inuit regions, it was more than 10 times the national rate (Government of Canada, 2006). Adolescents with Registered Indian status are far more likely to die by suicide than the average Canadian adolescent (five times more likely for males; 7.5 times, for females; Medical Services Branch Steering Committee on Native Mental Health, 1991). After age 70, the rate among status Indians then drops below that for the general population.

It is important to note that Aboriginal suicide rates may be underreported. Data collected by Statistics Canada pertain only to status Aboriginals, thus excluding nonstatus First Nations, Métis, and Inuit people from the Aboriginal suicide data. As well, the rate of accidental deaths among Aboriginal people is four to five times higher than in the general population, and up to 25% of these deaths (Royal Commission on Aboriginal Peoples, 1995) may be from suicide (White & Jodoin, 2003).

Although the rate of suicide is higher for Aboriginal people as compared with other Canadians, not every Aboriginal community in Canada experiences high rates

---

IN A LIFE

The Mushuau Innu of Davis Inlet

In 1993, the world was stunned to see a video of six children sniffing gas and screaming that they wanted to die. Combined with the report from the previous year of a house fire that had killed six children while their parents were drinking, long-needed attention was finally drawn to Davis Inlet and the plight of the Mushuau Innu who lived there. Prior to their relocation, approximately 680 Mushuau Innu lived in Davis Inlet, with 50% of the population being younger than 16 years of age. The community has one of the highest suicide rates in the world (178 per 100,000) and has been plagued with severe poverty, high infant mortality rates, alcohol and solvent abuse, violence, and parental neglect (Samson, 2003). The community is keenly aware of these problems and, for the past 30 years, has been working with other Innu communities, health care professionals, and government to address them.

In 2001, the Innu and federal and provincial governments jointly developed the Labrador Innu Comprehensive Healing Strategy, and, in December 2002, the community was relocated to Natuashish, Labrador. The relocation is said to have helped restore pride, cultural identity, and a sense of purpose to this Mushuau community, and there are new services within the community, including nursing. Progress has been slow, however, as all aspects of Mushuau Innu life, including education, governance, health, and spirituality, continued to be addressed.

of suicide (White & Jodoin, 2003). Marked differences can be noted between provinces, regions, and even between communities in the same geographic region (Suicide Information and Education Centre [SEIC], 2003). In studying suicide among British Columbia's Aboriginal communities, Chandler and Lalonde (1998) discovered that some communities have suicide rates 800 times the national average, while in other communities, suicide was virtually unknown. They also identified six protective factors that may explain the differences in suicidal rates between communities (see Box 38-2). According to a Health Canada (2003) report, community wellness strategies may have the best chance of making a difference in suicide rates between Aboriginal communities. Guidelines were suggested in developing such a strategy (see Box 38-3).

BOX 38.2

Community Protective Factors Against Risk for Suicide

Cultural continuity is identified in terms of six protective factors that may explain the differences in suicidal rates between Aboriginal communities. Those factors listed in terms of importance are

- Self-government
- Land claims
- Education services
- Police and fire services
- Health services
- Cultural Facilities

From Chandler, M. J., & Lalonde, C. (1998). Cultural continuity as a hedge against suicide in Canada's First Nations. *Transcultural Psychiatry, 35*(2), 191–219.

BOX 38.3

Aboriginal Community Wellness Strategies

- Develop locally initiated, owned, and accountable programs.
- Suicide prevention should be the responsibility of the entire community.
- Focus on behavioural patterns of children and young people is crucial and requires the involvement of family and community.
- Suicide prevention must be addressed from the biologic, psychological, sociocultural, and spiritual perspectives.
- Long-term crisis and intervention programs must be developed.
- Suicide intervention strategies must be evaluated as needed.

From Health Canada, First Nations and Inuit Health Branch. (2003). *A statistical profile on the health of First Nations in Canada.* Ottawa, ON: Government of Canada.

Sexual Orientation

In recent years, sexual orientation as a risk factor for suicide has been highly debated. Russell and Joyner (2001) point to the common belief that dealing with the stigma of homosexuality may lead gay, lesbian, bisexual, and transgendered (GLBT) people to depression or even suicide. During adolescence, when the major focus of a youth's life is on peers and sexuality, a GLBT youth's search for self-identity may heighten depression and suicidal behaviour (Rotheram-Borus & Fernandez, 1995). "Coming out" is a risk factor because of the possible negative reactions of others, particularly peers and family. Acknowledging one's sexual orientation at an early age or never disclosing one's sexual orientation can put GLBT youth at a higher risk of suicide (Remafedi, Farrow, & Deisher, 1991). Someone who comes out at an early age is at an increased risk for harassment and assaults, whereas someone who does not feel safe enough to disclose his or her sexual orientation may feel extremely isolated (Morrison & L'Heureux, 2001). In both cases, there can be feelings of helplessness, hopelessness, powerlessness, and isolation, which increase the risk for depression and suicide (Beck, Steer, Kovacs, & Garrison, 1985). GLBT youth are also at a higher risk for suicide if they self-present with high levels of gender nonconformity (Remafedi et al., 1991), report high levels of inner conflict regarding their sexual orientation (Savin-Williams, 1990), or report sexual abuse (Gibson, 1994). It is important to note that the risk factors associated with GLBT individuals are in addition to those common to all ages and sexual orientations.

Regional Variations

Provincial statistics from 2004 show varied rates of suicide across Canada (see Table 38-1). Eastern and central regions of the far north have some of the highest mortality rates from suicide in Canada (Statistics Canada, 2003). For instance, in 2001, Labrador had a rate of 27.0; Région du Nunavik in Quebec, 132.5; Northwestern Ontario, 26.7; Mamawetan/Keewatin/Athabasca, Saskatchewan, 19.0. These higher suicide rates may be due to a combination of factors. Most people in these regions live in rural or semirural environments where hunting (and ready access to firearms) is common; social isolation can occur due to low population per square mile; and the population is predominantly Aboriginal, a part of the Canadian population who have higher rates of suicide than the national average. Within each province, rates of suicide are not consistent because urban centres tend to have lower suicide rates than the national average, for example, Toronto (7.6), Winnipeg (10.5), and Vancouver (10.9). As with the north, various demographic, social, cultural, and geographic factors affect rates of suicide.

Table 38.1	Canadian Suicide Statistics (2004)
Province/Territory	**Suicide Rate***
Prince Edward Island	5.8
Ontario	8.2
Nova Scotia	9.6
Newfoundland and Labrador	10.2
British Columbia	11.1
Saskatchewan	11.2
Manitoba	11.3
New Brunswick	11.8
Alberta	14.0
Quebec	15.3
Yukon	19.4
Northwest Territories	25.7
Nunavut	80.9
National Average	11.3

*per 100,000 people.

Guns and Suicide

Almost 80% of all firearm deaths are suicides, and firearms are used in nearly 20% of all suicide fatalities (Canada Safety Council, 2004). Legislation by the Canadian government requiring the registration of all firearms is an attempt to decrease deaths (homicide and suicide) related to firearms. Research supports this legislation. A Québec study run by Le Centre de Prevention du Suicide (Simon, 1996) concluded that there is no evidence that if a firearm is not readily available, another method will be used. The Canadian Safety Council reported that, although the accessibility of firearms is usually associated with rural areas, urban areas show the highest rates of completed suicides by firearms.

Suicidal Ideation and Self-Harm

Rather than being seen as an overt expression of a desire to die, the majority of suicidal acts are seen as "cries for help" or attempts to postpone dealing with an unbearable situation (Health Canada, 1994). Understanding the motivation for such acts is important because 30% to 60% of suicides have been preceded by an attempt and 10% to 14% of those who attempt suicide eventually kill themselves (Tondo & Baldessarini, 2001). As well, long-term follow-up studies of people with parasuicidal behaviour found that 10% to 13% ultimately take their lives (Sakinofsky, Roberts, Brown, Cummings, & James, 1990).

Previous self-harm behaviour, then, is among the best predictors of future suicide attempts and completions. In addition, MDD and physical, cognitive, psychological, and social risk factors contribute to **suicidal ideation**. Physical factors include medical illness and alcohol and drug use (Grant & Hasin, 1999; Hendin,

1999; Kishi et al., 2001; Vilhjalmsson, Kristjansdottir, & Sveinbjarnardottir, 1998). Cognitive risk factors include problem-solving deficits and hopelessness (D'Zurilla, Chang, Nottingham, & Faccini, 1998). Psychological risk factors include internal distress and low self-esteem (Holden, Kerr, Mendonca, & Velamoor, 1998). Social risk factors include financial hardship, legal stress, family difficulties, and poor social support (Vilhjalmsson et al., 1998). Childhood trauma (including physical and sexual abuse) has been linked to both parasuicide and suicidal ideation in adulthood (Molnar, Berkman, & Buka, 2001).

Suicidal ideation and self-harm are more common among adolescents than other age groups. Contributing factors of such behaviour in adolescents include family discord, neglect, physical abuse, adolescent unemployment, residential transience, chronic behaviour problems, and recent interpersonal stress (Appleby, Cooper, et al., 1999; Grilo et al., 1999; Gunnell et al., 1999). Substance abuse increases the likelihood that suicidal ideation will result in parasuicide (Gould et al., 1998).

Self-harm behaviour in adolescents is often a way to communicate needs or wants, and often the need is for attention or care (Murray, 2003). As such, self-harm is an unacceptable means to acceptable ends and may communicate that the adolescent believes something is wrong, life is tough, and things are becoming unbearable. Parasuicide behaviour (e.g., cutting or self-mutilation) may also relieve or release certain emotions and feelings and may produce a tangible, physical pain to substitute for unfamiliar, unbearable psychological suffering (Harris, 2000; Levenkron, 1998; Machoian, 2001). In addition, such behaviours may be related to punishment of self or others (Rew, Thomas, Horner, Resnick, & Beuhring, 2001; Walsh & Rosen, 1988). Self-punishment is often identified with self-loathing, anger, guilt, and shame (Murray).

Behaviour escalates if the purpose of the self-harm is not achieved (Machoian, 2001). Therefore, feeling unheard or misunderstood often results in the escalation of self-harm behaviour. Furthermore, escalation occurs when self-harm behaviour is not understood in the context of why it is happening and when the purpose of the behaviour is not explored (Murray, 2003). Even if the purpose of self-harm behaviour is recognized, ignoring or minimizing the behaviour may escalate its intensity and frequency with increased attempts to get the message across (Murray).

■ ETIOLOGY OF SUICIDAL BEHAVIOUR

Suicidal behaviour occurs in the context of an individual's physiologic, psychological, and social situation and is usually triggered by stressors that are unmanageable and exceed typical coping efforts. Vulnerabilities are enhanced by engagement in risky behaviours, often used in an effort to cope with stress. Risky behaviours related to suicide include fast, dangerous driving; tempting death; promiscuity; use of alcohol or drugs; and purchase of a handgun. Appropriate interventions guided by a comprehensive assessment of risk at this point can reduce the likelihood of suicidal behaviour. Most who attempt suicide have seen a health care professional at least 1 month prior to the attempt (Blumenthal & Kupfer, 1990). Edwin Schneidman (1985), a clinical psychologist and leading authority on suicide, has described common characteristics of suicide in his book *Definition of Suicide* (see Box 38-4).

A comprehensive assessment identifies the physical, psychological, and social factors that contribute to feelings of self-harm (Fig. 38-1). These include changes in central nervous system neurotransmitters, engaging in negative thinking and risky behaviours, and deterioration of social relationships. The convergence of physiologic, psychological, social, and spiritual factors can be directly linked to suicidal behaviour. Most will agree that suicide, like many other aspects of humanness, does not solely lie within a single sphere of the bio/psycho/social/spiritual model. However, in order to facilitate learning, suicide will be discussed in relation to each of these spheres.

Biologic Theories

Biologic theories of suicide attempt to enlighten the phenomenon of suicide by recognizing and interpreting physiologic, neurophysiologic, and hormonal changes. Psychopathologic changes are evident in most suicidal people. MDD, sometimes comorbid with other psychiatric illnesses, is prevalent. Moreover, because suicide rates tend to be higher in families in which suicide has occurred, genetic and familial factors will be explored in this section. Finally, a biologic explanation of increased suicide risk among those who experienced childhood sexual abuse is considered.

MDD tends to develop when a person who is vulnerable to it (because of genetic or other factors) is subjected

---

BOX 38.4

Schneidman's Common Characteristics of Suicide

1. **The common stimulus for suicide is unendurable psychological pain.**
   Faced with intolerable emotion and unacceptable anguish, people will sometimes opt for a cessation of consciousness. The core ambivalence in suicide reflects the conflict between survival and unbearable stress. The main clinical rule is Reduce the suffering, often just a little bit, and the individual will choose to live.

2. **The common stressor in suicide is frustrated psychological needs.**
   Suicides are born, negatively, out of needs. Most suicides represent combinations of various needs. The clinical rule is Address the frustrated needs and the suicide will not occur.

3. **The common purpose of suicide is to seek a solution.**
   Suicide is not a random act. It is a way out of a problem, dilemma, or crisis. It is the answer—seemingly the only available answer—to a real puzzler: How to get out of this? It is important to view each suicidal act as an urgently felt effort to answer a question, to resolve an issue, to solve a problem.

4. **The common goal of suicide is "cessation of consciousness."**

5. **The common emotions in suicide are hopelessness and helplessness.**
   Often people on the edge of committing suicide would be willing to live if things—life—were only a little bit better, a just noticeable difference. The common fear is that the inferno is endless and that one has to draw the line on one's suffering somewhere.

6. **The common internal attitude toward suicide is ambivalence.**
   Something can be both "A" and "not A." We can both love and hate the same person. A prototypical suicidal state is one in which the individual feels that she or he has to do it, and simultaneously yearns, and even plans, for rescue and intervention.

7. **The common cognitive state in suicide is "constriction" (tunnel vision).**
   Suicide cannot be understood as a psychosis, a neurosis, or a character disorder. It is a transient psychological constriction of affect and intellect. It is a narrowing of the range of options that leads to either/or thinking.

8. **The common interpersonal act in suicide is communication of intention.**
   The communication of suicidal intention is not always a cry for help. First, it is not always a cry; it can be a shout or a murmur or the nonverbal communication of something unspoken. The communication is not always for help; it can be for autonomy or any number of needs. Nonetheless, in most cases of suicide there is some interpersonal communication related to that intended final act.

9. **The common action in suicide is egression or escape.**
   Suicide is a death in which the decedent removes himself or herself from intolerable pain and simultaneously from others in the world.

10. **Suicide is consistent with lifelong coping patterns.**
    "You can't fire me; I quit." "I'll leave her before she leaves me." Schneidman believes that suicide is not a random act, and sometimes is reasonably predictable.

From Schneidman, E. (1985) *Definition of suicide.* New York, NY: John Wiley & Sons.

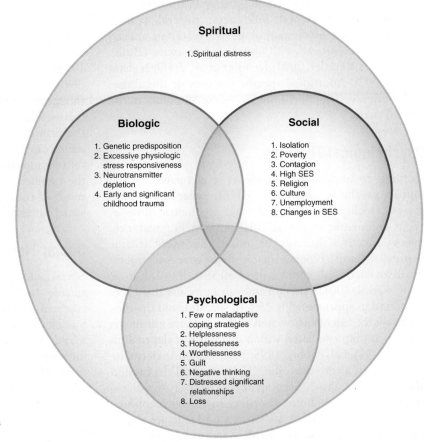

FIGURE 38.1 Bio/psycho/social/spiritual etiologies of suicide.

to repeated or sustained stress. Stress responsiveness in these people ultimately changes neurotransmitter and hormonal functioning to affect a depressed state (Hauenstein, 1996). Those who complete suicide have extremely low levels of the neurotransmitter serotonin, 5-hydroxytryptamine (5-HT; Mann, Oquendo, Underwood, & Arango, 1999) or lower levels of the neurotransmitter dopamine (Pitchot et al., 2001).

Considerable evidence exists showing a familial trend in suicide (McGuffin, Marusic, & Farmer, 2001; Qin, Agerbo, & Mortenson, 2003). First-degree relatives of individuals who have completed suicide have a two- to eight-times higher risk for suicide than do individuals in the general population (McGuffin et al.). Suicide of a first-degree relative is highly predictive of a medically serious suicide attempt in another first-degree relative (Modai et al., 1999). This risk is slightly heightened in females (Qin et al.). The children of depressed mothers with a history of suicide attempts have higher rates of suicidal behaviour (Klimes-Dougan et al., 1999; Pfeffer, Normandin, & Kakuma, 1998). The genetic link to suicide is evident in studies of twins. Qin et al. showed that suicidal behaviour in one monozygotic twin increased the risk 11-fold for suicidal behaviour in the co-twin. Another study showed that a serious attempt by one

twin increased the risk in a dizygotic co-twin more than twofold and in a monozygotic co-twin almost fourfold (Statham et al., 1998). In this study, genetic factors alone accounted for about half the increased risk for suicidal behaviour. Among adolescent female twins, genetic factors played a part in 35% of suicide attempts (Glowinski et al., 2001). Adoption studies have shown that among adults who experience mood disorders and were adopted as children, the suicide rate among the biologic relatives of the adoptees is much higher than the rate among the adoptive relatives. Genetic abnormalities in the serotonergic neurotransmitter system may be responsible for the heightened familial risk for suicide (Mann, Brent, & Arango, 2001). Collectively, these studies demonstrate that the biologic risk for suicide appears to be independent of environmental factors.

Child abuse has been described as a specific vulnerability for psychopathology and suicide (MacMillan et al., 2001). Enhanced vulnerability to MDD and suicide associated with child abuse are attributable to changes in the hypothalamic–pituitary–adrenal axis caused by intractable stress and altered serotonin and dopamine metabolism (Skodol, Siever, & Livesley, 2002). Evidence from twin studies suggests that the link between childhood sexual abuse and biologic alterations contributing to psychopathology may be independent of other environmental influences. Several studies show that adult psychopathology is greater in abused twins when compared with nonabused co-twins (Bulik, Prescott, & Kendler, 2001; Kendler et al., 2000; Nelson et al., 2002). Additional specific features of the abuse, including severity, contributed to worse outcomes in the abused twins.

Psychological Theories

Coming to understand suicide as it is related to the human psyche is important. MDD, generalized anxiety, personality disorders, and other psychiatric illnesses occur frequently in the suicidal person. For instance, major affective illnesses or mood disorders (major depressive and bipolar manic-depressive disorders) are associated with about half of all suicides (Tondo & Baldessarini, 2001). Alcohol and substance use disorders are found in approximately 25% of suicides, and the lifetime risk for suicide associated with substance abusers is similar to that associated with a diagnosis of depression (Clark & Goebel-Fabbri, 1998; Roy, 1989). Anxiety disorders, even after controlling for comorbid depression and substance abuse, account for 15% to 20% of suicides, whereas psychotic disorders such as schizophrenia account for a further 10% to 15% of suicides (Roy). Furthermore, the risk for suicide is increased by a factor of six in personality disorders like borderline and antisocial personality (Foster et al., 1999). Those with multiple comorbid problems such as affective or psychotic disorders combined with drug or alcohol abuse are at the highest risk for suicide (Angst et al., 1999; Appleby, Cooper, et al., 1999; Baldessarini, Tondo, & Hennen, 1999; Guze & Robins, 1970; Roy).

Psychodynamic theories designate conflicts, losses, and changes in relationships as contributors to suicidal risk and view suicide as a depressive or psychotic act, sometimes associated with fantasies of escape, reward, reunion, and resurrection (Hendin, 1991). Suicide can be conceptualized psychologically as an excessive reaction arising from intense preoccupation with humiliation and disappointment (Leenaars, 1998). It can be driven by intolerable aloneness and isolation (Adler & Buie, 1996); punitive and aggressive impulses of revenge, spite, or self-sacrifice; wishes to kill and be killed; or yearning for release into a better experience through death (Tondo & Baldessarini, 2001). Cognitive approaches also attribute suicide to learned helplessness and hopelessness as an automatic and pervasive pathologic scheme for organizing and interpreting experience (Beck, Kovacs, & Weissman, 1979; Rosenberg, 1993). The widely used cognitive theory of depression espoused by Aaron Beck and his associates (Beck, Rush, Shaw, & Emery, 1979) accounts for how negative thoughts occur, how they tend to be repetitive

and intrusive, and how they can lead to suicidal behaviour (see Chapter 15).

People who engage in suicidal behaviour often have difficult relationships with the people in their lives (Jamison, 1999). Attachment theory explains social isolation and disrupted interpersonal relationships as being a part of the spectrum of suicide (Lopez & Brennan, 2000). In this theory, adult behaviour is shaped by early interactions with the primary caregiver during infancy. Disturbed attachment results in the individual's inability to form meaningful relationships or in his or her constant concern about the viability of a lasting relationship. Suicide, then, is the result of conflicted or distant adult relationships and the social isolation that arises (Eng et al., 2002).

Social Theories

Social factors are particularly important to the etiology of suicide. As humans we are inherently a part of the social fabric in which we exist. To be alive is to be in the world. Suicide, then, is the desire to estrange oneself from the world. Some suicidal people describe a desire to "feel nothing for a while," a temporary respite from life and the world.

Studying the social factors that contribute to rates of suicide, Emile Durkheim, at the end the 19th century, developed a theoretical framework outlining the social causes of suicide. Durkheim (1897, 2006) classified suicide under four headings: egoistic suicide, altruistic suicide, anomic suicide, and fatalistic suicide. These classifications of suicide are based on the degree of imbalance between social integration and moral regulation (Kendall, Lothian-Murray, & Linden, 2004).

Durkheim believed that the degree of social integration was a variable affecting rates of suicide. *Egoistic suicide* occurs among individuals who are not significantly bound to society. Some believe that the social isolation of single people is causally related to their higher rates of suicide when compared with their married counterparts. Conversely, *altruistic suicide* occurs when individuals become overly connected to society, for example, a patriotic soldier who kills himself or herself after a defeated battle because he or she is shamed.

Durkheim also acknowledged that extreme cases of social stability and social consensus contribute to rises in suicide rates. A society lacking a sense of purpose, social regulation, or community values experiences *anomic suicide*. This type of suicide occurs during times of financial depression. Contrastingly, in areas of over-regulation and oppression, *fatalistic suicides* occur. Although Durkheim discussed little about fatalistic suicide, many use the suicide of slaves as an exemplar.

Contemporary sociologic investigations seek social structure models of influence on suicide. A theory explicated by Cohen et al. (2003) contends that socioeconomic status is a driving factor in what happens to an individual, affecting the physical and social structures available to him or her. For example, poverty represented by substandard housing affects other important neighbourhood social structures, such as schools, voluntary organizations, and jobs. People who may wish to teach in these schools, help out, or conduct business in the neighbourhood are deterred by the neighbourhood deterioration. Poverty also reduces exposure to opportunities for individual advancement. Poverty affects health outcomes directly, because of environmental hazards, or indirectly, through inadequate access to health care.

Substantial data exist to support this model of suicide. Cohen et al. (2003) found that the percentage of boarded-up buildings in a neighbourhood was positively associated with suicide. Socioeconomic deprivation and unemployment were found to be associated with suicide in several studies (Cubbin, LeClere, & Smith, 2000; Goodman, 1999; Hawton et al., 2001; Kposowa, 2001; Steenland, Halperin, Hu, & Walker, 2003). Unemployment may also pose an indirect risk for suicide through family tension arising from the loss of income and a normal social role. This loss may then lead to indignity, isolation, hopelessness, alcohol abuse, and violence (Platt, 1993).

Tondo and Baldessarini (2001) agree that rates of suicide are significantly higher at the poorer end of the socioeconomic continuum. However, they note increases in suicide among the extremely wealthy. Although this may appear paradoxical, wealth brings with it a distinct set of worries and concerns. Importantly, suicide is at its greatest rates when a substantial change in social status occurs.

Suicide and Religion

Research regarding the impact of religion on suicide has not yielded consistent results (Stack & Lester, 1991). It has been hypothesized that not only personal but also contextual differences in religious beliefs may determine an individual's willingness to consider suicide (Neeleman & Lewis, 1990). Greater moral objections to suicide in those with a religious affiliation may be protective against suicide attempts (Dervic et al., 2004). However, social scientists do not find that not believing in God or lack of religiosity are causative factors leading to suicide. Rather, it is likely that an individual's belief that suicide is wrong is a strong deterrent to the act of suicide (Hilton, 2002).

Suicide Contagion

A social phenomenon seen among adolescents is **suicide contagion**. Several studies have shown that when one teenager takes his or her life, several more may follow (Gould & Kramer, 2001; Poijula, Wahlberg, & Dyregrov, 2001). Poijula et al. found an increase in suicides in three secondary schools in the year after a suicide occurred. However, rates did not increase in schools that used crisis intervention at the time of the suicide.

Suicide by imitation seems to be influenced, in part, by its portrayal through mass media (Goldney, 1989; Phillips & Carstensen, 1986; Schmidtke & Hafner, 1988). However, mass media's influence can be minimized by avoiding sensationalized reports of suicide that supply details as to the methods used (Jobes, Berman, O'Carroll, Eastgard, & Knickmeyer, 1996). Key factors in imitative behaviour are identification with a victim by age, sex, and location, although other influences, such as economic status, attitudes toward suicide, and problem-solving strategies, affect imitative behaviour (Berman, 1988).

Social circumstances also affect parasuicidal behaviour. Research indicates that changes in the life circumstances of people with parasuicidal behaviour can reduce the risk for suicide. Sakinofsky et al. (1990) studied 228 parasuicidal people for 1 year to determine whether the resolution of their problems reduced further suicidal behaviour. Three months after their attempts, those who had overcome their difficulties were significantly less depressed and hostile and felt less isolated than they initially reported. Their self-esteem had risen, they did not feel as powerless as before, and they experienced significant improvements in marital and family relationships. Those who had not resolved their issues continued to fare poorly in all respects.

Spiritual Theories

Due to modern nursing's scientific orientation, spirituality has reemerged as an important component of nursing care only in the last decade (Tinley & Kinney, 2007). Increasingly, it is recognized as a key component of holistic care. Spirituality, which can mean a search for meaning, connectedness (both intrapersonal and interpersonal), energy, and a person's worldview (Pesut, 2003, 2008), is being recognized as a source of resilience and coping (Martin, 2002). Studies have shown that people with spiritual involvement were at a decreased risk of substance abuse, addiction, and suicide (Benson, 1992; Koenig & Larson, 2001) and that, for some people with mental illness, spirituality was used as a coping resource and lowered the risk of substance abuse and suicide (Larson & Larson, 2003).

▄▄▄ EFFECTS OF SUICIDE

Effect on Survivors

Worldwide, about 1 million people die from suicide each year (WHO, 2002). Each suicide has an impact on an average of six or seven survivors, meaning that approximately 6 to 7 million people lose someone close to them as a result of suicide each year (Tondo & Baldessarini, 2001). Suicide has devastating effects on everyone it touches, especially family and close friends. Undue and prolonged suffering can be caused by the sudden shock, the unanswered questions of "why," and potentially the discovery of the body (Knieper, 1999). Suicide bereavement is different than that experienced by families whose loved one's death is not self-inflicted. The grieving over the way the death occurred, the social processes affecting the survivors, and the effect of the suicide on the family converge to establish a grieving process that is unique (Jordan, 2001).

Often family survivors of suicide reported more stigmatization, shame, and rejection than did matched families whose family member died in other ways. They also reported that police, medical examiners, and the media exacerbated their grief by their insensitivity. For this reason, it is important for nurses to listen and be present, patient, compassionate, and understanding with survivors of suicide. Simplistic explanations and clichés should be avoided. Survivors of suicide need help in following their own search for an understanding of what has happened. In the end, their personal search for meaning regarding the death is important. Their coping abilities will mediate their grief responses. It is an ongoing task, but recovery from a loved one's suicide is made easier by good coping skills and social support that help one deal with the psychological trauma (Mitchell, Gale, Garand, & Wesner, 2003; Reed, 1998).

Economic Effects

Suicide affects society by consuming both human lives and economic resources (Clayton & Barceló, 2000). Estimating the cost of suicide is difficult. In Canada, the average cost of hospitalization for suicide and attempted suicide was $5,500 per admission, ranging from $3,000 to $31,000 (HereToHelp, 2003). In 1997, suicide and attempted suicide cost the Canadian health care system $100 million (HereToHelp). In New Brunswick in 1996, for the 94 reported suicide deaths, the direct costs were $535,158, including health care services, autopsies, and funerals. The indirect cost per suicide death due to lost productivity had a value of $79,353,354, a mean cost of $849,877 (Clayton & Barceló).

▬▬ LEGAL CONSIDERATIONS IN CARING FOR SUICIDAL PEOPLE

In Canada, evolving social and religious attitudes have been reflected in the decriminalization of attempted suicide. In 1972, attempted suicide was removed from the provisions of the Criminal Code. Counselling or assisting suicide, however, remains a criminal act (Section 241, *Criminal Code of Canada* [Government of Canada, 1985])

Canadians have legal rights that health care providers must consider during suicide prevention and treatment. Providers cannot deprive patients of their right to self-determination unless no other course is available to ensure a patient's safety. They must preserve rights to privacy and anonymity unless they cannot protect a patient without disclosing his or her suicidal intent to others. Patients have the right to be free from harm. Physically restraining or hospitalizing a patient against his or her will has the potential for both physical and emotional harm and should be used only under the threat of imminent suicide or psychosis. Nurses must understand patients' legal rights and be able to explain them clearly. This means that nurses need to be familiar with their provincial mental health legislation (see Chapter 3).

Confidentiality

Disclosing information without a patient's permission violates his or her rights to privacy and anonymity and may damage the therapeutic relationship. Patients lose trust when the nurse shares their suicidal intent with others unless the nurse has specifically explained the limits of confidentiality. When informing the patient of existing limits of confidentiality, the nurse must be very clear and specific. The Canadian Nurses Association (CNA) clearly articulates the concept of **confidentiality** as safeguarding information acquired within a professional relationship, except when doing so would cause significant harm (CNA, 2002).

The CNA code of ethics is consistent with provincial legislation. Namely, the patient has a right to confidentiality unless he or she is at risk for harming self or others or discloses any form of abuse of minors, including neglect, sexual, physical, psychological, and emotional abuses. In those situations, the nurse can enlist the help of others (e.g., outside of the health care team) to protect the patient's or others' safety.

Protecting the patient's right to confidentiality is a special concern when a minor child has suicidal intent. As with adult patients, the nurse is required to describe the right to confidentiality and its limits. The nurse must always consider informing parents or legal guardians of a child who has suicidal intent. The parents of a minor child retain the privilege to determine the right care for their child, and they need sufficient information to make good decisions. Before beginning any suicide risk assessment, nurses must let a child know that disclosure of self-harm may be shared with parents. Honesty about what the nurse can and cannot keep confidential ultimately increases a child's trust and often results in a more therapeutic relationship.

Informed Consent

Obtaining fully **informed consent** from the patient protects his or her right to self-determination. However, nurses must inform suicidal patients about limits to their self-determination and make efforts to obtain their cooperation. From the time that the nurse encounters a suicidal patient until a suitable placement is made in consultation with other members of the interprofessional team, the nurse must share with the patient his or her right to be placed in the **least restrictive environment** that will ensure safety. The least restrictive environment is the setting that puts the fewest constraints on the patient's rights while still ensuring the patient's safety. By informing a patient about his or her choices, the nurse gains the patient's trust and decreases the likelihood that involuntary hospitalization will be necessary.

The ethical requirement of **beneficence**, doing no harm, is critical when restraining patients against their will. Caring for patients who are suicidal and determined to get away is difficult without touching and actively restraining them. Still, nurses must do their best to disclose to patients the specifics of planned treatments, including restraints, and attempt to obtain their consent to proceed. Respect for the patient needs to be maintained throughout the process. (For further discussion of these issues, see Chapter 6.)

Documentation

The nurse must thoroughly document encounters with suicidal patients. This action is for the patient's ongoing treatment and the nurse's protection. The nursing notes must reflect that the nurse took every reasonable action to provide for the patient's safety. If a **no self-harm contract** has been instituted, the record must contain specific aspects of the contract.

Involuntary Admission and the Provincial Health Acts

When a patient will not or cannot (because of noncompetent status) agree to enter the hospital voluntarily, **involuntary hospitalization** may be initiated. Considerable controversy surrounds the notion of involuntary hospitalization and treatment. See Chapter 3 for a discussion of provincial legislation that empowers physicians and peace officers to detain, without consent, a person whom they consider to be of danger to themselves or others (Health Canada, 1994). Changing social attitudes toward human rights, together with the influence of the 1982 Canadian Charter of Rights and Freedoms, has led to more stringent criteria for involuntary committal. For example, Ontario's Mental Health Act requires that a physician assess the situation and state, in writing,

---

BOX 38.5

Child and Adolescent Hospitalization

Hospitalizing a child or adolescent is different from hospitalizing an adult. The decision to admit a child to the hospital rests with the parents and the mental health professional. The requirements for the least restrictive environment still pertain to children and adolescents, but minors do not have the same civil rights as adults. Moreover, making decisions about the safety of children and adolescents is frequently difficult. Their competence to enter into contracts is often questionable, and their ability to manage their own behaviour is hard to assess. For these reasons, many mental health professionals err on the side of hospitalization for young people with active suicidal ideation.

Hospitalization of suicidal children tends to be prolonged because many have underlying psychosocial issues. Childhood suicidal behaviour may occur in the context of extreme family discord, and children in these dysfunctional families may be the victims of abuse or neglect (Grilo et al., 1999; Lipschitz et al., 1999; Renaud et al., 1999). Nursing care is directed toward connecting with the child/adolescent and family in order to complete a comprehensive assessment of risk and family function. Interventions are then based on the results of the assessment and identifying what needs to change in the child/adolescent's life situation.

---

that because of a mental disorder, the individual is at risk for serious bodily harm to self or other unless admitted (Health Canada). Legislative changes in many provinces have reinforced the individual's right to refuse admission and treatment except in narrowly defined circumstances.

Special considerations for the hospitalization of children and adolescents are given in Box 38-5. Health care practitioners must make every effort to obtain the patient's permission to enter the hospital voluntarily, for both legal and therapeutic reasons. Legally, **voluntary hospitalization** protects the rights of patients, permitting them some freedom in negotiating discharge from the hospital. Therapeutically, voluntary admission reinforces patients' control of the situation as partners in their own care and preserves dignity.

■ NURSING ASSESSMENT AND INTERVENTIONS

Suicidal behaviours are seriously underreported and often not recognized by health care professionals. Estimates are that approximately 40% of people who complete suicide have visited a health care provider within 1 to 6 months of a suicide attempt (Foster et al., 1999; Link, Phelan, Bresnahan, Stueve, & Pescosolido, 1999). Nurses can play important roles in suicide prevention because they practice in diverse health care settings and thus work with many different kinds of patients. Acutely suicidal behaviour is a true psychiatric emergency. Nurses must act immediately and vigorously to prevent the patient's death.

Bio/psycho/social/spiritual Domains

Nursing interventions based on a comprehensive assessment of risk provide a holistic approach to nursing care of the suicidal patient. The process of risk assessment will be discussed, followed by a discussion of nursing interventions in relation to the biologic, psychological, and social aspects of the suicidal person.

Comprehensive Assessment of Risk

Comprehensive assessment provides a clear picture of self-harm behaviour and guides possible interventions. (See Box 38-6 for questions to guide a comprehensive assessment of risk.) A model developed by Murray integrates a number of theories to establish a comprehensive assessment of risk. The model emphasizes an approach that views patients in context of their family, their social world, and the broader community (Murray & Wright, 2006). It encourages engagement and the development of a connectedness with the patient and his or her family,

using the language of a Brief Solutions and Family Therapy approach (Berg, 1994; Corcoran, 1998; DeShazer, 1988; Eggert & Thompson, 2002; Minuchin & Fishman, 1981; O'Hanlon & Werner-Davis, 1989), emphasizing the power and resiliency of families as key components for change and resolution. An intergenerational perspective and use of the genogram (deGraaf, 1998; McGoldrick, 1992) are also an integral part of the approach. This perspective recognizes family patterns over time and traces the history of abuse, alcoholism, trauma, and loss (Gould & Kramer, 2001; Maine, Shute, & Martin, 2001). Recognition of developmental factors that contribute to individual and family struggles and of family interactional patterns and boundaries also assists in providing a broad and complete assessment. (See Chapter 17 for information on family assessment.)

Applied Suicide Intervention Skills Training (ASIST)/ Living Works Inc. (Ramsey, Tanny, Taierney, & Lang, 1994) provides the framework for risk assessment, emphasizing assessment of stressors, symptoms, prior suicidal behaviour, current plan, and resources and support. An overall Rogerian approach (Rogers, 1980) guides the interactions with the patient and their family with a nonblaming, nonjudgmental, and unconditional positive regard to understand and process what the suicidal ideation or behaviour is really about. The integration of the model also assists in understanding the onset, purpose, maintenance, and

---

BOX 38.6

Questions to Guide a Comprehensive Assessment of Risk

The most successful approach is to ask open-ended questions and explore further with curious questions.

STRESSORS
What is troubling you most at the moment?
  Explore with curious questions in terms of all areas of the patient's life.
  Explore each area, asking the patient to tell you more.
  The idea is to get a clear picture of the patient's life situation and presenting stressors as the patient perceives them.

SYMPTOMS
Can you tell me about your sleep patterns?
  Explore using curious questions:
  Are you having difficulty in sleeping?
  Do you want to stay in bed and sleep through the day?
Can you tell me about your eating habits?
  Explore using curious questions:
  Have you lost your appetite?
  Do you eat in an attempt to cope with difficulties?
What do you do for enjoyment?
  Explore with curious questions:
  Do you find you no longer enjoy activities you thought were enjoyable?
  How often do you use drugs or alcohol to cope?

PRIOR BEHAVIOUR
Have you ever thought of harming yourself?
  Explore with curious questions:
  Can you tell me about that? (time, place, situation, feelings, meaning)
  What was the self-harm about?
  What happened?
  What did you expect to happen?
  What did you want to happen?

CURRENT PLAN
  Do you currently have a plan to harm yourself?
  Explore with curious questions:
  What would you do?
  Do you have access to the pills? (other methods)
  Have you picked a specific day or time?

RESOURCES AND SUPPORT
Do you have someone you recognize as supportive?
  Explore with curious questions:
  Who can you talk to about your concerns?
  Who can you confide in?
  Offer suggestions of a number of people the patient may not have thought of (e.g., parent's friend, colleague, clergy, coach, etc.).

escalation of the suicidal behaviour and assesses specific risk factors related to the self-harm behaviour.

A comprehensive assessment of stressors is vital to guide appropriate interventions. Assessment includes collection of adequate data to provide a clear picture of the patient's life and relevant stressors. As much as possible, the patient's perspective of his or her stressors and life situations should be explored. This includes a good understanding of the patient's family, peers, and social relationships as well as workplace issues. Past loss issues need to be explored with the patient to identify any possible precipitating factors related to change or loss. It is also important to discuss issues of abuse and to be aware that these issues must be approached with the appropriate degree of sensitivity.

Symptoms may be explored in the context of a depression assessment, keeping in mind the broad spectrum of depressive symptoms. (See Chapter 20 for assessment of depression.) Such symptoms include isolating or withdrawing from friends and family, sleep and eating disturbances, and not enjoying or participating in activities that were enjoyed in the past. Engaging in risky behaviour such as rebellion, noncompliance, or drugs or alcohol use are commonly associated with suicide (Ramsey et al., 1994).

The nurse or another experienced professional should assess the patient for other psychiatric disorders, especially those most commonly associated with suicidal behaviour (e.g., MDD, panic disorder, severe anxiety disorder, schizophrenia, substance abuse, borderline personality disorder, and antisocial personality disorder; Brieger et al., 2002; Catallozzi, Pletcher, & Schwarz, 2001; Preuss et al., 2002; Prigerson & Slimack, 1999; Radomsky, Haas, Mann, & Sweeney, 1999). Severity of MDD is associated with a greater likelihood of suicide completion (Alexopoulos, Bruce, Hull, Sireej, & Kakumo, 1999; Grant & Hasin, 1999). For adolescents, a key question is whether any family member has attempted or completed suicide (Cerel, Fristad, Weller, & Weller, 1999; Klimes-Dougan et al., 1999; McKeown et al., 1998). Alcoholism is another prominent factor in suicide. Patients with alcoholism account for 25% of completed suicides (Berglund & Ojehagen, 1998).

In 1997, Beck revised the Scale for Suicide Ideation (Beck, Brown, & Steer, 1997; Beck, et al., 1979) to include only eight items, and renamed it the Suicide Intent Scale. This scale is short and useful in determining whether a patient has a strong intent to die. However, even with low levels of intent, a completed suicide may occur.

● CRNENOTE

A comprehensive suicide assessment is always a priority. Taking the time to engage and connect with the patient before the assessment is crucial (Murray, 2003). It is important for nurses to integrate an assessment process that delineates stressors, symptoms, prior suicidal behaviour, current plan, and available identified resources and support (Ramsey et al., 1994).

Assessing Self-Harm

Assessing the context of each act of prior self-harm behaviour begins to paint a picture of motivation behind the behaviour. An exploration of prior behaviour also gives a message of interest and concern on the part of the health professional. A nonblaming, nonjudgmental approach allows further exploration and understanding of the patient's situation as the patient begins to trust the therapeutic relationship.

Assessment also includes exploration of self-harm behaviour that has been observed by the patient. Self-harm behaviour can be imitative, especially if it is interpreted as a way of coping with frustration and anger or a way of punishing self or others (Rew et al., 2001). Depending on the reaction of others, people may misunderstand self-harm behaviour as an acceptable way to cope with a difficult or intolerable life. Others' reaction of self-harm behaviour needs to be explored, whether or not the response was the expected or desired one. Understanding this can be the first step in helping the patient meet needs and wants in more healthy ways.

Having a Current Plan

Suicide requires intent, a plan, knowledge of how to carry out the act, and few obstacles to completing it. Patients who complete suicide have developed a workable method of killing themselves. They are less likely to have young children or other immediate responsibilities and may not be concerned with religious prohibitions concerning the act. The relationship between the availability of a method of suicide and the suicide completion is strong (Cantor & Baume, 1998). It is important for the nurse to ask whether the patient has a current plan for suicide. Further exploration of the plan gives the nurse a more accurate assessment of risks and guides appropriate interventions.

In contrast to those who carefully prepare to take their own lives are those who decide impulsively to end their lives. The latter are usually adolescents, people who abuse alcohol or drugs, or people with personality disorders. Patients with psychoses may respond impulsively to "voices" that direct them to kill themselves. Patients with psychoses are at considerable risk because of their inability to separate psychotic thinking from reality.

Resources and Support

Lack of resources and support may put patients at the greatest risk for self-harm behaviour. Suicidal people often feel socially isolated and struggle to identify and accept support from people in their immediate environment; therefore, it is important to explore supportive people in the patient's life. Interest in the patient's life

BOX 38.7

Research for Best Practice:

Murray, B. L., & Wright, K. (2006). Integration of a suicide risk assessment and intervention approach: The perspective of youth. Journal of Psychiatric and Mental Health Nursing, 13(2), 157–164.

QUESTION: What is the experience of suicide assessment and intervention for an adolescent when it is conducted by a clinical nurse specialist (CNS) using a described risk assessment model?

METHOD: Adolescent participants were interviewed using a phenomenologic approach to explore their lived experience of suicide risk assessment and intervention.

FINDINGS: The major themes that emerged from the data were change, hope, and connection. Participants described the initial assessment interview as *helpful, beneficial, reducing their anxiety,* and giving them a sense of *getting things under control.* They described a change in their thinking, other intrapersonal changes, and a change in interpersonal relationships over time as a result of the assessment. They spoke of their *hope* that things could or would change and how they shifted from a sense of giving up hope to hopefulness. They also spoke of recognizing their ability to deal with problems and issues, and of the importance of not feeling alone. The participants spoke of feeling *connected* to the CNS and of feeling that someone cared.

IMPLICATIONS FOR PRACTICE: Nurses' use of an assessment model that focuses on understanding the suicidal person's world and the meaning of his or her behaviour was experienced as helpful by adolescents. The first step in establishing a meaningful relationship with the adolescent is connecting with them and engaging them in the relationship. This requires genuine interest on the part of the nurse and an ability to set aside one's own values and beliefs while allowing adolescents to tell their story from their point of view. Active listening and open-ended questioning are necessary for a meaningful exchange of ideas and solutions. The challenging behaviour of adolescents needs to be viewed in the context of their family, social and school environment, and broader community. A focus on the adolescent's strengths and resources often promotes a shift toward cooperation and away from problematic, inappropriate, self-harm behaviours. The nurse's expectation and confidence in the adolescent's ability to act appropriately promotes responsible participation, self-direction, and self-control.

and attention received during a thorough assessment are therapeutic and can also provide connectedness and engagement with the patient and family. This connectedness provides the therapeutic environment necessary to engage the patient and family in meaningful change (Jobes, 2000) (see Box 38-7).

Nursing Diagnoses and Outcome Identification

Several nursing diagnoses may be useful when dealing with a suicidal patient, including risk for suicide, interrupted family processes, ineffective health maintenance, risk for self-directed violence, impaired social interaction, ineffective coping, chronic low self-esteem, disturbed sleep pattern, social isolation, and spiritual distress.

Planning and Implementing Nursing Interventions

Thorough assessment becomes part of the intervention process. The health professional's genuine interest, concern, and exploration begin to establish a needed trusting relationship. Using this approach, health care professionals help patients identify what and who needs to change in their environment. This approach uncovers concrete areas of improvement or change. This empowerment addresses their feelings of hopelessness, helplessness, and powerlessness.

Understanding the purpose and meaning of the self-harm behaviour guides the intervention strategies. It also gives the patient and their family a sense of hope that things can change and that someone understands their situation and is willing to assist them in making changes. If behaviour is understood as a means of communication, then interventions need not only change behaviours, but also the "cry for help" that underpins the acts. Therefore, ignoring self-harm behaviour is not helpful, although family members may not know what to do and may hope it will go away (Hall, Oliver, & Murphy, 2001). This response may actually escalate the behaviour. Punishment and overreaction are also not helpful.

If some or many of the risk factors for suicide (see Box 38-1) are present in a member of a high-risk group, the nurse must determine what is necessary to ensure the patient's ongoing safety, which is the nurse's first priority. Until the nurse has identified a patient's safety needs and implemented a plan to ensure the patient's safety, the nurse must not leave the acutely suicidal person alone for any reason, not even briefly.

A nurse should not try to treat a potentially suicidal patient without help or consultation. Even the most experienced mental health professional may lose a patient in treatment because of suicide. The reader is referred to SEIC's (n.d.) "Suicide Helpcard" for a short checklist of things to do when a patient is suicidal.

No Self-Harm (Contracting for Safety)

The nurse should consider a no self-harm contract only after performing a thorough assessment of the patient (Simon, 1999). The nurse must consider several factors in making a no self-harm contract with a patient. The patient must be competent to enter into such a contract; patients under the influence of drugs or alcohol or experiencing psychoses are not competent enough to make no self-harm contracts. Patients who have made previous suicide attempts or who are extremely isolated are not good candidates for no self-harm contracts. Legal and professional scholars disagree on the ability of children and adolescents to make decisions of this gravity on their own behalf. Involving parents in the decision about the appropriate mode of environment for their suicidal child is important. Advantages and disadvantages of no self-harm contracts and several examples of contracts can be found in a review by Range and colleagues (2002).

Inpatient Care and Acute Treatment

Suicidal patients were once hospitalized for extended periods to ensure that the suicidal crisis had passed and to provide sufficient time to establish a solid base of treatment for the underlying psychiatric disorder. This is no longer the case. Hospitals are overly restrictive environments that may inhibit the patient's development of the self-reliance needed to return to the community. Objectives of hospitalization are to maintain the patient's safety, reduce or eliminate the suicidal crisis, decrease the level of suicidal ideation, initiate treatment for the underlying disorder, evaluate for substance abuse, and reduce the patient's level of social isolation.

If the nurse and another professional determine that the patient is acutely suicidal and at considerable risk for completing suicide, he or she must decide whether to hospitalize the patient for the patient's safety. Safety in such cases is commonly determined by whether a patient may be a threat to self or others. Provincial law requires the patient to be hospitalized only when he or she cannot make reasoned decisions to ensure his or her safety. The law also requires that the restriction of the patient occurs only when it provides a therapeutic effect. In considering the hospitalization of a patient, the nurse must consider how hospitalization will be useful in ensuring safety and relieving the patient's suicidal crisis.

Interventions for the Biologic Domain

Ensuring Safety

During the early part of the hospitalization, the most important way to reduce stress is to help the patient feel more secure and hopeful. Nurses can do so by ensuring the patient's safety with as little intrusion as possible on the person's exercise of free will. Achieving this goal can be difficult. The major deterrent to patients' completing suicide in psychiatric hospitals is their engagement in a therapeutic relationship and regular observation by nurses. Each hospital has its own specific protocol for maintaining patients' safety. In addition to nursing standards of care, hospital staffing and other policies that affect the degree to which a suicidal patient can be restrained may influence the procedures mandated for caring for patients.

Maintaining a safe environment includes observing the patient regularly for suicidal behaviour, removing dangerous objects, and providing counselling opportunities for the patient. Part of ensuring patient safety is helping patients to reestablish personal control by including them in decisions about their care and restricting their behaviour only as necessary. Ongoing and effective communication with the patient is key to allowing patients to disclose and discuss their life situation and the resulting emotions and behaviour. Patients often feel shaky in the first hours of psychiatric hospitalization, and it is comforting to know that a caring person is nearby. Observational periods can be used to help the patient express a broad range of feelings and strengthen their belief in their own abilities to keep themselves safe. The nurse can help the patient who is not skilled in self-expression or self-management skills to describe feelings more effectively and cite ways of managing safety needs. Then, at the next observation time, the nurse may have the opportunity to reinforce the patient's own safety behaviour. Thus, the observation period can be transformed from something negative (e.g., "The patient can't be trusted," "I am out of control") to something positive (e.g., "The patient is becoming safer," "Maybe I can keep myself safe after all"; Cardell & Pitula, 1999). As the patient becomes more confident in understanding and controlling self-harm behaviour, the frequency of observation periods can be reduced.

Seclusion and restraint are two modalities sometimes used in the inpatient settings to maintain patient safety. However, these restrictive interventions are extremely stressful for patients and may interfere with their recovery. Moreover, seclusion and restraint often are used to compensate for inadequate staffing numbers. Unduly restraining patients to prevent their suicide interferes with the development of trusting relationships between patients and health care providers. The stress associated with restraints contributes to the biochemical disarray of their underlying psychiatric disorders. Restraints prevent patients from managing their own dysphoric and anxiety symptoms and reinforce their sense of hopelessness and helplessness. Restraints also enhance patients' fears that they are "crazy" and incapable of controlling their impulses. These methods reinforce a patient's perception of being out of control and lessen his or her ability to form a partnership with mental health providers.

Assisting With Somatic Therapies

Suicidal patients who are seriously depressed will likely receive somatic therapies, and patients' response to them must be monitored. The major somatic therapies used in the treatment of suicidal behaviour are antidepressant medications and electroconvulsive therapy (ECT). ECT may be useful for selected patients with intractable suicidal ideation and severe depression. ECT may be used for people who do not experience response to medication or who do not tolerate antidepressant medications, such as older adults and those with comorbid medical disorders. Although the decision to use ECT must be made carefully, ECT can be a life-saving procedure for the acutely suicidal patient with depression. Nurses need to be able to support patients in accepting and understanding this treatment (see Chapter 14).

The objective of medication for suicidal behaviour is to raise serotonin rapidly to a level that reduces suicide risk (Nemeroff et al., 2001). To that end, third-generation and newer antidepressant medications should be used for those who are in imminent danger of harming themselves. These include fluoxetine (Prozac), sertraline (Zoloft), paroxetine (Serzone), bupropion (Wellbutrin), venlafaxine (Effexor), and citalopram (Celexa). These drugs generally are nontoxic and cause few side effects, especially after being taken for 1 to 2 weeks. They often are faster acting than the older drugs, but their onset of action varies. Especially useful are fluoxetine and paroxetine, which may be taken once a day. Sertraline also can be taken once a day, but achieving the proper dose can sometimes be difficult. Patients who take an overdose of these medications have much better outcomes than those who abuse first- and second-generation antidepressants.

The first- and second-generation antidepressants, including tricyclics and monoamine oxidase inhibitors, are equally effective for severe depression (Sutherland, Sutherland, & Hoehns, 2003). However, for those with suicidal behaviour, they may not be the best choice because these are highly toxic medications that people with suicidal intent can use to kill themselves. The resuscitation of a patient who has taken large amounts of one of these medications can be difficult because they are cardiotoxic. Medical sequelae may be long term if the patient is saved. Also, the side effects of these early antidepressants may result in the patient stopping the use of prescribed medication while still having suicidal thoughts. The need for laboratory assessment for therapeutic drug levels is another disadvantage of these drugs. Blood monitoring requires the patient's cooperation when his or her motivation may be at its lowest.

Assisting With Treatment for Substance Use

Suicidal behaviour is often associated with substance use disorders, especially among men. When substance use is an issue for the suicidal patient, the use must be addressed, or inpatient treatment of suicidal behaviour is only palliative, and the danger of the patient repeating a suicidal attempt is high. For men, substance use disorder may be the primary psychiatric disorder, with depression a side effect of it. For women, depression commonly is the primary psychiatric disorder, and substance use disorders result from attempts to medicate the underlying depressive condition. The nurse should help the patient understand the role that alcohol and drugs play in his or her suicidal behaviour. Treatment for substance use disorders should be part of the treatment plan, as appropriate, including referral to specific inpatient or community-based programs.

Interventions for the Psychological Domain

It is important for nurses to use the hospitalization period to find out what may have precipitated or contributed to the suicidal crisis. Often, the precipitating factors and how the patient's coping process began to break down become evident. After identifying extreme stressors experienced by the patient, the nurse and patient can help determine ways for the patient to avoid those stressors in the future or, if they cannot be avoided, to manage them more effectively.

During hospitalization, the nurse should evaluate the patient's ways of thinking about problems and generating solutions. Some patients, by virtue of their depressive illness or social learning, have an unusually negative view of life. They often think such thoughts as, "I am no good," "Everything I do is useless," "I have no future," or "Nobody has ever liked me, and nobody ever will." Often patients are unable to recognize the connection between their stressors and their suicidal behaviour. Many patients have had very difficult and abusive experiences in their lives, and their ability to cope is threatened. It is important for the nurse to help the patient identify what needs to change in his or her life and how that change can come about most effectively. The prevention of further suicidal behaviour is dependent on the patient's belief that he or she can make changes with the necessary support and resources and that there is hope for the future. (See Box 38-8 for examples of effective and ineffective dialogue with a patient.)

Interventions for the Social Domain

Improving Communication

Some suicidal patients can identify family and friends who are willing to help, but in many cases, patients are concerned about burdening these people or do not

BOX 38.8

Therapeutic Dialogue: *Suicide*

When Caroline sought medical care from her nurse practitioner for a cold, the nurse observed more than a cough and runny nose. Caroline appeared downcast and unusually sad. As the nurse and patient talked, the subject of family life came up, whereupon Caroline began to cry softly. As the words tumbled out, she said that she had been unhappy at home for a long time. When she was very young, she recalled being happy, but things changed when her brother was born, 4 years after her. Her father began to abuse her sexually, starting when Caroline was 5 years old and continuing until he moved out of the house when she was 12 years old. Caroline suspects her mother knew of the abuse, although she did nothing about it.

Two years ago, Caroline's father completed suicide. Caroline feels relieved about his death but frustrated that she never got a chance to tell him how angry she was with him. Caroline's relationship with her mother has not improved. Caroline says that her mother favours her brother and is always telling her she won't amount to anything. Caroline begins to cry harder.

INEFFECTIVE APPROACH

Nurse: Clearly, many things are troubling you. Don't you think that things seem worse now because you have a cold?

Caroline: Well, that could be. What are you going to do to make me feel better?

Nurse: Give you some medicine to help you sleep and clear your nose. I think you should see a psychiatrist, too.

Caroline: I don't need a psychiatrist. I came here for my cold.

Nurse: I know you did, but you seem to be depressed.

Caroline: What are you, some kind of social worker? I am just tired.

Nurse: I am a nurse, and you seem down to me. Are you thinking about suicide?

Caroline: I don't think you know what you're talking about. I want to go now. Could you give me my medicine?

EFFECTIVE APPROACH

Nonjudgmental, curious questions; painting a picture helps you and the patient.

Nurse: It seems as though many things have been piling up on you. Does it seem that way to you, too?

Caroline: It sure does. I've just been trying to get through one day at a time, but now with this cold and no sleep, I feel like I can't go on.

Nurse: When you say you can't go on, what do you mean by that?

Caroline: Lately, I have been thinking about running away to some place where I can't be found and maybe starting over. But then I think, where would I go? Where would I stay? Who would take care of me?

Nurse: When you think that your plan for escape won't work, what happens?

Caroline: (Starting to cry again.) Then I think that maybe it would be better if I just did what my father did. I really don't think anyone would miss me.

Nurse: So you think you might take your life, like your Dad did?

Caroline: Yeah, and what really scares me is lately I have been thinking about that a lot. I keep saying to myself, "You're just tired," but I am so exhausted now that I can't chase the thoughts away.

Nurse: So, do you think about suicide every day?

Caroline: It seems like I never stop thinking about it.

Nurse: Is there anything you can do to make the thoughts go away?

Caroline: Nothing. (Silence.)

Nurse: What would you do?

Caroline: I think I would get as many pills as I could find, drink a lot of alcohol, and maybe smoke some pot and just go to sleep.

Nurse: Do you have enough pills at home to kill yourself?

Caroline (wan smile): I was hoping that the sleeping medicine you would give me might do the job.

Nurse: It sounds like you need some help getting through this time in your life. Would you like some?

Caroline: I honestly don't know—I just want to sleep for a long time.

CRITICAL THINKING CHALLENGE

- In the first interaction, the nurse made two key blunders. What were they? What effect did they have on the patient? How did they interfere with the patient's care?
- What did Caroline do that might have contributed to the nurse's behaviours in the first interaction?
- In the second interaction, the nurse did several things that ensured reporting of Caroline's suicidal ideation. What were they? What differences in attitude might differentiate the nurse in the first interaction from the nurse in the second?

---

feel comfortable sharing their concerns with others. Helping the suicidal patient express these concerns and arrive at ways of reducing them is important. In other cases, because of trauma and abuse, the patient may have difficulty identifying anyone in his or her life as supportive. These patients are usually at a high risk for suicide because of their perception of aloneness and lack of connection with any significant other.

The nurse needs to assist the patient in identifying people in the patient's life that may be supportive and also by making appropriate referrals to professionals with expertise in the area. Within the confines of therapeutic boundaries, the nurse can also be one of the supportive people in the patient's life if the nurse is successful in establishing a professional relationship with the patient.

Networking and Discharge Planning

A final concern may be the patient's embarrassment about the hospitalization and his or her emotional state. Through education, the nurse can do much to destigmatize the situation for both the patient and significant others. Before discharge, it is ideal for the patient to be able to name people who can act as a support. When supportive people are present, with the patient's permission, the nurse can work with them to begin to develop a network for the patient to rely on to remain safe. It is important for the patient and supportive family and friends to have a plan to contact another person, either a confidante or a mental health care provider, when they have questions or distressing thoughts or feel unable to manage or control suicide thoughts and behaviours.

Educating the Patient and Family

The objectives of patient and family education are to increase the patient's understanding of the origins of his or her suicidal behaviour, establish effective treatment for depression, provide for ongoing and seamless outpatient treatment, devise a plan for managing future suicidal ideation, identify supportive others in the community, establish a plan to make contact with these people and community resources, and continue with drug and alcohol treatment. These objectives are demanding for both the nurse and patient during a brief hospitalization.

In addition to trying to reduce the stigma that the patient and family may associate with suicide, the nurse must educate them about depression, suicidal behaviour, and treatments. When possible, the nurse should schedule educational sessions to include significant others so that they will better understand the patient's illness and also learn what is necessary in providing outpatient care.

Interventions for the Spiritual Domain

There can be a gap between how a patient defines his or her spirituality and the ability of health care professionals to understand and participate in their patient's spirituality in a therapeutic way (Tacey, 2003; Webb, 2005). Nurses must not only understand the influences within the bio/psycho/social/spiritual domains on their patients' experiences but also must understand how a person's spirituality, their meaning and purpose of life, encompasses the other three domains. In order to understand suicide from the patient's perspective, it is important to be open to their concept of spirituality, their thoughts and feelings around the meaning of suicide, and what it is like to contemplate killing oneself (Tacey, 2003). The lived experience of suicide contemplation needs to be heard in a caring way. Nurses, by providing a patient with the time and space to explore their meaning of life, their spirituality, and their concept of death and dying, may gain insight into the factors that precipitate the patient's suicidal thoughts and behaviours.

Evaluation and Treatment Outcomes

The most desirable treatment outcome is the patient's return to the community. Because most hospitalizations for suicidal behaviour are brief, discharge planning must begin immediately after the patient is admitted. The nurse needs to explain to the patient that hospitalization is likely to be short term and should immediately begin to form a partnership with the patient and family to ensure a smooth transition to the community. *Partnering* means empowering the patient to engage in self-care as soon as possible by helping to provide the tools he or she needs to manage.

Identifying Continuing Sources of Social Support

Appropriate referrals to professionals in the community and available resources and support are important. The community nurse or therapist requires adequate information to continue with effective interventions after discharge. In addition, engaging family and friends in the patient's ongoing care and finding sources of help in the community, such as church groups, clubhouses, drop-in centres, or other social groups, is a necessary task. A patient's inability to name any significant others or social groups often means a poor outpatient course.

Establishing an Outpatient Care Plan

At the time of discharge, the patient is still considered very ill. Most suicides occur during the first week after discharge, and many happen within the first 24 hours (Appleby, Shaw, et al., 1999). Before the patient's release, a specific, concrete plan for outpatient care must be in place. The care plan includes scheduling an appointment for outpatient care, providing for continuing medication until the first outpatient treatment visit, ensuring postrelease contact between the patient and significant others, providing for access to emergency psychiatric care, and arranging the patient's environment so that it provides both structure and safety.

At discharge, the patient should have enough medication on hand to last until the first community nurse visit. At that time, the community nurse can assess the patient's level of stability and determine whether a full prescription can be given safely to the patient. At that visit, the patient and community nurse can establish a plan of care that specifies the intensity of outpatient care. Very unstable patients may need two to three outpatient visits per week in the early days after hospitalization to maintain their safety in the community.

The patient and significant others must have a plan for the patient's ongoing supervision. This plan must be established in such a way that the patient does not feel undermined in his or her ability to manage self-care but is reassured that help will be available when needed. The family members or friends involved must feel that they are resources for the patient but not responsible for the patient's life or death. In the end, it is the patient, not supporters, who must bear responsibility for his or her safety. The patient who feels connected to but not dependent on significant others will be most likely to maintain safety in the community.

The patient's outpatient environment should be made as safe as possible before discharge. The nurse must share the care plan with family members so that they can remove any objects in the patient's environment that could be of assistance in completing suicide. The nurse must explain this measure to the patient to reinforce his or her sense of self-control. It is important to be reasonable in deciding what to remove from the environment. Patients who are truly determined to kill themselves after discharge may ultimately complete suicide.

Finally, there should be some continuity between inpatient and outpatient care. The nurse must tell the patient specifically how to obtain emergency psychiatric care. He or she should place written instructions near the patient's telephone. It is helpful for the community nurse, in addition to visits, to call periodically during the few first weeks after discharge to determine whether the patient is improving. This contact will help the patient to feel valued and connected to others. Lack of continuity is thought to contribute to significant suicide mortality after hospital discharge (Hulten & Wasserman, 1998).

Short-Term Outcomes

Short-term outcomes for the suicidal patient include maintaining the patient's safety, averting suicide, and mobilizing the patient's resources. Whether the patient is hospitalized or cared for in the community, his or her emotional distress must be reduced. This often is accomplished in an environment that restricts suicidal behaviour and provides sustained emotional support. The treatment during the suicidal crisis should also set the stage for meeting long-term objectives.

Long-Term Outcomes

Long-term outcomes must focus on maintaining the patient in psychiatric treatment, enabling the patient and family to identify and manage suicidal crises effectively, and widening the patient's support network.

Avoiding Compassion Fatigue

There is a cost to caring. It can be difficult to listen and engage deeply with patients' stories of fear, pain, and suffering. Professional work centred on relief of emotional suffering involves empathy as a key tool. Over time, being empathetic can become exhausting, even when the caregiver is diligently maintaining self-care skills. Secondary traumatization and burnout, the two components of compassion fatigue, affect most caregivers at some point during their professional career, leaving them challenged to reach out for help (Figley, 1995).

Compassion fatigue is a very real concern and one that may result in diminished capacity to function at work, at home, and within personal relationships. Its symptoms can parallel patient symptoms of post-traumatic stress disorder (see Chapter 37). These symptoms include intrusive thoughts or images of patients' situations or trauma, difficulty separating work from personal life, lower frustration tolerance, hypervigilance, decreased feelings of confidence, diminished sense of purpose or enjoyment of career, and sleep disturbances or nightmares. The nurse may begin to avoid the stress through absenteeism. These symptoms signal that a nurse's mental health is at risk. Caring for suicidal patients who are close to one's own age or having a history of being abused or neglected in childhood enhances the risks. The suicidal behaviour of a patient with whom the nurse can particularly identify can be especially upsetting.

To care successfully for suicidal patients or others prone to crises, the nurse must engage in an active program of self-care, beginning with proper rest, exercise, and nutrition, which facilitates managing stress physiologically. Self-monitoring of symptoms is the next step. Like their patients, nurses need to develop cognitive coping skills and engage in stress reduction exercises. Debriefing (i.e., sharing experiences and feelings concerning caring for a suicidal patient with other care team members) can help alleviate symptoms of stress. Some health regions in Canada have organized Critical Incident Stress Management (CISM) teams to provide Critical Incident Stress Debriefing (CISD) education regarding compassion fatigue, as well as in-services regarding self-care and stress management strategies for their health professionals.

SUMMARY OF KEY POINTS

❑ Suicidal behaviour is a means of communication that something is wrong in one's life, that life is difficult or intolerable.

❑ Suicide is a common and major public health problem that accompanies 15% of all cases of major depression.

❑ More than half of all suicides are completed on the first attempt.

☐ Parasuicide is more common among women than men.

☐ Men have a higher rate of completed suicide because of the use of more lethal means (e.g., guns, hanging).

☐ People who attempt suicide most commonly do not seek medical or psychiatric assistance.

☐ People who engage in parasuicide are likely to do so repeatedly.

☐ Suicidal behaviour may be associated with genetic and biologic origins, as well as psychological, social, and spiritual factors.

☐ People who threaten suicide have rights that must be preserved.

☐ The no self-harm contract (i.e., contracting for safety) is one means of increasing the suicidal patient's safety in the community.

☐ When a patient must be hospitalized, voluntary hospitalization is the method of choice.

☐ The major objectives of brief hospital care are to maintain the patient's safety, reestablish the patient's biologic equilibrium, strengthen the patient's cognitive coping skills, and develop an outpatient support system.

☐ The nurse who cares for suicidal patients is vulnerable to compassion fatigue and must take steps to maintain personal mental health.

CRITICAL THINKING CHALLENGES

1 A religious woman who lives with her three children, husband, and mother in rural Québec comes to her primary care provider. She is tearful and very depressed. What factors should be investigated to determine her risk for suicide and the need for hospitalization?

2 You are the primary health care nurse on a First Nations reservation. You want to implement a youth suicide prevention program. Discuss how you would proceed and some potential problems you might face.

3 Analyse lyrics of popular music that have a message about suicide and consider their possible effects on listeners. For instance, REM's "Everybody Hurts" (*Automatic for the People*) and David Bowie's "Rock and Roll Suicide" (*Ziggy Stardust*).

WEB LINKS

www.daretolive.com This is the site of Dare to Live, a teen suicide prevention page that provides information about suicide that is written for and directed to helping teens who are considering suicide.

www.nimh.nih.gov This is the site of the U.S. National Institute of Mental Health, which provides statistical facts about suicide, recent reports on mental health and suicide, current research on suicide, and a bibliography.

www.save.org This is the site of Suicide Awareness Voices of Education (SAVE), which provides information about suicide and access to texts and books. It also provides information on what to do in the event a loved one is suicidal.

www.SEIC.ca This is the site of the Canadian-based Suicide Information and Education Centre (SEIC), which provides a link to the Suicide Prevention Training Program. The goal of this program is to provide skills and training to increase caregiver competence. This site provides a library and resource centre with information on suicide and suicidal behaviour.

www.casp-acps.ca This is the site of the Canadian Association for Suicide Prevention (CASP), which provides resources and information on mental health and suicide prevention in both French and English.

video.aol.com/video/music-good-charlotte-hold-on-aol-sessions/1201548 This is a link to a Good Charlotte video of the song "Hold On," which confronts the issue of suicide and provides a message of hope to those considering suicide.

MOVIES, NOVELS, AND BIOGRAPHIES

The Hours: 2003. This Oscar-winning movie encompasses one day in the life of three women from different eras: Clarissa (Meryl Streep) who lives today; Laura (Julianne Moore), a 1950s homemaker; and Virginia Woolf (Nicole Kidman), the author as she was in 1923. The themes of life and death found in Woolf's novel, Mrs. Dalloway, connect them across time. Virginia Woolf, who suffered from depression, killed herself in 1941 at the age of 59.

VIEWING POINTS: What similarities and differences do you identify among the three women? What does the movie seem to say about suicide? About finding meaning in life? About being unable to face life despite the genuine love of family and friends?

Dead Poets Society: 1989. An English teacher, Mr. Keating (played by Robin Williams), helps his students at a private school for boys awaken to the idea that one discovers one's identity within oneself, with others' (including those in authority) serving only as guides. This free thinking brings trouble for one of the boys, Neil, who decides to pursue acting, rather than medicine, the career his father chose for him. Neil eventually kills himself in his father's office when his father moves him from Welton to a military school. Mr. Keating is blamed for Neil's death by the school administration but not by his students, who find a way to show him that his messages about life have been understood.

VIEWING POINTS: How do life pressures and societal attitudes toward the successful life contribute to suicide? What are the particular pressures within your own school or local society?

Night Mother: 1986. Sissy Spacek stars as Jessie Cates, who has decided to end her desperately unhappy life by shooting herself with her father's gun. While putting her house in order, she tries to explain her decision to her mother, Thelma, played by Anne Bancroft. Thelma tries to talk Jessie out of suicide.

VIEWING POINTS: What factors have contributed to Jessie's decision to end her life? What approach would you have taken to help Jessie?

REFERENCES

Adler, G., & Buie, D. H., Jr. (1996). Aloneness and borderline psychopathology: Possible relevance of child development issues. In J. T. Maltsberger & M. J. Goldblatt (Eds.), *Essential papers on suicide* (pp. 356–378). New York, NY: New York University Press.

Alexander, J. (2001). Depressed men: An exploratory study of close relationships. *Journal of Psychiatric & Mental Health Nursing, 8*(1), 67–75.

Alexopoulos, G. S., Bruce, M. L., Hull, J., Sireej, J. A., & Kakumo, T. (1999). Clinical determinant of suicidal ideation and behaviour in geriatric depression. *Archives of General Psychiatry, 56*(11), 1048–1053.

Angst, J., Angst, F., & Stassen, H. S. (1999). Suicide risk in patients with major depressive disorder. *Journal of Clinical Psychiatry, 60*(Suppl. 2), 57–62.

Appleby, L., Cooper, J., Amos, T., & Faragher, B. (1999). Psychological autopsy study of suicides by people aged under 35. *British Journal of Psychiatry, 175,* 168–174.

Appleby, L., Shaw, J., Amos, T., McDonnell, R., Harris, C., McCann, K., et al. (1999). Suicide within 12 months of contact with mental health services: National clinical survey. *British Medical Journal, 318*(7193), 1235–1239.

Baldessarini, R. J., Tondo, L., & Hennen, J. (1999). Effects of lithium treatment and its discontinuation on suicidal behaviour in bipolar manic-depressive disorders. *Journal of Clinical Psychiatry 60*(Suppl. 2), 77–84.

Beck, A. T., Brown, G. K., & Steer, R. A. (1997). Psychometric characteristics of the scale for suicide ideation with psychiatric outpatients. *Behaviour Research and Therapy, 35,* 1039–1046.

Beck, A. T., Kovacs, M., & Weissman, A. (1979). Assessment of suicidal intention: The scale for suicidal ideation. *Journal of Consulting and Clinical Psychology, 47*(2), 343–352.

Beck, A. T., Rush, A. J., Shaw, B. F., & Emery, G. (1979). *Cognitive therapy in depression.* New York, NY: Guilford Press.

Beck, A. T., Steer, R. A., Kovacs, M., & Garrison, B. (1985). Hopelessness and eventual suicide: A 10 year prospective study of patients hospitalized with suicide ideation. *American Journal of Psychology, 142,* 559–563.

Benson, P. (1992). Religion and substance use. In J. E. Schumaker (Ed.), *Religion and mental health* (pp. 211–220). New York, NY: Oxford University Press.

Berg, I. K. (1994). *Family-based services: A solution-focused approach.* New York, NY: W. W. Norton.

Berglund, M., & Ojehagen, A. (1998). The influence of alcohol drinking and alcohol use disorders on psychiatric disorders and suicidal behaviour. *Alcoholism: Clinical & Experimental Research, 22*(Suppl. 7), 3335–3455.

Berman, A. L. (1988). Fictional depiction of suicide in television films and imitation effects. *American Journal of Psychiatry, 145,* 982–986.

Blumenthal, S. J., & Kupfer, D. J. (Eds.) (1990). *Suicide over the life cycle: Risk factors, assessment, and treatment of suicidal patients.* Washington, DC: American Psychiatric Press.

Brieger, P., Ehrt, U., Bloeink, R., & Marneros, A. (2002). Consequences of comorbid personality disorders in major depression. *Journal of Nervous and Mental Disease, 190*(5), 304–309.

Bulik, C. M., Prescott, C. A., & Kendler, K. S. (2001). Features of childhood sexual abuse and the development of psychiatric and substance use disorders. *British Journal of Psychiatry, 179,* 444–449.

Canada Safety Council. (2004). *Canada's silent tragedy.* Retrieved November 24, 2009, from http://archive.safety-council.org/info/community/suicide.html

Canadian Nurses Association. (2002). *Code of ethics for registered nurses.* Ottawa, ON: Author.

Cantor, C. H., & Baume, P. J. (1998). Access to methods of suicide: What impact? *Australian & New Zealand Journal of Psychiatry, 32*(1), 8–14.

Cardell, R., & Pitula, C. R. (1999). Suicidal inpatients' perceptions of therapeutic and non-therapeutic aspects of constant observation. *Psychiatric Services, 50*(8), 1066–1070.

Catallozzi, M., Pletcher, J. R., & Schwarz, D. F. (2001). Prevention of suicide in adolescents. *Current Opinion in Pediatrics, 13,* 417–422.

Cerel, J., Fristad, M. A., Weller, E. B., & Weller, R. A. (1999). Suicide-bereaved children and adolescents: A controlled longitudinal examination. *Journal of the American Academy of Child and Adolescent Psychiatry, 38*(6), 672–679.

Chandler, M. J., & Lalonde, C. (1998). Cultural continuity as a hedge against suicide in Canada's First Nations. *Transcultural Psychiatry, 35*(2), 191–219.

Clark, D. C., & Goebel-Fabbri, A. E. (1998). Lifetime risk of suicide in major affective disorders. In D. Jacobs (Ed.), *Harvard Medical School guide to assessment and intervention in suicide* (pp. 270–286). San Francisco, CA: Jossey-Bass.

Clayton, D., & Barceló, A. (2000). The cost of suicide mortality in New Brunswick, 1996. Retrieved November 24, 2009, from http://www.phac-aspc.gc.ca/publicat/cdic-mcc/20-2/e_e.html

Cohen, D. A., Mason, K., Bedimo, A., Sckibner, R., Basolo, V., & Farley, T. A. (2003). Neighborhood physical conditions and health. *American Journal of Public Health, 93*(3), 467–471.

Conwell, Y., & Duberstein, P. R. (2001). Suicide in elders. *Annals of the New York Academy of Sciences, 932,* 132–150.

Conwell, Y., Duberstein, P. R., & Caine, E. D. (2002). Risk factors for suicide in later life. *Biological Psychiatry, 52,* 193–204.

Corcoran, J. (1998). Solution-focused practice with middle and high school at-risk youths. *Social Work in Education, 20*(4), 232–242.

Coverdale, J., Naim, R., & Claasen, D. (2002). Depictions of mental illness in print media: A prospective national sample. *The Australian and New Zealand Journal of Psychiatry, 36*(5), 697–700.

Cubbin, C., LeClere, F. B., & Smith, G. S. (2000). Socioeconomic status and injury mortality: Individual & neighbourhood determinants. *Journal of Epidemiology & Community Health, 54*(7), 517–524.

Cvinar, J. (2005). Do suicide survivors suffer social stigma? A review of the literature. *Perspective in Psychiatric Care, 41*(1), 14–21.

Cutcliffe, J. R. (2003). Research endeavours into suicide: A need to shift the emphasis. *British Journal of Nursing, 12,* 92–99.

deGraaf, T. K. (1998). A family therapeutic approach to transgenerational traumatization. *Family Processes, 37,* 233–242.

Dervic, K., Oquendo, M. A., Grunebaum, M. F., Ellis, S., Burke, A. K., & Mann, J. J. (2004). Religious affiliation and suicide attempt. *American Journal of Psychiatry, 161,* 2303–2308.

DeShazer, S. (1988). *Clues: Investigating solutions in brief therapy.* New York, NY: W. W. Norton.

Durkheim, E. (1897, 2006). *On Suicide.* London, UK: Penguin.

D'Zurilla, T. J., Chang, E. C., Nottingham, E. J., & Faccini, L. (1998). Social problem-solving deficits and hopelessness, depression, and suicidal risk in college students and psychiatric inpatients. *Journal of Clinical Psychology, 54*(8), 1091–1107.

Edwards, M. J., & Holden, R. R. (2001). Coping, meaning in life, and suicidal manifestations: Examining gender differences. *Journal of Clinical Psychology, 57,* 1517–1534.

Eggert, L. L., & Thompson, E. A. (2002). Preliminary effects of brief school-based prevention approaches for reducing youth suicide: Risk behaviours, depression and drug involvement. *Journal of Child and Adolescent Psychiatric Nursing, 15*(2), 48–64.

Eng, P. M., Rimm, E. B., Fitzmaurice, G., & Kawachi, I. (2002). Social ties and change in social ties in relation to subsequent total and cause-specific mortality and coronary heart disease incidence in men. *American Journal of Epidemiology, 155*(8), 700–709.

Figley, C. (1995). *Compassion fatigue.* New York, NY: Brunnwe/Mazel.

Foster, T., Gillespie, K., McClelland, R., & Patterson, C. (1999). Risk factors for suicide independent of *DSM-III-R* Axis I disorder: Case-control psychological autopsy study in Northern Ireland. *British Journal of Psychiatry, 175,* 175–179.

Gibson, P. (1994). Gay male and lesbian youth suicide. In M. Feinleif (Ed.), *Report of the Secretary's Task Force on Youth Suicide* (pp. 131–142). Washington, DC: Department of Health and Human Services.

Glowinski, A. L., Bucholz, K. K., Nelson, E. C., Fu, Q., Madden, P., Reich, W., et al. (2001). Suicide attempts in an adolescent female twin sample. *Journal of the American Academy of Child and Adolescent Psychiatry, 40*(11), 1300–1307.

Goldney, R. D. (1989). Suicide: Role of the media. *Australian and New Zealand Journal of Psychiatry, 23*, 30–34.

Goodman, E. (1999). The role of socioeconomic status gradients in explaining differences in U.S. adolescents' health. *American Journal of Public Health, 89*, 1522–1528.

Gould, M. S., King, R., Greenwald, S., Fisher, P., Schwab-Stone, M., Kramer, R., et al. (1998). Psychopathology associated with suicidal ideation and attempts among children and adolescents. *Journal of the American Academy of Child & Adolescent Psychiatry, 37*(9), 915–923.

Gould, M. S., & Kramer, R. A. (2001). Youth suicide prevention. *Suicide and Life-Threatening Behaviour, 31*, 6–31.

Government of Canada. (1985). *Criminal code of Canada*. Ottawa, ON: Author.

Government of Canada. (2006). *The human face of mental health and mental illness in Canada 2006*. Ottawa, ON: Minister of Public Works and Government Services of Canada.

Grant, B. F., & Hasin, D. S. (1999). Suicidal ideation among the United States drinking population: Results from the National Longitudinal Alcohol Epidemiologic Survey. *Journal of Studies on Alcohol, 60*(3), 422–429.

Grilo, C. M., Sanislow, C. A., Fehon, D. C., Martino, S., & McGlashan, T. H. (1999). Psychological and behavioral functioning in adolescent psychiatric inpatients who report histories of childhood abuse. *American Journal of Psychiatry, 156*, 538–543.

Gunnell, D., Lopatatzidis, A., Dorling, D., Wehner, H., Southall, H., & Frankel, S. (1999). Suicide and unemployment in young people: Analysis of trends in England and Wales, 1921–1995. *British Journal of Psychiatry, 175*, 263–270.

Guo, B., Scott, A., & Bowker, S. (2003). *Suicide prevention strategies: Evidence from systematic reviews. HTA 28*. Edmonton, AB: Heritage Foundation for Medical Research.

Guze, S. B., & Robins, E. (1970). Suicide and primary affective disorders. *British Journal of Psychiatry, 117*, 437–438.

Hall, S., Oliver, C., & Murphy, G. (2001). Early development of self-injurious behaviour: An empirical study. *American Journal on Mental Retardation, 106*, 395–400.

Hall, R. C., Platt, D. E., & Hall, R. C. (1999). Suicide risk assessment: A review of risk factors for suicide in 100 patients who have made severe suicide attempts: Evaluation of suicide risk in a time of managed care. *Psychosomatics, 40*(1), 18–27.

Harris, J. (2000). Self-harm: Cutting the bad out of me. *Qualitative Health Research, 10*, 164–173.

Hauenstein, E. (1996). A nursing practice paradigm for depressed rural women: Theoretical basis. *Archives of Psychiatric Nursing, X*(5), 283–292.

Hawton, K., Harriss, L., Hodder, K., Simkin, S., & Gunnell, D. (2001). The influence of the economic and social environment on deliberate self-harm and suicide: An ecological and person-based study. *Psychological Medicine, 31*(5), 827–836.

Health Canada. (1994). *Suicide in Canada: Update of the Report of the Task Force on Suicide in Canada*. Ottawa, ON: Government of Canada.

Health Canada. (2003). *Acting on what we know: Preventing youth suicide in First Nations*. Retrieved November 24, 2009, from http://www.hc-sc.gc.ca/fniah-spnia/pubs/promotion/_suicide/prev_youth-jeunes/

Health Canada, First Nations and Inuit Health Branch. (2003). *A statistical profile on the health of First Nations in Canada*. Ottawa, ON: Government of Canada.

Hendin, H. (1991). Psychodynamics of suicide, with particular reference to the young. *American Journal of Psychiatry, 148*, 1150–1158.

Hendin, H. (1999). Suicide, assisted suicide, and medical illness. *Journal of Clinical Psychiatry, 60*(Suppl. 2), 46–50.

HereToHelp. (2003). *Economic costs of mental disorders and addictions*. Retrieved November 24, 2009 from http://www.heretohelp.bc.ca/publications/factsheets/costs

Hilton, S. C. (2002). Active Latter-day Saints seven times less likely to commit suicide. *American Journal of Epidemiology, 155*, 413–419.

Holden, R. R., Kerr, P. S., Mendonca, J. D., & Velamoor, V. R. (1998). Are some motives more linked to suicide proneness than others? *Journal of Clinical Psychology, 54*(5), 569–576.

Hulten, A., & Wasserman, D. (1998). Lack of continuity: A problem in the care of young suicides. *Acta Psychiatrica Scandinavica, 97*(5), 326–333.

Jamison, K. R. (1999). *Night falls fast: Understanding suicide*. New York, NY: Knopf.

Joachim, G., & Acorn, S. (2000). Stigma of visible and invisible chronic conditions. *Journal of Advanced Nursing, 32*(1), 243–248.

Jobes, D. (2000). Collaborating to prevent suicide: A clinical research perspective. *Suicide and Life-Threatening Behaviour, 30*, 164–173.

Jobes, D. A., Berman, A. L., O'Carroll, P. W., Eastgard, S., & Knickmeyer, S. (1996). The Kurt Cobain suicide crisis: Perspectives from research, public health, and the news media. *Suicide and Life-Threatening Behaviour, 26*, 260–271.

Jordan, J. R. (2001). Is suicide bereavement different? A reassessment of the literature. *Suicide and Life-Threatening Behaviour, 31*(1), 91–102.

Kendall, D., Lothian-Murray, J., & Linden, R. (2004). *Sociology: In our time* (3rd ed.). Scarborough, ON: Thompson Canada Inc.

Kendler, K. S., Bulik, C. M., Silberg, J., Hettema, J. M., Myers, J., & Prescott, C. A. (2000). Childhood sexual abuse and adult psychiatric and substance use disorders in women: An epidemiological and cotwin control analysis. *Archives of General Psychiatry, 57*(10), 953–959.

Kishi, Y., Robinson, R. B., & Kosier, J. (2001). Suicidal ideation among patients during the rehabilitation period after life threatening physical illness. *Journal of Nervous and Mental Disease, 189*(9), 623–628.

Klimes-Dougan, B., Free, K., Ronsaville, D., Stillwell, J., Welsh, C. J., & Radke-Yarrow, M. (1999). Suicidal ideation and attempts: A longitudinal investigation of children of depressed and well mothers. *Journal of the American Academy of Child & Adolescent Psychiatry, 38*(6), 651–659.

Knieper, A. J. (1999). The suicide survivor's grief and recovery. *Suicide and Life-Threatening Behaviour, 29*(4), 353–364.

Koenig, H. G., & Larson, D. B. (2001). Religion and mental health: Evidence for an association. *International Review of Psychiatry, 13*, 67–78.

Kohlmeier, R. E., McMahan, C. A., & DiMaio, V. J. M. (2001). Suicide by firearms: A fifteen year experience. *American Journal of Forensic Medicine and Pathology, 22*(4), 337–340.

Koplin, B., & Agathen, J. (2002). Suicidality in children and adolescents: A review: *Current Opinion in Pediatrics, 14*, 713–717.

Kposowa, A. J. (2001). Unemployment and suicide: A cohort analysis of social factors predicting suicide in the U.S. National longitudinal mortality study. *Psychological Medicine, 31*(1), 127–138.

Kreitman, N. S., Philip, A. E., Greer, S., & Bagley C. R. (1969). Parasuicide. *British Journal of Psychiatry, 115*, 1227–1228.

Kreitman, N. S. (1970). *Parasuicide*. New York, NY: John Wiley and Sons.

Langlois, S., & Morrison, P. (2002). Suicide deaths and suicide attempts. *Health Reports, 13*(2), 9–22.

Larson, D., & Larson, S. B. (2003). Spirituality's potential relevance to physical and emotional health: A brief review of quantitative research. *Journal of Psychology and Theology, 31*, 37–51.

Leenaars, A. A. (1998). *Suicide notes: Predictive clues and patterns*. New York, NY: Human Sciences Press.

Levenkron, S. (1998). *Cutting: Understanding and overcoming self-mutilation*. London, UK: W. W. Norton.

Link, B. G., Phelan, J. C., Bresnahan, M., Stueve, A., & Pescosolido, B. (1999). Public conceptions of mental illness: Labels, causes, dangerousness, and social distance. *American Journal of Public Health, 89*(9), 1328–1333.

Lipschitz, D. S., Winegar, R. K., Nicolaou, A. L., Hartnick, E., Wolfson, M. A., & Southwick, S. (1999). Perceived abuse and neglect as risk factors for suicidal behaviour in adolescent inpatients. *Journal of Nervous and Mental Disease, 187*, 32–39.

Lopez, F. G., & Brennan, K. A. (2000). Dynamic processes underlying adult attachment organization: Toward an attachment theoretical perspective on the health and effective self. *Journal of Counseling Psychology, 47*(3), 283–300.

Luoma, J., & Pearson, J. L. (2002). Suicide and marital status in the United States, 1991–1996: Is widowhood a risk factor? *American Journal of Public Health, 92*(9), 1518–1522.

Machoian, L. (2001). Cutting voices: Self-injury in three adolescent girls. *Journal of Psychosocial Nursing and Mental Health Services, 39*(11), 22–29.

MacMillan, H. L., Fleming, J. E., Streiner, D. L., et al. (2001). Childhood abuse and lifetime psychopathology in a community sample. *American Journal of Psychiatry, 158*(11), 1878–1883.

Maine, S., Shute, R., & Martin, G. (2001). Educating parents about youth suicide: Knowledge, response to suicidal statements, attitudes, and intention to help. *Suicide and Life-Threatening Behaviour, 31*(3), 320–332.

Mann, J. J., Brent, D. A., & Arango, V. (2001). The neurobiology and genetics of suicide and attempted suicide: A focus on the serotonergic system. *Neuropsychopharmacology, 24*(5), 467–477.

Mann, J. J., Oquendo, M., Underwood, M. D., & Arango, V. (1999). The neurobiology of suicide risk: A review for the clinician. *Journal of Clinical Psychiatry, 60*(Suppl. 2), 7–11.

Martin, G. (2002). Spirituality and suicide prevention. *Auseinetter, 15*(2), 3–4.

McGoldrick, M. (1992). The legacy of loss. In F. Walsh & M. McGoldrick (Eds.), *Living beyond loss: Death in the family* (pp. 104–129). New York, NY: Norton.

McGuffin, P., Marusic, A., & Farmer, A. (2001). What can psychiatric genetics offer suicidology. *Journal of Crisis Intervention and Suicide, 22*(2), 62–65.

McKeown, R. E., Garrison, C. Z., Cuffe, S. P., Waller, J. L., Jackson, K. L., & Addy, C. L. (1998). Incidence and predictors of suicidal behaviours in a longitudinal sample of young adolescents. *Journal of the American Academy of Child & Adolescent Psychiatry, 37*(6), 612–619.

Medical Services Branch Steering Committee on Native Mental Health. (1991). *Statistical profile on Native mental health: Background report #1.* Ottawa, ON: Health Canada.

Meehan, P. J., Lamb, J. A., Saltzman, L. E., & O'Carroll, P. (1992). Attempted suicide among young adults: Progress toward a meaningful estimate of prevalence. *American Journal of Psychiatry, 149*(1), 41–44.

Minuchin, S., & Fishman, C. (1981). *Family therapy techniques.* Cambridge, MA: Harvard University Press.

Mishara, B. L. (1999). Conceptions of death and suicide in children ages 6–12 and their implications for suicide prevention. *Suicide and Life-Threatening Behaviour, 29,* 105–119.

Mitchell, A. M., Gale, D. D., Garand, L., & Wesner, S. (2003). The use of narrative data to inform the psychotherapeutic process with suicide survivors. *Issues in Mental Health Nursing, 24,* 91–106.

Modai, I., Valevski, A., Solomish, A., Kurs, R., Hines, I. L., Ritsner, M., et al. (1999). Neural network detection of files of suicidal patients and suicidal profiles. *Medical Informatics & the Internet in Medicine, 24*(4), 249–256.

Molnar, B., Berkman, L. F., & Buka, S. L. (2001) Psychopathology, childhood sexual abuse and other childhood adversities: Relative links to subsequent suicidal behaviour in the U.S. *Psychological Medicine, 31*(6), 965–977.

Morrison, L. L., & L'Heureux, J. (2001). Suicide and gay/lesbian/bisexual youth: Implications for clinicians. *Journal of Adolescence, 24,* 39–49.

Murray, B. L. (2003). Self-harm among adolescents with developmental disabilities: What are they trying to tell us? *Journal of Psychosocial Nursing, 41*(11), 37–45.

Murray, B. L., & Wright, K. (2006). Integration of a suicide risk assessment and intervention approach: The perspective of youth. *Journal of Psychiatric Mental Health Nursing, 13*(2), 157–164.

NANYouth. (2004). Aboriginal suicide statistics. Retrieved August 10, 2005, from http://www.nandecade.ca/article/71.asp

Neeleman, J., & Lewis, G. (1990). Suicide, religion, and socioeconomic conditions. An ecological study in 26 countries. *Journal of Epidemiology and Community Health, 53,* 204–210.

Nelson, E. C., Heath, A C., Madden, P. A. F., Cooper, M. L., Dinwiddie, S. H., Bucholz, K. K., et al. (2002). Association between self-reported childhood sexual abuse and adverse psychosocial outcomes: Results from a twin study. *Archives of General Psychiatry, 59,* 139–145.

Nemeroff, C. B., Compton, M. T., & Berger, J. (2001). The depressed suicidal patient: Assessment and treatment. *Annals of American Academy of Sciences, 932,* 1–23.

Nisbet, P. A., Duberstein, P. R., Conwell, Y., & Seidlitz, L. (2000). The effect of participation in religious activities on suicide versus natural death in adults 50 and older. *The Journal of Nervous and Mental Disease, 188*(8), 543–546.

O'Connell, H., Chin, A., Cunningham, C., & Lawlor, B. A. (2004). Recent developments: Suicide in older people. *British Medical Journal, 329,* 895–899.

O'Connor, R. C., & Noel, P. S. (1997). Suicide and gender. *Mortality, 2*(3), 239–254.

O'Hanlon, W. H., & Werner-Davis, M. (1989). *In search of solutions: A new direction in psychotherapy.* New York, NY: W. W. Norton.

Ohberg, A., & Lonnqvist, J. (1998). Suicides hidden among undetermined deaths. *Acta Psychiatrica Scandinavica, 98*(3), 214–218.

Pesut, B. (2003). Developing spirituality in the curriculum: Intrapersonal connectedness, interpersonal connectedness. *Nursing Education Perspectives, 24,* 290–294.

Pesut, B. (2008). A conversation on diverse perspectives of spirituality in nursing literature. *Nursing Philosophy, 9,* 98–109.

Pfeffer, C. R., Normandin, L., & Kakuma, T. (1998). Suicidal children grow up: Relations between family psychopathology and adolescents' lifetime suicidal behaviour. *Journal of Nervous Mental Disease, 186,* 269–275.

Phillips, D. P., & Carstensen, L. L. (1986). Clustering of teenage suicides after television news stories. *New England Journal of Medicine, 315,* 685–689.

Pitchot, W., Hansenne, M., Moreno, A., Pinto, E., Reggers, J., Fuchs, S., et al. (2001). Reduced dopamine function in depressed patients is related to suicidal behaviour but not its lethality. *Psychoneuroendocrinology, 26,* 689–696.

Platt, S. (1993). The social transmission of parasuicide: Is there a modeling effect? *Crisis, 14,* 23–31.

Poijula, S., Walberg, K. E., & Dyregrov, A. (2001). Adolescent suicide and suicide contagion in three secondary schools. *International Journal of Emergency Mental Health, 3*(3), 163–168.

Preuss, U. W., Schuckit, M. A., Smith, T. L., Danko, G. P., Buckman, K., Bierut, L., et al. (2002). Comparison of 3190 alcohol-dependent individuals with and without suicide attempts. *Alcoholism: Clinical and Experimental Research, 26*(4), 471–477.

Prigerson, H. G., & Slimack, M. J. (1999). Gender differences in clinical correlates of suicidality among young adults. *Journal of Nervous and Mental Disease, 187*(1), 23–31.

Public Health Agency of Canada. (2000). *Leading causes of death and hospitalization in Canada.* Retrieved November 24, 2009, from http://www.phac-aspc.gc.ca/publicat/lcd-pcd97/index.html

Qin, P., Agergbo, E., & Mortensen, P. B. (2003). Suicide risk in relationship to socioeconomic, demographic, psychiatric, and familial factors: A national register-based study of all suicides in Denmark, 1981–1997. *American Journal of Psychiatry, 160*(4), 765–772.

Qin, P., Agerbo, E., Westergård-Nielson, N., Erikson, T., & Mortenson, P. B. (2000). Gender differences in risk factors for suicide in Denmark. *British Journal of Psychiatry, 177,* 546–550.

Quan, H., Arboleda-Flórez, J., Fick, G. H., Stuart, H. L., & Love, E. J. (2002). Association between physical illness and suicide among the elderly. *Social Psychiatry & Psychiatric Epidemiology, 37,* 190–197.

Radomsky, E. D., Haas, G. L., Mann, J. J., & Sweeney, J. A. (1999). Suicidal behaviour in patients with schizophrenia and other psychotic disorders. *American Journal Psychiatry, 156*(10), 1590–1595.

Ramsey, R. F., Tanny, B. L., Taierney, R. J., & Lang, W. A. (1994). *Suicide intervention handbook.* Calgary, AB: Living Works Education Inc.

Range, L. M., Campbell, C., Kovac, S. H., Marion-Jones, M., Aldridge, H., Kogos, S. & Crump, Y. (2002). No-suicide contracts: An overview and recommendations. *Death Studies, 26,* 51–74.

Reed, M. (1998). Predicting grief symptomology among the suddenly bereaved. *Suicide and Life Threatening Behavior, 28*(3), 285–301.

Remafedi, G., Farrow, J., & Deisher, R. (1991). Risk factors for attempted suicide in gay and bisexual youth. *Pediatrics, 87,* 869–875.

Renaud, J., Brent, D. A., Birmaher, B., Chiappetta, L., & Bridge, J. (1999). Suicide in adolescents with disruptive disorders. *Journal of the American Academy of Child & Adolescent Psychiatry, 38,* 846–851.

Rew, L., Thomas, N., Horner, S., Resnick, M., & Beuhring, T. (2001). Correlates of recent suicide attempts in a tri-ethnic group of adolescents. *Journal of Nursing Scholarship, 4,* 361–367.

Rihmer, Z., & Pestality, P. (1999). Bipolar II disorder and suicidal behavior. *Psychiatric Clinics of North America, 22*(3), 667–673.

Rogers, C. (1980). *A way of being.* Boston, MA: Houghton Mifflin.

Rosenberg, N. K. (1993). Psychotherapy of the suicidal patient. *Acta Psychiatrica Scandinavica, 371,* 54–56.

Rotheram-Borus, M. J., & Fernandez, M. I. (1995). Sexual orientation and developmental challenges experienced by gay and lesbian youths. *Suicide and Life-Threatening Behaviour, 23*(Suppl.), 26–34.

Roy, A. (1989). Suicide. In H. I. Kaplan & B. J. Sadock (Eds.), *Comprehensive textbook of psychiatry* (pp. 1414–1427). Baltimore, MD: Williams & Wilkins.

Royal Commission on Aboriginal Peoples. (1995). *Choosing life: Special report on suicide among Aboriginal people.* Ottawa, ON: Communication Group.

Russell, S. T., & Joyner, K. (2001). Adolescent sexual orientation and suicide risk: Evidence from a nation study. *American Journal of Public Health, 91*(8), 1276–1281.

Saarinen, P. I., Lehtonen, J., & Lonnqvist, J. (1999). Suicide risk in schizophrenia: An analysis of 17 consecutive suicides. *Schizophrenia Bulletin, 25*(3), 533–542.

Sakinofsky, I., Roberts, R. S., Brown, Y., Cummings, C., & James, P. (1990). Problem resolution and repetition of parasuicide: A prospective study. *British Journal of Psychiatry, 156*, 395–399.

Samson, C. (2003). Sexual abuse and assimilation: Oblates, teachers and the Innu of Labrador. *Sexualities, 6*(1), 46–53.

Savin-Williams, R. (1990). *Gay and lesbian youth: Expressions of identity.* New York, NY: Hemisphere.

Schmidtke, A., & Hafner, H. (1988). The Werther effect after television films: New evidence for an old hypothesis. *Psychological Medicine, 18*, 665–676.

Schneidman, E. (1985). *Definition of suicide.* New York, NY: John Wiley & Sons.

Simon, R. (1996, April). Suicide and firearms: Restricting access in Canada. Paper presented to the American Association of Suicidology, Washington, DC.

Simon, R. I. (1999). The suicide prevention contract: Clinical, legal and risk management issues. *Journal of the American Academy of Psychiatry & the Law, 27*(3), 445–450.

Skodol, A. E., Siever, L. J., & Livesley, W. J. (2002). The borderline diagnosis. II. Biology, genetics, and clinical course. *Biological Psychiatry, 51*, 951–963.

Stack, S., & Lester, D. (1991). The effect of religion on suicide ideation. *Social Psychiatry and Psychiatric Epidemiology, 26*, 168–170.

Statham, D. J., Heath, A. C., Madden, P. A., Bucholz, K. K., Bierut, L., Dinwiddie, S. H., et al. (1998). Suicidal behaviour: An epidemiological and genetic study. *Psychological Medicine, 28*(4), 839–855.

Statistics Canada. (2003). Depression. In *Health indicators: Highlights.* Retrieved November 24, 2009, from http://www.statcan.ca/english/freepub/82-221-XIE/01103/high/region/hdepres.htm

Statistics Canada. (2005). *Chapter XX: External causes of morbidity and mortality (V01-Y89), by age group and sex.* Retrieved November 24, 2009, from http://www.statcan.gc.ca/pub/84-208-x/2002/t/4152749-eng.htm

Statistics Canada. (2006). *Causes of death, 2003.* Ottawa, ON: Author.

Statistics Canada. (2007). *Suicides and suicide rate, by sex and by age group.* Retrieved November 24, 2009, from http://www40.statcan.gc.ca/l01/cst01/perhlth66a-eng.htm

Statistics Canada. (2008). *Selected leading causes of death, by sex.* Retrieved November 24, 2009, from http://www40.statcan.ca/l01/cst01/health36-eng.htm

Steenland, K., Halperin, W., Hu, S., & Walker, J. T. (2003). Deaths due to injuries among employed adults: The effects of socioeconomic class. *Epidemiology, 14*(1), 74–79.

Stewart, S. E., Manion, I. G., Davidson, S., & Cloutier, P. (2001). Suicidal children and adolescents with first emergency room presentations: Predictors of six-month outcome. *Journal of the American Academy of Child and Adolescent Psychiatry, 40*(5), 580–587.

Suicide Information and Education Centre. (2003). *Suicide among Canada's Aboriginal peoples.* Retrieved November 24, 2009, from http://www.suicideinfo.ca/csp/assets/Alert52.pdf

Suicide Information and Education Centre. (n.d.). *Suicide helpcard.* Retrieved March 24, 2009, from, http://www.suicideinfo.ca/csp/assets/helpcard.pdf

Sutherland, J. E., Sutherland, S. J., & Hoehns, J. D. (2003). Achieving the best outcome in treatment of depression. *Journal of Family Practice, 53*(3), 118–126.

Tacey, D. (2003). *The spirituality revolution.* Sydney, Australia: Harper Collins.

Tadros, G., & Jolley, D. (2001). The stigma of suicide. *British Journal of Psychiatry, 179*(2), 178. (correspondence).

Tinley, S. T., & Kinney, A. Y. (2007). Three philosophical approaches to the study of spirituality. *Advances in Nursing Science, 30*, 71–80.

Tondo, L., & Baldessarini, R. J. (2001). *Suicide: Historical, descriptive, and epidemiological considerations.* Retrieved November 24, 2009, from http://yenoh93.medceu.com/index/courses/suicide.htm

Vilhjalmsson, R., Kristjansdottir, G., & Sveinbjarnardottir, E. (1998). Factors associated with suicide ideation in adults. *Social Psychiatry and Psychiatric Epidemiology, 33*(3), 97–103.

Walsh, B. W., & Rosen, P. M. (1988). *Self-mutilation: Theory research and treatment.* New York, NY: Guilford Press.

Webb, D. (2005). Bridging the spirituality gap. *Australian e-Journal for the Advancement of Mental Health, 4*(1), 1–9. Retrieved November 24, 2009, from http://www.auseinet.com/journal/vol4iss1/webb.pdf

Welch, S., S. (2001). A review of the literature on the epidemiology of parasuicide in the general population. *Psychiatric Services, 52*(3), 368–375.

White, J., & Jodoin, N. (2003). *Aboriginal youth: A manual of promising suicide prevention strategies.* Retrieved November 24, 2009, from http://www.suicideinfo.ca/csp/go.aspx?tabid=144

World Health Organization. (2002). *Self-directed violence.* Retrieved August 10, 2005, from http://www.who.int/violence_injury_prevention/violence/world_ report/factsheets/en/selfdirectedviolfacts.pdf

Zor, F., Mustafa, D., Mehmet, B., Semih, D., Duman, H., & Sengezer, M. (2005). Psychological evaluation of self-inflicted burn patients: Suicide or parasuicide? *Burns, 31*, 178–181.

APPENDIX A

DSM-IV-TR Classification: Axes I and II Categories and Codes

■▬ DISORDERS USUALLY FIRST DIAGNOSED IN INFANCY, CHILDHOOD, OR ADOLESCENCE

Mental Retardation

Note: These are coded on Axis II.
- 317   Mild Mental Retardation
- 318.0   Moderate Mental Retardation
- 318.1   Severe Mental Retardation
- 318.2   Profound Mental Retardation
- 319   Mental Retardation, Severity Unspecified

Learning Disorders

- 315.00   Reading Disorders
- 315.1   Mathematics Disorders
- 315.2   Disorder of Written Expression
- 315.9   Learning Disorder NOS

NOS, not otherwise specified.

An X appearing in a diagnostic code indicates that a specific code number is required.

An ellipsis (…) is used in the names of certain disorders to indicate that the name of a specific mental disorder or general medical condition should be inserted when recording the name (e.g., 293 Delirium Due to Hypothyroidism).

*Indicate the General Medical Condition.

**Refer to Substance-Related Disorders for substance-specific codes.

***Indicate the Axis I or Axis II Disorder.

American Psychiatric Association. (2000). *Diagnostic and statistical manual of mental disorders* (4th ed., Text revision). Washington, DC: Author.

Motor Skills Disorder

- 315.4   Developmental Coordination Disorder

Communication Disorders

- 315.31   Expressive Language Disorder
- 315.32   Mixed Receptive-Expressive Language Disorder
- 315.39   Phonological Disorder
- 307.0   Stuttering
- 307.9   Communication Disorder NOS

Pervasive Developmental Disorders

- 299.00   Autistic Disorder
- 299.80   Rett's Disorder
- 299.10   Childhood Disintegrative Disorder
- 299.80   Asperger's Disorder
- 299.80   Pervasive Developmental Disorder NOS

Attention-Deficit and Disruptive Behaviour Disorders

- 314.xx   Attention-Deficit/Hyperactivity Disorder
  - .01   Combined Type
  - .00   Predominantly Inattentive Type
  - .01   Predominantly Hyperactive-Impulsive Type
- 314.9   Attention-Deficit/Hyperactivity Disorder NOS
- 312.8   Conduct Disorder
  - *Specify type*: Childhood-Onset/Adolescent-Onset

313.81	Oppositional Defiant Disorder
312.9	Disruptive Behaviour Disorder NOS

Feeding and Eating Disorders of Infancy or Early Childhood

307.52	Pica
307.53	Rumination Disorder
307.59	Feeding Disorder of Infancy or Early Childhood

Tic Disorders

307.23	Tourette's Disorder
307.22	Chronic Motor or Vocal Tic Disorder
307.21	Transient Tic Disorder
	Specify if: Single Episode/Recurrent
307.20	Tic Disorder NOS

Elimination Disorders

—.-	Encopresis
787.6	With Constipation and Overflow Incontinence
307.7	Without Constipation and Overflow Incontinence
307.6	Enuresis (Not Due to a General Medical Condition)
	Specify type: Nocturnal Only/Diurnal Only/ Nocturnal and Diurnal

Other Disorders of Infancy, Childhood, or Adolescence

309.21	Separation and Anxiety Disorder
	Specify if: Early Onset
313.23	Selective Mutism
313.89	Reactive Attachment Disorder of Infancy or Early Childhood
	Specify type: Inhibited/Disinhibited
307.3	Stereotypic Movement Disorder
	Specify if: With Self-Injurious Behaviour
313.9	Disorder of Infancy, Childhood, or Adolescence NOS

▰◗ DELIRIUM, DEMENTIA, AND AMNESTIC AND OTHER COGNITIVE DISORDERS

Delirium

293.0	Delirium Due to...*
—.-	Substance Intoxication Delirium**
—.-	Substance Withdrawal Delirium**
—.-	Delirium Due to Multiple Etiologies (code each of the specific etiologies)
780.09	Delirium NOS

Dementia

294.xx	Dementia of the Alzheimer's Type, With Early Onset
.10	Without Behavioural Disturbance
.11	With Behavioural Disturbance
294.xx	Dementia of the Alzheimer's Type, With Late Onset
.10	Without Behavioural Disturbance
.11	With Behavioural Disturbance
294.xx	Vascular Dementia
.40	Uncomplicated
.41	With Delirium
.42	With Delusions
.43	With Depressed Mood
	Specify if: With Behavioural Disturbance
294.1x	Dementia Due to HIV Disease
294.1x	Dementia Due to Head Trauma
294.1x	Dementia Due to Parkinson's Disease
294.1x	Dementia Due to Huntington's Disease
294.10	Dementia Due to Pick's Disease
290.10	Dementia Due to Creutzfeldt-Jakob Disease
294.1	Dementia Due to... [Indicate the General Medical Condition not listed above]
—.-	Substance-Induced Persisting Dementia**
—.-	Dementia Due to Multiple Etiologies (code each of the specific etiologies)
294.8	Dementia NOS

Amnestic Disorders

294.0	Amnestic Disorder Due to...*
	Specify if: Transient/Chronic
—.-	Substance-Induced Persisting Amnestic Disorder**
294.8	Amnestic Disorder NOS

Other Cognitive Disorders

294.9	Cognitive Disorder NOS

▰◗ MENTAL DISORDERS DUE TO A GENERAL MEDICAL CONDITION NOT CLASSIFIED ELSEWHERE

293.89	Catatonic Disorder Due to...*
310.0	Personality Change Due to...*

Specify type: Labile/Disinhibited/
Aggressive/Apathetic/Paranoid/Other/
Combined/Unspecified

293.9   Mental Disorder NOS Due to...*

▰ SUBSTANCE-RELATED DISORDERS

The following specifiers may be applied to Substance Dependence:

With Physiological Dependence/Without
   Physiological Dependence
Early Full Remission/Early Partial Remission
Sustained Full Remission/Sustained Partial Remission
On Agonist Therapy/In a Controlled Environment

*The following specifiers apply to Substance-Induced Disorders
as noted*:

With Onset During Intoxication/[W]With Onset
   During Withdrawal

Alcohol-Related Disorders

Alcohol Use Disorders

303.90   Alcohol Dependence
305.00   Alcohol Abuse

Alcohol-Induced Disorders

303.00   Alcohol Intoxications
291.8   Alcohol Withdrawal
        Specify if: With Perceptual Disturbances
291.0   Alcohol Intoxication Delirium
291.0   Alcohol Withdrawal Delirium
291.2   Alcohol-Induced Persisting Dementia
291.1   Alcohol-Induced Persisting Amnestic Disorder
291.x   Alcohol-Induced Psychotic Disorder
  .5   With Delusions[I,W]
  .3   With Hallucinations[I,W]
291.8   Alcohol-Induced Mood Disorder[I,W]
291.8   Alcohol-Induced Anxiety Disorder[I,W]
291.8   Alcohol-Induced Sexual Dysfunction[I]
291.   Alcohol-Induced Sleep Disorder[I,W]
291.9   Alcohol-Related Disorder NOS

Amphetamine (or Amphetamine-like)-Related Disorders

Amphetamine Use Disorders

304.40   Amphetamine Dependence*
305.70   Amphetamine Abuse

Amphetamine-Induced Disorders

292.89   Amphetamine Intoxication
        Specify if: With Perceptual Disturbances
292.0   Amphetamine Withdrawal

292.81   Amphetamine Intoxication Delirium
292.xx   Amphetamine-Induced Psychotic Disorder
  .11   With Delusions[I]
  .12   With Hallucinations[I]
292.84   Amphetamine-Induced Mood Disorder[I,W]
292.89   Amphetamine-Induced Anxiety Disorder[I]
292.89   Amphetamine-Induced Sexual Dysfunction[I]
292.89   Amphetamine-Induced Sleep Disorder[I,W]
292.9   Amphetamine-Related Disorder NOS

Caffeine-Related Disorders

Caffeine-Induced Disorders

305.90   Caffeine Intoxication
292.89   Caffeine-Induced Anxiety Disorder[I]
292.89   Caffeine-Induced Sleep Disorder[I]
292.9   Caffeine-Related Disorder NOS

Cannabis-Related Disorders

Cannabis Use Disorders

304.30   Cannabis Dependence*
305.20   Cannabis Abuse

Cannabis-Induced Disorders

292.89   Cannabis Intoxication
        Specify if: With Perceptual Disturbances
292.81   Cannabis Intoxication Delirium
292.xx   Cannabis-Induced Psychotic Disorder
  .11   With Delusions[I]
  .12   With Hallucinations[I]
292.89   Cannabis-Induced Anxiety Disorder
292.9   Cannabis-Related Disorder NOS

Cocaine-Related Disorders

Cocaine Use Disorders

304.20   Cocaine Dependence*
305.60   Cocaine Abuse

Cocaine-Induced Disorders

292.89   Cocaine Intoxication
        Specify if: With Perceptual Disturbances
292.0   Cocaine Withdrawal
292.81   Cocaine Intoxication Delirium
292.xx   Cocaine-Induced Psychotic Disorder
  .11   With Delusions[I]
  .12   With Hallucinations[I]
292.84   Cocaine-Induced Mood Disorder[I,W]
292.89   Cocaine-Induced Anxiety Disorder[I,W]
292.89   Cocaine-Induced Sexual Dysfunction[I]

292.89　Cocaine-Induced Sleep Disorder[I,W]
292.9　Cocaine-Related Disorder NOS

Hallucinogen-Related Disorders

Hallucinogen Use Disorders

304.50　Hallucinogen Dependence*
305.30　Hallucinogen Abuse

Hallucinogen-Induced Disorders

292.89　Hallucinogen Intoxication
292.89　Hallucinogen Persisting Perception
　　　　Disorder (Flashbacks)
292.81　Hallucinogen Intoxication Delirium
292.xx　Hallucinogen-Induced Psychotic Disorder
　.11　With Delusions[I]
　.12　With Hallucinations[I]
292.84　Hallucinogen-Induced Mood Disorder[I]
292.89　Hallucinogen-Induced Anxiety Disorder[I]
292.9　Hallucinogen-Related Disorder NOS

Inhalant-Related Disorders

Inhalant Use Disorders

304.60　Inhalant Dependence*
305.90　Inhalant Abuse

Inhalant-Induced Disorders

292.89　Inhalant Intoxication
292.81　Inhalant Intoxication Delirium
292.82　Inhalant-Induced Persisting Dementia
292.xx　Inhalant-Induced Psychotic Disorder
　.11　With Delusions[I]
　.12　With Hallucinations*
292.84　Inhalant-Induced Mood Disorder[I]
292.89　Inhalant-Induced Anxiety Disorder[I]
292.9　Inhalant-Related Disorder NOS

Nicotine-Related Disorders

Nicotine Use Disorder

305.10　Nicotine Dependence*

Nicotine-Induced Disorders

292.0　Nicotine Withdrawal
292.9　Nicotine-Related Disorder NOS

Opioid-Related Disorders

Opioid Use Disorders

304.00　Opioid Dependence*
305.50　Opioid Abuse

Opioid-Induced Disorders

292.89　Opioid Intoxication
　　　　Specify if: With Perceptual Disturbances
292.0　Opioid Withdrawal
292.81　Opioid Intoxication Delirium
292.xx　Opioid-Induced Psychotic Disorders
　.11　With Delusions[I]
　.12　With Hallucinations[I]
292.84　Opioid-Induced Mood Disorder[I]
292.89　Opioid-Induced Sexual Dysfunction[I]
292.89　Opioid-Induced Sleep Disorder[I,W]
292.9　Opioid-Related Disorder NOS

Phencyclidine (or Phencyclidine-like)-Related Disorders

Phencyclidine Use Disorders

304.90　Phencyclidine Dependence*
305.90　Phencyclidine Abuse

Phencyclidine-Induced Disorders

292.89　Phencyclidine Intoxication
　　　　Specify if: With Perceptual Disturbances
292.81　Phencyclidine Intoxication Delirium
292.xx　Phencyclidine-Induced Psychotic Disorders
　.11　With Delusions[I]
　.12　With Hallucinations[I]
292.84　Phencyclidine-Induced Mood Disorder[I]
292.89　Phencyclidine-Induced Anxiety Disorder[I]
292.9　Phencyclidine-Related Disorder NOS

Sedative-, Hypnotic-, or Anxiolytic-Related Disorders

Sedative-, Hypnotic-, or Anxiolytic Use Disorders

304.10　Sedative, Hypnotic, or Anxiolytic
　　　　Dependence*
305.40　Sedative, Hypnotic, or Anxiolytic Abuse

Sedative-, Hypnotic-, or Anxiolytic-Induced Disorders

292.89　Sedative, Hypnotic, or Anxiolytic
　　　　Intoxication
292.0　Sedative, Hypnotic, or Anxiolytic
　　　　Withdrawal
　　　　Specify if: With Perceptual Disturbances
292.81　Sedative, Hypnotic, or Anxiolytic
　　　　Intoxication Delirium
292.81　Sedative, Hypnotic, or Anxiolytic
　　　　Withdrawal Delirium

292.82   Sedative-, Hypnotic-, or Anxiolytic-Induced Persisting Delirium

292.83   Sedative-, Hypnotic-, or Anxiolytic-Induced Persisting Amnestic disorder

292.xx   Sedative-, Hypnotic-, or Anxiolytic-Induced Psychotic Disorder
.11   With Delusions[I,W]
.12   With Hallucinations[I,W]

292.84   Sedative-, Hypnotic-, or Anxiolytic-Induced Mood Disorder[I,W]

292.89   Sedative-, Hypnotic-, or Anxiolytic-Induced Anxiety Disorder[W]

292.89   Sedative-, Hypnotic-, or Anxiolytic-Induced Sexual Dysfunction[I]

292.89   Sedative-, Hypnotic-, or Anxiolytic-Induced Sleep Disorder[I,W]

292.9   Sedative-, Hypnotic-, or Anxiolytic-Induced Disorder NOS

Polysubstance-Related Disorder

304.80   Polysubstance Dependence*

Other (or Unknown) Substance-Related Disorders

Other (or Unknown) Substance Use Disorders

304.90   Other (or Unknown) Substance Dependence*

305.90   Other (or Unknown) Substance Abuse

Other (or Unknown) Substance-Induced Disorders

292.89   Other (or Unknown) Substance Intoxication
Specify if: With Perceptual Disturbances

292.0   Other (or Unknown) Substance Withdrawal
Specify if: With Perceptual Disturbances

292.81   Other (or Unknown) Substance-Induced Delirium

292.82   Other (or Unknown) Substance-Induced Persisting Dementia

292.83   Other (or Unknown) Substance-Induced Persisting Amnestic Disorder

292.xx   Other (or Unknown) Substance-Induced Psychotic Disorder
.11   With Delusions[I,W]
.12   With Hallucinations[I,W]

292.84   Other (or Unknown) Substance-Induced Mood Disorder[I,W]

292.89   Other (or Unknown) Substance-Induced Anxiety Disorder[I,W]

292.89   Other (or Unknown) Substance-Induced Sexual Dysfunction[I]

292.89   Other (or Unknown) Substance-Induced Sleep Disorder[I,W]

292.9   Other (or Unknown) Substance-Induced Disorder NOS

◼◼ SCHIZOPHRENIA AND OTHER PSYCHOTIC DISORDERS

295.xx   Schizophrenia

The following Classification of Longitudinal Course applies to all subtypes of Schizophrenia:

Episodic With Interepisode Residual Symptoms
   (*Specify if*: With Prominent Negative Symptoms)/
   Episodic With No Interepisode Residual
   Symptoms/Continuous
   (*Specify if*: With Prominent Negative Symptoms)
Single Episode in Partial Remission
   (*Specify if*: With Prominent Negative Symptoms)
Single Episode in Full Remission
Other or Unspecified Patterns

.30   Paranoid Type
.10   Disorganized Type
.20   Catatonic Type
.90   Undifferentiated Type
.60   Residual Type

295.40   Schizophreniform Disorder
   Specify if: Without Good Prognostic Features/With Good Prognostic Features

295.70   Schizoaffective Disorder
   Specify type: Bipolar/Depressive

297.1   Delusional Disorder
   Specify type: Erotomanic/Grandiose/Jealous/Persecutory Somatic/Mixed/Unspecified

298.8   Brief Psychotic Disorder
   Specify if: With Marked Stressor(s)/Without Marked Stressor(s)/With Postpartum Onset

297.3   Shared Psychotic Disorder

293.xx   Psychotic Disorder Due to...*
.81   With Delusions
.82   With Hallucinations

—.-   Substance-Induced Psychotic Disorder (refer to Substance-Related Disorders for substance-specific codes)
   Specify if: With Onset During Intoxication/With Onset During Withdrawal

298.9   Psychotic Disorder NOS

▰◗ MOOD DISORDERS

Code current state of Major Depressive Disorder or Bipolar I Disorder in fifth digit

1 = Mild
2 = Moderate
3 = Severe Without Psychotic Features
4 = Severe With Psychotic Features
   Specify if: Mood-Congruent Psychotic Features/ Mood-Incongruent Psychotic Features
5 = In Partial Remission
6 = In Full Remission
0 = Unspecified

The following specifiers apply (for current or most recent episodes) to Mood Disorders as noted:

[a]Severity/Psychotic/Remission Specifiers/[b]Chronic/[c]With Catatonic Features/[d]With Melancholic Features/[e]With Atypical Features/[f]With Postpartum Onset

The following specifiers apply to Mood Disorders as noted:

[g]With or Without Full Interepisode Recovery/With Seasonal Pattern/[i]With Rapid Cycling

Depressive Disorders

296.xx	Major Depressive Disorder
.2x	Mingle Episode[a,b,c,d,e,f]
.3x	Recurrent[a,b,c,d,e,f,g,h]
300.4	Dysthymic Disorder
	Specify if: Early Onset/Late Onset
	Specify if: With Atypical Features
311	Depressive Disorder NOS

Bipolar Disorders

296.xx	Bipolar I Disorder
.0x	Single Manic Episode[a,c,f]
	Specify if: Mixed
.40	Most Recent Episode Hypomanic[a,h,j]
.4x	Most Recent Episode Manic[a,c,f,g,h,i]
.6x	Most Recent Episode Mixed[a,c,f,g,h,i]
.5x	Most Recent Episode Depressed[a,b,c,d,e,f,g,h,i]
.7	Most Recent Episode Unspecified[g,h,i]
296.89	Bipolar II Disorder[a,b,c,d,e,f,g,h,i]
	Specify (current or most recent episode) if: Hypomanic/Depressed
301.13	Cyclothymic Disorder
296.80	Bipolar Disorder NOS
293.83	Mood Disorder Due to…*
	Specify type: With Depressive Features/ With Major Depressive-like Episode/ With Manic Features/With Mixed Features

—.—	Substance-Induced Mood Disorder**
	Specify type: With Depressive Features/ With Manic Features/With Mixed Features
	Specify if: With Onset During Intoxication/With Onset During Withdrawal
296.90	Mood Disorder NOS

▰◗ ANXIETY DISORDERS

300.01	Panic Disorder without Agoraphobia
300.21	Panic Disorder With Agoraphobia
300.22	Agoraphobia Without History of Panic Disorder
300.29	Specific Phobia
	Specify type: Animal Type/Natural Environment Type/Blood-Injection-Injury Type/Situational Type/Other Types
300.23	Social Phobia
	Specify if: Generalized
300.3	Obsessive-Compulsive Disorder
	Specify if: With Poor Insight
309.81	Posttraumatic Stress Disorder
	Specify if: Acute/Chronic
	Specify if: With Delayed Onset
308.3	Acute Stress Disorder
300.02	Generalized Anxiety Disorder
293.80	Anxiety Disorder Due to…*
	Specify if: With Generalized Anxiety/ With Panic Attacks/With Obsessive-Compulsive Symptoms…*
293.84	Substance-Induced Anxiety Disorder
	Specify if: With Generalized Anxiety/With Panic Attacks/With Obsessive-Compulsive Symptoms/With Phobic Symptoms
	Specify if: With Onset During Intoxication/ With Onset During Withdrawal
300.00	Anxiety Disorder NOS

▰◗ SOMATOFORM DISORDERS

300.81	Somatization Disorder
300.82	Undifferentiated Somatoform Disorder
300.11	Conversion Disorder
	Specify type: With Motor Symptom or Deficit/With Sensory Symptom or Deficit/With Seizures or Convulsions/ With Mixed Presentation
307.xx	Pain Disorder
.80	Associated With Psychological Factors
.89	Associated with Both Psychological Factors and a General Medical Condition
	Specify if: Acute/Chronic
300.7	Hypochondriasis
	Specify if: With Poor Insight

300.7   Body Dysmorphic Disorder
300.82   Somatoform Disorder NOS

◼◖ FACTITIOUS DISORDERS

300.xx   Factitious Disorder
   .16   With Predominantly Psychological Signs and Symptoms
   .19   With Predominantly Physical Signs and Symptoms
   .19   With Combined Psychological and Physical Signs and Symptoms
300.19   Factitious Disorder NOS

◼◖ DISSOCIATIVE DISORDERS

300.12   Dissociative Amnesia
300.13   Dissociative Fugue
300.14   Dissociative Identity Disorder
300.6   Depersonalized Disorder
300.15   Dissociative Disorder NOS

◼◖ SEXUAL- AND GENDER-IDENTITY DISORDERS

Sexual Dysfunctions

The following specifiers apply to all primary Sexual Dysfunctions:

Lifelong Type/Acquired
Generalized Type/Situational Type
Due to Psychological Factors/Due to Combined Factors

Sexual Desire Disorders

302.71   Hypoactive Sexual Desire Disorder
302.79   Sexual Aversion Disorder

Sexual Arousal Disorders

302.72   Female Sexual Arousal Disorder
302.72   Male Erectile Disorder

Orgasmic Disorders

302.73   Female Orgasmic Disorder
302.74   Male Orgasmic Disorder
302.75   Premature Ejaculation

Sexual Pain Disorders

302.76   Dyspareunia (Not Due to General Medical Condition)
306.51   Vaginismus (Not Due to a General Medical Condition)

Sexual Dysfunction Due to a General Medical Condition

625.8   Female Hypoactive Sexual Desire Disorder Due to...*
608.89   Male Hypoactive Sexual Desire Disorder Due to...*
607.84   Male Erectile Disorder Due to...*
625.0   Female Dyspareunia Due to...*
608.89   Male Dyspareunia Due to...*
625.8   Other Female Sexual Dysfunction Due to...*
608.89   Other Male Sexual Dysfunction Due to...*
—.-   Substance-Induced Sexual Dysfunction**
         Specify if: With Impaired Desire/With Impaired Arousal/With Impaired Orgasm/With Sexual Pain
         Specify if: With Onset During Intoxication
302.70   Sexual Dysfunction NOS

Paraphilias

302.4   Exhibitionism
302.81   Fetishism
302.89   Frotteurism
302.2   Pedophilia
         Specify if: Sexually Attracted to Males/Sexually Attracted to Females/Sexually Attracted to Both
         Specify if: Limited to Incest
         Specify type: Exclusive Type/Nonexclusive type
302.83   Sexual Masochism
302.84   Sexual Sadism
302.3   Transvestic Fetishism
         Specify if: With Gender Dysphoria
302.82   Voyeurism
302.9   Paraphilia NOS

Gender Identity Disorders

302.xx   Gender Identity Disorders
   .6   In Children
   .85   In Adolescents or Adults
         Specify if: Sexually Attracted to Males/Sexually Attracted to Females/Sexually Attracted to Both/Sexually Attracted to Neither
302.6   Gender Identity Disorder NOS
302.9   Sexual Disorder NOS

◼◖ EATING DISORDERS

307.1   Anorexia Nervosa
         Specify type: Restricting, Binge Eating/Purging

307.51	Bulimia Nervosa
	Specify type: Purging/Nonpurging
307.50	Eating Disorder NOS

▪◗ SLEEP DISORDERS

Primary Sleep Disorders

Dyssomnias

307.42	Primary Insomnia
307.44	Primary Hypersomnia
	Specify if: Recurrent
347	Narcolepsy
380.59	Breathing-Related Sleep Disorder
307.45	Circadian Rhythm Sleep Disorder
	Specify type: Delayed Sleep Phase/Jet Lag/ Shift Work/Unspecified
307.47	Dyssomnia NOS

Parasomnias

307.47	Nightmare Disorder
307.46	Sleep Terror Disorder
307.46	Sleepwalking Disorder
307.47	Parasomnia NOS

Sleep Disorders Related to Another Mental Disorder

307.42	Insomnia Related to…***
307.44	Hypersomnia Related to…***

Other Sleep Disorders

780.xx	Sleep Disorder Due to…*
.52	Insomnia Type
.54	Hyposomnia Type
.59	Parasomnia Type
.59	Mixed Type
—.-	Substance-Induced Sleep Disorder (refer to Substance-Related Disorders for substance-specific codes)
	Specify type: Insomnia/Hypersomnia/ Parasomnia/Mixed
	Specify if: With Onset During Intoxication/With Onset During Withdrawal

▪◗ IMPULSE-CONTROL DISORDERS NOT CLASSIFIED ELSEWHERE

312.34	Intermittent Explosive Disorder
312.32	Kleptomania
312.33	Pyromania
312.31	Pathological Gambling
312.39	Trichotillomania
312.30	Impulse-Control Disorder NOS

▪◗ ADJUSTMENT DISORDERS

309.xx	Adjustment Disorder
.0	With Depressed Mood
.24	With Anxiety
.28	With Mixed Anxiety and Depressed Mood
.3	With Disturbance of Conduct
.4	With Mixed Disturbance of Emotions and Conduct
.9	Unspecified
	Specify if: Acute/Chronic

▪◗ PERSONALITY DISORDERS

Note: These are coded on Axis II

301.0	Paranoid Personality Disorder
301.20	Schizoid Personality Disorder
301.22	Schizotypal Personality Disorder
301.7	Antisocial Personality Disorder
301.83	Borderline Personality Disorder
301.50	Histrionic Personality Disorder
301.81	Narcissistic Personality Disorder
301.82	Avoidant Personality Disorder
301.6	Dependent Personality Disorder
301.4	Obsessive-Compulsive Personality Disorder
301.9	Personality Disorder NOS

▪◗ OTHER CONDITIONS THAT MAY BE A FOCUS OF CLINICAL ATTENTION

Psychological Factors Affecting Medical Condition

316…	[Specified Psychological Factor] Affecting…*

Choose name based on nature of factors:

Mental Disorder Affecting Medical Condition
Psychological Symptoms Affecting Medical Condition
Personality Traits or Coping Style Affecting Medical Condition
Maladaptive Health Behaviours Affecting Medical Condition
Stress-Related Physiological Response Affecting Medical Condition
Other or Unspecified Psychological Factors Affecting Medical Condition

Medication-Induced Movement Disorders

332.1	Neuroleptic-Induced Parkinsonism
333.92	Neuroleptic Malignant Syndrome
333.7	Neuroleptic-Induced Acute Dystonia
333.99	Neuroleptic-Induced Acute Akathisia
333.82	Neuroleptic-Induced Tardive Dyskinesia
333.1	Medication-Induced Postural Tumor
333.90	Medication-Induced Movement Disorder NOS

Other Medical-Induced Disorder

995.2	Adverse Effects of Medication NOS

Relational Problems

V61.9	Relational Problem Related to a Mental Disorder or General Medical Condition
V61.1	Partner Relational Problem
V61.20	Parent-Child Relational Problem
V61.8	Sibling Relational Problem
V62.81	Relational Problem NOS

Problems Related to Abuse or Neglect

(code 995.5 if focus of attention is on victim)

V61.21	Physical Abuse of Child
V61.21	Sexual Abuse of Child
V61.21	Neglect of Child
V61.12	Physical Abuse of Adult
V61.1	Sexual Abuse of Adult
V62.83	Person Other Than Partner

Additional Conditions That May Be a Focus of Clinical Attention

V15.81	Noncompliance With Treatment
V65.2	Malingering
V71.01	Adult Antisocial behaviour
V71.02	Child or Adolescent Antisocial behaviour
V62.89	Borderline Intellectual Functioning *Note: Coded on Axis II.*
780.9	Age-Related Cognitive Decline
V62.82	Bereavement
V62.3	Academic Problem
V62.2	Occupational Problem
313.82	Identify Problem
V62.89	Religious or Spritual Problem
V62.4	Acculturation Problem
V62.89	Phase of Life Problem

◼◖ ADDITIONAL CODES

300.9	Unspecified Mental Disorder (nonpsychotic)
V71.09	No Diagnosis or Condition on Axis I
799.9	Diagnosis or Condition Deferred on Axis I
V71.09	No Diagnosis on Axis II
799.9	Diagnosis Deferred on Axis II

APPENDIX B

Brief Psychiatric Rating Scale

DIRECTIONS: Place an X in the appropriate box to represent the level of severity of each symptom.

	Not Present	Very Mild	Mild	Moderate	Mod. Severe	Severe	Extremely Severe
SOMATIC CONCERN—preoccupation with physical health, fear of physical illness, hypochondriasis.	☐	☐	☐	☐	☐	☐	☐
ANXIETY—worry, fear, overconcern for present or future, uneasiness.	☐	☐	☐	☐	☐	☐	☐
EMOTIONAL WITHDRAWAL—lack of spontaneous interaction, isolation deficiency in relating to others.	☐	☐	☐	☐	☐	☐	☐
CONCEPTUAL DISORGANIZATION—thought processes confused, disconnected, disorganized, disrupted.	☐	☐	☐	☐	☐	☐	☐
GUILT FEELINGS—self-blame, shame, remorse for past behaviour.	☐	☐	☐	☐	☐	☐	☐
TENSION—physical and motor manifestations of nervousness, overactivation.	☐	☐	☐	☐	☐	☐	☐
MANNERISMS AND POSTURING—peculiar, bizarre unnatural motor behaviour (not including tic).	☐	☐	☐	☐	☐	☐	☐
GRANDIOSITY—exaggerated self-opinion, arrogance, conviction of unusual power or abilities.	☐	☐	☐	☐	☐	☐	☐
DEPRESSIVE MOOD—sorrow, sadness, despondency, pessimism.	☐	☐	☐	☐	☐	☐	☐
HOSTILITY—animosity, contempt, belligerence, disdain for others.	☐	☐	☐	☐	☐	☐	☐
SUSPICIOUSNESS—mistrust, belief that others harbour malicious or discriminatory intent.	☐	☐	☐	☐	☐	☐	☐
HALLUCINATORY BEHAVIOUR—perceptions without normal external stimulus correspondence.	☐	☐	☐	☐	☐	☐	☐
MOTOR RETARDATION—slowed, weakened movements or speech, reduced body tone.	☐	☐	☐	☐	☐	☐	☐
UNCOOPERATIVENESS—resistance, guardedness, rejection of authority.	☐	☐	☐	☐	☐	☐	☐
UNUSUAL THOUGHT CONTENT—unusual, odd, strange, bizarre thought content.	☐	☐	☐	☐	☐	☐	☐
BLUNTED AFFECT—reduced emotional tone, reduction in formal intensity of feelings, flatness.	☐	☐	☐	☐	☐	☐	☐
EXCITEMENT—heightened emotional tone, agitation, increased reactivity.	☐	☐	☐	☐	☐	☐	☐
DISORIENTATION—confusion or lack of proper association for person, place, or time.	☐	☐	☐	☐	☐	☐	☐
Global Assessment Scale (Range 1–100)	☐	☐	☐	☐	☐	☐	☐

Reprinted with permission from Overall J. E. (1988). The Brief Psychiatric Rating Scale (BPRS): Recent developments in ascertainment and scaling. *Psychopharmacology Bulletin, 24,* 97–99.

APPENDIX C

Simpson-Angus Rating Scale

1. GAIT: The patient is examined as he walks into the examining room; his gait, the swing of his arms, and his general posture all form the basis for an overall score for this item. This is rated as follows:

   0 Normal.
   1 Diminution in swing while the patient is walking.
   2 Marked diminution in swing with obvious rigidity in the arm.
   3 Stiff gait with arms held rigidly before the abdomen.
   4 Stooped shuffling gait with propulsion and retropulsion.

2. ARM DROPPING: The patient and the examiner both raise their arms to shoulder height and let them fall to their sides. In a normal subject, a stout slap is heard as the arms hit the sides. In the patient with extreme Parkinson's syndrome, the arms fall very slowly.

   0 Normal, free fall with loud slap and rebound.
   1 Fall slowed slightly with less audible contact and little rebound.
   2 Fall slowed, no rebound.
   3 Marked slowing, no slap at all.
   4 Arms fall as though against resistance, as though through glue.

3. SHOULDER SHAKING: The subject's arms are bent at a right angle at the elbow and are taken one at a time by the examiner who grasps one hand and also clasps the other around the subject's elbow. The subject's upper arm is pushed to and fro, and the humerus is externally rotated. The degree of resistance from normal to extreme rigidity is scored as follows:

   0 Normal.
   1 Slight stiffness and resistance.
   2 Moderate stiffness and resistance.
   3 Marked rigidity with difficulty in passive movement.
   4 Extreme stiffness and rigidity with almost a frozen shoulder.

4. ELBOW RIGIDITY: The elbow joints are separately bent at right angles and passively extended and flexed, with the subject's biceps observed and simultaneously palpated. The resistance to this procedure is rated. (The presence of cogwheel rigidity is noted separately.) Scoring is from 0 to 4, as in the Shoulder Shaking test.

   0 Normal.
   1 Slight stiffness and resistance.
   2 Moderate stiffness and resistance.
   3 Marked rigidity with difficulty in passive movement.
   4 Extreme stiffness and rigidity with almost a frozen shoulder.

5. FIXATION OF POSITION OR WRIST RIGIDITY: The examiner holds the wrist in one hand and the fingers in the other hand, with the wrist moved to extension flexion and both ulnar and radial deviation. The resistance to this procedure is rated as in Items 3 and 4.

   0 Normal.
   1 Slight stiffness and resistance.
   2 Moderate stiffness and resistance.

981

3 Marked rigidity with difficulty in passive movement.

4 Extreme stiffness and rigidity with almost a frozen shoulder.

6. LEG PENDULOUSNESS: The patient sits on a table with his legs hanging down and swinging free. The ankle is grasped by the examiner and raised until the knee is partially extended. It is then allowed to fall. The resistance to falling and the lack of swinging form the basis for the score on this item.

   0 The legs swing freely.
   1 Slight diminution in the swing of the legs.
   2 Moderate resistance to swing.
   3 Marked resistance and damping of swing.
   4 Complete absence of swing.

7. HEAD DROPPING: The patient lies on a well-padded examining table and his head is raised by the examiner's hand. The hand is then withdrawn, and the head is allowed to drop. In the normal subject, the head will fall upon the table. The movement is delayed in extrapyramidal system disorder, and in extreme parkinsonism, it is absent. The neck muscles are rigid, and the head does not reach the examining table. Scoring is as follows:

   0 The head falls completely, with a good thump as it hits the table.
   1 Slight slowing in fall, mainly noted by lack of slap as the head meets the table.
   2 Moderate slowing in the fall, quite noticeable to the eye.
   3 The head falls stiffly and slowly.
   4 The head does not reach the examining table.

8. GLABELLA TAP: The subject is told to open his eyes wide and not to blink. The glabella region is tapped at a steady, rapid speed. The number of times the patient blinks in succession is noted:

   0 0 to 5 blinks
   1 6 to 10 blinks
   2 11 to 15 blinks
   3 16 to 20 blinks
   4 21 or more blinks

9. TREMOR: The patient is observed walking into the examining room and then is reexamined for this item:

   0 Normal.
   1 Mild finger tremor, obvious to sight and touch.
   2 Tremor of hand or arm occurring spasmodically.
   3 Persistent tremor of one or more limbs.
   4 Whole body tremor.

10. SALIVATION: The patient is observed while talking and then asked to open his mouth and elevate his tongue. The following ratings are given:

   0 Normal.
   1 Excess salivation to the extent that pooling takes place if the mouth is open and the tongue raised.
   2 When excess salivation is present and might occasionally result in difficulty in speaking.
   3 Speaking with difficulty because of excess salivation.
   4 Frank drooling.

Scoring: Each item is rated on a 5-point scale, with 0 meaning the complete absence of the condition, and 4 meaning the presence of the condition in extreme form. The score is obtained by adding the items and dividing by 10.

Reprinted with permission from Simpson, G. M., & Angus, J. W. S. (1970). A rating scale for extrapyramidal side effects. *Acta Psychiatrica Scondinovica, 212*(Suppl.), 11–19. Copyright 1970, Munksgaard International Publishers, Ltd.

Abnormal Involuntary Movement Scale (AIMS)

	None	Minimal	Mild	Moderate	Severe
Facial and Oral Movements					
1: Muscles of facial expression (e.g., movements of forehead, eyebrows, periorbital area, cheeks. Include frowning, blinking, smiling, grimacing)	0	1	2	3	4
2: Lips and perioral area (e.g., puckering, pouting, smacking)	0	1	2	3	4
3: Jaw (e.g., biting, clenching, chewing, mouth opening, lateral movement)	0	1	2	3	4
4: Tongue Rate only increase in movement both in and out of the mouth, NOT inability to sustain movement	0	1	2	3	4
Extremity Movements					
5: Upper (arms, wrists, hands, fingers) Include choreic movements (i.e., rapid, objectively purposeless, irregular, spontaneous), athetoid movements (i.e., slow, irregular, complex, serpentine) Do NOT include tremor (i.e., repetitive, regular, rhythmic)	0	1	2	3	4
6: Lower (legs, knees, ankles, toes) (e.g., lateral knee movement, foot tapping, heel dropping, foot squirming, inversion and eversion of the foot)	0	1	2	3	4
Trunk Movements					
7: Neck, shoulders, hips (e.g., rocking, twisting, squirming, pelvic gyrations)	0	1	2	3	4
8: Severity of abnormal movements	0	1	2	3	4
Global Judgment					
9: Incapacitation due to abnormal movements	0	1	2	3	4

Continued

10: Patient's awareness of abnormal movements Rate only the patient's report	No awareness	0
	Aware, no distress	1
	Aware, mild distress	2
	Aware, moderate distress	3
	Aware, severe distress	4

Global Judgment

11: Current problems with teeth and/or dentures	No	0
	Yes	1
12: Does the patient usually wear dentures?	No	0
	Yes	1

Examination Procedures for AIMS

Either before or after completing the examination procedure, observe the patient unobtrusively, at rest (e.g., in the waiting room). The chair to be used in this examination should be a hard, firm one without arms.

1: Ask patient whether there is anything in his/her mouth (i.e., gum, candy, etc.) and if there is, to remove it.

2: Ask the patient about the *current* condition of his/her teeth. Ask the patient if he/she wears dentures. Do teeth or dentures bother the patient *now?*

3: Ask the patient whether he/she notices any movements in the mouth, face, hands, or feet. If yes, ask the patient to describe and to what extent they *currently* bother him/her or interfere with his/her activities.

4: Have the patient sit in the chair with hands on knees, legs slightly apart, and feet flat on the floor. (Look at the entire body for movements while in this position.)

5: Ask the patient to sit with his/her hands hanging unsupported. If male, between legs; if female and wearing a dress, hanging over knees. (Observe hands and other body areas.)

6: Ask the patient to open his/her mouth. (Observe tongue at rest within the mouth.) Do this twice.

7: Ask the patient to protrude the tongue. (Observe tongue at rest within the mouth.) Do this twice.

*8: Ask the patient to tap the thumb, with each finger, as rapidly as possible for 10–15 seconds; separately with right hand, then with left hand. (Observe facial and leg movements.)

9: Flex and extend the patient's left and right arms (one at a time). (Note any rigidity and rate on NOTES.)

10: Ask the patient to stand up. (Observe in profile. Observe all body areas again, hips included.)

*11: Ask the patient to extend both arms outstretched in front with palms down. (Observe trunk, legs, and mouth.)

*12: Have the patient walk a few paces, turn, and walk back to the chair. (Observe hand and gait.) Do this twice.

*Activated movements.

Reprinted from Guy, W. (1976). ECDEU: Assessment manual for psychopharmacology (DHEW Publ No 76–338). Washington, DC: Department of Health, Education, and Welfare, Psychopharmacology Research Branch.

APPENDIX E

Simplified Diagnoses for Tardive Dyskinesia (SD-TD)

PREREQUISITES—The three prerequisites are as follows. Exceptions may occur.

1. A history of at least 3 months' total cumulative neuroleptic exposure. Include amoxapine and metoclopramide in all categories below as well.
2. **SCORING/INTENSITY LEVEL.** The presence of a **TOTAL SCORE OF FIVE OR ABOVE.** Also, be alert for any change from baseline or scores below five which have at least a "moderate" (3) or "severe" (4) movement on any item or at least two "mild" (2) movements on two items located in different body areas.
3. Other conditions are not responsible for the abnormal involuntary movements.

DIAGNOSES—The diagnosis is based upon the current exam and its relation to the last exam. The diagnosis can shift depending upon (a) whether movements are present or not, (b) whether movements are present for 3 months or more (6 months if on a semiannual assessment schedule), and (c) whether neuroleptic dosage changes occur and effect movements.

- **NO TD**—Movements **are not** present on this exam **or** movements are present, but some other condition is responsible for them. The last diagnosis must be NO TD, PROBABLE TD, or WITHDRAWAL TD.
- **PROBABLE TD**—Movements **are** present on this exam. This is the first time they are present, **or** they have never been present for 3 months or more. The last diagnosis must be NO TD or PROBABLE TD.
- **PERSISTENT TD**—Movements **are** present on this exam, **and** they have been present for 3 months or more with this exam or at some point in the past. The last diagnosis can be any except NO TD.
- **MASKED TD**—Movements **are not** present on this exam, **but** this is due to a neuroleptic dosage increase or reinstitution after a prior exam when movements were present. Also, use this conclusion if movements are not present due to the addition of a nonneuroleptic medication to treat TD. The last diagnosis must be PROBABLE TD, PERSISTENT TD, WITHDRAWAL TD, or MASKED TD.
- **REMITTED TD**—Movements **are not** present on this exam, **but** PERSISTENT TD has been diagnosed **and** nouroleptic dosage increase or reinstitution has occurred. The last diagnosis must be PERSISTENT TD or REMITTED TD. If movements reemerge, the diagnosis shifts back to PERSISTENT TD.
- **WITHDRAWAL TD**—Movements **are not seen while** receiving neuroleptics or at the last dosage level **but are seen within** 8 weeks following a neuroleptic reduction or discontinuation. The last diagnosis must be NO TD or WITHDRAWAL TD. If movements continue for 3 months or more after the neuroleptic dosage reduction or discontinuation, the diagnosis shifts to PERSISTENT TD. If movements do not continue for 3 months or more after the reduction or discontinuation, the diagnosis shifts to NO TD.

Instructions

1. The rater completes the Assessment according to the standardized exam procedure. If the rater also completes Evaluation items 1–4, he/she must also sign the preparer box. The form is given to the physician. Alternatively, the physician may perform the assessment.
2. The physician completes the Evaluation section. The physician is responsible for the entire Evaluation section and its accuracy.
3. It is recommended that the physician examines any individual who meets the three prerequisites or who has movements not explained by other factors. Neurological assessments or differential diagnostic tests which may be necessary should be performed.
4. File form according to policy or procedure.

Other Conditions (Partial List)

1. Age
2. Blind
3. Cerebral Palsy
4. Contact Lenses
5. Dentures/No Teeth
6. Down Syndrome
7. Drug Intoxication (specify)
8. Encephalitis
9. Extrapyramidal Side Effects (specify)
10. Fahr's Syndrome
11. Heavy Metal Intoxication (specify)
12. Huntington's Chorea
13. Hyperthyroidism
14. Hypoglycemia
15. Hypoparathyroidism
16. Idiopathic Torsion Dystonia
17. Meige Syndrome
18. Parkinson's Disease
19. Stereotypies
20. Sydenham's Chorea
21. Tourette's Syndrome
22. Wilson's Disease
23. Other (specify)

Sprague, R. L., & Kalachnik, J. E. (1991). Reliability, validity, and a total score cutoff for the Dyskinesia Identification System Condensed User Scale (DISCUS) with mentally ill and mentally retarded populations. Psychopharmacology Bulletin, 27(1), 51–58.

APPENDIX F

Hamilton Rating Scale for Depression

Clinic No._____ Date_____ Rating No._____ Code Number_____

Sex_____ Age_____ Patient's Name_____

Patient's Address_____ Tel_____

Item	Range	Score
1. Depressed mood	0–4	
2. Guilt	0–4	
3. Suicide	0–4	
4. Insomnia initial	0–2	
5. Insomnia middle	0–2	
6. Insomnia delayed	0–2	
7. Work and interest	0–4	
8. Retardation	0–4	
9. Agitation	0–4	
10. Anxiety (psychic)	0–4	
11. Anxiety (somatic)	0–4	
12. Somatic gastrointestinal	0–2	
13. Somatic general	0–2	
14. Genital	0–2	
15. Hypochondriasis	0–2	
16. Insight	0–4	
17. Loss of weight	0–2	
	Total Score	
Diurnal variation (M.A.E.)	0–2	
Depersonalization	0–4	
Paranoid symptoms	0–4	
Obsessional symptoms	0–4	

The scale is designed to measure the severity of illness of patients already diagnosed as suffering from depressive illness. It is obviously not a diagnostic instrument because that requires much more information (e.g., previous history, family history, precipitating factors).

As far as possible, the scale should be used in the manner of a clinical interview. The first time, the interview should be conducted in a relaxed, free, and easy manner, giving the patients time to unburden themselves and giving them the opportunity to speak of their problems and ask whatever questions they wish. It may then be necessary to obtain further information by asking them questions. At subsequent assessments, the interview can be briefer and more to the point.

An observer rating scale is not a checklist in which each item is strictly defined. The raters must have sufficient clinical experience and judgment to be able to interpret the patients' statements and reticences about some symptoms and to compare them with other patients. They should use all sources of information (e.g., from relatives and nurses).

The scale consists of 17 items, the scores of which are summed to give a total score. These are four other items, one of which (diurnal variation) is excluded on the grounds that it is not an additional burden on the patient. The last three are excluded from the total score because they occur infrequently, although information on them may be useful for other purposes.

The method of assessment is simple. For some symptoms, it is difficult to elicit such information as will permit of full quantification. If present, score 2; if absent, score 0; and if doubtful or trivial, score 1. For those symptoms where more detailed information can be obtained, the score of 2 is expanded into 2 for mild, 3 for moderate, and 4 for severe. In case of difficulty, the raters should use their judgment as clinicians.

Hamilton, M. (1960). A rating scale for depression. *Journal of Neurology, Neurosurgery and Psychiatry, 23*, 56.

APPENDIX G

Clinical Institute Withdrawal Assessment of Alcohol Scale, Revised (CIWA-Ar)

Patient: _____ **Date:** _____ **Time:** _____ (24 hour clock, midnight = 00:00)

Pulse or heart rate, taken for one minute: _____ **Blood pressure:** _____

NAUSEA AND VOMITING — Ask "Do you feel sick to your stomach? Have you vomited?" Observation.

  0 no nausea and no vomiting
  1 mild nausea with no vomiting
  2
  3
  4 intermittent nausea with dry heaves
  5
  6
  7 constant nausea, frequent dry heaves and vomiting

TREMOR — Arms extended and fingers spread apart. Observation

  0 no tremor
  1 not visible, but can be felt fingertip to fingertip
  2
  3
  4 moderate, with patient's arms extended
  5
  6
  7 severe, even with arms not extended

TACTILE DISTURBANCES — Ask "Have you any itching, pins and needles sensations, any burning, any numbness, or do you feel bugs crawling on or under your skin?" Observation.

  0 none
  1 very mild itching, pins and needles, burning or numbness
  2 mild itching, pins and needles, burning or numbness
  3 moderate itching, pins and needles, burning or numbness
  4 moderately severe hallucinations
  5 severe hallucinations
  6 extremely severe hallucinations
  7 continuous hallucinations

AUDITORY DISTURBANCES — Ask "Are you more aware of sounds around you?" "Are they harsh?" "Do they frighten you?" "Are you hearing anything that is disturbing to you?" "Are you hearing things you know are not there?" Observation.

  0 not present
  1 very mild harshness or ability to frighten
  2 mild harshness or ability to frighten
  3 moderate harshness or ability to frighten
  4 moderately severe hallucinations
  5 severe hallucinations
  6 extremely severe hallucinations
  7 continuous hallucinations

PAROXYSMAL SWEATS — Observation.

0 no sweat visible
1 barely perceptible sweating, palms moist
2
3
4 beads of sweat obvious on forehead
5
6
7 drenching sweats

ANXIETY — Ask "Do you feel nervous?" Observation.

0 no anxiety, at ease
1 mild anxious
2
3
4 moderately anxious, or guarded, so anxiety is inferred
5
6
7 equivalent to acute panic states as seen in severe delirium or acute schizophrenic reactions

AGITATION — Observation.

0 normal activity
1 somewhat more than normal activity
2
3
4 moderately fidgety and restless
5
6
7 paces back and forth during most of the interview, or constantly thrashes about

VISUAL DISTURBANCES — Ask "Does the light appear to be too bright?" "Is its color different?" "Does it hurt your eyes?" "Are you seeing anything that is disturbing to you?" "Are you seeing things you know are not there?" Observation.

0 not present
1 very mild sensitivity
2 mild sensitivity
3 moderate sensitivity
4 moderately severe hallucinations
5 severe hallucinations
6 extremely severe hallucinations
7 continuous hallucinations

HEADACHE, FULLNESS IN HEAD — Ask "Does your head feel different?" "Does it feel like there is a band around your head?" Do not rate for dizziness or lightheadedness. Otherwise, rate severity.

0 not present
1 very mild
2 mild
3 moderate
4 moderately severe
5 severe
6 very severe
7 extremely severe

ORIENTATION AND CLOUDING OF SENSORIUM — Ask "What day is this?" "Where are you?" "Who am I?"

0 oriented and can do serial additions
1 cannot do serial additions or is uncertain about date
2 disoriented for date by no more than 2 calendar days
3 disoriented for date by more than 2 calendar days
4 disoriented for place/or person

Total **CIWA-Ar** Score _____
Rater's Initials _____
Maximum Possible Score 67

---

*The **CIWA-Ar** is not* copyrighted and may be reproduced freely. This assessment for monitoring withdrawal symptoms requires approximately 5 minutes to administer. The maximum score is 67 (see instrument). Patients scoring less than 10 do not usually need additional medication for withdrawal.

Sullivan, J. T., Sykora, K., Schneiderman, J., Naranjo, C. A., & Sellers, E. M. (1989). Assessment of alcohol withdrawal: The revised Clinical Institute Withdrawal Assessment for Alcohol scale (CIWA-Ar). *British Journal of Addiction*, 84, 1353–1357.

APPENDIX H

Specific Defence Mechanisms and Coping Styles*

Defence Mechanism	Definition	Example
Acting out	Using actions rather than reflections or feelings during periods of emotional conflict	A teenager gets mad at his or her parents and begins staying out late at night.
Affiliation	Turning to others for help or support (sharing problems with others without implying that someone else is responsible for them)	An individual has a fight with his or her spouse and turns to his or her best friend for emotional support.
Altruism	Dedicating life to meeting the needs of others (receives gratification either vicariously or from the response of others)	After being rejected by her boyfriend, a young girl joins the Peace Corps.
Anticipation	Experiencing emotional reactions in advance or anticipating consequences of possible future events and considering realistic, alternative responses or solutions	A parent cries for 3 weeks before the last child leaves for college. On the day of the separation, the parent spends the day with friends.
Autistic fantasy	Excessive daydreaming as a substitute for human relationships, more effective action, or problem solving	A young man sits in his room all day and dreams about being a rock star instead of attending a baseball game with a friend.
Denial	Refusing to acknowledge some painful aspect of external reality or subjective experience that would be apparent to others (*psychotic denial* used when there is gross impairment in reality testing)	A teenager's best friend moves away, but the adolescent says he does not feel sad.
Devaluation	Attributing exaggerated negative qualities to self or others	A boy has been rejected by his longtime girlfriend. He tells his friends that he realizes that she is stupid and ugly.
Displacement	Transferring a feeling about, or a response to, one object onto another (usually less threatening), substitute object	A child is mad at her mother for leaving for the day but says she is really mad at the sitter for serving her food she does not like.
Dissociation	Experiencing a breakdown in the usually integrated functions of consciousness, memory, perception of self or the environment, or sensory and motor behaviour	An adult relates severe sexual abuse experienced as a child but does it without feeling. She says that the experience was as if she were outside her body watching the abuse.
Help rejecting/ complaining	Complaining or making repetitive requests for help that disguise covert feelings of hostility or reproach toward others, which are then expressed by rejecting the suggestions, advice, or help that others offer (complaints or requests may involve physical or psychological symptoms or life problems)	A college student asks a teacher for help after receiving a bad grade on a test. Every suggestion the teacher has is rejected by the student.

Continued

Specific Defence Mechanisms and Coping Styles* *(Continued)*

Defence Mechanism	Definition	Example
Humour	Emphasizing the amusing or ironic aspects of the conflict or stressor	A person makes a joke right after experiencing an embarrassing situation.
Idealization	Attributing exaggerated positive qualities to others	An adult falls in love and fails to see the negative qualities in the other person.
Intellectualization	Excessive use of abstract thinking or the making of generalizations to control or minimize disturbing feelings	After rejection in a love relationship, the rejected explains about the relationship dynamics to a friend.
Isolation of affect	Separation of ideas from the feelings originally associated with them	The individual loses touch with the feelings associated with a rape while remaining aware of the details.
Omnipotence	Feeling or acting as if one possesses special powers or abilities and is superior to others	An individual tells a friend about personal expertise in the stock market and the ability to predict the best stocks.
Passive aggression	Indirectly and unassertively expressing aggression toward others. There is a facade of overt compliance masking covert resistance, resentment, or hostility.	Passive aggression often occurs in response to demands for independent action or performance or the lack of gratification of dependent wishes but may be adaptive for individuals in subordinate positions who have no other way to express assertiveness more overtly.
Projection	Falsely attributing to another one's own unacceptable feelings, impulses, or thoughts	A child is very angry at a parent, but accuses the parent of being angry.
Projective identification	Falsely attributing to another one's own unacceptable feelings, impulses, or thoughts. Unlike simple projection, the individual does not fully disavow what is projected. Instead, the individual remains aware of his or her own affect or impulses but misattributes them as justifiable reactions to the other person. Not infrequently, the individual induces the very feelings in others that were first mistakenly believed to be there, making it difficult to clarify who did what to whom first.	A child is mad at a parent, who in turn becomes angry at the child, but may be unsure of why. The child then feels justified at being angry with the parent.
Rationalization	Concealing the true motivations for one's own thoughts, actions, or feelings through the elaboration of reassuring or self-serving but incorrect explanations	A man is rejected by his girlfriend but explains to his friends that her leaving was best because she was beneath him socially and would not be liked by his family.
Reaction formation	Substituting behaviour, thoughts, or feelings that are diametrically opposed to one's own unacceptable thoughts or feelings (this usually occurs in conjunction with his or her repression)	A wife finds out about her husband's extramarital affairs and tells her friends that she thinks his affairs are perfectly appropriate. She truly does not feel, on a conscious level, any anger or hurt.
Repression	Expelling disturbing wishes, thoughts, or experiences from conscious awareness (the feeling component may remain conscious, detached from its associated ideas)	A woman does not remember the experience of being raped in the basement but does feel anxious when going into that house.
Self-assertion	Expressing feelings and thoughts directly in a way that is not coercive or manipulative	An individual reaffirms to another that going to a ball game is not what he or she wants to do.
Self-observation	Reflecting feelings, thoughts, motivation, and behaviour and responding to them appropriately	An individual notices an irritation at his friend's late arrival and decides to tell the friend of the irritation.
Splitting	Compartmentalizing opposite affect states and failing to integrate the positive and negative qualities of the self or others into cohesive images.	Self and object images tend to alternate between polar opposites: exclusively loving, powerful, worthy, nurturant, and kind or exclusively bad, hateful, angry, destructive, rejecting, or worthless. One friend is wonderful and another former friend, who was at one time viewed as being perfect, is now believed to be an evil person.
Sublimation	Channeling potentially maladaptive feelings or impulses into socially acceptable behaviour	An adolescent boy is very angry with his parents. On the football field, he tackles someone very forcefully.
Suppression	Intentionally avoiding thinking about disturbing problems, wishes, feelings, or experiences	A student is anxiously awaiting test results but goes to a movie to stop thinking about it.
Undoing	Words or behaviour designed to negate or to make amends symbolically for unacceptable thoughts, feelings, or actions	A man has sexual fantasies about his wife's sister. He takes his wife away for a romantic weekend.

*These defence mechanisms and coping styles are identified in the DSM-IV TR as being used when the individual deals with emotional conflict or stressors (either internal or external).

Adapted from the American Psychiatric Association. (2000). *Diagnostic and statistical manual of mental disorders* (4th ed., Text revision, pp. 811–814). Washington, DC: Author.

Glossary

absorption Movement of drug from the site of administration into plasma.

acetylcholine (ACh) An important neurotransmitter associated with cognitive functioning, and disruption of cholinergic mechanisms damages memory in animals and humans.

acetylcholinesterase (AChE) Key enzyme that inactivates the neurotransmitter acetylcholine. AChE is found in high concentrations in the brain and is one of two cholinesterase enzymes capable of breaking down ACh.

acetylcholinesterase inhibitors (AChEIs) Mainstay of pharmacologic treatment of dementia; these drugs inhibit AChE, resulting in an enhancement of cholinergic activity. AChEIs have been shown to delay the decline in cognitive functioning but generally do not improve cognitive function once it has declined; therefore, it is important that this medication be started as soon as the diagnosis is made.

active listening Focusing on what the patient is saying in order to interpret and respond to the message in an objective manner, while using techniques such as open-ended statements, reflection, and questions that elicit additional responses from the patient.

acute stress disorder (ASD) A mental disorder characterized by persistent, distressing stress-related symptoms that last between 2 days and 1 month and that occur within 1 month after a traumatic experience.

adaptability Capacity of a person to survive and flourish.

adaptive inflexibility Rigidity in interactions with others, achievement of goals, and coping with stress.

addiction A chronic, relapsing brain disorder that results from the prolonged effects of exposure of the brain to drugs (substances or chemicals).

adherence A patient's maintenance of the therapeutic regimen, includes self-administering medications as prescribed, keeping appointments, and following other treatment suggestions; it exists on a continuum and can be conceived of as full, partial, or nil.

adverse reactions Unwanted medication effects that may have serious physiologic consequences.

affect An expression of mood manifest in a pattern of observable behaviours.

affective blunting Flat or blunted emotion.

affective instability Rapid and extreme shifts in mood, erratic emotional responses to situations, and intense sensitivity to criticism or perceived slights; one of the core characteristics of borderline personality disorder.

affective lability Abrupt, dramatic, unprovoked changes in the types of emotions expressed.

afferent Toward the central nervous system or a particular structure.

affinity Degree of attraction or strength of the bond between a drug and its receptor.

aggression Behaviours or attitudes that reflect rage, hostility, and the potential for physical or verbal destructiveness; usually occurs if the person believes someone is going to do him or her harm.

agitation Inability to sit still or attend to others, accompanied by heightened emotions and tension.

agnosia Failure to recognize or identify objects despite intact sensory function, or a disturbance in executive functioning (ability to think abstractly, plan, initiate, sequence, monitor, and stop complex behaviour).

agonists Chemicals producing the same biologic action as the neurotransmitter.

agoraphobia Anxiety about being in places from which escape might be difficult or embarrassing, or about being in places in which help may not be readily available if a panic attack should occur.

akathisia A medication-related, involuntary movement disorder characterized by the inability to sit still; may be experienced as "jitteriness" without obvious motor behaviour.

alexithymia Inability to experience and communicate feelings consciously.

allodynia Lowered pain threshold.

allostasis Adaptive processes that maintain homeostasis through the production of various brain and peripheral stress-related chemicals and promote adaptation to perceived threat or stress.

alogia Brief, empty verbal responses; often referred to as *poverty of speech*.

ambivalence Presence and expression of two opposing forces, leading to inaction.

amino acids Building blocks of proteins that have different roles. Amino acids function as neurotransmitters in as many as 60% to 70% of synaptic sites in the brain.

amygdala A bulb-like structure attached to the tail of the caudate and often considered part of the limbic system.

anger An affective state experienced as the motivation to act in ways that warn, intimidate, or attack those who are perceived as challenging or threatening.

anhedonia Inability to gain pleasure from activities.

anorexia nervosa A life-threatening eating disorder characterized by refusal to maintain body weight appropriate for age, intense fear of gaining weight or becoming fat, a severely distorted body image, and refusal to acknowledge the seriousness of weight loss.

antagonists Chemicals blocking the biologic response at a given receptor site.

anticholinergic crisis A potentially life-threatening medical emergency that occurs as a result of overdose or sensitivity to drugs with anticholinergic properties.

anxiety Apprehension or dread in response to internal or external stimuli that can be experienced in physical, emotional, cognitive, and/or behavioural ways.

anxiolytics Drugs that reverse or diminish anxiety.

apathy Reactions to stimuli that are decreased, along with a diminished interest and desire.

aphasia Alterations in language ability.

apraxia Impaired ability to execute motor activities despite intact motor functioning.

ascertainment bias Bias that occurs in research when the method of identifying cases creates a sample that differs from the population it purports to represent.

assertiveness A set of behaviours and a communication style that is open, honest, direct, and confident that enables the expression of emotions, including anger, in a manner that assumes responsibility.

assessment The purposeful and systematic collection, evaluation and documentation of a client's health–illness information.

assortative mating Tendency for individuals to select mates who are similar in genetically linked traits such as intelligence and personality styles.

attachment Emotional bond between the infant and parental figure.

autism A pervasive developmental disorder (PDD) that is distinguished from other PDD by early age of onset (before age 30 months) and severe disturbance in social relatedness.

Children with autism appear indifferent to others and to prefer inanimate objects.

automatic thoughts Spontaneous words and images generated in a particular situation that may be illogical and/or difficult to stop.

autonomic nervous system Part of the nervous system that regulates involuntary vital functions including cardiac muscle, smooth muscles, and glands. It is composed of the sympathetic and parasympathetic systems.

autonomy Concept that each person has the fundamental right of self-determination.

avolition Inability to complete projects, assignments, or work.

basal ganglia One set of structures in each hemisphere; areas of gray matter containing many cell bodies or nuclei.

behaviour modification A specific, systematized behaviour therapy technique that can be applied to individuals, groups, or systems.

behaviour therapy Interventions that reinforce or promote desirable behaviours or alter undesirable ones.

behaviourism A paradigm shift in understanding human behaviour that was initiated by Watson, who theorized that human behaviour is developed through a stimulus–response process rather than through unconscious drives or instincts.

beneficence The ethical principle of "try to do good"; promote benefit.

bereavement The objective event or occurrence of having suffered a loss.

best practice guidelines (BPGs) Clinical practice recommendations based on the best current evidence.

bibliotherapy The use of books and other reading materials to help individuals cope with various life stressors.

binge eating Episodes of uncontrollable, ravenous eating of large amounts of food within discrete periods of time, usually followed by feelings of guilt that result in purging.

bioavailability The amount of the drug that actually reaches systemic circulation; affected significantly by the route by which a drug is administered.

biogenic amines Small molecules manufactured in the neuron that contain an amine group. These include dopamine, norepinephrine, and epinephrine (all synthesized from the amino acid tyrosine), serotonin (from tryptophan), and histamine (from histidine).

biologic markers Physical indicators of disturbances within the central nervous system that differentiate one disease state from another.

biotransformation (metabolism) The process by which a drug is altered, often broken down into smaller substances known as *metabolites*.

body dissatisfaction The body becomes overvalued as a way of determining one's worth. Body dissatisfaction has been related to low self-esteem, depression, dieting, bingeing, and purging.

body image Self-perception of one's body. Extreme discrepancy between body image and others' perceptions of one's body indicates a *body image distortion*.

boundary violation Behaviour by a professional that has violated the limits (what is and is not permitted) in a professional-client relationship.

boundaries   The defining limits of individuals, objects, or relationships.

bradykinesia   An extrapyramidal condition characterized by a slowness of voluntary movement and speech.

brain stem   Area of the brain containing the midbrain, pons, and medulla, which continues beneath the thalamus.

breach of confidentiality   Release of patient information without the patient's consent in the absence of legal compulsion or authorization to release information.

Broca's area   A section of the left frontal lobe of the brain thought to be responsible for the articulation of speech.

bulimia nervosa   An eating disorder in which the individual engages in recurrent episodes of binge eating and compensatory behaviour to avoid weight gain through purging methods such as self-induced vomiting, or use of laxatives, diuretics, enemas, or emetics, or through nonpurging methods such as fasting or excessive exercise.

bullying   Persistent physical or psychological harm that is intentionally inflicted on an individual who feels unable to avoid or stop the harm.

burnout   Psychological exhaustion, detachment, and loss of sense of accomplishment related to chronic work-related stress.

butyrylcholinesterase (BuChE)   A nonspecific cholinesterase found in the brain and especially in the glial cells. Both acetylcholinesterase and BuChE work in the gastrointestinal tract. If these enzymes are inhibited, the breakdown of acetylcholine will be delayed, resulting in an increase in acetylcholine activity.

case management   Problem solving and coordinating services for the patient to ensure continuity of services and overcome system rigidity, fragmentation of services, misuse of facilities, and inaccessibility.

catatonic excitement   Hyperactivity characterized by purposeless activity and abnormal movements like grimacing and posturing.

central sulcus   Posterior boundary of the frontal lobe that separates it from the parietal lobe.

cerebellum   Part of the brain that is responsible for controlling movement and postural adjustments; it receives information from all parts of the body.

cerebrospinal fluid   Cushioning fluid that circulates around the brain beneath the arachnoid layer in the subarachnoid space; it is colourless and contains sodium chloride and other salts.

chemical restraints   Use of medication to control patients or manage behaviour.

cholecystokinin   A neuropeptide found in high levels in the cerebral cortex, hypothalamus, and amygdala; it is also excreted by the gastrointestinal system in response to food intake, which is believed to play a role in the control of eating and satiety by controlling the release of dopamine.

chronobiology   Study and measure of time structures or biologic rhythms.

circadian rhythm (cycle)   From the Latin *circa* and *dies*, meaning "about a day"; refers to a biologic system that fluctuates or oscillates in a pattern that repeats itself in about a day.

circumstantiality   Occurs when an individual takes a long time to make a point because his or her conversation is indirect and contains excessive and unnecessary detail.

clang association   Repetition of word phrases that are similar in sound but in no other way, for example, "right, light, sight, might."

classical conditioning   A learning situation in which an unconditioned stimulus initially produces an unconditioned response; over time, a conditioned response is elicited for a specific stimulus (Pavlov).

clearance   Total amount of blood, serum, or plasma from which a drug is completely removed per unit of time.

clinical domain outcome statements   Statements that indicate a reduction in symptoms of illness or cure of a specific mental illness.

closed group   A group in which all the members begin at one time. New members are not admitted after the first meeting.

cognition   A system of interrelated abilities, such as perception, reasoning, judgment, intuition, and memory, that allow one to be aware of oneself and one's surroundings. Impairments in these abilities can result in a failure of the afflicted person to recognize that he or she is not well and is in need of treatment.

cognitive restructuring   A process in which cognitions (automatic thoughts, intermediate and core beliefs) are identified, analyzed, and modified to effect positive change in mood and behaviour.

cognitive schema (core beliefs)   Basic beliefs so fundamental that they are accepted as absolute truths; assist in evaluating and assigning meaning to events and influence subsequent affective and behavioural responses.

cognitive-behavioural model   A model of perception that includes emotion, cognition, environment, and physical and psychological factors.

cognitive-behavioural therapy   Psychotherapy focused on identifying, analyzing, and ultimately changing the habitually inflexible and negative cognitions about oneself, others, and the world that contribute to distress and problematic behaviours.

communication triad   A technique used to provide a specific syntax and order for patients to identify and express their feelings and seek relief. The "sentence" consists of three parts: (1) an "I" statement to identify the prevailing feeling, (2) a nonjudgmental statement of the emotional trigger, and (3) a statement of what the person would like differently or what would restore comfort to the situation.

community treatment orders (CTOs)   A type of mandatory outpatient treatment, usually initiated by a physician, that can require an individual with a mental illness who does not meet provincial involuntary admission criteria to comply with stipulated treatment.

comorbidity (comorbid)   Disease that coexists with the primary disease.

compassion fatigue   Disengagement on the part of caregiving professionals; frequently equated with burnout.

compassionate release   *Parole by exception* for incarcerated offenders, allowed under the Corrections and Conditional Release Act, and considered on an individual basis (e.g., for palliative care due to a terminal illness).

competence   The degree to which the patient is able to understand and appreciate the information given during the consent process; the patient's cognitive ability to process information at a specific time; the patient's ability to gather and interpret information and make reasonable judgments based on that information to participate fully as a partner in treatment.

compulsions   Behaviours that are performed repeatedly, in a ritualistic fashion, with the goal of preventing or relieving anxiety and distress caused by obsessions.

concordant   Used in genetics to indicate that both members of twins have same trait.

concrete thinking   Lack of abstraction in thinking, in which people are unable to understand punch lines, metaphors, and analogies.

confabulation   False memories, perceptions, or beliefs that are the consequence of neurological dysfunction or damage.

confidentiality   An ethical duty of nondisclosure; the patient has the right to disclose personal information without fear of it being revealed to others.

conflict resolution   A specific type of counselling in which the nurse helps the patient resolve a disagreement or dispute.

conservation   The child's awareness that a quantity remains the same despite its shape.

content themes   Repetition of concerns or feelings that occur within the therapeutic relationship. Themes may emerge as symbolic representations of fears.

continuum of care   The integrated health system of supports and services that is provided by professional health care clinicians (some who offer specialized services, such as psychiatric and mental health services), as well as by non-professional caregivers, designed to maximize people's health and well-being.

coping   An individual's constantly changing cognitive and behavioural efforts to manage specific external or internal demands that are appraised as taxing or exceeding the individual's resources.

corpus callosum   Functional link between the two hemispheres of the brain, made up of a thick band of fibres.

cortex   Outer surface of the mature brain.

cortical dementia   A type of dementia that is characterized by amnesia, aphasia, apraxia, and agnosia.

counselling interventions   Specific time-limited interactions between a nurse and a patient, family, or group experiencing intermediate or ongoing difficulties related to their health or well-being.

countertransference   The nurse's reactions to a patient that are based on the nurse's unconscious needs, conflicts, problems, and views of the world. It can significantly interfere with the nurse–patient relationship.

crisis   A severely stressful experience for which coping mechanisms fail to provide any adaptation, whether the experience is positive or negative.

crisis intervention   A specialized short-term (usually no longer than 6 hours) goal-directed therapy designed to assist patients in an immediate manner, after which they are usually transferred to an inpatient unit or an intensive outpatient setting.

crisis response   Occurs when an individual encounters an obstacle or problem important to life goals that cannot be solved by customary problem-solving methods; acute, time-limited, and may be developmental, situational, or interpersonal in nature.

cultural brokering   Act of bridging, linking, or mediating between groups or individuals of different cultural systems for the purpose of reducing conflict or producing change.

cultural competence   The ability to give care and services appropriate to the cultural characteristics of the person, family or community receiving them.

culture   A way of life that is the totality of learned, socially transmitted beliefs, values, and behaviours emerging from interpersonal transactions of people who identify or associate with one another on the basis of a common purpose, need, or similarity of background.

cycle of violence   A three-phase pattern of tension, abuse, and kindness in which the abuser engages first in abuse and then in seemingly sincere expressions of love, contrition, and remorse.

cyclothymic   A term used to describe periods of hypomanic and depressive episodes that do not meet full criteria for a major depressive episode.

de-escalation   An interactive process of calming and redirecting a patient who has an immediate potential for violence directed at others or self.

defence mechanisms   Coping styles; the automatic psychological process protecting the individual against anxiety and creating awareness of internal or external dangers or stressors.

defining characteristics   Key signs and symptoms that relate to each other and inform a nursing diagnosis.

deinstitutionalization   Downsizing or elimination of psychiatric hospitals with a new orientation to community-based services.

delirium   A disorder of physical origin that develops over a short period of time and is characterized by fluctuating consciousness and attention. *Hyperactive delirium* involves behaviours such as being overly alert, exhibiting psychomotor hyperactivity, and marked excitability (may hallucinate). *Hypoactive delirium* is marked by lethargy, sleepiness, apathy, and psychomotor slowing; *mixed delirium* involves behaviour that fluctuates between the hyperactive and hypoactive states over brief or long periods.

delirium tremens   An acute syndrome related to alcohol withdrawal that is characterized by gross tremulousness, disorientation, delusions, hallucinations (auditory, visual or tactile), tachycardia, sweating, hypertension, irregular tremor, and severely agitated behaviour.

delusion   A false, fixed belief, based on an incorrect inference about reality, not shared by others, inconsistent with the individual's intelligence or cultural background and which cannot be corrected by reasoning. *Delusions of control* are about one's thoughts, feelings, or will being controlled by outside forces; *delusions of grandeur*, one's importance or power; *paranoid delusions*, being the focus of others' harmful intent; *religious delusions*, being an agent of or favoured by a greater being; and *somatic delusions* involving the body or bodily functions.

delusional disorder   A disorder in which there is the presence of nonbizarre delusions; includes several subtypes: erotomania, grandiose, jealous, somatic, mixed, and specified.

dementia   A state characterized by chronic cognitive impairment; differentiated by underlying cause, not by symptom patterns, which are often similar; can be further classified as cortical or subcortical to denote the location of the underlying pathology.

denial Refusal to acknowledge some painful aspect of external reality or subjective experience that would be apparent to others. *Psychotic denial* is when there is gross impairment in reality testing.

deontology The approach to ethics that sets duty or obligation as the basis of doing right.

depersonalization A nonspecific experience in which the individual loses a sense of personal identity and feels strange or unreal.

depressive episode In a major depressive episode, either a depressed mood or a loss of interest or pleasure in nearly all activities must be present for at least 2 weeks. Four of seven additional symptoms must be present: disruption in sleep, appetite (or weight), concentration, energy; psychomotor agitation or retardation; excessive guilt or feelings of worthlessness; suicidal ideation.

desensitization A rapid decrease in drug effects that may develop within a few minutes or over a period of days, months, years, or lifetime of exposure to a drug.

detoxification Process of safely and effectively withdrawing a person from an addictive substance, usually under medical supervision.

developmental delay The impairment of normal growth and development that may not be reversible.

diagnosis-specific outcomes Outcomes based on nursing diagnoses.

dialectical behaviour therapy (DBT) An important biosocial approach to treatment that combines numerous cognitive and behaviour therapy strategies. It requires patients to understand their disorder by actively participating in formulating treatment goals by collecting data about their own behaviour, identifying treatment targets in individual therapy, and working with the therapists in changing these target behaviours.

diathesis Constitutional predisposition or vulnerability to a disorder.

dichotomous thinking Tendency to view things as absolute, either black or white, good or bad, with no perception of compromise.

disaster A sudden, overwhelming, and catastrophic event that causes widespread damage, social disorganization, mass casualties, and human suffering.

discrimination The differential treatment of others because they are members of a particular group.

disinhibition A concept borrowed from physics and biology and based on the idea of a dynamic, self-regulatory model of equilibrium in which equilibrium is defined (Piaget) as compensation for external disturbance; a mechanism for providing the self-regulation by which intelligence adapts to internal and external changes.

disordered water balance A state of chronic fluid imbalance, vacillating between normal and hyponatremic, that commonly occurs in psychiatric patients with chronic illnesses.

disorganized symptoms Symptoms of schizophrenia that make it difficult for the person to understand and respond to the ordinary sights and sounds of daily living; include *confused speech and thinking* and *disorganized behaviour*.

dissociation A disruption in the normally occurring linkages among subjective awareness, feelings, thoughts, behaviour, and memories.

dissociative identity disorder (DID) A mental disorder characterized by the existence of two or more distinct identities with unique personality characteristics and the inability to recall important information about oneself or events.

dissupport Term for the opposite of support in a relationship, such as verbal, physical, or emotional abuse; discounting an individual's opinions, feelings, behaviours, or values; blocking access to resources; or consuming an individual's material resources.

distraction The purposeful focusing of attention away from undesirable sensations.

distribution The amount of a drug that may be found in various tissues at the site of the drug action for which it is intended.

disturbances of executive functioning Problems in the ability to think abstractly, plan, initiate, sequence, monitor, and stop complex behaviour.

dual diagnosis Presence of both substance-related disorder and mental illness.

dyad A group of only two people who are usually related, such as a married couple, siblings, or parent and child.

dynamic security Security awareness that is concerned with institutional policies, staffing patterns, methods of operation, and relational security.

dysfunctional family A family whose interactions, decisions, or behaviours interfere with the positive development of the family and its individual members.

dyslexia Significantly lower score for mental age on standardized test in reading that is not due to low intelligence or inadequate schooling.

dysphagia Difficulty swallowing.

dysthymic disorder A milder but more chronic form of major depressive disorder.

dystonia An impairment in muscle tone that is generally the first extrapyramidal symptom to occur, usually within a few days of initiating an antipsychotic. Dystonia is characterized by involuntary muscle spasms, especially of the head and neck muscles.

echolalia Parrot-like repetition of another's words; inappropriate choice of topics.

echopraxia Involuntary imitation of another person's movements and gestures; regressed behaviour that is childlike or immature.

efferent Away from the central nervous system or other particular structure.

efficacy Ability of a drug to produce a response as a result of the receptor or receptors being occupied.

egocentrism Tendency to view the world as revolving around oneself.

emotion The psychophysiologic reaction that shapes the individual's experience of a feeling state.

emotional circuit The interrelationship between the emotional processes of the limbic system and the neurocognitive processes of the frontal lobe and other parts of the cortex. It is hypothesized that the functioning of this system determines the meaning a person gives to a particular situation.

emotional dysregulation Inability to control emotion in social interactions.

emotional vulnerability   Sensitivity and reactivity to environmental stress.

emotion-focused coping   Coping strategies directed at managing one's emotional distress (e.g., through exercise, prayer/meditation, expressing emotions, talking to friends, etc.).

empathic linkage   Ability to feel in oneself the feelings being expressed by another person or persons.

empathy   The experience of putting oneself in another person's circumstances and imagining his or her feelings.

encopresis   Soiling clothing with feces or depositing feces in inappropriate places.

endorphins   Neurotransmitters that have opiate-like behaviour and produce an inhibitory effect at opiate receptor sites; probably responsible for pain tolerance.

enmeshment   An extreme form of intensity in family interactions.

enuresis   Involuntary excretion of urine after the age at which a child should have attained bladder control.

epidemiology   The study of patterns of disease distribution in time and space that focuses on the health status of population groups or aggregates, rather than on individuals, and involves quantitative analysis of the occurrence of illnesses in population groups; basic science of public health.

epigenesis   A concept borrowed from embryology: if a particular part does not manifest itself during the appropriate phase, it cannot reach full development because the moment for doing so has passed; each developmental stage must be completed at the appropriate time, or successful completion of the stage will not occur.

episode   A period of a minimal duration of 2 weeks during which an individual experiences symptoms that meet the diagnostic criteria for that disorder.

equilibration   Compensation for external disturbances; a mechanism for providing the self-regulation by which intelligence adapts to external and internal changes (Piaget).

erotomania   The belief that someone (often a public figure) is in love with one or involved with one in a relationship when, in reality, one is a stranger to him or her.

ethnocentrism   The notion that one's own culturally learned ideas and values are central and correct for everyone.

excretion   The elimination of drugs from the body either unchanged or as metabolites. *Clearance* refers to the total volume of blood, serum, or plasma from which a drug is completely removed per unit of time.

exhibitionism   A behaviour associated with paraphilias involving exposing one's genitals to strangers, with occasional masturbation.

existential anxiety   The foreboding that arises from an awareness of human mortality. Also referred to as *angst*.

exposure therapy   The treatment of choice for agoraphobia that puts the patient into contact with the feared situations until the stimuli no longer produce anxiety.

expressed emotion   Family members' responses that include one or more of the following dynamics: critical comments, hostility, or emotional over involvement.

extended family   Several nuclear families who may or may not live together and function as one group.

externalizing disorders   Disorders that are characterized by acting-out behaviour.

extinction   Elimination of a classically conditioned response by the repeated presentation of the conditioned stimulus without the unconditioned stimulus, or elimination of an operantly conditioned response by no longer presenting the reward after the response.

extrapyramidal motor system   Collection of neuronal pathways that provides significant input in involuntary motor movements.

factitious disorder   A type of psychiatric disorder characterized by somatization, in which the person intentionally causes an illness for the purpose of becoming a patient.

factitious disorder by proxy   (Münchausen syndrome by proxy) The intentional production or feigning of physical or psychological signs or symptoms in one person by another who desires to indirectly assume the sick role.

family development   A broad term that refers to all the processes connected with the growth of a family, including changes associated with work, geographic location, migration, acculturation, and serious illness.

family dynamics   The patterned interpersonal and social interactions that occur within the family structure over the life of a family.

family life cycle   A process of expansion, contraction, and realignment of relationship systems to support the entry, exit, and development of family members.

family structure   According to Minuchin, the organized pattern within which family members interact.

fetal alcohol syndrome   A group of non-curable growth, mental, and physical problems that may occur in a baby when a mother ingests alcohol during pregnancy.

first-pass effect   Loss of orally administered drugs prior to entering the systemic circulation due to metabolism in the gastrointestinal wall.

fissures   The grooves of the cerebrum.

flight of ideas   Repeated and rapid changes in the topic of conversation, generally within just one sentence or phrase.

flooding   A type of therapy for agoraphobia in which highly anxiety-provoking stimuli are presented to the patient in vivo or with imagery, with no relaxation until the anxiety dissipates.

forensic nursing   Nursing practice in which psychiatric and mental health nursing philosophy and skills are integrated within a sociocultural context that includes the criminal justice system in order to provide comprehensive care to clients, families, and communities.

formal group roles   The designated leader and members of a group.

formal operations   The period of cognitive development, described by Piaget, characterized by the ability to use abstract reasoning to conceptualize and solve problems.

functional activities   Activities of daily living necessary for self-care (i.e., bathing, toileting, dressing, and transferring).

functional status   Extent to which a person has the ability to carry out independent personal care, home management, and social functions in everyday life that has meaning and purpose.

gate-control model   Pain response based on the model that pain perception involves pathways in the dorsal horn of the spinal column that relay noxious stimuli to the brain and that certain other nerve fibres function as an antagonistic "gate" to augment or dampen the subjective experience of pain.

gender role How one functions and behaves as a male or a female in relation to others in society, also referred to as *sex role identity*.

genogram A multigenerational schematic diagram that lists family members and their relationships.

genome The complete set of human genes.

genomics The study of the complete DNA structure or genome.

gerotranscendence A psychosocial theory of aging that regards aging as the final stage in a natural progression towards maturation and wisdom that generally results in increased satisfaction and meaning in life.

glia (white matter) A fatty or lipid substance with a white appearance that surrounds the pathways of the cell body axons.

gray matter The cortex, with its gray-brown colour due to the capillary blood vessels.

grief The subjective experience (e.g., thoughts, feelings, behaviours, and body sensations) that accompanies the perception of a loss.

group An open or closed social system with structures, norms, and customary ways of acting.

group cohesion Forces that act on the members to stay in a group.

group dynamics Interactions within groups.

group process The "what is happening" in the group; how members are interacting and relating as individuals and as a whole group, including nonverbal communications.

groupthink The tendency of many groups to avoid conflict and adopt a normative pattern of thinking that is often consistent with the group leader's ideas.

guided imagery The purposeful use of imagination to achieve relaxation or direct attention away from undesirable sensations; especially useful in stress management.

gyri Bumps and convolutions in the brain.

half-life The time required for plasma concentrations of a drug to be reduced by 50%.

hallucinations Perceptual experiences that occur in the absence of actual external sensory stimuli and may be auditory, visual, tactile, gustatory, or olfactory.

hallucinogen A class of drug that produces euphoria or dysphoria, altered body image, distorted or sharpened visual and auditory perception, confusion, uncoordination, and impaired judgment and memory.

hallucinogen persisting perception disorder A transient and intermittent disorder associated with the longterm use of hallucinogens; includes depression, prolonged psychosis, and flashbacks.

harm reduction A community health intervention designed to reduce the harm (consequences) of substance use to the individual, the family, and society by reducing the risk for adverse consequences arising from substance use without necessarily reducing its use.

helplessness The perception of having limited ability or ambition to change one's current life situation; characterized by a sense of being unable to help oneself and a sense that there is a lack of support or protection.

hippocampus Subcortical gray matter embedded within each temporal lobe that may be involved in determining the best way to store information or memory; "time-dating" memory.

HIV-1-associated cognitive-motor complex Neurologic complications that occur with HIV-1 that are directly attributable to infection of the brain and include impaired cognitive and motor function.

home visits Delivery of nursing care in a patient's living environment.

homeostasis The body's ability to maintain a stable internal environment despite changing environmental conditions.

hopelessness A perception of having no hope that one's life situation or circumstance will change or improve; characterized by feelings of inadequacy and an inability to act on one's own behalf.

hyperactivity Excessive motor activity, movement, and/or utterances that may be either purposeless or aimless.

hyperalgia Increased nociceptor sensitivity.

hyperesthesia Increased sensation of pain.

hypervigilance Sustained attention to external stimuli as if expecting something important or frightening to happen.

hypofrontality Reduced cerebral blood flow and glucose metabolism in the prefrontal cortex of people with schizophrenia.

hypomanic episode Mildly dysphoric mood that meets the same criteria as for a manic episode except that it lasts at least 4 days rather than 1 week and no marked impairment in social or occupational functioning is present.

hyponatremia Decreased sodium concentration in the blood.

hypothalamus Immediately ventral and slightly anterior to the thalamus, forming the floor and part of the walls of the third ventricle.

hypothalamic–pituitary–adrenal (HPA) axis Neurotransmitters responsible for behavioural responses to fear and anxiety that are usually held in balance until information from the sensory processing areas in the thalamus and cortex alerts the amygdala. If events are interpreted as threatening, this axis is activated, initiating the stress response.

ideas of reference False belief that other people, objects, and events are related to or have a special significance for oneself (e.g., a person on television is sending one signals).

identity An integration of a person's social and occupational roles and affiliations, self-attributed personality traits, attitudes about gender roles, beliefs about sexuality and intimacy, long-term goals, political ideology, and religious beliefs.

identity diffusion Occurs when parts of a person's identity are absent or poorly developed; a lack of consistent sense of identity.

illogical thinking A thinking error that occurs when a person draws a faulty conclusion; for example, a university student equates failure on an examination with loss of future career.

illusions Disorganized perceptions that create an oversensitivity to colours, shapes, and background activities, which occur when the person misperceives or exaggerates stimuli in the external environment.

impulsivity Acting without considering the consequences of the act or alternative actions.

incidence A rate that includes only new cases that have occurred within a clearly defined time period.

indicators Representation of the dimension of outcome; data or information to answer the question of how close the patient is coming toward an outcome.

individual roles Group roles that either enhance or detract from the group's functioning but have nothing to do with either the group task or maintenance.

individual treatment plan A plan of care that identifies the patient's problems, outcomes, interventions, the individuals assigned to implement interventions, and evaluation criteria.

informal group roles Positions in the group with rights and duties directed toward other group members. These positions are not formally sanctioned.

informal support systems Family members, friends, and neighbours who can provide care and support to the individual.

informed consent Consent for treatment given by a competent adult after being provided the available information necessary for making an informed choice; based on the ethical principle of autonomy.

inhalants Organic solvents, also known as volatile substances, that are central nervous system depressants and when inhaled cause euphoria, sedation, emotional lability, and impaired judgment.

inhibited grieving Inability to fully experience and personally integrate or resolve significant traumatic events and loss.

insight The ability of the individual to be aware of his or her own thoughts and feelings and to compare them with the thoughts and feelings of others.

insomnia Inability to fall or remain asleep throughout the night.

instrumental activities Activities that facilitate or enhance the performance of activities of daily living (e.g., shopping, using the telephone, transportation). These aspects are critical to consider for any older adult living alone.

interdisciplinary approach Interventions from different disciplines integrated into the delivery of patient care.

interdisciplinary treatment plan A plan of care that identifies the patient's problems, outcomes, interventions, and members of different disciplines assigned to implement interventions, and evaluation criteria.

intermediate beliefs Attitudes, rules or expectations, and assumptions that influence one's perceptions, affect, and behaviours; often take the form of "should" statements that are rigid and unrealistic.

internalizing disorders Anxiety disorders and depression in which the symptoms tend to be within the individual.

interoceptive awareness Term used to describe the sensory response to emotional and visceral cues, such as hunger.

intrinsic activity The ability of a drug to produce a biologic response when it becomes attached to its receptor.

invalidating environment A highly personal social situation that negates the individual's emotional responses and communication.

invincibility fable The egocentric phenomenon seen in adolescence where the individual views his or herself as unique, invulnerable and immune to death.

ischemic cascade Cell breakdown resulting from brain cell injury.

judgment The ability to reach a logical decision about a situation and to choose a course after looking at and analyzing various possibilities.

kindling Repetitive stimulation of certain tracts may facilitate conduction of impulses in the future and lead to enhancement of intense behaviours after even mild stimulation.

kleptomania A disorder in which the patient is unable to resist the urge to steal and independently steals items that he or she could easily afford. These items are not particularly useful or wanted. The underlying issue is the act of stealing.

Korsakoff's syndrome An amnestic syndrome in which there is a profound deficit in the ability to form new memories; associated with a variable deficit in recall of old memories despite a clear sensorium. Confabulation is a key feature.

lability of mood Rapid alternations of mood, usually between euphoria and irritability.

lateral ventricles The horn-shaped first and second ventricles that are the largest of the brain's ventricles.

learning disorder A discrepancy between actual achievement and expected achievement that is based on a person's age and intellectual ability.

least restrictive environment The patient has the right to treatment in an environment that restricts the exercise of free will to the least extent; an individual cannot be restricted to an institution when he or she can be successfully treated in the community.

level of consciousness An individual's level of arousal or wakefulness.

limbic system (limbic lobe) Structures including the septum and the fornix, as well as the amygdala, hippocampus, cingulate, parahippocampal gyrus, epithalamus, portions of the basal ganglia, paraolfactory area, and the anterior nucleus of the thalamus.

longitudinal fissure The longest and deepest groove of the cerebrum, separating the right and left hemispheres.

loose associations Absence of the normal connectedness of thoughts and ideas; sudden shifts without apparent relationship to preceding topic.

magical thinking The belief that one's thought, words, or actions have the power to cause or prevent things happening; similar to Piaget's preoperational thinking in young children.

maintenance function A term used to describe the informal role of group members that encourages the group to stay together.

malingering The production of illness symptoms intentionally with an obvious self-serving goal such as being classified as disabled and avoiding work.

mandatory outpatient treatment (MOT) Legal provisions that can require an individual with a mental illness to comply with a treatment plan while living in the community.

mania A state characterized by an abnormally and persistently elevated, expansive, or irritable mood.

manic episode A distinct period during which there is an abnormally and persistently elevated, expansive, or irritable mood.

manipulation Influencing others or a situation for one's own benefit.

maturation The process of completing a state of development; a ripening.

memory A facet of cognition concerned with retaining and recalling past experiences, whether they occurred in the physical environment or internally as cognitive events.

meningeal layer   The inner layer of dura mater that becomes continuous with the spinal dura mater and sends extensions into the brain for support and protection of the different lobes or structures.

mental disorder   Health condition characterized by alterations in a variety of factors that include mood and affect, behaviour, thinking and cognition.

mental health act   A law that gives certain powers, and sets the conditions (including time limits) for those powers, to stipulated health care professionals and designated institutions regarding the admission and treatment of individuals with a mental disorder.

mental health problem   A term used when signs and symptoms of mental illnesses occur but do not meet specified criteria for a disorder.

mental illness   A term used to mean all diagnosable mental disorders.

mental retardation   Significantly below-average intelligence accompanied by impaired adaptive functioning.

mental status examination   Systematic assessment of an individual's appearance, affect, behaviour, and cognitive processes, reflecting the examiner's observations and used in clinical settings to evaluate developmental, neurologic, and psychiatric disorders.

mesocortical   Medial aspects of the cortex.

metabolism   Biotransformation, or the process by which a drug is altered.

milieu therapy   An approach using the total environment to provide a therapeutic community; a therapeutic environment.

misidentification   Delusions in which the person believes that a familiar person is replaced by an impostor.

mixed episode   Irritability or excitement and depression occurring at the same time.

mobbing   Occurs when several people gang up and bully an individual.

mood   A pervasive, sustained emotion that influences one's perception of the world and can be described as *euthymic* (normal), *euphoric* (elated), or dysphoric (depressed, disquieted, restless). Normal variations in mood (e.g., sadness, euphoria, anxiety) occur as responses to specific life experiences, are time limited, and are not associated with significant functional impairment.

mood disorder   Recurrent disturbances or alterations in mood that cause psychological distress and behavioural impairment.

moral dilemma   The need to make a morally relevant choice between conflicting options.

moral distress   The anger, frustration, or anguish felt when one is unable to fulfill ethical obligations in the way one believes that one should.

moral treatment   An approach to curing mental illness, popular in the 1800s, which was built on the principles of kindness, compassion, and a pleasant environment.

motivational interviewing   (MI; motivational enhancement therapy) A directive, client-centred style of psychotherapy that helps clients to explore and resolve their ambivalence about changing.

mourning   The external manifestation of grief, which is highly influenced by gender, ethnicity, culture, religion, and the cause of death.

multiaxial diagnostic system   A diagnostic structure that includes more than one domain of information, such as the psychiatric diagnoses of the *DSM-IV-TR*.

multidisciplinary approach   Several disciplines providing services to a patient at one time.

multigenerational transmission process   The transmission of emotional processes from one generation to the next.

music therapy   The controlled use of music to promote physiologic or psychological well-being.

myoclonus   Twitching or clonic spasms of a muscle group.

myoglobinuria   The presence of myohemoglobin in the urine due to sustained muscular rigidity and necrosis.

negative symptoms   Symptoms of schizophrenia that reflect a lessening or loss of normal functions, such as restriction or flattening in the range and intensity of emotion (*affective flattening* or *blunting*); reduced fluency and productivity of thought and speech (*alogia*); withdrawal and inability to initiate and persist in goal-directed activity (*avolition*); and inability to experience pleasure (*anhedonia*).

neglect   Failure to protect from injury or to provide for the physical, psychological, and medical needs of a child or dependent elder.

neologisms   Words that are made up that have no common meaning and are not recognized.

neuritic plaques   Extracellular lesions consisting of β-amyloid protein and apolipoprotein A (apoA) cores that form in the nucleus basalis of Meynert, gradually increase in number, and are abnormally distributed throughout the cholinergic system.

neurochemical modulation   Maintenance of a balance in the essential levels of the neurotransmitters that influence mood, perceptions, and emotional interpretation.

neurofibrillary tangles   Fibrous proteins, or *tau proteins*, that are chemically altered and twisted together and spread throughout the brain, interfering with nerve functioning in cholinergic neurons. It is hypothesized that formation of these neurofibrillary tangles are related to the apolipoprotein E_4 (apoE$_4$).

neurohormones   Hormones produced by cells within the nervous system, such as antidiuretic hormone (ADH).

neuroleptic malignant syndrome   A syndrome caused by neuroleptic medications that are dopamine receptor blockers. The classic signs and symptoms include hyperthermia, lead-pipe rigidity, changes in mental status, and autonomic nervous system changes.

neuropeptide Y   A recently discovered 36-amino-acid peptide that is a potent stimulator of feeding behaviour especially selective for foods heavy in carbohydrates.

neuropeptides   Short chains of amino acids that exist in the central nervous system and have a number of important roles, including as neurotransmitters, neuromodulators, or neurohormones.

neurotransmitters   Chemicals circulating in the synaptic areas of neurons that initiate, block, or modulate nerve signal transmission and ultimately control neural function.

nihilism   A psychiatric term for the belief that one is dead or nonexistent.

nociceptive   Pertaining to a neural receptor for painful stimuli.

nonverbal communication   The gestures, expressions, and body language used in communications between the nurse and the patient.

normalization Teaching individuals and families about normal development, behaviours, and responses that can be expected (e.g., child development, the grieving process).

no-suicide contract Written or verbal agreement between the health care professional and the patient that the patient will not engage in suicidal behaviour for a specific period of time.

nuclear family Two or more people related by blood, marriage, or adoption.

nurse–patient relationship A time-limited interpersonal process with definable phases during which the patient is able to consider alternative behaviours, try new health care strategies, and discuss complex health problems.

nursing diagnosis A clinical judgment about an identified problem/need that requires nursing interventions; based on nursing assessment.

nursing intervention Nursing activities that promote and foster health, assess dysfunction, assist patients to regain or improve their coping abilities, or prevent further disabilities.

nursing process Problem-solving method used by nurses that involves assessment, planning, implementation, and evaluation.

object relation The psychological attachment to another person or object.

observation Ongoing assessment of the patient's mental and health status to identify and subvert any potential problems.

obsessions Unwanted, intrusive, and persistent thoughts, impulses, or images that are incongruent with the patient's usual thought patterns.

obsessive-compulsive disorder (OCD) A disorder characterized by intrusive thoughts that are difficult to dislodge (obsessions) and ritualized behaviours that the person feels driven to perform (compulsions).

oculogyric crisis A medication side effect resulting from an imbalance of dopamine and acetylcholine, in which the muscles that control eye movements tense and pull the eyeball so that the patient is looking toward the ceiling; may be followed by torticollis or retrocollis.

open group A group in which new members can join at any time.

operant behaviour A type of learning that is a consequence of a particular behavioural response, not a specific stimulus.

opiate Any substance that binds to an opiate receptor in the brain to produce an agonist action, causing central nervous system depression, sleep or stupor, and analgesia.

orientation An individual's ability to perceive and grasp the significance of environmental information related to time, place, and person.

orientation phase The first phase of the nurse–patient relationship in which the nurse and the patient get to know each other. During this phase, the patient develops a sense of trust.

othering The way one perceives and engages with another person that can be exclusionary and negative (i.e., the other is different from and thus "less than" me) or inclusionary and tolerant or accepting (i.e., the other is different from me, so I need to learn about his or her world view).

outcomes Patient response to nursing care at a given point in time consisting of the patient's state, behaviour, or perception that is variable and can be measured.

panic A normal but extreme overwhelming form of anxiety often experienced when an individual is placed in a real or perceived life-threatening situation.

panic attacks Discrete periods of intense fear or discomfort that are accompanied by significant somatic or cognitive symptoms.

panic control treatment Systematic structured exposure to panic-invoking sensations such as dizziness, hyperventilation, tightness in chest, and sweating.

panicogenic Substances that produce panic attacks.

paranoia Suspiciousness and guardedness that is unrealistic and often accompanied by grandiosity.

parasomnia Disorders of abnormal physiologic or behavioural events that occur in relationship to sleep, specific sleep stages, or during transition from sleep to wakefulness.

parasuicide Intentional self-injurious behaviour.

parietal-occipital sulcus Separates the occipital lobe from the parietal lobe.

passive listening A nontherapeutic mode of interaction that involves sitting quietly and allowing the patient to talk without focusing on guiding the thought process; includes body language that communicates boredom, indifference, or hostility.

perceptions The awareness reached as a result of sensory inputs of real stimuli that are usually altered.

persecutory delusions Delusions in which the person believes that he or she is being conspired against, cheated, spied on, followed, poisoned, drugged, maligned, harassed, or obstructed in the pursuit of long-term goals.

personality A complex pattern of characteristics, predominately outside the person's awareness, that compose a person's distinctive pattern of perceiving, feeling, thinking, and behaving.

personality disorder An enduring pattern of inner experience and behaviour that deviates markedly from the expectations of the individual's culture; is pervasive and inflexible; has an onset in adolescence or early adulthood; is stable over time; and leads to distress or impairment.

personality traits Prominent aspects of personality that are exhibited in a wide range of important social and personal contexts.

person-environment relationship The interaction between the individual and the environment that changes throughout the stress experience.

pet therapy The therapeutic use of animals as pets to promote physical, psychological, or social well-being.

pharmacodynamics The study of the biologic actions of drugs on living tissue and the human body in general.

pharmacogenomics The science of pharmacology combined with genetic knowledge.

pharmacokinetics The study of how the human body processes a drug, including absorption, distribution, metabolism, and elimination.

phobia Persistent, unrealistic fear of situations, objects, or activities that often leads to avoidance behaviours.

phonologic processing Thought to be the cause of reading disability; a process that involves the discrimination and interpretation of speech sounds. Reading disability is believed to be caused by some disturbance in the development of the left hemisphere.

phototherapy Also known as *light therapy*; involves exposing the patient to an artificial light source during winter months to relieve seasonal depression.

physical restraints   The application of wrist, leg, and body straps made of leather or cloth for the purpose of controlling or managing behaviour.

pia mater   The third layer of the central nervous system, in Latin, "soft mother."

pineal body   Located in the epithalamus; contains secretory cells that emit the neurohormone melatonin (as well as other substances), which has been associated with sleep and emotional disorders and modulation of immune function.

plasticity   Capability to change or adapt in form or physiology.

point prevalence   Basic measure that refers to the proportion of individuals in a population who have a particular disorder at a specified point in time.

polydipsia   Excessive thirst that can be chronic in patients with severe mental illness.

polypharmacy   Use of several different medications at one time.

polysomnography   A special procedure that involves the recording of the electroencephalogram throughout the night. This procedure is usually conducted in a sleep laboratory.

polyuria   Excessive excretion of urine.

positive self-talk   Countering fearful or negative thoughts by using preplanned and rehearsed positive coping statements.

positive symptoms   Symptoms of schizophrenia that reflect an excess or distortion of normal functions, including delusions and hallucinations.

posttraumatic stress disorder   A mental disorder characterized by persistent, distressing symptoms lasting longer than 1 month after exposure to an extreme traumatic stressor.

poverty   The state when income and/or level of consumption are below what is necessary to meet basic needs; measured as absolute (comparison of total income against the cost of goods and services essential to daily life) or relative (comparison of total income and spending with the general population).

powerlessness   The perception of having no power or control over one's life circumstance; feeling that the world will never be fair; feeling helpless and totally ineffectual; or feeling one lacks legal or other authority.

prejudice   The preconceived, unreasonable judgment of others, usually negative, based solely on their membership in a particular group.

pressured speech   A speech pattern in which the person is talkative due to a sense of pressure to speak; a symptom of manic episodes of bipolar disorder.

prevalence   The total number of people who have a particular disorder within a given population at a specific time.

prevention   Interventions used before the initial onset of a disorder that become distinct from the treatment.

principlism   The approach to ethics that uses common principles or ethical norms as the basis for ethical decision-making. In health ethics the principles used include *nonmaleficence* (do no harm), *beneficence* (promote benefit), *respect for autonomy* (the right to make one's own decisions) and *justice* (fairness in the distribution of risks and benefits).

problem-focused coping   Coping comprised of inner- or outer-directed coping strategies. Outer-directed strategies attempt to eliminate or alter a situation or another's behaviour, while inner-directed strategies aim at altering one's own beliefs, attitudes, skills, responses, etc.

process recording   A verbatim transcript of a verbal interaction usually organized according to the nurse-patient interaction. It often includes analysis of the interaction.

projective identification   A psychoanalytic term used to describe behaviour of people with borderline personality disorder when they falsely attribute to others their own unacceptable feelings, impulses, or thoughts.

pseudodementia   Memory difficulties in older adults with major depression (may be mistaken for early signs of dementia).

pseudologia fantastica   False stories of personal triumph that are a core symptom of factitious disorders.

pseudoneurologic symptoms   Somatic symptoms of conversion disorders that pertain to neurologic conditions affecting voluntary motor or sensory function (e.g., impaired balance, paralysis, blindness, deafness). The symptoms do not follow neurologic paths, but rather follow the individual's conceptualization of the problem.

pseudoparkinsonism   Sometimes referred to as *drug-induced parkinsonism*; presents identically as Parkinson's disease without the same destruction of dopaminergic cells.

psychoanalytic movement   Freud's radical approach to psychiatric mental health care, which involved using a new technique called *psychoanalysis* based on unconscious motivations for behaviour, or drives.

psychodrama   A group role-playing technique used to encourage expression of emotion and exploration of problems.

psychoeducation   An educational approach used to enhance knowledge and shape behaviour so that coping skills are learned or enhanced.

psychoendocrinology   The study of the relationships among the nervous system, endocrine system, and behaviour.

psychoimmunology   The study of immunology as it relates to emotions and behaviour.

psychopathy   Refers to individuals who behave impulsively and are interpersonally irresponsible, act hastily and spontaneously, are shortsighted, and fail to plan ahead or consider alternatives. Equated with antisocial personality disorder.

psychopharmacology   A subspecialty of pharmacology that studies medications that affect the brain and behaviour and that are used to treat psychiatric and neurodegenerative disorders.

psychosis   A state in which the individual is experiencing hallucinations, delusions, or disorganized thoughts, speech, or behaviour.

psychosomatic   Conditions in which a psychological state contributes to the development of a physical illness.

purging   A compensatory behaviour to rid oneself of food already eaten by means of self-induced vomiting or the use of laxatives, enemas, or diuretics.

pyromania   An irresistible impulse to start fires.

rapidly cycling bipolar disorder   The occurrence of four or more mood episodes during the past 12 months.

rapport   Interpersonal harmony characterized by understanding and respect.

rate   A proportion of the cases in the population compared to the total population.

reaction time   The lapse of time between stimulus and response.

receptor   Site where a substance can specifically interact with the cell membrane to produce a change; biologic action of a drug depends on how its structure interacts with a specific receptor.

recovery model An approach that supports individual potential for recovery, focusing on the personal journey involved, the upholding of human rights, a positive culture of healing, and recovery-oriented services.

regressed behaviour Behaving in the manner of a less mature life stage; childlike and immature.

relapse Return of symptoms after a period of remission.

relational ethics The approach to ethics that situates ethical action in relationship, recognizing that complexity, vulnerability, and the environment are important considerations.

relaxation A mental health intervention that promotes comfort, reduces anxiety, alleviates stress, reduces pain, and prevents aggressive behaviour.

religiosity A psychiatric symptom characterized by excessive or affected piety.

REM sleep A sleep cycle state of rapid eye movement.

reminiscence Thinking about or relating past experiences.

reminiscence therapy The healing process of looking back on specific times or events in one's life.

remission A period when the symptoms of a disease are abated.

resilience The capacity to overcome adversity in spite of extreme stress; involves the balancing of risk and protective factors.

resolution phase The termination phase of the nurse-patient relationship that lasts from the time the problems are resolved to the close of the relationship.

restraint The use of any manual, physical, or mechanical device or material, which when attached to the patient's body (usually the arms and legs) restricts the patient's movements.

retrocollis The neck muscles pull the head back.

risk factors Characteristics that do not cause the disorder or problem and are not symptoms of the illness, but rather are factors that have been shown to influence the likelihood of developing a disorder.

role An individual's social position and function within an environment.

ruminations Repetitive thoughts that are forced into a patient's consciousness even when unwanted; when a person goes over and over the same ideas endlessly; part of an obsessive style of thinking.

satiety Internal signals that indicate one has had enough to eat.

schema A cognitive structure that screens, codes, and evaluates the incoming stimuli through which the individual interprets events.

schizoaffective disorder An interrupted period of illness during which at some point there is a major depressive, manic, or mixed episode, along with two of the following symptoms of schizophrenia: delusions, hallucinations, disorganized speech, disorganized or catatonic behaviour, or negative symptoms (affective flattening, alogia, or avolition).

school phobia Anxiety in which the child refuses to attend school in order to stay at home and with the primary attachment figure. School phobia is a common presenting complaint in child psychiatric clinics and may be part of separation anxiety, general anxiety, social phobia, obsessive-compulsive disorder, depression, or conduct disorder.

seclusion The involuntary confinement of a person in a room which the person is physically prevented from leaving for the purposes of safety or behavioural management.

sedative-hypnotics Medications that induce sleep and reduce anxiety.

selectivity The ability of a drug to be specific for a particular receptor.

self-awareness Being cognizant of one's own beliefs, thought motivations, biases, physical and emotional limitations, and the impact one may have on others.

self-concept The sum of beliefs about oneself, which develops over time.

self-disclosure The act of revealing personal information about oneself.

self-efficacy Self-effectiveness.

self-esteem The way one feels about oneself; components are self-acceptance, self-worth, self-love, and self-nurturing.

self-identity Formed through the integration of social and occupational roles and affiliations, self-attributed personality traits, attitudes about gender roles, beliefs about sexuality and intimacy, long-term goals, political ideology, and religious beliefs. Without an adequately formed identity, goal-directed behaviour is impaired and interpersonal relationships are disrupted.

self-monitoring Observing and recording one's own information, usually behaviour, thoughts, or feelings.

separation-individuation A process during which the child develops a sense of self, a permanent sense of significant others (object constancy), and an integration of both bad and good as components of the self-concept.

serotonin Centrally mediates the release of endorphin. Along with histamine and bradykinin, serotonin stimulates the pain receptors to generate experienced pain. Serotonin is involved in inhibiting gastric secretion, stimulating smooth muscle, and serving as a central neurotransmitter.

serotonin syndrome A toxic side effect that occurs as a result of the newer serotonergic drugs; this syndrome is thought to be caused by hyperstimulation of the 5-HT receptor in the brain stem and spinal cord.

severe and persistent mental illness Mental disorders that are long term and have recurring periods of exacerbation and remission.

sexual abuse Sexual misconduct toward another person.

sexuality Basic dimension of every individual's personality, undergoing periods of growth and development, and influenced by biologic and psychosocial factors.

sibling position A child's place in the family based on birth order (e.g., first born, youngest).

side effects Unwanted or untoward effects of medications.

social change The structural and cultural evolution of society; is constant and, at times, erratic.

social distance Degree to which the values of a formal organization and its primary group members differ.

social functioning Performance of daily activities within the context of interpersonal relations and family and community roles.

social network Linkages among a defined set of people, among whom there are personal contacts.

social skills training A psychoeducational approach that involves instruction, feedback, support, and practice with learning behaviours, it helps people interact more effectively with peers, and also children with adults.

social support Resources provided to an individual by others that may moderate the adverse effects of stress.

somatoform disorder One in which the patient experiences physical symptoms as a result of psychological stress.

somatization The manifestation of psychological distress as physical symptoms.

somatization disorder A polysymptomatic disorder that begins before age 30 years, extends over a period of years, and is characterized by a combination of pain and gastrointestinal, sexual, and psychoneurologic symptoms.

speech The motor aspects of speaking.

spinal cord A long, cylindrical collection of neural fibres continuous with the brain stem, housed within the vertebral column.

spirituality A complex, even mysterious, concept related to one's connection to the sacred and to the beliefs and values that give meaning to one's life.

splitting A primitive defence mechanism involving the compartmentalization of opposite and conflicting affect states so that self, others, and events are understood as all one way or all another (e.g., viewing a particular person as being all good or all bad).

static security Security awareness focused on structural or environmental artefacts common to secure environments, for example, the use of two-way radios, personal protection alarms, video monitoring, electronic door locks, internal barriers, and perimeter fences or walls.

stereotypic behaviour Repetitive, driven, nonfunctional, and potentially self-injurious behaviour, such as head banging, rocking, and hand flapping, seen in autistic disorder, with an extraordinary insistence on sameness.

stereotyping The expectation that an individual will act in a characteristic manner that conforms to a perception, usually negative, of their cultural group.

stereotypy Repetitive, purposeless movements that are idiosyncratic to the individual and to some degree outside of the individual's control.

stigma The mark of a spoiled identity or disgrace.

stigmatization A process of assigning negative characteristics and identity to a person or group and causing that person or group to feel unaccepted, devalued, ostracized, and isolated from the larger society.

stress The relationship between the person and the environment that is appraised as exceeding the person's resources and endangering his or her well-being.

stressors Events that initiate a stress response; can be physical, psychological, or social; can be short-term (acute) or long-term (chronic).

stress-diathesis model An explanation about the relationship between stress and mental health-illness that proposes that pre-existing genetic, biologic, and psychological vulnerabilities interact with negative or stressful life events to cause illness; an inverse relationship between vulnerability and stress is predicted (i.e., the more vulnerable the individual, the less stress is required to cause illness).

structured interaction Purposeful interaction that allows patients to interact with others in a way that is useful to them.

subcortical Structures inside the hemispheres and beneath the cortex.

subcortical dementia Dementia that is caused by dysfunction or deterioration of deep gray-or white-matter structures inside the brain and brain stem.

substance abuse A maladaptive use of chemical substance(s) leading to clinically significant outcomes or distress (e.g., recurrent legal problems, failure to perform, engaging in physically hazardous behaviour). Criteria for abuse do not include tolerance, withdrawal, or compulsive use.

substance dependence Continued use of a substance despite significant substance-related problems, along with a pattern of repeated self-administration that can result in tolerance, withdrawal, and compulsive drug-taking behaviour.

substance P The most common nociceptive transmitter that is released and transported along the central and peripheral pain synapses in the presence of noxious stimuli.

subsystems A systems term used by family theorists to describe subgroups of family members who join together for various activities.

suicidal ideation Thinking about and planning one's own death without actually engaging in self-harm.

suicidal contagion A social phenomenon seen among adolescents: when one teenager takes his or her life, others may follow.

suicide The act of killing oneself voluntarily.

symbolism The use of a word or a phrase to represent an object, event, or feeling.

symptom expression The behavioural symptoms of mental illness linked to their neurobiologic basis.

synapse The region across which nerve impulses are transmitted through the action of a neurotransmitter.

systematic desensitization A method used to desensitize patients to anxiety-provoking situations by exposing the patient to a hierarchy of feared situations. Patient is taught to use muscle relaxation as levels of anxiety increase through multisituational exposure.

tangentiality When the topic of conversation changes to an entirely different topic that is within a logical progression but causes a permanent detour from the original focus.

tardive dyskinesia A late-appearing extrapyramidal side effect of antipsychotic medication that includes abnormal involuntary movements of the mouth, tongue, and jaw such as lip smacking, sucking, puckering, tongue protrusion, the bon-bon sign, athetoid (worm-like) movements of the tongue, and chewing.

target symptoms Specific symptoms for which psychiatric medications are prescribed, such as hallucinations, delusions, paranoia, agitation, assaultive behaviour, bizarre ideation, social withdrawal, disorientation, catatonia, blunted affect, thought blocking, insomnia, and anorexia.

task function The group role that focuses on the task of the group.

temperament A person's characteristic intensity, rhythmicity, adaptability, energy expenditure, and mood.

tenuous stability Fragile personality patterns that lack resiliency under subjective stress.

thalamus Thought to play a role in controlling electrical activity in the cortex; provides the relay mechanism for information to and from the cerebrum.

therapeutic communication The ongoing process of interaction, verbal and nonverbal, through which meaning emerges.

therapeutic index A ratio of the maximum nontoxic dose to the minimum effective dose.

thought broadcasting Belief that one's thoughts are open to others or are being broadcast to the world.

thought insertion Belief that thoughts or ideas are being inserted into one's mind by someone or something external to one's self.

thought stopping A practice in which a person identifies negative feelings and thoughts that exist together, says "stop," and then engages in a distracting activity.

thymoleptic Mood stabilizing.

tidal model A theory-based approach to mental health nursing that emphasizes empowering collaboration between nurse and the person receiving nursing care.

token economy Applies behaviour modification techniques to multiple behaviours; clients are rewarded with tokens for selected desired behaviours.

tolerance Increased amounts of a substance are needed to achieve intoxication or desired effect, or there is diminished effect with the same amount of the substance.

torticollis The neck muscles pull the head to the side.

toxicity The point at which concentrations of a drug in the blood stream become harmful or poisonous to the body.

transference The unconscious assignment to others of feelings and attitudes that were originally associated with important figures such as parents or siblings.

transitional object A symbolic attachment figure, such as a blanket or a stuffed animal, that a child may cling to when a parent is not available.

transition times A term used to describe times of addition, subtraction, or change in status of family members.

traumatic bonding A strong emotional attachment between an abused person and his or her abuser, formed as a result of the cycle of violence.

triad A group consisting of three people.

trichotillomania Chronic, self-destructive hair pulling that results in noticeable hair loss, usually in the crown, occipital, or parietal areas, though sometimes of the eyebrows and eyelashes.

unipolar A term used to describe depression where the affected person has never experienced a manic episode. When a manic episode has been experienced, the depression is termed *bipolar*.

universal preventive interventions Preventive interventions that are targeted to everyone within a general public or whole population group.

urine specific gravity A measure of the degree of concentration of solutes in urine.

utilitarianism The approach to ethics that sets what is right to do as being what gives the best consequences (happiness, pleasure, preference, satisfaction) for the greater number of people.

ventricles The four cavities of the brain.

verbal communication The use of the spoken word, including its underlying emotion, context, and connotation.

verbigeration Purposeless repetition of words or phrases.

vicious circles of behaviour A term used to describe the tendency to become trapped in rigid and inflexible patterns of behaviour that are self-defeating.

violence (violent behaviour) A physical act of force intended to cause harm to a person or an object and to convey the message that the perpetrator's, and not the victim's, point of view is correct.

voluntary admission The legal status of a patient who has consented to being admitted to the hospital for treatment, during which time he or she maintains all civil rights and is free to leave at any time, even if it is against medical advice.

water intoxication A severe state of fluid overload occurring when large amounts of water are ingested and serum sodium levels rapidly fall to a level below 120 mEq/L.

waxy flexibility Posture held in an odd or unusual fixed position for extended periods of time.

well-being The state of contentment and positive sense that one's existence is as it should be. It is connected with one's self-identity and relationships.

Wernicke's area An area in the left superior temporal gyrus of the brain thought to be responsible for comprehension of speech.

Wernicke's syndrome An alcohol-induced amnestic disorder caused by a thiamine-deficient diet and characterized by diplopia, hyperactivity, ataxia, and delirium.

withdrawal The adverse physical and psychological symptoms that occur when a person ceases to use a substance.

word salad A string of words that are not connected in any way.

working phase The second phase of the nurse-patient relationship, in which patients can examine specific problems and learn new ways of approaching them.

work-life balance Achieved when an individual finds a satisfactory interaction among all the domains of his or her life.

xerostomia Dry mouth.

zeitgebers Specific events that function as time givers or synchronizers and that result in the setting of biologic rhythms.

Index

Page numbers followed by "b" indicate boxed materials; page numbers followed by "f" indicate figures; page numbers followed by "t" indicate tables.